Robert R. Cardell, Jr.
Professor and Chairman
Anatomy and Cell Biology
University of Cincinnati
Cincinnati, Ohio 45267

D1788718

CLINICAL AND FUNCTIONAL
HISTOLOGY
FOR MEDICAL STUDENTS

BY THE SAME AUTHOR

An Atlas of Normal Radiographic Anatomy (with Alvin C. Wyman, M.D.), 1976
Atlas of Clinical Anatomy, 1978
Gross Anatomy Dissector: A Companion for Atlas of Clinical Anatomy, 1978
Clinical Neuroanatomy for Medical Students, 1980
Clinical Anatomy for Medical Students, Second Edition, 1981
Clinical Embryology for Medical Students, Third Edition, 1983

RICHARD S. SNELL, M.D., Ph.D.

Professor and Chairman, Department of Anatomy,
The George Washington University School of Medicine
and Health Sciences, Washington, D.C.

LITTLE, BROWN AND COMPANY *Boston/Toronto*

CLINICAL AND FUNCTIONAL HISTOLOGY FOR MEDICAL STUDENTS

Copyright © 1984 by Little, Brown and Company (Inc.)

First Edition

All rights reserved. No part of this book may be reproduced in any form or by any electronic or mechanical means, including information storage and retrieval systems, without permission in writing from the publisher, except by a reviewer who may quote brief passages in a review.

Library of Congress Catalog Card No. 83-80487

ISBN 0-316-80216-6

Printed in the United States of America

HAL

For Maureen

CONTENTS

Preface *xi*

Introduction *1*

1. Organization of the Human Body *21*
2. The Cell *29*
3. Epithelial Tissue *85*
4. Connective Tissue *107*
5. Blood and Bone Marrow *155*
6. Muscle Tissue *195*
7. Nerve Tissue *225*
8. Cardiovascular System *291*
9. Lymphatic System *333*
10. Respiratory System *365*
11. Digestive Tract *409*
12. Liver, Bile Ducts, Gallbladder, and Pancreas *477*
13. Urinary System *503*
14. Male Reproductive System *539*
15. Female Reproductive System *571*
16. Endocrine System *631*
17. Skin and Its Appendages *689*
18. Special Sense Organs *729*

Answers to Clinical Problems *781*

Index *829*

PREFACE

Histology is the study of the normal microscopic structure of the body. A medical student must master this subject, because only by doing so will he be able to understand how the different tissues function. Moreover, histology is basic to the understanding of cell and tissue disease; it is impossible to study the abnormal before the normal is known.

Most existing textbooks are either too long and too detailed for present-day curricula or too short and only superficially concerned with those tissues that are commonly diseased.

The primary objective of this book is to provide the student with a basic understanding of the structure and function of those tissues of the body that are often diseased. Throughout the book, the practical application of histological and physiological facts to clinical medicine is stressed. At the end of each chapter is a series of clinical problems that require histological knowledge for their solution; the answers are placed at the back of the book.

The illustrations consist of photomicrographs of different tissues, taken at various magnifications, and simple explanatory line diagrams. It is recommended that the student have access to histological slides and to an atlas of histology to provide further examples of tissue structure.

The writing of this book would not have been possible without the work of anatomists, physiologists, and physicians too numerous to mention, and I gratefully acknowledge their assistance.

I thank the many medical students, clinical colleagues, and friends who stimulated me to write this book. I am most grateful to my colleagues in anatomy and cell biology in this country and other parts of the world who provided me with photographic examples of histological material.

I also thank Mrs. Mike Barnard and Lois Gottlieb for their invaluable technical assistance in preparing the hundreds of histology slides examined during the preparation of this book. I thank the staff of the audiovisual service of the George Washington University School of Medicine and Health Sciences, and in particular Jill Weinstein, B.S., for her skillful preparation of the many photomicrographs. I extend my sincere appreciation to my artist, Myra Feldman, for the very fine drawings. Special acknowledgment is due to Michele Boyd, Sandra Kosha, and Patricia Keogh for their skill and patience in typing the manuscript. Finally, to the staff of Little, Brown and Company go my gratitude and appreciation for their friendly assistance throughout the preparation of this book.

R. S. S.

CLINICAL AND FUNCTIONAL
HISTOLOGY
FOR MEDICAL STUDENTS

INTRODUCTION

Before beginning the study of histology, a freshman medical student should first become familiar with the general structure and use of a microscope. The student should also understand the basic principles involved in the preparation and staining of tissues so that he or she will be able to interpret histological sections more accurately. It has been my experience that many students are so awed by the fact that they have at last gained entrance into medical school after years of hard work that they are tempted to plunge immediately into the subject with little knowledge of the "tools of the trade."

LIGHT MICROSCOPE

A *simple microscope* has a single lens and produces only a moderately magnified image of the object you are studying. A *compound microscope* consists of a series of lenses and produces a far greater magnification. You will be using a compound microscope in your histology course.

The compound microscope (Fig. I-1) consists of mechanical and optical parts. The mechanical part has a *base*, which provides a stable foundation for the microscope, a *pillar*, which extends upward from the base, and a *stage*, on which the object to be studied is placed. The optical parts are attached to the pillar above and below the stage. They consist of the eyepieces or oculars, the objectives, the condenser, and the mirror. In many microscopes, the mirror and the illuminator are securely housed in the base of the instrument.

The *eyepieces* consist of a combination of lenses, which are inserted into the upper end of the tube of the microscope. The engraved value, such as "12.5×," indicates the magnification of the eyepiece. The *objectives* (there may be three, four, or five) are a combination of lenses attached to the lower end of the tube of the microscope. The engraved value, such as "10×," indicates the magnification of the objective. A 10× objective used with a 12.5× eyepiece gives a total magnification of 125×. The different objectives are attached to the *nosepiece,* which in turn is attached to the lower end of the microscope tube. One changes from one objective to another by rotating the nosepiece so that one objective is moved away and another is moved into position.

The *condenser* is a combination of lenses situated below the stage. It projects a cone of light onto the object being observed. The condenser can be raised

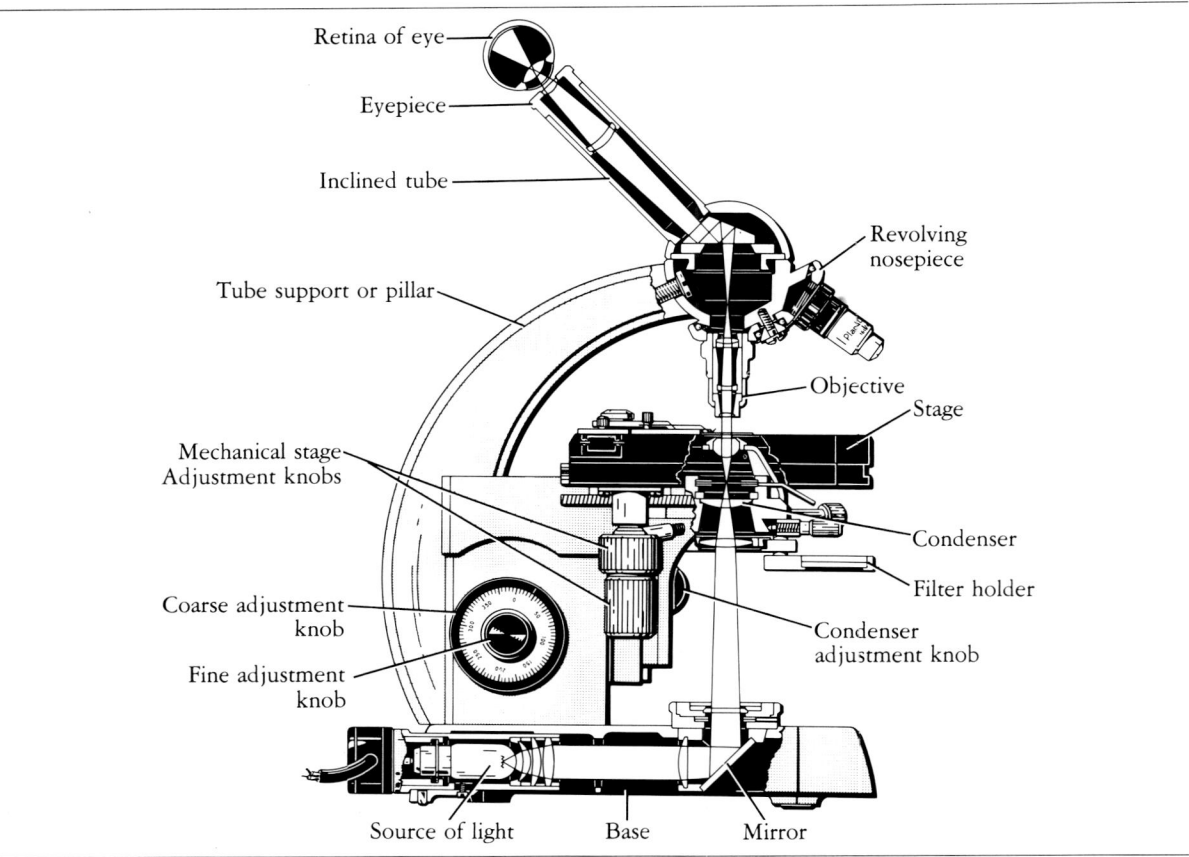

Fig. I-1. *A student's light microscope and its main parts. The pathway of the light from the lamp in the base to the eye of the observer is shown. (Courtesy of Carl Zeiss Co.)*

or lowered by a rack-and-pinion mechanism so that the light can be focused on the object. The passage of marginal rays into the condenser is prevented by the *iris diaphragm*.

The *mirror* that is situated below the condenser reflects light rays coming from the light source. Situated between the mirror and the condenser there is usually a swing-out holder for *light filters*.

How Does the Light Microscope Work?

The object to be studied is mounted on a glass slide, which is placed on the stage of the microscope. The object is moved into position beneath the objective either by hand or by using a *mechanical stage*. The object is brought into correct focus either by raising or lowering the stage or by raising or lowering the microscope tube, to which are attached the eyepieces and the objective. The light rays originating from the light bulb in the illuminator are reflected from the mirror and pass through the condenser. Here they are bent so that they converge on the object. The light rays then enter the objective and pass through its lenses, which cause them to converge and cross. From this point the light rays pass through the lenses of the eyepiece, where they are again bent. Having emerged from the eyepiece, the light rays are directed toward the pupil of the eye; they then impinge on the retina. If the eye is relaxed, as in long-distance vision, a clear image of the object should be obtained when the objective is in the position of exact focus. The position of the lenses of the microscope in relation to the object can be changed by adjusting the coarse and fine adjustments. The *coarse adjustment* brings about long-range movements, whereas the *fine adjustment* is a delicate mechanism bringing about small movements.

The compound light microscope is thus a two-stage magnifying system. The object is magnified first by the lenses in the objective and then again by a second set of lenses in the eyepiece. The total magnification is the product of the magnifications of the objective and the eyepiece. A compound microscope produces an image that is upside down and laterally reversed. The reversal is easily demonstrated: if you move the specimen to one side, the image moves in the opposite direction.

Magnification, Definition, Resolution, and Depth of Focus

Magnification is the increased size of the image as compared with the object. The total magnification of a compound microscope, as explained previously, is the degree of image magnification produced by the objective lenses multiplied by the magnification produced by the lenses of the eyepiece. Always use a low-power objective when you begin your examination of an object; it permits you to observe a wider field, and it is useful for scanning.

Definition is the sharpness of the image when the lens system has been adjusted correctly. A blurred image usually means that the lenses have been adjusted incorrectly or that they are dirty. Another common cause is inadvertently placing the glass slide on the stage with the wrong side up.

Resolution is the ability of a lens to visualize separately two points that appear as a single point when seen with a lower magnification. A good objective has the ability to separate adjacent points and thereby to permit minute details to be seen distinctly. An objective with a high resolving power has lenses that have been carefully made so that the rays of light passing through a given point do not get mixed up with rays passing through adjacent points.

The resolving power of an objective depends on an important factor called the *numerical aperture*.

This may be defined as the angle between the light rays entering the center of the objective and those entering its outer, peripheral margin. The magnitude of this angle is not indicated in degrees but in the form of a sine value, that is, a numerical value. The numerical aperture (NA) of the lens is engraved on each objective, beside the magnification. The numerical aperture determines the ability of the objective to collect diffracted light from fine details in the object.

Depth of focus is the ability of the lens to show structures that are related to one another but lie at different levels in the specimen. The depth of focus diminishes as the magnifying power and the numerical aperture of the objective increase.

Objective Lenses and the Oil-Immersion Objective

The ordinary compound microscope is equipped with three or four objective lenses: $2.5\times$ (low power), $10\times$ (medium power), $40\times$ (high dry objective), and $100\times$ (oil immersion). These lenses will, for example, give magnifications of $25\times$, $100\times$, $400\times$, and $1000\times$, respectively, when combined with a $10\times$ eyepiece. A wider range of magnification can be obtained by replacing the $10\times$ eyepiece with others ranging from $5\times$ to $20\times$.

To change objectives, rotate the nosepiece until the new objective clicks into position. Even though the objectives are parafocal, slight focusing may be necessary with the fine adjustment. With the high-power objectives, extreme care should be exercised to prevent damage to the thin glass coverslip covering the specimen or to the objective. Using the coarse adjustment, move the specimen (or objective) until the objective almost touches the coverslip. Then look through the eyepiece and use the fine adjustment to bring the object into focus.

The oil-immersion objective is used as follows: First, the area of the specimen to be examined is brought to the center of the field of vision with the use of a low-magnification objective. The stage of the microscope is lowered, and the nosepiece is rotated to swing the oil-immersion objective into place. A small drop of immersion oil is then placed on the coverslip above the object. The stage of the microscope is then gradually raised until the objective just touches the drop of oil. Looking through the eyepiece, you then gradually raise the stage, using the fine adjustment, until the object comes into view and is in focus. When you are examining tissues with oil-immersion objectives, repeated focusing is necessary, because of the extremely shallow depth of focus.

The immersion oil tends to cling to the lower end of the objective, so the slide may be moved about on the stage as different fields of vision are explored. After you have completed your examination, the oil should be removed from the objective and the coverslip. Wipe the surfaces with lens paper or a soft cloth moistened with 90% alcohol.

PHASE CONTRAST MICROSCOPE

When a piece of unstained tissue is examined with an ordinary light microscope, the detailed structure cannot be visualized. The reason for this is that the refractive indices of the cellular components are very similar, resulting in a lack of contrast. The phase contrast microscope is an instrument that converts small differences in refractive index that cannot be seen into differences in intensity that are visible.

Light waves traveling through cellular components of different optical densities will do so at different speeds. Thus, light waves traversing nuclei, mitochondria, and cell inclusions will emerge at different times, out of phase with one another. There are special apertures with absorbing and phase-shifting plates situated within the condenser and the objective lenses of the phase contrast microscope that convert phase differences into intensity differences. The phase contrast microscope is particularly useful in studying unstained tissues and living cells.

INTERFERENCE MICROSCOPE

The interference microscope uses two separate beams of light that pass through the specimen. One beam passes through the object being studied, and the second passes through another, neutral area. The two separate beams are then combined in the image plane. Because the object being studied has a greater optical density than the neutral area, the beam of light passing through it will have been retarded or interfered with to a greater extent than the beam passing through the neutral area. The degree of interference can be used to measure the refractive index, the thickness, and the dry mass per unit area of the object.

POLARIZING MICROSCOPE

Polarization is a phenomenon that occurs when light passes through certain substances, such as crystals, and is divided so that two light rays emerge that are derived from one. These substances have two refractive indices and are said to be *birefringent*. In the polarizing microscope, the light is polarized below the stage of the microscope by a Nicol quartz prism called the *polarizer*. The polarized light then passes through the specimen. A second prism, called the *analyzer*, is located next to the eyepiece within the microscope tube. When the position of the analyzer and polarizer prisms is adjusted so that the two polarized light beams are traveling in parallel directions, a normal image can be seen through the eyepiece. If the analyzer is then rotated so that its axis lies at right angles to the polarizer, no light reaches the eyepiece and nothing can be seen. The placing of an amorphous (monorefringent) object on the microscope stage with the prisms in the same right-angle position will result in nothing being seen, because the light rays have not been split by the object. If now a crystalline or birefringent object is placed on the stage, a light image will appear on a dark background. Thus, for biological materials to alter the direction of polarized light, and thus be visualized with a polarized microscope, their submicroscopic structure must consist of oriented, asymmetrical molecules. Muscle fibers, connective tissue fibers, and lipid droplets exhibit birefringence and have been studied extensively using polarizing microscopes.

FLUORESCENCE MICROSCOPE

In this form of microscopy, ultraviolet light is used to illuminate the specimen. Certain biological substances emit visible light when they absorb ultra-

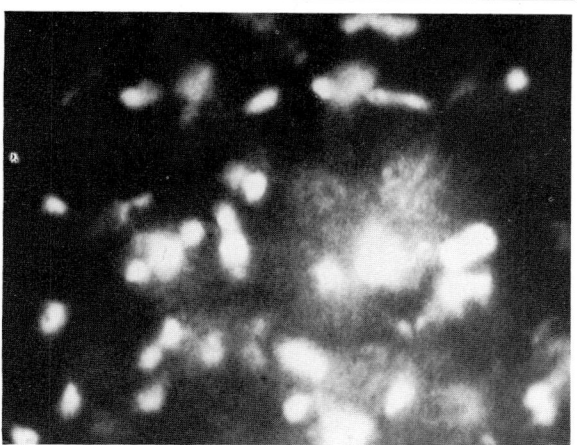

Fig. I-2. Photomicrograph of Kupffer cells of liver that have phagocytosed fluorescent latex particles. (Courtesy of Dr. R. S. McCuskey.)

violet light and are said to exhibit fluorescence. The observed image gives the appearance of being self-luminous. Fluorescence may take place with naturally occurring compounds such as vitamin A. Also, fluorescent dyes can be introduced into the specimen (Fig. I-2), where they may bind to specific compounds or be coupled with specific antibodies.

TRANSMISSION ELECTRON MICROSCOPE

The transmission electron microscope (TEM) differs from the light microscope in that it uses a beam of electrons rather than a beam of visible light (Fig. I-3). One of the great disadvantages of the light microscope is the long wavelength of visible light, which limits the maximum resolving power to about 0.2 μm. A stream of electrons has a very short wavelength, and resolutions of about 0.2 nm can be obtained with modern electron microscopes.

In the electron microscope, the electrons are emitted by a heated tungsten filament called the *cathode*. Because electrons are charged particles and would collide with air molecules and thus be absorbed and deflected, the entire optical system of an electron microscope must operate in a vacuum. The *anode* is a metallic plate with a small hole in its center. A potential difference of 40 to 100 kV between

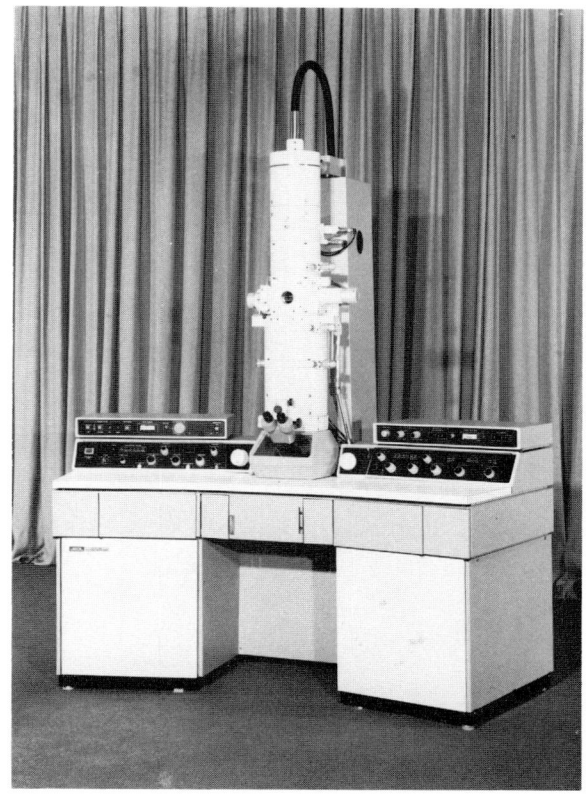

Fig. I-3. The JEOL model JEM-100 CX transmission electron microscope. (Courtesy of JEOL, Ltd.)

the cathode and the anode accelerates the electrons as they pass from the cathode to the anode. On reaching the anode, many of the electrons pass through the hole in its center to form a beam. The electron beam then passes through a series of electromagnetic lenses similar to the glass lenses found in the light microscope (Fig. I-4). The electromagnetic lenses serve to focus the beam of electrons, and the strength of the magnetic field produced by the lenses can be changed by altering the amount of current passing through the coils of wire in the lenses. In this way the condenser focuses the beam on the object. As the electrons leave the object, they are focused by the objective lens, and a magnified image is obtained. The image is further enlarged by one or two projection lenses. Because

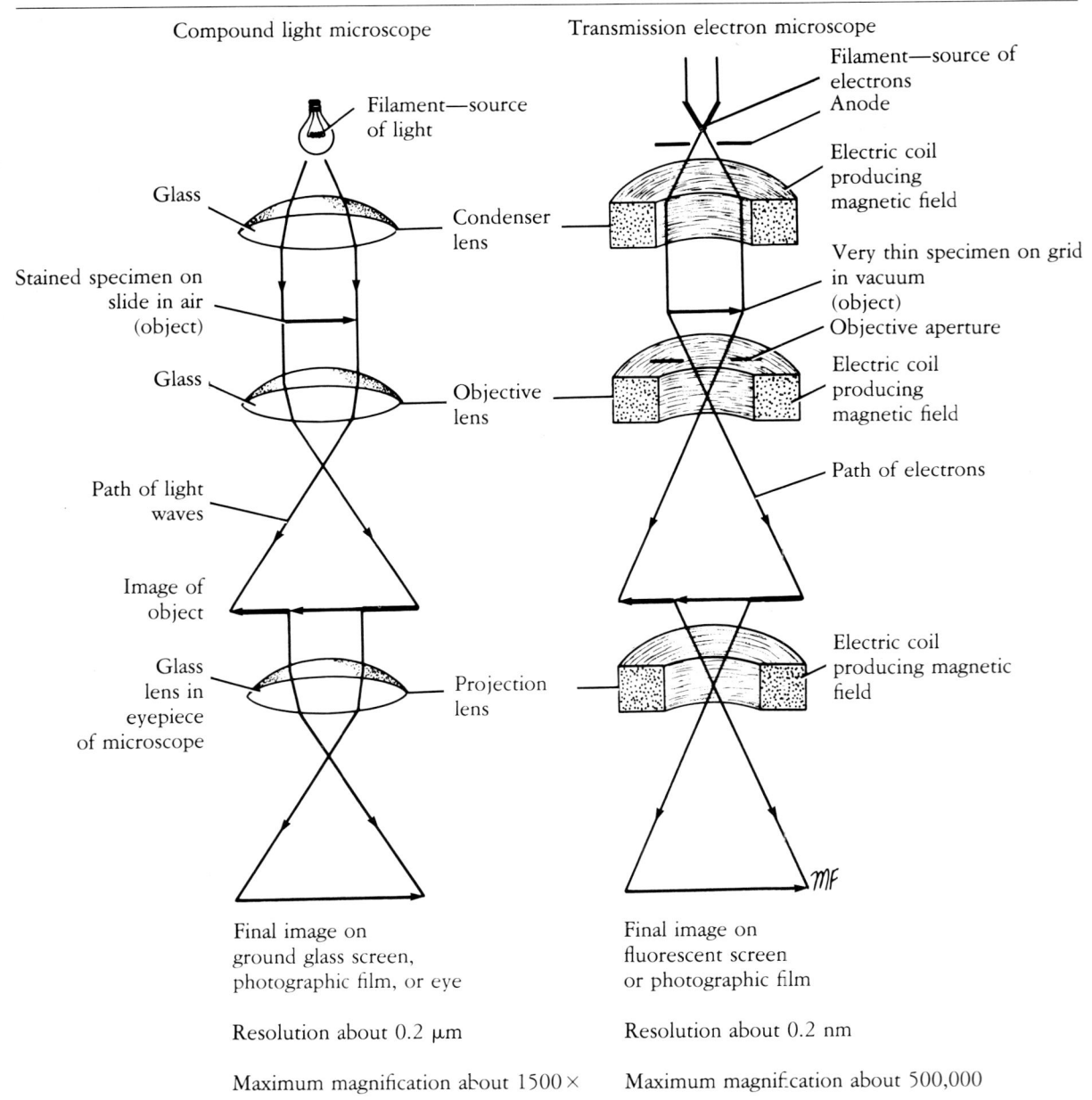

Fig. I-4. Comparison of the paths taken by a beam of light in a compound light microscope and a beam of electrons in a transmission electron microscope.

electron beams are invisible to the eye, the image is revealed by causing the electrons to project onto a fluorescent screen or photographic film.

Unfortunately, electron beams have a very poor penetrating power, so specimens must be cut in extremely thin slices (0.02–0.1 µm). Because the thin sections have very little contrast, they have to be stained with heavy electron-absorbing metals (such as uranium and lead) to increase the contrast.

The penetrating power of electrons is augmented by increasing the accelerating voltage. It is now possible with accelerating voltages of a million volts to use thicker sections (1–5 µm) and at the same time have a higher resolution.

SCANNING ELECTRON MICROSCOPE

The scanning electron microscope (SEM) examines the surface of the tissue; the electron beam does not pass through the specimen (Fig. I-5). A narrow electron beam is directed onto the surface of the specimen and scans back and forth in a regular manner. As the electron beam strikes the surface of the specimen, secondary electrons are emitted from the surface. The secondary electrons are caught by detectors, creating an electrical signal, which is displayed on a television screen. The scanning beam of electrons impinging on the specimen travels in synchrony with the image-producing beam on the television screen. In this way, a three-dimensional image of the surface of the specimen can be built up on the television screen. Micrographs can be obtained by photographing the image.

The tissue is prepared for SEM first by fixation and then by careful dehydration. The surface of the specimen is then coated with a thin layer of metal, such as gold, gold-palladium, or carbon, to assist in the scatter of the electrons.

PREPARATION OF TISSUES FOR LIGHT MICROSCOPIC EXAMINATION

Obtaining the Specimen

Human tissues to be examined are usually from surgical specimens that include normal as well as dis-

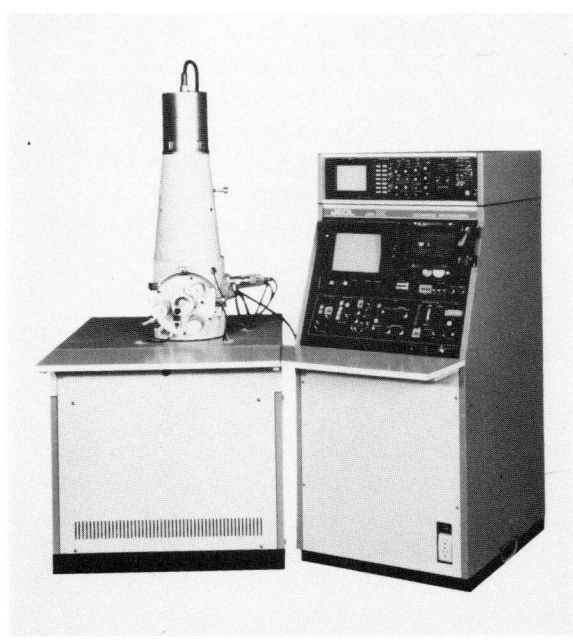

Fig. I-5. The JEOL model JSM-35 scanning electron microscope. (Courtesy of JEOL, Ltd.)

eased tissue. Small samples of normal tissue, only a few millimeters thick, are carefully cut from the specimen by using a pair of forceps and a sharp razor blade. It is important at this stage that the tissue not be damaged or distorted by excessive handling or by using dull cutting instruments.

Fixation

The tissue block is then rapidly immersed in a solution of chemicals to preserve the protoplasm. The chemical substances used to preserve tissues are called *fixatives*. Fixatives cause the precipitation of proteins, and most inactivate cell enzymes and inhibit autolysis. Tissues become harder as a result of fixation. Tissues removed from the body should be rapidly fixed, and this is best accomplished by using a small block of tissue and a large volume of fixative. This ensures a quick penetration of the tissue by the fixative. Failure to fix the tissue adequately permits intracellular enzymes to continue to function and to break down the cellular structure, a condition known as *postmortem degeneration.*

There are many different fixatives, and the choice among them will depend on the particular structures you wish to study. Not all fixatives are compatible with all staining methods. For example, one fixative may act as a mordant for staining, whereas others inhibit staining. The fixative that preserves glycogen and allows it to be stained is absolute alcohol; the fixative of choice for fat is formalin. The most commonly used fixative is a 10% solution of formalin in saline.

Processing

After the tissue has been preserved, the next step is to prepare it for microscopic examination. In order to permit light to pass through the tissue, very thin sections of the tissue must be cut. Unfortunately, although the process of fixation does harden the tissue, the material does not become sufficiently firm or cohesive to permit perfect thin sections to be cut. For this degree of firmness to be achieved, the tissue must be completely impregnated with some supporting medium that will hold the cells and intercellular structures together. The supporting materials used are referred to as *embedding materials.*

Some embedding materials, such as Carbowax and gelatin, are water-soluble, and tissues do not have to be dehydrated before their use. The most commonly used embedding materials are paraffinlike substances that are not miscible with water; when they are to be used, tissues must be dehydrated prior to impregnation. Examples of such substances are Paraplast and Tissue Prep.

Dehydration

Before an embedding material such as paraffin can penetrate fixed tissue, the water content must be removed. Dehydration is carried out by immersing the tissue block in increasing concentrations of ethyl alcohol. The use of graded strengths of alcohol gradually removes the water from the tissue without causing cellular damage and replaces the water with alcohol. Alcohol has the advantage of further hardening the tissue.

Clearing

Impregnating the tissue with an embedding medium is impossible at this stage, because the paraffinlike substances used for embedding are immiscible in alcohol. The tissue must therefore be immersed in a chemical in which both alcohol and paraffin are soluble. The chemical xylene is commonly used. Such a chemical is often referred to as a *clearing agent,* because it makes the tissue transparent as a result of its high refractive index. The block of tissue is removed from the absolute alcohol and passed through successive changes of xylene until all the alcohol is replaced with xylene.

Embedding

Once the tissue is impregnated with the clearing agent, the block of tissue is placed in melted paraffin. The tissue is transferred through two changes of paraffin to ensure the replacement of all the clearing agent with paraffin. The tissue block and the paraffin are then poured into a mold and allowed to harden. Excess paraffin is then trimmed away.

Sectioning

The small block of paraffin containing the tissue is then mounted on an instrument that is designed to cut thin tissue slices. The instrument, called a *microtome,* has a sharp steel knife, capable of regularly cutting paraffin sections 4 to 6 μm thick (Fig. I-6). The paraffin sections are caused to flatten by floating them on warm water; they are then transferred to glass slides coated with adhesive.

Staining

Most unstained tissues are almost transparent, and the recognition of structures under the light microscope is difficult, if not impossible, in such tissues. Staining methods were introduced in the middle of the nineteenth century, and their use immediately led to enormous advances in our knowledge of histology.

The different staining techniques result in the differential dyeing or metallic coating of the various

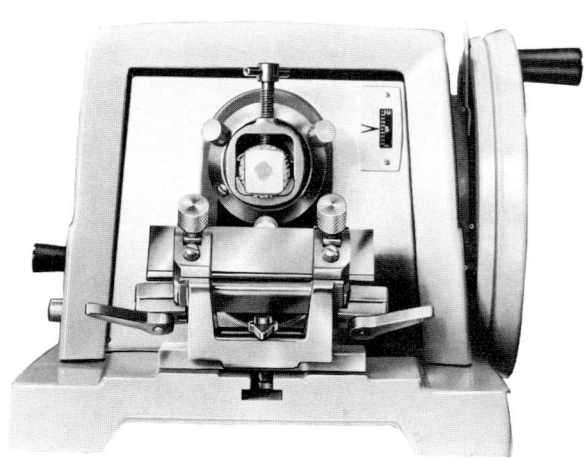

Fig. I-6. Microtome for cutting paraffin-embedded tissues. Each turn of the wheel seen at the right advances the specimen block, which then strikes the knife edge, cutting the sections. (Courtesy of American Optical Corporation.)

tissue components. Unfortunately, the chemistry involved in the majority of techniques is not understood, and many staining techniques were discovered by accident. There are three broad groups of biological stains. The first consists of the general tissue stains, which use one or two dyes to differentiate the nucleus from the cytoplasm of cells. The second group involves special staining procedures, for example, those used to demonstrate collagen and elastin in connective tissue. The third group includes heavy metal impregnation methods, in which metal salts are deposited on tissues and the salts are then converted to metal.

It is unnecessary for a medical student to have an encyclopedic knowledge of the different staining techniques now available to make different tissue components visible under the light microscope. Table I-1 summarizes some of the common techniques used in the preparation of microscope slides. Examples are shown in Figure I-7.

The most common combination of dyes used for histology and histopathology is *hematoxylin* and *eosin* (H&E). Hematoxylin is a natural dye obtained from the bark of logwood trees. It is not a dye as such, and must be oxidized to hematein to become a stain. Furthermore, the resulting dye (hematoxylin-hematein) has no affinity for tissues. A mordant, such as aluminum or iron, must be used with the hematoxylin mixture before it can stain tissues. The dye mixture stains a purple-blue color. Eosin is a synthetic dye and gives a pink to red color.

In cells stained with H&E, the nucleic acids present in the nucleus are stained with hematoxylin, giving the nucleus a purple-blue color. Eosin is attracted to the basic elements of protein in the cell cytoplasm, staining the cytoplasm pink to red. Tissue components that stain readily with basic dyes are called *basophilic*; those with an affinity for acid dyes are termed *acidophilic*. Hematoxylin behaves as a basic stain and therefore stains nuclei basophilically. Eosin is an acid dye and stains the basic protein elements in the cytoplasm acidophilically.

Metachromasia

Certain dyes react with tissue components and stain them a different color from that of the dye solution. The color change in the dye is called *metachromasia*. Examples of single dyes that exhibit metachromasia are methylene blue, toluidine blue, and thionin. With blue dyes, the color shift is toward red. A good example is the staining of mast cells with methylene blue. The cytoplasmic granules will stain purple-red, whereas the remainder of the tissue will be blue. The cause of metachromasia is not fully understood, but it has been suggested that polymerization of the dye molecules is responsible. The presence of macromolecules with electronegative radicals in the tissue is thought to facilitate the polymerization and bring about a color change.

Process of Staining and Mounting Sections

Before a tissue section can be stained, the paraffin in which the tissue is embedded must be removed. The section, which is adherent to the glass slide, is passed through xylene, and this dissolves the paraffin. Because many stains are dissolved in water, it is now necessary to remove the xylene from the

Table I-1. Stains commonly used in histology

Method	Composition	Result
Hematoxylin and eosin (H&E)	Hematoxylin, hematein, metal mordant	Nucleus—blue; cytoplasm—varying shades of red; collagen—very pale pink; cartilage and calcium deposits—dark blue; red blood cells—bright red
Heidenhain's iron hematoxylin	Iron alum, hematoxylin	Muscle striations—blue-black; nuclei—blue-black; mitochondria—blue-black
Masson's trichrome stain	Iron hematoxylin, Biebrich scarlet, acid fuchsin, phosphomolybdic-phosphotungstic acid, aniline blue	Nuclei—black; cytoplasm, keratin, muscle fibers—red; collagen, mucin—blue
Mallory's aniline blue collagen stain	Acid fuchsin, aniline blue, orange G	Nuclei—red; collagen—blue; ground substance, cartilage, mucin—blue; red cells, myelin—yellow; elastic fibers—pink, yellow, or unstained
Verhoeff's elastic stain	Hematoxylin, ferric chloride, iodine, sodium thiosulfate	Elastic fibers—blue-black to black
Orcein elastic stain	Orcein, alcohol, hydrochloric acid	Elastic fibers—dark brown
Weigert's elastic stain	Hematoxylin, resorcin-fuchsin	Elastic fibers—blue-black to black
Metallic impregnation of reticular fibers	Silver nitrate or silver hydroxide	Reticular fibers—black
Wright and Giemsa stains for blood	Methylene blue, methylene violet, azure A, azure B, eosin	Nuclei of white cells—purple; basophilic cytoplasm of lymphocytes, monocytes—blue; eosinophilic granules—pink to orange; neutrophilic granules—pink to purple; basophils—dark blue cytoplasmic granules; red blood cells—pink

tissue and replace it with water. The section is immersed in a series of diminishing concentrations of ethyl alcohol until it is filled with water. After the section has been stained with the appropriate dye solution, it is passed through alcohols of increasing concentration to remove all the water once again. Finally, the section is immersed in xylene before being mounted in a mounting medium soluble in xylene. A thin glass coverslip is then placed over the section to protect it and to make a permanent preparation.

PREPARATION OF TISSUES FOR ELECTRON MICROSCOPY

The same general principles are involved in the preparation of tissues for electron microscopy as for light microscopy, with the following important differences.

Fixation

Most fixatives used for light microscopy produce a coarse precipitation of protein and loss of ultrastructural detail; they are therefore unsatisfactory for electron microscopy. A double fixation process is

Fig. I-7. Photomicrographs of sections, showing the use of common stains. (A) Transverse section of esophagus stained with hematoxylin alone; the nuclei are blue. (B) Transverse section of esophagus stained with eosin alone; the cell cytoplasm shows varying shades of red. (C) Transverse section of esophagus stained with hematoxylin and eosin (H&E); the nuclei are blue, and the cytoplasm is red. (D) Transverse section of esophagus stained with Mallory's stain; cytoplasm is pink, the collagen is blue. (E) Transverse section of small artery stained with Weigert's elastic stain; elastic fibers are black. (F) Section of lymph node, showing reticular fibers impregnated with silver; reticular fibers are black.

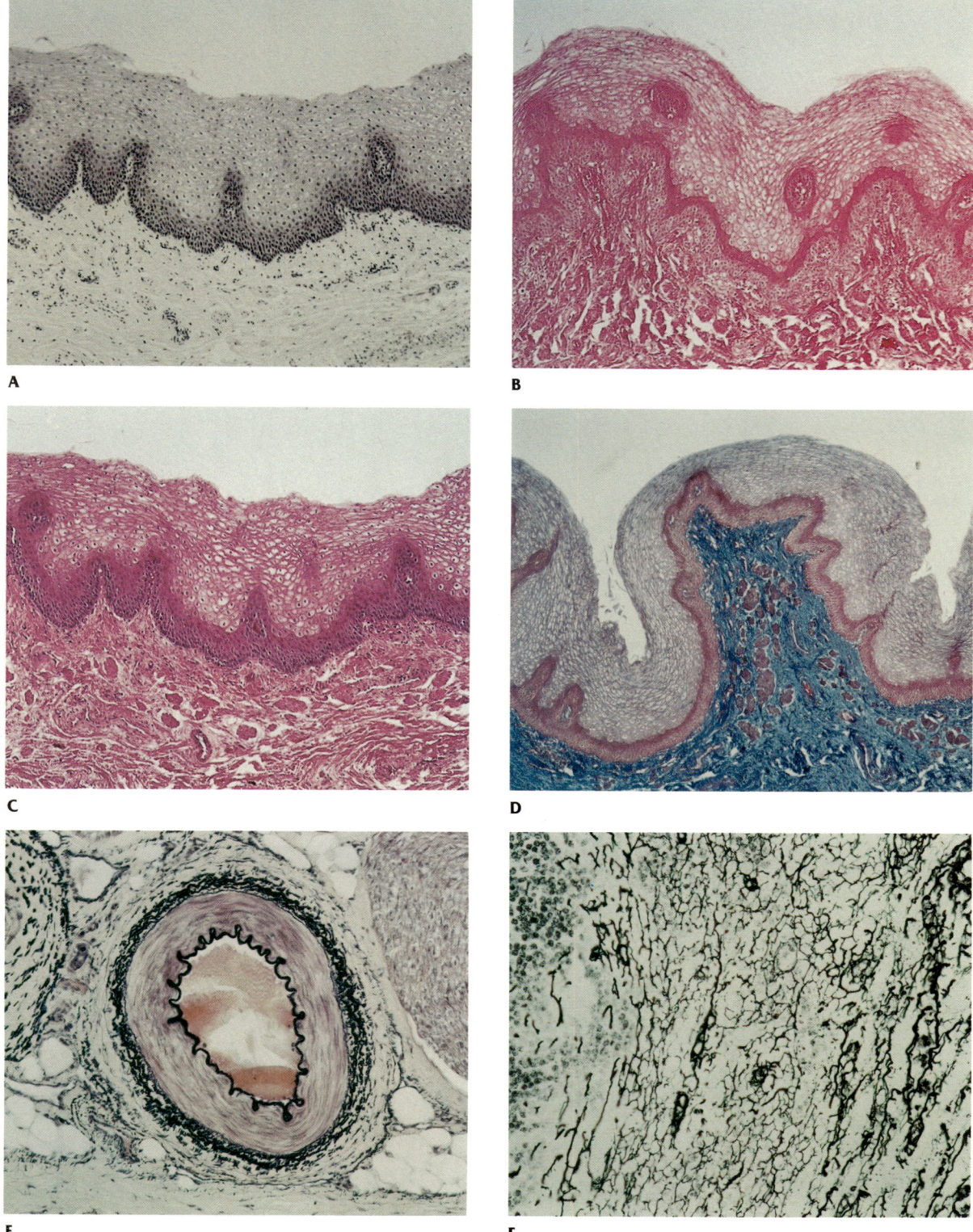

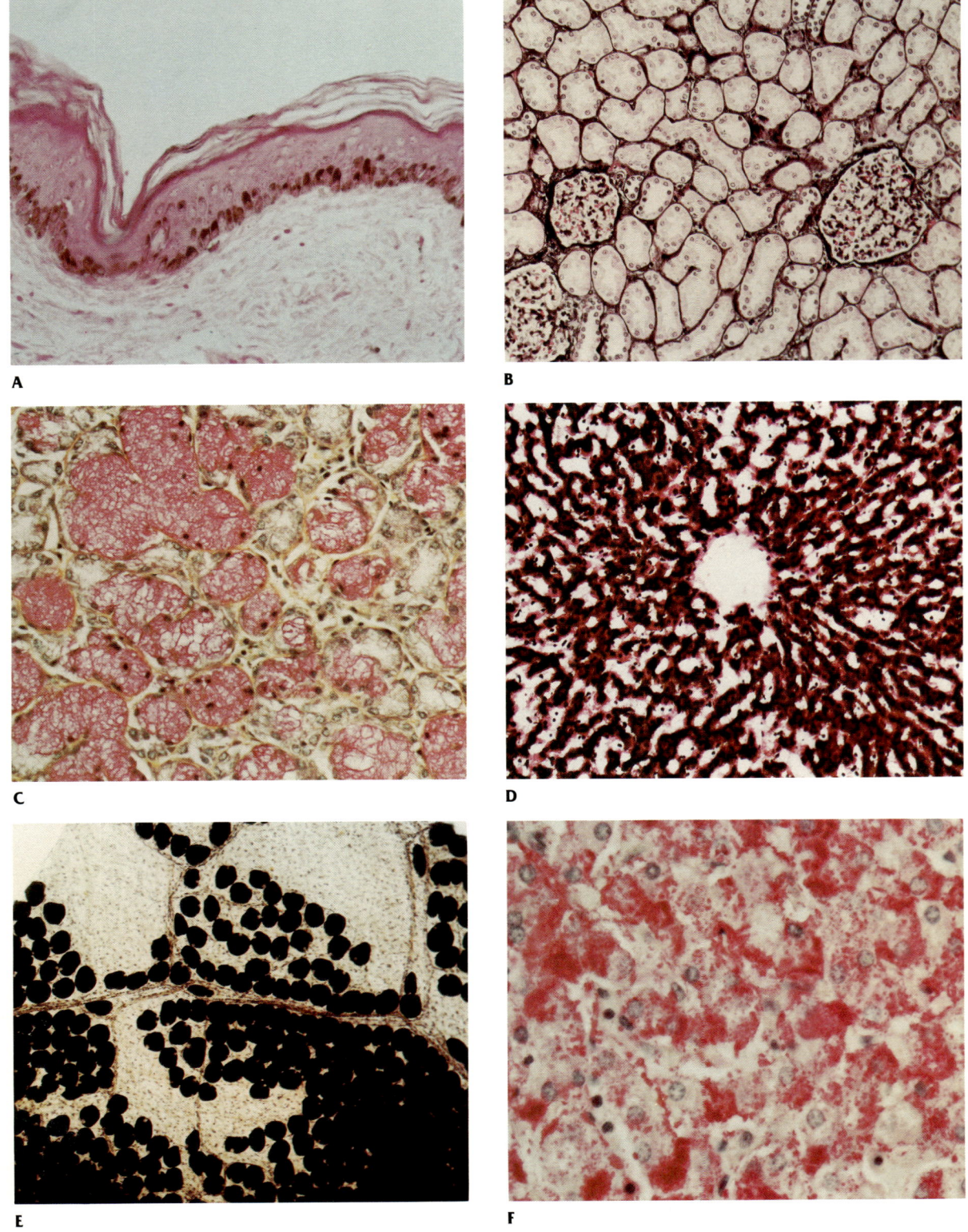

now commonly employed. First, a very small piece of tissue (just a few cubic millimeters) is fixed in buffered glutaraldehyde solution. In the case of animal tissues, it is sometimes preferable to perfuse the organ before death to ensure that the minimum of postmortem degeneration occurs. The tissue is then exposed to a second fixative of buffered osmium tetroxide. Osmium tetroxide not only fixes the tissue but also "stains" many of its components. Staining here means that the reduced osmium becomes adherent to some of the cell components and, because of its density, increases the contrast of the image.

Embedding

Because electrons have very little penetrating power and are scattered by passing through a specimen, electron microscopy requires that very thin sections be used. For this to be possible, the tissue must be embedded in material that is harder than paraffin. The epoxy resins Epon and Araldite are commonly used.

Sectioning

Ultrathin sections, 50 to 100 nm thick, are necessary for electron microscopy. Compare this thickness with the 5 to 10 μm required for the light microscope. The very thin sections are cut on an ultramicrotome (Fig. I-8) with a knife made of plate glass or diamond. The sections are floated on water and mounted on copper grids. The grids support the delicate sections and permit the passage of the electrons through those portions of the section that lie suspended over the grid perforations.

Staining

Staining is a misnomer in electron microscopy, because colored dyes are not used. In order to obtain a greater contrast in the black-and-white images of tissue components on the fluorescent screen or photographic film, however, substances are used that adhere to the different cellular components and make them more electron-dense. Solutions of salts of heavy metals such as uranyl acetate or lead citrate are commonly used for this purpose.

Freeze-Fracture Etching

Freeze-fracture etching is a method of preparing tissues for electron microscopy without using chemical fixatives or dehydrating and embedding agents. The tissue is rapidly frozen at very low temperatures ($-160°C$) and then fractured with a metal blade. The cut surface of the tissue is not produced by the metal blade cutting through the tissue; rather, the striking of the frozen tissue by the blade initiates a fracture line that spreads across the tissue, much like a fracture line running across broken glass. The exposed surface of the tissue is then kept in a vacuum at a low temperature, which permits the frozen water on the surface of the tissue to sublimate into the vacuum. This is the etching phase of the process, and it leaves the various cell components standing out in relief on the frozen surface (Fig. I-9). Carbon and platinum are then deposited on the frozen-fractured-etched surface of the tissue at an angle to produce a shadowed effect, similar to the way driven snow is blown over a group of houses: the snow piles up on the near sides of the houses but leaves clear spaces or shadows on the far sides of the houses. The tissue is now brought back to normal atmospheric pressure and temperature. The carbon-platinum replica is placed on a copper grid after the tissue has been digested by a strong acid and can then be examined with a transmission electron microscope. Freeze-fracture etching has been most useful in the study of cell membranes and their junctional complexes.

Fig. I-10. Photomicrographs of sections, showing the use of some common histochemical stains. (A) Vertical section of white skin treated with dopa reagent and counterstained with eosin; the melanin granules are brown. (B) Section of cortex of kidney, Jones's periodic acid–methenamine silver stain; the basement membrane is black. (C) Section of submandibular salivary gland, mucicarmine stain; the mucin is red. (D) Section of liver, acid phosphatase stain; black lead phosphate precipitate at site of enzyme activity. (E) Adipose tissue cells, osmic acid stain; fat is stained black. (F) Liver hepatocytes, Best's carmine stain; glycogen is red.

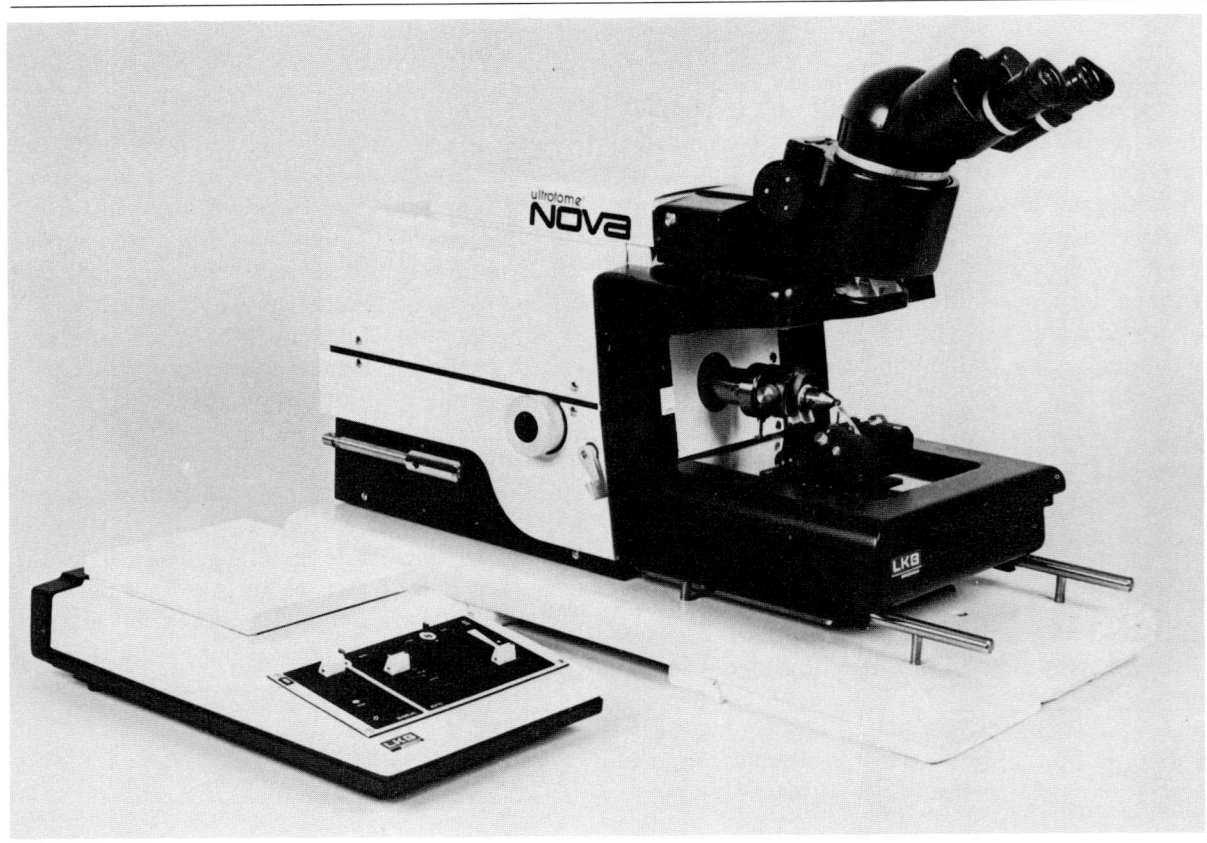

Fig. I-8. *Ultramicrotome for cutting epoxy-embedded tissues. The knife is plate glass or diamond, and the sections are floated on water. The tissue block is advanced by heat expansion of a metal rod or by a delicate mechanical mechanism. The cutting procedure is closely watched through a low-power binocular microscope. (Courtesy of LKB.)*

HISTOCHEMISTRY AND CYTOCHEMISTRY

Histochemistry and cytochemistry are the study of the chemical processes that take place within cells and tissues and the identification of the structural sites where these chemical reactions take place. Using a tissue section, one attempts to localize a particular chemical component by means of a chemical reaction whose end product is visible with the microscope. At first, the use of histochemistry was limited to light microscopy, but the methods have been so refined that, for example, it is now possible to localize glucose-6-phosphate in the rough and smooth endoplasmic reticulum with the electron microscope.

At this point you may ask yourself what the difference is between a histochemical staining method and a morphological staining method that has been used traditionally by histologists for demonstrating such structures as nuclei, Golgi complexes, and nerve fibers. A histochemical technique is one based on fully understood inorganic or organic chemical reactions, whereas the use of ordinary dyes for staining involves reactions that are not always understood and may involve a multitude of physicochemical phenomena.

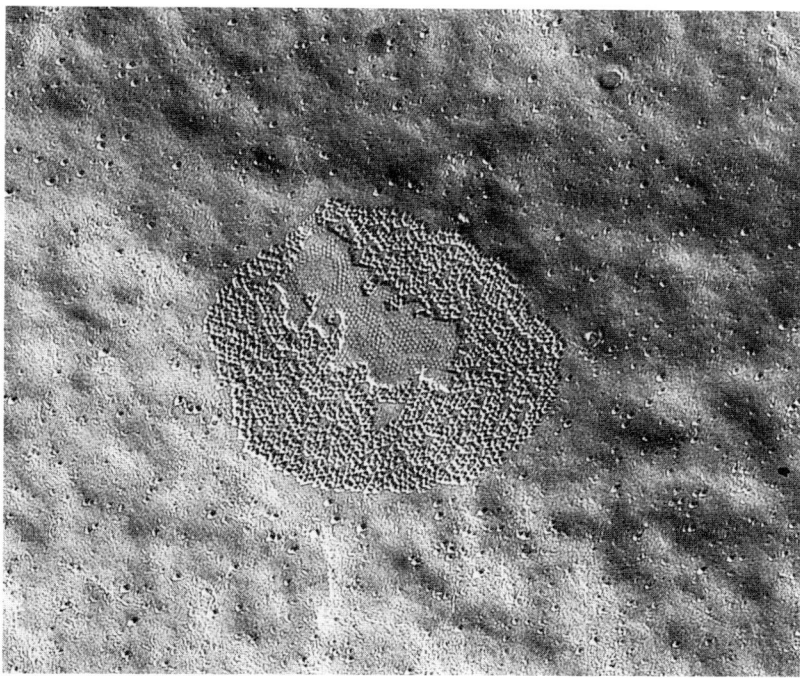

Fig. I-9. Electron micrograph of a freeze-fracture replica view of the P-face (see Ch. 2, p. 70) of an ovarian granulosa cell gap junction. The direction of the shadowing is toward the top of the photograph. The outwardly directed half membrane shows an aggregation of globular intramembrane particles at the gap junction. (Courtesy of Dr. D. Albertini.)

General Requirements for Histochemical Techniques

Requirements for histochemical techniques are much more rigorous than those for ordinary staining. Some of the more important are as follows:

1. *The chemical substance and the tissue must be preserved.* One of the most important first steps in histochemistry is the preservation of both the chemical substance being studied and the structure of the tissue in which it resides. Enzymes, which are proteins, are inactivated if exposed for long periods to fixatives. Fixatives are, however, necessary for the preservation of structure. The process of fixation is thus to some extent a compromise between preserving chemical activity and maintaining structural integrity. Formaldehyde is a common fixative used in light microscopy; glutaraldehyde is often used in electron microscopy.

2. *Diffusion of the chemical substances from their morphological sites must be prevented.* Chemicals with large molecules tend to remain stationary. Other substances, such as amino acids, sugars, and electrolytes, are water-soluble and quickly diffuse from their morphological sites, making accurate localization of these substances very difficult or impossible. Lipids are soluble in organic solvents such as xylene and chloroform; consequently, these solvents must be avoided.

3. *The histochemical technique must yield an insoluble end product.* The end product must be insoluble so that it does not diffuse from the site of the chemical reaction. Moreover, it should be colored or sufficiently opaque to be recognizable with a light microscope or sufficiently electron-dense to be identifiable with a transmission electron microscope.

Table I-2. Common histochemical reactions used in histology

Method	Components	Result
Periodic acid–Schiff (PAS) reaction	Periodic acid; leucofuchsin or fuchsin–sulfurous acid	Glycogen, epithelial mucins, Golgi complex, cell coats, basement membranes, proteoglycans in connective tissue ground substance—purple-red
Feulgen reaction for deoxyribonucleic acid	Mild hydrolysis with hydrochloric acid, Schiff reagent	Deoxyribonucleic acid (DNA) in nuclear chromatin—magenta
Sudan black for lipids	Sudan black B	Lipid—blue-black
Osmium tetroxide for lipids	Osmium tetroxide	Lipid—black
Azodye methods for phosphatases	Naphthol AS-B1 phosphate, diazonium salt, fast red violet LB; pH 9–9.6 alkaline phosphatase; pH 4.5–6 acid phosphatase	Sites of enzyme activity—pink-red
DOPA reaction for tyrosinase in melanocytes	3,4-Dihydroxyphenylalanine	Granules of melanin—brown-black; nonspecific, because other oxidizing systems, such as cytochromes and peroxidases, cause nonspecific staining reactions

4. *The histochemical reaction must be specific for the chemical being studied.* This requirement may be satisfied by using control sections that are subjected to the same chemical procedures as the test specimen but with one of the important reagents omitted. In enzyme histochemistry, for example, the specific substrate may be omitted or the control sections may be exposed to specific inhibitors of the enzyme being studied. In all histochemical techniques, it is important that the control and the test sections are processed at the same time under identical conditions of pH and temperature.

Some histochemical reactions that are frequently used in histology are shown in Table I-2; some examples are shown in Figure I-10.

IMMUNOCYTOCHEMISTRY

Immunocytochemistry is a very sensitive method for localizing specific proteins or polysaccharides. The method depends on the fact that the body produces specific proteins, called *antibodies,* in response to injected foreign proteins, called *antigens.* The antibodies then react with the antigens and inactivate them. Fluorescent dye molecules can be linked chemically to antibody molecules so that the sites

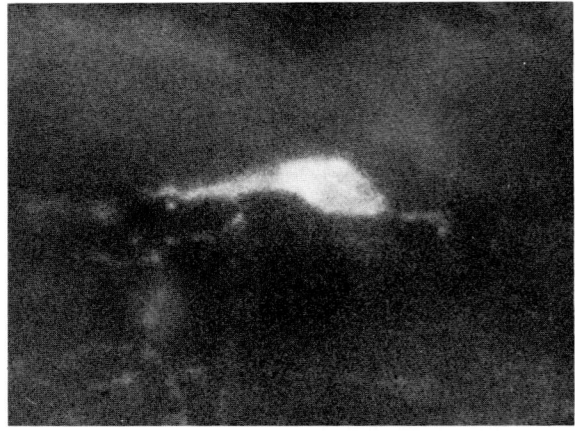

Fig. I-11. Photomicrograph of a retinal somatostatin-containing neuron. The cell was identified by the use of an indirect immunofluorescence technique. The labeled cell is situated in layer VIII of the retina. (Courtesy of Dr. J. P. Ellis.)

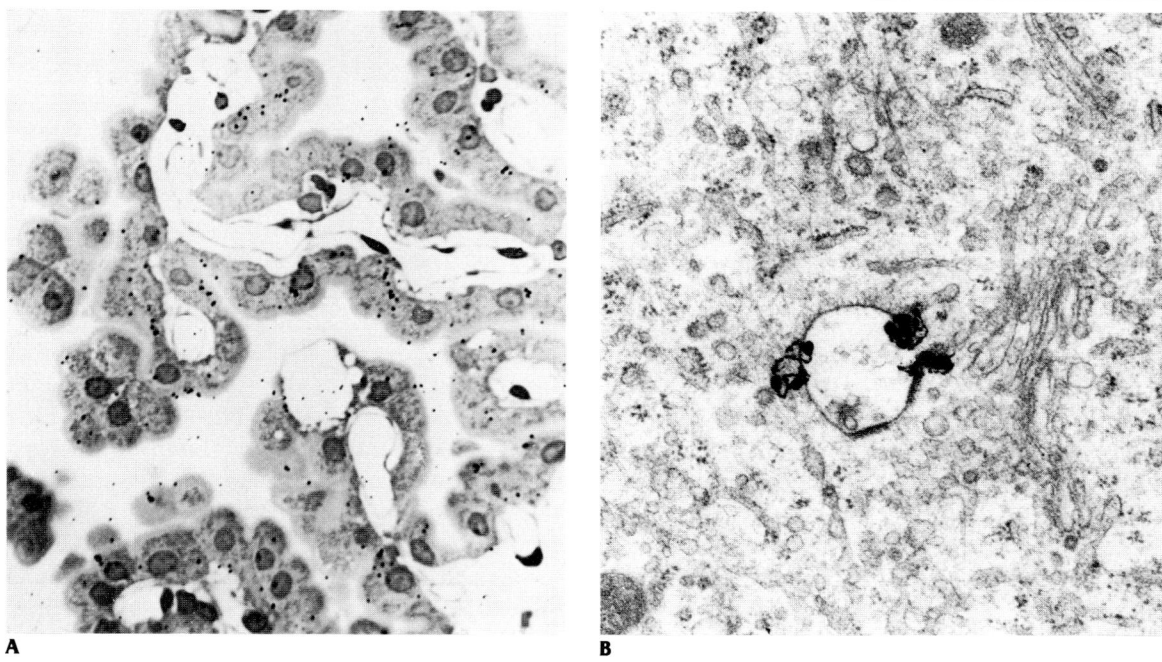

Fig. I-12. Radioautographs of epithelial cells of choroid plexus in lateral ventricle of brain. (A) Light micrograph, showing silver grains depicting position of iodine 125 prolactin in cytoplasm. (B) Electron micrograph, showing filamentous silver grains in multivesicular body in cytoplasm. (Courtesy of Dr. R. Walsh.)

where the antibodies react with the antigens can be localized with a fluorescent microscope (Fig. I-11). Immunocytochemistry techniques have been used with great success in the localization of myosin in muscle fibers and the localization of the cells of origin of hormones in endocrine glands. In many instances, it has been possible to couple the antibody protein with an iron-rich protein called *ferritin* in place of the fluorescent dye. This substance is electron-dense and permits the ferritin-bound antibody-antigen reaction to be localized accurately with the electron microscope.

RADIOAUTOGRAPHY (AUTORADIOGRAPHY)

Radioautography is very valuable in the localization of specific chemical substances within the body. This method can also be used to study dynamic biological events taking place within cells. It is now possible to obtain synthetic radioactive isotopes of many normal tissue metabolites you may wish to study. The tracer isotope is injected into an animal, and the tissue to be investigated is removed and processed for light or electron microscopy in the usual manner. The tissue section, on a slide, is then placed in contact with a photographic emulsion and stored in a lightproof box for a period of days or weeks.

Over time, the radiation emitted by the isotope at its site within the tissue will act on the silver bromide crystals in the overlying photographic emulsion. The site of the isotope in the tissue will be seen as small black granules on the developed photograph. The quantity of the granules is proportional to the strength of the radioactivity. To assist in the localization of the specific chemical in relation to cellular components, the tissue section can be stained and mounted in the usual manner (Fig. I-12). You can also use the method with the electron microscope, using ultrathin sections. Because a resolution of about 0.2 nm can be obtained, accurate localization of chemical substances within cells is possible. The black granules on an electron micrograph appear as short, coiled filaments.

Radioautography has been used with great success to study the dynamics of chemical reactions in the metabolism of carbohydrates, lipids, and proteins. One of the first important uses of this technique was to determine the turnover of cell populations and trace their migration from their sites of origin. For this purpose, tritiated thymidine is used. This compound is incorporated into deoxyribonucleic acid (DNA) when it is synthesized in the nuclei of cells about to divide. As a result, the nuclei of these cells and their daughter cells are labeled and thus easily identified wherever they move, whereas the nuclei of nondividing cells remain unlabeled.

INTERPRETATION OF TISSUE SECTIONS

1. Make sure that your microscope is in good working order and that the lenses are clean. The eyepiece lens nearest the eye tends to become greasy from the oil on your eyelashes. The lower objective lens should be cleaned periodically to remove traces of immersion oil or grease from your fingers. Always use the objective with the lowest possible magnification first in order to identify the main structures on a histological slide; after all, when you examine a road map, you obtain a general idea of the major land masses and roads before you examine the detail of the minor roads, streams, and houses. In other words, the high-power objectives should be used only for detail work.

2. Hold up your histological slide to the light and examine the section with the naked eye. Get some appreciation of the general shape and size of the tissue section. Many organs and tubular structures have characteristic shapes that enable you, after practice, to recognize them before you actually use the microscope. What has the section been stained with?

3. Understand that you are about to look at a slice of tissue that may measure several millimeters in diameter but only about 7 μm in thickness. Realize that the section in most cases is less than one cell thick. Realize also that the slice of tissue was cut by a machine in one plane only, and that the direction of the cut through the tissue block was determined by the histology technician to reveal to the best advantage only certain structures. Try to imagine what you would see in the sections taken above and below the section on your slide. Structures such as blood vessels and nerves often take a wavy path through tissues, so that when they are identified in a particular plane of section, they may be cut across several times, sometimes in cross section, sometimes obliquely, and sometimes longitudinally.

4. Understand that if you examine a section cut across a cell, the plane of section may miss the nucleus altogether, so that the cell looks empty (Fig. I-13). The same observation can be made when you cut across an egg with a knife; you may section the yolk, or you may miss it completely.

5. Sections across tubular structures like blood vessels and air passages often are difficult for the student to interpret (see Fig. I-13), especially if the section goes through a curved part of the tube or if the wall of the tube shows infolding.

6. Try to convert what you see in two planes on a section into three planes in your mind's eye. In other words, think about what you are looking at and at the same time combine this information with what you have read about the tissue or organ so that you can construct in your mind a three-dimensional picture.

7. Appreciate the relative sizes of the different components of the tissue or organ that you are examining. A red cell, which can be found in most sections, measures about 7 μm across and is a useful reference for measurement.

8. Read the label on your slide and determine which stains have been used. Ask yourself what structures have been stained with the different dyes. Has metachromasia taken place?

9. Never regard your section as merely a pretty image of a dead piece of tissue. Remember that the image represents the moment in time when the tissue was fixed and all metabolic activities suddenly ceased. A second or two before fixation, the activities of the cells may have been different, and consequently the cells may have had a different appear-

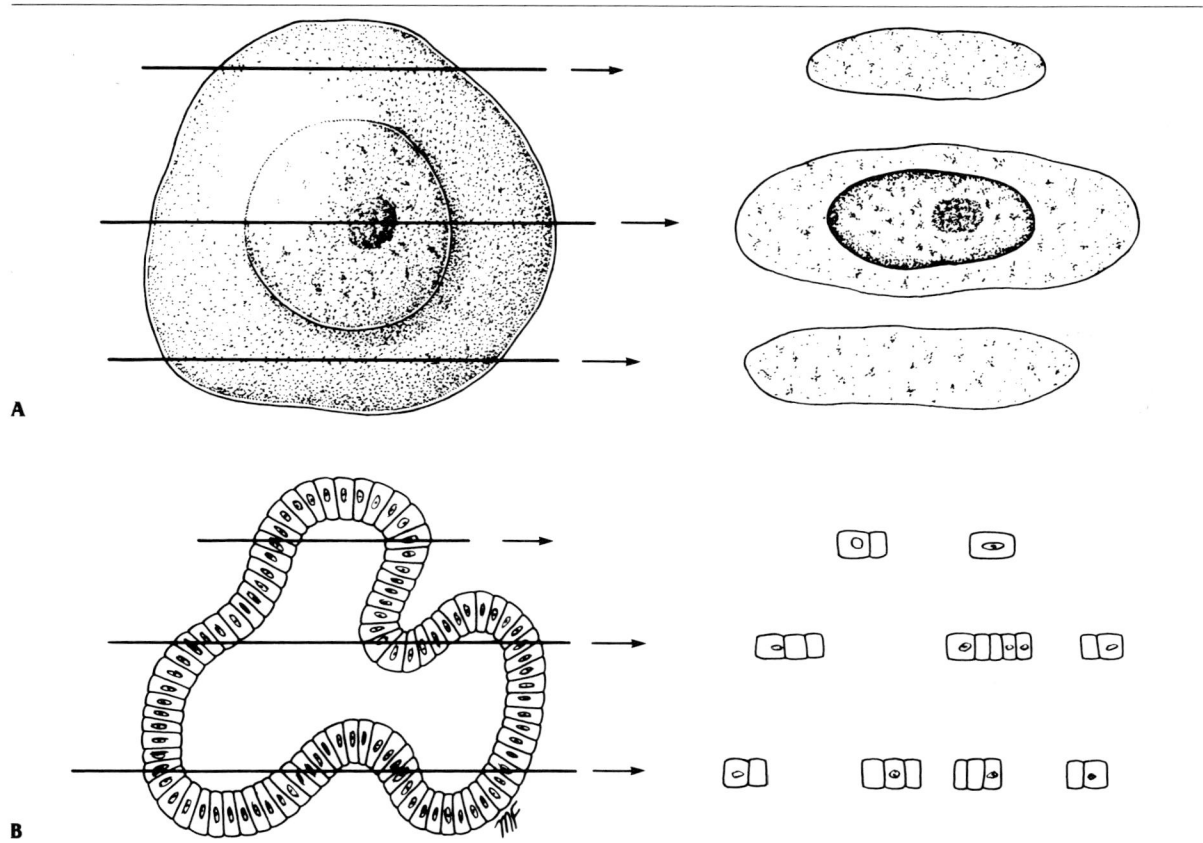

Fig. I-13. *Different appearances of sections cut in different planes. (A) shows a cell cut across at different levels; (B) shows a much-infolded single layer of cells cut across at three sites. Note that the size and shape of the cells and the presence or absence of their nuclei will depend on the plane of section through each cell. Note also how the curving and infolding of the layer of cells may give the impression that the layer is discontinuous.*

ance. There may have been fewer or more secretory granules present in the cytoplasm, for example. Regard your section as a living tissue. Identify each structure present on the slide with care and ask yourself what its function is. If you read the Clinical Notes sections of this book, you should also have some idea of the diseases that commonly can affect the tissue or organ. Furthermore, you might be able to speculate on the clinical consequences to the patient of a particular disease process.

10. Before returning the slide to your slide collection, make sure that you have recognized three or four significant structures that clearly identify the tissue or organ. Ask yourself, for example, why this is a section of the appendix and not a section of the tonsil, the thymus, a lymph node, or the spleen. If you do this with every section, you will quickly be able to recognize a given tissue when you view it again.

11. Beware of the situation in which you examine a section and you start to feel that you are unable to recognize anything on the slide. This experience is a common one for the beginner and also may occur with more practiced students under examination conditions. Don't panic. We have all had the experience at some time in our lives. Slowly and meth-

odically scan your section with the low-power and possibly the medium-power objectives. Identify structures that you can easily recognize, such as blood vessels, nerves, or ducts. Gradually collect your data and consciously assemble the facts. To your surprise, you will suddenly recognize the tissue or organ. In class you should always follow this procedure. Never get into the habit of raising your hand for assistance before using your eyes and your brain. The recognition of a tissue or organ on which you have had to work painstakingly to identify will give you ample reward: not only will you understand the structure and function of the tissue or organ; more important, you will never forget it.

UNITS OF MEASURE USED IN LIGHT AND ELECTRON MICROSCOPY

When you examine histological sections or electron micrographs, it is important to have some idea of size. You should become familiar with the following units of measure:

METRIC UNITS OF LENGTH

centimeter (cm)	$= 0.01\ (10^{-2})$ meter
millimeter (mm)	$= 0.001\ (10^{-3})$ meter
micrometer (μm)	$= 0.000001\ (10^{-6})$ meter
nanometer (nm)	$= 0.000000001\ (10^{-9})$ meter

OLD TERMINOLOGY	NEW TERMINOLOGY
1 micron (μ)	= 1 micrometer (μm)
1 millimicron (mμ)	= 1 nanometer (nm)
1 Ångström unit (Å)	= 0.1 nm

In practical terms, the red cell is a useful reference for measurement when you are looking through a light microscope, as stated previously, because it measures about 7 μm across; when you are examining an electron micrograph, a ribosome, which measures about 15 nm, can be used in the same way.

ADDITIONAL READING

Bancroft, J. D., and Stevens, A. (eds.). *Theory and Practice of Histological Techniques.* Edinburgh: Churchill Livingstone, 1977.

Barer, R. *Lecture Notes on the Use of the Microscope.* Oxford: Blackwell, 1968.

Barka, T., and Anderson, P. J. *Histochemistry: Theory, Practice, and Bibliography.* New York: Hoeber Medical Division, Harper & Row, 1963.

Baserga, R., and Malamud, D. *Autoradiography: Techniques and Application.* New York: Harper & Row, 1969.

Bullivant, S. Freeze-etching and freeze fracturing. In Koehler, J. (ed.), *Advanced Techniques in Biological Electron Microscopy.* New York: Springer-Verlag, 1973, p. 66.

Coons, A. H. Fluorescent antibody methods. In Danielli, J. F. (ed.), *General Cytochemical Methods.* New York: Academic, 1958, p. 400.

Davenport, H. A. *Histological and Histochemical Technics.* Philadelphia: Saunders, 1960.

Everhart, T. E., and Hayes, T. L. The scanning electron microscope. *Sci. Am.* 226:54, 1972.

Fawcett, D. W. Electron microscopy in histology and cytology. In Siegel, B. M. (ed.), *Modern Developments in Electron Microscopy.* New York: Academic, 1963.

Glauert, A. M. Fixation, dehydration and embedding of biological specimens. In Glauert, A. M. (ed.), *Practical Methods in Electron Microscopy.* Vol. 3, Part 1. Amsterdam: North Holland, 1975.

Hale, A. J. *The Interference Microscope in Biological Research.* Edinburgh and London: Churchill Livingstone Inc., 1958.

Hall, C. A. *How to Use the Microscope* (4th ed.). New York: Macmillan, 1955.

Hama, K., and Porter, K. R. An application of high voltage electron microscopy to the study of biological materials. *J. Microsc.* 8:149, 1969.

Hayat, M. A. *Basic Electron Microscopy Technics.* New York: Van Nostrand Reinhold, 1972.

Hayat, M. A. *Principles and Techniques of Electron Microscopy.* New York: Van Nostrand Reinhold, 1972.

Hayat, M. A. *Introduction to Scanning Electron Microscopy.* Baltimore: University Park Press, 1978.

Hollenburg, M. J., and Erickson, A. M. The scanning electron microscope: Potential usefulness to biologists. A review. *J. Histochem. Cytochem.* 21:109, 1973.

Kimoto, S., and Russ, J. C. The characteristics and applications of the scanning electron microscope. *Am. Sci.* 57 (1):112, 1969.

Koehler, J. K. The technique and application of freeze-etching in ultrastructure research. *Adv. Biol. Med. Phys.* 12:1, 1968.

Lillie, R. D. *Histopathologic Technique and Practical Histochemistry* (2nd ed.). New York: Blakiston, 1954.

McManus, J. F. A., and Mowry, R. W. *Staining Methods: Histologic and Histochemical.* New York: Hoeber, 1960.

Pearse, A. G. E. *Histochemistry: Theoretical and Applied* (3rd ed.). Boston: Little, Brown, 1968.

Pease, D. C. *Histological Techniques for Electron Microscopy.* New York: Academic, 1960.

Pelc, S. R., Appleton, T. C., and Wilton, M. E. State of light autoradiography. In Leblond, C. P., and Warren, K. B. (eds.), *The Use of Radioautography in Investigating Protein Synthesis.* New York: Academic, 1965.

Porter, K. R. Ultramicrotomy. In Siegel, B. M. (ed.), *Modern Developments in Electron Microscopy.* New York: Academic, 1963.

Reid, N. Ultramicrotomy. In Glauert, A. M. (ed.), *Practical Methods in Electron Microscopy.* Vol. 3, Part 2. Amsterdam: North Holland, 1975.

Rogers, A. W. Recent developments in the use of autoradiography techniques with electron microscopy. *Philos. Trans. R. Soc. Lond. {Biol.}* 261:159, 1971.

Rogers, A. W. *Techniques of Autoradiography.* New York: American Elsevier, 1973.

Saltpeter, M. M., and Bachmann, L. Assessment of technical steps in electron microscope autoradiography. In Leblond, C. P., and Warren, K. B. (eds.), *The Use of Radioautography in Investigating Protein Synthesis.* New York: Academic, 1965.

Scarpelli, D. G., and Kanczak, N. M. Ultrastructural cytochemistry: Principles, limitations and applications. *Int. Rev. Exp. Pathol.* 4:55, 1965.

Sheehan, D. C., and Hrapchak, B. B. *Theory and Practice of Histotechnology* (2nd ed.). St. Louis: Mosby, 1980.

Sjöstrand, F. S. *Electron Microscopy of Cells and Tissues.* Vol. 1, *Instrumentation and Techniques.* New York: Academic, 1967.

Staehelin, L. A. The interpretation of freeze-etched artificial and biological membranes. *J. Ultrastruct. Res.* 22:326, 1968.

Sternberger, L. A. Electron microscopic immunocytochemistry: A review. *J. Histochem. Cytochem.* 15:139, 1967.

Weinstein, R. S., and Someda, K. The freeze-cleave approach to the ultrastructure of frozen tissues. *Cryobiology* 4:116, 1967.

Williams, M. A. Autoradiography and immunocytochemistry. In Glauert, A. M. (ed.), *Practical Methods in Electron Microscopy.* Vol. 6, Part 1. Amsterdam: North Holland, 1978.

Wischnitzer, S. *Introduction to Electron Microscopy* (2nd ed.). New York: Pergamon, 1970.

ORGANIZATION OF THE HUMAN BODY

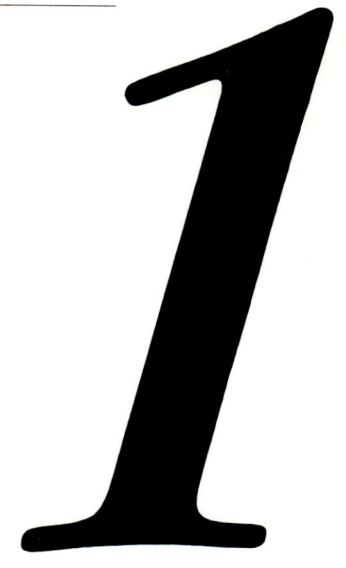

Anatomy is the study of the structure of the body and the relationship of its constituent parts to one another. Anatomy can be subdivided into the study of that which is visible to the naked eye, *gross anatomy,* and that which can be seen only with the help of a microscope, *microscopic anatomy* or *histology.* Clinical and functional histology is the study of those aspects of microscopic structure and function that are essential for patient care.

The human body is a highly complex organism which may be broken down into four structural subunits: cells, tissues, organs, and systems.

CELLS

These are the smallest structural and functional units in the body. They vary in size from 8 to 200 μm (1 μm equals 1/1,000 mm); thus, to study cells, one must view them under a microscope.

Cells vary in shape. Those that line blood vessels and body cavities are flattened, those that line ducts of glands are cuboidal, and those that line most of the digestive tract are rectangular or columnar. Some cells are shaped like biconcave discs, such as the red cells of the blood; others are elongated and fusiform, such as the cells of skeletal muscle. Nerve cells are irregular in shape and possess elongated processes.

All cells, whatever their size or shape, are simple units of living matter and exhibit fundamental metabolic activities. Each cell takes up oxygen and other basic materials from its environment, metabolizes those materials, and excretes carbon dioxide and other waste substances. Many cells are capable of reproduction by cell division; others have become highly specialized and have lost this ability.

As will be seen in the next chapter, the delicate protoplasm that constitutes the interior of a cell is constantly carrying out chemical reactions that are essential to life. This watery intracellular material is separated from the extracellular fluid by a plasma membrane (Fig. 1-1). In a complex multicellular organism, such as a human being, only the surface cells are directly in contact with the external environment. The internal cells are bathed in fluid from which they obtain their nutrients and into which they excrete waste products. For a human cell to be able to function normally, the composition of this surrounding fluid (*internal environment*) must be kept as constant as possible. As a result, in large multicellular organisms, many cells specialize and

21

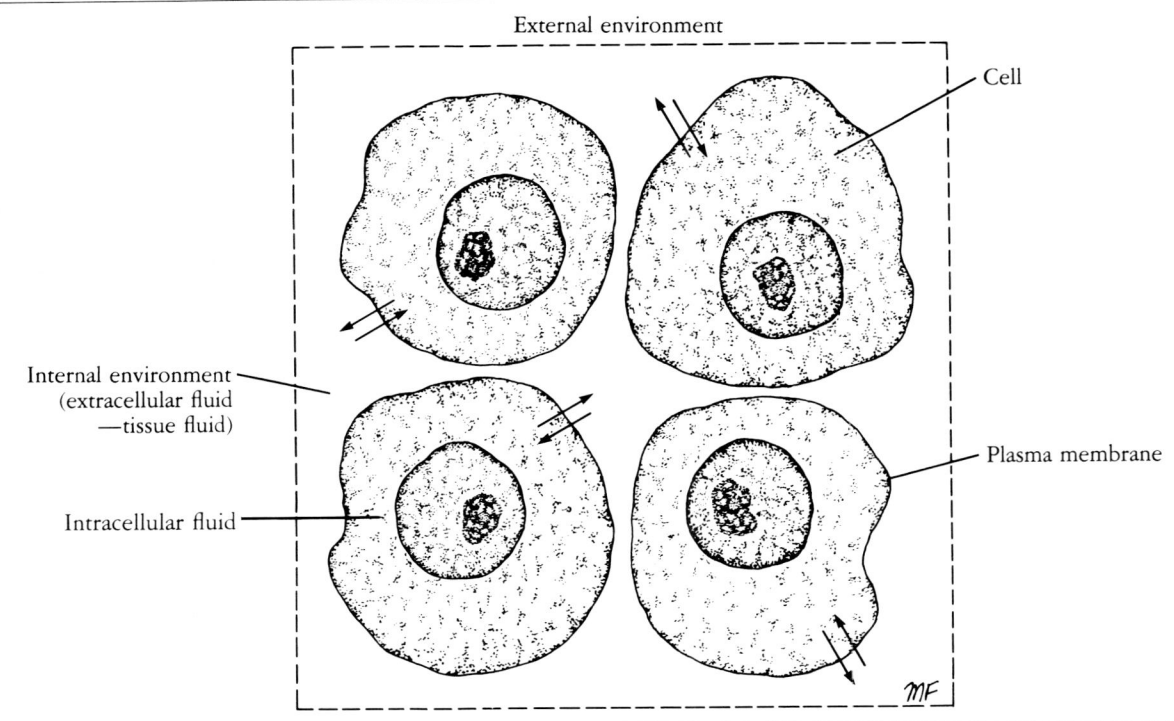

Fig. 1-1. *The cells of the body and their relationship to the internal and external environment. Note that the plasma membrane separates the intracellular fluid from the extracellular fluid.*

become grouped together as functional units in order to assist the body as a whole to maintain a stable environment for its cells. For example, some cells become grouped together to form the respiratory system, so that oxygen can be taken up from the atmosphere and carbon dioxide be excreted. Other cells form the circulatory system, so that these gases can be transported to and from the deeply placed cells.

TISSUES

Tissues are composed of groups of cells performing a similar function. There are four main types of tissues: (1) epithelial tissue, (2) connective tissue, (3) muscular tissue, and (4) nervous tissue.

Epithelial tissue is protective and covers the surfaces of the body and lines tubes and ducts that communicate with the surface. The cells may be arranged in a single layer or may be stratified. The one feature common to all epithelial tissue is that the cells are situated close to one another.

Connective tissues serve as supporting and strengthening material and connect other tissues with one another. The cells are usually widely separated by large amounts of matrix. The matrix consists of an amorphous jelly in which are embedded long, slender fibers. It is the intercellular matrix that holds the body together.

Muscular tissue consists of long, slender muscle cells that are positioned side by side to form long and short chains. The cells have the ability to shorten and thicken, a process known as *contraction*.

Nervous tissue rapidly conducts information from one part of the body to another and is receptive to various types of stimuli that occur either outside or inside the body. The cells are irregular in shape and are functionally connected. Information can be transmitted from one nerve cell to another at specialized sites known as *synapses*.

ORGANS

An organ is an organization of several different kinds of tissues that together perform a special function. The kidney, for example, is composed of epithelial tissue, connective tissue, and nervous tissue. The function of the kidney is the separation from the blood of water and certain materials to form urine.

SYSTEMS

A system is an organization of different organs that together perform the more complex functions of the body. The human body is composed of ten major systems: (1) skeletal, (2) muscular, (3) nervous, (4) endocrine, (5) cardiovascular, (6) lymphatic, (7) respiratory, (8) digestive, (9) urinary, and (10) reproductive.

The *skeletal system* is composed of the bones, cartilages, and joints of the body. The system serves to support and protect the body and provide it with levers for movement. It also serves as a site for the formation of blood cells and as a reservoir for calcium salts.

The *muscular system* is composed of all the muscles of the body and includes skeletal, smooth (visceral), and cardiac muscle. The function of the system is to bring about movements in the different parts of the body, to maintain the attitude or position of the body (posture), and to produce heat.

The *nervous system* comprises the brain, spinal cord, nerves, and sense organs, such as the nose, the eye, and ear. The system coordinates and integrates the activities of the different parts of the body by means of nerve impulses that travel along nerve cells and their processes and by chemicals that are discharged at the ends of the nerve processes.

The *endocrine system* is composed of a number of glands that release chemical substances directly into the bloodstream to control the activities of various bodily organs and tissues. The endocrine system and the nervous system assist each other, and together they govern the activities of the body.

The *cardiovascular system* consists of the blood, heart, and blood vessels. It is the body's transportation system. For example, the blood picks up oxygen and the products of digestion from the respiratory and digestive systems and delivers them to the cells of the body. From the cells, the blood carries the products of metabolism, such as carbon dioxide and lactic acid, and delivers them to the excretory organs. In addition, blood transports hormones, maintains the acid-base balance of the body, protects against disease, and assists in regulating body temperature.

The *lymphatic system* is composed of lymph, lymphatic vessels, and lymphatic tissues, such as lymph nodes, the spleen, and the thymus. It serves to return tissue fluid and proteins to the cardiovascular system, produce blood cells, filter the blood, and protect the body against disease.

The *respiratory system*—the lungs and the air passages leading into them—supplies oxygen to the body and removes carbon dioxide. It also assists in regulating the acid-base balance of the body.

The *digestive system* consists of a long tube (and its associated glands) that extends from the mouth to the anus. The system breaks down the complex molecules of food, which are then absorbed into the blood and lymph and distributed for use by the cells. It also eliminates unabsorbed food residues and waste products from the body.

The *urinary system* comprises the kidneys, which produce urine; the ureters, which convey the urine to the bladder; the urinary bladder, which serves as a reservoir; and the urethra, which discharges the urine to the exterior. The system controls the chemical composition of the blood and regulates the fluid and electrolyte balance within the body. It assists in maintaining the acid-base balance of the blood and excretes waste products and excess salts in the urine.

The *reproductive system* is formed by the testes or ovaries, which produce the reproductive cells (spermatozoa or ova), and the passages and glands that transport and nourish the reproductive cells. The function of the system is to reproduce and pass on

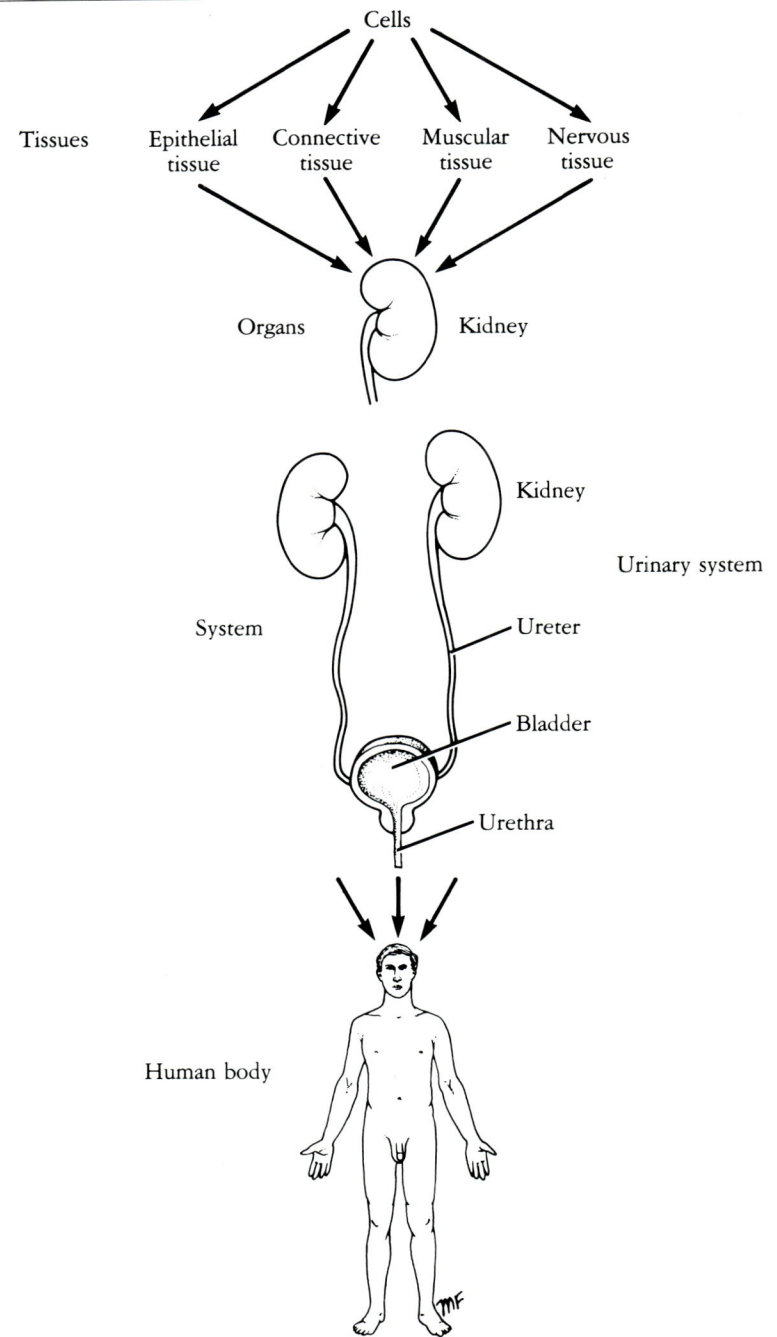

Fig. 1-2. The organization of the body into structural subunits: cells, tissues, organs, and systems.

genetic material so that a new individual can be formed and the species continued.

Thus, the body is made up of many trillions of cells grouped together as tissues and organs to perform specific functions. Collections of organs (systems) are necessary to perform some of the more complicated functions (Fig. 1-2).

HOMEOSTASIS

All cells function normally provided that their environment remains constant within narrow limits. The maintenance of a constant cellular environment is referred to by physiologists as *homeostasis*. The mechanisms responsible for the maintenance of such a state are known as *homeostatic mechanisms*. The need for homeostasis means that the temperature, osmotic pressure, hydrogen ion concentration, and chemical composition of the tissue fluid bathing the cells must be carefully regulated. Small deviations from normal result in cell malfunction; large deviations may cause cell death.

CLINICAL NOTES

EFFECTS OF SEX, RACE, AND AGE ON BODY STRUCTURE AND FUNCTION

Physicians must always remember that there are sexual and racial differences and that the body's structure and function changes as a person grows and ages.

The adult male tends to be taller than the adult female and to have longer legs; his bones are bigger and heavier, and his muscles are larger. He has less subcutaneous fat, which makes his appearance more angular. His larynx is larger and his vocal cords are longer, so that his voice is deeper. He has a beard and coarse body hair. He possesses axillary and pubic hair, with the latter extending up to the region of the umbilicus.

The adult female tends to be shorter than the adult male and to have smaller bones; her muscles are less bulky. She has more subcutaneous fat, with accumulations in the breasts, buttocks, and thighs giving her a more rounded appearance. Her head hair is finer, and her skin is smoother in appearance. She has axillary and pubic hair, but the latter does not extend up to the umbilicus. Women have larger breasts and a wider pelvis.

Until the age of about 10 years, boys and girls grow at roughly the same rate. At about age 12, boys start to grow faster than girls, so that the majority reach adulthood taller than women.

Puberty begins between ages 10 and 14 in girls and 12 and 15 in boys. In the girl, the breasts enlarge and the pelvis broadens. At the same time, a boy's penis, testes, and scrotum enlarge, and in both sexes axillary and pubic hair appears.

Racial differences may be seen in the color of the skin, hair, and eyes and in the shape and size of the eyes, nose, and lips. Africans and Scandinavians tend to be taller, because of longer legs, whereas Orientals are shorter, with shorter legs. The heads of central Europeans and Orientals tend to be rounder and broader.

The fact that the structure and functions of the human body change with age may seem obvious, but it is often overlooked. A few examples of such changes follow:

1. The bones of the skull are more resilient in the infant than in the adult; for this reason, fractures of the skull are very common in the adult and much less so in the young child.
2. At birth, all bone marrow is red marrow. With advancing age, the red marrow recedes up the bones of the limbs, so that in the adult it is confined largely to the bones of the head, thorax, and abdomen.
3. Lymphatic tissues reach their maximum development at puberty and atrophy thereafter, so that in old age the volume of lymphatic tissue is considerably reduced.
4. After birth and during childhood, bodily functions become progressively more efficient and reach their maximum efficiency during young adulthood. During late adulthood and old age,

many bodily functions become less efficient. The ability to metabolize drugs is maximal during early and middle adult life. Therefore, much smaller doses of drugs, such as anesthetic agents, may be used in the young and old to produce the same effect.

DISEASE AND THE HUMAN BODY

We have seen that the body is a highly organized structure consisting of cells, tissues, organs, and systems. The student must not forget, however, that it is the whole patient who consults the physician, and the person should not be regarded merely as a disordered stomach, a kidney tumor, or a case of heart failure.

Our ideas about diseases have changed drastically in recent years. Former, the medical profession tended to be preoccupied with studying the lesion, that is, the structural changes that had taken place within the patient. Now, we recognize disease as disordered function and know that it is the disturbed function that is responsible for the patient's symptoms.

It is also becoming increasingly evident that many diseases whose causes were previously unknown stem from cellular malfunctions. Recent technological advances have shown that patients' symptoms may be attributed to abnormalities at the molecular level. For example, in sickle cell anemia, there is an abnormal hemoglobin molecule, which is genetically inherited. Familial goitrous cretinism, juvenile diabetes mellitus, and cystic fibrosis are other examples of genetic cellular defects. There are also a considerable number of inheritable diseases characterized by abnormalities in the metabolism of amino acids; phenylketonuria is an example. Further clinical examples of diseases connected with cellular abnormalities are given on page 72.

ALTERED HOMEOSTASIS

As we have seen, the body is made up of trillions of cells, which are teeming with enzymes and other chemical substances necessary for carrying out the various life processes. None of these cells would be able to function normally without a constant internal environment, which can be likened to a miniature water bath that surrounds each cell and protects it against the constantly changing external environment.

The complex organs of the body have been developed with the main objective of preserving the constancy of the water content, the electrolyte concentration, the glucose concentration, the hormone concentration, and similar balances of the internal environment. The lungs, the cardiovascular system, the kidneys, and the endocrine glands all play a leading role in this process. Disease of those organ systems can therefore profoundly affect the general metabolic activity of cells. Diabetes insipidus, Addison's disease of the adrenal cortex, diabetic acidosis, and myxedema are examples of endocrine disturbances that upset the homeostatic mechanisms.

In patients who have experienced excessive vomiting or in whom the salt and water balance of the body has been changed following major intestinal surgery, the disturbed internal environment can be corrected by the introduction of suitable intravenous fluids by the physician. In these circumstances, the patient's fluid input (drink, intravenous fluid) and output (urine, vomit, and so forth) have to be monitored carefully. It is very easy to introduce too much fluid and greatly upset the internal environment of the patient. If this fluid imbalance is not corrected, death will result.

CLINICAL PROBLEMS

For the answers to these problems, see page 781.

1. Define the term *homeostasis*. Name three organ systems that are involved in maintaining normal homeostasis. Name three diseases that may profoundly affect the homeostatic mechanisms.

2. Carcinomas are malignant neoplasms arising in epithelial tissues; sarcomas are malignant neoplasms arising in connective tissues. Before we can study these tumors, we must know the essential structural

differences between these tissues. What are these structural differences?

3. The symptoms and signs of disease may be caused by altered function at the cellular level. Give three examples of genetic cellular defects.

4. At which period during life do the cells and tissues function most efficiently?

5. Give examples of tissues whose structure changes with age.

ADDITIONAL READING

Adolph, E. F. *Origins of Physiological Regulations.* New York: Academic, 1968.

Borow, M. *Fundamentals of Homeostasis: A Clinical Approach to Fluid Electrolyte Acid-Base Energy Metabolism in Health and Disease.* Flushing, N.Y.: Medical Examination Publishing Co., 1977.

Frisancho, A. R. *Human Adaptation.* St. Louis: Mosby, 1979.

Guyton, A. C., et al. *Dynamics and Control of the Body Fluids.* Philadelphia: Saunders, 1975.

Jones, R. W. *Principles of Biological Regulation: An Introduction to Feedback Systems.* New York: Academic, 1973.

Sweetser, W. *Human Life (Aging and Old Age).* New York: Arno, 1979.

Toates, F. M. *Control Theory in Biology and Experimental Psychology.* London: Hutchinson Education, 1975.

THE CELL

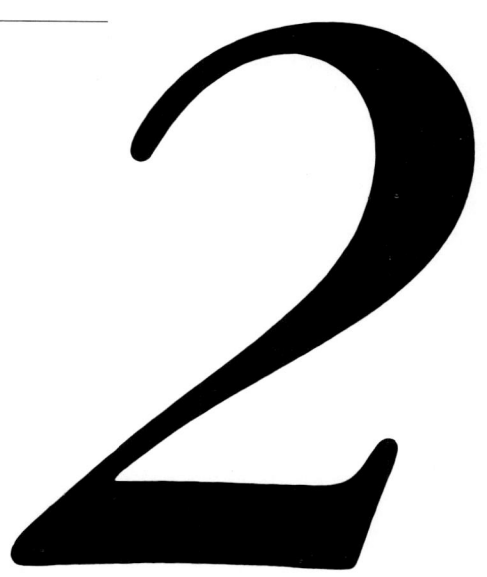

The cell is the smallest organized unit of the body. The various tissues of the body are made up of different kinds of cells and of extracellular material produced by the cells. The cells of the human body are so small that they cannot be seen without the aid of a microscope, with the exception of the fertilized ovum (200 μm in diameter),* which is seen as a tiny speck with the naked eye.

Cells are made up of a living substance called *protoplasm*. This is a complex aqueous gel chemically composed of protein, carbohydrate, fat, and nucleic acids, as well as inorganic materials.

CELL STRUCTURE

Each cell is composed of two parts, the nucleus and the cytoplasm (Figs. 2-1 and 2-2).

Nucleus

In a cell that is not undergoing division, the nucleus is a large, rounded structure that usually occupies the central portion of the cell. Most cells possess only one nucleus, but there are exceptions. For example, osteoclasts, foreign body giant cells, and hepatocytes may possess several nuclei. Some cells that have become highly developed lose their nuclei, for example, the red blood cells and the keratinized cells of the skin. The nucleus is made up of (1) a nucleolus, (2) chromatin, (3) nuclear sap, and (4) a nuclear membrane (Fig. 2-3; see Fig. 2-2).

Nucleolus

The nucleolus can be single or double and is the most prominent structure seen in the nucleus (see Fig. 2-3). It is composed largely of protein and RNA (ribonucleic acid). Nucleoli are not surrounded by a membrane. Two types of ribonucleic acid (RNA), *ribosomal RNA* and *messenger RNA*, are synthesized in the nucleolus. In fact, the major function of nucleoli is the synthesis of ribosomal RNA. Because, as we shall see later, ribosomes are active sites of protein synthesis within cells, it follows that cells making greater amounts of protein (for example, the cells of the pancreas) will have larger nucleoli. In contrast, in cells with a low level of protein synthetic activity—for example, muscle cells and spermatocytes—the nucleoli may be small or absent.

The nucleolus in a section stained with hematoxy-

---

*Metric units of measurement: micrometer (μm) = micron (μ); nanometer (nm).

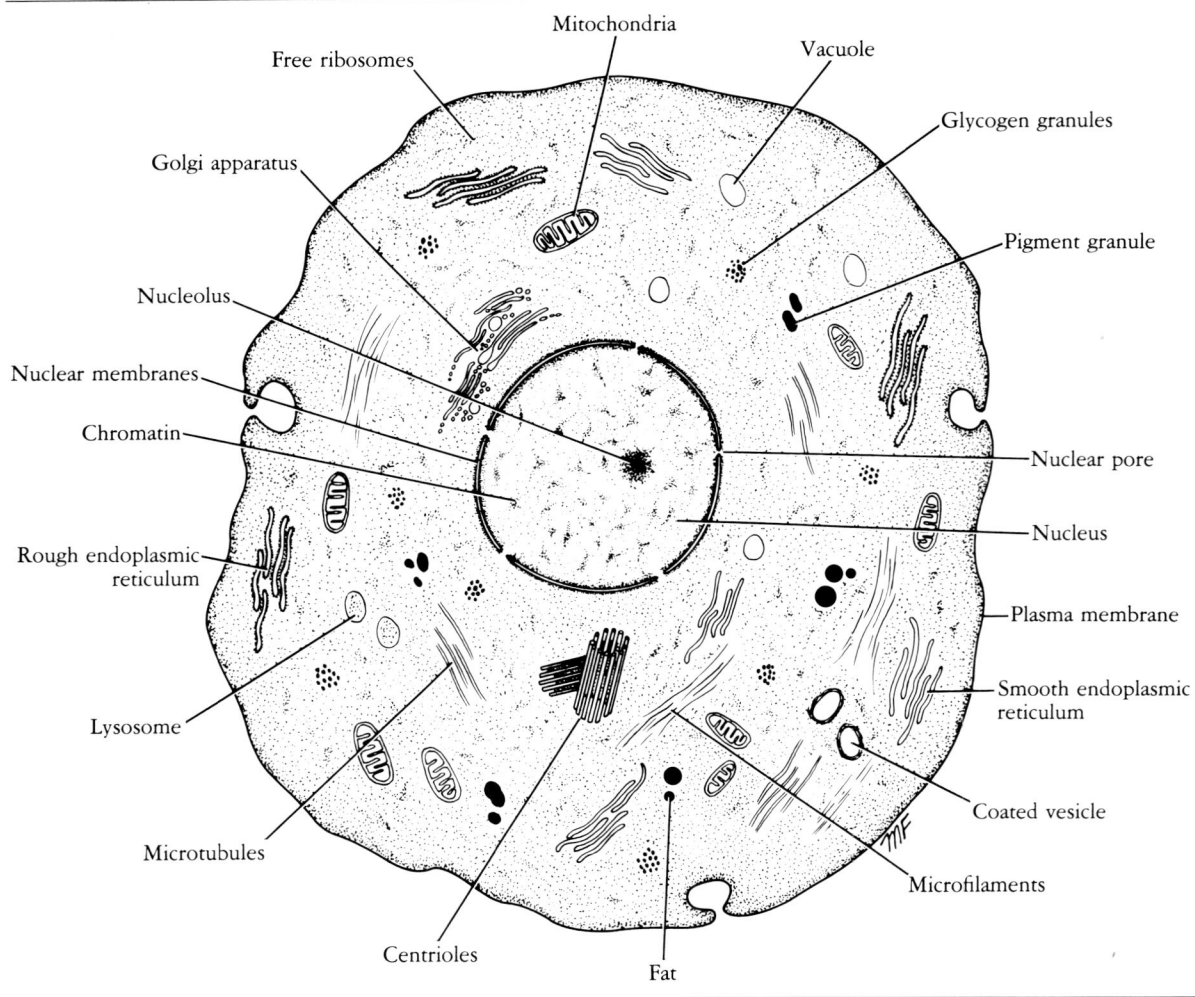

Fig. 2-1. General structure of a cell.

lin and eosin will appear, when the section is viewed through a light microscope, darkly stained with hematoxylin: it is basophilic because of its RNA content.

Chromatin

Under a light microscope, chromatin has the appearance of small clumps or masses within the nucleus (Fig. 2-4; see Fig. 2-3). The chromatin is composed of *deoxyribonucleic acid* (DNA) and protein. The DNA-protein complex is sometimes referred to as DNP. The chromatin clumps comprise tangled masses of threadlike structures, the *chromosomes*. When a cell is about to divide, each chromosome becomes highly coiled, shorter, and thicker and can be seen more easily through the light microscope. In female cells, a large mass of chromatin containing one of the female sex chromosomes may be seen lying against the nuclear membrane. It is called the *sex chromatin,* or *Barr body* (Figs. 2-5 and 2-6).

HETEROCHROMATIN AND EUCHROMATIN. *Heterochromatin* is that part of the chromatin that can be

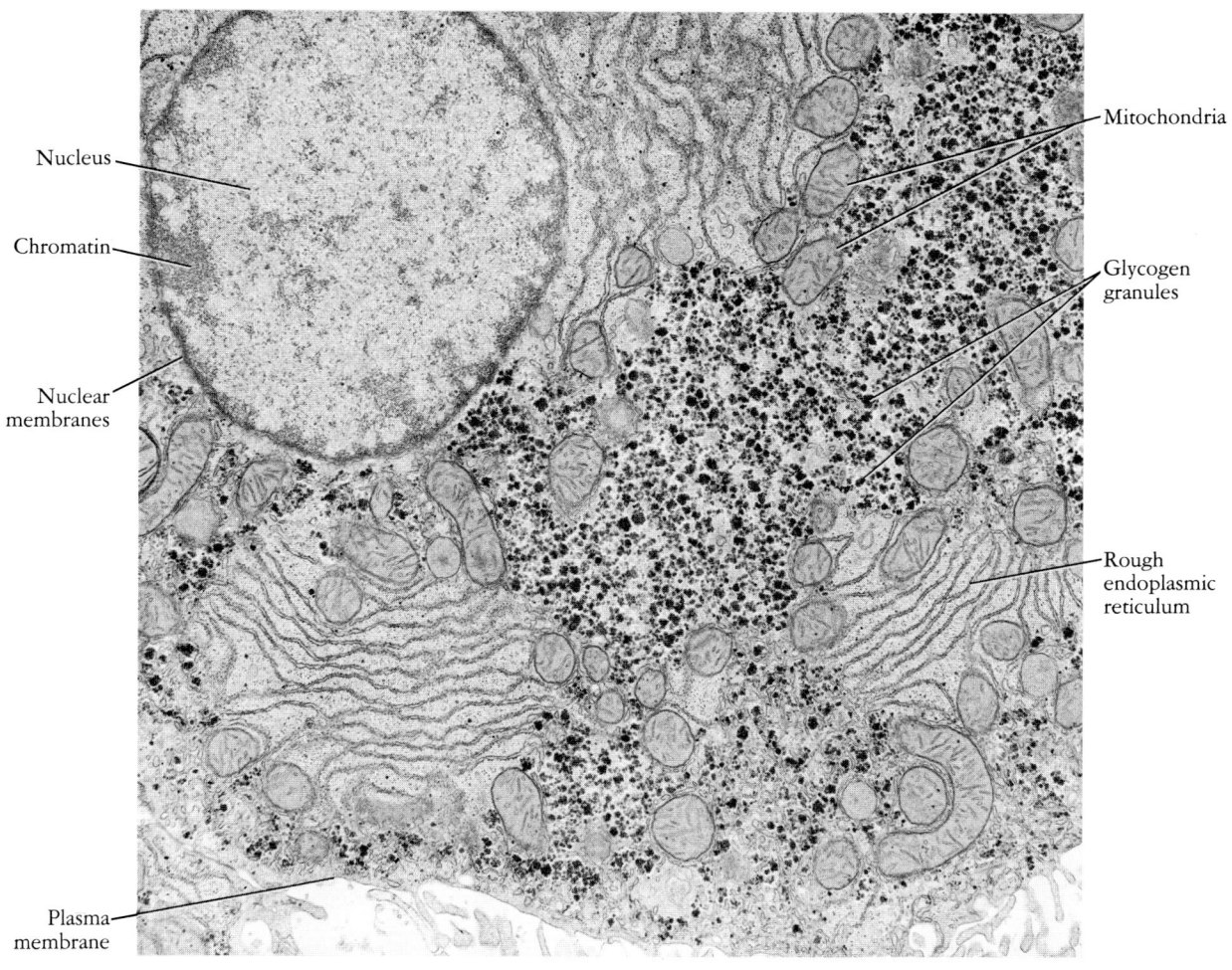

Fig. 2-2. Electron micrograph of a hepatic cell showing the nucleus, numerous mitochondria, and rough endoplasmic reticulum. Glycogen inclusions appear as groups of electron-dense particles. (Courtesy of Dr. A. L. Jones.)

seen in the resting interphase nucleus of a cell with a light microscope. It is strongly basophilic, staining deeply with hematoxylin, and is formed by the tight coiling of the chromosomes. Because of the tight coiling, the genes are not available for the transcription of messenger RNA.

Parts of the chromosomes are uncoiled and extended and, because they are fine threads, they are invisible with the light microscope. The chromatin forming these parts of the chromosomes is known as *euchromatin*. Here the genes are readily available for the transcription of messenger RNA.

The amounts of heterochromatin and euchromatin present in a nucleus vary in different cells. In those cells that are actively engaged in protein synthesis, a large amount of invisible euchromatin will be present and the nuclei will have an open appearance (see Fig. 2-2). In those cells that are not producing much protein, a large amount of visible heterochromatin will be present and the nuclei will be densely stained.

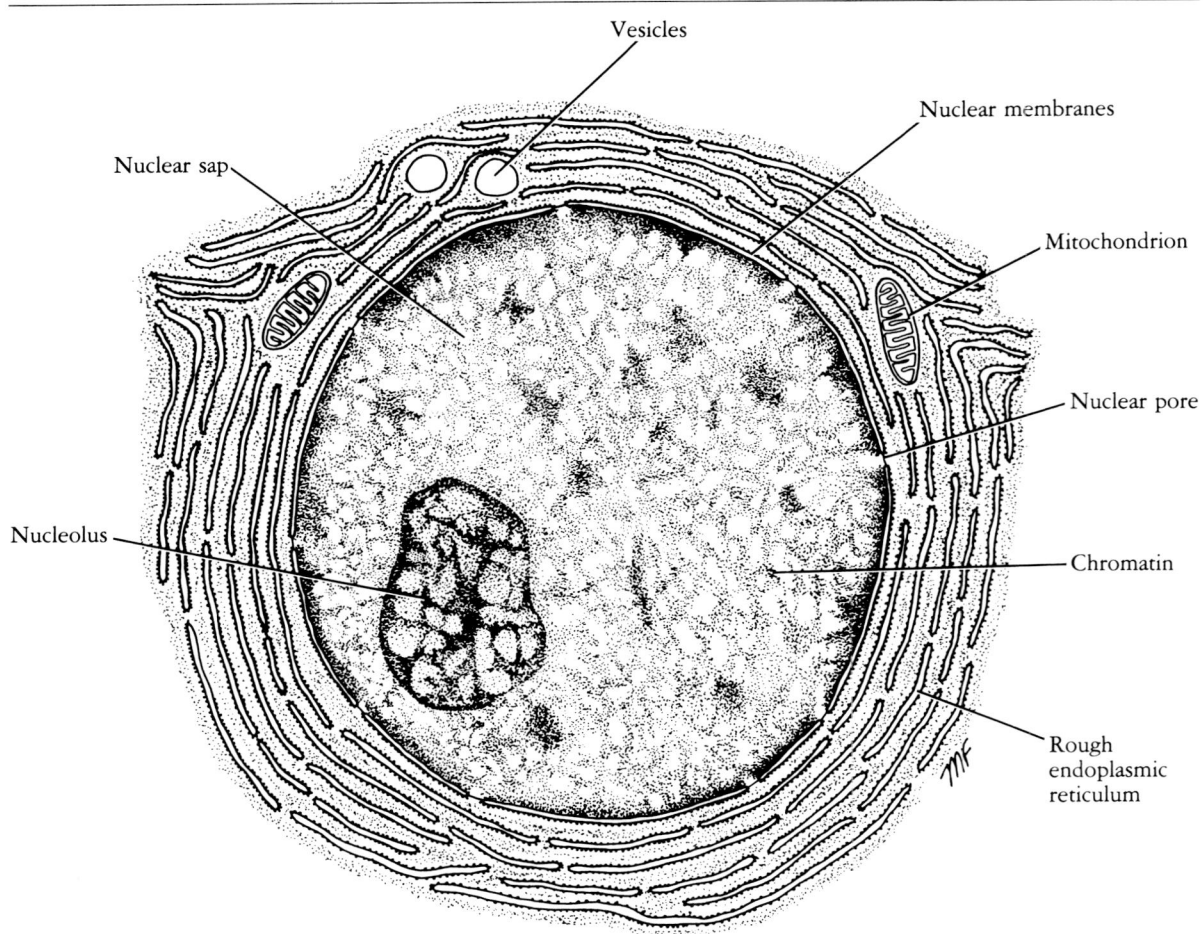

Fig. 2-3. Structure of a typical interphase nucleus with a prominent nucleolus. Note the presence of clumps of chromatin lying against the nuclear membranes and the existence of numerous nuclear pores. The nucleus is surrounded by cytoplasm containing high concentrations of rough endoplasmic reticulum.

Nuclear Sap

The nuclear sap lies in the spaces between the chromatin (heterochromatin) and the nucleolus (see Fig. 2-3). It is made up of a semifluid colloidal solution and contains the invisible (euchromatin) portions of the chromosomes.

Nuclear Membrane

The nuclear membrane forms an envelope around the nucleus and is composed of two layers with a small space between them (see Fig. 2-3). The outer nuclear membrane is often seen to be continuous with the endoplasmic reticulum of the cytoplasm and may have an accumulation of ribosomes on its outer surface. Following cell division, the nuclear membranes are re-formed from the rough endoplasmic reticulum.

There appear to be small passageways between the nucleus and the cytoplasm scattered along the nuclear membrane. These are known as *nuclear pores* (see Fig. 2-3) and measure about 70 nm in diameter.

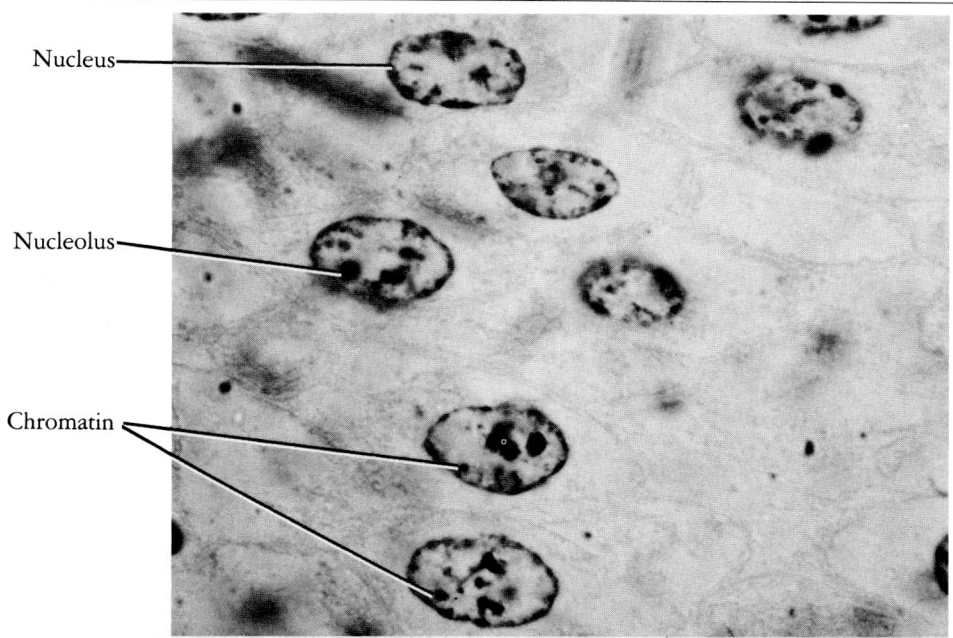

Fig. 2-4. Photomicrograph of epithelial cells stained to show nuclear structure. ($\times 1,000$.)

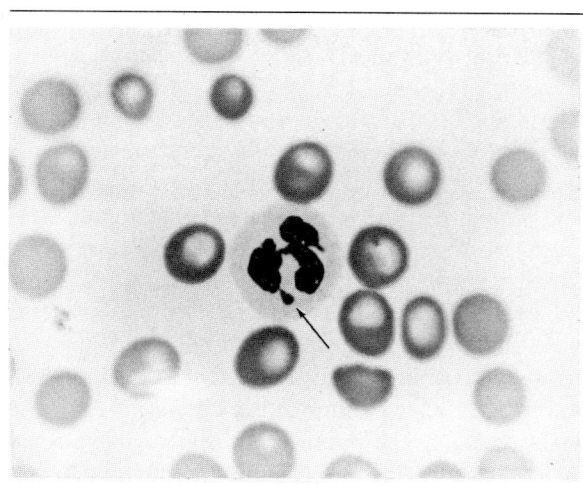

Fig. 2-5. Photomicrograph of a polymorphonuclear leukocyte from a human female. The sex chromatin, or Barr body, has a drumstick shape (arrow). *($\times 510$.) (Courtesy of Dr. M. L. Barr.)*

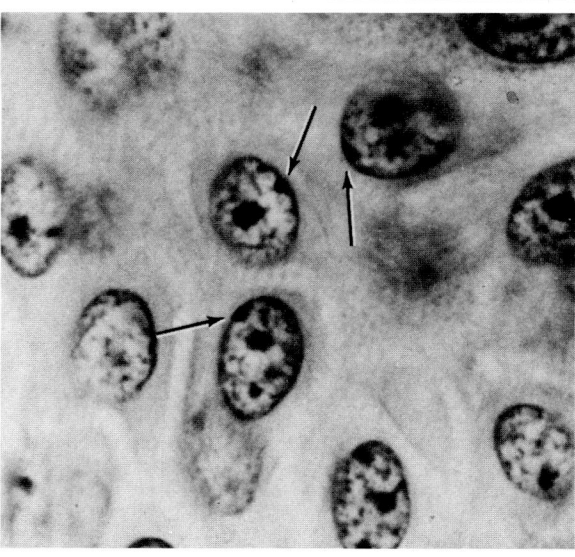

Fig. 2-6. Photomicrograph of epithelial cells from a human female. The sex chromatin, or Barr body, is seen as a peripherally located mass of chromatin within the nucleus (arrows). *($\times 950$.) (Courtesy of Dr. M. L. Barr.)*

At these sites, the outer and inner nuclear membranes come together and form the boundary of each nuclear pore. The "opening" of the pore is closed by a thin membrane that is semipermeable and allows the passage of messenger RNA, transfer RNA, and ribosomal RNA from the nucleus to the cytoplasm; it also permits the entrance of other molecules from the cytoplasm to the nucleus.

Functions of the Nucleus

The nucleus has two chief functions: (1) it plays the major role in reproduction of the cell and maintenance of hereditary characteristics of the cell, and (2) it controls the work that is performed by the interphase cell (nondividing cell).

CELL DIVISION. The multiplication of cells is essential for the growth of the body and the replacement of those cells with a short life-span, for example, the cells of the blood and those of the skin and the lining of the intestinal tract, which are constantly wearing away. Multiplication is also necessary for the repair of tissues following injury. The process of cell multiplication is called *cell division*. Cells that are not dividing are said to be in a resting phase or *interphase*.

Two distinct forms of cell division can take place, *mitosis* and *meiosis*. Mitotic division occurs in the majority of cells and results in the replication of cell hereditary material and the equal distribution of chromosomes (46 in number) to the resulting new cells. Meiotic division is restricted to the cells in the gonads responsible for the formation of the sex cells. In this form of division, the number of chromosomes is halved, so that each new sex cell has only 23 chromosomes. When fertilization takes place, the full complement of 46 chromosomes is restored.

Meiosis consists of two divisions in quick succession, so that each cell gives rise to four new sex cells. In meiosis, an exchange of genes occurs between chromosomes, which leads to a wide range of genetic variability in the offspring of the parents. The details of meiosis are considered on pages 543 and 578.

Mitosis. For purposes of description, mitosis can be divided into four phases: prophase, metaphase, anaphase, and telophase (Fig. 2-7).

Prophase. As mitosis begins, the nuclear membrane and the nucleolus disappear. The chromatin becomes condensed as each chromosome becomes coiled, shorter, and thicker. Each of the 46 chromosomes now splits longitudinally into two chromatids, which are attached to each other at a *centromere*.

During the resting phase of the cell (interphase), the DNA molecule, which has many thousands of genes, is duplicated. Thus, as a cell begins to divide, each chromosome has two sets of genes. Later, when each chromosome splits, each chromatid will thus have one complete set.

The centrosome now undergoes changes. It is a condensed area of cytoplasm that contains two hollow, cylindrical structures known as *centrioles*. During early prophase, the centrioles begin to diverge around the nucleus to take up positions at opposite poles of the cell (see Fig. 2-7). From each centriole, there is seen radiating toward the center of the cell into and around the mass of chromosomes a system of poorly stained microtubules known as the *spindle*. Some of the tubules are attached to the centromeres of the chromosomes, and others run directly between the centrioles without chromosomal attachment.

Metaphase. The chromosomes now become gathered in the middle of the cell; more precisely, the centromeres come to lie in the equatorial plane but the limbs of the chromosomes extend in all directions. The limbs of the chromosomes meanwhile continue to shorten (see Fig. 2-7).

Anaphase. During this phase, the centromeres split and the two chromatids of each chromosome become separated from each other. The separated chromatids now pass to the opposite poles of the cell (see Fig. 2-7). Precisely how this is accomplished is not known. The presence of the contractile elements *actin* and *myosin*, in association with the microtubules of the spindle, may play a part. Each chromatid is now referred to as a chromosome. The cell at this stage has become elongated.

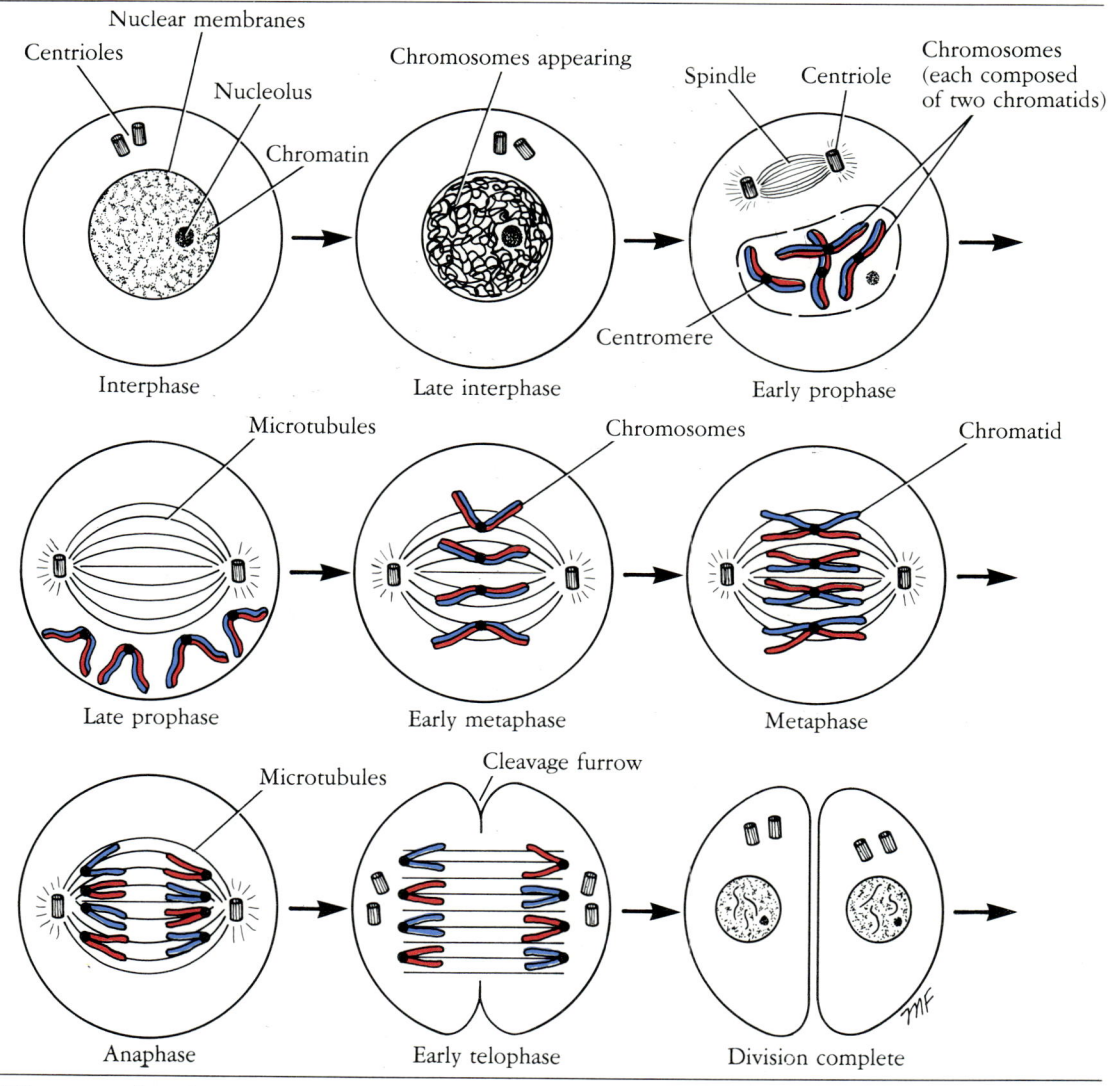

Fig. 2-7. The main nuclear changes in mitotic division.

Telophase. A constriction begins to develop at the midpoint of the elongated cell called the *cleavage furrow*. Beneath the furrow there is a contractile ring of actin and myosin, which eventually splits the cell into two new cells. The nuclear membranes begin to form from the rough endoplasmic reticulum, and the chromosomes become less coiled. The nucleolus appears in each nucleus.

Chromatin and Chromosomes

As has been explained previously, chromosomes can be seen with the light microscope during mitosis and are formed of chromatin. The name *mitotic figure* is given to a nucleus that is undergoing mitosis and is displaying its chromosomes. Mitotic figures are commonly seen in tissues in which cell division is required to maintain the cell population, such as

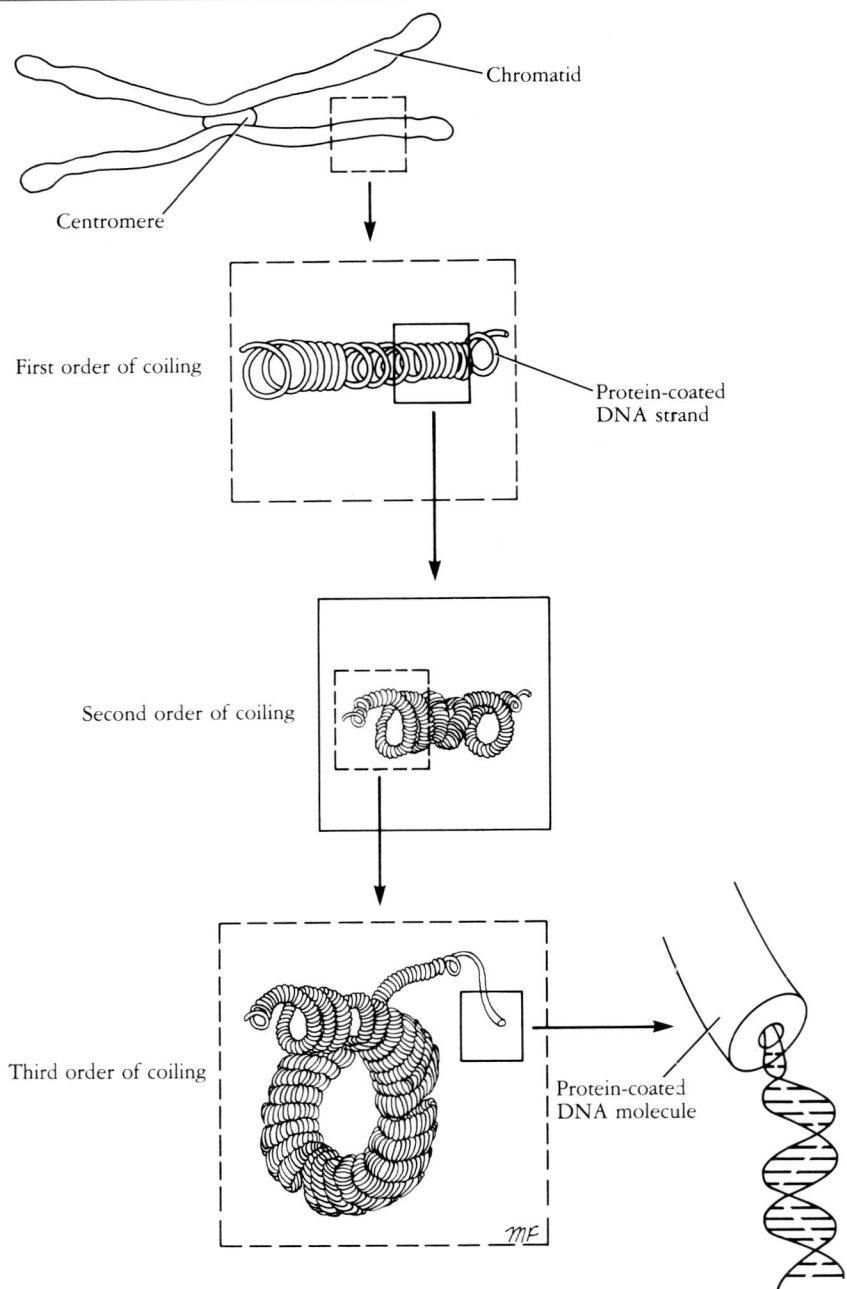

Fig. 2-8. The organization of DNA and protein during metaphase in mitosis. A portion of a single chromatid has been enlarged in a series of diagrams passing from the chromatid to the DNA molecule.

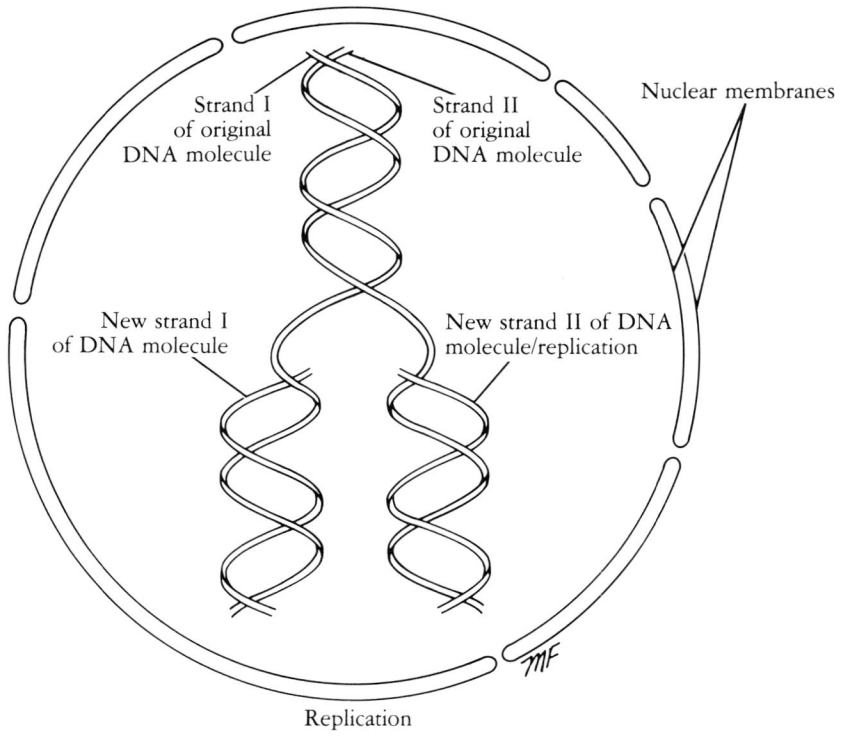

Fig. 2-9. Replication. The two strands of a DNA molecule first separate, and a new strand is then synthesized alongside each of the separate strands. The result is that each newly formed double-stranded molecule is identical to the original molecule whose strands became separated.

the lining of the gastrointestinal tract, the bone marrow, and the epidermis.

Each chromosome is a long thread of chromatin material and is composed of DNP, that is, DNA and protein (Fig. 2-8). The genes are contained in and distributed along each chromosome. They are composed of DNA. DNA is the hereditary material of cells and is capable of replicating itself (Fig. 2-9). In this way it provides precise copies of the genetic code, which are then passed on to daughter cells during cellular division.

The DNA molecules of human chromosomes each consist of two long, thin strands arranged as a double helix or twisted ladder (Fig. 2-10). The sides of the ladder are composed of sugar (deoxyribose) and phosphate. The rungs of the ladder are composed of the nitrogenous bases *adenine* and *thymine* or *cystosine* and *guanine*. There may be as many as 40 million deoxyribonucleotides in sequence along one strand of a DNA molecule. The genetic information contained in a single DNA molecule depends on the number and order of the amino acids along its strands. It is important to realize that each strand complements the other and each strand can serve as a template or pattern by which a new strand of DNA can be synthesized during the interphase.

Genes exert their control on the protein manufactured within a cell in the following manner. The long DNA molecules serve as templates for the long molecules of messenger RNA synthesized beside them. The messenger RNA molecules leave the nucleus and move to sites of protein synthesis within the cytoplasm (Fig. 2-11). We know that those sites are the ribosomes (see p. 49) and it is here that the amino acids are strung together, with

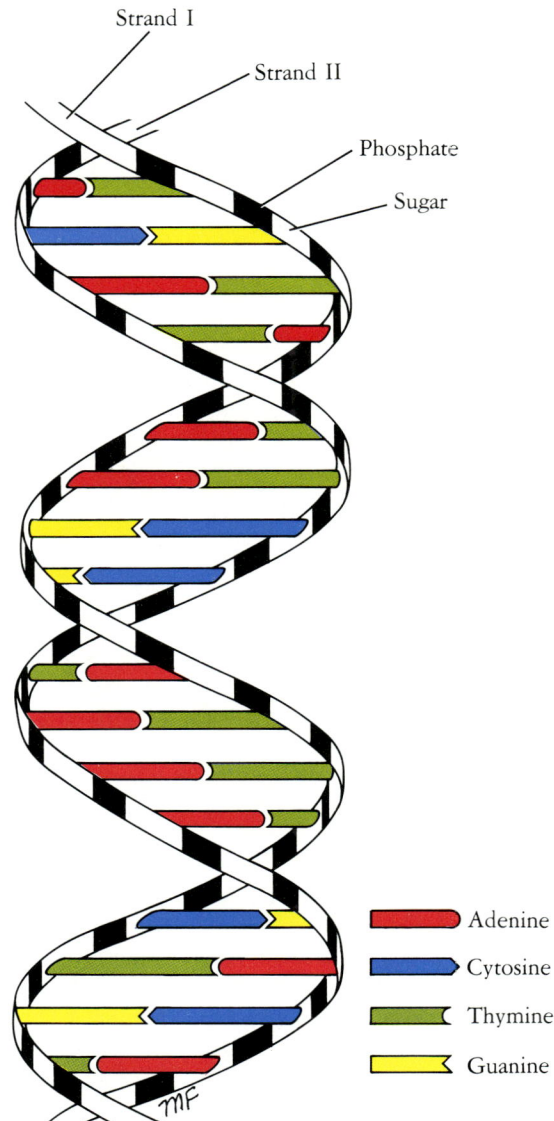

Fig. 2-10. Part of a double-stranded DNA molecule, showing the deoxyribonucleotides of one strand joined to those of the second strand. Note that adenine is joined to thymine and cytosine is joined to guanine.

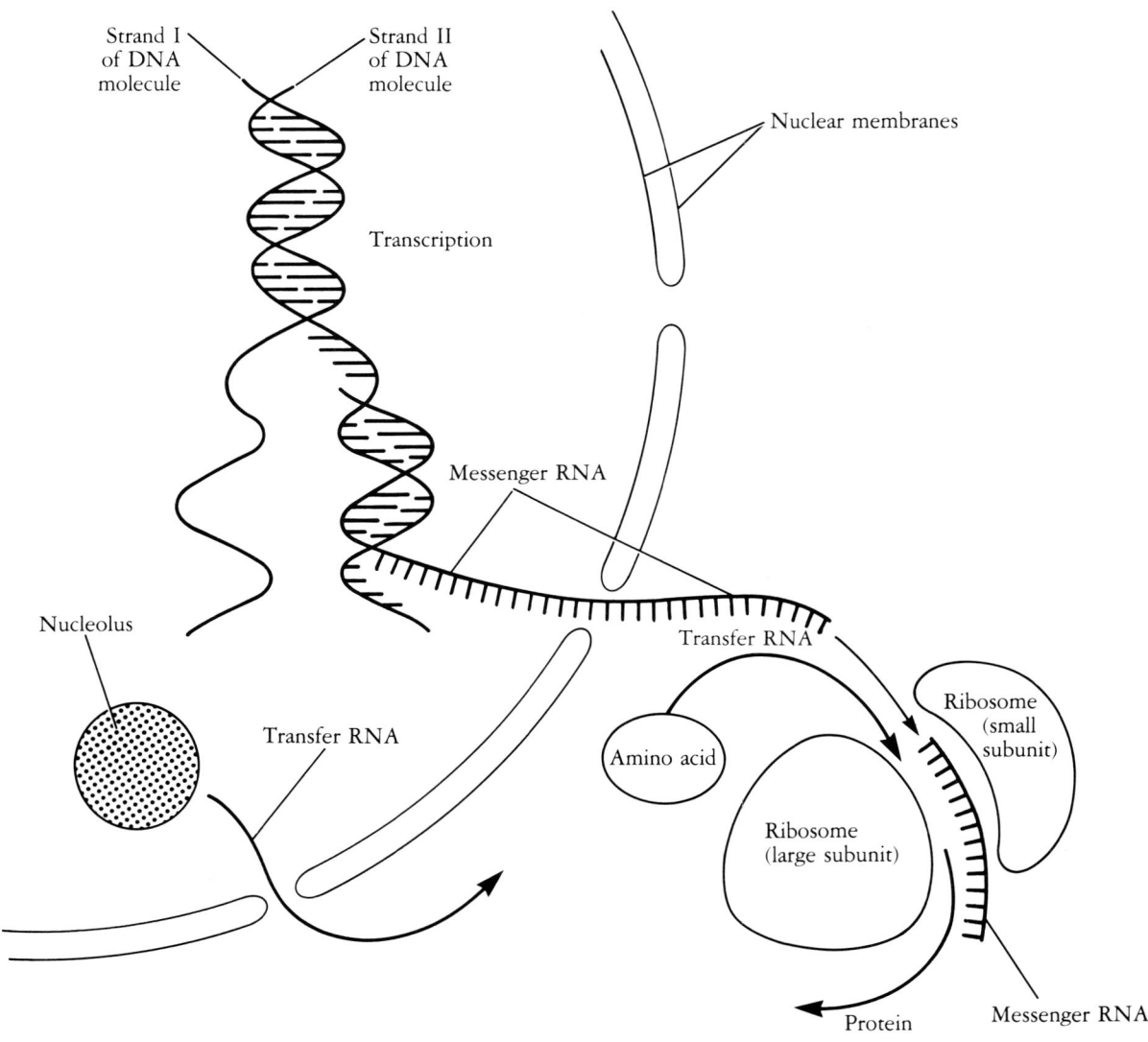

Fig. 2-11. The process of transcription.

the help of transfer RNA, into protein macromolecules that are synthesized in a particular cell.

CLASSIFICATION OF CHROMOSOMES. Chromosomes can be classified into groups according to their shape and size, and this classification assists the clinician in detecting anomalies. Colchicine, an alkaloid chemical, when added to cultures of cells that are growing and dividing in nutritive media, arrests the process of mitosis at metaphase by interfering with the formation of spindle microtubules. Under those circumstances, the chromatids do not separate from one another. If the cells are spread out on a slide and stained, the chromosomes can be easily counted and identified. The process by which the chromosomes of a cell from a given individual are classified is called *karyotyping.*

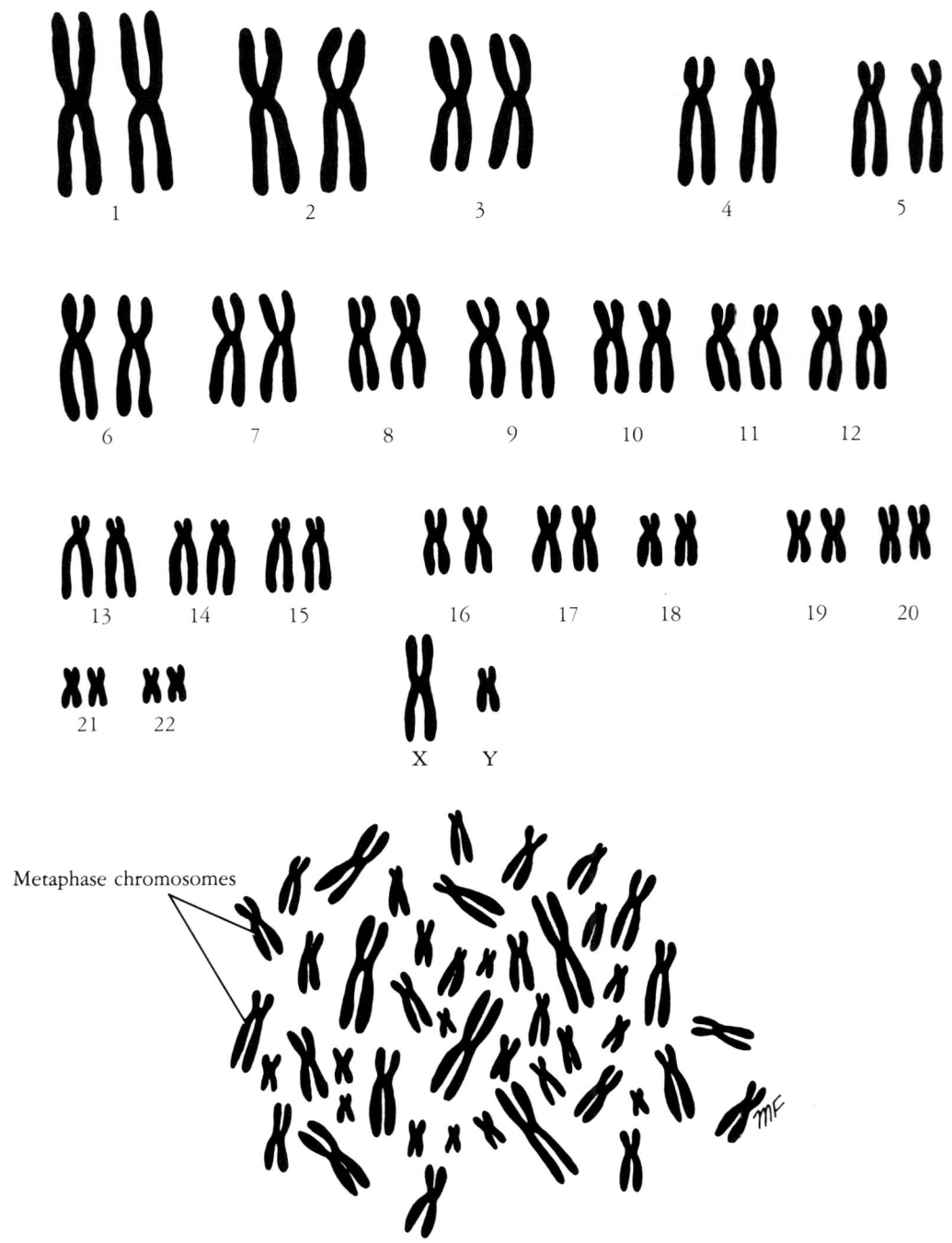

Fig. 2-12. *A human male karyotype. Note the presence of the X and Y sex chromosomes.*

Examination of a metaphase chromosome following colchicine treatment shows the unseparated chromatids attached to one another at the centromere (Fig. 2-12). The centromere in some chromosomes is at the midpoint of the chromosome; in others, it is nearer one end of the chromosome. A particular chromosome is identified on the basis of its length and the position of the centromere.

The human nucleus contains 46 chromosomes, paired as 23 homologs. Twenty-two pairs are almost identical and are known as *autosomes*. The remaining two chromosomes in the female are also alike; they are the X *sex chromosomes*. In the male, however, these two chromosomes are not alike and are the X and Y *sex chromosomes*.

It is important to remember that chromosomes are present in the nucleus at all times. In the interphase nucleus, they are long, very thin, and coiled and form the heterochromatin and euchromatin referred to previously. During mitosis, the chromosomes shorten and thicken and when suitably stained can easily be seen with the light microscope.

Cytoplasm

The cytoplasm surrounds the nucleus and is bounded by the *plasma membrane*. The cytoplasm is the region of the cell responsible for the formation and release of energy, for the synthesis of proteins, for growth and motility, and for many other functions. It is the area of the cell where most of the work is accomplished. The activities of the cytoplasm are, however, under the direction and control of the nucleus. The components of the cytoplasm may be divided into three groups: (1) organelles, (2) inclusions, and (3) matrix.

Cytoplasmic Organelles

An organ may be defined as a particular part of the body that is responsible for a special function. An *organelle* may be defined as a particular part of the cytoplasm that is responsible for a special function or functions. The most important cytoplasmic organelles are (1) mitochondria, (2) rough endoplasmic reticulum, (3) smooth endoplasmic reticulum, (4) the Golgi apparatus, (5) lysosomes, (6) coated vesicles, (7) free ribosomes, (8) microtubules, (9) centrioles and basal bodies, and (10) microfilaments.

The metabolic activity within the cytoplasm is possible only if the various enzymes and chemical substances are prevented from mixing freely by the presence of plasma membranes. It is thus found that the majority of organelles have membranous walls, which allow the chemical composition within an organelle to be different from that of the surrounding cytoplasmic matrix. Moreover, because the membrane is semipermeable, it permits the passage of certain ions through the membrane but restricts the passage of others. The membrane also serves as a scaffolding that supports the enzyme molecules. The structure of the plasma membrane will be discussed on page 55.

MITOCHONDRIA. Mitochondria contain the enzymes that are responsible for cellular respiration and are the chief sites within the cells for the formation of chemical energy. They are often referred to as the "powerhouses" of the cells. Under a light microscope, mitochondria are seen as thin rods measuring about 2 to 6 μm long and about 2 μm wide. Under an electron microscope, mitochondria are seen to be essentially vesicular structures bounded by two membranes (Figs. 2-13 and 2-14). The outer membrane is smooth and completely surrounds the mitochondrion. It is freely permeable to small molecules. The inner membrane is formed into folds that project toward the center of the mitochondrion. These folds are called *cristae* (see Fig. 2-14). The inner membrane is semipermeable, and its inner surface is studded with large numbers of small particles called *elementary particles*. Each particle has a globular head and a stalk that is attached to the inner membrane. The interior of each mitochondrion is filled with *matrix*.

The size and shape of the mitochondria and their cristae vary considerably in different cell types. Mitochondria can be found scattered throughout the cytoplasm but are usually concentrated in those areas that have high energy requirements, such as between the myofibrils in muscle.

The mitochondrial enzymes that are associated

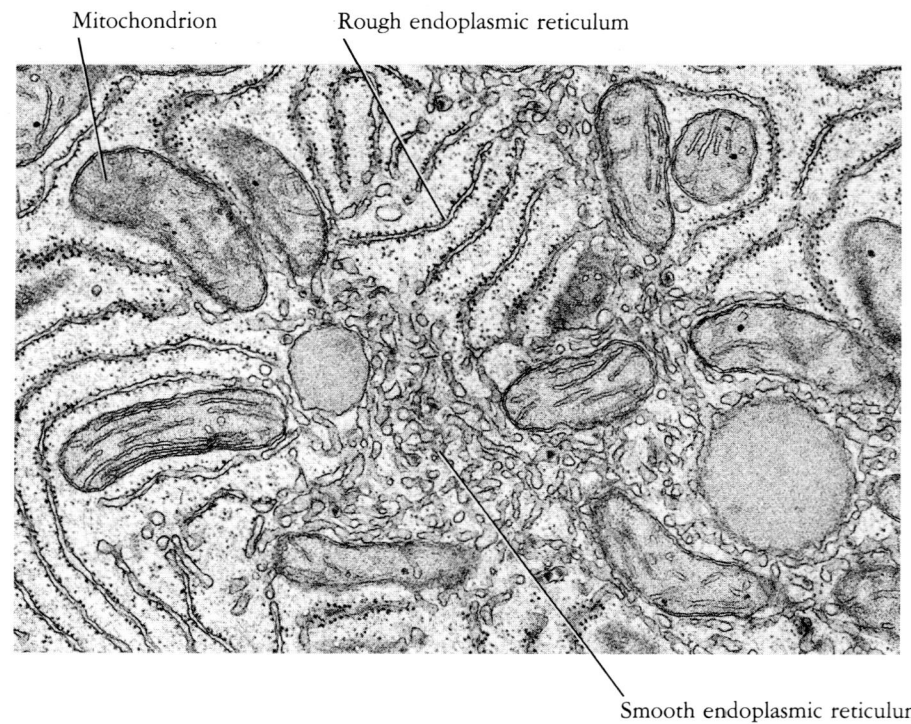

Fig. 2-13. Electron micrograph of a hepatocyte, showing numerous mitochondria, rough endoplasmic reticulum, and smooth endoplasmic reticulum. (× 27,000.) (Courtesy of Dr. R. P. Bolender.)

with electron transport and oxidative phosphorylation are situated on the inner mitochondrial membrane and its cristae. The elementary particles that are the sites of the enzymes concerned with electron transport, such as succinic dehydrogenase and cytochrome oxidase, are thought to be situated within the inner mitochondrial membrane.

Small molecules pass into the mitochondria from the cytoplasmic matrix. The enzymes dissolved in the mitochondrial matrix, together with the enzymes present on the mitochondrial cristae, catalyze their oxidation to a high-energy compound called adenosine triphosphate (ATP). The energy-rich ATP is released from the mitochondria and enters the cytoplasmic matrix. Here it provides energy to different parts of the cell by transferring one of its terminal phosphate groups to another molecule. In this manner, ATP is changed to *adenosine diphosphate* (*ADP*). The energy released permits other compounds essential for cell metabolism to be synthesized. Meanwhile, the ADP returns to the interior of the mitochondria and is converted back to ATP by the addition of a phosphate group.

Mitochondria are in a continuous state of change in volume and shape and are capable of reproducing by simple binary fission. For this purpose, they contain their own supply of DNA, in the form of closed loops in the mitochondrial matrix. Also present in the matrix are calcium salts, ribosomes, and RNA. Thus, mitochondria possess many of the enzymes necessary to carry out a semiautonomous existence. In fact, it has been suggested that in the evolutionary past, mitochondria were symbiotic bacteria that, having gained entrance to cells, lost their capability

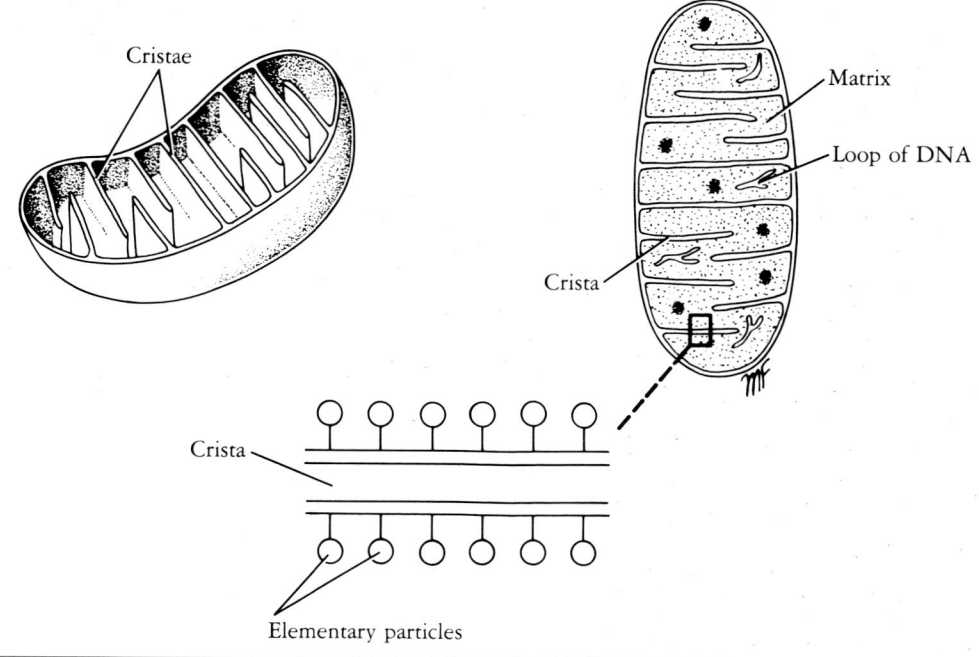

Fig. 2-14. The electron microscopic structure of a mitochondrion.

for an independent existence. It is important to remember that most of the mitochondrial enzymes and proteins are controlled not by mitochondrial DNA but by nuclear genes and are synthesized by cytoplasmic ribosomes and then passed into the mitochondrion.

ROUGH ENDOPLASMIC RETICULUM. Rough endoplasmic reticulum functions in the synthesis of protein. With the light microscope, it is easily recognizable as clumps of basophilic material within the cell cytoplasm. When viewed with the electron microscope, the rough endoplasmic reticulum consists of a network of interconnected, flattened sacs, or cisternae, whose walls are formed of a single membrane (Figs. 2-15 and 2-16). The sacs are packed close together and are often parallel to one another. The outer surface of the walls is studded with small particles called ribosomes, which are responsible for the designation *rough*. The ribosomes, which will be described later, are composed of protein and ribosomal RNA; it is the RNA that is responsible for the basophilic staining seen with the light microscope.

The function of the ribosomes is to synthesize proteins from amino acids. The proteins are immediately discharged into the interior of the sacs and thus are separated from the cytoplasmic matrix. The amino acids, the *transfer RNA*, and the *messenger RNA* are available in the cytoplasmic matrix and take part in the reaction with the ribosomes to form the protein. In secretory cells, such as those of the pancreatic acini, the proteins formed are enzymes. These are packaged in membranes by the rough endoplasmic reticulum, and the membrane-bound enzymes travel through the cytoplasm to the Golgi apparatus. Here the material is concentrated and further transported in vacuoles, to be released from the cell surface by a process of exocytosis (see p. 64). Some of the enzymes produced for use by the

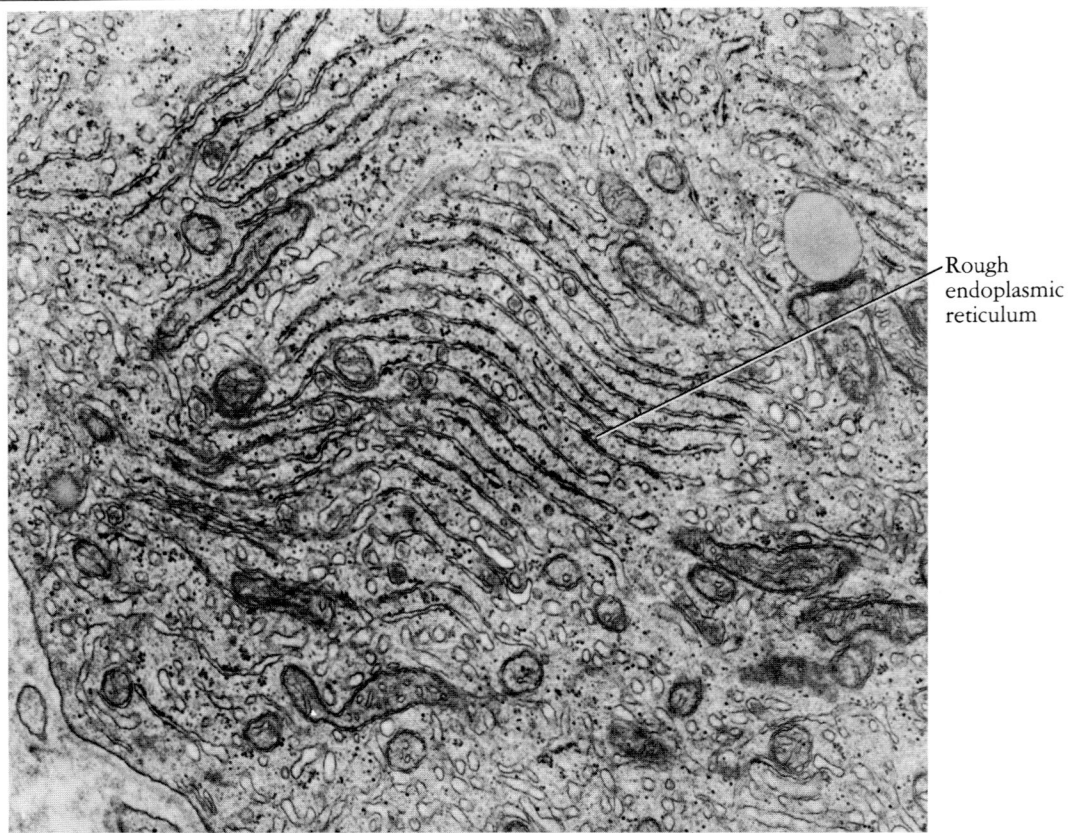

Fig. 2-15. Electron micrograph of a cell of the corpus luteum of the ovary, showing the rough endoplasmic reticulum. ($\times$ 17,050.) (Courtesy of Dr. M. J. Koering.)

cell, if released into the cytoplasm, would quickly result in the breakdown of the cell. It is therefore not surprising to find that the enzymes produced for lysosomes, for example, are enclosed by membranes produced by the rough endoplasmic reticulum.

Other cells that are very active in the formation of proteins are hepatocytes, which are responsible for the production of plasma proteins. Plasma cells actively form immunoglobulins. Both hepatocytes and plasma cells contain large amounts of rough endoplasmic reticulum.

SMOOTH ENDOPLASMIC RETICULUM. Smooth endoplasmic reticulum is similar in appearance to rough endoplasmic reticulum, but its outer surface is not studded with ribosomes (Fig. 2-17). Because it does not possess ribosomes, it is not involved in the synthesis of protein. In the cells of the suprarenal cortex, its function is to synthesize lipids, lipoproteins, and steroid hormones. In the hepatocytes of the liver, the smooth endoplasmic reticulum synthesizes glycogen and adds lipid to protein to form lipoprotein; hepatocytes also take part in drug detoxification, especially that of barbiturates. In skeletal muscle cells, the smooth endoplasmic reticulum participates in the binding of calcium and is associated with the process of contraction.

The cells lining the small intestine that are concerned with the absorption of fat contain smooth

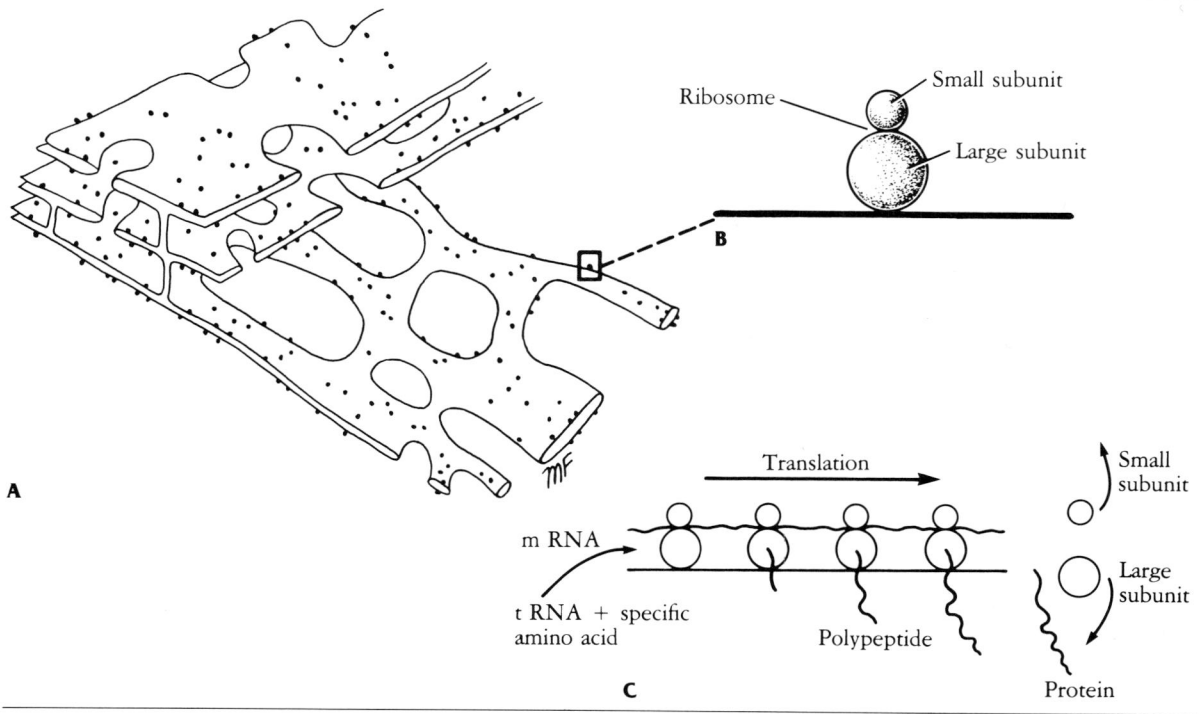

Fig. 2-16. The electron microscopic structure of rough endoplasmic reticulum. (A) shows the general configuration of the reticulum, (B) shows the structure of a ribosome, and (C) shows the part played by ribosomes in the formation of protein.

endoplasmic reticulum. In order to be absorbed, the fat is broken down within the lumen of the intestine by intestinal enzymes. Later, the enzymes associated with the smooth endoplasmic reticulum re-form the fat within the cell.

Close examination of a cell with an electron microscope shows that in many areas the smooth endoplasmic reticulum is continuous with the rough endoplasmic reticulum. It is believed that the latter produces the former by simply shedding its ribosomes.

THE GOLGI APPARATUS. With the light microscope and the use of silver-impregnated specimens, one sees the Golgi apparatus as a network of channels situated close to the nucleus. When viewed with the electron microscope, the apparatus consists of flattened, membranous sacs that are usually stacked close together (Figs. 2-18 and 2-19). The outer surface of the membrane is not studded with ribosomes. The stack of sacs is curved like a bowl, so that the Golgi apparatus has a concave and a convex surface.

The Golgi apparatus performs a number of important functions; it (1) adds carbohydrate to the protein molecules brought to it, (2) packages products for export from the cell, and (3) forms cell membranes. In a mucus-secreting cell, for example, the newly synthesized protein formed by the rough endoplasmic reticulum is passed to the Golgi apparatus by means of small, smooth membrane–bound vesicles that have budded off from the ends of the rough endoplasmic reticulum. The vesicles move through the cytoplasm to the outer, convex side of the Golgi apparatus and discharge their contents into the lumen of the sac of the apparatus, the membrane of the vesicle being added to the mem-

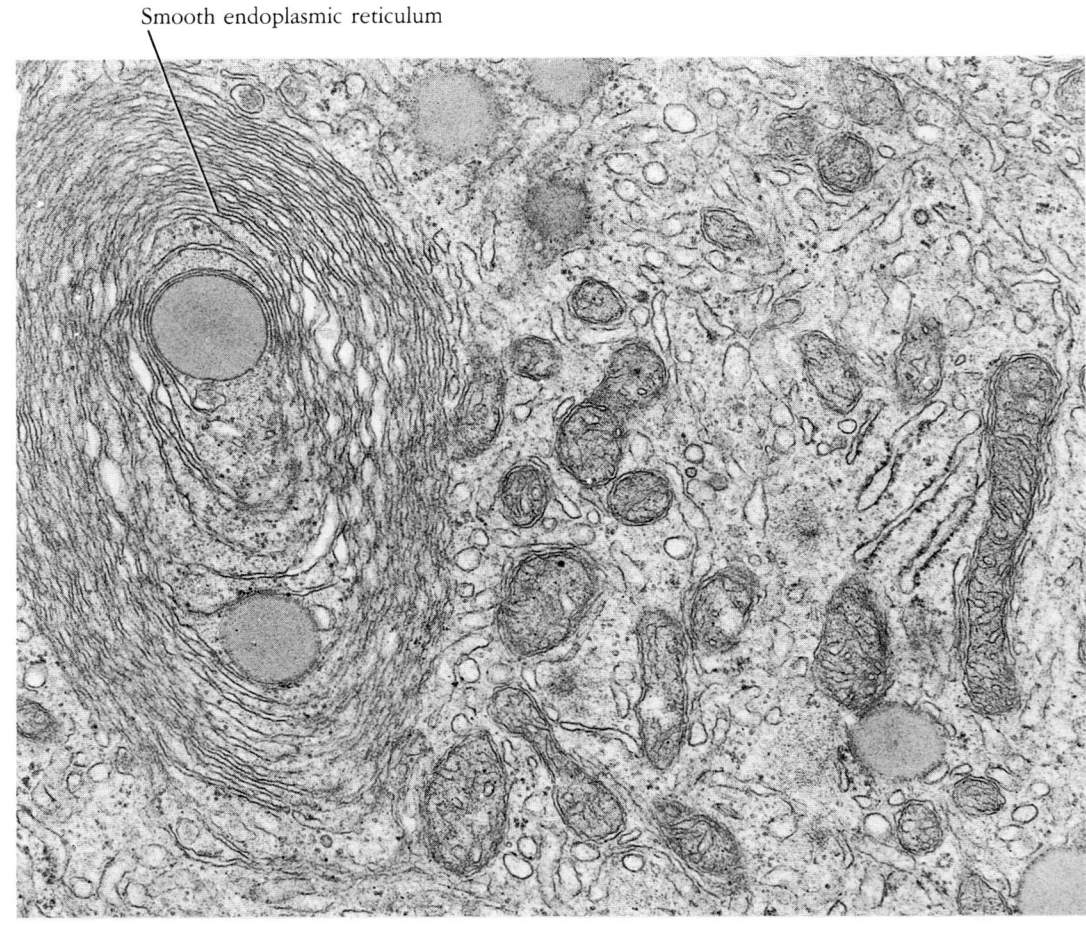

Fig. 2-17. Electron micrograph of a cell of the corpus luteum of the ovary, showing extensive smooth endoplasmic reticulum. (×24,362.) (Courtesy of Dr. M. J. Koering.)

brane of the sac of the apparatus. The Golgi apparatus is rich in sugar transferases, enzymes that add the carbohydrate to the proteins, forming mucus. The changed protein now travels through the stack of membranous sacs and leaves the apparatus on its concave surface in the form of a *secretory vesicle*. As the secretory vesicle travels through the cytoplasm, its contents become concentrated. Finally, the secretory vesicles pass to the surface of the cell, where the mucus is discharged.

It is important to realize that the Golgi apparatus is not responsible for the formation of new membrane in the apparatus itself. The vesicles carrying protein to the apparatus from the rough endoplasmic reticulum arrive at the same rate at which the secretory vesicles leave the apparatus (Fig. 2-19). As a result, the flattened, membranous sacs remain approximately constant in size.

Once the secretory vesicle reaches the cell surface, it discharges its contents by a process known as *exocytosis*. The membrane that surrounds the secretion is added to plasma membrane as the secretion leaves the cell. In this way, the Golgi apparatus continuously supplies new membrane to the plasma membrane.

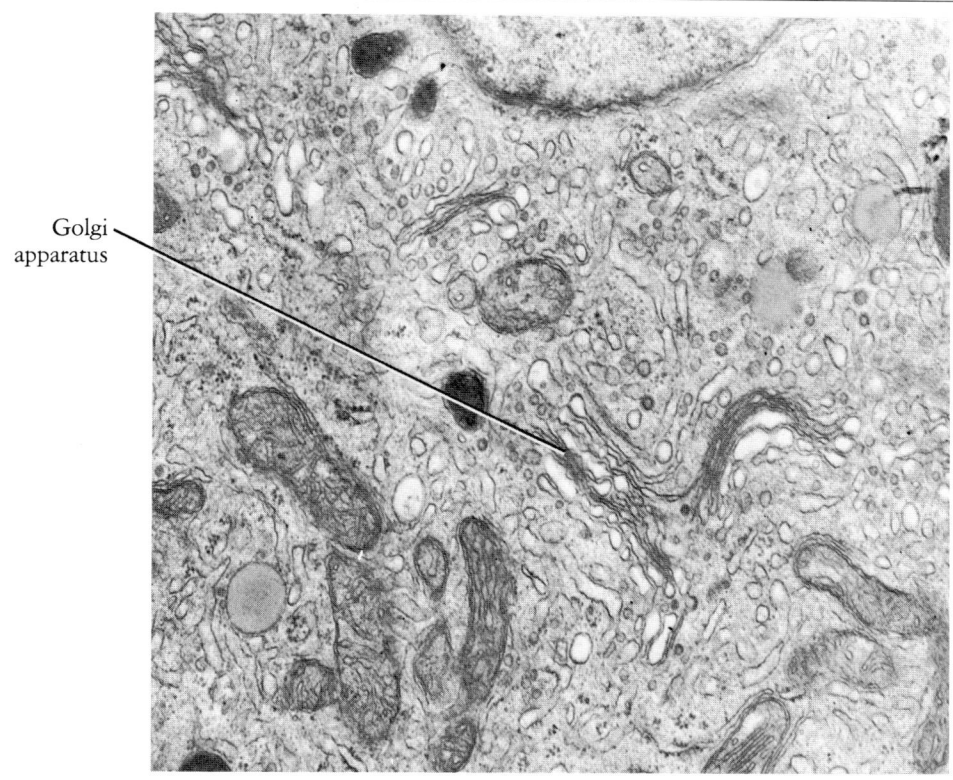

Fig. 2-18. Electron micrograph of a cell of the corpus luteum of the ovary, showing part of the nucleus, numerous mitochondria, vesicles, and the Golgi apparatus. ($\times 22{,}680$.) (Courtesy of Dr. M. J. Koering.)

LYSOSOMES. Lysosomes are membrane-bound, spherical bodies measuring about 8 nm in diameter. They contain hydrolytic enzymes that are active at acid pH. With the light microscope, they may be identified by using the acid phosphatase reaction, causing them to appear as very small, rounded structures. Because the hydrolytic enzymes are capable of breaking down the cytoplasmic matrix, it is not surprising that lysosomes are separated from the surrounding cytoplasm by membranous walls. The enzymes of lysosomes are originally formed in the rough-surfaced endoplasmic reticulum. They are transferred to the Golgi apparatus, where carbohydrate may be added. The Golgi apparatus then buds off a vesicle containing the hydrolytic enzyme and glycoproteins, thereby forming a lysosome (Fig. 2-20).

Lysosomes exist in three functional states: (1) *primary lysosomes,* which have just been formed by the Golgi apparatus and contain no digested material; (2) *secondary lysosomes,* containing partially digested material, which in this form may have the appearance of membranous whorls of *myelin figures;* and (3) *residual bodies,* which have evolved from secondary lysosomes. The enzymes in residual bodies are probably inactive, but the vesicle is filled with indigestible materials such as pigment, myelin figures, and lipid. These bodies may accumulate within the cell over the years or may be expelled through the plasma membrane on the cell surface.

A foreign substance of macromolecular dimensions is taken into a normal cell by a process known

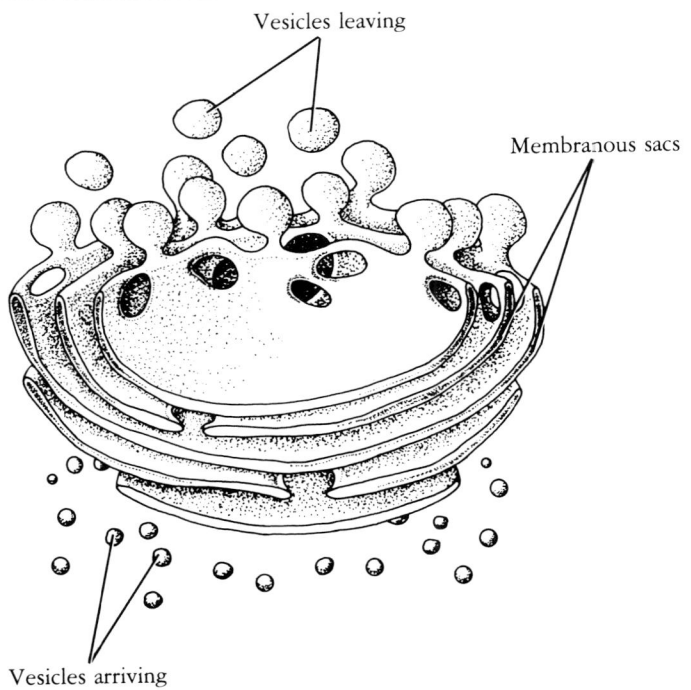

Fig. 2-19. *The electron microscopic structure of a Golgi apparatus. The cytoplasmic vesicles are shown arriving at the apparatus, while new vesicles are budding off and leaving the opposite surface of the apparatus. The process is discussed in the text.*

as *phagocytosis*. In short, the foreign material becomes surrounded by a section of the plasma membrane to form a vesicle. This membrane-bound vesicle is called a *phagosome*. If a phagosome contacts a lysosome, the membranes of the two vesicles fuse at their point of contact and the foreign material becomes exposed to the hydrolytic enzymes and is digested.

In a similar manner, worn-out mitochondria and other cell organelles that are functionless become fused to lysosomes and undergo digestion. The results of digestion of phagosomes or worn-out organelles may later be ejected from the cell by the process of *exocytosis* (see Fig. 2-20). Although lysosomes should be regarded as the general cleaners of the cell in that they dispose of unwanted absorbed foreign particles and worn out cellular contents, they may also play a leading role in cellular metabolism. For example, in liver cells, lysosomes are important in the breakdown of intracellular glycogen. In the thyroid gland, lysosomes are responsible for the breakdown of thyroglobulin into globulin and the hormone thyroxin.

Peroxisomes, or *microbodies*, have a structure similar to that of lysosomes. They contain a number of oxidases that can reduce hydrogen peroxide to oxygen and water. Peroxisomes control hydrogen peroxide metabolism within cells and assist in the formation of keto acids.

Multivesicular bodies are found in liver cells and are possibly modified lysosomes. They are larger than lysosomes and consist of a number of small vesicles lying within a larger vesicle. Their function is unknown.

COATED VESICLES. Coated vesicles are rounded in shape and lie free in the cytoplasm. Covering the outer surface of the membrane is a fuzzy coat. It has

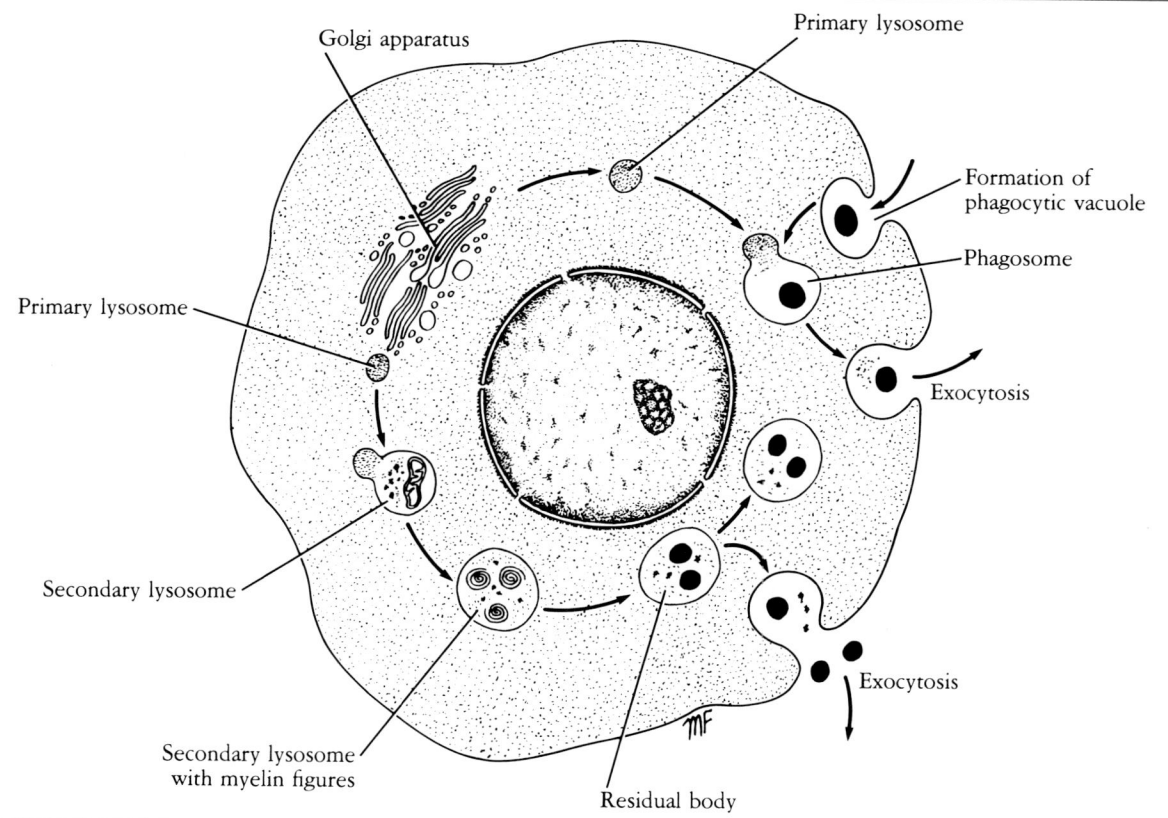

Fig. 2-20. The part played by lysosomes in the breakdown of a foreign particle that has been phagocytosed by a cell or the breakdown of cell organelles or inclusions that are no longer required by a cell. The end products finally leave the cell by a process of exocytosis. The processes involved are discussed in the text.

been shown that these vesicles can arise from the plasma membrane, the Golgi apparatus, rough endoplasmic reticulum, and secretory vesicles. The significance of the coat is not understood. It is believed to be formed from material in the cytoplasmic matrix. The function of these vesicles is not known.

FREE RIBOSOMES. Ribosomes either are found scattered diffusely throughout the cytoplasm, where they are referred to as *free ribosomes,* or they are attached to the outer surface of membranous structures, where they form part of the rough endoplasmic reticulum and are called *attached ribosomes.* The principal function of free ribosomes is to synthesize the protein necessary for the cell's own existence. For example, they produce enzymes, produce protein to replace worn-out organelles, and are particularly important in providing new protein during the process of cell growth and division. The main function of attached ribosomes is to provide new protein that will be secreted by the cell.

Ribosomes each consist of a large and a small subunit (see Fig. 2-16). The units contain *ribosomal RNA* and protein. Ribosomes are usually linked together like beads on a thread in groups of three to thirty. Each group is called a *polyribosome,* and the thread is a long molecule of *messenger RNA.* You will remember that the messenger RNA, which is formed in the nucleolus in close contact with the

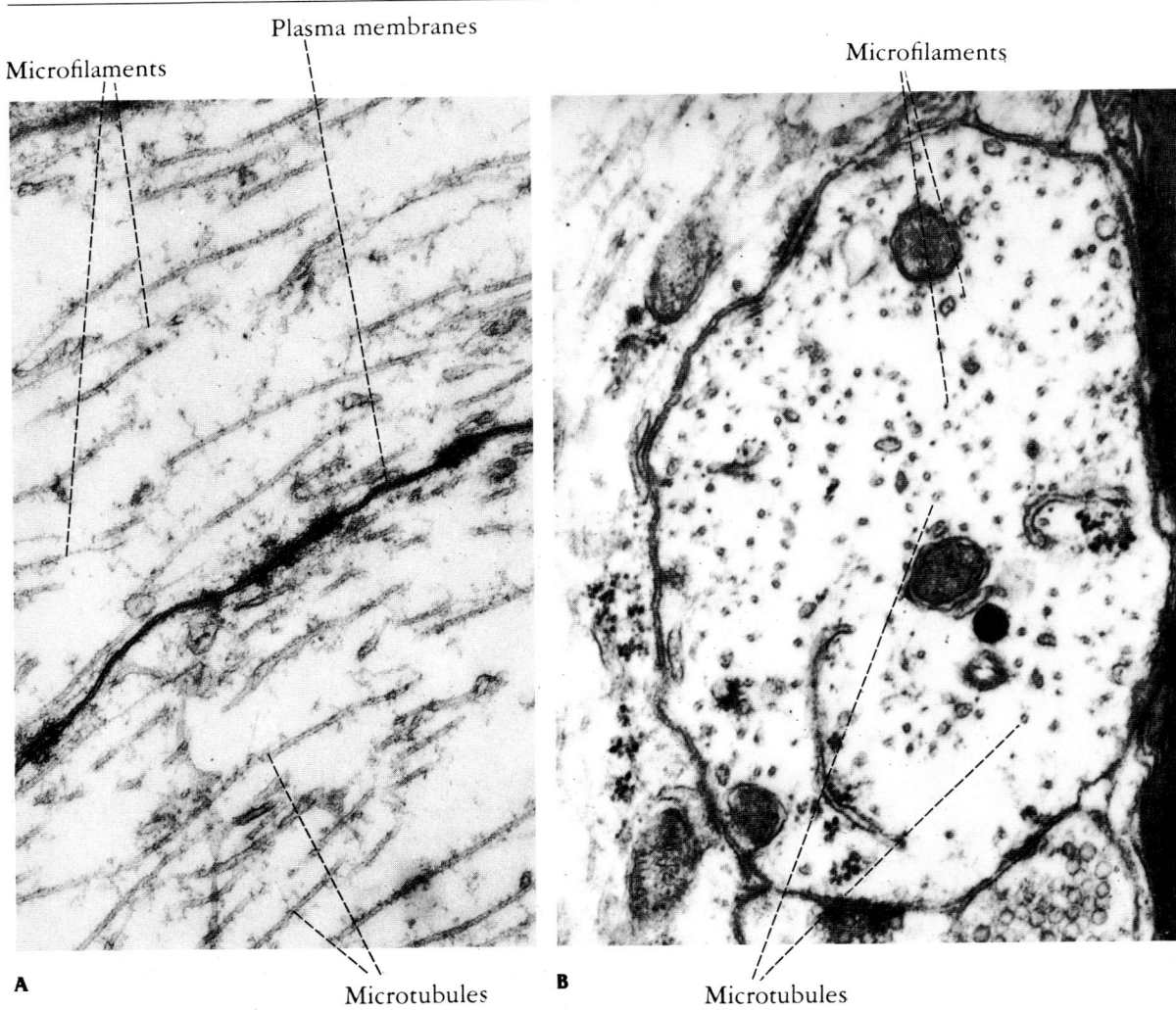

Fig. 2-21. Electron micrograph of dendrites of a nerve cell, showing the presence of microfilaments and microtubules within their cytoplasm. (A) Longitudinal section of two adjacent dendrites; (B) transverse section of a dendrite. (Courtesy of Dr. J. M. Kerns.)

chromosomes, passes out of the nucleus into the cytoplasm, carrying with it information that will determine the sequence of amino acids to be used to synthesize a specific protein. The amino acids in the cytoplasmic matrix first become oriented by *transfer RNA*. On reaching the ribosomes, which serve as a physical support, the amino acids are linked together to form polypeptides or proteins, the arrangement being determined by the messenger RNA. Once the new protein is formed, it is re-

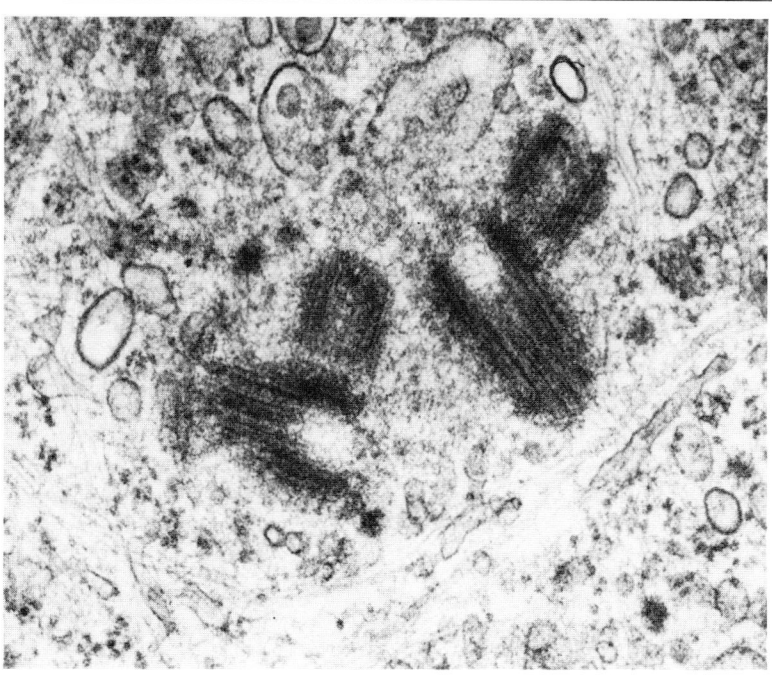

Fig. 2-22. Electron micrograph of a pair of centrosomes. Each centrosome consists of two centrioles oriented at right angles to each other. (Courtesy of Dr. J. B. Rattner.)

leased, and the ribosomes become detached from the thread of messenger RNA.

MICROTUBULES. Microtubules are relatively straight, long, slender tubules that in cross section appear as minute circles on an electron micrograph (Fig. 2-21). They are present in most cells and exist as single units scattered throughout the cytoplasm or in groups in parallel array. Microtubules are formed from the protein *tubulin.*

Microtubules serve as an internal skeleton for a cell, preserving its size and shape. In mitosis, microtubules form the cell spindle and appear to guide the movement of the chromosomes. This process can be halted by the administration of colchicine, which causes the microtubules to disappear and the cell spindle not to be formed. In cilia and flagella, microtubules show a sliding motion that causes the movement of these structures. Microtubules also play a role in the transport of substances within the cytoplasm. In this respect, they appear to determine the direction taken by the substances, rather like railway lines determining the direction taken by trains. In nerve cells, for example, chemical substances appear to be directed by microtubules away from the center of the cell body along the cell processes to their terminations. In a similar manner, pigment granules in pigment cells move along the cell processes in close association with the microtubules.

CENTRIOLES AND BASAL BODIES. Centrioles are small, paired structures found in every cell that has the ability to divide. The two centrioles are short rods oriented at right angles to each other and together known as the *centrosome* (Fig. 2-22). Each centriole is a hollow cylinder whose wall is formed of bundles of microtubules (Fig. 2-23).

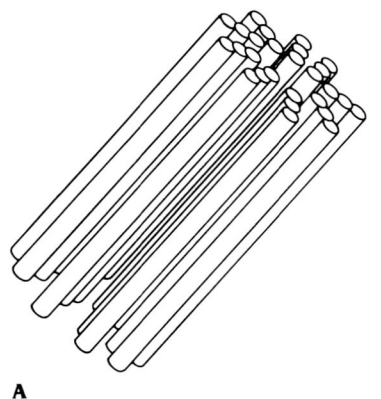
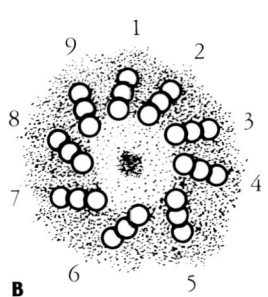

Fig. 2-23. *The structure of a centriole. (A) shows the nine bundles of microtubules forming the wall of the centriole; (B) shows a centriole in cross section and indicates that each bundle is made up of three microtubules.*

Centrioles are associated with cell division. During early prophase, the two centrioles diverge and take up positions at opposite poles of the cell. The two centrioles now become connected by a system of microtubules known as the *spindle* (see p. 34).

Centrioles are also associated with the formation of cilia (see p. 66). In the formation of a ciliated cell, the centrioles multiply, and large numbers appear in the cytoplasm, one for each cilium to be formed. The centrioles migrate toward the free surface of the cell and line up close to the plasma membrane. Microtubules now grow out from each centriole toward the cell surface and, carrying a covering of plasma membrane, project from the cell surface. A cilium is thus established. It is usual to refer to the centriole at the base of the cilium as the *basal body* (Fig. 2-24). It is believed that the movement of the microtubules upon one another is responsible for the bending movement of each cilium.

MICROFILAMENTS AND FIBRILS. Microfilaments are present in most cells and can be seen only with an electron microscope (see Fig. 2-21). They measure about 4 to 15 nm in diameter. A fibril is composed of a bundle of filaments and can be seen with the light microscope (Fig. 2-25). It measures about 0.2 to 1 μm in diameter.

Microfilaments can be divided into two types, supportive and contractile. The *supportive microfilaments* are larger in cross section and are present in the cytoplasm of motile and nonmotile cells. In some cells, they are attached to the cytoplasmic surface of desmosomes and appear to brace the cells against forces that will change their shape. In epidermal cells, they are present in very large numbers and serve to stiffen the cells. In columnar cells, the fine filaments form a network called the *terminal web* that crosses the cells near their free surface and provides support for microvilli or cilia.

The *contractile microfilaments* are smaller in cross section and are composed of the contractile proteins actin, myosin, tropomyosin, and α-actinin. They are present in many types of cells and are believed to be responsible for the movement of cells or the movement of parts of cells, such as ruffling of the plasma membrane or invagination of the cell membrane or indentation of the cell membrane during cell division. They are also responsible for the movement of microvilli. These contractile microfilaments are most highly developed in muscle cells, where the actin and myosin filaments are arranged in parallel bundles (see p. 197). It is the chemical reaction between the actin and myosin filaments that makes them slide upon one another and thus cause shortening of the cell.

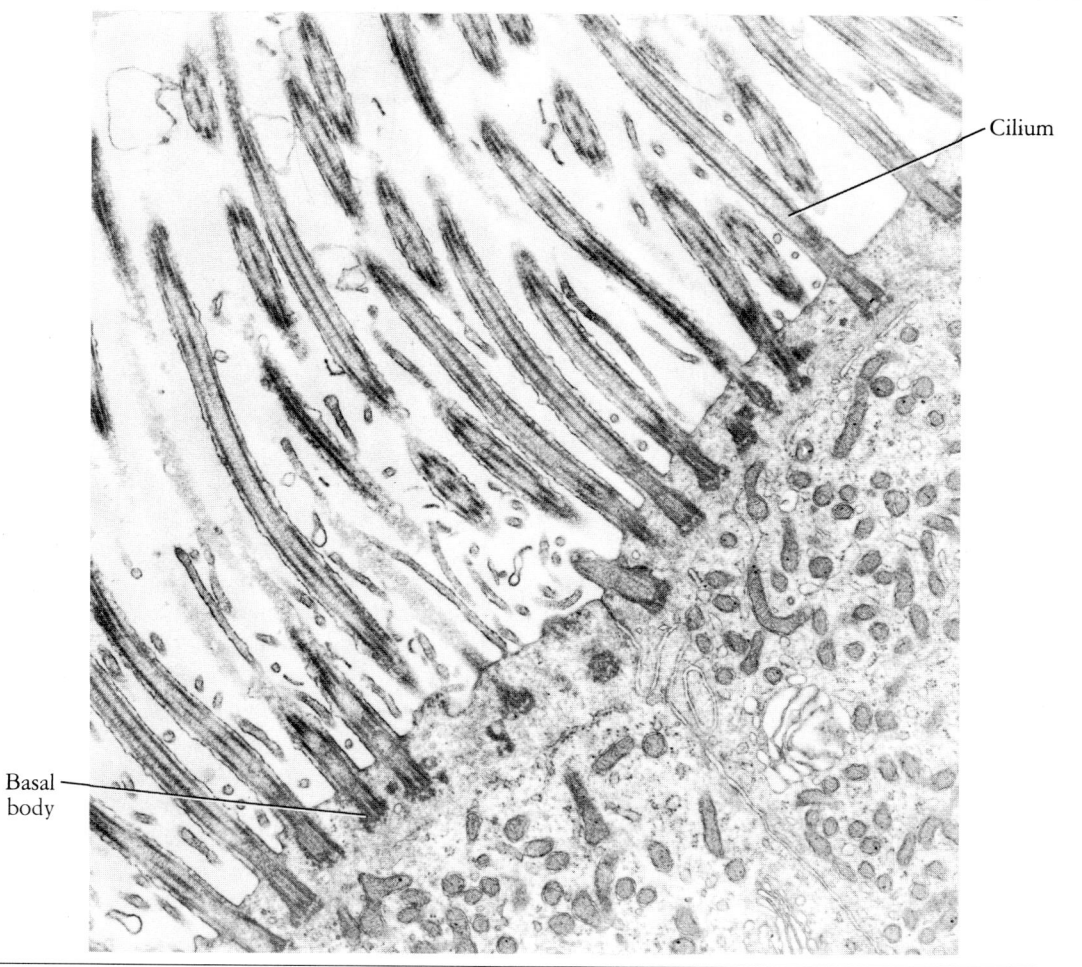

Fig. 2-24. Electron micrograph of the columnar ciliated epithelium lining the uterine tube, showing the internal structure of cilia and the position of the basal bodies. (× 16,600.) (Courtesy of Dr. M. J. Koering.)

Cytoplasmic Inclusions

Inclusions are inanimate substances that are found in cell cytoplasm and either have been produced by the cell or have been taken into the cell from the outside (Figs. 2-26 and 2-27).

FOOD SUBSTANCES. Carbohydrate is found stored in the cytoplasm of the liver and other cells in the form of glycogen granules (see Fig. 2-26). Unfortunately, glycogen is water-soluble, and in ordinary slide preparations used for light microscopy, the glycogen has been removed, leaving irregular spaces in the cytoplasm. If the specimen is specially prepared using the periodic acid–Schiff reagent, the glycogen granules are stained bright red. With the electron microscope, glycogen can be seen as fine particles that may be clumped together in rosettes (see Fig. 2-2).

Fat is stored in large amounts in the cytoplasm of connective tissue cells (see Fig. 4-5). Connective tis-

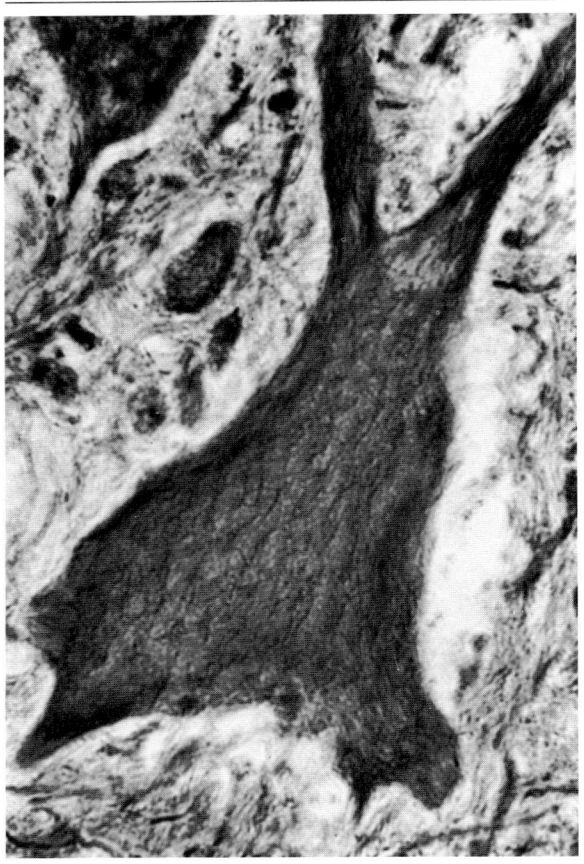

Fig. 2-25. Photomicrograph of a silver-stained section of a nerve cell, showing large numbers of neurofibrils in the cytoplasm of the cell body and the nerve processes.

sue containing many of these fat-laden cells is referred to as *adipose tissue.* Fat is also present in the cytoplasm of other cells, for example, those of the suprarenal cortex and the liver. The fat stored in adipose tissue cells is in the form of *triglycerides.* Liver cells contain large quantities of *phospholipids* and *cholesterol* in addition to triglycerides. In the suprarenal cortex, the fat droplets in the cytoplasm are composed of cholesterol.

In ordinary light microscope preparations, the fat is dissolved by organic solvents, leaving round, empty spaces. Fat can, however, be easily demonstrated by using osmium tetroxide as a fixative, causing the droplets to appear brown or black (see Fig. 4-7). With the electron microscope, fat droplets appear round and black.

PIGMENTS. *Carbon* or other dust particles are phagocytosed by macrophages in the respiratory system (see Fig. 9-17). *Carotene,* a pigment present in large amounts in carrots and tomatoes, is soluble in fat and may give the tissues a yellow coloration. *Silver* and *lead* can gain entrance to cells, should they be ingested, and can be regarded as cytoplasmic inclusions.

The blood pigments *hemosiderin* and *bilirubin* are derived from the hemoglobin of worn-out red blood cells. The red cells are phagocytosed by reticuloendothelial cells in the bone marrow, liver, and spleen, and the iron-containing hemoglobin is broken down into a iron-containing pigment called hemosiderin and a non-iron-containing pigment called bilirubin. Hemosiderin forms insoluble brown granules within the cytoplasm, but bilirubin is soluble and quickly leaves the cytoplasm and enters the bloodstream, where it is taken to the liver to be excreted with the bile.

Melanin is a pigment formed in the cytoplasm of melanocytes (see Fig. 17-9). It varies in color from orange to brown to black. The pigment, as seen with the electron microscope, is contained within membrane-bound granules called *melanosomes.* It is responsible for the color of the skin and hair, the color of the iris of the eye, and the pigmentation of the retina. In the skin, it serves to protect the deeper tissues from the harmful effects of ultraviolet light; in the eye, it prevents problems of internal reflection of light.

Lipofuscin is a golden-brown pigment that is found in liver, heart, and nerve cells and is visible with the light microscope (see Fig. 7-15). It increases in amount with age. It represents the accumulated undigested residue found in old lysosomes.

Cytoplasmic Matrix

The term *matrix* is applied to the colloidal solution that lies between the organelles and inclusions. It

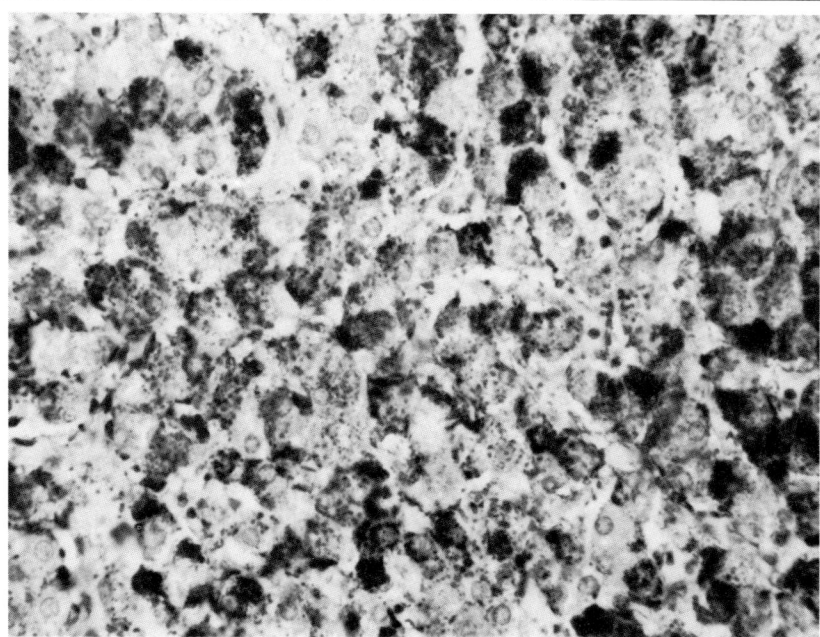

Fig. 2-26. Photomicrograph of a section of the liver, showing intracellular deposits of glycogen. The glycogen appears as fine or coarse black granules. (Best's carmine stain; × 400.)

contains many proteins, some of which are enzymatic, and soluble substances that either have been absorbed by the cell from the tissue fluid or have been formed within the cell.

PLASMA MEMBRANE

The plasma membrane (cell membrane) encloses the cell and separates the cytoplasm from the exterior (see Figs. 2-1, 2-2, and 2-28). The membrane is only about 8 nm thick and is therefore too thin to be seen with the light microscope. The dark boundary line that one sees at the margin of a cell with the light microscope is the edge of the cell, or the plasma membrane, seen in oblique section. When viewed under the electron microscope in ultrathin sections, the plasma membrane appears as two dark lines with a light line between them (Fig. 2-28).

Plasma membranes are composed of proteins (about 60 percent), lipids (about 30 percent), and carbohydrates (less than 10 percent). The proteins give the membrane structural stability and are sites of high metabolic activity. The lipids provide an entrance for fat-soluble compounds. The carbohydrates may serve as receptor molecules for the attachment of substances such as hormones, antibodies, or even viruses.

The precise structure of the plasma membrane has long fascinated cell biologists and is still not fully known. It is generally agreed that the plasma membrane is composed of an inner and an outer layer of very loosely arranged protein molecules, each layer about 2.5 nm thick, separated by a middle layer of lipid about 3 nm thick. The lipid layer is made up of two rows of phospholipid molecules arranged so that their hydrophobic ends are in contact with each other and their polar ends are in contact with the protein layers. It has been suggested that certain protein molecules lie within the phospholipid layer like islands in a lipid sea. Moreover, some of those intrinsic protein molecules are longer than the width of the membrane and therefore protrude from its outer and inner surfaces (Fig. 2-29). The carbohydrates are attached to the outside of the plasma

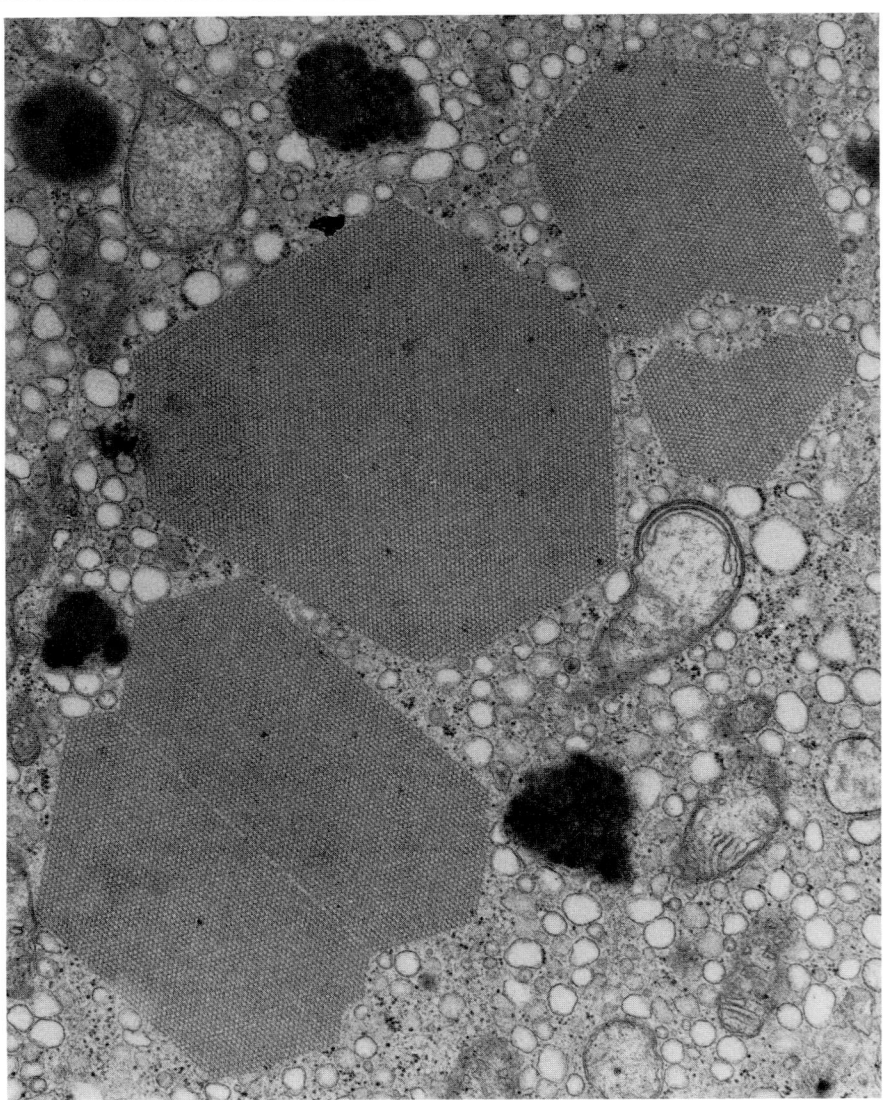

Fig. 2-27. Electron micrograph of Sertoli cell of testis, showing crystalline inclusions (crystals of Reinke) that are believed to be protein. (×17,335.) (Courtesy of Dr. T. Nagano.)

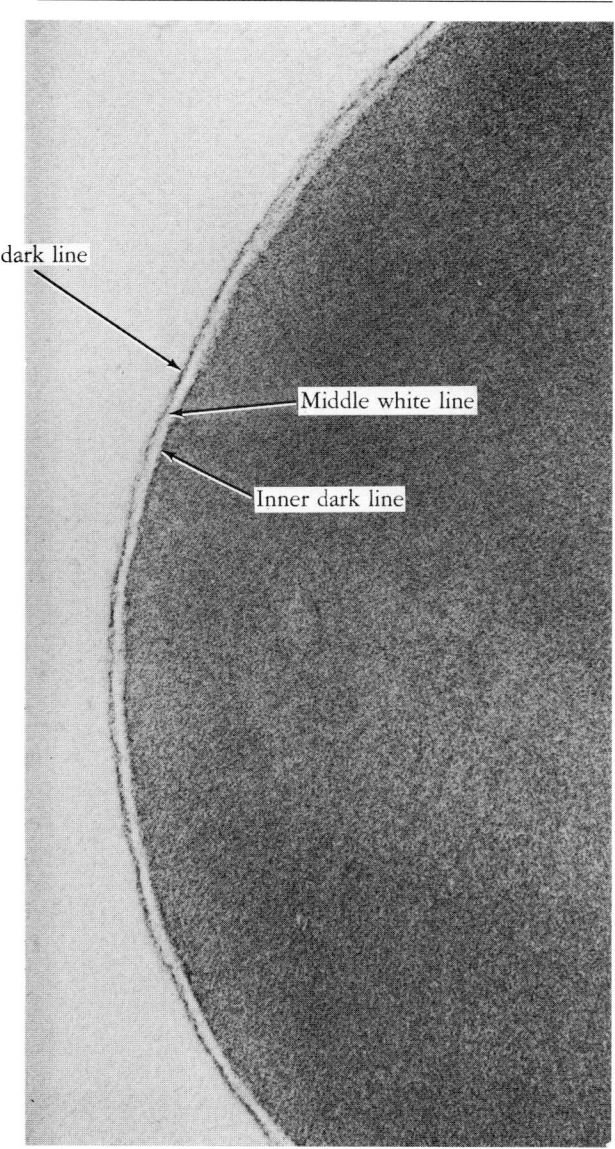

Fig. 2-28. Electron micrograph of a red blood cell, showing the structure of the plasma membrane. The outer and inner dark lines are probably produced by the deposition of the stain on the polar ends of the phospholipids. (Uranyl acetate and lead citrate stain; ×160,000.) (Courtesy of Dr. J. D. Robertson.)

membrane and are linked to the proteins or the lipids.

Recent research has revealed that the plasma membranes are not static structures and that the protein molecules have lateral mobility on the cell surface. It is thought that the actin and myosin filaments of the cytoplasm may be involved in this motility.

Cell Coat (Glycocalyx)

Every cell is believed to be surrounded by a cell coat composed of sialic acid (a carbohydrate) and glycoproteins or mucoproteins that are attached to the outside of the plasma membrane. In certain cells, for example, the columnar absorptive cells of the small intestine, the coat is very thick and can be seen with the light microscope as a fuzzy layer. The basal laminae of epithelium may be regarded as a form of glycocalyx. The function of the cell coat is not fully understood, although it is thought to act as an adhesive that holds cells together. It may also bind various molecules to the cell surface or serve as an area where ions may be concentrated prior to their absorption and passage through the plasma membrane. The cell coat is the site of the ABO blood groups and the receptors for hormones and enzymes. It is formed by the cells it surrounds.

Cytoplasmic Membranes

The membranes of cytoplasmic organelles such as mitochondria, the Golgi apparatus, and the endoplasmic reticulum have a structure similar to that of the plasma membrane. They are, however, a little thinner. Their chemical composition may also vary, and the enzymes attached to their inner surfaces are different in different organelles.

Physical Properties of Cell Membranes

Membranes are vital to cells. Not only do they enclose the cell, but they compartmentalize it so that different units can perform chemical reactions independently of one another. Thus, the cell is separated from the surrounding tissue fluid by the plasma membrane, the nucleus is separated from the cyto-

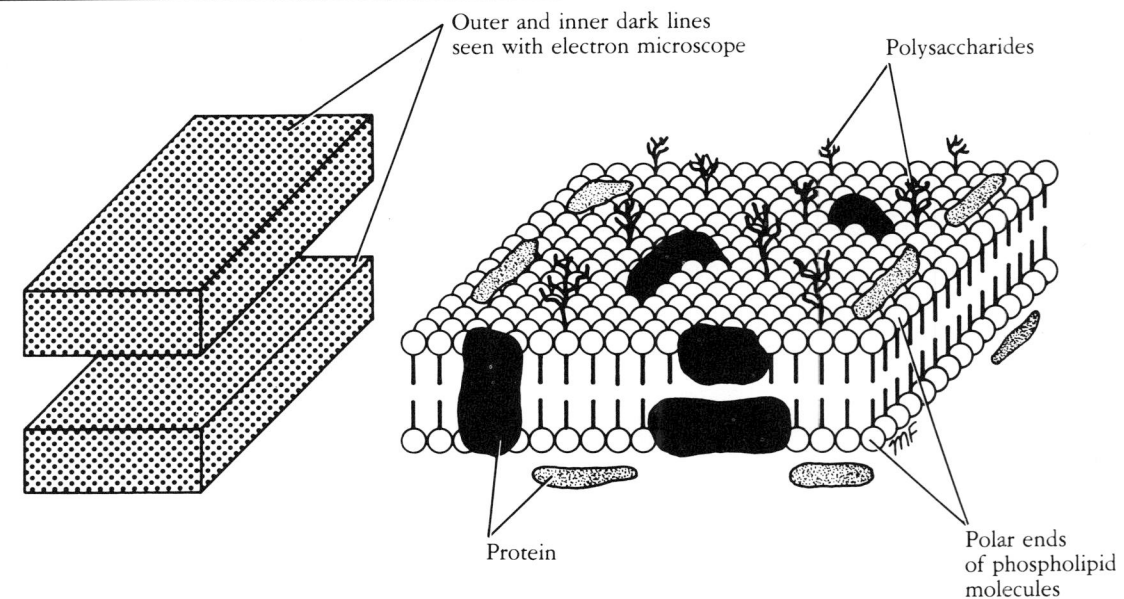

Fig. 2-29. *The probable structure of a plasma membrane. Note that the outer and inner dark lines, seen with the electron microscope, are probably produced by the deposition of the stain on the polar ends of the phospholipids.*

plasm by the nuclear membrane, and so on. The different functional activities that occur in different cytoplasmic organelles depend on the different enzymes that are present within the organelles and on the separation of the organelles from the cytoplasmic matrix by their bounding membranes.

Substances pass into or out of a cell through the plasma (cell) membrane by a variety of methods. Simple passage through the membrane is accomplished by (1) diffusion, (2) osmosis, (3) facilitated diffusion, or (4) active transport. Bulk passage through the membrane occurs by (1) pinocytosis or (2) phagocytosis.

Diffusion

Diffusion is the tendency for a substance to scatter or spread itself out equally so that eventually its molecules will be dispersed evenly throughout any space they occupy. When applied to the passage of a substance through a plasma membrane, this statement means that, provided the molecules of the substance in question are small enough and the plasma membrane does not serve as a barrier, the concentration of the molecules eventually will be equal on both sides of the membrane (Fig. 2-30). The molecules of some substances, such as proteins, are very large, however, and the plasma membrane has only small "openings," so the membrane is impermeable to such substances. Thus, certain substances, such as sodium ions, can diffuse rapidly through a membrane, whereas the macromolecules of protein cannot. This differential diffusion occurs because of the selective permeability of the cell membrane (see Fig. 2-30).

Osmosis

Osmosis is a passive process by which small molecules move across semipermeable membranes. If two solutions of different concentrations of large molecules are separated from each other by a semipermeable membrane with small pores, the solvent, consisting of small molecules, diffuses through the semipermeable membrane from the less concentrated solution into the more concentrated solution

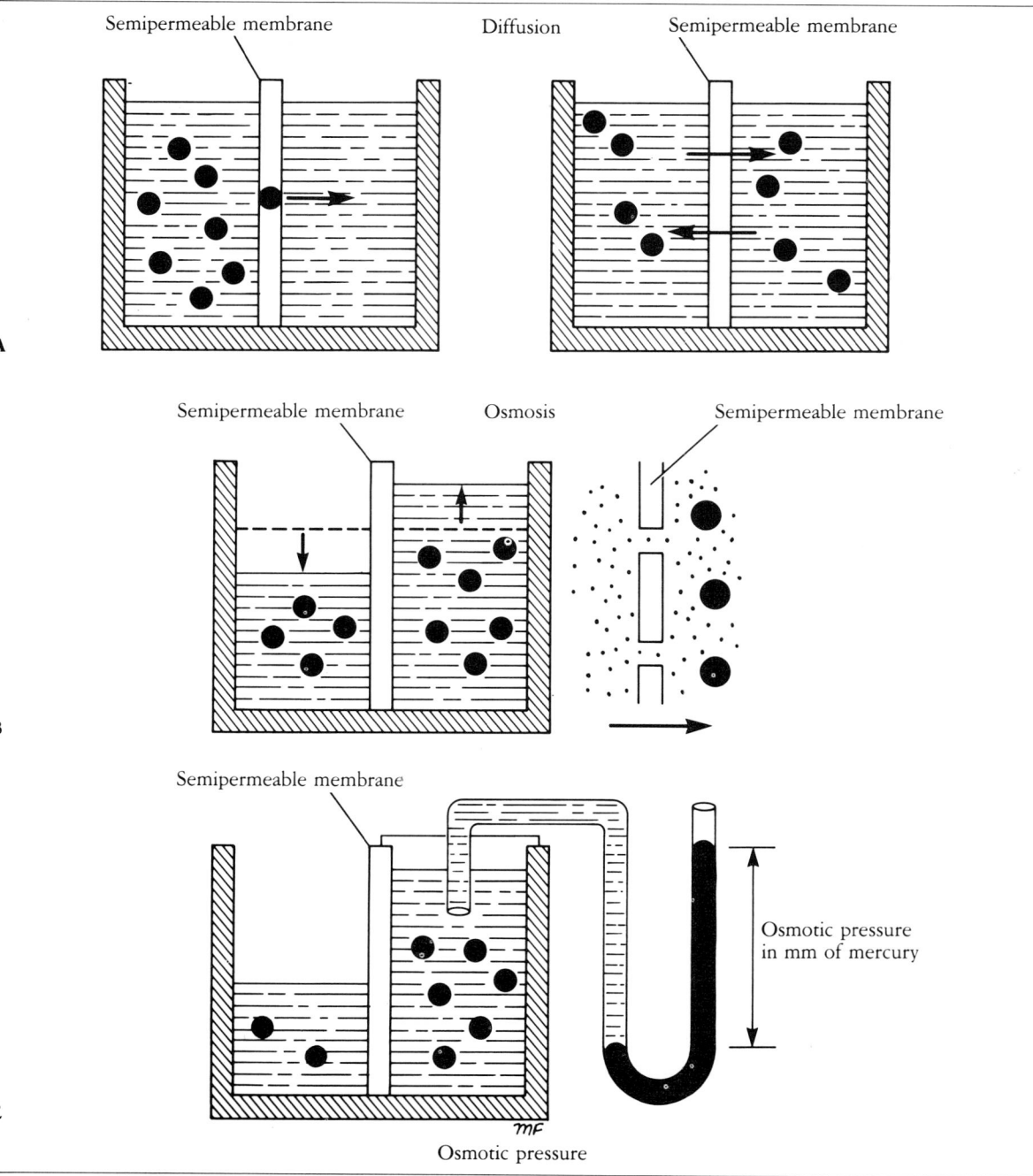

Fig. 2-30. Two mechanisms for the passage of substances through a plasma membrane: (A) diffusion and (B) osmosis. (C) shows a simple method of measuring osmotic pressure.

(see Fig. 2-30). This process is osmosis. In this situation, the membrane allows the small molecules to pass through freely but forms a barrier to the large molecules. As the solvent passes into the more concentrated solution, there is an increase in the volume of that solution. The pressure that is necessary to oppose the diffusion of the solvent through the semipermeable membrane is known as osmotic pressure (see Fig. 2-30). The diffusion of the solvent will continue until the concentrations of the solutions on the two sides of the membrane are equal.

In the living body, the solvent is water and the semipermeable membrane is a cellular (plasma) membrane. It should be pointed out that if the concentrations of the solutions on the two sides of a cell membrane are equal, no movement of water will take place and the solutions are said to be *isotonic*. For example, if a normal cell is placed in a solution of 0.9% sodium chloride or 5% glucose, either of which is isotonic with the intracellular fluid, water will not diffuse through the plasma membrane and the cell will not swell or shrink. If, however, a cell is placed in a solution of sodium chloride with a concentration of less than 0.9%, water will enter the cell and it will swell. Such a solution is said to be *hypotonic*. If a cell is placed in a solution of sodium chloride with a concentration greater than 0.9%, water will leave the cell and enter the solution, causing the cell to shrink. Such a salt solution is said to be *hypertonic*.

Facilitated Diffusion

Because the plasma membrane contains a double row of phospholipid molecules, substances that are soluble in lipids diffuse through the membrane easily, whereas those that are not soluble in lipids pass through the membrane with great difficulty. It is known, however, that some substances, such as sugars, pass through cell membranes very rapidly even though they are highly insoluble in lipids. This process of facilitated diffusion (Fig. 2-31) is able to occur because the transported substance—for example, glucose—combines reversibly with a specific membrane component or *carrier* at the outer surface of the plasma membrane. The carrier complex is soluble in the lipid part of the membrane and moves across to the inner surface of the membrane, where it dissociates, releasing the substance to the interior of the cell. The carrier then moves back across the membrane to the outer surface, where it can repeat the process. This transport mechanism can act in both directions, and only a relatively small number of carrier molecules is required to transport large amounts of a substance. Moreover, no metabolic energy is required during facilitated diffusion, because the movement of the substance is passive and from a region of higher concentration to one of lower concentration. The important fact is that the carrier makes the glucose soluble in the membrane. Without it, the glucose could not pass through the membrane.

Active Transport

In many instances, the concentration of a substance inside the cell is much higher than that outside the cell, yet it is important for the metabolism of the cell for more of the substance to enter. Such a substance is potassium, which is present in higher concentrations within cells. Clearly, the process of simple diffusion cannot achieve this objective, because no substance can diffuse against a concentration gradient. Energy must be imparted to the molecules if they are going to pass through a cell membrane from a dilute solution to a concentrated solution. This process is known as active transport. Substances commonly transported in this manner are sodium ions, potassium ions, chloride ions, sugars, and amino acids.

Active transport closely resembles facilitated transport in that the substance combines reversibly with a *carrier* at the outer surface of the plasma membrane. The carrier complex is soluble in the lipid part of the membrane and moves across to the inner surface of the membrane, where it dissociates, releasing the substance to the inner surface of the cell. It is believed that in this form of transport, the dissociation and release of the substance from the carrier require an enzyme-catalyzed reaction us-

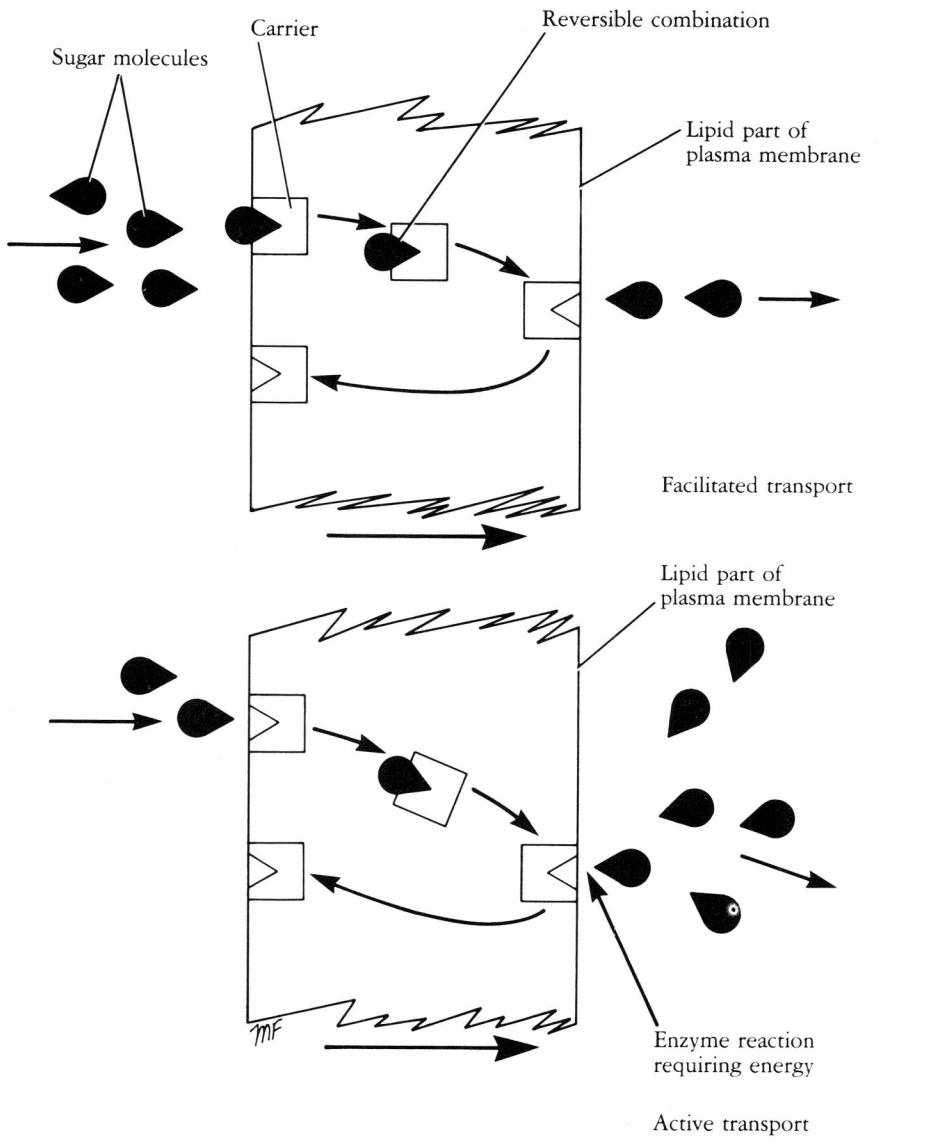

Fig. 2-31. The processes of facilitated transport and active transport of sugar molecules through the lipid layer of a plasma membrane.

ing energy from adenosine triphosphate (ATP) (see Fig. 2-31). It is interesting to note that it is possible to saturate this mechanism by having too high a concentration of the substance to be transported. Saturation can occur because of limitations in the amount of carrier available or the supply of enzymes that are necessary for the reaction.

THE SODIUM-POTASSIUM PUMP. Normally, the concentration of sodium outside the cell is higher than that inside the cell. Conversely, the concentration of potassium is higher inside the cell than outside it. The mechanism responsible for these different concentrations of sodium and potassium on the two sides of the cell membrane is referred to as the sodium-potassium pump. If the pump failed, the two ions would diffuse through the cell membrane until their concentrations on the two sides of the membrane were equal.

The sodium-potassium pump is situated in the cell membrane, and its energy is provided by ATP. The enzyme responsible is Na^+-K^+ ATPase, and it hydrolyzes ATP to adenosine diphosphate (ADP). It is believed that sodium on the outside of the cell membrane combines with a carrier and together they cross the membrane to the interior of the cell; here, the carrier is released.

It should be pointed out that although the movements of sodium and potassium across the cell membrane are coupled, there is not always a one-to-one relationship between them. In fact, the coupling ratio can fall anywhere between 1:1 and 1:4 or more. When the coupling ratio is 1:1, there is no change in the electrical charge across the membrane. When the amount of sodium pumped out of the cell is greater than the amount of potassium pumped in, however, the cell membrane becomes hyperpolarized.

It should be noted that the activity of the sodium-potassium pump is reduced by chemical poisons that interfere with the oxidative metabolism of the cell, namely, dinitrophenol and cyanide. In contrast, ouabain, which is chemically related to digitalis, inhibits the sodium-potassium pump but leaves the oxidative metabolism of the cell intact. It is believed that ouabain has a direct inhibitory action on ATPase.

Membrane "Pores"

Water and many dissolved ions can pass rapidly through a plasma membrane by diffusion. It has been suggested that the membrane possesses minute holes, called membrane pores, that permit this form of transport. Unfortunately, morphologists, even with the aid of the electron microscope, have been unable to demonstrate the existence of these pores. The protein molecules that cross the lipid layers and bridge the outer and inner protein layers may be the site of such openings.

The degree of permeability will depend on the size of the pores. Molecules of water, urea molecules, and chloride ions are small and can pass through a cell membrane rapidly. Glucose molecules and those of other sugars are large and have great difficulty passing through the pores. This is why the processes of facilitated diffusion and active transport are necessary in membrane transport.

Electrically Charged Ions and the Effect of Electrical Potential Difference across a Cell Membrane

Positively charged ions, such as potassium and sodium, have difficulty passing through a plasma membrane. The explanation suggested is that the protein, which forms islands within the lipid layers of the plasma membrane and is probably associated with the so-called pores of the membrane, is positively charged and repels these ions. Negatively charged ions, such as chloride, rapidly pass through the membrane.

If an electrical gradient is created across a cell membrane so that one side is positively charged and the other side is negatively charged, the positive charge attracts the negative ions (Fig. 2-32) and the negative charge attracts the positive ions. Moreover, the positive charge will repel the positive ions and the negative charge will repel the negative ions. As a result, the ions will move across the membrane even though no concentration difference exists to cause

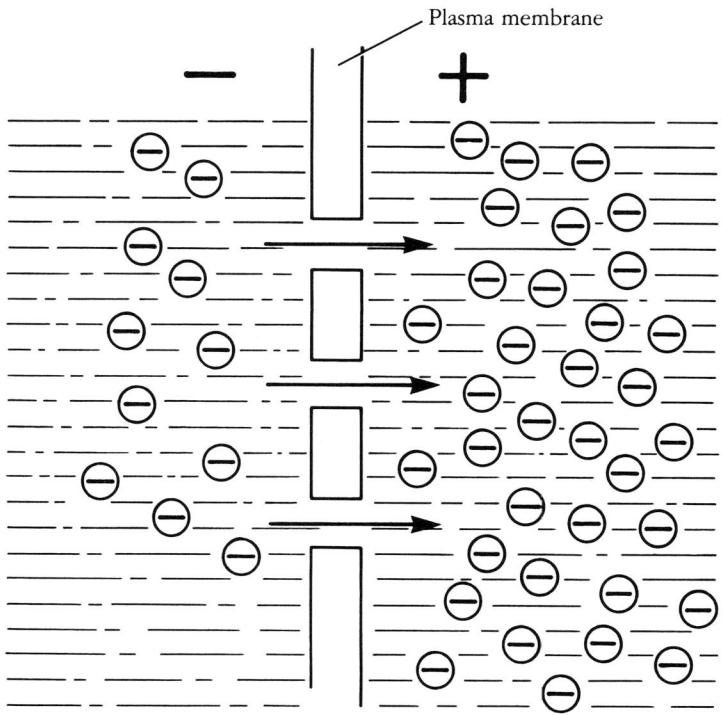

Fig. 2-32. The effect of an electrical potential difference on the diffusion of molecules and ions through a plasma membrane.

their movement. This phenomenon is of particular importance in the transmission of nerve impulses in nerve cells.

Pinocytosis

Pinocytosis is the process by which small amounts of substances that have a high molecular weight and are dissolved in solution are taken in through the plasma membrane (Fig. 2-33). Essentially, the substance in solution becomes engulfed by the cell membrane and moves into the cell, totally surrounded by a membranous bag called a *pinocytotic vesicle*. The vesicle then becomes detached from the cell membrane and lies free in the cytoplasmic matrix.

Phagocytosis

Phagocytosis is the process by which large particles are taken into the cell (see Fig. 2-33). Essentially, portions of the plasma membrane protrude from the cell surface or a small pocket occurs on the cell surface, and the particle becomes surrounded by the plasma membrane. The large, fluid-filled vesicle containing the particle then becomes detached from the plasma membrane and lies free in the cytoplasmic matrix. This phenomenon is similar to pinocytosis but is on a much larger scale.

In both pinocytosis and phagocytosis, the ingested substance is surrounded by a membrane. Pinocytosis is a method used to transport proteins across cell membranes, whereas phagocytosis tends to be restricted to certain cells, such as reticuloendothelial cells (mononuclear phagocytic cells) and polymorphonuclear leukocytes, which rid the body

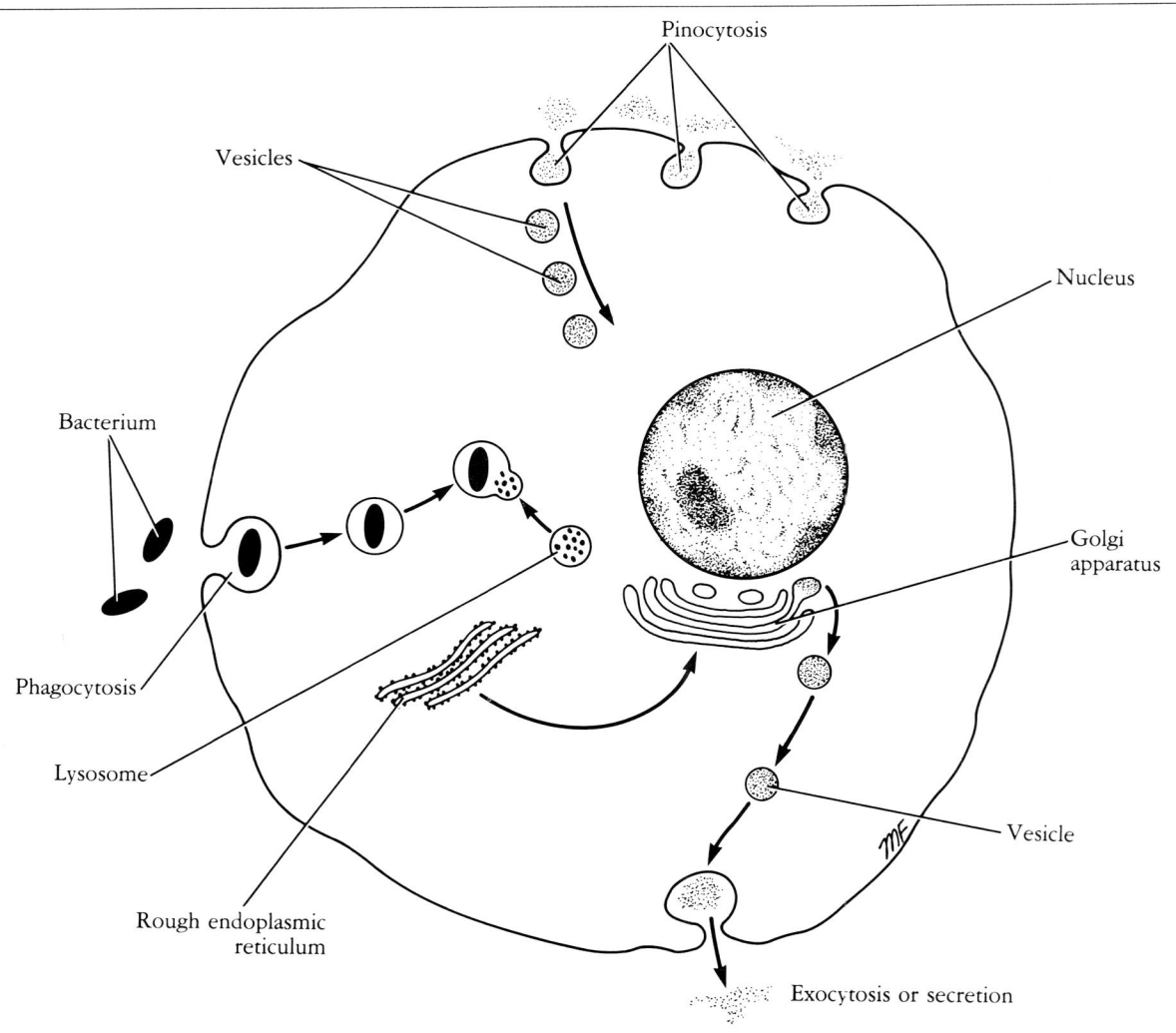

Fig. 2-33. *The processes of phagocytosis, pinocytosis, and exocytosis.*

of unwanted cellular debris and bacteria. Both pinocytosis and phagocytosis require energy.

Exocytosis

Exocytosis is the reverse of pinocytosis and phagocytosis. A vesicle containing a substance moves to the surface of the cell, where the membranous envelope fuses with the plasma membrane and opens to the exterior, discharging its contents (see Fig. 2-33). Secretory granules leave the cell by this mechanism.

Cell Membrane Specializations
Microvilli

Microvilli occur on the free surface of many cells, especially those whose main function is absorption (Fig. 2-34), such as the cells lining the small intestine and the convoluted tubules of the kidney. They consist of minute extensions of the plasma membrane from the free surface of the cell. Each possesses a

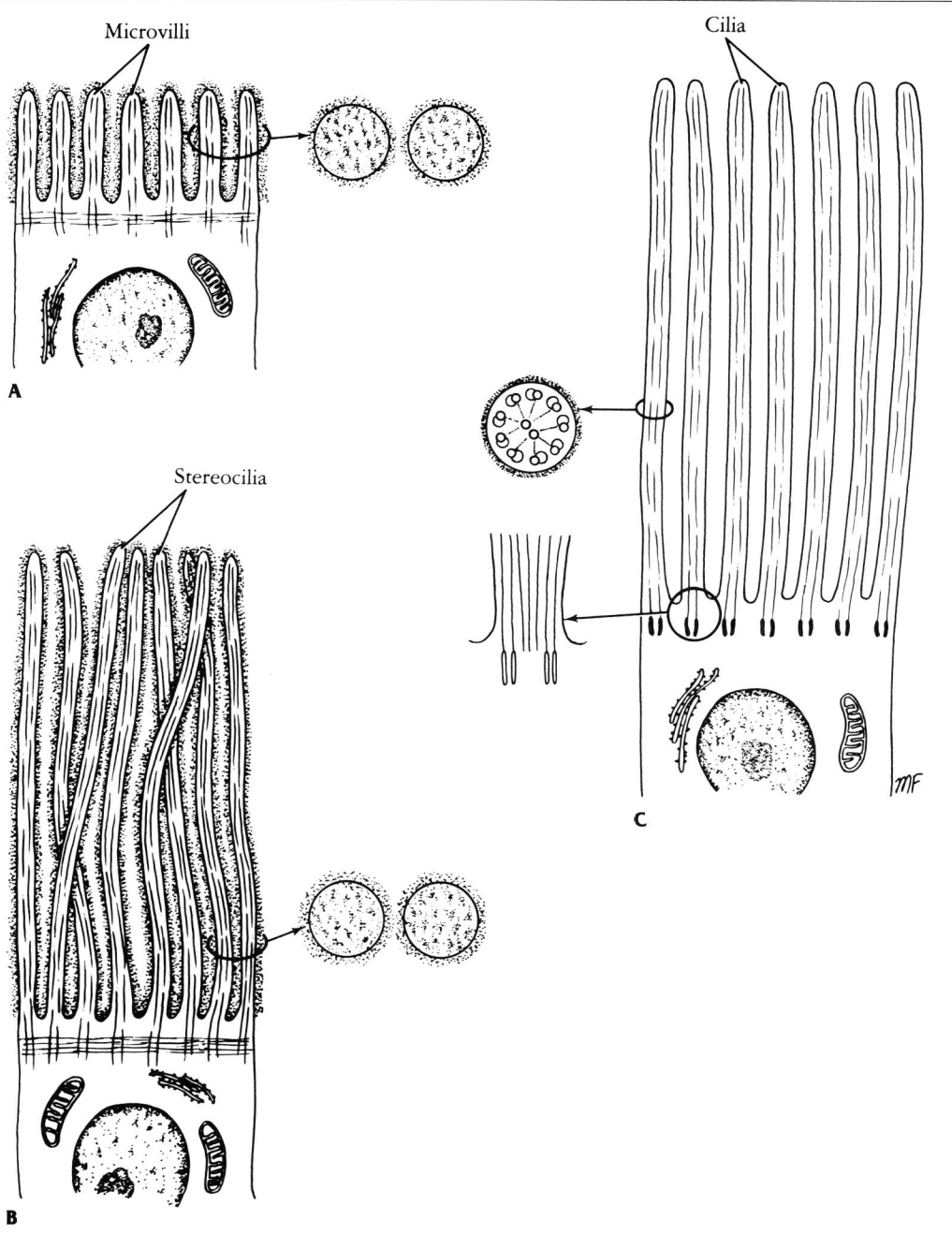

Fig. 2-34. The different forms of plasma membrane specialization: (A) microvilli, (B) stereocilia, and (C) cilia.

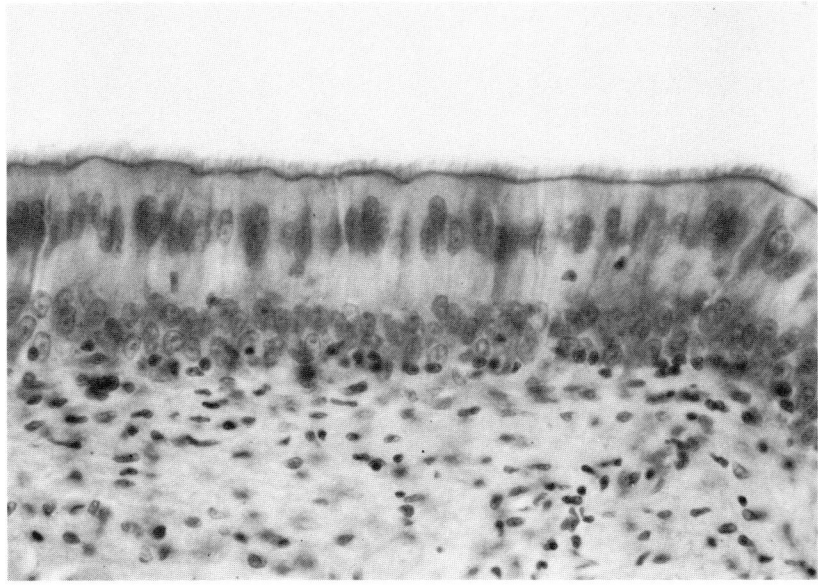

Fig. 2-35. Photomicrograph of ciliated columnar epithelium lining the trachea. (H&E; ×400.)

core of cytoplasm, which contains a bundle of microfilaments composed of actin. These microfilaments extend into the cytoplasm of the cell for a short distance and are attached to the terminal web. The microfilaments strengthen the villus and may bring about movement of the villus.

Situated in the cytoplasm of the microvilli of intestinal epithelia are enzymes capable of hydrolyzing disaccharides to monosaccharides. The function of microvilli is to increase greatly the absorptive surface of the columnar cells and, in the small intestine, to participate in the digestion of carbohydrates.

Stereocilia

Stereocilia are very long microvilli (see Fig. 2-34) and occur on the free surface of the columnar cells lining the epididymis (see Fig. 14-18). Stereocilia adjacent to one another tend to become entwined. They are nonmotile and increase the surface area of the cell to further absorption.

Cilia

Cilia are motile, hairlike processes extending from the free surface of cells (see Figs. 2-24 and 2-34). They are larger and have a more complex structure than either microvilli or stereocilia. They are seen easily with the light microscope (Fig. 2-35). Cells bearing cilia are found in the respiratory system and in parts of the female and male reproductive tracts. The cilia are immersed in mucus, which is moved in one direction by the bending of the cilia.

One cell may have several hundred cilia extending from its free surface. The shaft of each cilium is covered with a plasma membrane and possesses a core of cytoplasm. Within the cytoplasm are microtubules that extend from a centriole found close to the base of the cilium. This modified centriole is called a *basal body*. The beating action of the cilia is thought to be the result of the microtubules within them sliding upon one another. A cilium moves first with a rapid forward stroke, in which the cilium remains stiff (Fig. 2-36); this is followed by a slower recovery stroke, during which the cilium bends.

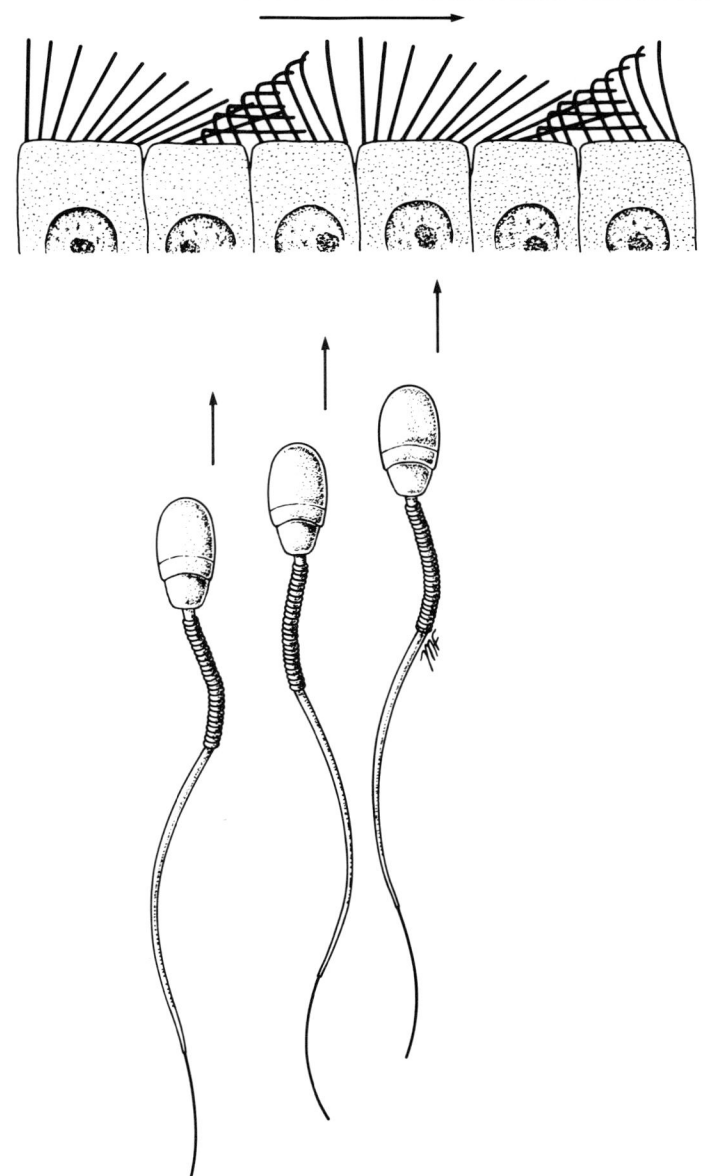

Fig. 2-36. (A) The process by which the bending of a group of cilia causes movement of material, such as mucus (in this case, toward the right). (B) The process by which the undulating movement of a flagellum of a spermatozoon causes the cell to move forward.

When viewed from the free surface of the epithelium, the cilia are seen to move in waves in one direction, similar to the movement of corn before the wind blowing across a cornfield. The energy necessary for the movement of cilia is derived from ATP.

Flagella

A flagellum is a very long cilium (see Fig. 2-36). In the human, the only cell to have a functional, motile flagellum is the spermatozoon. Unlike the cilium, which moves in forward and recovery strokes, the flagellum exhibits an undulation that extends from its base to its tip and propels the spermatozoon forward.

Occasionally, other cells show short flagella projecting from their surfaces: for example, cells lining ducts, smooth muscle cells, and even cells forming the anterior lobe of the pituitary. The function of these cell projections is unknown.

Cell Junctions

Three mechanisms are involved in holding cells together: (1) the presence of glycoproteins in the cell coats, causing plasma membranes of neighboring cells to adhere to each other; (2) the wavy course of plasma membranes of adjacent cells permits the tonguelike processes of one cell to fit into the groovelike depressions of the next cell, thus holding the cells together like a jigsaw puzzle; and (3) various types of cell junctions, which are seen only with the electron microscope. Junctions are localized modifications of plasma membranes of adjacent cells and tend to hold the cells together.

Zonula Occludens (Tight Junction)

The zonula (girdle) occludens (closed off) is a girdle of fused plasma membranes that surrounds each cell near its free surface (Fig. 2-37). It is formed by the fusion of the outer lamellae of adjacent plasma membranes and thus holds the cells tightly together and prevents the passage of molecules between them. The existence of the zonula occludens between the cells lining the intestine is of great importance, because it prevents harmful substances from leaking from the intestinal lumen into the tissues of the body. These junctions are also present in the cells of the renal tubules and the vascular endothelium of the brain, where they are responsible for the blood-brain barrier.

Fascia Occludens and Macula Occludens

The fascia (band) occludens is a site of a patchy fusion of the outer lamellae of adjacent plasma membranes (see Fig. 2-37).

The macula (spot) occludens is a site of spotlike fusion of the outer lamellae of adjacent plasma membranes (see Fig. 2-37).

Examples of the fascia occludens and macula occludens are found between adjacent endothelial cells lining blood and lymphatic capillaries. Because the areas are patchy or spotlike, gaps exist that allow fluid or cells to pass between adjacent cells.

Macula Adherens (Desmosome)

The macula (spot) adherens (stick), or desmosome (*desmos,* bond or fastening), is a special type of cell junction where the plasma membranes of adjacent cells do not come into close contact but are held strongly together by a special area of the cell coat formed of protein. This area of the cell coat is seen as an intermediate line of dense material (Fig. 2-37). At these sites, the plasma membrane is thickened by a condensation of cytoplasm to which are attached bundles of tonofilaments. This form of junction is found in many locations within the body, including epidermis and cardiac muscle.

Communicating or Gap Junctions

Communicating junctions are spotlike areas where the outer lamellae of adjacent plasma membranes come very close together but are not fused; in other words, a gap remains. Recent research has revealed that minute bridges composed of protein and lipid exist in the gap and extend from one cell membrane to the other. Moreover, the bridges penetrate both plasma membranes, so that there is a continuous communication between the cytoplasms of adjacent

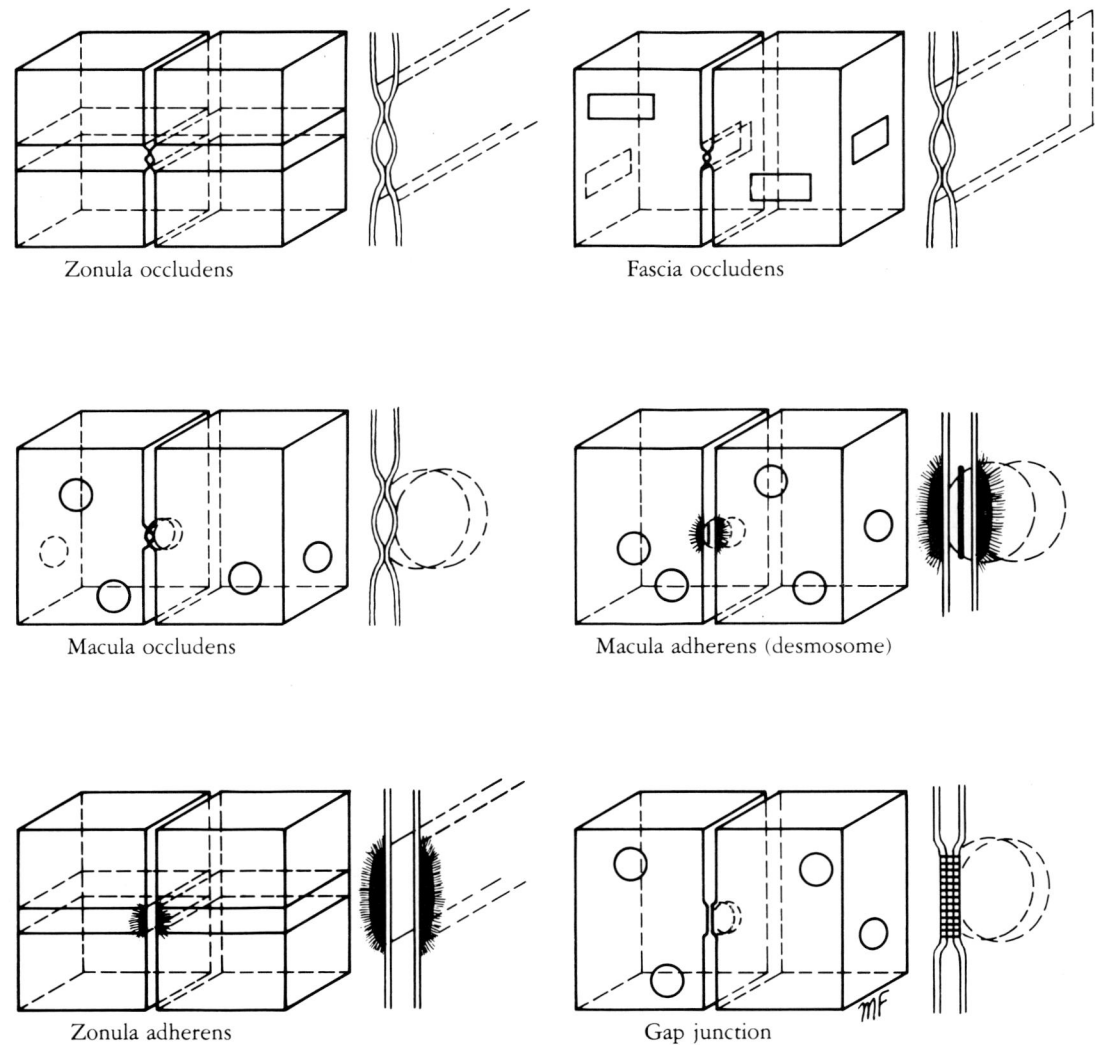

Fig. 2-37. The different types of cell junctions. Note that the zonula occludens not only holds adjacent cells together but provides an effective barrier to the passage of fluids between the cells.

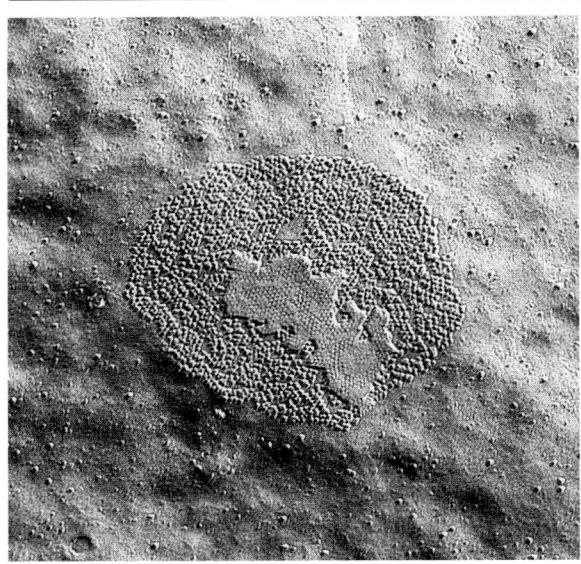

Fig. 2-38. Electron micrograph of a freeze-fracture replica view of the P-face of an ovarian granulosa cell gap junction. The outwardly directed half membrane shows an aggregation of globular intramembrane particles at the gap junction. (Courtesy of Dr. D. Albertini.)

cells (Figs. 2-38; see Fig. 2-37).* These bridges permit not only the passage of ions from one cell to another but also the passage of small molecules.

Communicating junctions are found between smooth and cardiac muscle fibers, where it is important that a wave of excitation pass quickly from one cell to another.

Junctional Complex

A dark area, sometimes called the *terminal bar,* can be seen with the light microscope along the lateral boundaries of cells in certain epithelia near their apices. The best examples are seen in the columnar cells lining the intestine. With the electron microscope, this area can be seen to comprise the zonula

---

*Replicas of freeze-fractured (split) plasma membranes present two distinct surfaces, or faces, called the P-face and the E-face. The P-face is the outwardly directed inner half membrane; the E-face is the inwardly directed outer half membrane. (See examples in Figure 2-39.)

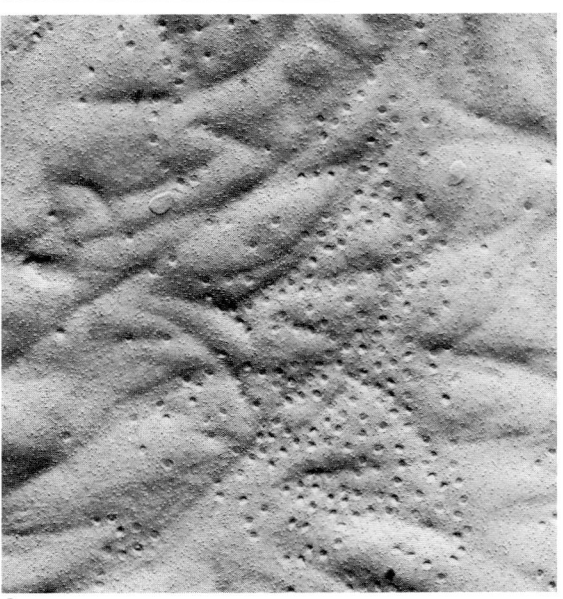

A

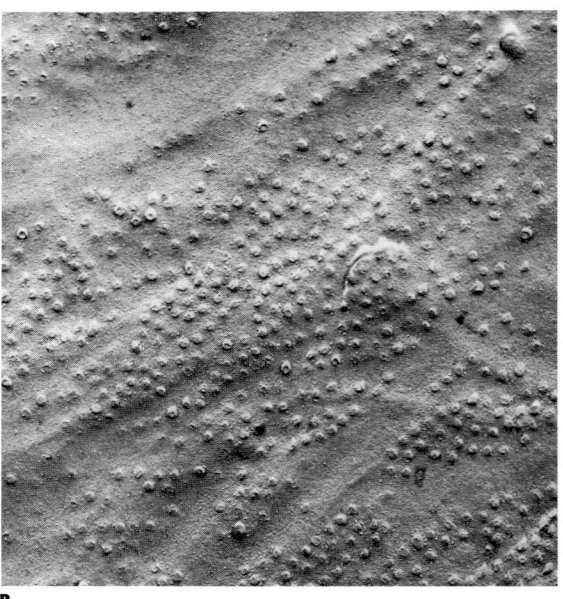

B

Fig. 2-39. Electron micrograph of a freeze-fracture replica view of the P-face (A) and E-face (B) of the plasma membrane of endothelial cells of the eye. The very fine intramembrane particles (probably protein) remain preferentially associated with the P-face of the plasma membrane. The larger structures correspond to the openings of the plasmalemma vesicles. ($\times 22,600$.) (Courtesy of Dr. G. Raviola.)

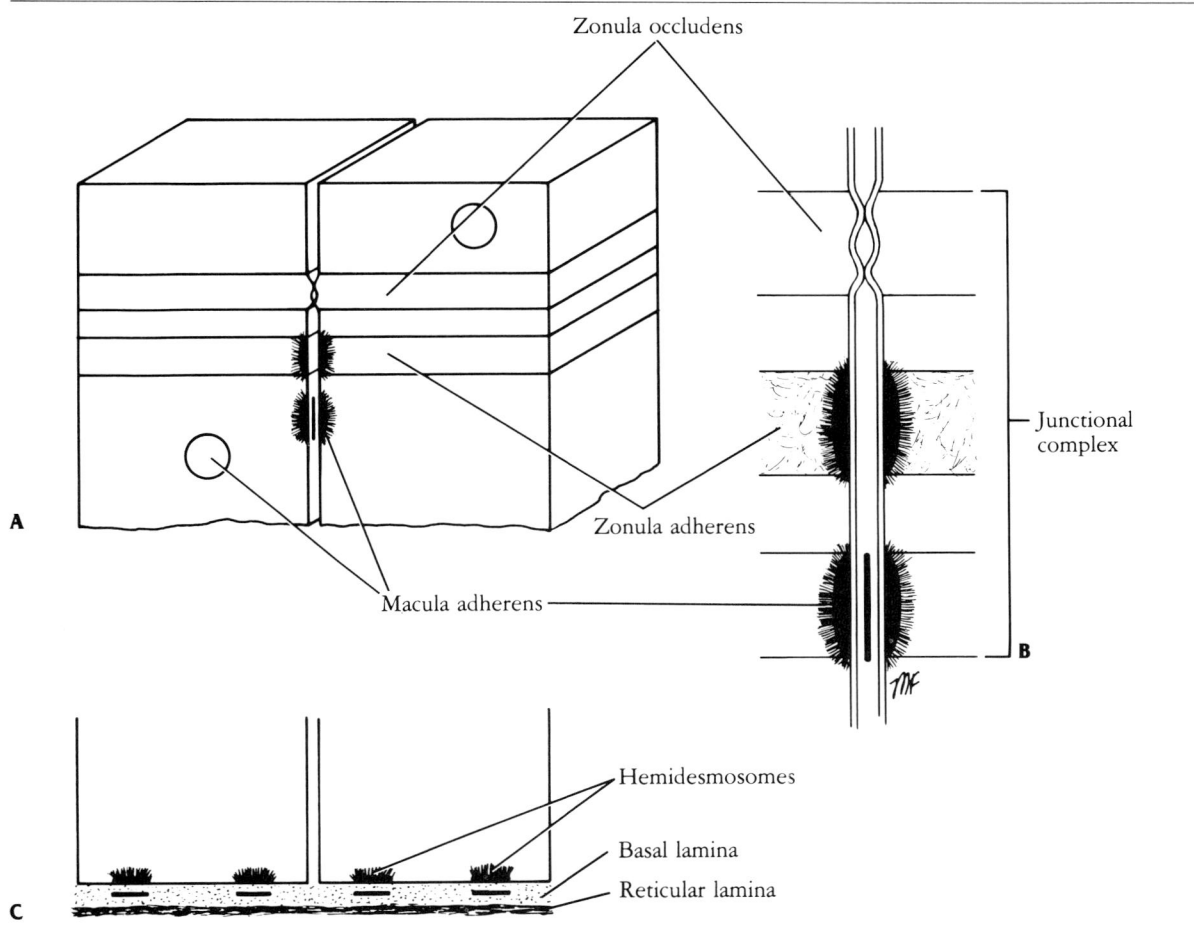

Fig. 2-40. (A and B). The structure of a junctional complex. The structure of a hemidesmosome is shown in (C).

occludens, the zonula adherens, and the macula adherens (Fig. 2-40). Collectively, these junctions are referred to as a *junctional complex*.

Specializations of the Basal Surface of Cells
Basement Membrane
The basement membrane consists of two parts: the basal lamina and the reticular lamina. The *basal lamina* lies closer to the epithelium and is composed of glycoprotein. It is produced by the overlying epithelial cells. The *reticular lamina* is composed of bundles of reticular fibers embedded in a matrix of polysaccharide. It is formed from the underlying connecting tissue.

The basement membrane serves two functions: (1) It connects the epithelial cells to the underlying connective tissue and thus stabilizes the basal end of the cell. This function is demonstrated clearly in the epidermis, where the basement membrane is very well developed. (2) It serves as a semipermeable membrane. This function is very important in the glomerulus of the kidney, where the basement membrane serves as a filter.

In many stratified epithelia, the basal plasma membrane of the cells is strongly adherent to the underlying basement membrane at sites known as *hemidesmosomes* (see Fig. 2-40). As the name implies, only half the desmosome is present; only one cell is participating, the second cell being represented by the basement membrane.

The basement membrane can be demonstrated easily histochemically with the light microscope. The glycoproteins and the polysaccharides give a positive periodic acid–Schiff reaction, and the reticular fibers can be revealed with silver stains.

CLINICAL NOTES

EVOLUTION OF THE CELL

The basic living unit of the human body is the cell. Although many cells differ from one another, they all have certain similar characteristics.

The cell is often mistakenly regarded as the lowest form of life. A small virus is the lowest form of life, and, although it consists of nothing more than a nucleic acid surrounded by protein, it is capable of metabolic activity and can reproduce itself if it is in a suitable environment in a living cell.

Evolutionary changes resulted in the formation of a cell membrane around the virus; later, enzymes and other chemicals appeared in a primitive cytoplasm. In this manner, bacteria evolved: highly complicated structures containing enzymes within their cytoplasm so that chemical reactions can take place inside the organism.

Developmentally higher forms of the cell contain the highly complex organelles that turn the cell cytoplasm into a complicated chemical factory. Most important, these higher forms contain a nucleus, which serves as a control center for all the chemical activities of the cell and controls the reproductive process, enabling the cell to produce, through cell division, new daughter cells with exactly the same structure as the mother cell.

THE CELL AND DISEASE

There was a tendency in the past to concentrate on the cellular changes that accompany disease. Investigators were preoccupied with recording the morphological changes that took place in cells as a disease progressed. Now, all interest is centered on determining the cellular malfunction that has produced a particular condition. Many pathologists believe it will not be long before most diseases are classified according to the biochemical derangement or molecular defect present in cells.

If we are to treat malfunctioning cells successfully by the administration of drugs, it is clearly important for us as physicians to understand, when possible, how a particular drug acts on a cell and where in the cell the biochemical or molecular change takes place.

The diagnosis, treatment, and prognosis of disease cannot be comprehended fully until the normal structure and function of cells and their ability to adapt to altered homeostasis are understood.

CELLULAR ADAPTATION TO ALTERED HOMEOSTASIS

Cells are capable of modifying their metabolic activities within certain limits when challenged by changes in their environment. This ability varies with different cell types and is greatest in a simple cell, such as a squamous epithelial cell, and least in a highly specialized cell, such as a neuron. Should the cell be unable to adapt to this altered activity, however, it will be injured and may die. Cells exhibit a number of adaptive changes, which include atrophy, hypertrophy, hyperplasia, metaplasia, and dysplasia.

Atrophy

Atrophy is a reduction in the size of a cell resulting from a loss of cell substance. The smaller cell contains fewer organelles, such as mitochondria and endoplasmic reticulum. In some cells, there is an increase in the number of secondary lysosomes and residual bodies as a consequence of organelle degeneration. When a large number of cells in an organ shows atrophy, the whole organ becomes smaller. It is important to realize that an atrophied cell is alive; it has merely reduced the size of its activities as an adjustment to the changes in its environment.

The possible causes of atrophy are (1) diminished workload, (2) loss of stimulation as the result of denervation or reduced hormonal control, and (3) diminished nutrition as the result of a reduced blood supply. Diminished workload occurs, for example, when a limb is immobilized in a plaster cast for a bone fracture. The muscles are unable to contract, and the muscle cells become reduced in size. Denervation of muscles, as the result of a peripheral nerve injury, will also lead to a reduction in the size of muscle cells. Following the menopause, the ovarian cells undergo atrophy because of the cessation of hormonal stimulation from the anterior lobe of the pituitary. The brain becomes reduced in size with advancing age as a result of neuronal atrophy following a reduction in arterial supply caused by arteriosclerosis.

It is interesting to note that should a specialized tissue, like skeletal muscle, be unable to adapt to, for example, a reduced arterial supply, it may be replaced by a less specialized tissue, such as connective tissue, whose cells can survive in the altered environment (see Metaplasia, below on this page).

Hypertrophy

Hypertrophy is an increase in the size of a cell that results from an increase in cell substance. The larger cell contains more cell organelles, such as mitochondria and endoplasmic reticulum. When large numbers of cells in an organ show hypertrophy, the organ becomes enlarged.

The possible causes of hypertrophy are increased workload and increased hormonal stimulation. Increased workload occurs, for example, in skeletal muscle in athletes. The organelles, particularly the myofilaments, increase in number to deal effectively with the increased metabolic activity of the muscle that occurs with training. In patients with hypertension (high blood pressure), the cardiac muscle cells of the left ventricle hypertrophy to enable the heart to pump the blood out of the heart into the aorta against an increased blood pressure. In pregnancy, the smooth muscle cells of the uterus undergo hypertrophy (and hyperplasia) as the result of increased hormonal stimulation by estrogen.

It is interesting to note that the hypertrophy of muscle cells is limited by the amount of blood supplied to the muscle and by the oxidative phosphorylation abilities of the mitochondria in the hypertrophied cells.

Hypertrophy of a Cell Organelle

It is possible for hypertrophy to occur in one cell organelle and not in others. For example, the smooth-surfaced endoplasmic reticulum may become hypertrophied in hepatocytes of the liver in response to increasing doses of barbiturate drugs. This increased ability to metabolize barbiturates results in the need for an increasing dose in order to maintain the desired effect.

Hyperplasia

Hyperplasia is an increase in the number of cells. When large numbers of cells in an organ show hyperplasia, the organ becomes enlarged.

In many instances, hypertrophy and hyperplasia occur simultaneously, but not all adult cells can undergo hyperplasia. The cells of the epidermis of the skin, the lining cells of the intestine, bone marrow cells, hepatocytes, and fibroblasts can all undergo hyperplasia. Nerve cells and cardiac and skeletal muscle cells cannot become hyperplastic.

The causes of hyperplasia may be physiological or pathological. Hyperplasia of the smooth muscle cells of the uterus in response to estrogen during pregnancy is an example of physiological hyperplasia. The increase in the number of cells in lymphatic tissue in response to infection is an example of pathological hyperplasia.

Metaplasia

Metaplasia is a reversible change in which one type of adult cell is replaced by another type. As an adaptation to changes in the environment, often a highly specialized, sensitive cell is replaced by a less specialized, tougher cell that is better able to withstand stress.

In the respiratory tract of a heavy cigarette smoker, for example, the specialized ciliated columnar cells are replaced by simple squamous cells better able to withstand chronic irritation. Unfortunately, the mucus-secreting ability of the lining of the bronchi is lost, as well as the ability to move the mucus produced by other, normal cells. These changes cause pooling of the mucus, which quickly becomes infected.

Another example occurs in the pelvis of the ureter, where the transitional epithelial cells are replaced by squamous cells in response to irritation caused by a renal stone. Squamous metaplasia can also occur in the gallbladder in response to irritation produced by gallstones. In connective tissues that have been injured, fibroblasts may be replaced by chondrocytes or osteoblasts.

It should be noted that in many situations, if the irritation is chronic, metaplasia may continue into neoplasia.

Dysplasia

Dysplasia is an alteration in the size, shape, and organization of the cell in response to chronic irritation or inflammation. Such changes are commonly seen in the cells lining the uterine cervix and the bronchi of the respiratory tract. In some instances, dysplasia will continue into neoplasia, but should the chronic irritation be removed, the cells may revert to normal.

CELL GROWTH AND REPRODUCTION

Cells usually grow prior to reproduction. Little is known about what controls cell growth and reproduction. Some cells grow and continue to multiply, such as the cells of the epidermis of the skin, the intestinal epithelium, and the bone marrow. Other cells, such as cardiac muscle cells and neurons, do not divide once the body has reached its full growth. Some cells, such as those of the liver, bone, and connective tissue, do not divide for long periods but can be made to reproduce by the application of suitable stimulants. Surgical removal of part of the liver results in the renewed division of the liver cells, and this process continues until the normal mass of the liver is restored. One must assume that a chemical feedback mechanism exists whereby reproduction continues until the inhibiting chemical suppresses further cell division. It is possible that the establishment of electrical coupling between newly formed cells at gap junctions inhibits further growth and cell division.

Neoplasms

A neoplasm is an uncontrolled new growth of cells that perform no useful function. Cancer is a malignant form of neoplasm. If normal human cells are removed from the body, they can be made to grow and reproduce in tissue culture. Moreover, they will continue to grow and reproduce as long as adequate amounts of suitable culture medium are provided and continually replenished. Growth and reproduction cease once the products of metabolism are allowed to collect in the medium. Chemical substances, therefore, can limit the growth and reproduction of normal cells both in the body and in tissue culture.

Cancer cells in the body grow and divide unchecked and thus ignore the chemical suppressants that normally limit cell growth. It is now believed that many cancer cells have a genetic makeup different from that of normal cells that allows them to ignore the chemical feedback mechanisms. Heredity, ionizing radiation, chemical irritants, and viruses may cause mutation of the chromosomes in the nucleus or alter the stability of the messenger RNA, permitting unlimited cell growth and reproduction.

It is interesting to note that cancer cells form fewer or abnormal intercellular junctions. As a result, these cells are held less securely in position and have greater freedom to invade surrounding tissues.

Cancer Cells

Cancer cells differ from normal cells in that (1) their size is very variable; (2) their nuclei vary in shape, size, and staining ability; and (3) they show an increase in the frequency of mitosis. Once cells become malignant, they multiply rapidly and invade surrounding tissues. Later, the proliferative cells gain access to the lymph or bloodstreams and spread to tissues some distance from their site of origin.

Because cancer cells continue to multiply indefinitely, they compete with normal cells for nourishment. Eventually, the demand for such nutrients is so great that normal cells are adversely affected and finally die.

It is not uncommon for cells that are about to become cancerous to pass through an incipient stage before they become truly malignant. In this condition, which is known as *carcinoma in situ*, the cells appear malignant on microscopic examination but have not yet started to multiply rapidly and to break through their basement membranes to invade neighboring tissues. If the cells showing carcinoma in situ are removed, cure is certain.

Diagnosis of Cancer

The only certain way to diagnose cancer is to examine under a microscope a histological section of a small piece of tissue that has been adequately stained. The taking of such a piece of tissue from a lesion is known as a *biopsy*. The early diagnosis of cancer arising from cells exposed to the surface of the body may be carried out by a careful cytological examination of cells that have exfoliated from the surface. The cells of the cervix of the uterus (Papanicolaou smear) and the lining of the bronchi can be studied by this method. Cells washed off the surface of the pleura or peritoneum can be studied similarly. The presence of large cells with large, irregularly shaped, deeply staining (hyperchromatic) nuclei is highly suggestive of malignancy.

Laboratory detection of the excessive production of substances normally produced by cells may also assist in diagnosis. For example, *acid phosphatase* produced by acinar cells in the prostate escapes into the bloodstream in excessive amounts when the prostate becomes cancerous. In a similar manner, *alkaline phosphatase* in large amounts escapes into the blood in cancer of the liver. The hormone *chorionic gonadotropin* is produced in high concentrations in *choriocarcinoma* of the uterus. The detection of large amounts of this hormone in the blood can be of great help in making the diagnosis. After the uterus has been removed, the level of this hormone in the blood should return to zero. If the hormone level remains high, it indicates that the tumor has already spread beyond the uterus.

CELL INJURY

Chemical poisons, physical trauma, bacteria, viruses, lack of oxygen (anoxia), dehydration, and excessive heat or cold are all agents that may cause cell injury. There has been a failure in homeostasis, and the cell will either recover or die.

In cell injury, the biochemical mechanisms within the cell are interfered with, and this interference in turn leads to an impairment of cell function. There are four sites of biochemical activity that are particularly susceptible to injury when a cell is damaged: (1) sites of oxidative phosphorylation reactions that produce ATP; (2) the plasma membrane, damage to which completely alters the ionic and osmotic homeostasis within the cell; (3) sites of formation of structural and enzymatic proteins; and (4) nuclear DNA and RNA.

Under the light microscope, an injured cell is seen to enlarge and the cytoplasm is seen to become granular. Under the electron microscope, the mitochondria are seen to swell and the endoplasmic reticulum and ribosomes are seen to change in appearance. Later, lipid droplets appear in the endoplasmic reticulum, because the cell is unable to manufacture the protein part of the lipoprotein molecule. Later still, the lysosomes start to engulf the degenerating mitochondria. As a result, curious, dense cytoplasmic inclusions of cellular debris appear. Meanwhile, the nucleus becomes smaller and denser (*pyknosis*), later breaks up (*karyorrhexis*), and finally disappears (*karyolysis*). The disruption of the nucleus is thought to be caused by the breakdown and liberation of enzymes by the cytoplasmic lysosomes. Finally, the cell dies and disintegrates.

In some cases, an injured cell recovers; the structural changes we have noted are reversed, and the cellular structure returns to normal.

Can a dead cell still function and contribute to the well-being of the body? Removal of the nucleus from the cell means that the cell has lost its control center and the genetic information necessary for normal reproduction. We know that such a cell may continue certain activities involving highly complex chemical reactions. For example, a red blood cell carries out important functions for about 120 days after the nucleus has been lost. The surface cells of the epidermis of the skin are dead, but their very presence protects the underlying cells from dehydration, excessive hydration, and physical trauma.

AGING OF CELLS

There is no single cause of cellular aging. Rather, it occurs as the result of genetic, metabolic, hormonal, and immunological influences. Some believe that there is a built-in genetic program that limits the life-span of cells. With advancing years, the individual is increasingly exposed to outside agents such as ultraviolet light, x-rays, and noxious chemicals that eventually may bring about structural and functional changes leading to cell death.

As the result of the normal wear and tear of life, cells gradually accumulate structural evidence of injuries. White blood cells, for example, often show evidence of broken-down mitochondria and the accumulation of dense cytoplasmic inclusions. In the central nervous system, aging is accompanied by a loss of neurons and degeneration of the neurofibrils within the neuronal cytoplasm. In many cells, there is an accumulation of lipofuscin granules in old lysosomes. Finally, with the onset of nuclear degeneration, cell death occurs.

CHROMOSOME ABNORMALITIES

Relatively simple techniques have now been established for the examination of human chromosome structure (see p. 39). It is now apparent that a relationship exists between specific congenital malformations and certain abnormalities of chromosome number and structure. The addition of a chromosome to a pair is known as *trisomy*. If the additional chromosome is not free but attached to another chromosome, the condition is known as *translocation*. The absence of one chromosome of a pair is rare and is known as *monosomy*. It is important that chromosome examinations be carried out not only on affected infants but also on their parents, so that accurate information can be obtained about risks of recurrence.

Trisomy 21 (Down's syndrome, mongolism) is the most common form of trisomy, occurring in Western countries once in about every 600 births. The incidence varies with maternal age, rising steeply in infants born to mothers more than 35 years old. It is believed that the chromosome abnormality occurs during the formation of the female germ cell. In complete Down's syndrome, the eyes are small and the palpebral fissures slant downward at the medial ends. The mouth is small and the tongue protrudes and is fissured. The hands are short and broad, with a deep, transverse crease on the palms. Those affected are mentally retarded and exhibit generalized poor muscle tone and retardation of physical development. Most die young.

Trisomy 17–18, trisomy 13–15, cri du chat syndrome, Klinefelter's syndrome, and *Turner's syndrome* are other, less common congenital anomalies associated with abnormal chromosomes.

GENE ABNORMALITIES

It is now known that some congenital malformations are caused by defects in the genes. It is important to realize that a single defective dominant gene can produce a multiplicity of effects involving many different tissues. *Retinitis pigmentosa, lobster-claw hand, achondroplasia, osteogenesis imperfecta, congenital cataract, albinism, deaf-mutism, fibrocystic disease of the pancreas, hydrocephalus, hemophilia,* and *adrenogenital syndrome* are some genetic defects.

THE ROLE OF LYSOSOMES IN DISEASE

Lysosomes contain enzymes that are capable of breaking down proteins, carbohydrates, and some lipids. Fortunately, under normal conditions, the membrane surrounding the lysosome is impermeable and keeps these enzymes from digesting cellular contents. If, however, there is serious injury to the cell, the permeability of the membrane increases. The enzymes are released and effect cellular destruction and, later, removal of the dead cell.

In some congenital metabolic defects, cells synthesize compounds that they cannot metabolize. The lysosomes of these cells accumulate these compounds and become filled with them.

The granules seen in the cytoplasm of polymorphonuclear leukocytes are lysosomes, and it is these structures that are responsible for bringing about the removal of bacteria that have been phagocytosed by these cells.

THE ROLE OF MICROTUBULES AND MICROFILAMENTS IN DISEASE

The spontaneous movement of polymorphonuclear leukocytes toward invading organisms, a process known as *diapedesis* (see p. 188), is believed to be the activity of the microtubules and microfilaments. In diabetes mellitus, there is a defect in leukocytic motility, probably caused by abnormal functioning of microtubules and microfilaments.

DEFECTS IN PLASMA MEMBRANES

In hereditary spherocytosis, the patient's red cells are spherical instead of the normal biconcave disk shape. This disease is probably caused by a protein abnormality of the plasma membrane of the red cells that renders the cells excessively permeable to water and sodium ions.

A fatal disease of childhood is caused by a defect in lysosome membranes. The polymorphonuclear white cells can phagocytose bacteria normally, but the lysosomes are unable to fuse with the vacuoles containing the bacteria. The result is that the bacteria are not destroyed even though the lysosomes contain a normal amount of bactericidal enzymes.

MOVEMENT OF SUBSTANCES THROUGH A CELL MEMBRANE

Knowledge of the mechanisms that operate in the passage of substances through cell membranes is basic to an understanding of cell physiology, and these mechanisms have been dealt with in some detail in this chapter. In clinical practice, knowledge of these same mechanisms is important when one is administering different concentrations of substances in intravenous fluids to a patient. In human blood, the red blood cells are suspended in plasma and the fluid inside the cells is of the same osmotic pressure as the plasma. A solution commonly given intravenously is 0.9% sodium chloride in water, referred to as *isotonic saline*. *Isotonic* means that it is of the same osmotic pressure as the fluid within red cells; when it is given intravenously, fluid will diffuse neither in nor out of the red cells, and the volume of the red cells therefore will remain unchanged (Fig. 2-41). Five percent dextrose (glucose) in water is another intravenous solution. It is of value as a nutrient.

If, however, a saline solution of lower osmotic pressure—for example, 0.45% sodium chloride—were given intravenously, water would rapidly pass into the red cells and they would swell. Such an intravenous solution is said to be *hypotonic*. If this therapy were continued, many of the red cells would rupture or burst, a condition known as *hemolysis* (see Fig. 2-41).

Should a strong salt solution, such as 5% sodium chloride, be given intravenously, the red cells would lose large quantities of water because of the passage of water through the cell membrane to the exterior. The salt solution is *hypertonic* compared with the fluid within the red cells. With very strong salt solutions, the red cells shrink and collapse, a condition known as *crenation* (see Fig. 2-41).

Dialysis

Hemodialysis and peritoneal dialysis in patients with renal failure are clinical applications of the principles governing the passage of substances across membranes. Dialysis takes place when a solution of both crystalloids and colloids is separated from water by a membrane that is impermeable to colloids and is permeable to crystalloids.

In *hemodialysis*, the patient's bloodstream is connected to a machine called a *hemodialyzer* (artificial kidney), by means of which dialysis occurs between the blood and the dialyzing solution, which are separated from each other by an artificial, semipermeable membrane. The products of metabolism, such as urea and uric acid, diffuse across the membrane from the blood, leaving the colloidal plasma proteins to circulate back into the patient's body.

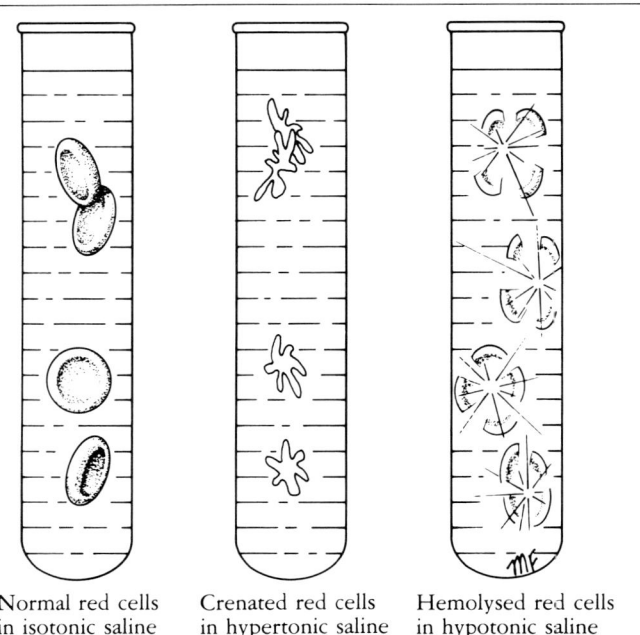

Fig. 2-41. *The effects of different concentrations of saline on red blood cells.*

In *peritoneal dialysis,* a watery solution, the dialysate, is introduced through a catheter into the patient's peritoneal cavity. The products of metabolism, such as urea, diffuse through the peritoneal lining cells from the blood vessels into the dialysate and are removed from the patient. In this instance, the dialyzing membrane is natural, formed by the cells lining the peritoneal cavity.

MICROORGANISMS THAT INVADE THE HUMAN BODY

In our discussion of the detailed structure of the cells that make up the human body, it seems appropriate to consider briefly the structure of microorganisms that invade the body and cause infection. Only by doing so can we understand the action of antibiotics and other chemotherapeutic agents.

Eukaryotic Cells

These microorganisms include the algae, protozoa, fungi, and slime molds. They all possess the same general cell structure found in human cells, in that each cell has a true nucleus with a set of chromosomes, a nuclear membrane, and cell organelles, including mitochondria. These cells may also possess cilia or flagellae.

Prokaryotic Cells

Prokaryotic cells include the bacteria and blue-green algae (cyanobacteria) and are primitive in structure. The cells have no true nuclei, but each possesses a single continuous strand of chromatin (that is, one chromosome). There is no nuclear membrane, and there are no cell organelles, such as mitochondria. Many enzymes are localized in the plasma membrane surrounding the cell.

Bacterial Cell Membrane

The plasma membrane closely resembles that found in human cells and consists of lipid and protein molecules.

Bacterial Cell Wall

Outside the plasma membrane, bacteria possess a strong cell wall composed of *peptidoglycan.* This wall is necessary because, unlike human cells, bacteria have an internal osmotic pressure as much as twenty times higher than atmospheric pressure; without the bacterial cell wall, the bacteria would burst. The different layers of the cell wall also serve as sites of major antigens on the cell surface.

Bacterial Capsule

Many bacteria excrete a polysaccharide slime that surrounds the outside of the cell wall and protects the cell against phagocytosis and penetration by viruses.

Bacterial Division

Bacteria multiply by simple binary fission. The cell elongates, the single chromosome divides into two, and a transverse cell membrane is formed that pushes the chromosomes apart so that each comes to reside in a new daughter cell. This simple arrangement is necessary because there is no mitotic spindle.

Actions of Chemotherapeutic Agents against Bacteria

For a chemotherapeutic agent to be used clinically, it must be bacteriostatic (able to inhibit bacterial multiplication) or bactericidal (able to kill the bacteria) without having an injurious effect on the patient's cells.

The common chemotherapeutic drugs exert their selective toxic action on bacteria in the following ways:

1. They inhibit the formation of the bacterial cell wall, causing the bacterial cell to burst. This type of action is seen with *penicillin* and the *cephalosporins,* for example.

2. They change the permeability of the cell membrane. The plasma membranes of bacteria and fungi, because of slight structural differences, are destroyed more readily by certain drugs than are those of human cells. This destruction results in the escape of nucleotides and proteins from the cell, and death follows. *Amphotericin B* and *nystatin,* for example, exert this type of action.

3. They inhibit the translation and transcription of genetic material. Bacterial ribosomes differ in structure from human ribosomes. Their structure permits certain chemotherapeutic drugs to inhibit bacterial protein synthesis without having a great effect on human ribosomes. This form of action is seen with the *chloramphenicols,* the *erythromycins, streptomycin,* and the *tetracyclines.*

4. They inhibit nucleic acid synthesis. Some of the drugs used form complexes with DNA and block the formation of messenger RNA; *actinomycin,* for example, acts in this way. Other drugs, such as the *mitomycins,* block DNA replication. Still others compete with p-aminobenzoic acid in the formation of folic acid, a substance necessary for the synthesis of nucleic acids. The *sulfonamides,* among other substances, exert this action.

Viruses

Viruses differ from all other cellular forms of life in that they consist merely of a molecule of nucleic acid, either DNA or RNA, surrounded by a protein envelope. Viruses can replicate only within living cells. Once a virus gains entrance to a cell, the nucleic acid can program the infected cell to synthesize, by means of its enzymes, specific macromolecules for the formation of new viruses. The new nucleic acid and specific viral proteins are assembled into new viral particles, which are then extruded from the cell into the tissue fluid.

Actions of Chemotherapeutic Agents against Viruses

Viruses multiply only in living cells, and the energy and synthetic enzymes needed for the synthesis of viral proteins and nucleic acid, as well as the precursors of this process, must be provided by the host cells.

It is interesting to note that the antibacterial antibiotics and the sulfonamides have no effect on viruses. *Actinomycin,* however, inhibits the replication of virus DNA, and *rifampin* inhibits virus multiplication by blocking the assembly of poxviruses.

PASSAGE OF DRUGS ACROSS CELL MEMBRANES

Because drugs generally pass through cells rather than between them, it is important to understand how drugs cross plasma membranes. Clearly, the size and shape of the drug molecule, its degree of ionization, and its solubility in lipid are important factors in the process. Simple diffusion, osmosis, facilitated diffusion, active transport, and pinocytosis, which have been fully described on pages 58–63, can all contribute to the passage of drugs across membranes. For example, drugs that are weak electrolytes cross plasma membranes by simple diffusion in the nonionized form in proportion to their lipid/water partition coefficient and are distributed in proportion to the pH differences between the intracellular and extracellular fluids.

Nonelectrolytes cross plasma membranes by diffusion in proportion to their solubility in the lipid of the membrane. Small molecules, however, such as those of urea, are thought to cross the membrane through the membrane pores. Drugs that are strong acids or alkalis and are completely ionized will cross the plasma membrane according to the potential difference across the membrane and the permeability of the membrane.

ACTION OF DRUGS ON CELLS

Drugs produce their effects on cells by combining with the functional components of the cells, especially the plasma membranes and the enzymes, thereby bringing about biochemical and physiological changes in the activity of the cell. The cell structure that is initially involved with the action of the drug is called the *receptor,* and the chemical groups of the cell that are involved in the combination of the drug with the receptor are called *receptor sites.* There are often many cell components that combine with the drug but are not involved in the drug action; these are called *secondary receptors.* The receptors for the majority of drugs have not been identified, but the concept of receptors provides a useful theory upon which to base drug action.

The nature of the drug action will be determined by the receptor site within the cell and the concentration of the drug at that site. The drug action may be spread throughout the body if the receptor is nonspecific and is present in many cell types. The action may be very specific if the receptor is located in only certain types of cells.

Many drugs apparently do not combine with macromolecules at receptor sites but exert their action by combining with small chemical molecules within cells and thus indirectly modify a cell's activity. Other drugs act by impersonating chemicals used by cells in the construction of their internal components. Once incorporated into the cell structure, the drug can bring about a functional change. Still other drugs are thought to act not by chemical combinations per se but by bringing about an altered biophysical state within the cell. For further discussion of this interesting subject, the student should consult a textbook of pharmacology.

CLINICAL PROBLEMS

For the answers to these problems, see page 781.

1. A mitochondrion is a cell organelle, and a virus is a microorganism that invades cells. Compare their structures. Can they live independently of the cell? Can they undergo division within the cell?

2. Mitochondria are often described as the powerhouses of cells. Where in a mitochondrion are the enzymes located that are concerned with electron transport and oxidative phosphorylation? What are the elementary particles?

3. Stereocilia and cilia are cell membrane specializations. Compare and contrast their structure and functions.

4. Drugs move across cell membranes by passive or active transfer processes. Using your knowledge of the structure and physiology of cell membranes, discuss these processes.

5. A gap junction is a form of cell junction. How does it differ in structure from a tight junction (zonula occludens)? What is the physiological significance of a gap junction? What possible role do gap junctions play in cell reproduction in wound healing? Do neoplastic cells possess normal cell junctions?

6. Many drugs used in clinical practice are weak

acids or weak bases and are present in solutions in both ionized and nonionized forms. The nonionized form is generally lipid soluble, whereas the ionized form usually has a low lipid solubility. Which form is likely to diffuse across the plasma membrane more rapidly?

7. Many drugs are metabolized by enzymes situated in the smooth endoplasmic reticulum of the hepatocytes of the liver. Describe the structure of the smooth endoplasmic reticulum. Where is this form of reticulum produced? Name some other functions of this smooth endoplasmic reticulum.

8. Describe the structure and function of lysosomes. What role may they play in disease?

9. Define atrophy, hypertrophy, and hyperplasia. Give physiological and pathological examples of each.

10. The penicillin antibiotics exert their antibacterial action by inhibiting mucopeptide synthesis in the bacterial cell wall; they have no effect on the boundary membranes of human cells. What is the explanation for this selective action? Do you think viruses would be affected by penicillin?

11. Streptomycin exerts its antibacterial activity on certain organisms by combining with the ribosomes and interfering with the translation of the genetic code. This results in the wrong amino acids being incorporated into the protein molecule, so that protein synthesis is interfered with and bacterial cell death occurs. What are ribosomes? What is the difference between ribosomal RNA and messenger RNA? What is transfer RNA?

12. Define the following terms: (a) membrane pores, (b) drug receptor site, (c) centromere, (d) metaplasia, (e) prokaryotic cell, (f) basement membrane, and (g) desmosome.

13. The nucleus of a cell is said to have two main functions. What are these functions? Can a human cell perform a useful function without a nucleus? Name three types of cells that may possess more than one nucleus.

14. A 55-year-old man consults a surgeon because he has a slow-growing, painless ulcer on his lower lip. The surgeon performs a biopsy and sends the tissue to a pathologist for a histological report. A diagnosis of epithelial carcinoma is made. What common histological changes occur in cells that become cancerous that enable a pathologist to diagnose cancer?

15. Name four sites of biochemical activity that are particularly susceptible to injury when a cell is damaged. Describe the main structural changes that take place in a cell when it is injured.

16. A 33-year-old woman is admitted to the hospital suffering from acute severe ulcerative colitis of the descending colon. For the past 3 weeks she has found it necessary to defecate six or seven times a day. The feces passed are semiliquid and accompanied by large quantities of pinkish-white mucus. On examination, she is found to be very dehydrated, and blood studies show evidence of slight salt loss. Bearing in mind the importance of preserving body homeostasis, select one or more of the following solutions for intravenous administration to this patient: (a) 0.45% sodium chloride; (b) 5% dextrose; (c) 0.9% sodium chloride; (d) 15% sodium chloride.

17. Clinically you will be using chemotherapeutic agents or drugs. The following is a list of a few chemotherapeutic agents and their actions. Can you explain why each action would prove fatal to a cell? (a) Vincristine is used in the treatment of Hodgkin's disease and other lymphomas. It damages the cell spindle. (b) Adriamycin (doxorubicin hydrochloride) is used in the treatment of lymphosarcoma. It binds with DNA to block messenger RNA production. (c) Cytosine arabinoside is used in the treatment of leukemia. It blocks the formation of DNA by inhibiting DNA polymerase, an enzyme concerned with DNA synthesis.

18. Having examined a 10-month-old child, a pediatrician makes a diagnosis of Down's syndrome. What chromosomal abnormality exists in this condition? Should the parents of children with congenital anomalies have their chromosomes examined?

19. A patient is suspected of having carcinoma of the uterine cervix. She is advised to have a Papanicolaou test ("Pap smear"). What is this test, and can it assist the physician in making a firm diagnosis?

20. Chronic bronchitis is usually associated with heavy cigarette smoking. Histological examination of the cells lining the bronchi shows that many of the ciliated cells have been replaced by flattened, nonciliated cells. What is the name given to this change in cell type? What is the structure of a cilium? How does the structure of a cilium differ from a flagellum? How may the loss of the ciliated cells in the respiratory tract affect the patient's health?

21. A newborn child is found to have external genitalia that are characteristic of neither the male nor the female. The pediatrician advises that an oral smear be taken and carefully examined cytologically so that the sex of the child can be determined. What are the morphological characteristics of the cells of a smear that enable one to identify accurately the sex of an individual?

ADDITIONAL READING

Allison, A. Lysosomes and disease. *Sci. Am.* 217(5):62, 1967.

Axline, S. G., and Cohn, Z. A. In vitro induction of lysosomal enzymes by phagocytosis. *J. Exp. Med.* 131:1239, 1970.

Bajer, A., and Mole-Bajer, J. Architecture and function of the mitotic spindle. *Adv. Mol. Biol.* 1:213, 1971.

Bangham, A. D. Lipid bilayers and biomembranes. *Annu. Rev. Biochem.* 41:753, 1972.

Barr, M. L. Sex chromatin and phenotype in man. *Science* 130:679, 1959.

Baudhuin, P. Liver peroxisomes: Cytology and function. *Ann. N.Y. Acad. Sci.* 168:214, 1969.

Beams, H. W., and Kessel, R. G. The Golgi apparatus: Structure and function. *Int. Rev. Cytol.* 23:209, 1968.

Bennett, G., Leblond, G. P., and Haddad, A. Migration of glycoprotein from the Golgi apparatus to the surface of various cell types as shown by radioautography after labeled fructose injection into rats. *J. Cell Biol.* 60:258, 1974.

Bessis, M. Cell death. *Triangle* 9:191, 1970.

Black, W. H. The development of smooth surfaced endoplasmic reticulum in adrenal cortical cells of fetal guinea pig. *Am. J. Anat.* 135:381, 1972.

Borgers, M., and DeBrander, M. (eds.). *Microtubules and Microtubule Inhibitors*. Amsterdam: North Holland, 1975.

Brökelmann, J. On the fine structure of polyribosomes. *Cell Tissue Res.* 179:531, 1977.

Burger, M. Surface properties of neoplastic cells. *Hosp. Pract.* 8(7):55, 1973.

Busch, H., and Smetena, K. *The Nucleolus*. New York: Academic, 1970.

Cardell, R. R. Smooth endoplasmic reticulum in rat hepatocytes during glycogen deposition and depletion. *Int. Rev. Cytol.* 48:221, 1977.

Caro, L. G., and Palade, G. E. Protein synthesis, storage, and discharge in the pancreatic exocrine cell. *J. Cell Biol.* 20:473, 1964.

Chambers, R. The relation of the extraneous coats to the organization and permeability of cell membranes. *Cold Spring Harbor Symp. Quant. Biol.* 8:144, 1940.

Chapman, D. Lipid dynamics in cell membranes. *Hosp. Pract.* 8(2):79, 1973.

Clark, B. F. C., et al. (eds.). *Gene Expression: Protein Synthesis and Control, RNA Synthesis and Control, Chromatin Structure and Function*. New York: Pergamon, 1978.

Cohen, A. H., and Sundeen, M. R. The nuclear fibrous lamina in human cells: Studies on its appearance and distribution. *Anat. Rec.* 186:471, 1976.

Cohen, S. N. The manipulation of genes. *Sci. Am.* 233(1):24, 1975.

Cummings, D. J., et al. (eds.). *Extrachromosomal DNA*. New York: Academic, 1979.

Danielli, J. F., and Davson, H. A contribution to the theory of permeability of thin films. *J. Cell. Comp. Physiol.* 5:495, 1935.

DeDuve, C., and Baudhuin, P. Peroxisomes (microbodies and related particles). *Physiol. Rev.* 46:323, 1966.

DePierce, J. W., and Karnovsky, M. L. Plasma membranes of mammalian cells: A review of methods for their characterization and isolation. *J. Cell Biol.* 56:275, 1973.

De Robertis, E. D., Nowinski, W. W., and Saez, F. A. *Cell Biology* (5th ed.). Philadelphia: Saunders, 1970.

Dingle, J. T., and Fell, H. B. (eds.). *Lysosomes in Biology and Pathology.* Vols. I and II. Amsterdam: North Holland, 1969.

Dirksen, E. R., and Crocker, T. T. Centriole replication in differentiating ciliated cells of mammalian respiratory epithelium. *J. Microscopie* 5:629, 1965.

Dowben, R. M. *Cell Biology.* New York: Harper & Row, 1971.

Dustin, P. *Microtubules.* Berlin: Springer-Verlag, 1978.

Erickson, H. P. Microtubule surface lattice and subunit structure and observations of reassembly. *J. Cell Biol.* 60:153, 1974.

Farber, E., Verbin, R. S., and Lieberman, M. Cell suicide and cell death. In Aldridge, W. N. (ed.), *Mechanisms of Toxicity.* London: Macmillan, 1971, p. 163.

Favard, P. The Golgi apparatus. Chapter 41 in Lima de Faria, A. (ed.), *Handbook of Molecular Biology.* Vol. 15. Amsterdam: North Holland, 1969, p. 1130.

Fawcett, D. W. *The Cell* (2nd ed.). Philadelphia: Saunders, 1981.

Flickinger, D. J., Brow, J. C., Kutchai, H. C., and Ogilvie, J. W. *Medical Cell Biology.* Philadelphia: Saunders, 1979.

Fox, C. F. The structure of cell membranes. *Sci. Am.* 226(2):30, 1972.

Franke, W. W. Structure, biochemistry and functions of the nuclear envelope. *Int. Rev. Cytol.* [Suppl.] 4:72, 1974.

Frankel, E. *DNA, The Ladder of Life.* New York: McGraw-Hill, 1978.

Friend, D. S., and Farquhar, M. G. Functions of coated vesicles during protein absorption in the rat vas deferens. *J. Cell Biol.* 35:337, 1967.

Friend, D. S., and Gilula, N. B. Variation in tight and gap junctions in mammalian tissues. *J. Cell Biol.* 53:758, 1972.

Ghosh, S. The nucleolar structure. *Int. Rev. Cytol.* 44:1, 1976.

Grisham, J. W. Cellular proliferation in the liver. In Fry, R. J. M., Griem, M. L., and Kirsten, W. H. (eds.), *Normal and Malignant Cell Growth.* New York: Springer-Verlag, 1969.

Hackenbrock, C. R. Ultrastructural bases for metabolically linked mechanical activity in mitochondria. I. Reversible ultrastructural changes with change in metabolic state in isolated liver mitochondria. *J. Cell Biol.* 30:269, 1966.

Hay, E. D. Structure and function of the nucleolus in developing cells. In Dalton, A. J., and Haguenau, F. (eds.), *The Nucleus.* Vol. 2. New York: Academic, 1968.

Hayfick, L. The cell biology of human aging. *N. Engl. J. Med.* 295:1302, 1976.

Hiatt, H. H., et al. (eds.) *Origins of Human Cancer.* Cold Spring Harbor, N.Y.: Cold Spring Harbor Laboratory, 1977.

Hirsch, J. G. Lysosomes and mental retardation. *Q. Rev. Biol.* 47:303, 1972.

Hopkins, C. R. *Structure and Function of Cells.* Philadelphia: Saunders, 1978.

Hsu, T. C. Longitudinal differentiation of chromosomes. *Annu. Rev. Genet.* 7:153, 1974.

Hughes, A. *The Mitotic Cycle.* New York: Academic, 1952.

Hughes, R. C. Glycoproteins as components of cellular membranes. *Prog. Biophys. Mol. Biol.* 26:189, 1973.

Ito, S. The enteric surface coating of cat intestinal microvilli. *J. Cell Biol.* 27:475, 1965.

Jamieson, J. D. Role of the Golgi complex in the intracellular transport of secretory proteins. In Clementi, F., and Ceccarelli, B. (eds.), *Advances in Cytopharmacology.* Vol. 1. New York: Raven Books, Abelard-Schuman, 1971, p. 83.

Jones, K. W. The role of the nucleolus in the formation of ribosomes. *J. Ultrastruct. Res.* 13:257, 1965.

Kappas, A., and Alvares, A. P. How the liver metabolizes foreign substances. *Sci. Am.* 232(6):22, 1975.

Kornberg, A. *DNA Replication.* San Francisco: Freeman, 1980.

Kornberg, R. D. Structure of chromatin. *Annu. Rev. Biochem.* 46:931, 1977.

LaFond, R. E. (ed.). *Cancer, the Outlaw Cell.* Washington: American Chemical Society, 1978.

Lagunoff, D. Macrophage pinocytosis: The removal and resynthesis of a cell surface factor. *Proc. Soc. Exp. Biol. Med.* 138:118, 1971.

Lazarides, E., and Revel, J. P. The molecular basis of cell movement. *Sci. Am.* 240(5):100, 1979.

Leblond, C. P., and Bennett, G. Role of the Golgi apparatus in terminal glycosylation. In Brinkley, B. R., and Porter, K. R. (eds.), *International Cell Biology 1976–1977*. New York: Rockefeller University Press, 1977.

Lucy, J. A. The fusion of cell membranes. *Hosp. Pract.* 8(9):93, 1973.

Maniatis, T., and Ptashne, M. A DNA operator-repressor system. *Sci. Am.* 234(1):64, 1976.

Margolis, R. L., Wilson, L., and Keifer, B. I. Mitotic mechanism based on intrinsic microtubule behavior. *Nature* 272:450, 1978.

Martin, G. M. Cellular aging. *Am. J. Pathol.* 89:484, 1977.

Maul, G. G., Price, J. W., and Lieberman, M. W. Formation and distribution of nuclear pore complexes in interphase. *J. Cell Biol.* 51:405, 1971.

Neutra, M., and Leblond, C. P. The Golgi apparatus. *Sci. Am.* 220(2):100, 1969.

Nicolson, G. L. Cancer metastasis. *Sci. Am.* 240(3):66, 1979.

Nicolson, G. L., Giotta, G., Lotan, R., Neri, A., and Poste, G. The membrane glycoproteins of normal and malignant cells. In Brinkley, B. R., and Porter, K. R. (eds.), *International Cell Biology 1976–1977*. New York: Rockefeller University Press, 1977.

Novikoff, A. B., and Holtzman, E. *Cells and Organelles.* New York: Holt, Rinehart and Winston, 1970.

Paine, P. L., and Feldherr, C. M. Nucleocytoplasmic exchange of macromolecules. *Exp. Cell. Res.* 74:81, 1972.

Palade, G. E. Intracellular aspects of the process of protein secretion. *Science* 189:347, 1975.

Parsons, D. S. (ed.). *Biological Membranes.* Oxford, Clarenden Press, 1975.

Pollard, T. D. Cytoplasmic contractile proteins. In Brinkley, B. R., and Porter, K. R. (eds.), *International Cell Biology 1976–1977*. New York: Rockefeller University Press, 1977.

Porter, K. R., and Bonneville, M. A. *An Introduction to the Fine Structure of Cells and Tissues* (4th ed). Philadelphia: Lea & Febiger, 1973.

Resibois, A., et al. Lysosome and storage diseases. *Int. Rev. Exp. Pathol.* 9:93, 1970.

Revel, J. P., Henning, V., and Fox, C. F. (eds.). *Cell Shape and Surface Architecture. Progress in Clinical and Biological Research*, Vol. 17. New York: Liss, 1977.

Robertson, J. D. The unit membrane. In Boyd, J. D., Johnson, F. R., and Lever, J. D. (eds.), *Electron Microscopy in Anatomy.* Baltimore: Williams & Wilkins, 1961.

Schopf, J. W. The evolution of the earliest cells. *Sci. Am.* 239(3):110, 1978.

Singer, S. J., and Nicolson, G. L. The fluid mosaic model of the structure of cell membranes. *Science* 175:720, 1972.

Sjöstrand, F. S. The structure of mitochondrial membranes: A new concept. *J. Ultrastruct. Res.* 64:217, 1978.

Sleigh, M. A. (ed.). *Cilia and Flagella.* London: Academic, 1974.

Söll, D., et al. (eds.). *Transfer RNA: Biological Aspects.* Cold Spring Harbor, N.Y.: Cold Spring Harbor Laboratory, 1979.

Spooner, B. S., Yamada, K. M., and Wessels, N. K. Microfilaments and cell locomotion. *J. Cell Biol.* 49:595, 1971.

Staehelin, L. A., and Hull, B. E. Junctions between living cells. *Sci. Am.* 238(5):41, 1978.

Stein, G. S., et al. Chromosomal proteins and gene regulation. *Sci. Am.* 232(2):46, 1975.

Tedeschi, H. *Mitochondria: Structure, Biogenesis and Transducing Functions. Cell Biology Monographs*, Vol. 4. Vienna: Springer-Verlag, 1976.

Trump, B. F., and Arstila, A. V. Cellular reactions to injury. In LaVia, M., and Hill, R. (eds.), *Principles of Pathobiology*. Vol. 9. New York: Oxford University Press, 1975.

Weissman, G., and Claiborne, R. (eds.). *Cell Membranes: Biochemistry, Cell Biology and Pathology.* New York: HP Publishing Company, 1975.

Wessels, N. K. How living cells change their shape. *Sci. Am.* 225(4):76, 1971.

Whaley, W. G., Dauwalder, M., and Kephart, J. E. Golgi apparatus: Influence on cell surfaces. *Science* 175:596, 1972.

Williams, R. C., Jr., and Fudenberg, H. H. (eds.). *Phagocytic Mechanisms in Health and Disease.* New York: Intercontinental Medical Book, 1972.

Yamamoto, T. On the thickness of the unit membrane. *J. Cell Biol.* 17:413, 1963.

EPITHELIAL TISSUE

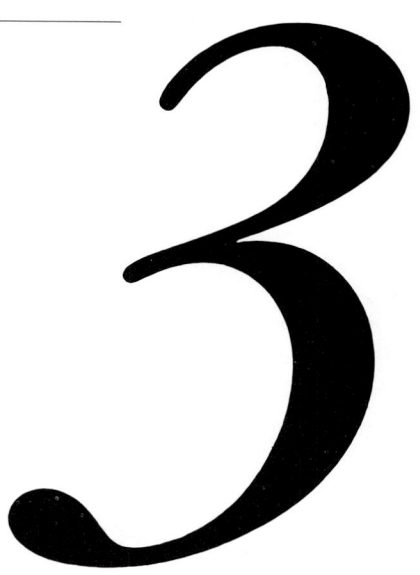

Tissues are composed of groups of cells performing similar functions. There are four main tissues: (1) epithelial tissue (epithelium), (2) connective tissue, (3) muscular tissue, and (4) nervous tissue. The epithelial tissue will be described in this chapter.

The epithelial tissue forms a barrier that covers the surfaces of the body and lines tubes and ducts that communicate with the surface. It also lines body cavities, namely, the pleural, pericardial, and peritoneal cavities; it lines the heart, the blood and lymphatic vessels, and the digestive and genitourinary tracts. The secretory cells of many glands are also epithelial tissue. The functions of epithelial tissue are protection, secretion, and absorption.

The cells of an epithelial tissue are held in close contact by a small amount of intercellular material and by cell junctions. All epithelial cells lie on a condensation of intercellular material called a *basement membrane* (Fig. 3-1). The basal lamina of the basement membrane is rich in glycoproteins and serves to anchor the cells. Epithelial tissue is nourished by diffusion of food substances from the blood vessels situated in the underlying connective tissue.

Epithelial tissue may be subdivided into (1) surface epithelium, (2) glandular epithelium, and (3) special epithelium.

SURFACE EPITHELIUM

Surface epithelium is classified according to the shape of the cells and the number and arrangement of the layers (Fig. 3-2). Cells specialized for absorption or filtration are arranged in a single layer. This arrangement is called *simple epithelium*. Cells exposed to a great deal of wear and tear are arranged in many layers; the arrangement is called *stratified epithelium*.

Surface epithelium may be classified as follows:

1. Squamous epithelium
   a. Simple
   b. Stratified
2. Cuboidal epithelium
   a. Simple
   b. Stratified
3. Columnar epithelium
   a. Simple
   b. Stratified

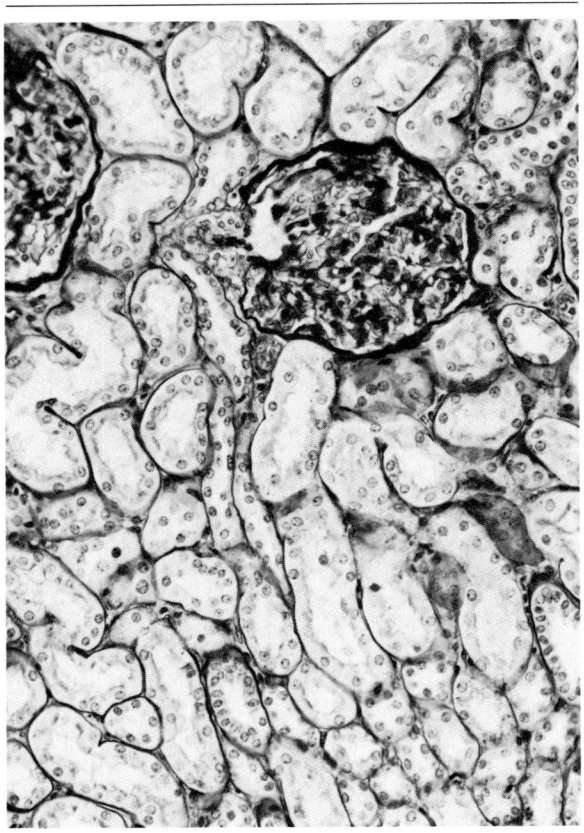

Fig. 3-1. Photomicrograph of kidney, showing cross sections of renal tubules and renal corpuscles. Note the dark, homogeneous basement membrane that surrounds those structures. (Periodic acid–Schiff stain; ×200.)

    c. Pseudostratified
    d. Specialized
4. Transitional epithelium

Squamous Epithelium

Simple squamous epithelium consists of a single layer of flat cells (Figs. 3-3 and 3-4; see Fig. 3-2) that resemble the tiles on a floor. The nucleus of each cell is centrally placed and is rounded or oval. The flat, thin cells are ideally suited to performing the functions of diffusion and filtration and line the alveoli of the lungs and the glomeruli of the kidneys. The simple squamous epithelium that forms the lining of the heart and the blood and lymphatic vessels is given the special name of *endothelium* (Fig. 3-5); that lining the pleural, pericardial, and peritoneal cavities is called *mesothelium* (Fig. 3-6).

    Stratified squamous epithelium consists of many layers of cells; the surface cells are flattened, and the deeper cells are thicker (see Fig. 3-2). By convention, stratified epithelium is named by the form of the surface cells. Stratified squamous epithelia can resist wear and tear, and protect the underlying tissues. The deeper, or basal, cells are continually undergoing cell division; the new cells are pushed upward toward the surface, where they are worn off. As the cells rise to the surface, they move farther from their nourishment, which is derived from the blood vessels in the underlying connective tissue. As a consequence, the cells shrink, become harder, and finally die. On dry surfaces, such as the skin (Fig. 3-7), the surface cells contain a tough protein material called *keratin*. This material resists trauma and bacterial and fungus infections and is watertight. This type of stratified squamous epithelium is called *keratinized stratified squamous epithelium*.

    On wet surfaces, such as those that line the mouth, esophagus (Fig. 3-8), and vagina (Fig. 3-9), the stratified cells do not contain keratin; this epithelium is known as *nonkeratinized stratified squamous epithelium*.

Cuboidal Epithelium

Simple cuboidal epithelium consists of a single layer of cells shaped like cubes (Fig. 3-10; see Fig. 3-2). The nucleus of each cell is round and centrally placed. This type of epithelium lines the small ducts of certain glands, such as the salivary glands, and forms the secretory units of other glands, such as the thyroid. Simple cuboidal cells perform the functions of secretion and absorption. Stratified cuboidal epithelium is relatively rare and is found lining ducts (see Fig. 3-2).

Columnar Epithelium

Simple columnar epithelium consists of a single layer of cells shaped like columns standing on end (see Fig. 3-2). The end of each cell that rests on the

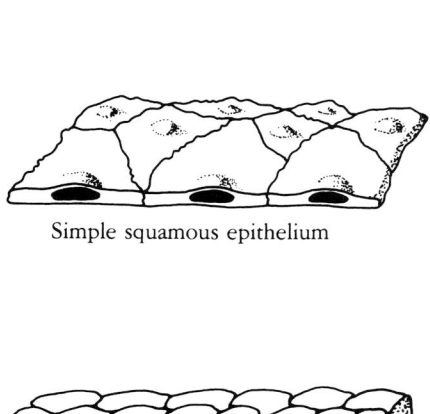
Simple squamous epithelium

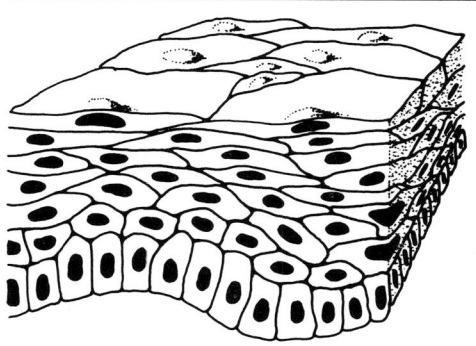
Stratified squamous epithelium

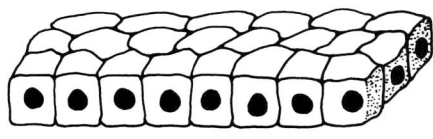
Simple cuboidal epithelium

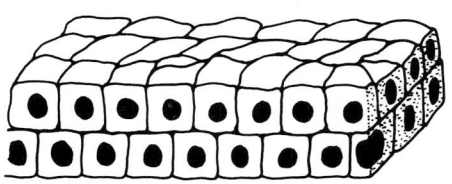
Stratified cuboidal epithelium

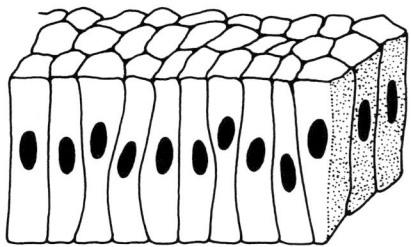
Simple columnar epithelium

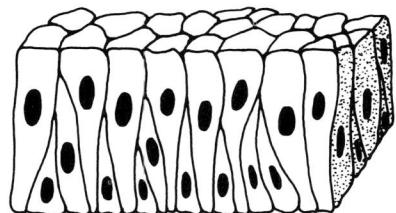
Pseudostratified columnar epithelium

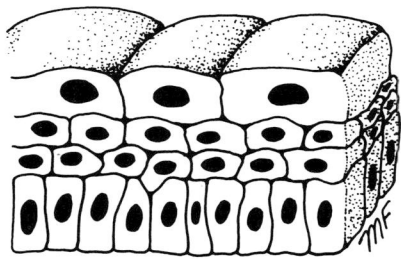
Transitional epithelium

Fig. 3-2. Different types of epithelium.

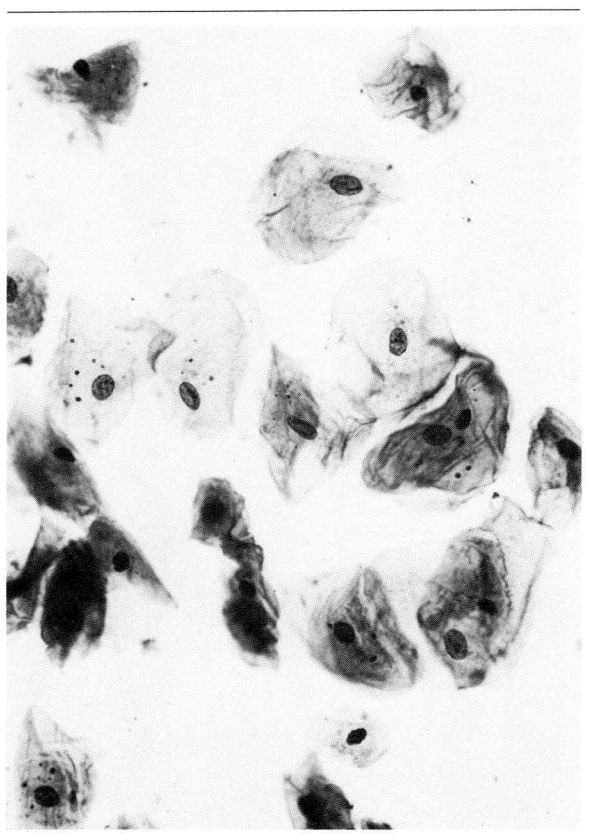

Fig. 3-3. Photomicrograph of squamous epithelial cells removed from the lining of the mouth (buccal smear). (H&E; ×100.)

basal lamina is known as the basal part of the cell. The nuclei are centrally placed or are located near the bases of the cells. Simple columnar cells line the stomach and intestines (Fig. 3-11). Simple columnar cells perform the functions of secretion and absorption. Stratified columnar epithelium is found in only a few places in the body, in the lining of the larger ducts of certain glands, such as the mammary glands.

Pseudostratified columnar epithelium is epithelium that gives the appearance of being stratified but is actually a simple epithelium with all its cells resting on a basal lamina (see Fig. 3-2). The stratified appearance results from the fact that the cells vary in height and not all of them reach the surface. Moreover, because the cells are of different heights, their nuclei occur at different levels, furthering the illusion that the epithelium is stratified. This epithelium is found on the surfaces of the upper part of the respiratory system (Fig. 3-12).

Specialized Columnar Cells

The structure of many columnar cells has been adapted to perform special functions. *Goblet cells* are actually unicellular glands whose function is to produce thick mucus (Fig. 3-13). The mucous secretion accumulates in the distal portion of the cell, causing the cell to assume the form of a goblet. The cytoplasm is displaced to the sides of the cell. The narrow stem of the goblet is formed by the basal part of the cell, and it is here that the nucleus and the rest of the cytoplasm are found. Goblet cells are present in large numbers in the epithelium lining the intestinal (Figs. 3-14 and 3-15) and respiratory systems.

Absorptive cells are cells whose free surface has a brushlike or striated border (see Fig. 3-13). When the cells are examined under the electron microscope, the striated border is seen to be composed of *microvilli*. This arrangement greatly increases the area of the free surface of the cell, furthering absorption. These cells are found lining the stomach, the small and large parts of the intestine (see Fig. 3-15), and the convoluted tubules of the kidney.

The epithelial cells lining the duct of the epididymis and the vas deferens of the male reproductive system have very long microvilli (Fig. 3-16), which are called *stereocilia* (see p. 66).

Ciliated columnar cells are cells whose free surface possesses a number of motile processes, the cilia, that have a coordinated beat (see Fig. 3-13). They occur on the epithelium lining the bronchi of the lungs and in the uterine tubes (Fig. 3-17) and uterus of the female reproductive system; they also occur in the efferent ducts of the testes in the male reproductive system. The cilia move the mucus or other fluid that covers the surface of the epithelium in a definite direction. In the respiratory system, the mucus, containing trapped foreign particles that

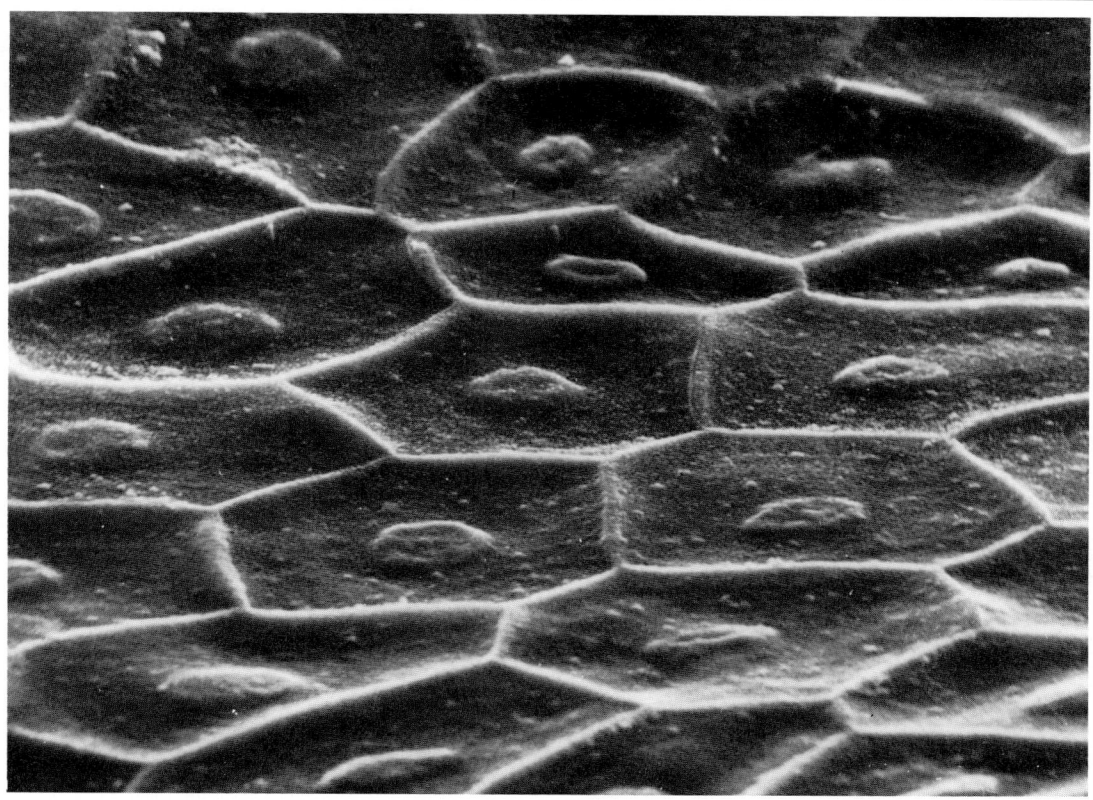

Fig. 3-4. Scanning electron micrograph of simple squamous epithelium, showing cell nuclei and cell boundaries. The small granular structures represent some of the cell organelles and inclusions that are present in the cytoplasm and produce bulges on the plasma membranes. (Courtesy of Dr. W. J. Krause.)

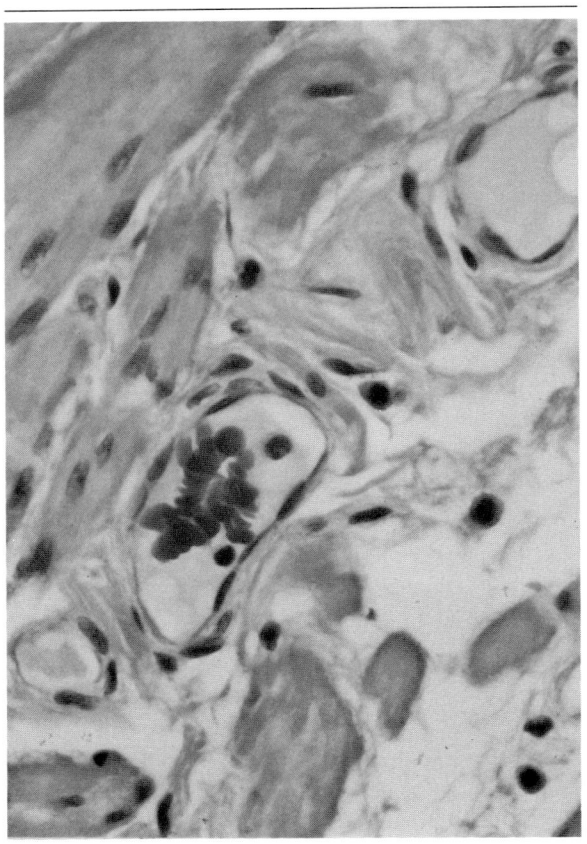

Fig. 3-5. Photomicrograph showing a cross section of a blood capillary and two lymph capillaries. Note that the small vessels are lined with flattened endothelial cells. (H&E; ×560.)

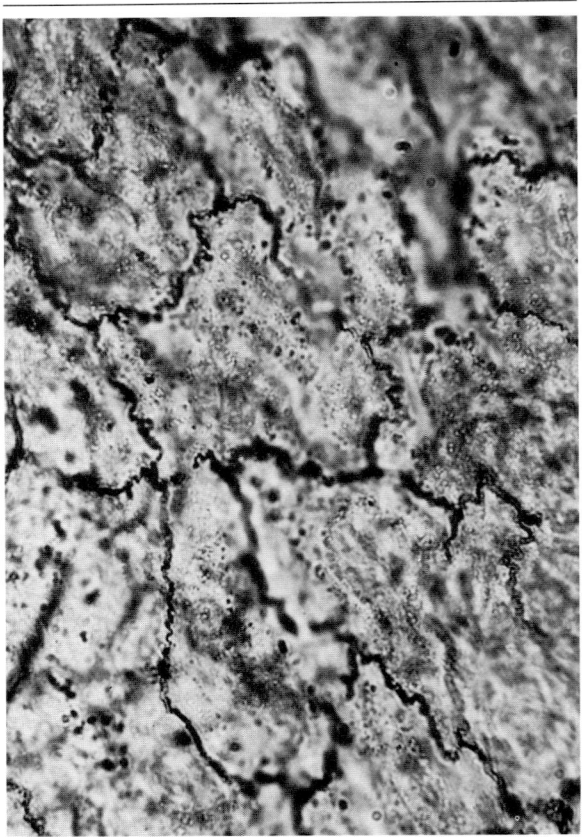

Fig. 3-6. Photomicrograph of the mesothelial cells of the peritoneum. On surface view, the mesothelial cells are irregular in shape. The intercellular substance is stained black with silver nitrate. (×1,000.)

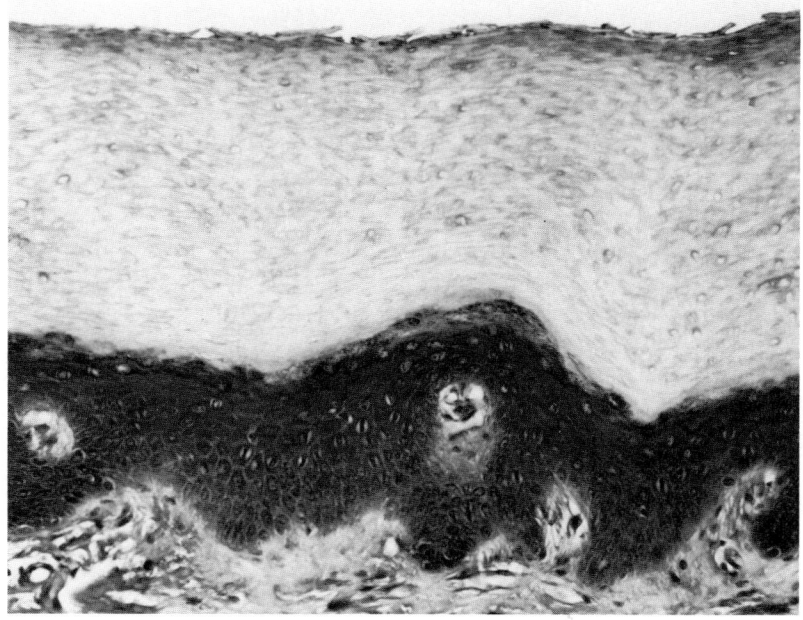

Fig. 3-7. Photomicrograph of a section of thick skin from the palm of the hand, showing the keratinized stratified squamous epithelium that forms the various layers of the epidermis. The deeper, more rounded cells are deeply stained; the superficial, flattened keratinized cells are lightly stained. (H&E; ×200.)

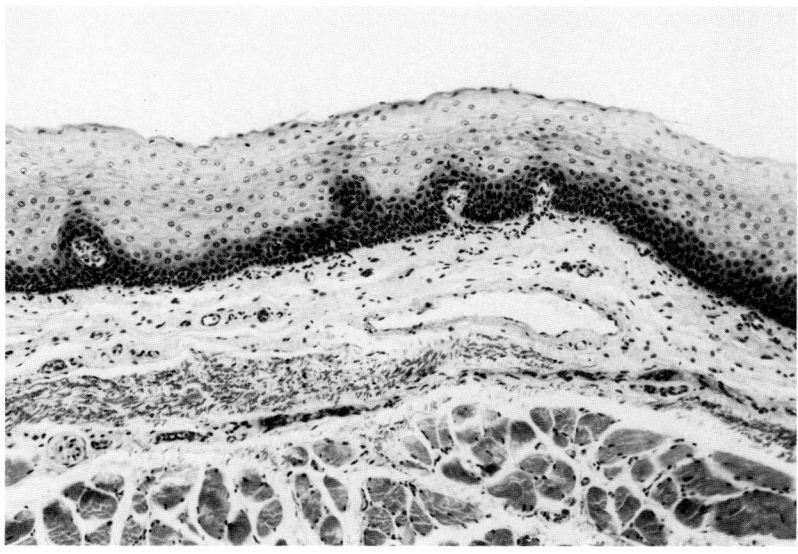

Fig. 3-8. Photomicrograph of a longitudinal section of the esophagus, showing the lining of nonkeratinized stratified squamous epithelium. (H&E; ×100.)

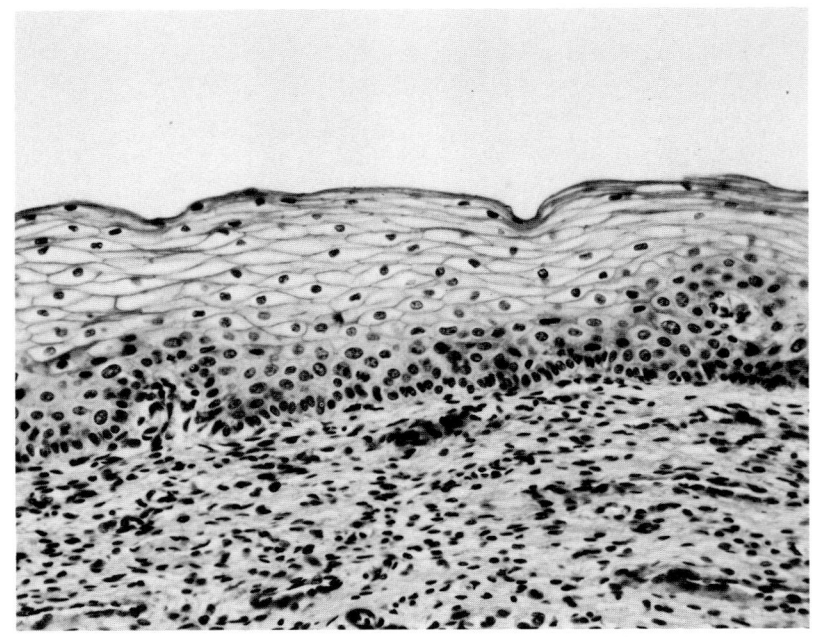

Fig. 3-9. Photomicrograph of a section of the vagina, showing the lining of nonkeratinized stratified squamous epithelium. (H&E; ×200.)

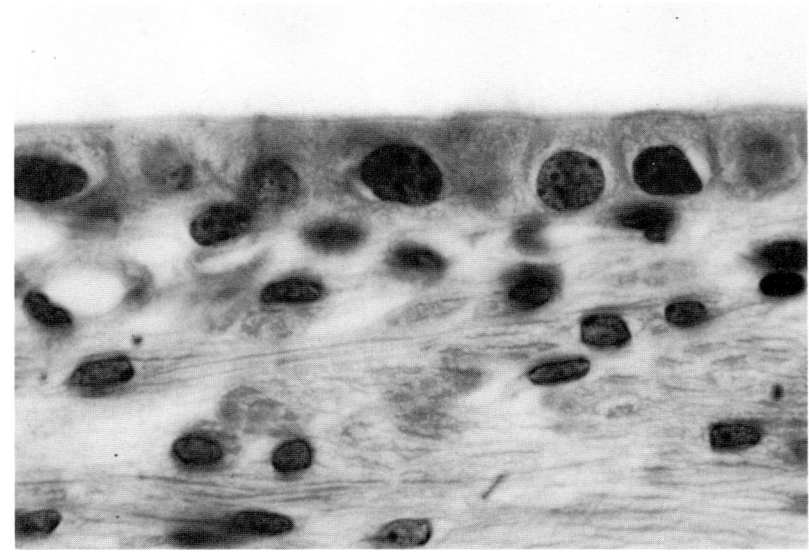

Fig. 3-10. Photomicrograph of a section of a renal tubule, showing the lining of cuboidal epithelium. (H&E; ×1,000.)

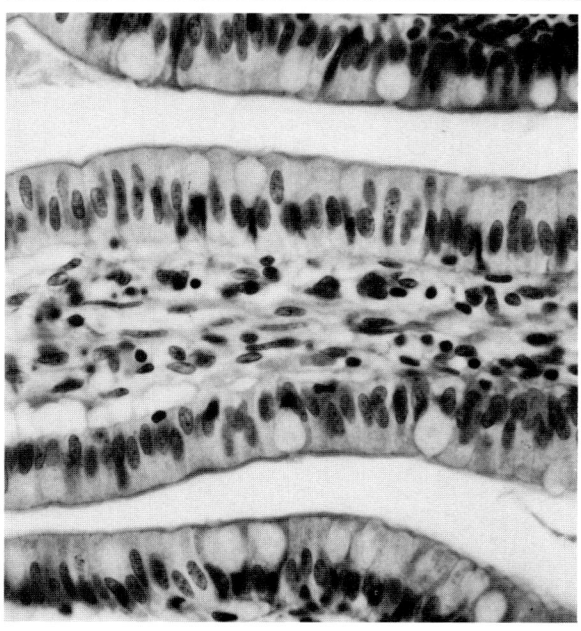

Fig. 3-11. Photomicrograph of a longitudinal section of villi of the small intestine. The villi are covered with tall columnar cells, many of which are goblet cells. The goblet cells are recognizable by the presence of pale-colored mucus in the cell cytoplasm. (H&E; ×400.)

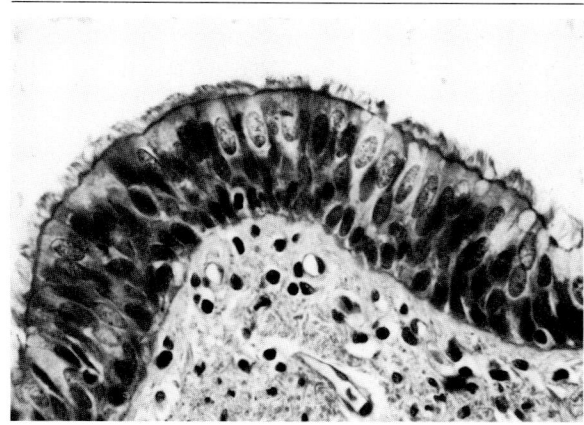

Fig. 3-12. Photomicrograph of the mucous membrane lining the trachea. The surface is covered with pseudostratified ciliated columnar epithelium. (H&E; ×426.)

have been inhaled, is moved toward the pharynx by the cilia, where the material is expectorated or swallowed.

Transitional Epithelium

Transitional epithelium is a stratified epithelium that occurs exclusively in the urinary system (Fig. 3-18; see Fig. 3-2). The number of layers varies, depending on whether the organ is contracted or distended. In the contracted state, this epithelium has several layers and the surface cells are large and round and bulge into the lumen. In the distended state, there may be two or three layers of cells and the surface cells become stretched and flattened. The arrangement of the epithelium allows hollow organs, such as the urinary bladder, to be distended without rupturing or separating the lining cells.

GLANDULAR EPITHELIUM

Glands are formed of groups of specialized cells whose function is secretion. *Secretion* is the production and release by cells of a fluid that contains a number of substances, such as mucus, enzymes, or a hormone. The secretory cells of the gland are referred to as the *parenchyma*. The connective tissue within the gland, which supports the secretory cells, is called the *stroma*. The stroma also supports the blood supply, nerve supply, and lymphatic drainage of the gland. There are two main types of glands, exocrine glands and endocrine glands. Exocrine glands possess ducts that convey the glandular secretions to the surface of the body or into the cavity (lumen) of a hollow organ. Examples of exocrine glands are sweat glands, salivary glands, and intestinal glands.

Endocrine glands have no ducts and pour their secretions directly into the bloodstream, where they are distributed throughout the body. The secretions of endocrine glands contain chemical substances called *hormones,* which regulate the activities of cells, usually at some distance from their glands of origin.

Exocrine Glands

A *simple gland* is one in which the duct is unbranched (see Fig. 3-13). A *compound gland* is one in

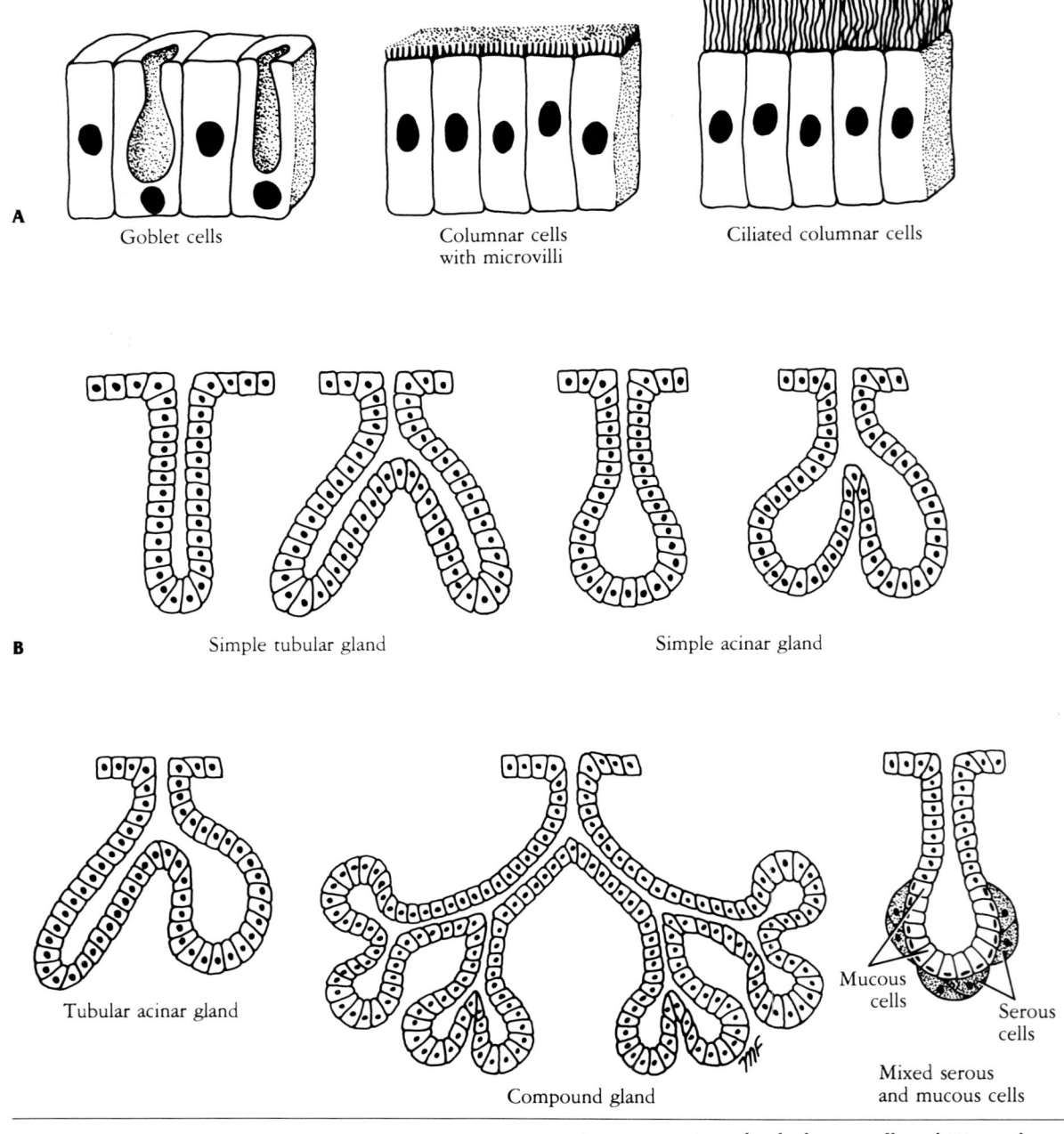

Fig. 3-13. (A) Specialized columnar cells and (B) simple tubular and compound exocrine glands.

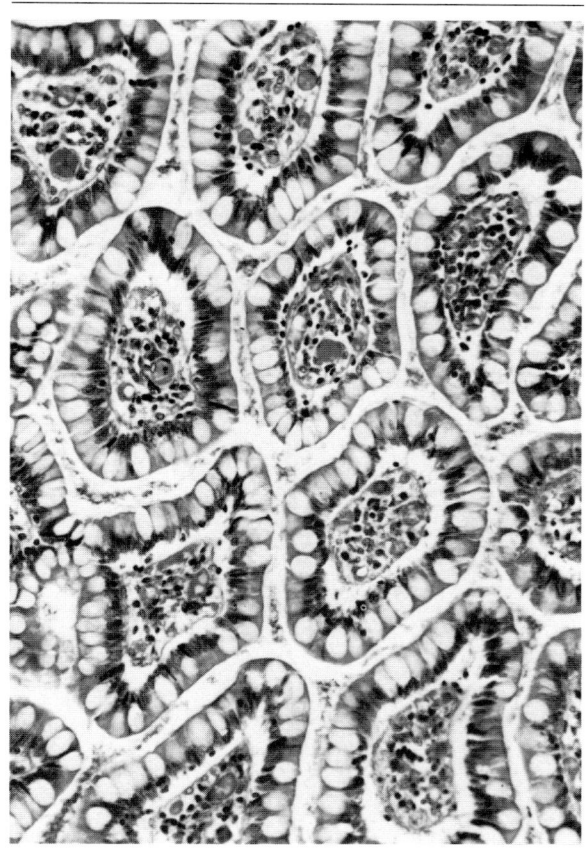

Fig. 3-14. Photomicrograph of cross sections of numerous villi of the small intestine. Large numbers of goblet cells filled with clear mucus are visible. (H&E; ×200.)

which the duct branches, often many times (see Fig. 3-13). An example of a simple gland is a sweat gland (Fig. 3-19); an example of a compound gland is the pancreas. If the secretory unit of the gland is tubular, the gland is called a *tubular gland*. If the secretory unit is rounded, the gland is referred to as *acinous* (see Fig. 3-13). *Serous glands* are those that secrete a watery fluid (Fig. 3-20). *Mucous glands* are those that secrete a thick, viscid fluid of glycoprotein called *mucus* (Fig. 3-21). Some glands, the *seromucous glands,* are composed of a mixture of serous and mucous secretory units (Fig. 3-22; see Fig. 3-13).

In many exocrine glands, there is a special type of branched contractile cell between the secretory cells and the basement membrane called a *myoepithelial cell*. These cells contain myofibrils and assist in the expression of the secretion from the acini into the ducts. The mammary, salivary, and sweat glands are examples of glands in which this type of cell is found (Fig. 3-23).

Exocrine glands can be classified, according to the means by which they release their secretions, as merocrine, apocrine, and holocrine glands.

Merocrine Glands

In these glands, the secretion is transported through the plasma membrane of the free surface in membranous vesicles by the process of exocytosis, with no resultant loss of cytoplasm (Fig. 3-24). An example of a merocrine gland is the exocrine part of the pancreas.

Apocrine Glands

In these glands, the secretion and possibly a part of the cytoplasm of the secretory cell is discharged from the free surface of the cell (see Fig. 3-24).* The remaining part of the cell then repairs itself. Examples of apocrine glands are the axillary sweat gland and the mammary gland.

Holocrine Glands

In these glands, entire cells become detached and die and form the secretion of the gland (see Fig. 3-24). The detached cells are replaced by division of neighboring cells. The sebaceous glands of the skin are examples of holocrine glands.

Endocrine Glands

Endocrine glands have no ducts. The secretory cells are arranged in straight or irregular cords or clumps that are separated from one another by a network of small blood vessels (see Fig. 3-24). The glands are usually highly vascular, and the secretion is passed directly into the bloodstream. The pituitary, thy-

---

*Electron microscopic studies have recently shown that many of these glands do not lose part of their structure in the formation of a secretion, as previously believed, and that in fact they are merocrine glands.

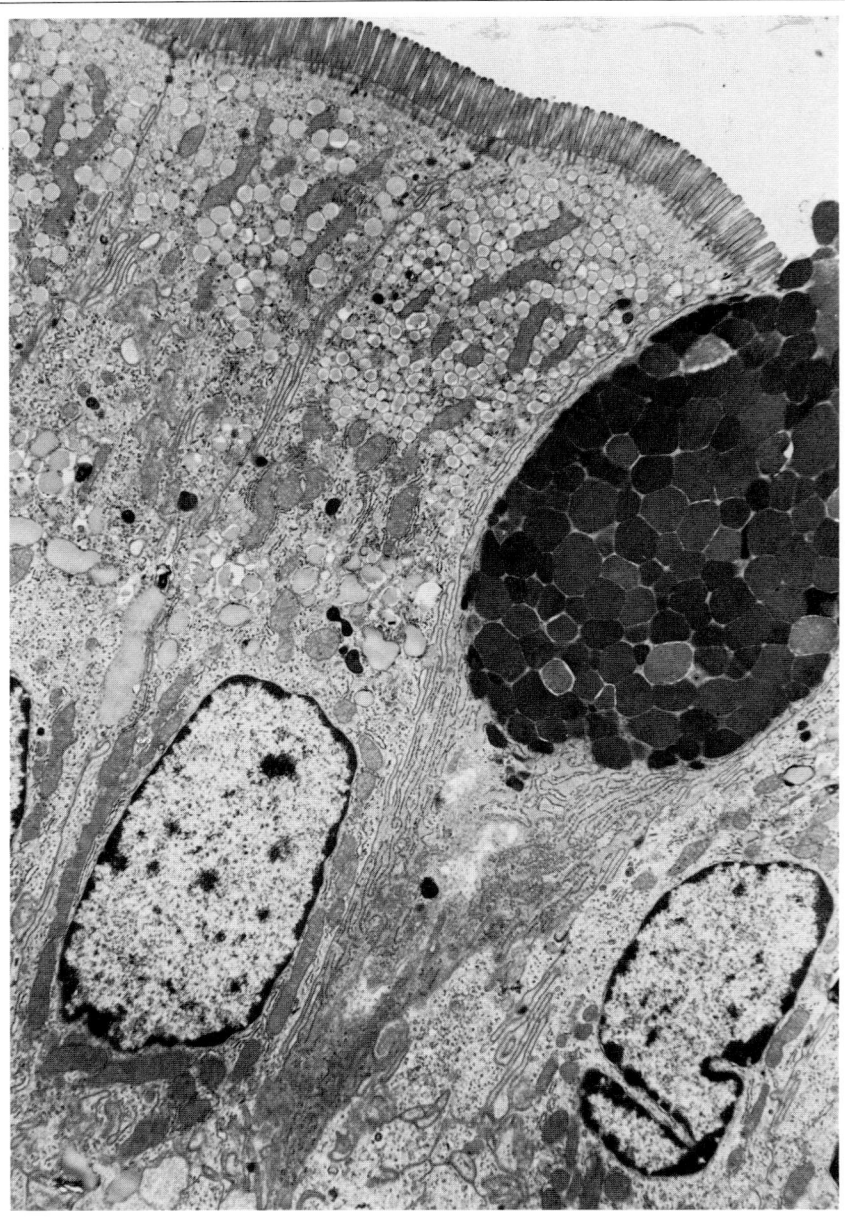

Fig. 3-15. Electron micrograph of columnar cells covering a villus of the small intestine. Part of a goblet cell filled with dark-staining mucous granules is clearly visible, as are parts of three absorptive cells with microvilli on their free borders. ($\times 4,000$.) (Courtesy of Dr. H. Friedman.)

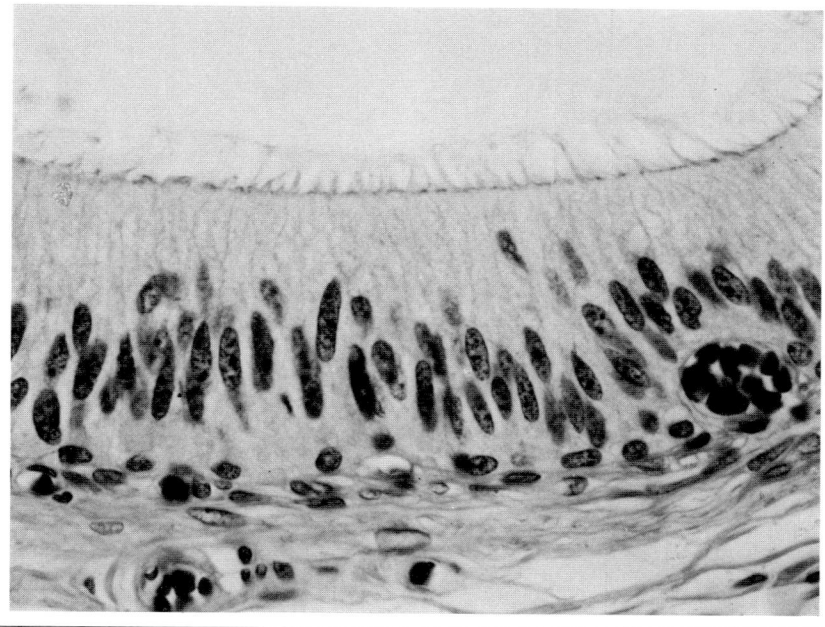

Fig. 3-16. Photomicrograph of a cross section of the duct of the epididymis. The duct is lined with tall principal cells with long, nonmotile microvilli called stereocilia. Small, rounded basal cells can also be seen between the bases of adjacent principal cells. (H&E; ×520.)

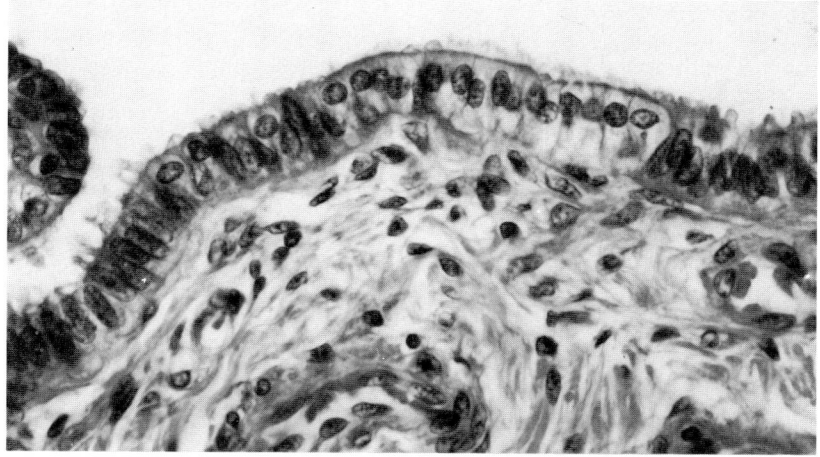

Fig. 3-17. Photomicrograph of a section of uterine tube. The tube is lined with ciliated columnar epithelial cells. (H&E; ×520.)

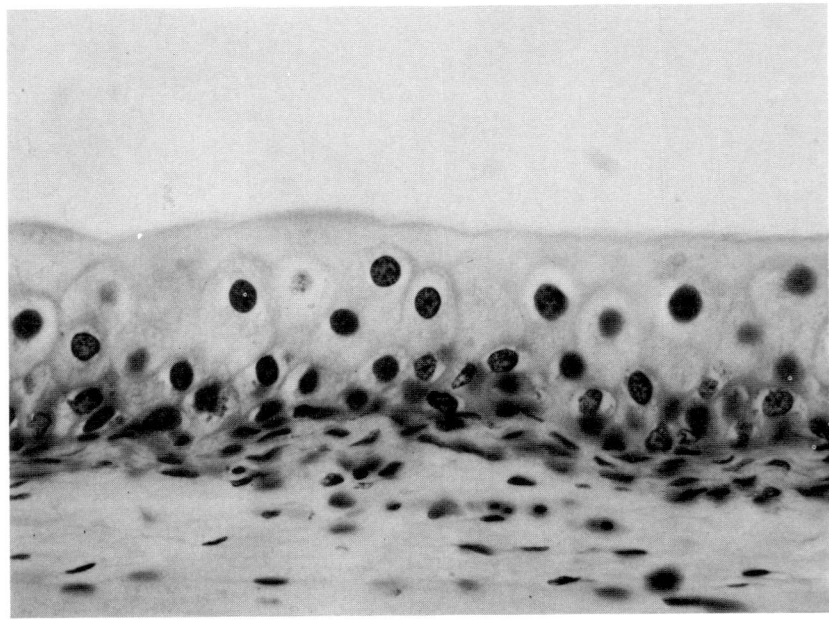

Fig. 3-18. Photomicrograph of a section of the urinary bladder, showing the lining of transitional epithelium. (H&E; ×400.)

roid, and suprarenal (adrenal) glands (Fig. 3-25) are examples of endocrine glands.

SPECIAL EPITHELIA

The cells in this group of epithelia are highly specialized and are concerned with sensory perception and reproduction. The rods and cones of the retina, the auditory epithelial cells, and the olfactory and gustatory cells are examples of such sensory receptor cells. The cells lining the seminiferous tubules of the testes are examples of such reproductive cells.

CLINICAL NOTES

REGENERATION OF EPITHELIAL CELLS

The ability of an epithelial tissue to regenerate is of great practical importance following injury or surgical interference. Epithelial cells may be divided into (1) labile cells, (2) stable cells, and (3) permanent cells.

Labile cells, under normal conditions, continue to multiply throughout life. The cells of the epidermis and of the mucous membranes of the gastrointestinal, urinary, and respiratory tracts are good examples. Red bone marrow cells are also labile cells, because they are actively hematopoietic throughout life. *Stable cells* cease multiplication about the time of puberty but can start to multiply again in special circumstances, for example, in case of tissue injury. The epithelial cells of the parenchyma of the liver, thyroid, pancreas, and kidney are examples of stable cells. It is important to note that, although the cells of the liver can replace themselves, they will resemble the normal structure of the liver only if the connective tissue framework is intact. Otherwise, disorganized groups of cells will be formed. The

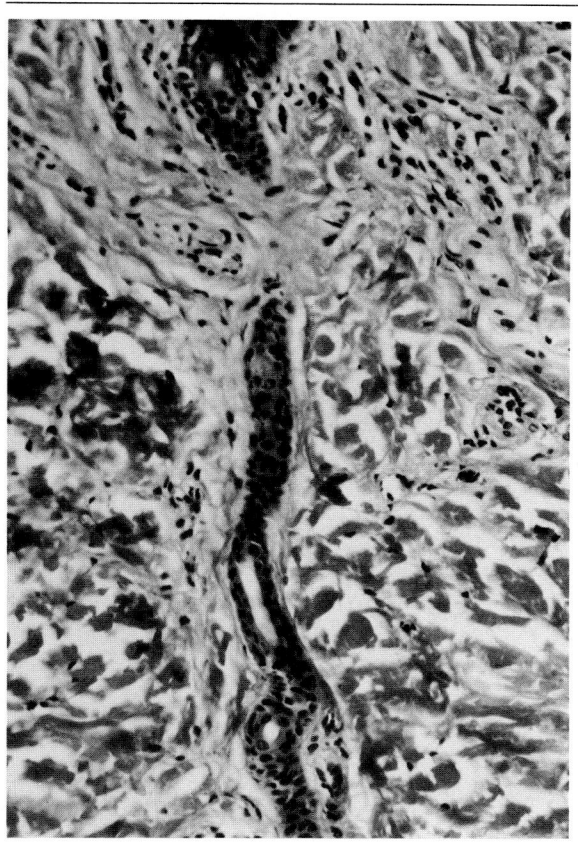

Fig. 3-19. Photomicrograph of a section of part of a sweat gland. The gland has the shape of a simple, unbranched tube. (H&E; ×200.)

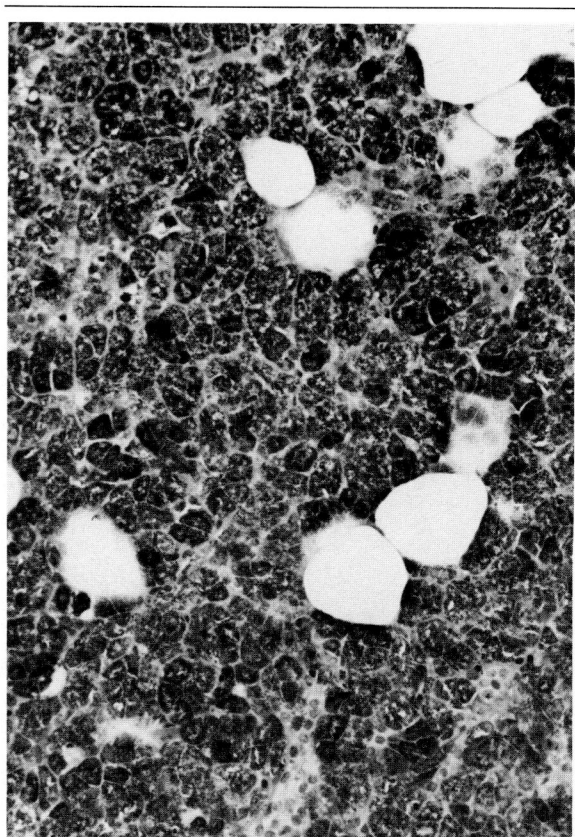

Fig. 3-20. Photomicrograph of a section of the parotid salivary gland, showing numerous dark-staining serous acini. The clear white spaces represent fat cells. (H&E; ×200.)

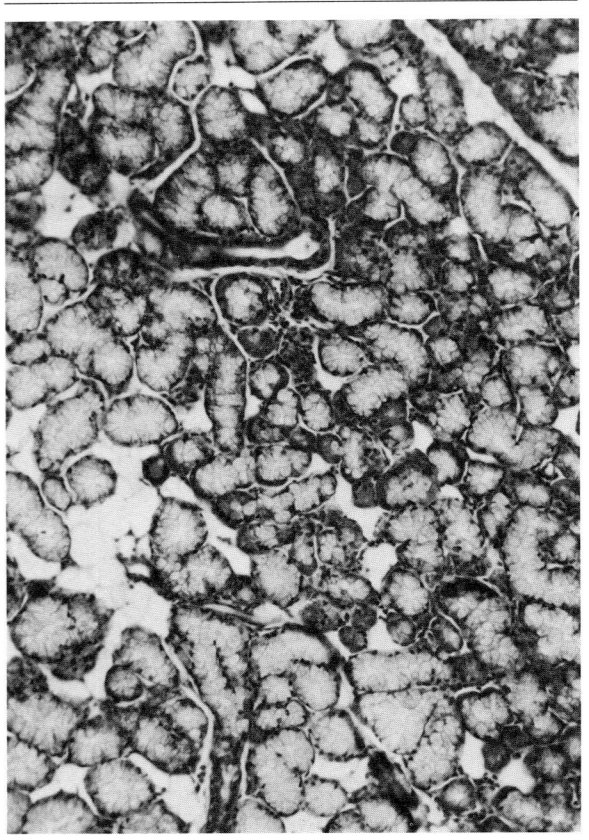

Fig. 3-21. Photomicrograph of a section of the sublingual salivary gland, showing numerous lightly stained mucous acini. The clear white spaces represent fat cells. (H&E; × 100.)

basement membrane appears to play an important role in the organization of regenerating epithelial cells. *Permanent cells* cease multiplication at birth, and nothing can stimulate them to multiply afterward. The neurons of nervous tissue are a good example.

It should be clearly understood that the different powers of regeneration possessed by different cells determine pratical medical and surgical treatment. We know, for example, that a wound or burn of the skin or a surgical wound or ulcer of the mucous membrane of the intestinal tract is quickly followed by cell regeneration. In contrast, the highly specialized nerve and muscle cells fail to regenerate when they die. This is the reason treatment of many diseases of the nervous system is ineffective. To be more specific, we know that if a neuron in the central nervous system dies, there is no cell division in the neighboring nerve cells. The only reaction is a multiplication of the supporting neuroglial cells, which fill in the space left by the dead neuron. If, however, the processes of nerve cells that extend into the peripheral nervous system are destroyed, the nerve cells possess the ability throughout life to replace their axons and dendrites and so to restore sensory and motor function to some extent.

CLASSIFICATION OF TUMORS ACCORDING TO THE TISSUE OF ORIGIN

Tumors arise by an irreversible change in the cells of the tissue of origin. The histological appearance of *benign tumors* closely resembles that of the parent tissue. *Malignant* and *rapidly growing tumors* less closely resemble their tissue of origin. It should be pointed out that although most tumors can be classified as benign or malignant, a few are borderline and possess the morphological features of both.

Benign epithelial tumors are of two types: those that arise from a surface epithelium, called *papillomas,* and those that arise from a glandular epithelium, called *adenomas*. A malignant tumor arising from a surface epithelium is called a *carcinoma;* one arising from a glandular epithelium is called an *adenocarcinoma*.

CLINICAL PROBLEMS

For the answers to these problems, see page 785.

1. Define the term *epithelial tissue* and give the special name that is applied to the cells that line the heart and the blood and lymphatic vessels. Name the cells that line the thoracic and abdominopelvic cavities.

2. Chemotherapeutic agents are used in the treatment of malignant disease. These agents have a toxic effect on cells that are multiplying rapidly. Because cancer cells constantly are undergoing mitotic division at a more rapid rate than are most normal cells,

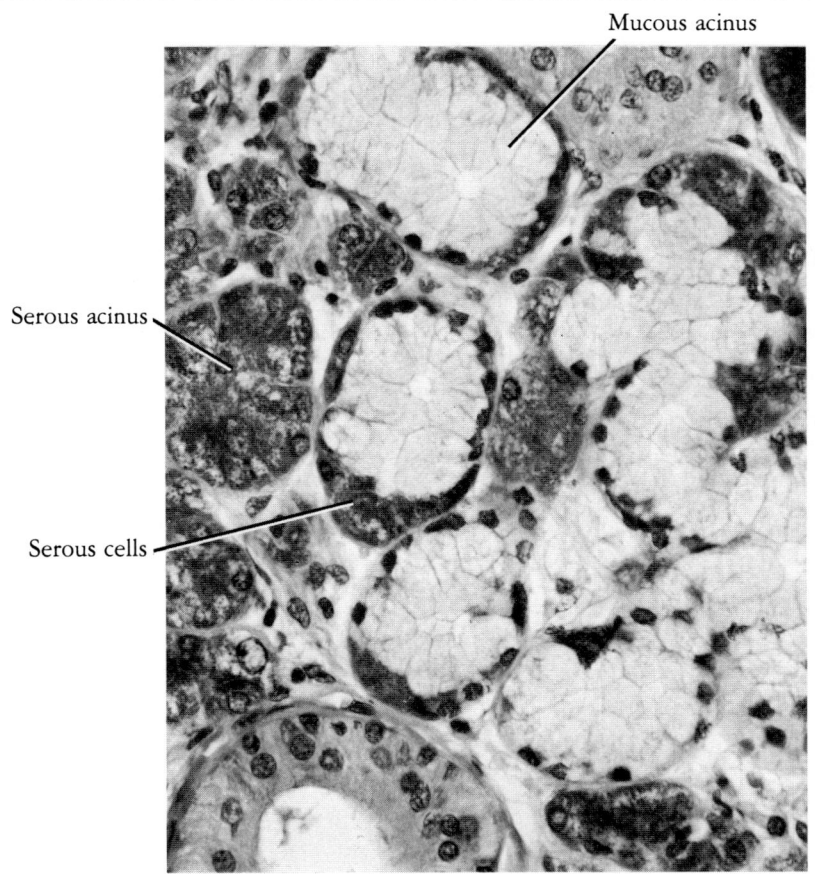

Fig. 3-22. Photomicrograph of a section of the submandibular salivary gland, showing a mixture of serous and mucous acini. (H&E; ×400.)

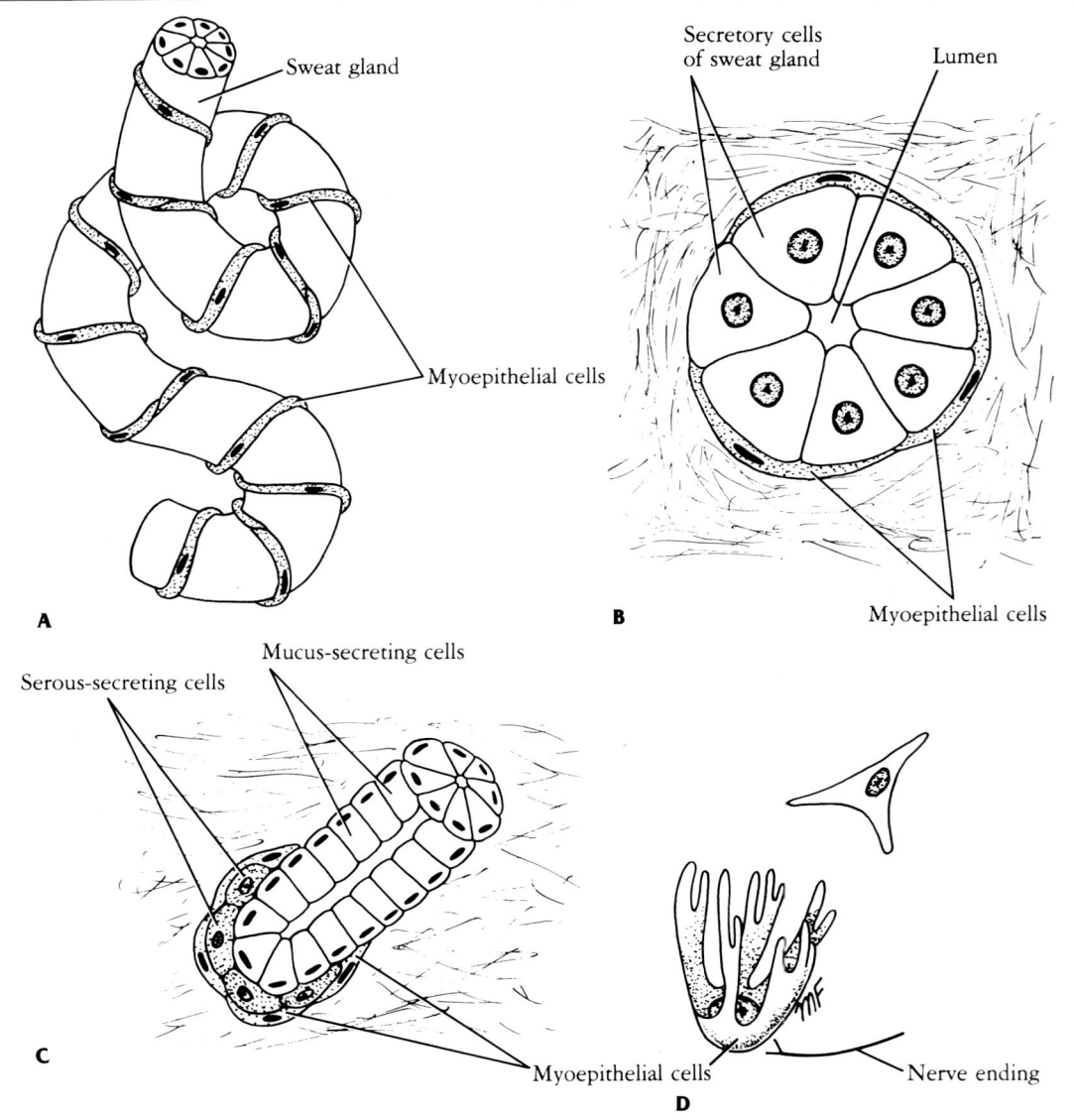

Fig. 3-23. (A and B) The position of the contractile myoepithelial cells in relation to the secretory cells of a sweat gland. (C) The position of myoepithelial cells in a seromucous gland. (D) The general shape of a myoepithelial cell and its close relationship to an autonomic nerve fiber.

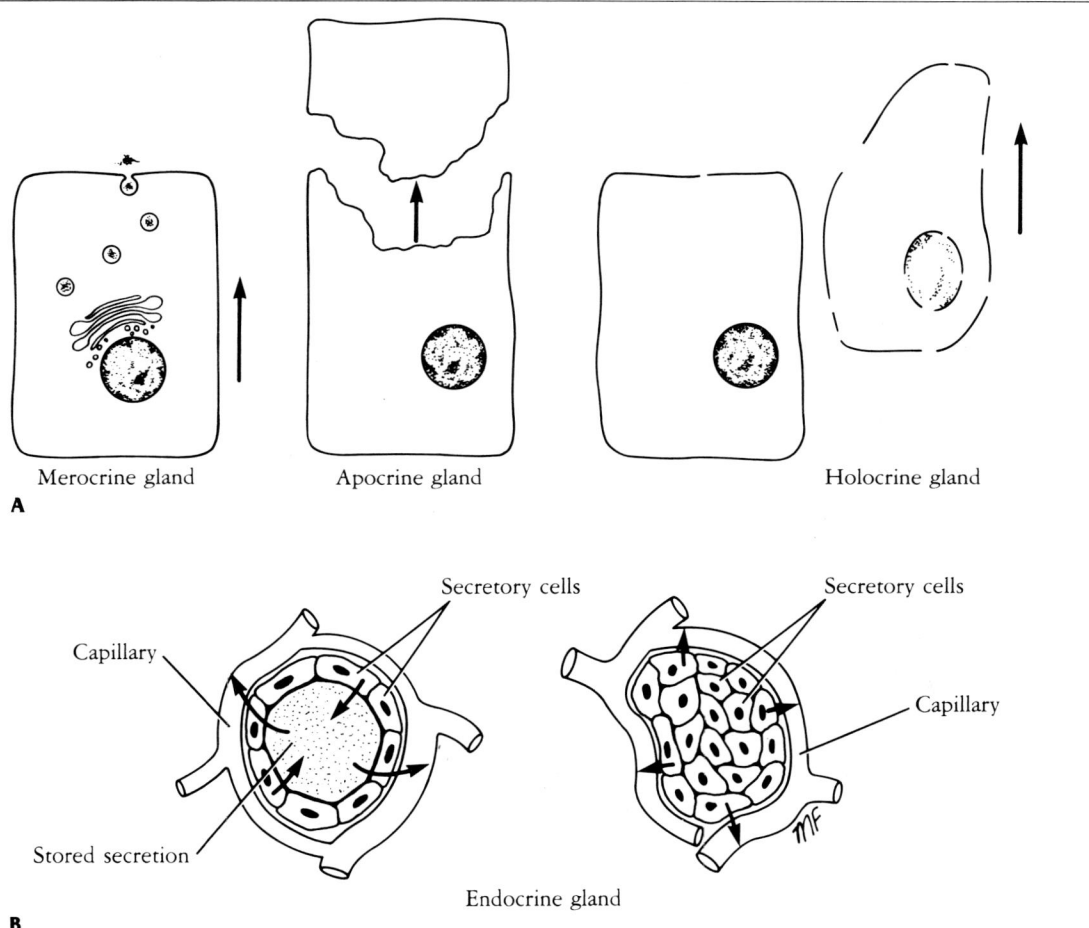

Fig. 3-24. (A) Secretory cells in a merocrine, an apocrine, and a holocrine gland; (B) two types of endocrine glands.

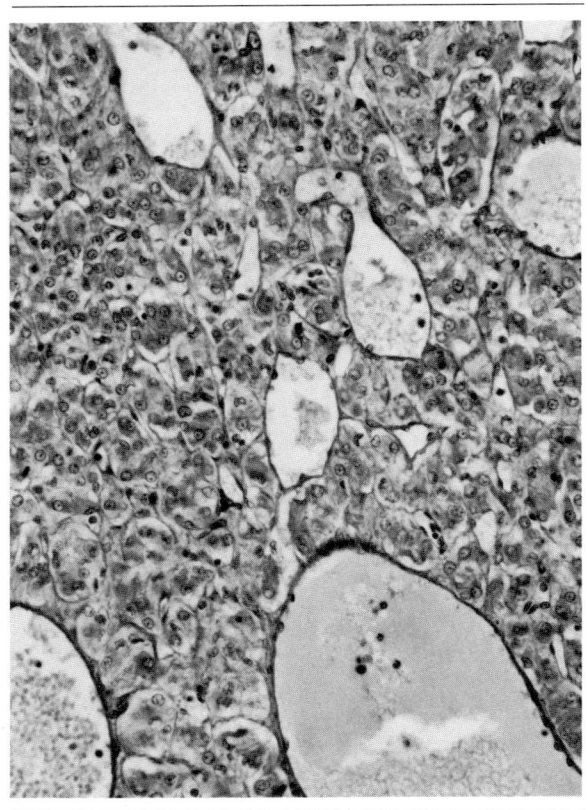

Fig. 3-25. Photomicrograph of a section of the suprarenal medulla. As in all endocrine glands, the secretory cells are arranged in cords or clumps that are separated by numerous capillaries. There are no ducts in an endocrine gland. (H&E; ×200.)

these toxic agents are likely to kill large numbers of malignant cells and leave most normal tissue cells unaffected. Can you explain why the cells of the bone marrow and those lining the gastrointestinal tract are also susceptible to chemotherapeutic agents?

3. Describe the ways in which an epithelial tissue differs from a connective tissue. Classify the different types of epithelium, and give examples of locations in the body where they may be found.

4. A 78-year-old man visits his physician because of a large, hard, painless ulcer of his upper lip, which he has had for 2 years. The patient is concerned because the ulcer shows no signs of healing. A biopsy specimen is taken from the edge of the ulcer, and a diagnosis of squamous cell carcinoma is made. What is meant by the term *squamous cell*? What is a carcinoma?

5. Discuss the specialized types of columnar epithelial cells. Indicate their functions and give examples of locations where they may be found.

6. A 48-year-old man has a history of repeated pain over his right kidney. A radiograph of the abdomen shows the presence of a large calculus (stone) in the right kidney. After examining the radiograph, the physician says to a medical student, "There is almost certainly metaplasia of the transitional epithelium around the renal stone." What does he mean by the term *metaplasia*?

7. Classify the different types of exocrine glands. What is the basic difference between an exocrine gland and an endocrine gland?

8. What is meant by irreversible and reversible injury to epithelial cells? Give some examples of the causes of epithelial injury. What are the differences among labile, stable, and permanent epithelial cells?

ADDITIONAL READING

Berridge, M. J., and Oschman, J. L. *Transporting Epithelia.* New York: Academic, 1972.

Botelho, S. Y., Brooks, F. P., and Shelley, W. B. *Symposium on the Exocrine Glands.* Philadelphia: University of Pennsylvania Press, 1969.

Bowen, R. H. The cytology of glandular secretion. *Q. Rev. Biol.* 4:299, 1929.

Busch, H. A general concept for molecular biology of cancer. *Cancer Res.* 36:4291, 1976.

De Bradander, M., et al. (eds.). *Cell Movement and Neoplasia.* New York: Pergamon, 1980.

Fawcett, D. W. Surface specializations of absorbing cells. *J. Histochem. Cytochem.* 13:75, 1965.

Fawcett, D. W., Long, J. A., and Jones, A. L. The ultrastructure of endocrine glands. *Recent Prog. Horm. Res.* 25:315, 1969.

Freeman, J. A. Goblet cell fine structure. *Anat. Rec.* 154:121, 1966.

Gabe, M., and Arvy, L. Gland cells. In Brachet, J., and Mirsky, A. E. (eds.), *The Cell.* Vol. 5. New York: Academic, 1961, p. 2.

Hennings, H., and Boutwell, R. K. Studies on the mechanism of skin tumor production. *Cancer Res.* 30:312, 1970.

Jamieson, J. D., and Palade, G. E. Intracellular transport of secretory protein in the pancreatic exocrine cell. 4. Metabolism requirements. *J. Cell Biol.* 39:589, 1968.

Krstic, R. V. *Ultrastructure of the Mammalian Cell.* New York: Springer-Verlag, 1979.

Mukherjee, T. M., and Williams, A. W. A comparative study of the ultrastructure of microvilli in the epithelium of small and large intestines of mice. *J. Cell Biol.* 34:447, 1967.

Neutra, M., and Leblond, C. P. Synthesis of the carbohydrate of mucus in the Golgi complex as shown by electron microscope radioautography of goblet cells from rats injected with glucose-^{3}H. *J. Cell Biol.* 30:119, 1966.

Pitot, H. C. The natural history of neoplasia. *Am. J. Pathol.* 89:402, 1977.

Revel, J. P., and Ito, S. The surface components of cells. In Davis, B. D., and Warren, L. (eds.), *The Specificity of Cell Surfaces.* Englewood Cliffs, N.J.: Prentice-Hall, 1967, p. 211.

Satir, P. How cilia move. *Sci. Am.* 231(4):44, 1974.

Schultz, S. G. Principles of electrophysiology and their application to epithelial tissues. *Int. Rev. Physiol.* 4:69, 1974.

Smith, A. D. Storage and secretion of hormones. *Sci. Basis Med. Ann. Rev.* 74:74, 1972.

Staehelin, L. A., and Hull, B. E. Junctions between living cells. *Sci. Am.* 238(5):140, 1978.

Tamarin, A. Myoepithelium of the rat submaxillary gland. *J. Ultrastruct. Res.* 16:320, 1966.

CONNECTIVE TISSUE

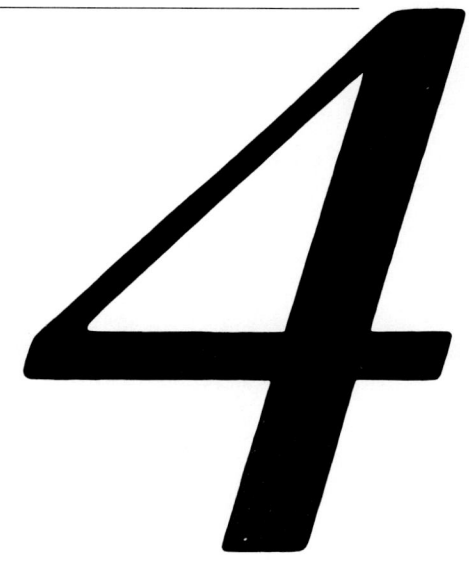

As its name implies, connective tissue connects, holds, and supports other body tissues. The cells of connective tissue are characteristically separated from one another by large amounts of intercellular material. It is the nonliving intercellular material that gives connective tissue its strength.

There are two main components of the intercellular material, fibers and amorphous material. The fibers are of three types: (1) collagenous, which is strong, inelastic, and composed of the protein *collagen;* (2) elastic, which is strong, elastic, and composed of the protein *elastin;* and (3) reticular, which is arranged in the form of a fine network and composed of collagen and a carbohydrate material. The amorphous material is in the form of a sol or a gel. It itself has very little strength, but it functions as a medium through which nutrients can diffuse from blood vessels to nourish the cells.

Although all connective tissues have the same basic structure, their physical properties depend on the composition of the intercellular material. For example, at one extreme is loose connective tissue, in which the fibers of the intercellular material are loosely arranged in a watery amorphous material. At the other extreme is bone, in which fibers are embedded in an amorphous material that is not only solidified but calcified. Blood may be regarded as a special form of connective tissue, in which the intercellular material is a liquid, the plasma.

Connective tissue may be classified as (1) loose connective tissue, (2) dense connective tissue, (3) supporting connective tissue, and (4) blood.

LOOSE CONNECTIVE TISSUE

Loose connective tissue is soft and pliable and serves as a kind of packing material between other tissues and organs (Figs. 4-1 and 4-2). It is found between muscles, allowing one to move freely over the other. It fills the spaces between the secretory units of glands and supports small blood vessels, lymphatic vessels, and nerves. Its structure consists of a number of different types of cells and fibers suspended in a semifluid intercellular material.

Cells

Six types of cells are present in loose connective tissue: (1) fibroblasts, (2) fat (adipose) cells, (3) plasma cells, (4) mast cells, (5) histiocytes, and (6)

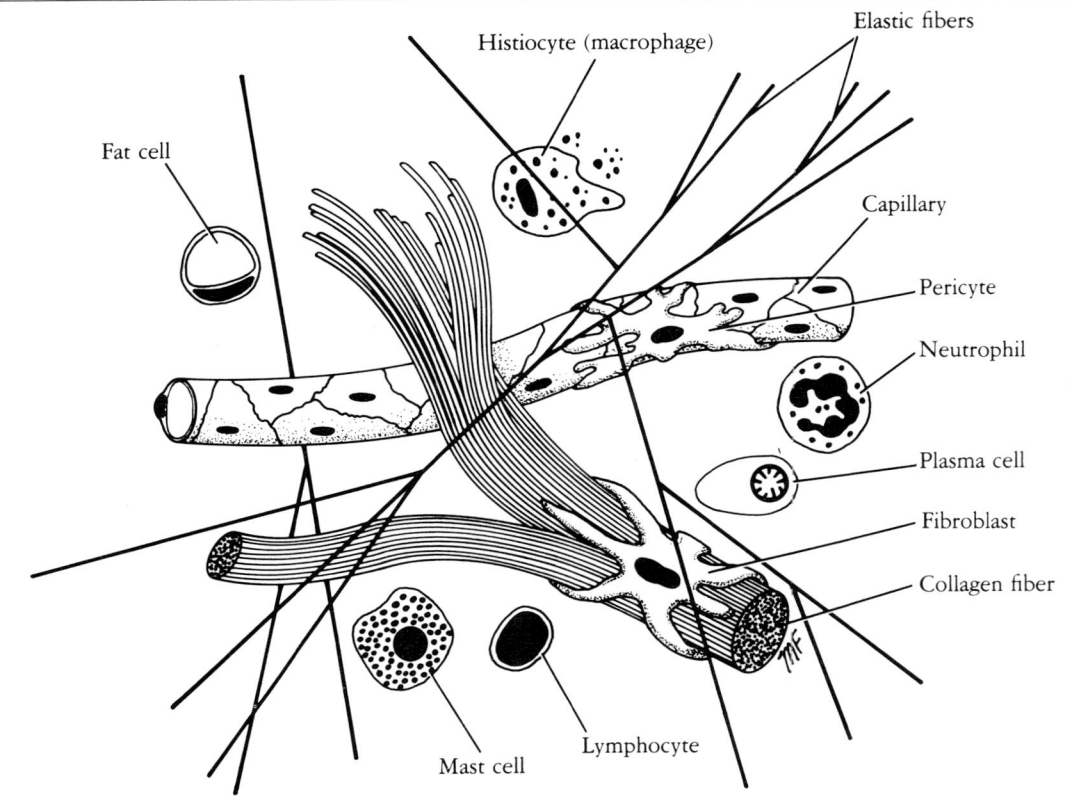

Fig. 4-1. Loose connective tissue. The different types of cells and fibers are illustrated.

uncommitted mesenchymal cells. In addition, certain cells emigrate from the blood and wander through the connective tissue: neutrophils, eosinophils, lymphocytes, and monocytes. It is the wandering cells that protect the tissue against invasion from microorganisms.

Fibroblasts

Fibroblasts are responsible for the formation of collagen, elastic, and reticular fibers and the amorphous material (Figs. 4-3 and 4-4). The older, nonproductive cells are commonly called *fibrocytes*. Fibroblasts are the most numerous cells seen in loose connective tissue. They are irregularly shaped or fusiform. In microscopical preparations stained with hematoxylin and eosin, the outlines of the cells appear indistinct. The cytoplasm stains weakly pink with eosin, but the spindle-shaped nucleus stains deeply with hematoxylin. Young, active fibroblasts have an abundant cytoplasm, and their nuclei have prominent nucleoli. Fibrocytes, in contrast, have little cytoplasm.

Fat Cells

Fat cells may have only a few droplets of fat within their cytoplasm, or there may be so much fat within them that the droplets have fused to form one large drop of fat (Fig. 4-5). When such fusion occurs, the drop of fat may greatly expand the cell from within and displace the cytoplasm and nucleus to the edge of the cell. The cell on cross section then has a "signet ring" appearance (see Fig. 4-5). In most his-

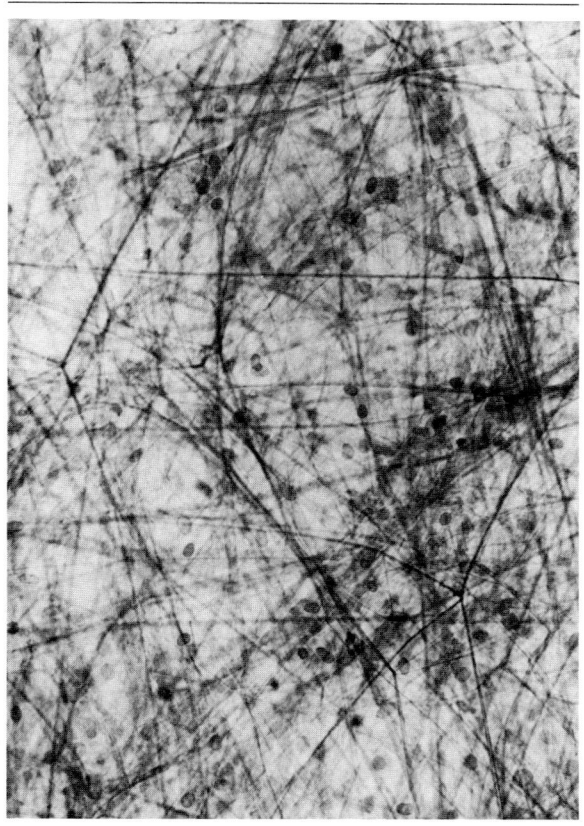

Fig. 4-2. Photomicrograph of a teased preparation of loose connective tissue. The elastic fibers are visible as thin, dark, branching filaments. The collagen fibers are lighter in color and cannot be seen clearly. Numerous nuclei of connective tissue cells are also visible. (H&E; ×200.)

tological sections, the fat has been dissolved, leaving only the empty space and the surrounding cytoplasm (Fig. 4-6). If the specimens are fixed and stained with osmic acid, the fat appears as black or brown globules (Fig. 4-7). In frozen sections, the fat stains orange with Sudan III.

Fat cells are found scattered throughout the body in loose connective tissue. In certain locations, such as under the skin, within the greater omentum, behind the peritoneum, around the kidneys, and around the heart, the connective tissue becomes dominated by fat cells. This form of connective tissue is referred to as *adipose tissue.*

The distribution of adipose tissue in the body differs in the two sexes. In the male, it is found in large quantities in the nape of the neck and in the subcutaneous tissue over the deltoid and triceps muscles. It is also present in large amounts in the subcutaneous tissue of the buttocks. In the female, adipose tissue is abundant in the mammary glands, the buttocks, and the thighs.

The fat present in fat cells has been formed within the cells and is derived from the fat in an individual's diet and from carbohydrate and protein. The storage of fat and the mobilization of fat is regulated by hormones. For example, insulin stimulates fat storage and inhibits fat mobilization, whereas adrenocorticotropic hormone (ACTH), thyroxin, and glucagon have the reverse effect.

Adipose tissue serves as a storehouse for fat; it may act as an insulator, protecting the individual from excessive heat loss. It also serves to support and protect organs from physical trauma.

Mature fat cells are incapable of division, and it is believed that new fat cells are derived from mesenchymal cells.

Brown adipose tissue is a special form of adipose tissue, which should be distinguished from the white adipose tissue forming almost all the adipose tissue of the body. Its brown color is caused by pigment in the fat and the high vascularity of this tissue. Brown fat differs from white adipose tissue in that the fat cells contain numerous fat droplets that do not coalesce, and the cells are directly innervated by sympathetic nerve fibers. It is present in large amounts in human fetuses and neonates and is then gradually replaced by white fat. Brown fat can be mobilized rapidly if the individual is exposed to cold. Starvation, however, fails to mobilize brown fat.

Plasma Cells

These cells are commonly rounded and possess abundant cytoplasm (see Fig. 4-5C). The nucleus is round and often eccentrically placed. Most of the

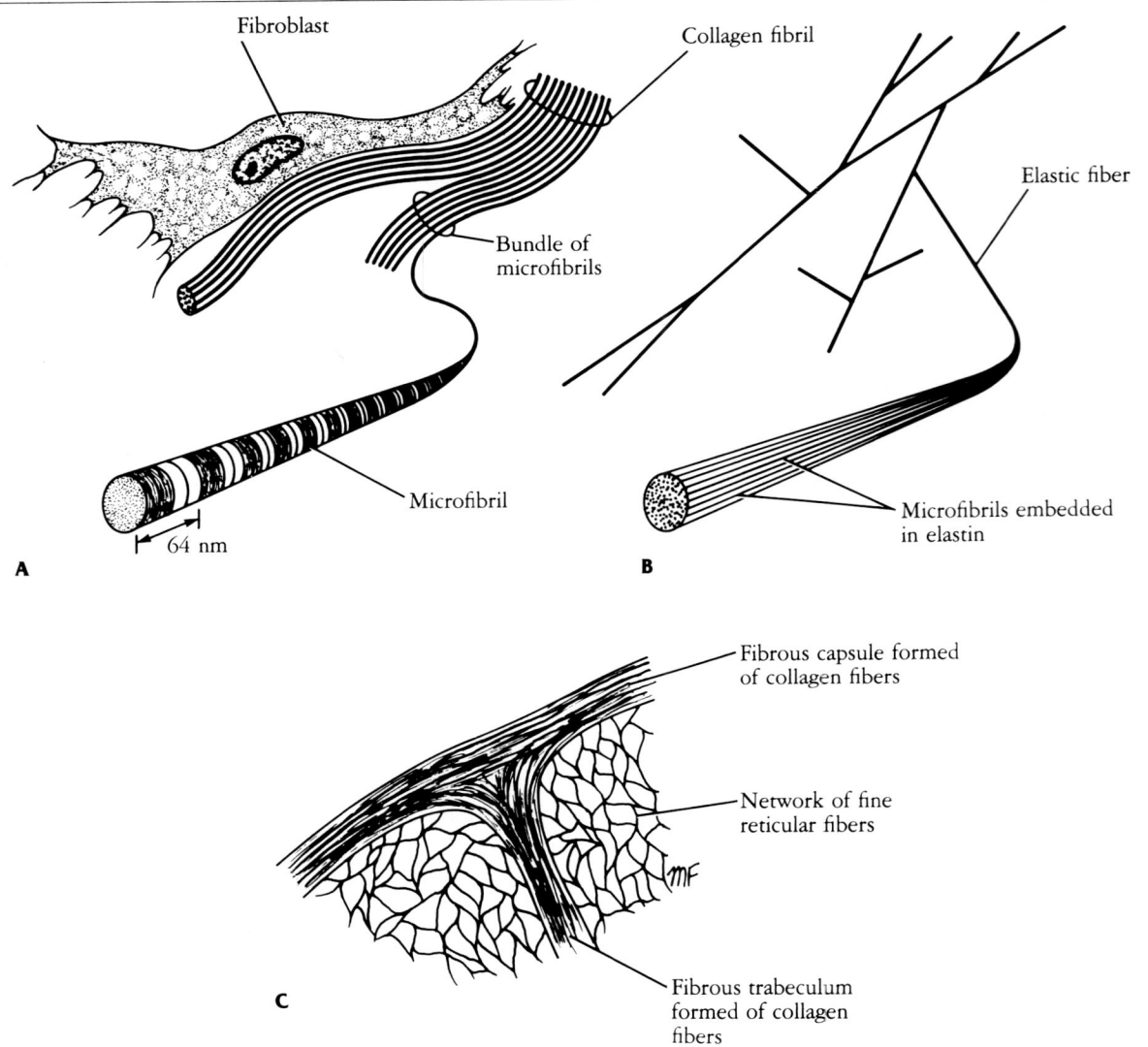

Fig. 4-3. (A) Fibroblast with exploded view of collagen microfibril. (B) Elastic fiber with exploded view of microfibril. (C) Fibrous capsule and trabeculum of lymph node formed of collagen fibers; a network of fine reticular fibers is suspended from these structures.

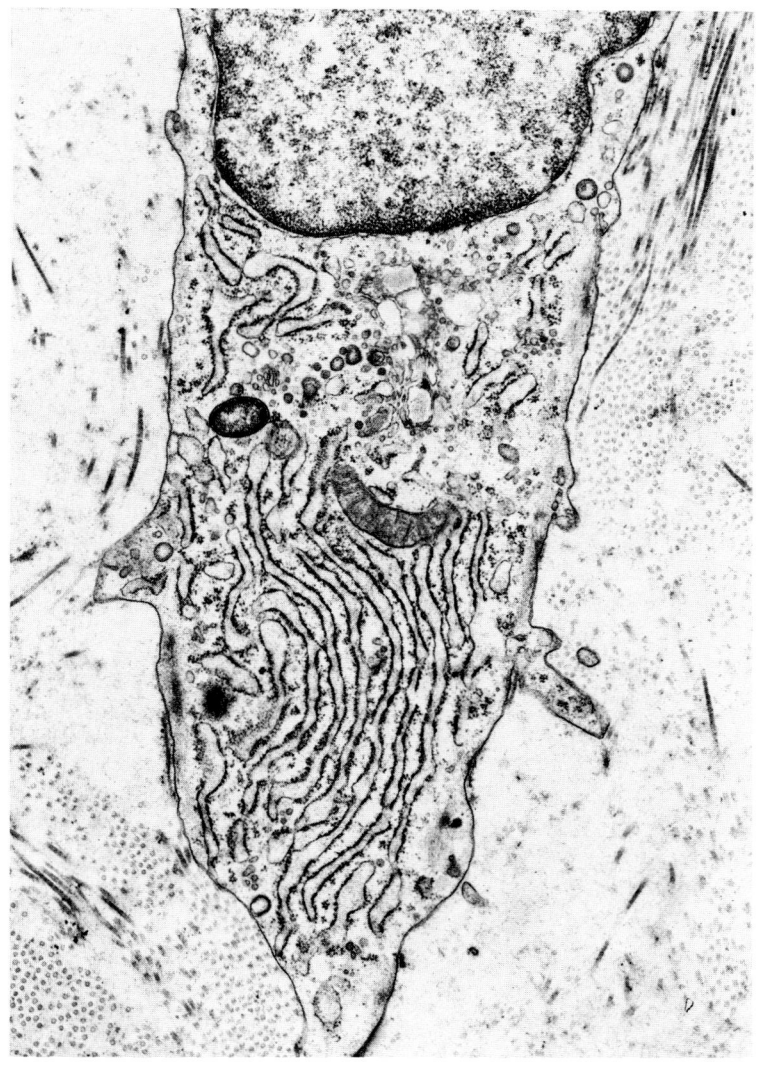

Fig. 4-4. Electron micrograph of a fibroblast actively forming collagen fibrils. Note the well-developed rough endoplasmic reticulum within the cytoplasm. (Courtesy of Dr. R. Ross.)

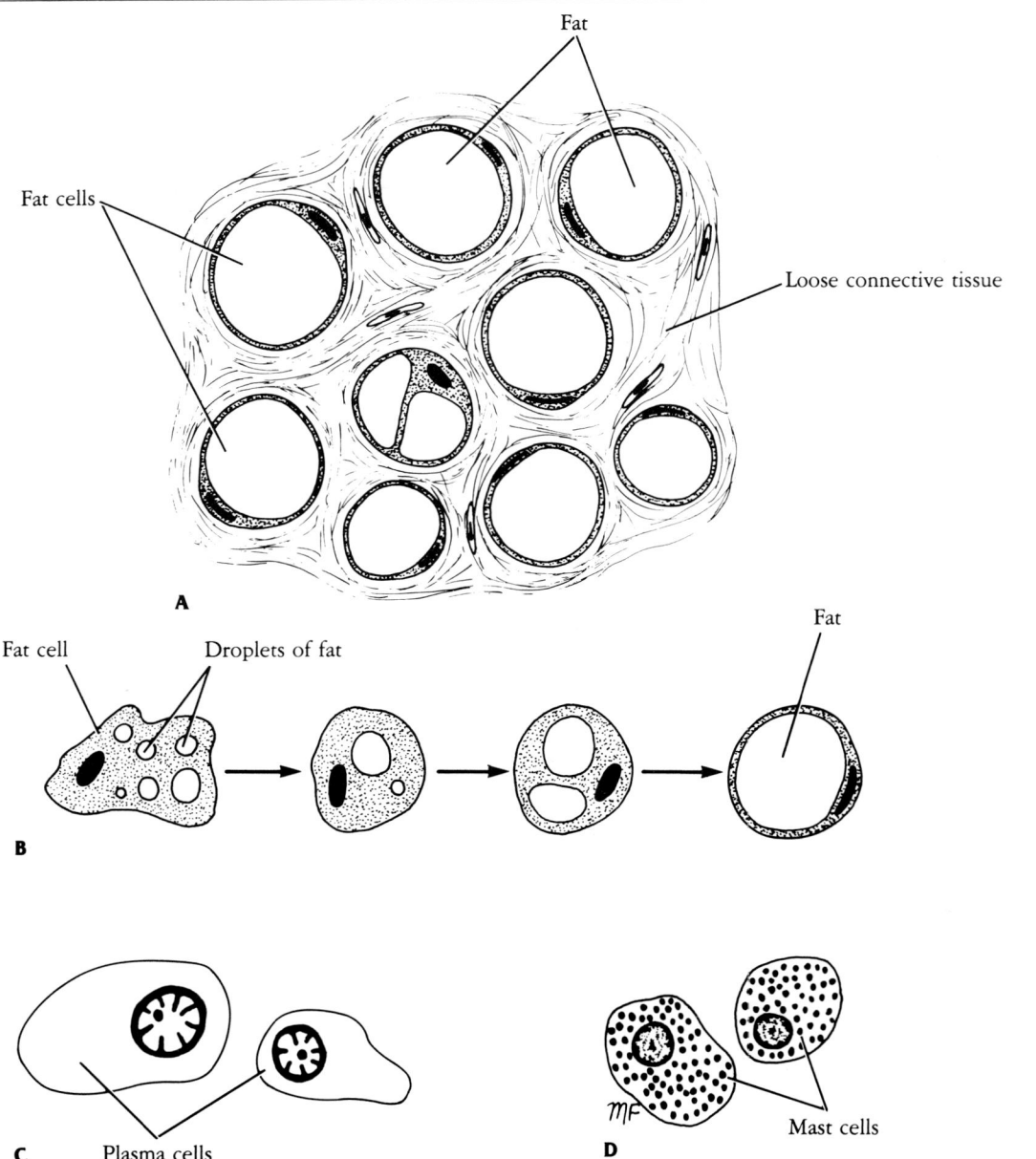

Fig. 4-5. (A) Adipose tissue; (B) a fat cell in the process of storing fat; (C) plasma cells, showing the "clock face" arrangement of the nuclear chromatin; (D) mast cells, showing the prominent cytoplasmic granules containing heparin and histamine.

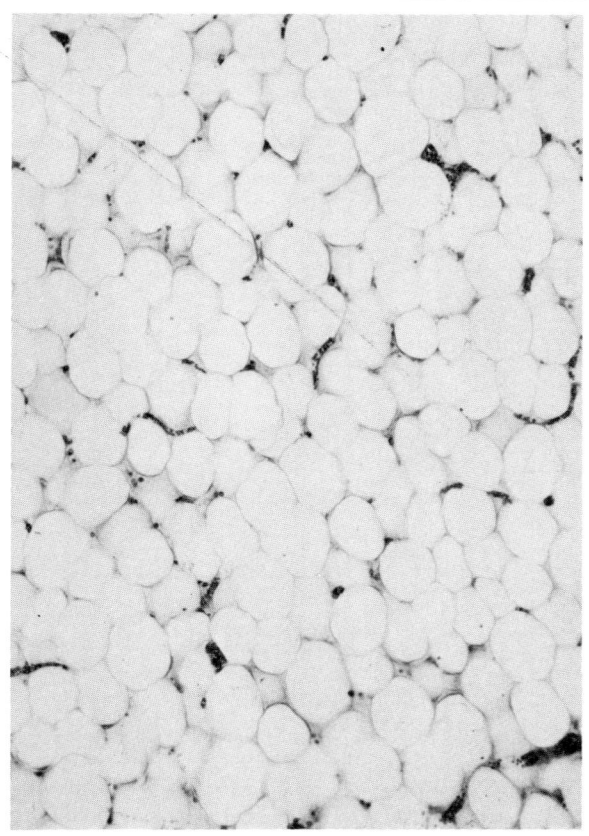

Fig. 4-6. Photomicrograph of a section of adipose tissue. The fat has been dissolved out of the section during the preparation of the slide, leaving large, empty spaces in the cytoplasm. (H&E; ×100.)

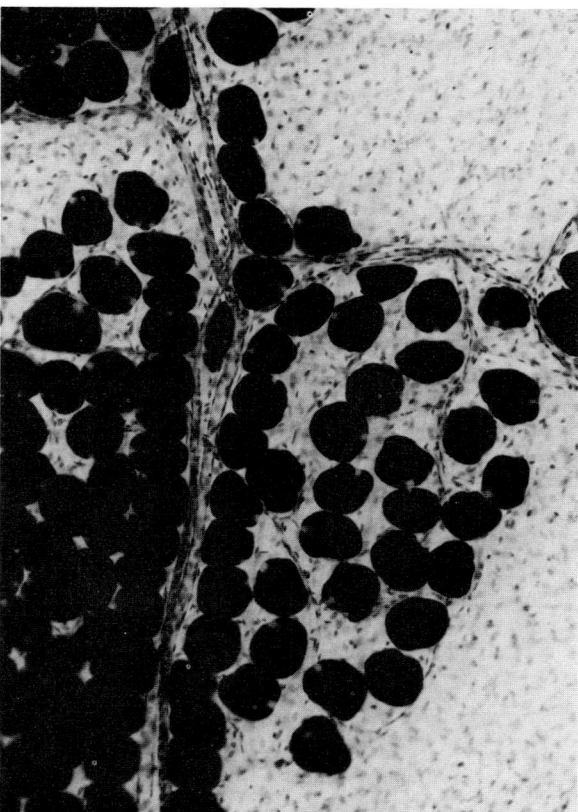

Fig. 4-7. Photomicrograph of a group of fat cells in the mesentery of the small intestine. The fat has been stained with osmic acid and looks black. (×100.)

chromatin of the nucleus is condensed into flakes that are arranged in the nucleus like the numbers on a clock face (Fig. 4-8).

Plasma cells are not present in large numbers in general connective tissue but are found in the connective tissue of the lining of the gastrointestinal tract and in lymphatic tissues.

Plasma cells are formed from B lymphocytes of the blood (see p. 341). The lymphocytes enter the connective tissue and differentiate into plasma cells. The function of plasma cells is to produce antibodies, which are released locally and circulate in the blood. Plasma cells therefore play an important role in defending the body against infection.

Mast Cells

Mast cells are rounded or spindle-shaped, and their cytoplasm is packed with granules that stain metachromatically with basic aniline dyes (Figs. 4-9 and 4-10). The nucleus is relatively small and is obscured by the granules. Mast cells are distributed throughout connective tissues and tend to be situated close to small blood vessels.

The granules of mast cells contain *heparin* and

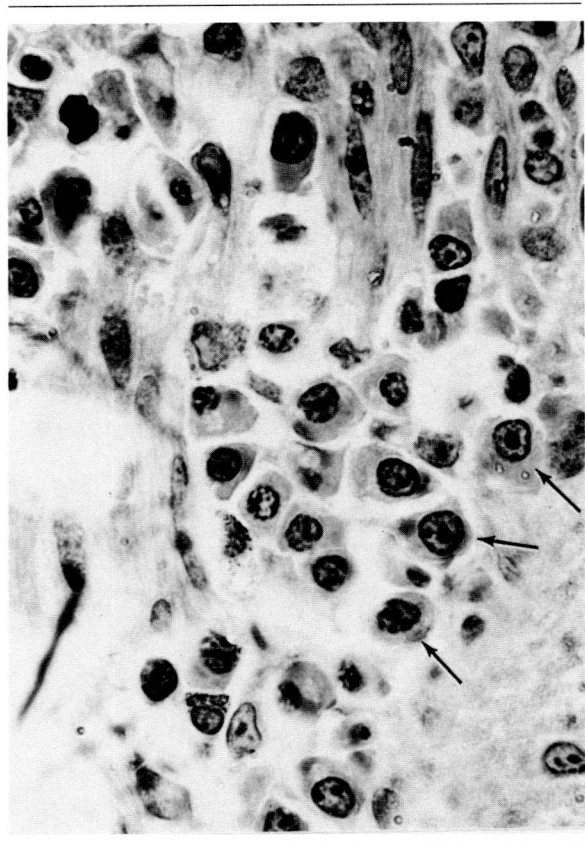

Fig. 4-8. Photomicrograph of a plastic section of loose connective tissue in the wall of the small intestine. Numerous plasma cells and the "clock face" arrangement of their nuclear chromatin (arrows) are visible. (H&E; ×1,000.)

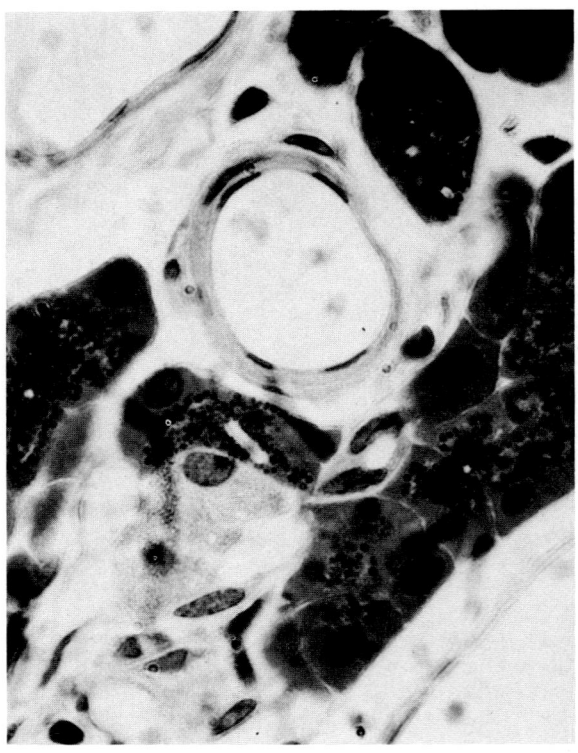

Fig. 4-9. Photomicrograph of a plastic section of loose connective tissue in the wall of the small intestine, showing many mast cells with prominent cytoplasmic granules grouped around a blood capillary. (Toluidine blue; ×1,000.)

histamine (see Fig. 4-5D). Heparin is known to prevent blood clotting and the agglutination of platelets. The cells release histamine in anaphylaxis in response to an antigen. The signs and symptoms of anaphylaxis (exaggerated reaction to foreign protein) are caused by the actions of histamine on blood vessels. Histamine causes arteriolar and capillary dilatation and increased capillary permeability, which in turn produce a drop in blood pressure. Respiratory distress may also occur, caused by edema of the mucous membrane of the respiratory tract and constriction of the smooth muscle of the bronchi.

Although mast cells resemble the basophils of the blood, which also possess metachromatic granules, they are believed to be unrelated.

Histiocytes

Histiocytes, or macrophages, are found scattered throughout the connective tissue (Fig. 4-11; see Fig. 4-1). They are very mobile cells and are capable of phagocytosing and digesting foreign and other particulate matter. This capability is evidenced by the numerous vacuoles, lysosomes, and residual bodies in their cytoplasm. They may be irregularly shaped or oval and usually possess an oval or indented nucleus. Their cytoplasm stains pink with eosin. Histiocytes have a protective function: they rid the body of foreign matter and debris from worn-out

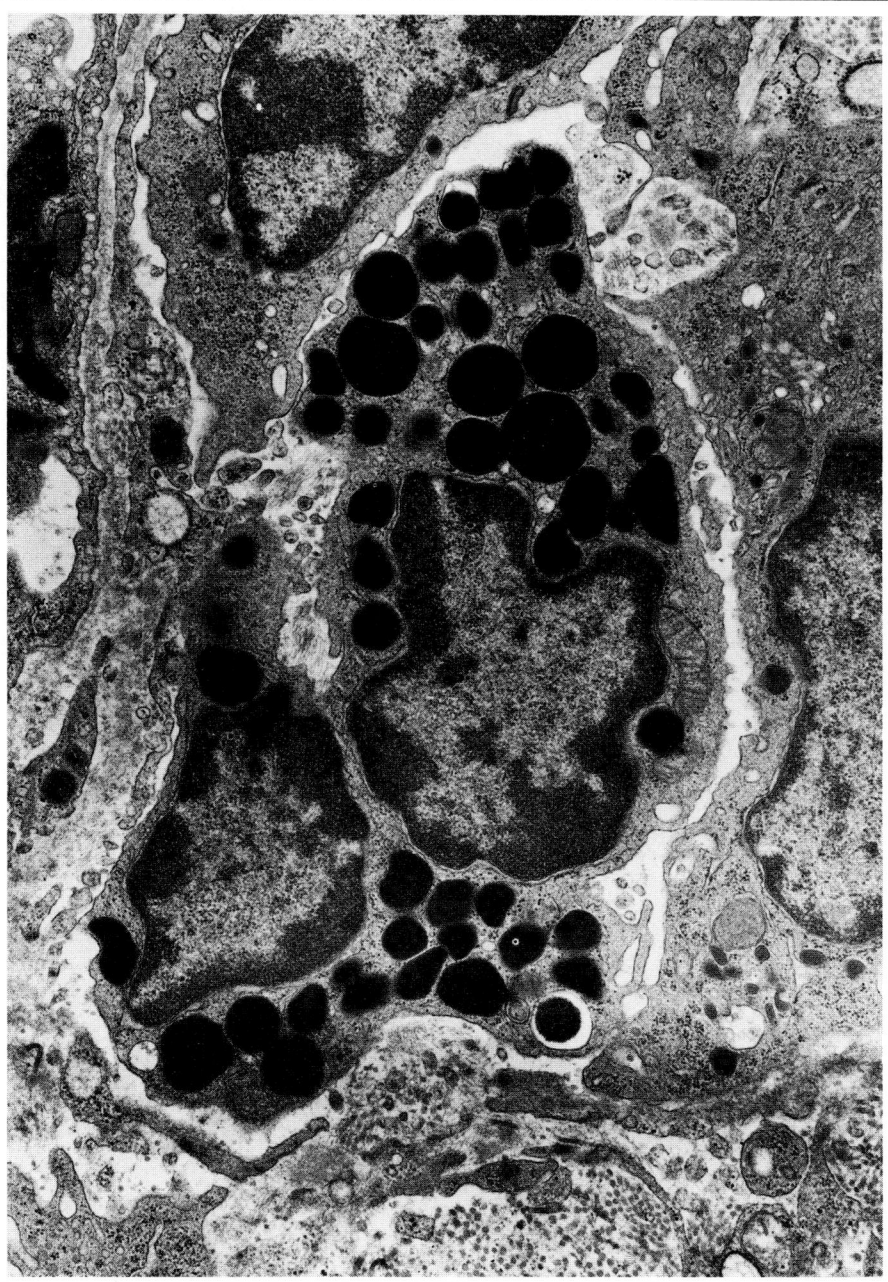

Fig. 4-10. Electron micrograph of a mast cell with a lobed nucleus. The cell contains numerous dark, membrane-bound granules within its cytoplasm. (× 17,000.) (Courtesy of Dr. V. W. Dimlich.)

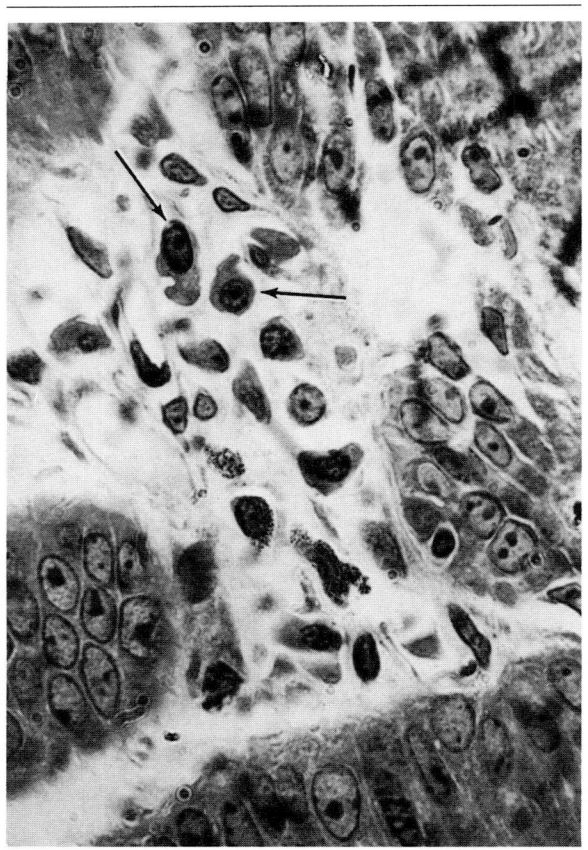

Fig. 4-11. Photomicrograph of a plastic section of loose connective tissue in the wall of the small intestine, showing two histiocytes (arrows). (H&E; ×1,000.)

cells. They also secrete a number of enzymes, including *elastase, collagenase,* and *lysozyme.* They are involved in the production of proteins in the complement system and the formation of *interferon,* an antiviral substance.

It is now believed that histiocytes are associated with the formation of specific antibodies by lymphocytes. The antigen is phagocytosed in the foreign material by the histiocyte. In this manner, the antigen is liberated, inducing the lymphocytes to react and become plasma cells. The plasma cells in turn form antibodies.

Histiocytes are formed from monocytes in the blood that have entered the connective tissue; they may also be formed from undifferentiated mesenchymal cells. Histiocytes, together with other cells in the body that have the ability to phagocytose particulate matter, belong to the *mononuclear phagocytic system,* the *reticuloendothelial system* (see p. 358).

Foreign body giant cells are very large cells with multiple nuclei that have formed from the fusion of several histiocytes (Fig. 4-12). They are formed when very large particles of foreign material, such as a wooden splinter, are introduced into connective tissue. Once formed, such a cell can enclose or phagocytose a large particle in an attempt to remove it from the body (see Fig. 4-12).

Uncommitted Mesenchymal Cells

These cells closely resemble fibroblasts and can give rise to other normal connective tissue cells, such as fat cells or fibroblasts. Their name stems from the fact that they retain the developmental multipotentiality of embryonic mesenchymal cells. They are thought to be important in forming new fibroblasts in the process of wound healing and may form other cell types, such as osteoblasts, in certain circumstances. The latter capability would explain the occasional appearance of bone in a healing wound.

Fibers

Three types of fibers are present in loose connective tissue: (1) collagen fibers, (2) elastic fibers, and (3) reticular fibers.

Collagen Fibers

Collagen fibers are composed of the protein *collagen.* They have great tensile strength and are inelastic. In sections stained with hematoxylin and eosin, they stain weakly pink with eosin; they stain red with van Gieson's stain, blue with Mallory's connective tissue stain, and green with Masson's trichrome stain. The fibers measure between 1 and 10 μm in thickness and are of indefinite length. They occur singly or in bundles and have a straight or slightly wavy course (Figs. 4-13 and 4-14).

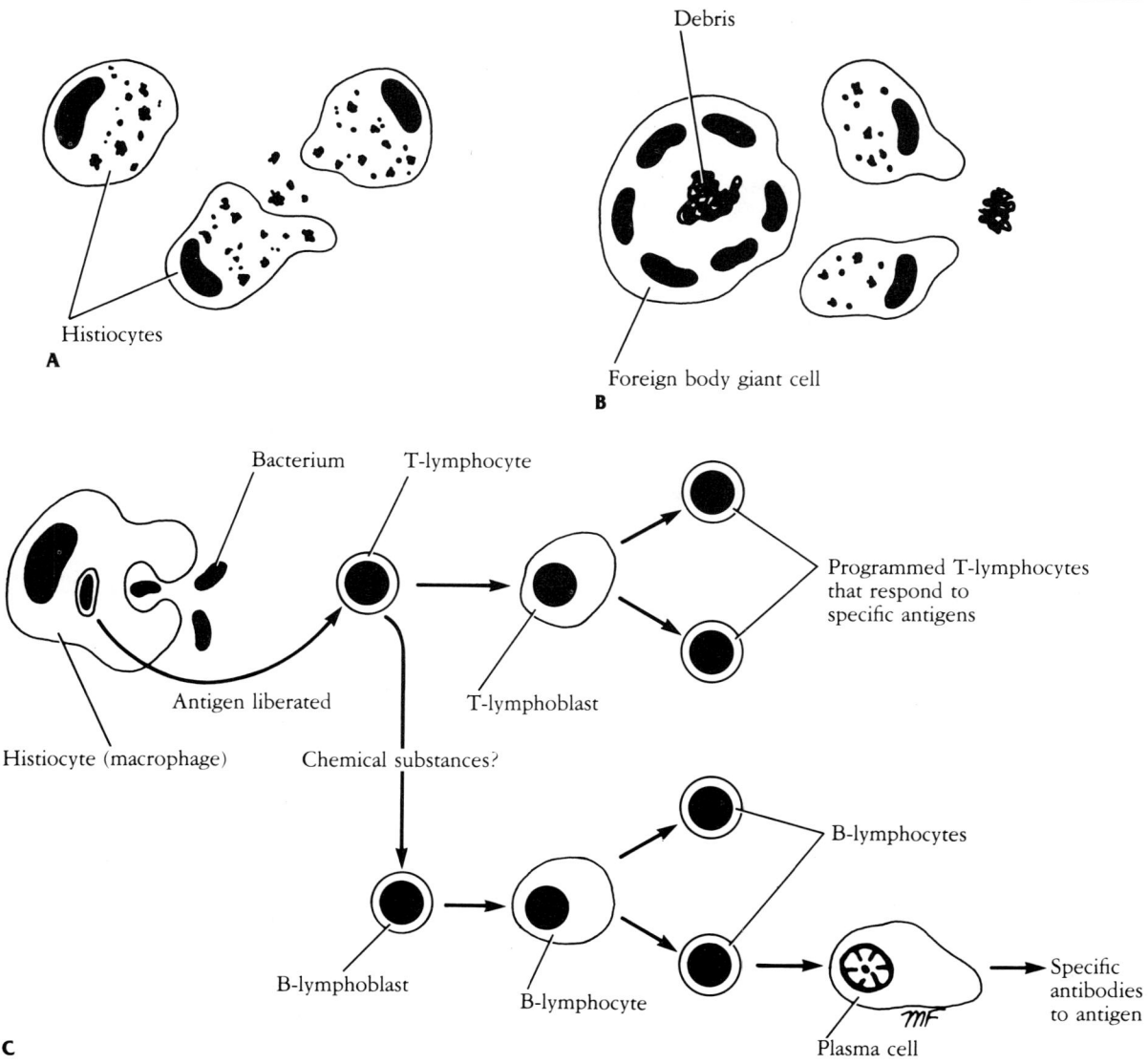

Fig. 4-12. (A) Histiocytes (macrophages) phagocytosing and digesting foreign particulate matter. (B) A foreign body giant cell and two histiocytes. (C) A histiocyte liberating antigens from a bacterium; the antigens then activate the T and B lymphocytes.

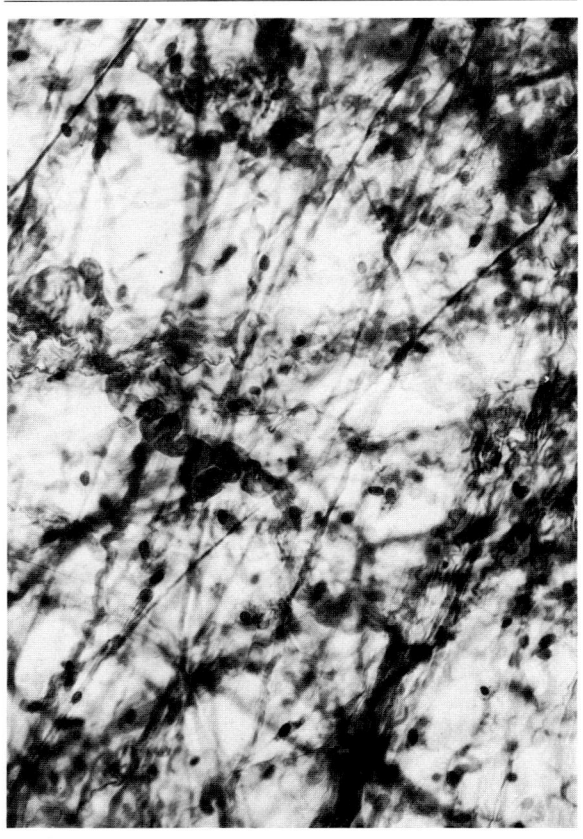

Fig. 4-13. Photomicrograph of a teased preparation of loose connective tissue, showing wavy bundles of collagen fibers and some thin, dark-staining elastic fibers. (H&E; ×200.)

Each collagen fiber is composed of parallel aggregations of many *fibrils* (Fig. 4-15). In turn, each fibril is composed of bundles of parallel *microfibrils*. The microfibrils can be seen only with the electron microscope and measure between 20 and 100 nm in thickness. They show characteristic major crossbanding with a periodicity of 64 nm; several minor crossbands can be seen between the major bands (Figs. 4-16 and 4-17).

Each microfibril is composed chemically of molecules of *tropocollagen,* each of which is about 260 nm long and 1.5 nm thick (see Fig. 4-15). Each tropocollagen molecule is made up of three polypeptide chains, called *alpha* units, that have a helical configuration and are coiled around one another in a right-handed direction; they are connected by cross links. Each polypeptide chain is rich in *glycine* and contains the amino acids *hydroxyproline* and *hydroxylysine*. It is interesting that the crossbanding of the microfibrils just discussed is caused by the overlapping of the parallel-running tropocollagen molecules along one-quarter of their length.

The collagen fibers found in loose connective tissue are formed by fibroblasts that secrete tropocollagen in its monomeric form. Polymerization of the tropocollagen takes place outside the cell. It should be pointed out that the collagen fibers of cartilage are formed by the chondroblasts and those in bone by the osteoblasts. In some organs, smooth muscle cells can synthesize collagen.

Collagen fibers are important mechanically in loose connective tissue, because they are flexible but strongly resist a pulling force.

Elastic Fibers

There are fewer elastic fibers than collagen fibers in loose connective tissue (Fig. 4-18). Elastic fibers are composed of the protein *elastin*. They are not as strong as collagen fibers. They stretch easily but return to their original length when the stretching force is removed. They stain a weak pink in sections stained with hematoxylin and eosin. They stain brown with orcein and blue-purple with resorcin-fuchsin. The fibers measure about 0.2 to 1.0 μm in thickness and branch and anastomose to form networks (see Fig. 4-18).

With the electron microscope, each elastic fiber is seen to be composed mainly of amorphous material (Fig. 4-19). At the periphery of each fiber, *microfibrils* measuring about 11 nm in thickness can be seen. There is no crossbanding.

Elastic fibers are formed by fibroblasts and smooth muscle cells. It is thought that a precursor is

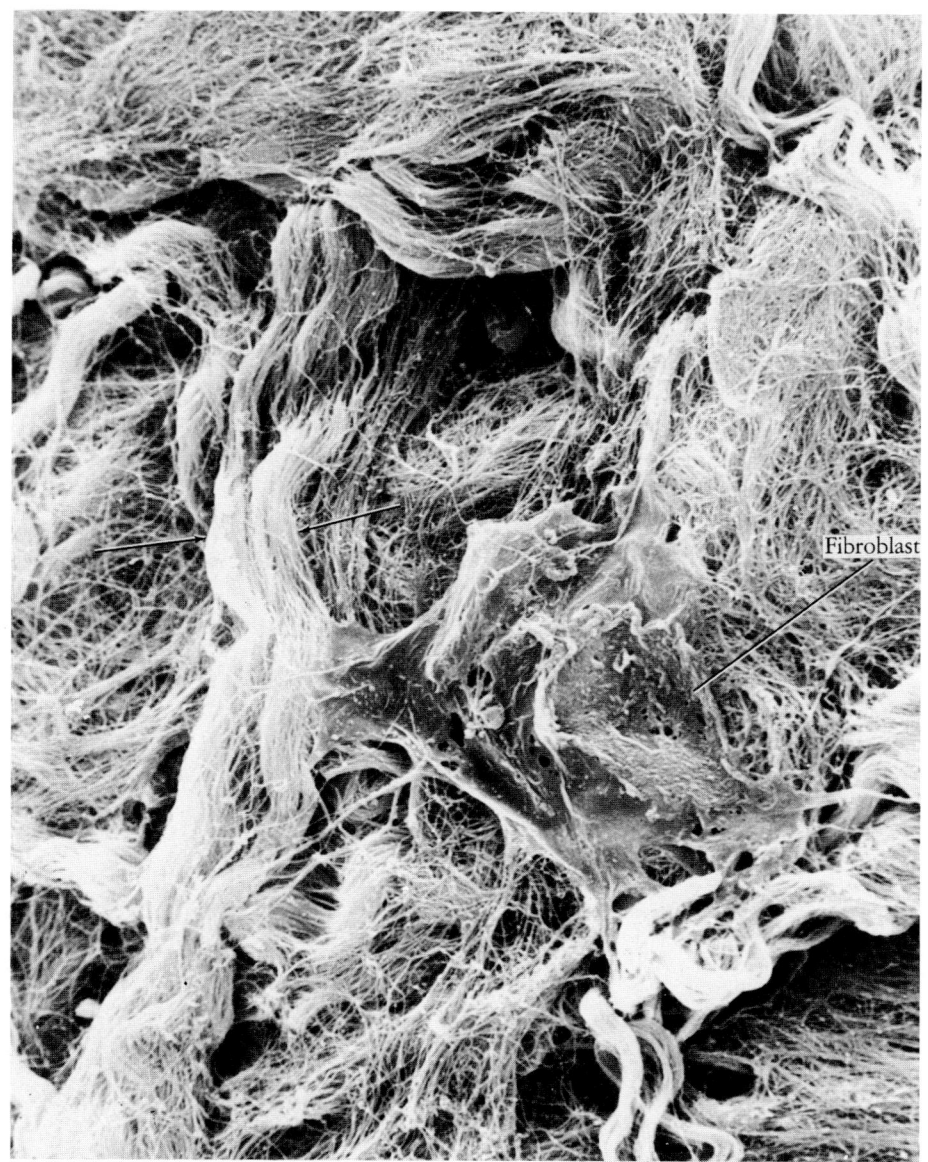

Fig. 4-14. Scanning electron micrograph of connective tissue, showing **bundles of collagen fibers** (between arrows) *close to a fibroblast.* (×1,134.) *(Courtesy of Dr. P. Andrews.)*

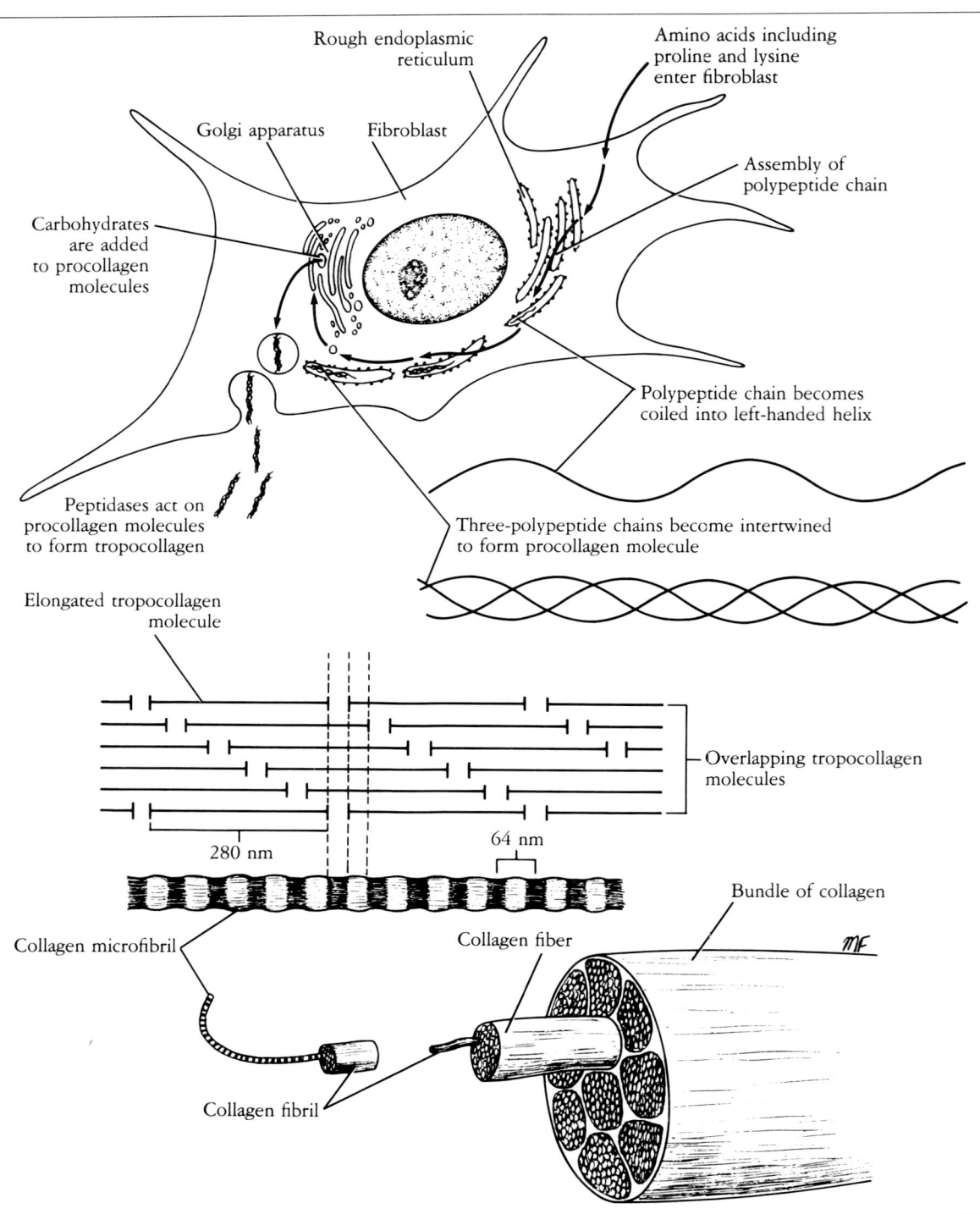

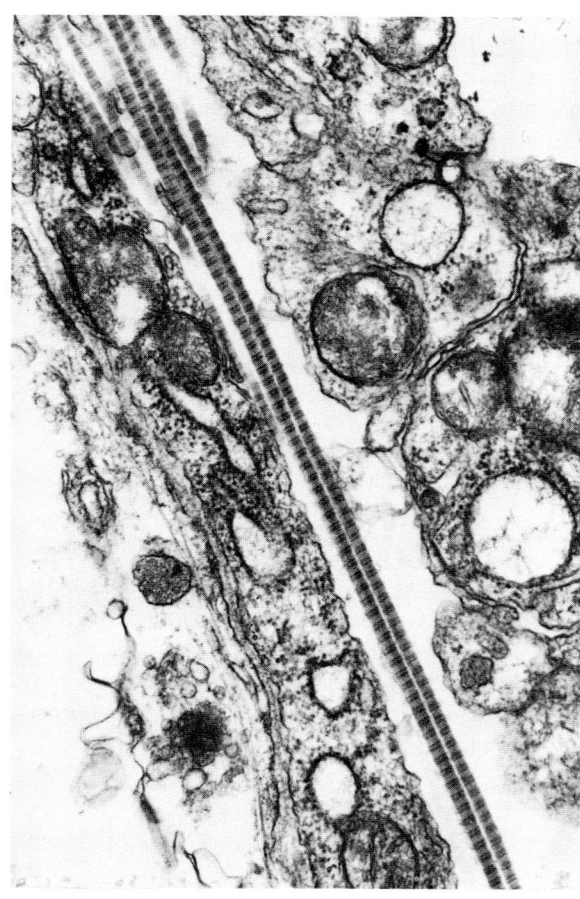

Fig. 4-16. Electron micrograph of a longitudinal section of a microfibril, showing the repeating periodicity characteristic of individual fibrils. (×13,774.) (Courtesy of Drs. D. E. Morse and F. N. Low.)

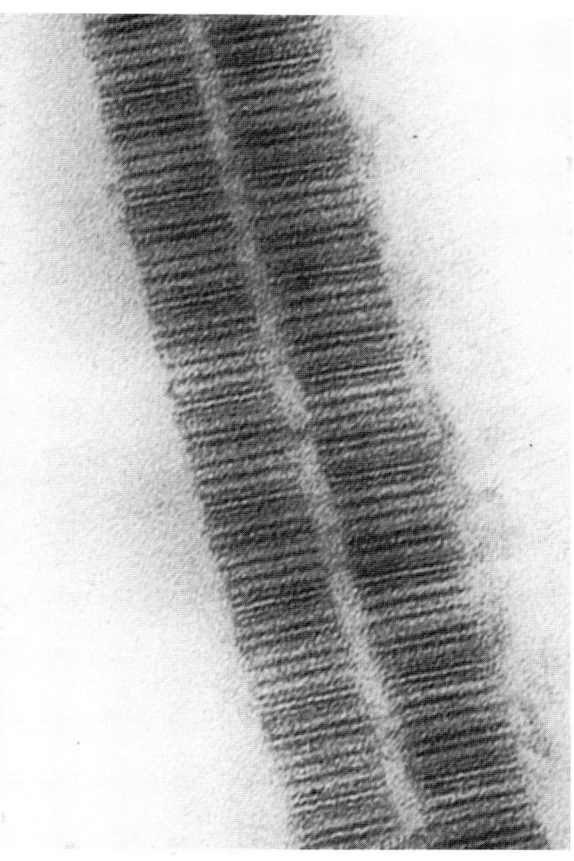

Fig. 4-17. Electron micrograph of a high-power view of a longitudinal section of a microfibril, showing the major and minor crossbands. (×103,360.) (Courtesy of Drs. D. E. Morse and F. N. Low.)

Fig. 4-15. The stages in the formation of collagen by fibroblasts. The dark and light crossbands of the collagen microfibrils seen in electron micrographs are produced by the overlapping of the rodlike tropocollagen subunits, each of which measures 280 nm. The gaps between the ends of the adjacent tropocollagen molecules hold more stain; this is thought to be the explanation for the dark bands. Note how the collagen microfibrils are collected to form collagen fibrils; these in turn become assembled to form collagen fibers and, finally, bundles of collagen fibers.

secreted by those cells and the elastic fibers are assembled outside the cells.

Reticular Fibers

Reticular fibers are very thin collagen fibers and have similar periodic crossbanding. They cannot be seen in ordinary histological sections stained with hematoxylin and eosin. They can be demonstrated by silver impregnation methods, with which they are seen as thin, dark lines (Fig. 4-20). Reticular fibers are often found to be continuous with collagen fibers. Like collagen fibers, they are formed by fibro-

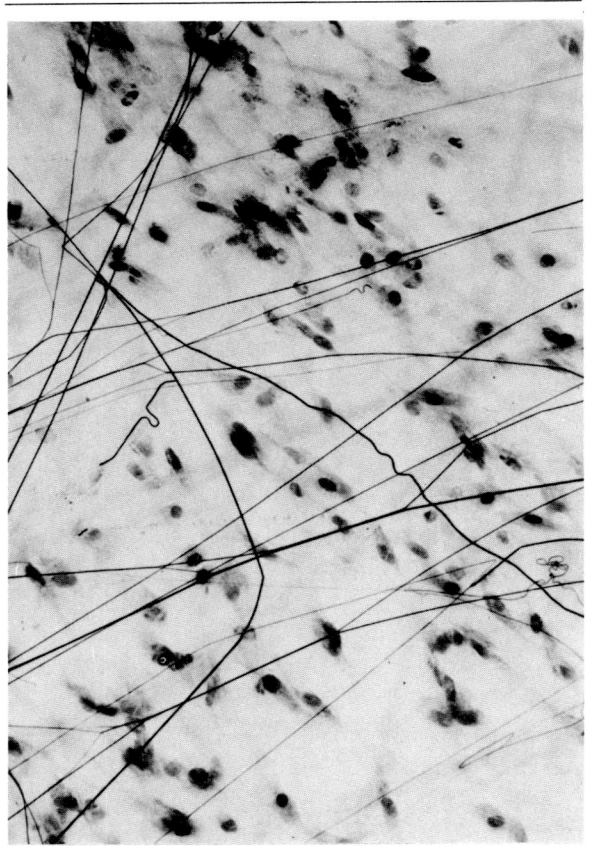

Fig. 4-18. Photomicrograph of a preparation of loose connective tissue, showing elastic fibers as thin, dark, branching filaments. Numerous connective tissue cells can be seen in the background. (H&E; ×200.)

blasts, chondroblasts, osteoblasts, and epithelial cells.

Reticular fibers form delicate networks around blood vessels and adipose tissue cells and are present in the endoneurium of nerves. They provide a supporting framework for lymphoid and blood-forming organs.

Amorphous Material

The amorphous material, or ground substance, is the material between the cells in which the fibers we have described are embedded. It permits the diffusion of tissue fluid containing nutrients and waste products between the blood and lymphatic capillaries and the cells. The gel-like nature of the material provides support for the tissue and serves as a physical barrier to the spread of microorganisms. Apart from water and salts, the amorphous material is composed of different types of mucopolysaccharides, including hyaluronic acid and chondroitin-sulphuric acid; there are also variable amounts of tropocollagen and glycoproteins. Fibroblasts are responsible for the synthesis of the amorphous material in loose connective tissue; it is also produced by chondroblasts and osteoblasts in cartilage and bone, respectively.

DENSE CONNECTIVE TISSUE

Dense connective tissue differs from loose connective tissue in that it possesses a far greater number of collagen fibers in the intercellular substance. In fact, the fibers are so densely packed together that there are only a few cells and only a small amount of amorphous intercellular material. Dense connective tissue is found in tendons, ligaments, aponeuroses, the capsules of organs, and the deep fasciae.

Tendons and Fibrous Ligaments

These structures consist of dense, regularly arranged bundles of collagen fibers, all of which run in the same basic direction (Fig. 4-21). Because the bundles run in the same direction, tendons and ligaments have great tensile strength (Fig. 4-22). The majority of the cells are fibrocytes that are situated between the bundles of collagen fibers. Tendons must have great tensile strength, because they join muscles to bones; so must ligaments that join bones to bones.

Fig. 4-19. Electron micrograph of elastic fibers and collagen fibrils in the wall of an artery. The elastic fibers (EF) are seen in longitudinal and transverse sections; microfibrils (M) are situated in association with the amorphous elastin. The collagen fibrils (CF) are also clearly visible. (×72,000.) (Courtesy of Drs. R. Ross and P. Bornstein.)

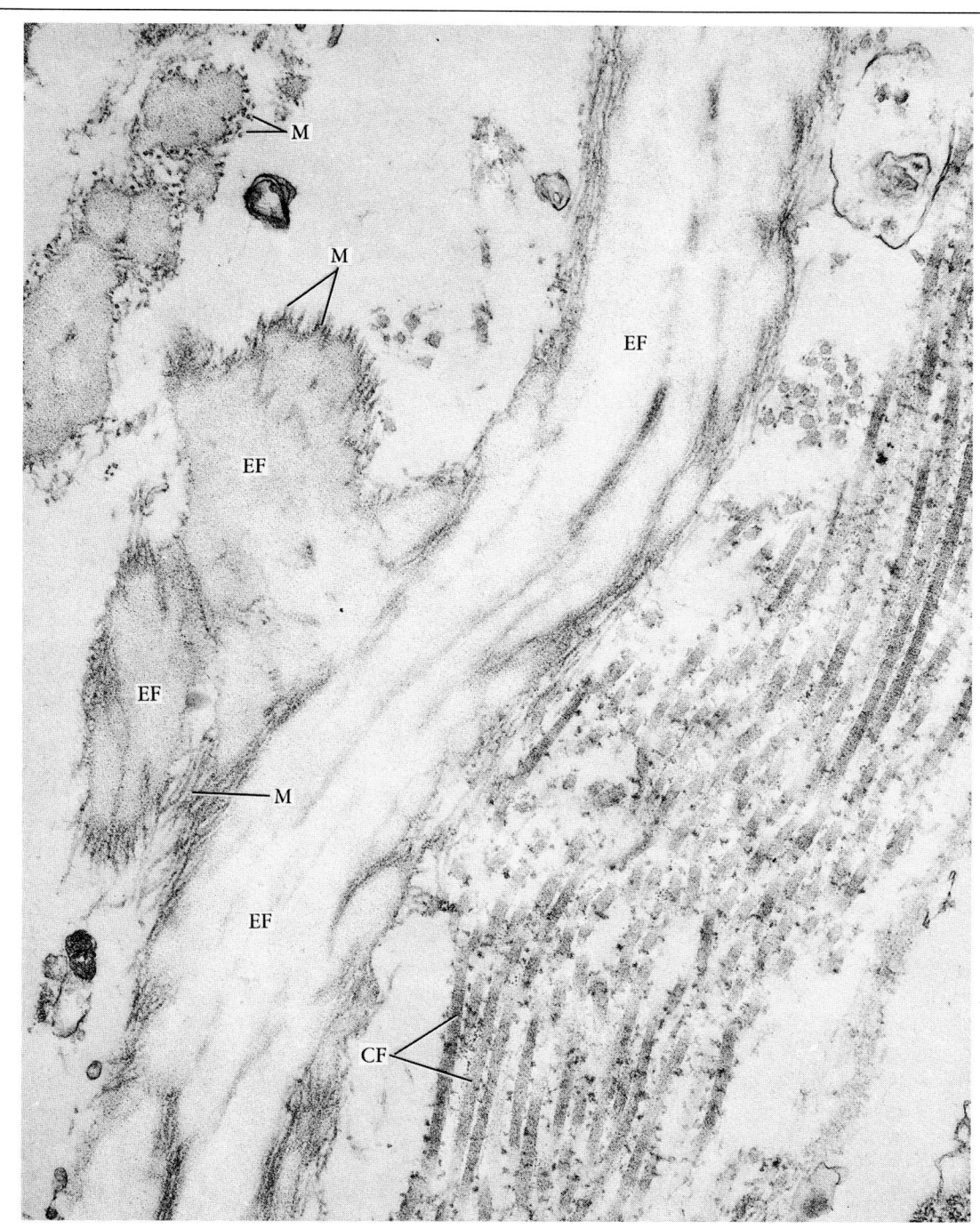

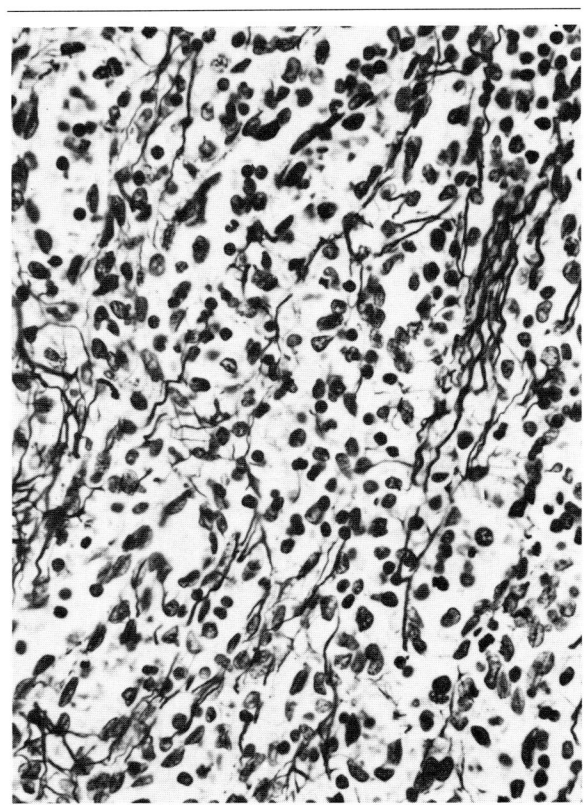

Fig. 4-20. Photomicrograph of reticular fibers in the medulla of a lymph node. The reticular fibers are seen as a network of thin, dark, wavy fibers supporting the lymphatic tissue. (Silver stain; ×400.)

Aponeuroses and Capsules of Organs

These structures consist of dense, irregularly arranged bundles of collagen fibers that run in different directions and often in different planes (see Fig. 4-21). Here also, the cells are few in number and are situated between the bundles of collagen fibers. Aponeuroses are flattened sheets connecting muscles with one another or with bones. Capsules are fibrous coverings of certain organs, such as the lymph nodes and the testes.

Elastic Ligaments

Certain ligaments, such as the important *ligamentum nuchae* on the back of the neck (Figs. 4-23 and 4-24) and the *ligamentum flavum* between adjacent vertebrae, are composed almost entirely of elastic tissue. They will therefore return to their original length after stretching. The fibroblasts that produce the elastic fibers are few in number and are situated between the fibers.

Fasciae

The fasciae of the body can be divided into two types, the *superficial* and the *deep.* They lie between the skin and the underlying muscles and bones.

The *superficial fascia,* or subcutaneous tissue, is a mixture of loose connective tissue and adipose tissue that unites the dermis of the skin with the underlying deep fascia (see Fig. 4-21).

The *deep fascia* is a membranous layer of dense connective tissue that invests the muscles and other deep structures (see Fig. 4-21). In the neck, it forms well-defined layers that support the muscles and viscera. It may play an important role in determining the route taken by pathogenic organisms during the spread of infection. In the thorax and abdomen, it is merely a thin film of loose connective tissue that covers and lies between the muscles, permitting them to move easily upon one another. In the limbs, the deep fascia forms a definite sheath around muscles and other structures, holding them in place. Fibrous septa extend from the deep surface of the membrane, between the groups of muscles, and, in many places, divide the interior of the limbs into compartments.

SUPPORTING CONNECTIVE TISSUE

Cartilage and bone are connective tissues in which the amorphous intercellular substance is hardened to provide rigidity, support, and attachment for tissues.

Cartilage

Cartilage is a form of connective tissue that is much firmer than dense connective tissue. It consists of a dense network of collagen and elastic fibers embedded in a gel-like intercellular material. This intercellular material is responsible for its firmness but also permits it to remain flexible. The main constituent

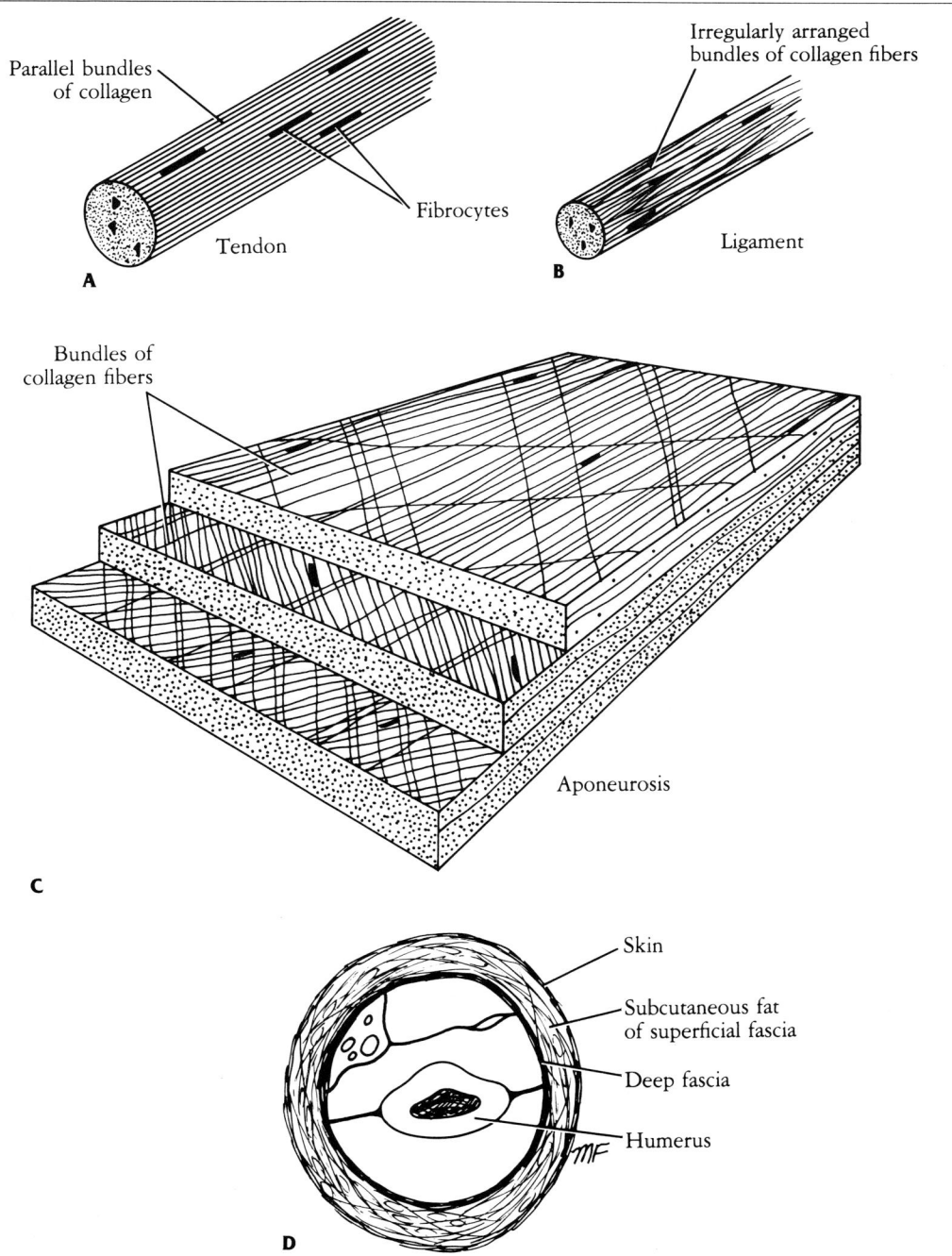

Fig. 4-21. The structure of dense connective tissue. (A) Tendon; (B) ligament; (C) aponeurosis. (D) shows arrangement of superficial and deep fasciae in a cross section of the arm.

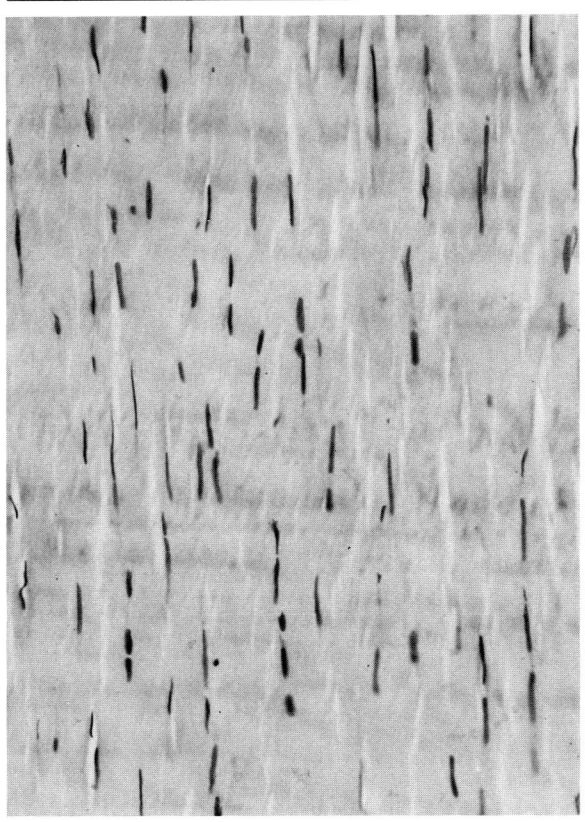

Fig. 4-22. Photomicrograph of longitudinal section of a tendon, showing tightly packed bundles of collagen fibers running in one direction. The nuclei of the flattened fibroblasts can be seen between the collagen bundles. (H&E; ×260.)

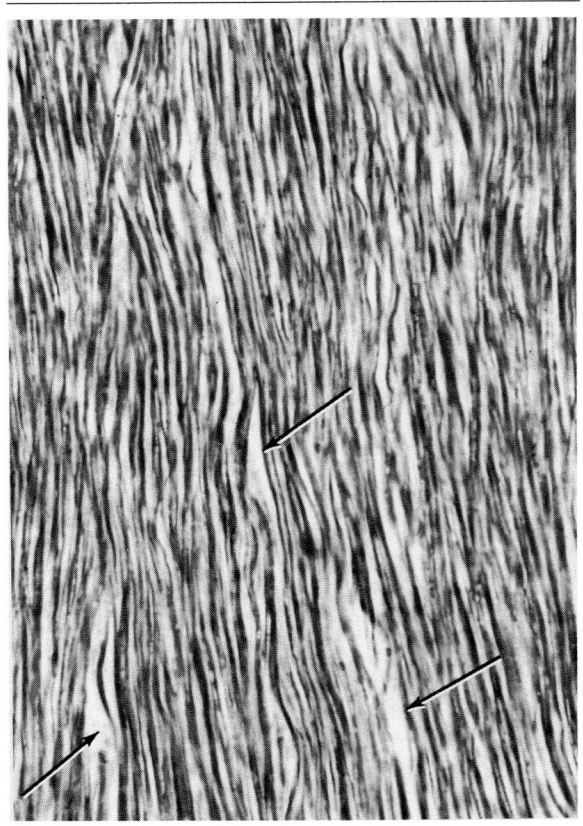

Fig. 4-23. Photomicrograph of a longitudinal section of an elastic ligament, the ligamentum nuchae. The darkly stained elastic fibers can be seen clearly. The flattened fibroblasts, which are unstained, occupy the clear spaces (arrows). (Verhoeff's stain; ×260.)

of the intercellular material is *chondromucoprotein,* which is a polymer of protein and the *chondroitin sulfates,* which are polysaccharides. The acid sulfate groups (glycosaminoglycans) are responsible for the basophilic staining of the material.

The cells of cartilage are called *chondrocytes;* they are situated in spaces in the intercellular material called *lacunae.* The intercellular material or matrix immediately surrounding the lacunae stains more deeply than that elsewhere, probably because of the higher concentration of chondroitin sulfates in this area. The darkly staining area is referred to as the *territorial matrix.* Cartilage has no blood vessels passing through its substance. Except on the exposed surfaces in joints, it is covered by a membrane called the *perichondrium.* The perichondrium consists of an outer protective, vascularized layer of fibrous tissue and an inner cellular layer, which is capable of forming new cartilage.

Nutrients and oxygen reach the chondrocytes by leaving the blood vessels in the perichondrium and diffusing through the intercellular material. In cartilage covering the surfaces of bone inside a joint (articular cartilage), the cells are nourished by the synovial fluid.

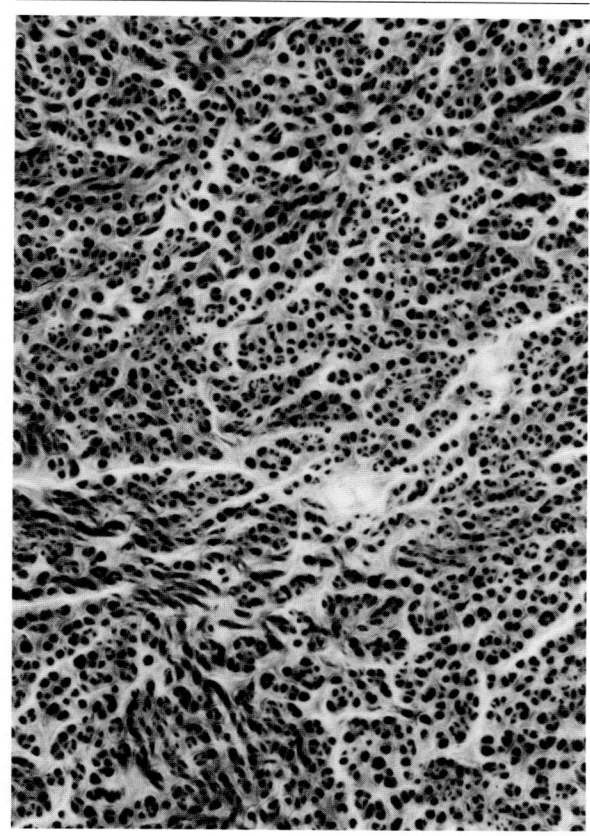

Fig. 4-24. Photomicrograph of a transverse section of an elastic ligament, the ligamentum nuchae. The darkly stained elastic fibers can be seen clearly. (Verhoeff's stain; ×260.)

Types of Cartilage

There are three types of cartilage: hyaline, fibrous, and elastic. These types of cartilage differ from one another mainly by the type of fiber embedded in the intercellular material (Fig. 4-25).

HYALINE CARTILAGE. Hyaline cartilage is the most widely distributed type of cartilage found in the body (Figs. 4-26 and 4-27). It has a glassy, translucent appearance, because the amorphous intercellular material of the matrix has the same refractive index as the collagen and the few elastic fibers embedded in it. Hyaline cartilage is firm and yet flexible and forms the greater part of the cartilaginous skeleton in the embryo. It forms the costal cartilages (see Figs. 4-26 and 4-27) and supports the nose, larynx, trachea, and bronchi of the respiratory system. It has great resistance to wear and covers the articular surfaces of nearly all synovial and cartilaginous joints. Because it forms the *epiphyseal plates,* which are the sites of active bone growth in children, it plays an important part in the growth in length of long bones throughout childhood and adolescence.

Adult hyaline cartilage is incapable of repairing itself when damaged, because adult chondrocytes cannot undergo mitosis. The best result that one can hope for is that a cartilage tear will be repaired with fibrous tissues.

FIBROCARTILAGE. Fibrocartilage has a large number of collagen fibers embedded in a small amount of amorphous intercellular material (Fig. 4-28). It is firm and yet flexible and is found in discs within joints, such as the pubic symphysis, the intervertebral joints between the bodies of the vertebrae (see Fig. 4-28), the knee joint, and the temporomandibular joint. If damaged, it repairs itself slowly in a manner similar to that of fibrous tissue elsewhere.

ELASTIC CARTILAGE. Elastic cartilage has a large number of elastic fibers embedded in a small amount of amorphous intercellular material (Figs. 4-29 and 4-30). As would be expected, it is very flexible; it is found in the auricle of the ear and the epiglottis of the larynx. If damaged, it repairs itself with fibrous tissue.

Hyaline cartilage and fibrocartilage tend to calcify and even ossify in later life. The chondrocytes are then cut off from their nourishment and die.

Development and Growth of Cartilage

During the fifth week of embryonic development, local mesenchyme condenses in areas where cartilage will be formed (Fig. 4-31). The mesenchymal cells enlarge and proliferate to form a compact mass

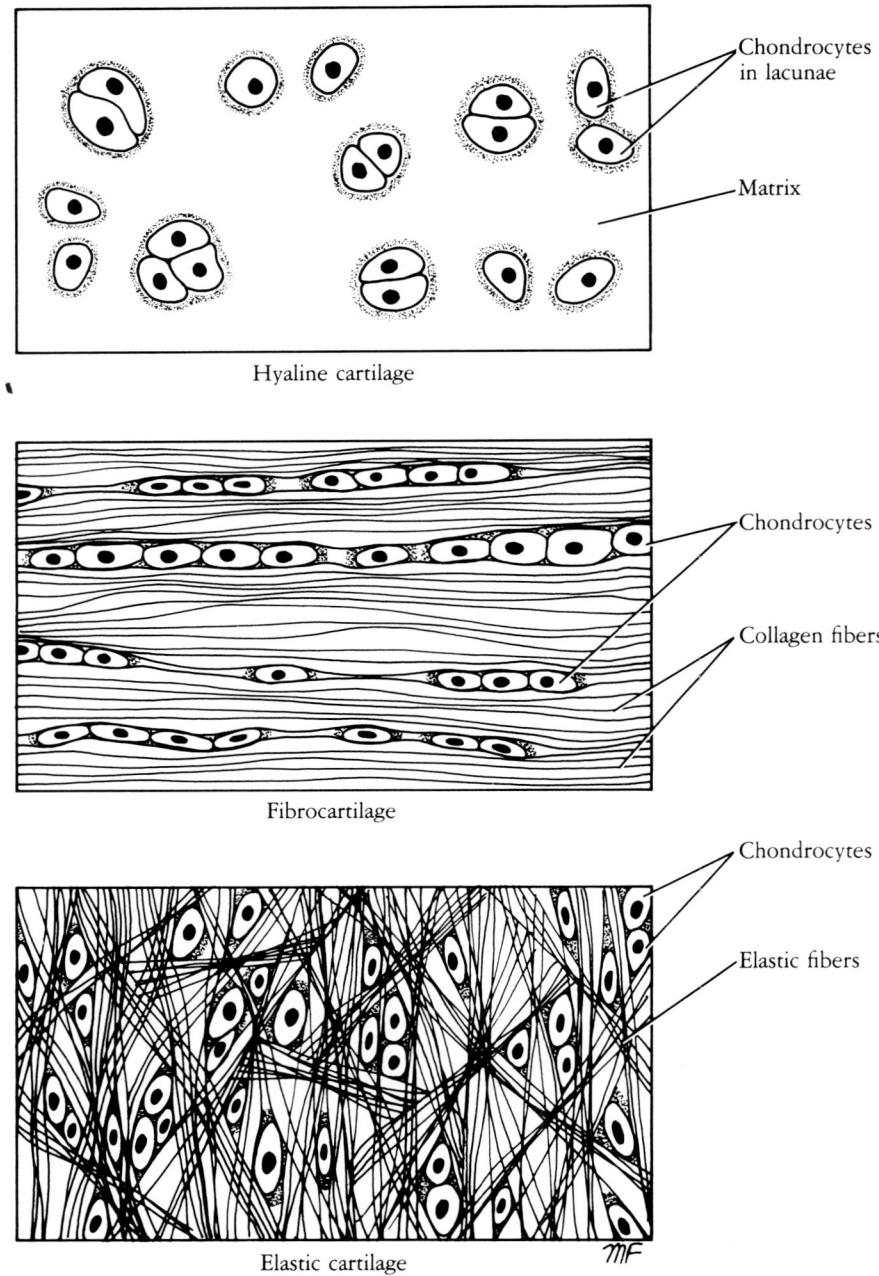

Fig. 4-25. The main differences in structure among the three types of cartilage.

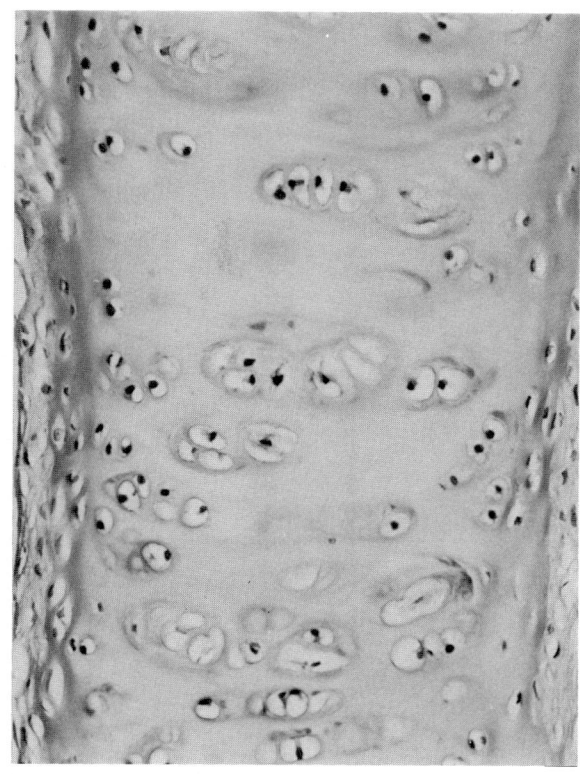

Fig. 4-26. Photomicrograph of section of hyaline cartilage taken from a piece of costal cartilage, showing groups of chondrocytes lying within their lacunae. The perichondrium is present on both sides of the figure. (H&E; ×239.)

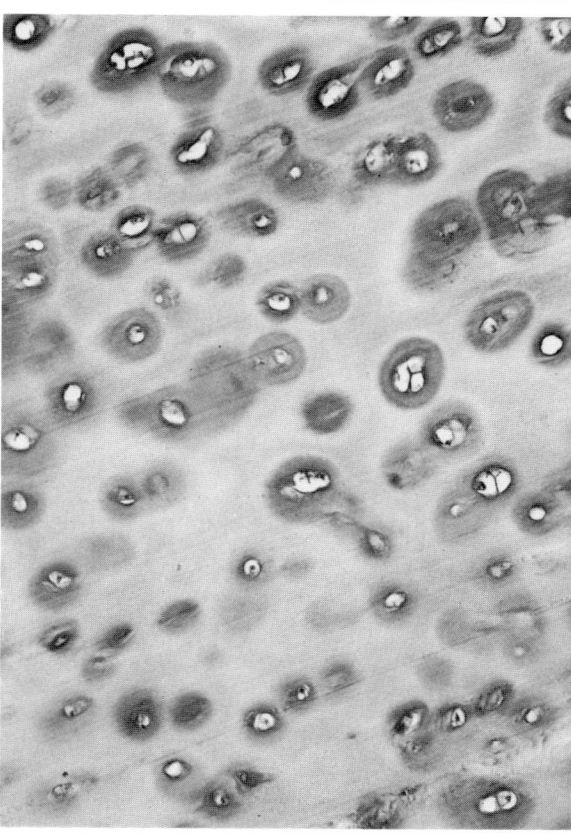

Fig. 4-27. Photomicrograph of section of hyaline cartilage, showing the intense staining of the matrix around each chondrocyte. The more darkly stained area is a zone of the cartilage matrix that is rich in glycosaminoglycans. (H&E; ×130.)

that assumes the shape of the future cartilage. The cells now become rounded and secrete a basophilic intercellular material in which the collagenous and elastic fibers lying between them become embedded. The cells, now known as *chondrocytes,* continue to produce new matrix and push themselves apart. The mesenchyme surrounding the cartilage, except at the joint surfaces, forms the perichondrium.

Cartilage grows by *interstitial growth* and *appositional growth.* Interstitial growth occurs as the result of the division of chondrocytes within the cartilage and the secretion of more intercellular material. Appositional growth occurs as the result of the differentiation of the inner cells of the perichondrium into chondroblasts. The cells develop into chondrocytes that secrete intercellular material. By these two methods, new cartilage is formed in the interior and on the outer surface.

Bone

Bone is a rigid form of connective tissue and is much firmer than cartilage. It consists of cells and intercellular material; the latter consists of formed collagen fibers and amorphous intercellular substance. The

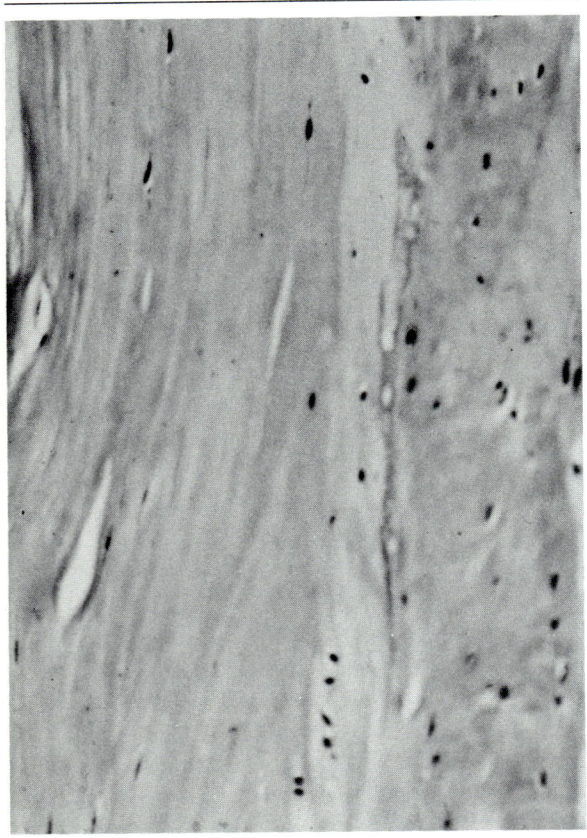

Fig. 4-28. Photomicrograph of a section of fibrocartilage from an intervertebral disk, showing concentric rings of tightly packed bundles of collagen fibers. The nuclei of chondrocytes can also be seen. (H&E; ×260.)

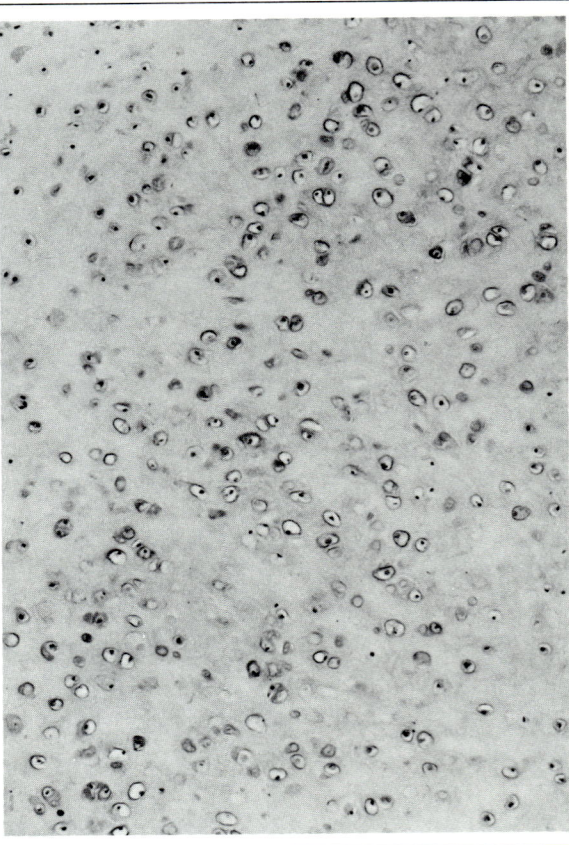

Fig. 4-29. Photomicrograph of a section of elastic cartilage from the auricle of the external ear, showing numerous chondrocytes scattered throughout the matrix. Note that the elastic fibers present in the matrix have not been stained. (H&E; ×100.)

collagen fibers make up about 95 percent of the organic matrix and are responsible for the pink staining with eosin. They are embedded in the amorphous intercellular substance, which is rich in mucopolysaccharides. Mineral salts that consist mainly of a crystalline form of calcium phosphate called *hydroxyapatite* are located between the collagen fibers and account for 65 percent of bone weight. The hardness of a bone (equal to that of cast iron) is caused by the presence of calcium phosphate; the certain degree of elasticity possessed by bone is caused by the presence of organic collagen fibers.

The cells of bone are known as *osteocytes* and are contained in small spaces in the matrix called lacunae (Fig. 4-32). Small tubular canals, the *canaliculi*, connect adjacent lacunae. They contain the slender processes of the osteocytes. The canaliculi permit tissue fluid to flow from one lacuna to another and bathe the osteocytes.

Types of Bone

Bone exists in two forms, *compact* and *spongy* (*cancellous*). Compact bone appears as a solid mass, but spongy bone is extremely porous, being composed

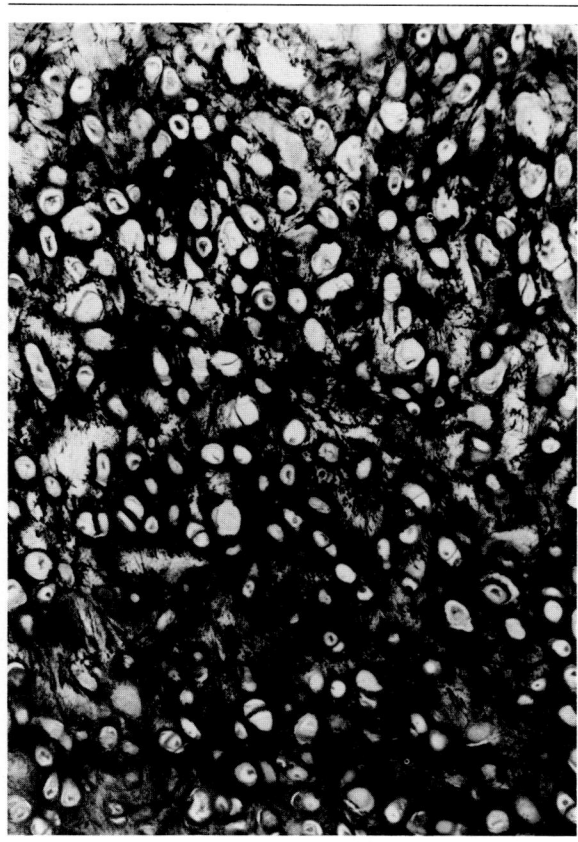

Fig. 4-30. Photomicrograph of elastic cartilage from the auricle of the external ear. The black-stained elastic fibers are clearly visible in the matrix between the chondrocytes. (Verhoeff's stain; ×130.)

of slender trabeculae (strands) that branch and join to form a delicate bony meshwork (Fig. 4-33; see Fig. 4-32). The spaces of the network are filled with bone marrow.

COMPACT BONE. Compact bone is found in the shafts of long bones (see Fig. 4-33). In flat bones, it forms two plates of bone, separated by a middle layer of spongy bone. Irregularly shaped bones are formed of spongy bone covered by a thin outer shell of compact bone.

The structural units of compact bone are called *haversian systems*. These are cylindrical structures whose long axes are parallel to the long axis of a long bone. Running through the center of a haversian system is a *haversian canal* (Fig. 4-34; see Fig. 4-32), which contains blood vessels and occasional nerves. The haversian canals are connected with one another, with the exterior of the bone, and with the interior of the bone (the marrow cavity) by transverse canals called *Volkmann's canals* (see Fig. 4-32). The haversian canals are surrounded by intercellular material deposited in successive layers known as *concentric lamellae*. Thus, each lamella consists of a layer of closely packed collagen fibers embedded in amorphous intercellular substance. The osteocytes in their lacunae lie between adjacent lamellae (Fig. 4-35). These cells receive their nourishment from the blood vessels in the haversian and Volkmann's canals by way of the tissue fluid that permeates the canaliculi.

The irregular spaces lying between the haversian systems are filled with the fragments of older haversian systems that have been partially destroyed during the internal reorganization of bone during bone growth. These fragments of lamellae are known as *interstitital lamellae.*

Surrounding the outer and inner surfaces of compact bone and, as it were, holding the many haversian systems together, there are a number of lamellae called the *outer* and *inner circumferential lamellae.*

SPONGY BONE. Spongy (cancellous) bone is found at the ends of long bones and in the center of flat and irregular bones. It is made up of branching trabeculae, each of which is composed of irregularly arranged lamellae (see Figs. 4-32 and 4-33). There are no haversian systems, and the osteocytes in their lacunae are nourished by the diffusion of tissue fluid through the canaliculi from the marrow cavity.

Macroscopic Structure of Bone

A typical long bone, such as the femur, has a *shaft,* or *diaphysis,* consisting of a hollow cylinder of compact bone that contains a central *marrow cavity* filled with *bone marrow.* The ends of long bones are composed largely of spongy bone surrounded by a thin cortex of compact bone (see Fig. 4-33).

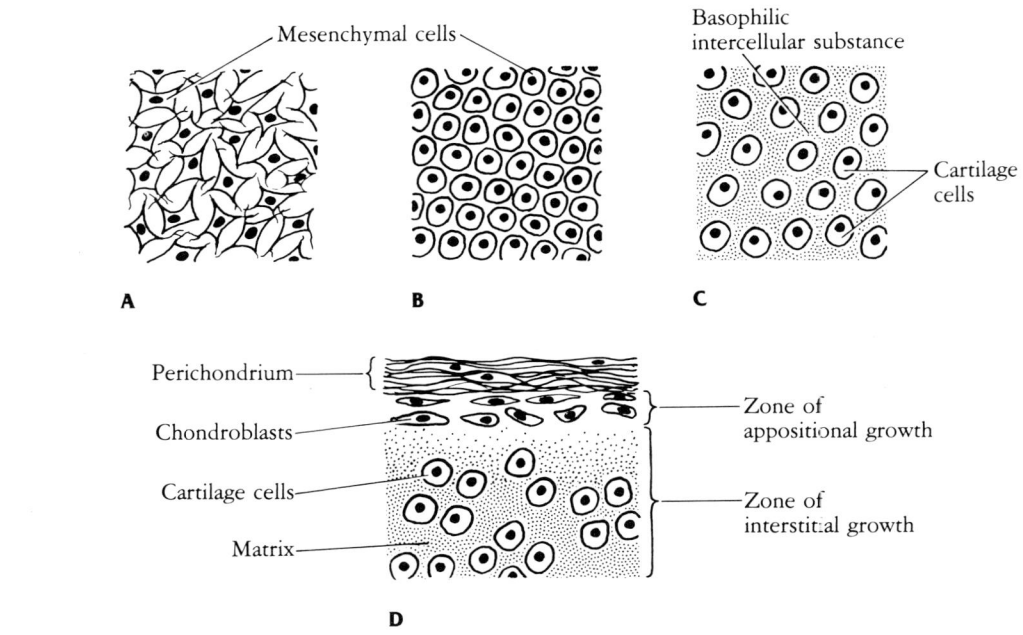

Fig. 4-31. The histogenesis of cartilage. (A) Loose mesenchyme with cells having long processes. (B) Compact mesenchyme; the cells have become rounded and have proliferated and now lie close together. (C) Cartilage cells secrete basophilic intercellular substance rich in glycosaminoglycans. (D) Mature cartilage; cells are surrounded by matrix in which collagenous fibers are embedded; the perichondrium is formed from surrounding mesenchyme.

Where long bones articulate with one another at joints, their outer surfaces are usually covered with hyaline cartilage. Elsewhere, the outer surface of bones is completely covered by a layer of connective tissue called *periosteum*. The periosteum is composed of an outer vascular, fibrous coat and an inner cellular coat, which has the ability to form bone. The periosteum has a rich nerve supply and is very sensitive. The marrow cavity of the shaft, the cavities of the spongy bone, and the haversian and Volkmann's canals are lined by *endosteum*, which has a structure similar to that of periosteum. The endosteum, however, has no connective tissue layer; the cells have an osteogenic potential.

Tendons and ligaments are attached to the periosteum. Here, bundles of collagen fibers extend from the periosteum into the bone matrix. These tethering fibers are called *Sharpey's fibers*.

Long bones receive their blood supply by three routes: (1) the *nutrient artery* perforates the shaft to enter the marrow cavity through a foramen called the *nutrient canal;* (2) *periosteal arteries* penetrate and supply the outer part of the compact bone through Volkmann's canals; and (3) arteries supply the epiphyseal ends of the bone. Nerves and possibly lymphatic vessels accompany these arteries.

Classification of Bones

Bones can be classified, according to their general shape, as (1) long and short bones, (2) irregular bones, (3) flat bones, and (4) sesamoid bones. The long and short bones are found in the limbs; the irregular and flat bones, in the skull, vertebral column, and the limb girdles; and the sesamoid bones, in certain tendons (such as those of the quadriceps femoris and flexor hallucis brevis muscles).

Bone marrow occupies the marrow cavity (see Fig.

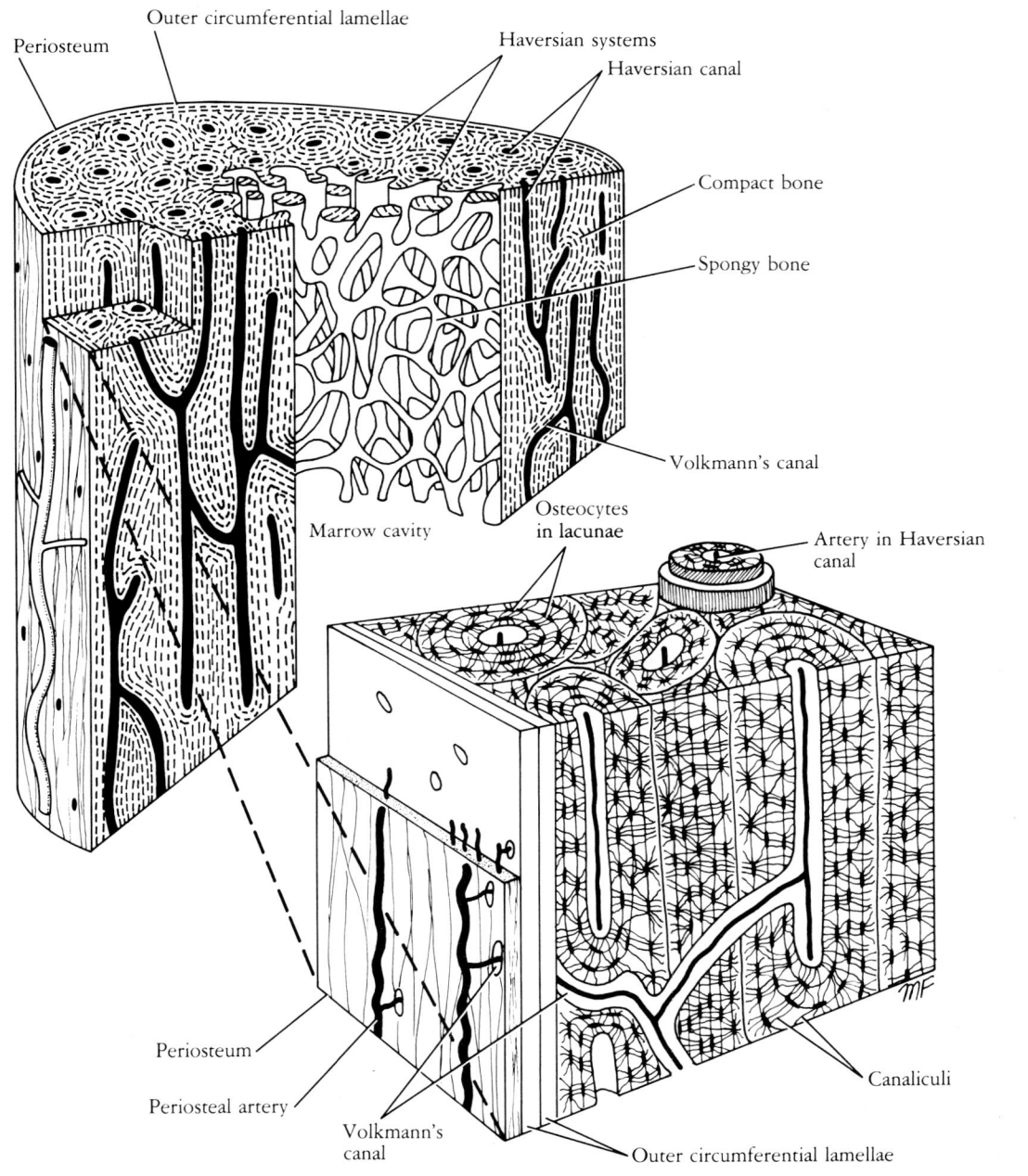

Fig. 4-32. Microscopic structure of bone, shown in both transverse and longitudinal sections. Note the presence of compact and spongy bone. The Haversian systems—the Haversian and Volkmann's canals and their contents—are visible, as are the osteocytes in their lacunae.

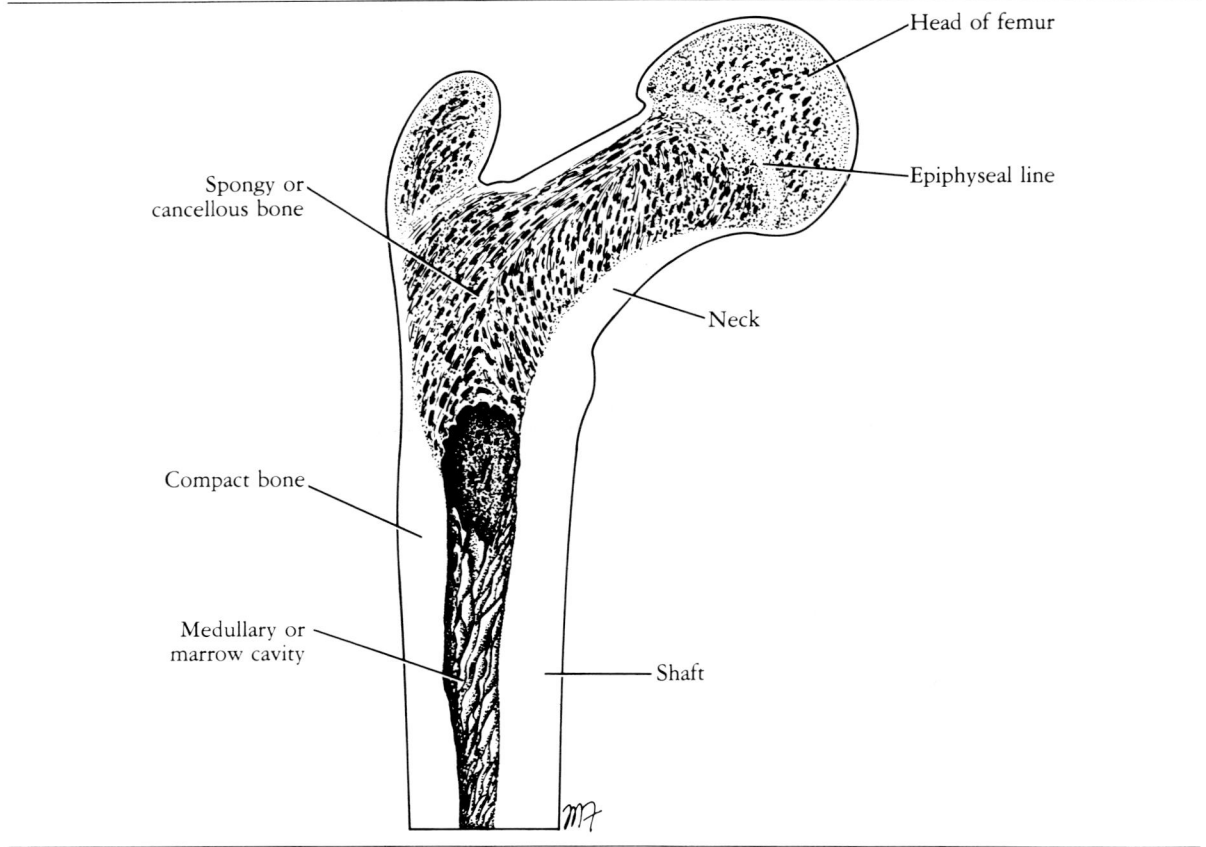

Fig. 4-33. *Longitudinal section of the upper end of the femur, showing the distribution of the compact and spongy bone. Note the medullary or marrow cavity and the epiphyseal line.*

4-33) in long and short bones and the spaces of the spongy bone in flat and irregular bones. At birth, the marrow of all the bones of the body is red and hematopoietic. This blood-forming activity gradually lessens with age, and the red marrow is replaced by yellow marrow, which is composed largely of fat cells. When the individual reaches 7 years of age, yellow marrow begins to appear in the distal bones of the limbs. This replacement of marrow gradually moves proximally, so that by the time the person reaches adulthood, the red marrow is restricted to the bones of the skull, the vertebral column, the thoracic cage, the girdle bones, and the head of the humerus and femur.

Examination of Bone

Because of the presence of calcium salts, it is impossible to cut routine histological sections of bone. Two methods are used to prepare sections: (1) The bone is decalcified in an acid solution. The bone can then be embedded, sectioned, and stained in the usual way. The osteocytes, however, tend to be deformed as a result of the acid used. (2) The bone is cut with a saw into thin pieces, which are then ground down between glass plates with abrasives. When a section is thin enough to be viewed with a light microscope, it is mounted. The structure of the haversian system

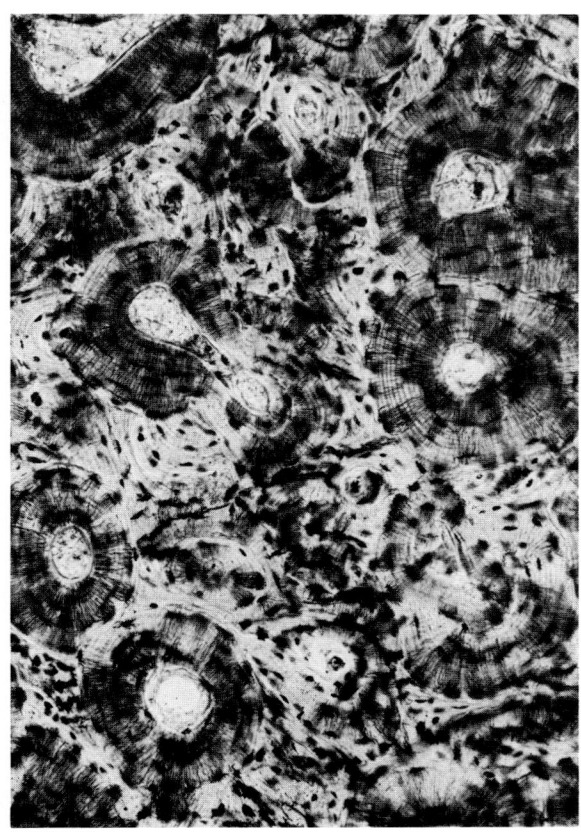

Fig. 4-34. Photomicrograph of a thick ground section of bone. The haversian systems, the lacunae, and the canaliculi have become filled with black debris during the grinding process. (Unstained; ×100.)

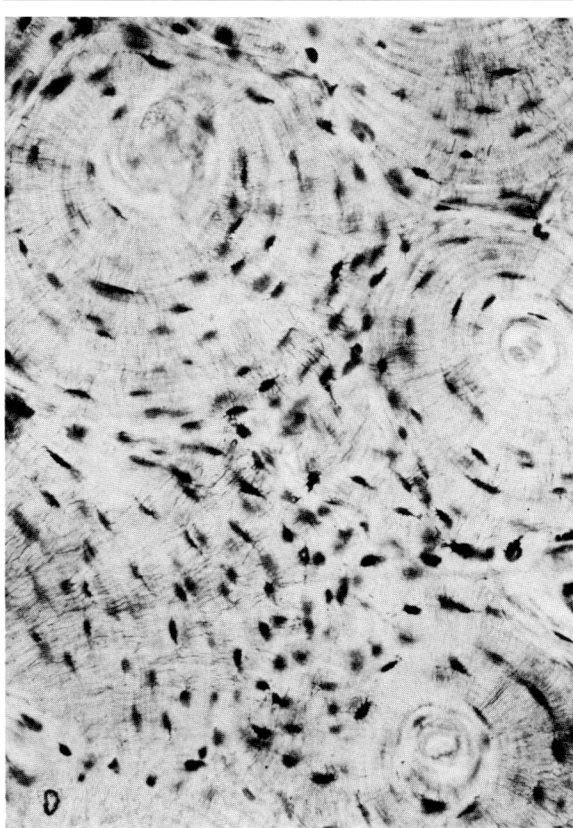

Fig. 4-35. Photomicrograph of a thin ground section of bone. The detailed structure of the haversian systems is clearly visible. Note that the black material filling the lacunae and canaliculi is debris formed during the grinding process; the osteocytes have been destroyed. (Unstained; ×200.)

is clearly visualized, but the cells are destroyed and the lacunae and canaliculi are filled with debris (see Figs. 4-34 and 4-35).

Bone Formation

In the embryo, bone is formed by two methods: intramembranous ossification and endochondral ossification. Intramembranous ossification takes place in the bones of the vault of the skull and the clavicle. Endochondral ossification forms the remainder of the skeleton.

INTRAMEMBRANOUS OSSIFICATION. A condensation of mesenchyme occurs in the area in which bone formation is to take place (Fig. 4-36). The cells are small and spindle-shaped; they begin to lay down collagenous fibers, and the area comes to resemble a fibrous membrane. The cells now become known as *osteoblasts,* and they continue to produce large amounts of collagenous material and amorphous intercellular substance that fills the intercellular spaces and is known as *osteoid* (see Fig. 4-36). At this stage, no calcium salts have been deposited in the intercel-

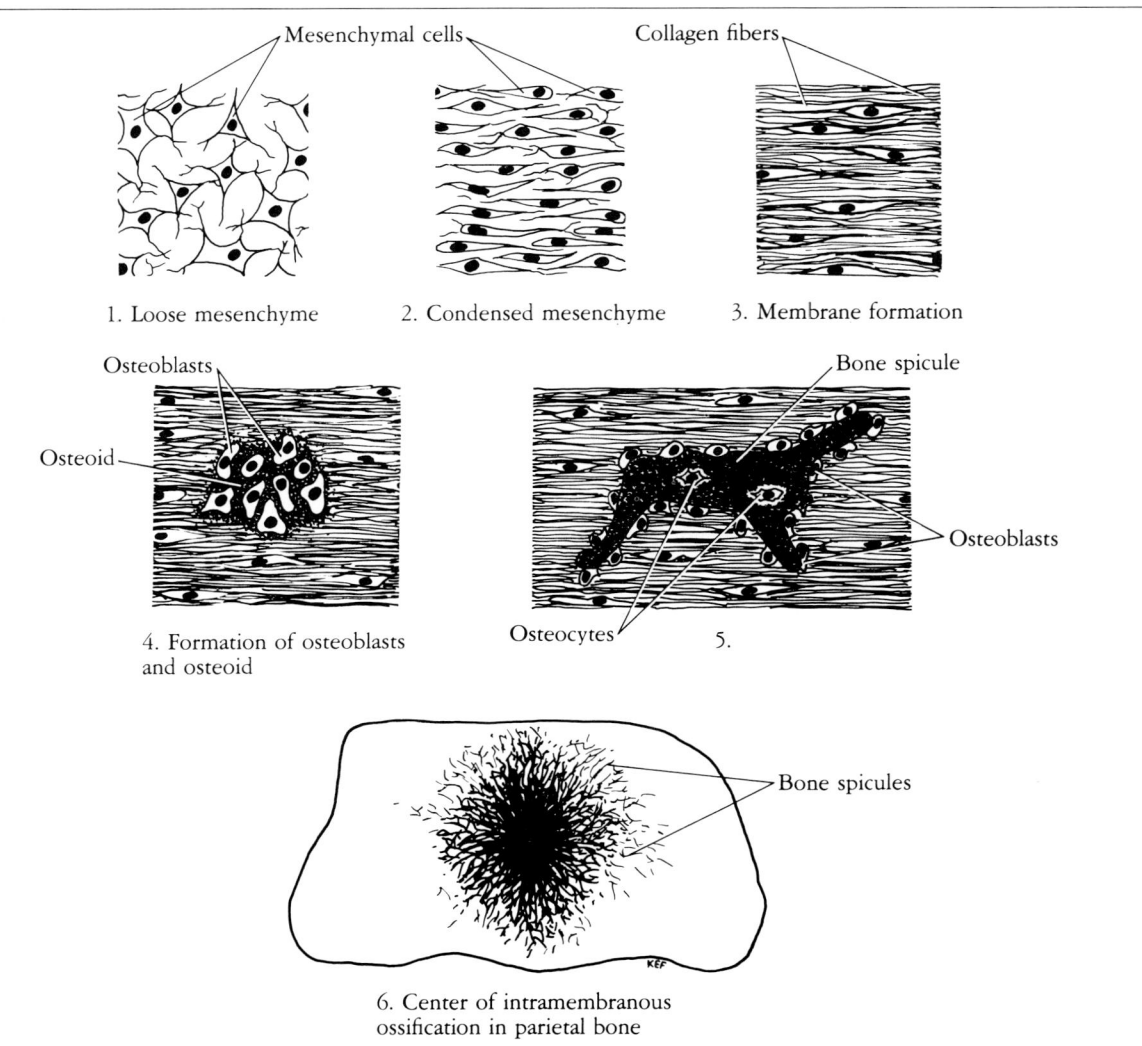

Fig. 4-36. *The stages in intramembranous ossification.*

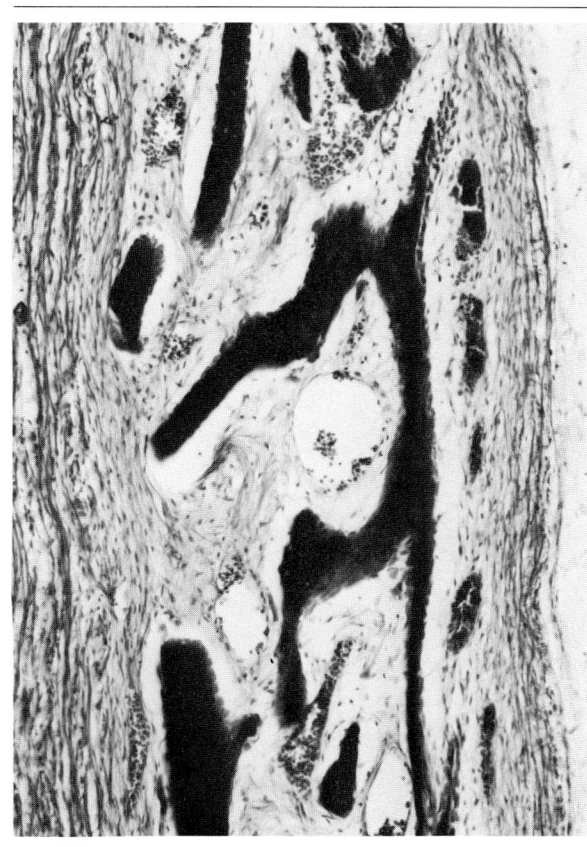

Fig. 4-37. Photomicrograph of a section through a skull bone from an embryo, showing intramembranous bone formation. Note the newly formed, dark-staining bone spicules. Around the spicules are many osteoblasts and osteoclasts. The periosteum is seen on the right and left margins of the photograph. (H&E; ×100.)

lular substance and the osteoid is still a pliable membrane.

The osteoblasts now start to secrete *alkaline phosphatase,* resulting in the deposition of calcium salts in the form of minute crystals of *apatite* that are deposited on and obscure the fibrils of the matrix. In this manner, the osteoid is converted into bone matrix. As more and more bone matrix is produced, some osteoblasts become trapped within it; they are known as *osteocytes* (see Fig. 4-36). The space within the bone matrix that is occupied by an osteocyte is known as a *lacuna*. Gradually, the bone matrix grows in amount and extends in all directions within the membrane as *bone spicules* (Fig. 4-37). A center of ossification has now been established.

Meanwhile, a layer of vascular mesenchyme has condensed on the outside of the membrane to form the *periosteum.* The periosteum consists of an outer fibrous layer and an inner layer composed of cells that differentiate into osteoblasts. These new osteoblasts now start to lay down bone in the form of parallel plates of lamellae, known as *compact bone,* just beneath the periosteum.

In a flat bone, such as that found in the vault of the skull, the original center of ossification in the middle of the membrane lays down vascular *spongy* or *cancellous bone,* while the periosteal osteoblasts lay down relatively avascular compact bone on the surface of the membrane (Fig. 4-38). The compact bone forms the *inner* and *outer tables* of the skull bone; the central spongy bone is known as the *diploë*. The vascular tissue that fills the spaces of the cancellous bone differentiates into *red bone marrow* and becomes hematopoietic.

As development proceeds and the new bone grows, the shape of the bone is continually being changed. Much of the original matrix laid down by the osteoblasts is resorbed by multinucleated giant cells called *osteoclasts.* These cells are thought to be formed either from osteoblasts or from undifferentiated mesenchymal cells. While bony resorption is taking place, new bone is being laid down by osteoblasts.

ENDOCHONDRAL OSSIFICATION. The long bones of the body are formed by endochondral ossification. First, the long bone is represented by a model of condensed mesenchyme, which is soon replaced by a model of hyaline cartilage formed as previously described (Fig. 4-39). During the eighth week of embryonic life, ossification begins in the middle of the cartilaginous shaft. The cartilage cells in the region increase in size (Fig. 4-40), and calcium salts are deposited in the intercellular matrix. The enlarged

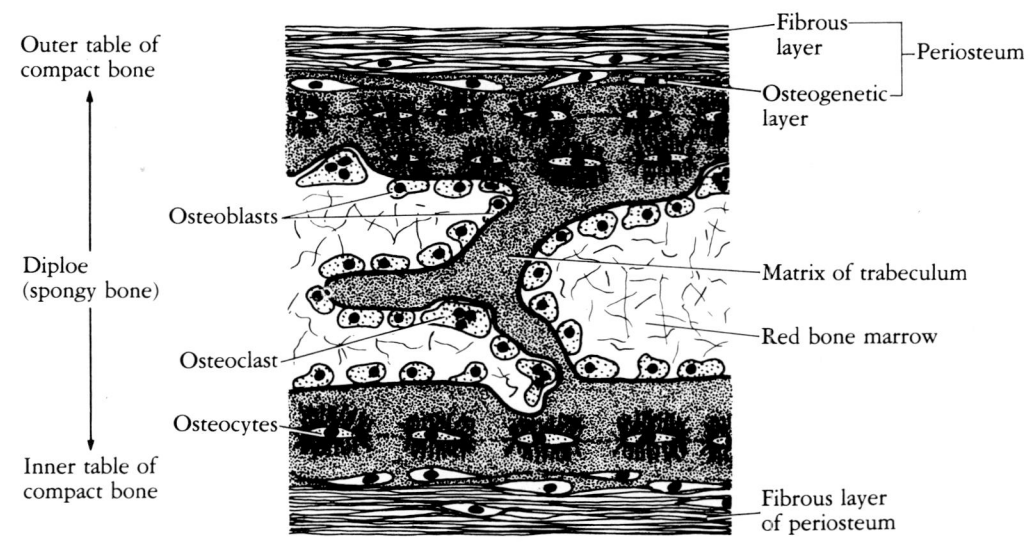

Fig. 4-38. *A section of developing parietal bone of the vault of the skull, showing the inner and outer tables of compact bone and the central spongy bone.*

cartilage cells now degenerate and disappear, leaving empty cavities (Figs. 4-41 and 4-42). Meanwhile, the perichondrium becomes active and is now known as *periosteum*. The cells of its inner layer differentiate into osteoblasts that start to lay down a collar of compact bone around the shaft. This formation of subperiosteal new bone is a compensatory protective mechanism, because it will strengthen the developing bone at a time when the middle zone of the cartilage model is about to be broken down.

A bud of vascular tissue formed from the inner layer of the periosteum now grows inward. Accompanying the actively growing capillaries are osteoclasts and chondroclasts derived from mesenchymal cells. The osteoclasts break down areas in the newly formed periosteal bone and allow the vascular bud to invade the underlying calcified cartilaginous matrix. The chondroclasts break down the walls of the lacunae previously occupied by the dead chondrocytes, forming irregular spaces (see Fig. 4-39). Osteoblasts that have accompanied the vascular bud now start to lay down bone on the walls of the spaces (Fig. 4-43). Gradually, as the result of bone resorption by the osteoclasts and bone deposition by the osteoblasts, spongy bone is formed in the center of the shaft, surrounded by compact bone (Fig. 4-44). Later, a large *marrow cavity* occupied by *red marrow* appears in the center of the bone.

The primary center of ossification has now been established in the center of the shaft of the cartilaginous model. This region of the developing bones is referred to as the *diaphysis*. Growth of the cartilaginous model continues by the proliferation of the chondrocytes and the deposition of further cartilaginous matrix. An examination of the cartilage in the region of the primary center of ossification shows three regions of differentiation (see Figs. 4-40, 4-41, and 4-42). In the region closest to the center, the chondrocytes are enlarged and degenerating and calcium salts are being deposited in the matrix. In the second region, farther away from the center, the chondrocytes are enlarged but otherwise appear normal. In the third region, which extends toward the ends of the cartilage model, the chondrocytes are actively dividing and becoming ar-

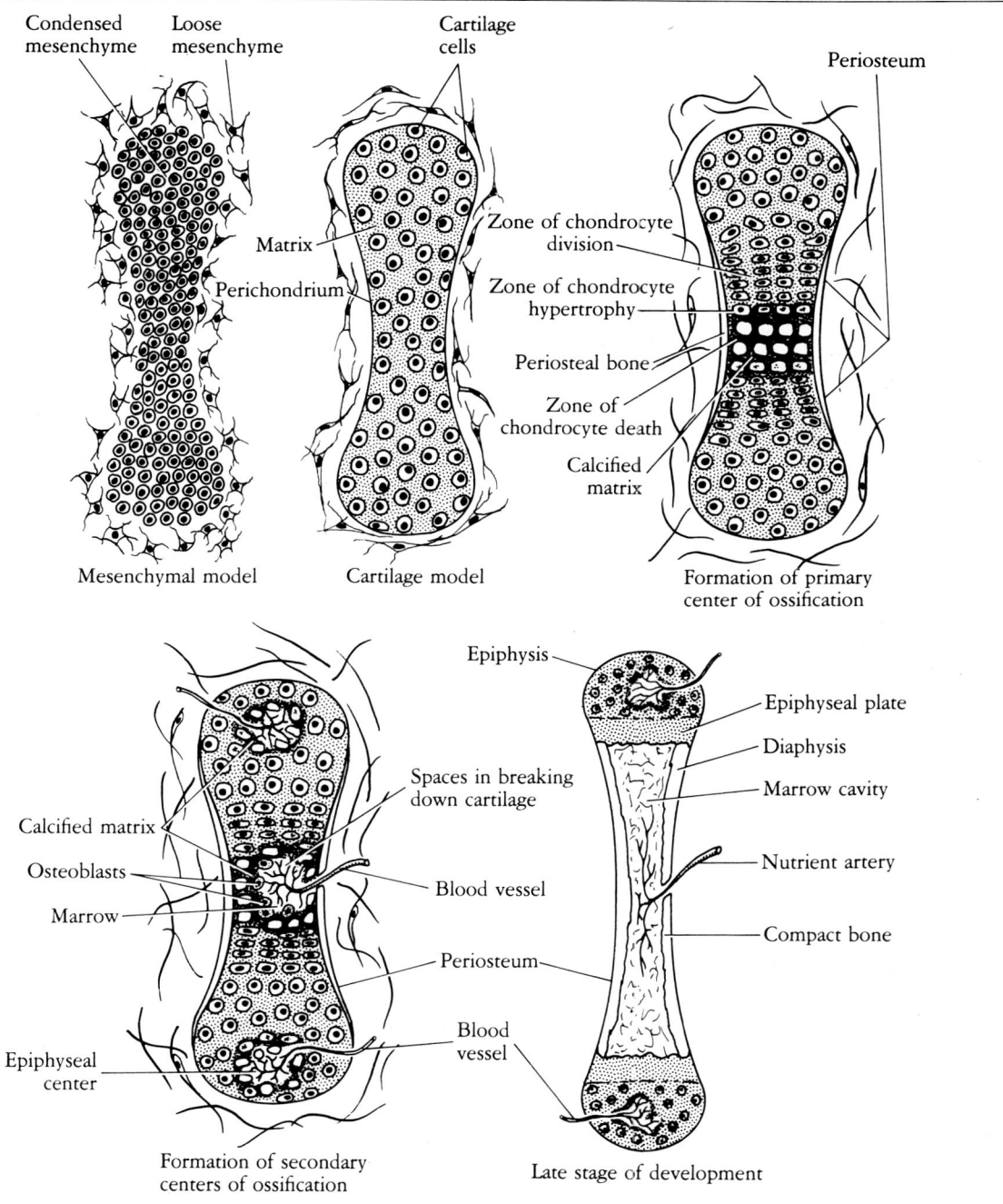

Fig. 4-39. The stages in endochondral ossification, shown in longitudinal sections of a long bone.

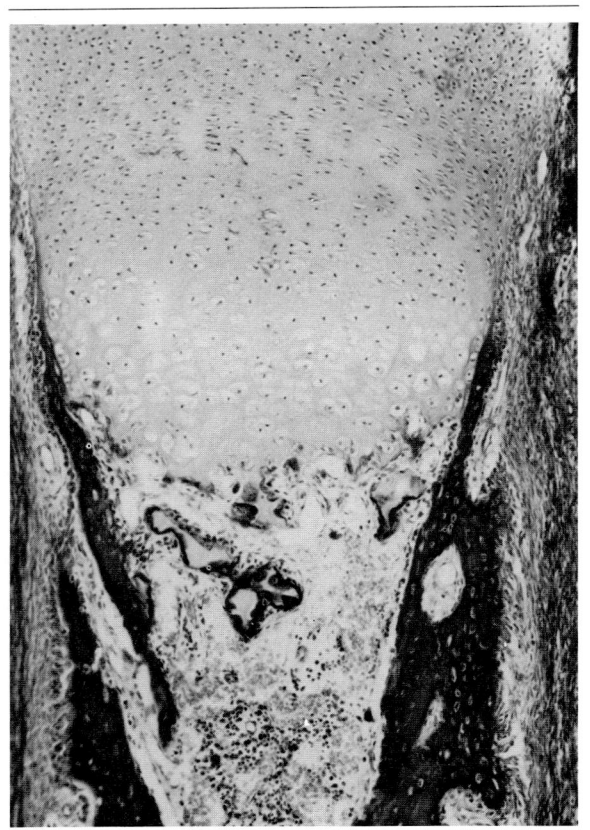

Fig. 4-40. Photomicrograph of a longitudinal section of the developing phalanx of a finger, showing endochondral ossification taking place at the primary center of ossification. The cartilage has disappeared from the central part of the developing bone and has been replaced by dark-staining bone spicules and bone marrow. A thick layer of subperiosteal bone has also been formed. Note that chondrocytes in the epiphyseal cartilage at the top of the photograph are enlarging and becoming arranged in columns. (H&E; ×100.)

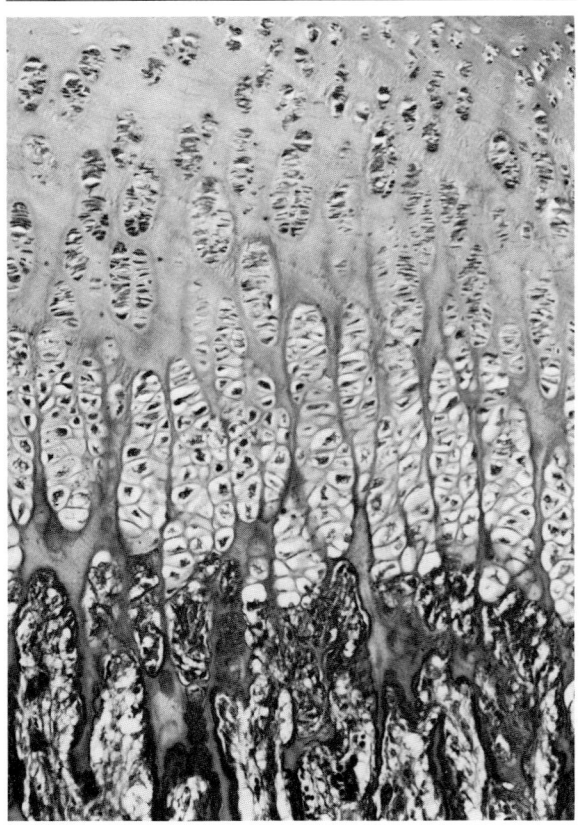

Fig. 4-41. Photomicrograph of a longitudinal section of the developing phalanx of a finger, showing endochondral ossification taking place in the epiphyseal plate. Note that the chondrocytes have undergone division and have become arranged in parallel columns. Many of the chondrocytes are enlarged, and some are in the process of dying. The diaphyseal side of the epiphyseal plate is seen in the lower part of the photograph. Note the presence of cartilaginous trabeculae on which dark-staining bone has been deposited. (H&E; ×100.)

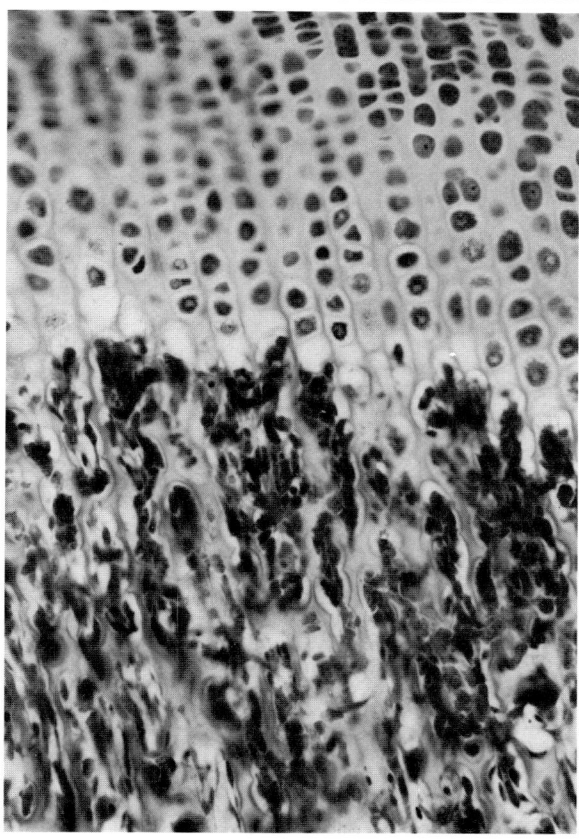

Fig. 4-42. Photomicrograph of a longitudinal section of the developing phalanx of a finger. At the top, the chondrocytes of the epiphyseal cartilage are shown to be enlarged and arranged in columns. Note that some of the chondrocytes have died, leaving empty spaces in the calcified matrix. The lower part of the photograph shows the formation of bony trabeculae. (H&E; ×200.)

ranged in parallel rows. As new cartilage is formed, the center of ossification extends toward each end of the model.

At birth, the long bone has a bony shaft, the *diaphysis,* with two cartilaginous ends, the *epiphyses* (see Fig. 4-39). Later, one or more secondary centers of ossification appear in each epiphysis. Now, bone formation takes place in three areas: at the center of the shaft and in each extremity. The continuous growth in length of the cartilage model occurs as a result of the division of the chondrocytes in the epiphyseal cartilage, which, as development continues, is reduced to a thin plate, the *epiphyseal plate.* Growth in length of a long bone ceases when the chondrocytes in the epiphyseal cartilage cease to divide and to form new cartilage. The epiphyseal plates now disappear, and the epiphyses fuse with the diaphysis.

Meanwhile, the diameter of the long bone has been increasing as a result of the continued deposition of new compact bone under the periosteum and the resorption of old bone in the center of the shaft. The marrow cavity also increases in size in this way. In the epiphyseal region, the transverse diameter increases as a result of the growth of the epiphyseal ossification center.

In the long bones, at least one epiphyseal center is found at each end; in the smaller bones, such as the phalanges and metacarpals, one epiphyseal center is found at the proximal end; in irregular bones, such as the scapula and vertebrae, one or more primary centers are formed, and several secondary centers appear. In most bones, the epiphyses have fused with the diaphyses by the twentieth year. The clavicle is one important exception: its shaft is formed by intramembranous ossification, and fusion with the epiphysis at the sternal end does not occur until the twenty-fifth year.

Joints

The site where two or more bones come together, whether or not there is movement between them, is called a *joint.* Joints are classified, according to the tissues that lie between the bones, as fibrous joints, cartilaginous joints, and synovial joints.

FIBROUS JOINTS. The articulating surfaces of the bones at these joints are joined by fibrous tissue (Fig. 4-45). The degree of movement possible depends on the length of the collagen fibers uniting the bones. The sutures of the vault of the skull and the inferior tibiofibular joints are examples of fibrous joints.

CARTILAGINOUS JOINTS. Cartilaginous joints can be divided into two types, *primary* and *secondary.* A pri-

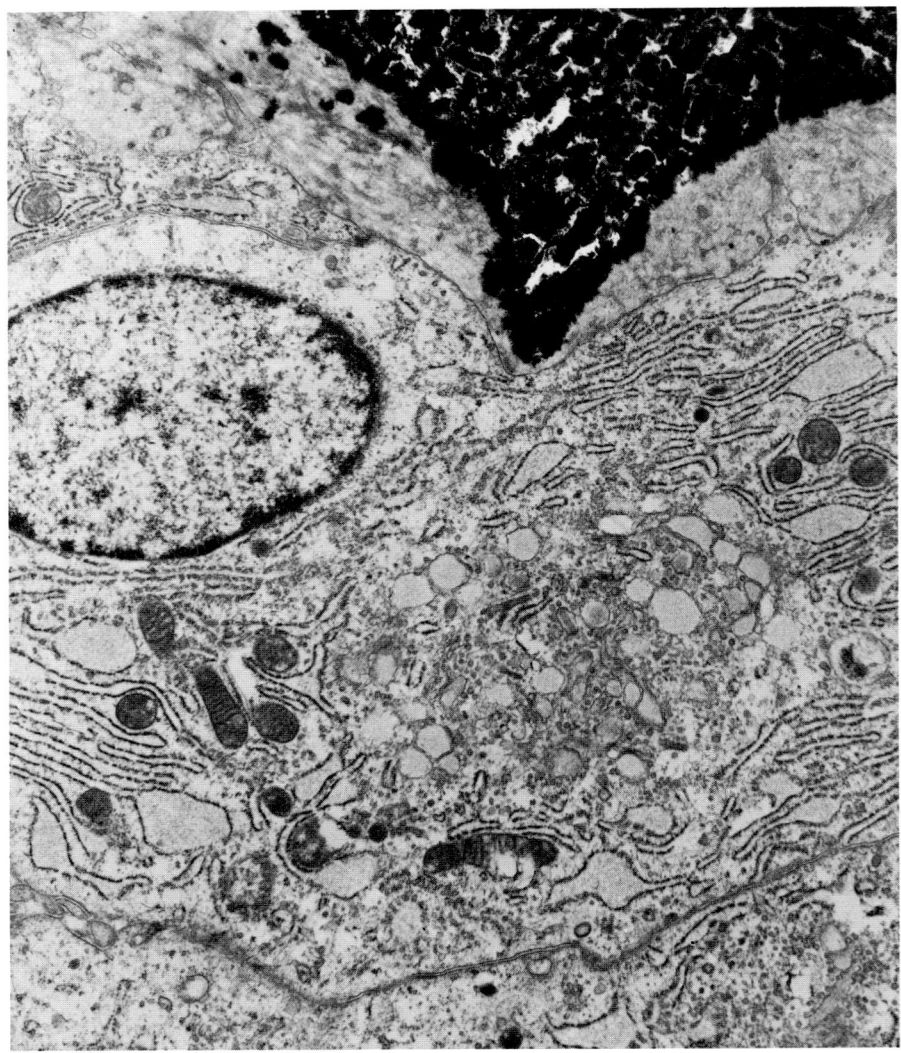

Fig. 4-43. Electron micrograph of part of an osteoblast. At the top is a dark-staining area of calcified bone matrix. Between the bone matrix and the plasma membrane of the osteoblast is osteoid tissue containing collagen fibrils. Note the nucleus, the mitochondria, and the extensive rough endoplasmic reticulum. Numerous vesicles containing procollagen are also present within the cytoplasm. (Courtesy of Drs. J. A. Maynard and R. R. Cooper.)

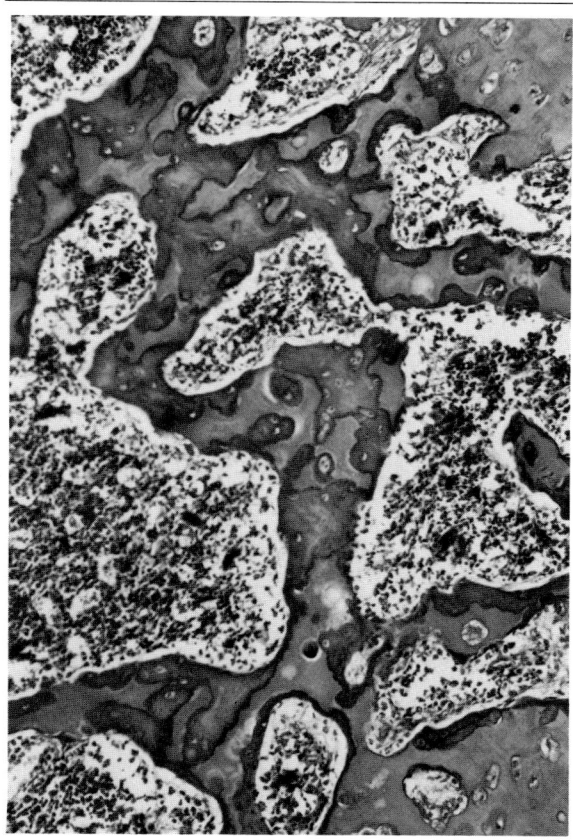

Fig. 4-44. Photomicrograph of endochondral ossification in a developing phalanx of a finger, showing trabeculae of calcified cartilage matrix on which dark-staining new bone has been deposited. Between the trabeculae is developing bone marrow. Note the presence of osteocytes in the new bone. (Mallory's trichrome; × 100.)

mary cartilaginous joint is one in which the bones are united by a plate or bar of hyaline cartilage. Thus, the union between the epiphysis and the diaphysis of a growing bone and that between the first rib and the manubrium sterni are examples of such joints. No movement is possible.

In a secondary cartilaginous joint, the bones are united by a plate of fibrocartilage; the articular surfaces of the bones are covered by a thin layer of hyaline cartilage (see Fig. 4-45). Examples are the intervertebral joints (see Fig. 4-28) and the symphysis pubis. The amount of movement possible is dependent on the physical qualities of the fibrocartilage.

SYNOVIAL JOINTS. The articular surfaces of the bones at synovial joints are covered by a thin layer of hyaline cartilage separated by a synovial joint cavity (see Fig. 4-45). This arrangement permits a great degree of freedom of movement. The cavity of the joint is lined with *synovial membrane,* which extends from the margins of one articular surface to those of the other. The synovial membrane is composed of loose connective tissue whose surface cells are formed of fibroblasts that are also called *synovial cells.*

The synovial membrane is protected on the outside by a tough, fibrous membrane referred to as the *capsule* of the joint. The articular surfaces are lubricated by a viscous fluid called *synovial fluid.* The synovial fluid is thought to be an exudate of the blood to which mucopolysaccharides have been added by the secretory activity of the cartilage cells covering the articular surfaces and by the fibroblasts of the synovial membrane.

In certain synovial joints, such as the knee joint, disks or wedges of fibrocartilage are interposed between the articular surfaces of the bones. These are referred to as *articular discs.*

The degree of movement in a synovial joint is limited by the shape of the bones participating in the joint, the coming together of adjacent anatomical structures (for example, the thigh and the anterior abdominal wall upon flexion of the hip joint), and the presence of fibrous *ligaments* uniting the bones. Most ligaments lie outside the joint capsule, but in the knee some important ligaments, the cruciate ligaments, lie within the capsule.

Bursae and Synovial Sheaths. A bursa is a lubricating device consisting of a closed, fibrous sac lined with a form of synovial membrane. Its walls are separated by a film of viscous fluid. Bursae are found wherever tendons rub against bones, ligaments, or other tendons. They are commonly found close to

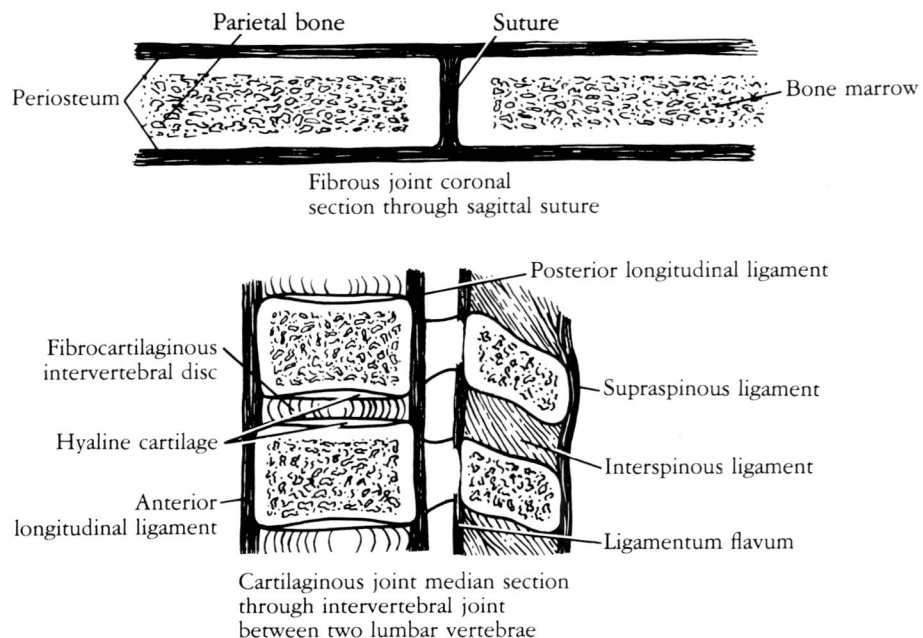
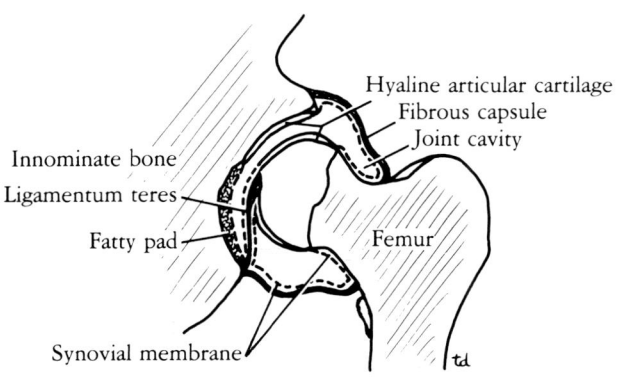

Fig. 4-45. *Fibrous, cartilaginous, and synovial joints.*

joints where the skin rubs against underlying bony structures, for example, the *prepatellar bursa*. Occasionally, the cavity of a bursa communicates with the cavity of a synovial joint. For example, the *suprapatellar bursa* communicates with the knee joint.

A synovial sheath is a tubular bursa that surrounds a tendon. The tendon invaginates the bursa from one side, and the tendon becomes suspended within the bursa by a *mesotendon*.

BLOOD

The structure of blood will be considered in Chapter 5.

CLINICAL NOTES

REGENERATION OF CONNECTIVE TISSUES

Following the destruction of connective tissue, whether by infection or by trauma, a number of changes take place in the surrounding tissue that are at first protective and then reparative. Once the protective or inflammatory reactions have subsided, the local fibroblasts and capillary endothelial cells play a major role in the reparative process. The fibroblasts lay down the connective tissue matrix, and the endothelial cells form a new capillary bed. Whether the damaged tissue is a pure connective tissue or a mixture of connective tissue and epithelial tissue, the resulting reparative process almost invariably leads to an excess of fibrous tissue termed a *scar*.

Repair of a Surgical Incision

The reparative process following a surgical incision is the least complicated form of wound healing and is sometimes referred to as *primary union* or *healing by first intention*.

In an aseptic surgical wound, where the edges of the wound have been drawn together by sutures, the interval between the two edges of the wound is filled by a thin layer of coagulated blood. Dehydration of the surface clot forms the *scab*, which covers and protects the underlying wound from contamination by environmental microorganisms.

The trauma of the surgical knife has caused the death of or injury to a number of cells, which in turn release chemotactic agents that serve to attract neutrophil leukocytes and macrophages to the area. The neutrophils phagocytose and destroy any pathogenic bacteria that are present, and the macrophages phagocytose the red cells and cell debris in the blood clot.

Within 24 to 48 hours, the epithelial cells of the epidermis undergo rapid cell division and start to migrate across the narrow wound beneath the surface scab. Within 48 hours, epidermal continuity is complete.

Later, the surrounding fibroblasts at the sides of the wound enlarge and divide and migrate into the blood clot. At the same time, the endothelial cells of the local blood capillaries start to divide and to form small buds of cells, which grow into the blood clot. These buds join with one another and become canalized to form a capillary network. This vascularization of the blood clot and the proliferation of the fibroblasts form a pink soft tissue that has a granular appearance when seen from the surface and is known as *granulation tissue*. The endothelial cells of the capillaries of granulation tissue are loosely attached to one another, permitting blood cells and plasma to leak into the surrounding tissue.

By the third day, the fibroblasts have started to lay down fine collagen fibers, which at first run in all directions; later, they become oriented along the lines of mechanical stress. By the fifth day, the collagen fibers extend across the wound, and the surface epidermis has reached its normal thickness. The normal maturation of the collagen fibers is dependent on an adequate supply of vitamin C (see p. 149); wounds heal more rapidly, with the formation of strong scars, if patients are provided with an adequate amount of vitamin C in their diets.

During the second week of the repair process, more collagen fibers are laid down along the lines of tension within the scar. The blood supply to the area becomes reduced, and the neutrophils and macrophages disappear. During the next few months, the number of fibroblasts becomes reduced, and those that remain in the scar become fibrocytes. As the scar becomes progressively devascularized, it loses its pink color and becomes white. The sweat glands, hair follicles, and sebaceous glands that were destroyed by the incision are permanently lost.

In the dermis of the skin the bundles of collagen fibers are arranged mostly in parallel rows. A surgical incision through the skin made along or between these rows causes minimal collagen disruption, and the resulting wound heals with the minimum of scar tissue. An incision made across the rows of collagen disrupts and disturbs the collagen, resulting in the massive production of fresh collagen and the formation of a broad, ugly scar. The direction of the rows of collagen is known as the *lines of cleavage;* these lines tend to run longitudinally in the limbs and circumferentially in the neck and trunk.

Repair of a Wound with a Large Amount of Tissue Loss

Wounds of this nature may occur on the surface of the body, the surface of mucous membranes (for example, peptic ulcers), or within an abscess. Repair of such wounds is called *secondary union* or *healing by secondary intention.*

Because of the large amount of tissue damage, there is a strong inflammatory response, with a resultant invasion of the area by large numbers of neutrophils and macrophages. Once the debris has been removed, the defect is filled with granulation tissue, which grows in from the normal tissue at the margins of the wound.

As the fibroblasts lay down collagen within the granulation tissue, large surface wounds undergo a reduction in size of as much as 90 percent. This phenomenon is called *wound contraction* and is thought to be caused by contraction of the fibroblasts and shortening of the collagen fibers. The epithelial defect in surface wounds is filled as a result of the mitotic activity in the surrounding normal epithelial cells and the migration of these cells over the surface of the granulation tissue.

In some individuals with large wounds, the formation of granulation tissue may be excessive, so that the tissue protrudes above the surrounding surface. This so-called proud flesh may interfere with the normal covering of the surface with epithelium and may have to be removed surgically.

Occasionally, in the repair of surgical as well as large wounds, the scar tissue formation is excessive and produces a large, unsightly scar known as a *keloid.* This condition occurs more commonly in blacks and is difficult to treat because it may recur following excision.

Repair of a Fractured Bone

Fracture of a bone is accompanied by a considerable hemorrhage of blood between the bone ends and into the immediate surrounding tissue. Three main cells take part in the repair process: (1) capillary endothelial cells, (2) fibroblasts, and (3) osteoblasts from the deeper layers of the periosteum and the haversian systems.

The capillary endothelial cells grow into the clotted blood and form a vascular network. The fibroblasts and osteoblasts accompany the capillary vessels and displace the blood clot that fills the interval between the bone fragments.

The osteoblasts that have followed the capillaries and lie between the bone fragments become surrounded by deposited calcium salts. This new, hard tissue is known as *callus.* Callus is much wider than the normal bone and extends for some distance beyond the fractured ends, forming a splint for the broken bone. The osteoblasts that lie away from the capillaries form a tissue that resembles cartilage; it later becomes ossified. Thus, the bone fragments at first are temporarily held together by a mass of callus. Later, the callus becomes modified by the activities of the osteoblasts and the osteoclasts. The osteoclasts, which arrive late in the process, remove the excess material on the outside of the bone. They also remove the excess material from the inside of the bone and thus reconstruct the marrow cavity. The osteoblasts not only deposit new bone matrix but also organize the formation of the haversian systems and the trabeculae of the spongy bone. Over a period of months, the callus and, later, the bone fragments are remodeled as a result of the stimulation provided by mechanical forces and muscular activity.

CONNECTIVE TISSUE TUMORS

The names of benign connective tissue tumors are formed by adding the suffix -*oma* to a prefix based on the name of the tissue of origin: a tumor of fibrous tissue is called a *fibroma;* of cartilage, a *chondroma;* and of bone, an *osteoma.* All malignant tumors of connective tissue are called *sarcoma.* Thus, a malignant tumor of fibrous tissue is a *fibrosarcoma;* of cartilage, a *chondrosarcoma;* and of bone, an *osteogenic sarcoma.* In addition, there is a small group of specialized tumors that may arise from other tissues in the body. For example, lymphoid tissue gives rise to a *lymphosarcoma* and neuroglial tissue can form an *astrocytoma.*

FASCIAE

A knowledge of the arrangement of the deep fasciae is emphasized by surgeons, because the arrangement will often explain the path taken by an infection when it spreads from its primary site. The density of the feltwork of collagen fibers making up the fascia provides an impermeable barrier to an inflammatory exudate or frank pus. In the neck, for example, the arrangement of various fascial planes explains how infection can extend from the region of the floor of the mouth to the larynx.

BURSAE AND SYNOVIAL SHEATHS

Bursae and synovial sheaths are commonly the site of traumatic and infectious disease. For example, the extensor tendon sheaths of the hand may become inflamed following excessive or unaccustomed use; an inflammation of the prepatellar bursa may occur as the result of trauma from repeated kneeling on a hard surface.

IMMUNOLOGICAL PROCESSES

Plasma Cells in Antibody Production

The role of plasma cells in the formation of antibodies will be discussed at length in Chapter 9. It is sufficient here to state that once a foreign antigen enters the lymphoid tissue, it is engulfed by macrophages, which then present it to the B lymphocytes. The B lymphocytes, often assisted by the T lymphocytes, then proliferate and mature into plasma cells. The plasma cells produce a specific antibody to the antigen. Plasma cells thus play a vital role in the production of humoral immunity.

In chronic inflammation, such as tuberculosis or syphilis, lymphocytes and plasma cells appear in the lesion. It is thought that this may result from a local immunological reaction.

Plasma Cell Neoplasms

Multiple myeloma is a malignant neoplasm of plasma cells of the skeleton. The malignant plasma cells invade the bones and produce large quantities of immunoglobulins in the blood and urine. The neoplasm may arise from a group of B lymphocytes that have been stimulated chronically by long-standing infection.

Mast Cells and Anaphylactic Hypersensitivity

An anaphylactic reaction to an antigen may be general, producing a state of shock, or local, producing such conditions as hives, hay fever, bronchial asthma, and food allergies. The antigen, on first entering the body, stimulates the production of IgE antibody by the lymphocytes and plasma cells. This antibody now attaches itself to the plasma membranes of mast cells (and the basophils of the blood). Reexposure of the body to the antigen causes the antigen to bind to the antibody on the mast cell (and the basophil cell). Immediately, these cells release histamine, which causes contraction of the smooth muscle of the bronchi, increased permeability of the capillaries, and increased gastric secretion. A factor is also released that attracts eosinophils to the site. It is thought that the eosinophils release substances that counteract histamine and limit the reaction.

Macrophages: Their Role as Phagocytes and the Development of Immunity

Macrophages are distributed throughout the body and are given a variety of names. In connective tissues, they are called *histiocytes;* in the blood, *monocytes;* in the lungs, *alveolar macrophages;* and in the liver, *Kupffer cells.* This mononuclear group of cells is collectively known as the *mononuclear phagocytic system* or *reticuloendothelial system,* and most of these cells are believed to be derived from the blood monocytes. The cells are large and have one common distinguishing feature: they engulf and digest foreign particles, a process known as *phagocytosis.* They must be distinguished from the smaller, more mobile phagocytosing cells found in the blood, the *neutrophils.*

Recently, macrophages have been shown to play a fundamental role in the development of immunity, in that they make available to the lymphocyte the antigen present in the foreign material that has invaded the body. It has also been shown that T lymphocytes can produce substances, called *lymphokines,* that can inhibit or activate macrophages in response to specific antigens.

In inflammation, macrophages appear late, when the battle between the invading and defensive forces is nearly over. They actively phagocytose dead and dying cells and foreign material, thus clearing the area and allowing the healing process to begin. It must not be forgotten that some of the macrophages may fall victim to the invaders and die, liberating highly potent enzymes that may bring about a local breakdown of normal tissues and so slightly delay the healing process. They will certainly release antigens and substances that will produce leukocytosis and fever.

FAT CELLS

The Fat Cell and Fat Embolism

Fat embolism occurs in patients who have suffered severe traumatic injuries to adipose tissue, such as that found in the yellow marrow of long bones, or extensive injury to subcutaneous tissue. Fat globules enter the blood circulation through ruptured venules and may obstruct the pulmonary circulation or circulation in the central nervous system. The clinical signs and symptoms, and the outcome, will depend on the size and number of fat globules that enter the bloodstream and the severity of the obstruction to the circulation in the lungs and the nervous system.

The Fat Cell and Fat Necrosis

Localized fat necrosis occasionally occurs in the breast following trauma. The fat cells undergo necrosis and become surrounded by macrophages that contain lipid globules in their cytoplasm. Later, the area is invaded by lymphocytes and fibroblasts. The latter lay down collagen, and the lesion is thus replaced by a localized area of scar tissue. The clinical importance of the mass of scar tissue lies in the possibility of its being mistaken for a neoplasm.

The Fat Cell as a Storehouse of Energy

Fat is a very efficient form in which to store energy. About 9 calories can be liberated for every gram of adipose tissue. Unfortunately, in Western society, the average individual overeats. This excessive consumption leads to obesity, which is a risk to health.

Obesity and the Fat Cell

Obesity may be defined as the presence of excess body fat that is inconsistent with good health. Clinical observation has shown that obese individuals are more likely to suffer from such diseases as high blood pressure (hypertension), diabetes mellitus, respiratory disease, and cerebrovascular hemorrhages. The hypertension is probably caused by the increased blood volume required to serve the increased volume of adipose tissue, and the cerebrovascular hemorrhages may be secondary to the hypertension. The respiratory disease is secondary to the reduced efficiency of respiratory movement following accumulations of fat in the thorax and abdomen. In the majority of patients with diabetes mellitus, there is a significant increase in obesity that greatly influences carbohydrate metabolism. Varicose veins are aggravated by obesity, possibly because of pooling of excess blood and reduced efficiency of the thoraco-abdominal pump that aids venous return to the right side of the heart. Osteoarthritis of the joints of the lower limbs is exacerbated by the increased workload secondary to an individual's increase in weight.

Because obesity is caused by the ingestion of more calories than the body requires for metabolism, it would seem a simple matter to prevent obesity by eating less. This is easier said than done, as many individuals who have excessive weight problems well know. Hereditary, cultural, psychological, and hormonal factors, among others, have been implicated as causing obesity. One theory is that the number of fat cells in the body is important because the cells exert some form of control on the feeding center in the hypothalamus. It has been suggested that there are three periods in the life cycle when new fat cells are formed in connective tissue: the last 3 months of fetal life, the first 5 years of life, and the period immediately after puberty. It follows that the accumulation of excessive fat during these periods will lead to lifelong obesity.

Another possibility is that excess body fat is acquired at some period during life and does not stem from heredity or other predisposing causes, and once acquired it is very difficult to lose permanently. This suggestion is supported by the fact that very few individuals who successfully lose weight are able to maintain the weight loss.

BONE DISORDERS

Osteogenesis Imperfecta: A Defect in Collagen Synthesis

Osteogenesis imperfecta is a hereditary bone disease caused by a defect in collagen synthesis that results in the formation of an abnormal bone matrix. The bones are thin and subject to multiple fractures, and the individual is loose-jointed. Those affected also have thin skin and blue sclerae because of the lack of normal collagen.

Achondroplasia: A Defect in the Cartilage Cells of Long Bones

Achondroplasia is a hereditary disease affecting the cartilage cells of long bones. The cartilage cells fail to proliferate in the epiphyseal cartilages, and there is premature fusion of the epiphyses with the diaphysis. Because the bones of the face and vault of the skull are produced by membrane bone formation, they are not affected. The individual is thus a dwarf, having a head and trunk of normal size and short arms and legs.

Rickets, Osteomalacia, and Vitamin D Deficiency

Rickets and osteomalacia are disorders of bone in which there is a defective mineralization of the matrix. In rickets, it is the growing bones that are involved, and there is also a defect in the mineralization of the matrix around the cartilage cells in the epiphyseal plates.

Adequate amounts of vitamin D are necessary for the normal mineralization of bone matrix. Vitamin D is normally absorbed from the diet in the small intestine and is produced in the skin by the photoconversion of sterols. The metabolites of vitamin D control the absorption of calcium in the small intestine, the renal reabsorption of calcium in the tubules, and the mobilization of calcium from bone. By these means, vitamin D is able to sustain a normal calcium level in the blood.

In rickets, the failure of mineralization of cartilage results in a persistence of the cartilage cells, which continue to grow, producing excess cartilage and a widening of the epiphyseal plates. The poorly mineralized cartilaginous matrix and the osteoid matrix are soft, and they bend under the stress of weight bearing.

In osteomalacia, which occurs in adults, the normally mineralized bone is replaced with soft, poorly mineralized osteoid matrix. Deformity may follow.

COLLAGEN AND VITAMIN C DEFICIENCY (SCURVY)

Human beings are unable to synthesize ascorbic acid and, consequently, require vitamin C in the diet to prevent scurvy. Ascorbic acid is vital for collagen formation. It is essential for the hydroxylation of proline to hydroxyproline. Nonhydroxylated collagen is unstable and cannot form the triple helix required for normal collagen structure. As a result, there is a disruption of the tunica adventitia, media, and basal laminae of blood vessels and a delay in wound healing, with low tensile strength in the resulting scar. It is interesting to note that in scurvy, old scars frequently break down. This deterioration can be explained by the constant remodeling that occurs in scar tissue: old collagen is being broken down, and new collagen is being formed. It is the new collagen that is weak in ascorbic acid deficiency.

The clinical manifestations of scurvy include hemorrhages into the skin, joints, and muscles and loosening of the teeth. The disease rapidly responds to the ingestion of ascorbic acid. Although scurvy is now rare in the United States, it still may occur in infants whose milk formulas are not supplemented by vitamin C. It also occurs in the elderly who neglect to eat adequate amounts of fruits and fresh vegetables.

CLINICAL PROBLEMS

For the answers to these problems, see page 786.

1. An 8-year-old girl is run over by an automobile as she crosses a road on her way to school. She sustains severe lacerations of her right hand with extensive skin loss, which requires a full-thickness skin graft. It is decided to perform a pedicle graft of skin from her right thigh. The plastic surgeon asks a third-year medical student whether the subcutaneous fat of the thigh might later present problems in this patient if transplanted to the hand. How would you answer that question?

2. A 23-year-old man is admitted to the emergency room in anaphylactic shock following an injection of penicillin at the doctor's office. The patient complains of tightness in the chest and exhibits difficulty in breathing, accompanied by a wheezing noise. On examination, he has a rapid pulse rate and a low blood pressure. He has three large hives on the skin of the anterior abdominal wall. On questioning, the patient admits that he has suffered from hay fever all his life. Patients with hypersensitivity reactions have elevated levels of IgE. What is IgE? To which cells in connective tissue and blood does this substance become attached? What chemical is released by these cells to produce the signs and symptoms of anaphylaxis?

3. One characteristic is common to all the cells of the reticuloendothelial system (mononuclear phagocytic system). What is that characteristic? Give examples of cells that belong to the reticuloendothelial system. What role do these cells play in the healing of a wound?

4. A medical student is involved in a motorcycle accident that results in the fracture of the lower third of the left tibia. After prolonged immobilization of the fracture, it is found that healing is not taking place. The orthopedic surgeon explains to the student that the vascularization of the fractured area is poor because of the large area of soft tissue destroyed at the time of the accident. Proper union of a fracture is very dependent on the blood supply to the bone. Describe how a long bone receives its blood supply.

5. A 35-year-old woman has a papilloma removed from her right armpit. The surgeon makes an elliptical incision on both sides of the stalk of the tumor and removes the tumor, together with a small amount of normal skin. He then sutures the skin edges together. Twelve months later, the scar is seen as a fine white line. What is a papilloma? Describe the process of wound healing after a clean surgical incision. Name a vitamin necessary for the formation of a strong scar. What is a keloid scar?

6. After sustaining a severe knee injury in a football match, a man is told by the orthopedic surgeon that he has a torn medial cartilage within the joint. Does a torn cartilage in the knee heal by regeneration?

7. What role do plasma cells play in the defense of the body against infection?

8. A 9-year-old boy is examined by a pediatrician and found to have cleidocranial dysostosis. This is a congenital condition in which the clavicles are partially or completely absent and the transverse diameter of the skull is greater than normal. The physician informs the parents that this condition affects bones that are formed from membrane. What does he

mean by this statement? Describe how these particular bones are formed from membrane.

9. A black woman aged 45 years undergoes a partial thyroidectomy for removal of a thyroid adenoma. The surgeon is particularly careful to make the incision in the line of cleavage in the neck skin. What is meant by the term *line of cleavage*? Is this woman likely to develop a keloid scar?

10. During the course of a lecture on connective tissues, the professor of pathology continually refers to "fixed" cells, which remain stationary in connective tissue, and "freely mobile" cells, which enter and leave connective tissue via the capillaries of blood and lymph vessels. Make a list of the so-called fixed and free cells found in loose connective tissue, for example.

11. A plastic surgeon, while reconstructing a patient's nose, makes the comment that the plates of hyaline cartilage must be preserved so that the nose will retain its shape and flexibility. What is the structure of hyaline cartilage? Why is it firm and yet flexible? How does it differ in structure from elastic cartilage?

12. Granulation tissue is vitally important in the healing of a large open wound of the skin, for example. What is granulation tissue? Why does it provide an effective barrier against wound infection? What is wound contraction? How does it differ from wound contracture?

13. A 50-year-old man decides to start jogging; everyone in his neighborhood seems to be doing it. After 5 minutes of jogging, he experiences a sudden, severe pain over his right calf and becomes unable even to walk. The orthopedic surgeon tells him that he has ruptured his right tendo calcaneus (tendo Achillis) and that it requires immediate operation. The tendo calcaneus is composed of bundles of collagen fibers. Which cell or cells in the body are capable of forming collagen? Describe the stages in the formation of collagen. At what point is vitamin C essential for the normal formation of collagen?

14. A 5-year-old boy is admitted to the hospital with a tuberculous osteomyelitis of the distal end of the diaphysis of the right radius. What is the diaphysis?

15. A junior resident is shown the radiograph of the right humerus of a 10-year-old boy and asked to point out the epiphysis. What is the epiphysis? What is an epiphyseal plate? What part does an epiphyseal plate play in the growth of a long bone?

16. A surgeon, while carrying out a ward round with his staff, says to his senior resident, "This patient may well develop a pyogenic arthritis in one of her synovial joints." What is a synovial joint? Give an example of a synovial joint.

17. Following a skiing accident, a 25-year-old woman is examined by an orthopedic surgeon. A diagnosis of a spiral fracture of the right tibia is made. Two months later, the surgeon examines radiographs of the healing fracture and tells the patient that good callus formation is visible on the radiographs. What is callus?

18. A 25-year-old pregnant woman has had a problem with obesity all her life. She reads in a magazine article that some authorities believe that the center in your brain that controls your eating habits is regulated by the number of fat cells laid down at certain periods in life. Are there certain periods in life when fat cells can be produced in large quantities? If many fat cells are produced at these times, is the resulting obesity permanent? What is the structure of a fat cell? What is the calorific value of fat? What is the function of adipose tissue?

19. After a severe automobile accident, a 45-year-old man is admitted to the hospital with a comminuted fracture of the shaft of the left femur. The patient dies suddenly 36 hours later with acute pulmonary insufficiency. At postmortem examination, a diagnosis of fat embolism is made. Can you explain the diagnosis?

20. A 19-year-old mother who is mentally retarded takes her 3-year-old son to a pediatrician for a physical examination. The doctor is distressed to find that the child has severe rickets. The child's forehead is enlarged, and the bones of the lower limbs are bent

and deformed. The child is treated with large amounts of vitamin D added to his diet, and the mother is advised to take the child out into the sunlight as much as possible. Why are adequate amounts of vitamin D and sunlight necessary for the normal formation of bone? Why are the epiphyseal cartilages thickened in rickets?

ADDITIONAL READING

Anderson, D. R. The ultrastructure of elastic and hyaline cartilage in the rat. *Am. J. Anat.* 114:403, 1964.

Anderson, H. C. Calcium-accumulating vesicles in the intercellular matrix of bone. In Elliott, K., and Fitzsimmons, D. W., *Hard Tissue Growth, Repair and Remineralization. Ciba Foundation Symposium II.* Amsterdam: ASP (Elsevier-North Holland), 1973, p. 213.

Alpert, E. N. Developing elastic tissue. *Am. J. Pathol.* 69:89, 1972.

Burwen, S. J., and Satir, B. H. Plasma membrane folds on the mast cell surface and their relationship to secretory activity. *J. Cell Biol.* 74:690, 1977.

Carr, I. *The Macrophage: A Review of Ultrastructure and Function.* New York: Academic, 1973.

Chvapil, M. *Physiology of Connective Tissue.* Washington, D.C.: Butterworth, 1967.

Clark, I. C. Articular cartilage: A review and scanning electron microscope study. II. The territorial fibrillar architecture. *J. Anat.* 118:261, 1974.

Combs, J. W. An electron microscope study of mouse mast cells arising *in vivo* and *in vitro*. *J. Cell Biol.* 48:676, 1971.

Cushman, S. W. Structure-function relationship in the adipose cell. I. Ultrastructure of the isolated adipose cell. *J. Cell Biol.* 46:326, 1970.

De Petris, S., Karlsbad, G., and Pernis, B. Localization of antibodies in plasma cells by electron microscopy. *J. Exp. Med.* 117:849, 1963.

Dunphy, J. E. (ed.). *Wound Healing.* New York: Medcom, 1974.

Gay, S., and Miller, E. J. *Collagen in the Physiology and Pathology of Connective Tissue.* Stuttgart: Fischer, 1978.

Goel, S. C. Electron microscopic studies on developing cartilage. I. The membrane system related to the synthesis and secretion of extracellular materials. *J. Embryol. Exp. Morphol.* 23:169, 1970.

Haines, R. W. The histology of epiphyseal union in mammals. *J. Anat.* 120:1, 1975.

Hall, D. A. *The Aging of Connective Tissue.* New York: Academic, 1976.

Hall, R. W. The origin and fate of osteoclasts. *Anat. Rec.* 183:1, 1975.

Ham, A. W., and Harris, W. R. Repair and transplantation of bone. In Bourne, G. H. (ed.), *The Biochemistry and Physiology of Bone.* Vol. 3. New York: Academic, 1972, p. 338.

Hancox, N. M. *Biology of Bone.* New York: Cambridge University Press, 1972.

Holtrop, M. E. The ultrastructure of bone. *Ann. Clin. Lab. Sci.* 5:264, 1975.

Jande, S. S. Fine structural study of osteocytes and their surrounding bone matrix with respect to their age in young chicks. *J. Ultrastruct. Res.* 37:279, 1971.

Jones, S. J., and Boyde, A. Some morphologic observations on osteoclasts. *Cell Tissue Res.* 185:387, 1977.

Kewley, M. A., Stevens, F. S., and Williams, G. The presence of fine elastin fibrils within the elastin fibre observed by scanning electron microscopy. *J. Anat.* 123:129, 1977.

Merklin, R. J. Growth and distribution of human fetal brown fat. *Anat. Rec.* 178:637, 1974.

Morse, D. E., and Low, F. N. The fine structure of developing unit collagenous fibrils in the chick. *Am. J. Anat.* 140:237, 1974.

Nelson, D. S. (ed.). *Immunobiology of the Macrophage.* New York: Academic, 1976.

Owen, M. The origin of bone cells. *Int. Rev. Cytol.* 28:213, 1970.

Page, R. C. The macrophage as a secretory cell. *Int. Rev. Cytol.* 52:119, 1978.

Papadimitriov, J. M., and Archer, M. The morphology of foreign body multinucleate giant cells. *J. Ultrastruct. Res.* 49:372, 1974.

Peacock, E. E., Jr., and Van Winkle, W., Jr. *Surgery and Biology of Wound Repair.* Philadelphia: Saunders, 1970.

Pritchard, J. J. The osteoblast. In Bourne, G. H. (ed.), *The Biochemistry and Physiology of Bone* (2nd ed.). Vol. 1. New York: Academic, 1972, p. 21.

Revel, J. P. Role of the Golgi apparatus of cartilage cells in the elaboration of matrix glycosaminoglycans. In Balazs, E. A. (ed.), *Chemistry and Molecular Biology of the Intercellular Matrix.* Vol. 3. New York: Academic, 1970, p. 1485.

Robert, A. M., Robert, B., and Robert, L. Chemical and physical properties of structural glycoproteins. In Balazs, E. A. (ed.), *Chemistry and Molecular Biology of the Intercellular Matrix.* Vol. 1. New York: Academic, 1970, p. 237.

Ross, R. The fibroblast and wound repair. *Biol. Rev.* 43:51, 1968.

Ross, R. The elastic fiber: A review. *J. Histochem. Cytochem.* 21:199, 1973.

Ross, R., and Bornstein, P. Elastic fibers in the body. *Sci. Am.* 224(6):44, 1971.

Selye, H. *The Mast Cells.* Washington, D.C.: Butterworth, 1965.

Slavin, B. G. The cytophysiology of mammalian adipose cells. *Int. Rev. Cytol.* 33:297, 1972.

Steer, H. W. Mast cells of the human stomach. *J. Anat.* 121:385, 1976.

Trelstad, R. L., et al. Isolation of two distinct collagens from chick cartilage. *Biochemistry* 9:4993, 1970.

Vaughan, J. M. *The Physiology of Bone.* London: Oxford University Press, 1970.

Wright, V., Dowson, D., and Kerr, J. The structure of joints. In Hall, D. A., and Jackson, D. S. (eds.), *International Review of Connective Tissue Research.* Vol. 6. New York: Academic, 1973, p. 105.

BLOOD AND BONE MARROW

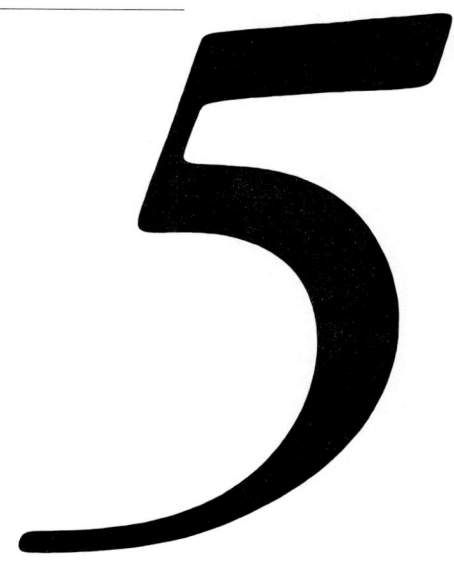

BLOOD

Blood is a viscous, opaque fluid that when oxygenated is scarlet and when deoxygenated is dark red or purple. It is actually a fluid connective tissue in which the blood cells are suspended in a fluid matrix called *plasma*. The blood transports oxygen from the lungs, the products of digestion from the digestive system, hormones from the endocrine glands, and enzymes and many other chemical substances from widely scattered organs. The blood carries these substances to tissues all over the body, where the substances pass out of the capillaries and enter the tissue fluid. The tissue fluid then carries them to the cells, where they are metabolized. The waste products of metabolism then enter the blood via the tissue fluid. The blood transports the waste materials to the lungs, kidneys, and sweat glands, where they are excreted from the body.

The major functions of the blood are (1) transport of oxygen, carbon dioxide, and hormones; (2) maintenance of acid-base balance; (3) removal of waste products of cellular metabolism; (4) maintenance of cellular homeostasis; (5) temperature control of the body; and (6) defense against infection.

Blood Volume

Blood is contained in a closed system of tubes that together with the heart is known as the cardiovascular system. The volume of blood in a healthy individual is surprisingly constant. In a normal adult it is about 5,000 ml, and is greater in men than in women.

Composition of Blood

If fresh blood is placed in a centrifuge tube and rotated rapidly, the blood will separate into its component parts. The cells are thrown down by centrifugal force to the bottom of the tube. The clear, light amber fluid lying above the cells is called *plasma* and forms about 55 percent of the volume of the blood sample. The packed mass of blood cells (or formed elements) at the bottom of the tube forms about 45 percent of the volume of the sample (Fig. 5-1A). *Erythrocytes* or *red blood cells* form about 44 percent, and the remaining 1 percent is formed of *leukocytes* or *white blood cells*. The thin layer of white cells lies on top of the red cells and is known as the *buffy coat*.

If fresh blood is placed in a test tube and allowed

155

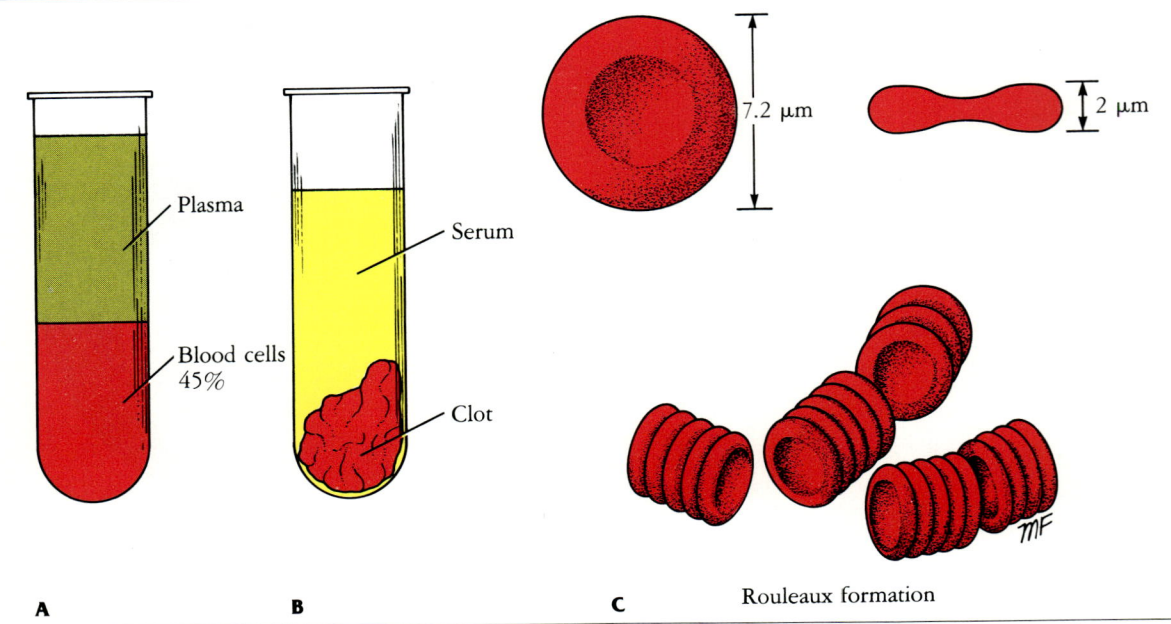

Fig. 5-1. (A) Hematocrit tube after centrifugation of whole blood. (B) The formation of serum from clotted blood. (C) Red blood cells, or erythrocytes.

to stand, it soon clots. Eventually the blood clot begins to contract and expresses a straw-colored fluid called *serum* (Fig. 5-1B). Serum is in fact plasma from which the protein *fibrinogen* has been removed by clotting.

Microscopic examination enables one to distinguish between the erythrocytes and the different types of leukocytes. The Romanovsky methods of staining are commonly used for this purpose. The Giemsa and Leishman stains are among those used in these methods and consist of mixtures of methylene blue and eosin. The stains are applied to a thin, dried film of blood on a glass slide (Fig. 5-2).

Blood is composed of the following elements:

1. Cells
   a. Red cells, or erythrocytes
   b. White cells, or leukocytes
   c. Platelets, or thrombocytes
2. Plasma
   a. Water
   b. Solids
      i. Organic substances, including proteins and other compounds
      ii. Inorganic substances
      iii. Gases
      iv. Hormones and enzymes

Hematocrit

The hematocrit is the percentage of red blood cells in the blood, as determined by centrifugation of whole blood in a hematocrit tube. The percentage of the red cells is determined by measuring the level of the packed red cells at the bottom of the tube (see Fig. 5-1A). The normal hematocrit for a man is about 40 to 45; that for a woman, about 35 to 40.

Red Blood Cells

Red blood cells or erythrocytes are small, disc-shaped cells that have no nuclei (Figs. 5-3 and 5-4; see Fig. 5-1). Just before a red cell reaches maturity and enters the blood from the red bone marrow, the nucleus is pushed through the cell membrane. As a result, the cell collapses inward and assumes the shape of a biconcave disc. This peculiar shape gives

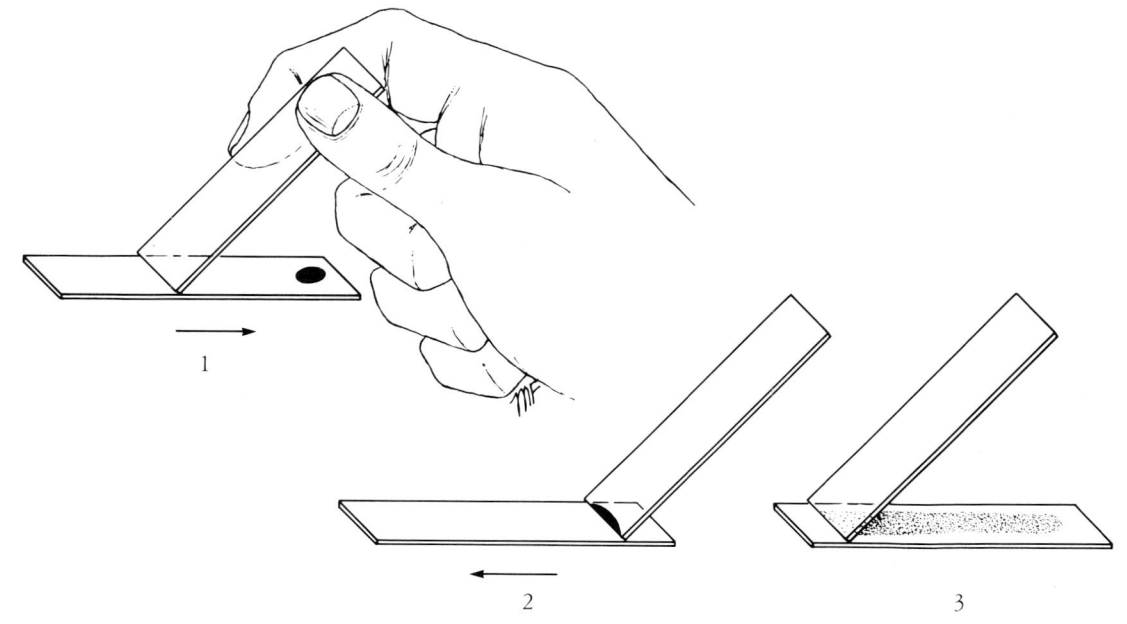

Fig. 5-2. The three stages in the preparation of a blood film.

it a very large surface area relative to its volume, ideal for the exchange of gases, but the loss of the nucleus prevents the cell from reproducing and restricts its metabolic activities.

Red blood cells have a mean diameter of approximately 7.2 μm and a thickness at the thickest part of about 2 μm. The red cell is soft and elastic and can be deformed into almost any shape as it passes through small capillaries. It gets its red color from the large amount of the conjugated protein *hemoglobin* in its cytoplasm. Hemoglobin is called a conjugated protein because it consists of a protein called *globin* united to the red pigment *heme*. In blood that has been removed from the body and allowed to stagnate, the red cells tend to stick together on their broad surfaces like a pile of coins. This arrangement is known as *rouleaux formation* (Fig. 5-5; see Fig. 5-1). Sometimes rouleaux formation takes place in the bloodstream when the circulation is not rapid. Rouleaux formation is not permanent and does no harm to the red blood cells.

In the normal male the average number of red blood cells per cubic millimeter of blood is about 5 *million;* in the female, it is about 4.7 *million*.

FUNCTION. The chief function of the red cells is to transport oxygen from the lungs to the tissues and, indirectly, to transport carbon dioxide from the tissues to the lungs. The red cell is able to carry oxygen in large amounts because of the *hemoglobin* within its cytoplasm. Hemoglobin combines rapidly with oxygen to form the compound *oxyhemoglobin*. When the oxyhemoglobin reaches the tissues of the body, oxygen is released rapidly, and the hemoglobin that remains is called *reduced hemoglobin*.

The presence of large quantities of the enzyme *carbonic anhydrase* within the red cell cytoplasm makes it possible for large quantities of carbon dioxide to combine with water and thereby be transported from the tissues to the lungs in the form of bicarbonate.

Hemoglobin, like other proteins, is an excellent acid-base buffer, and, because there are so many red cells in the blood, the hemoglobin plays a large role in controlling the hydrogen ion concentration of the blood.

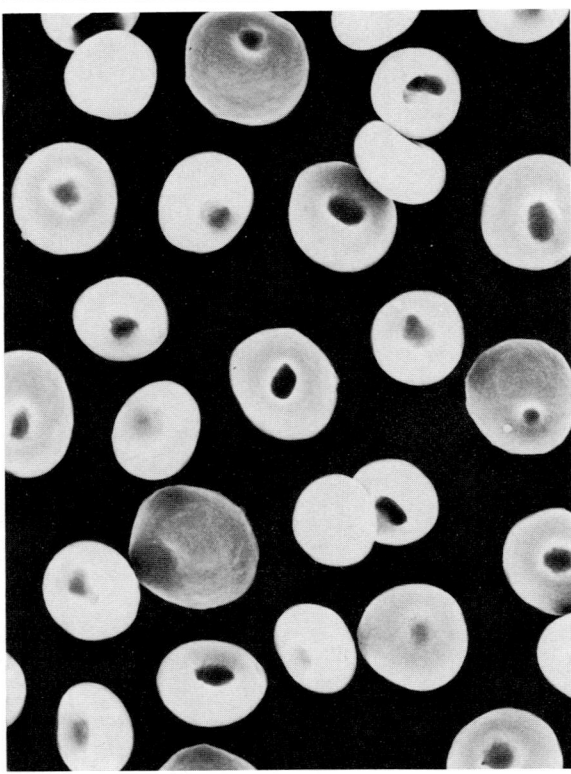

Fig. 5-3. Scanning electron micrograph of a blood film, showing numerous erythrocytes exhibiting their biconcave disc shape. (×2,304.) (Courtesy of F. G. Lightfoot.)

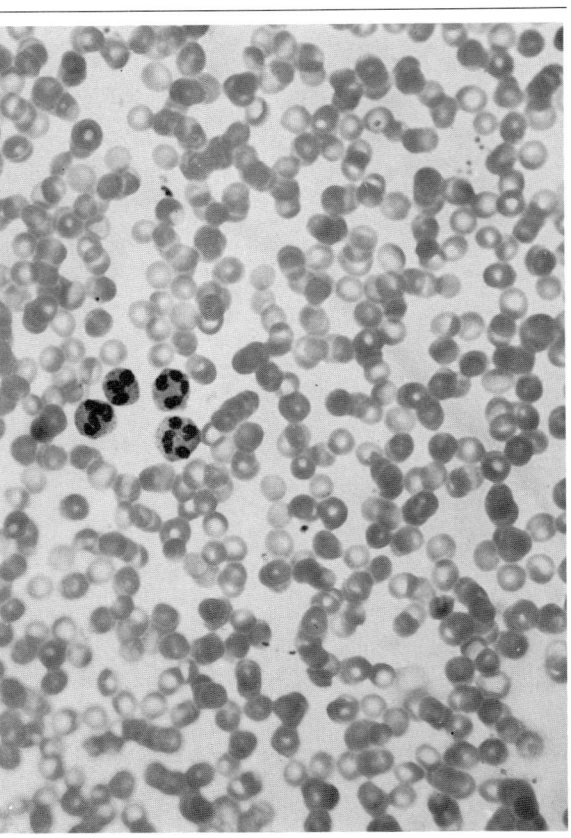

Fig. 5-4. Photomicrograph of a blood film, showing numerous erythrocytes; four polymorphonuclear leukocytes can also be seen. (Leishman stain; ×655.)

The biconcave shape of the red cell permits the maximum surface area of the cell membrane per unit of hemoglobin to be exposed to the plasma. The surface area is greater than it would be if, for example, the red cell were a sphere.

Hemoglobin. Hemoglobin, as stated previously, is a conjugated protein composed of a pigment *heme* and a protein known as *globin.* Heme is a porphyrin combined with iron. The whole blood of men contains about *15 gm of hemoglobin per 100 ml,* and that of women, about *14 gm per 100 ml.*

The volume of oxygen that blood has taken up when its hemoglobin is fully saturated is called the *oxygen capacity* of blood. Because each gram of hemoglobin combines with 1.34 ml of oxygen, 100 ml of blood in a healthy male will have an oxygen capacity of 15 × 1.34, or 20.1 ml. It follows that a patient with a low hemoglobin level will have a low oxygen-carrying capacity.

FORMATION OF RED BLOOD CELLS. After birth, red blood cell formation, *erythropoiesis,* takes place exclusively in the red bone marrow. The red cells pass through several stages of development (Fig. 5-6) before they escape from the marrow into the general circulation.

The process of red cell formation starts with *stem cells* located throughout the bone marrow. These cells are continually dividing, and the most primitive

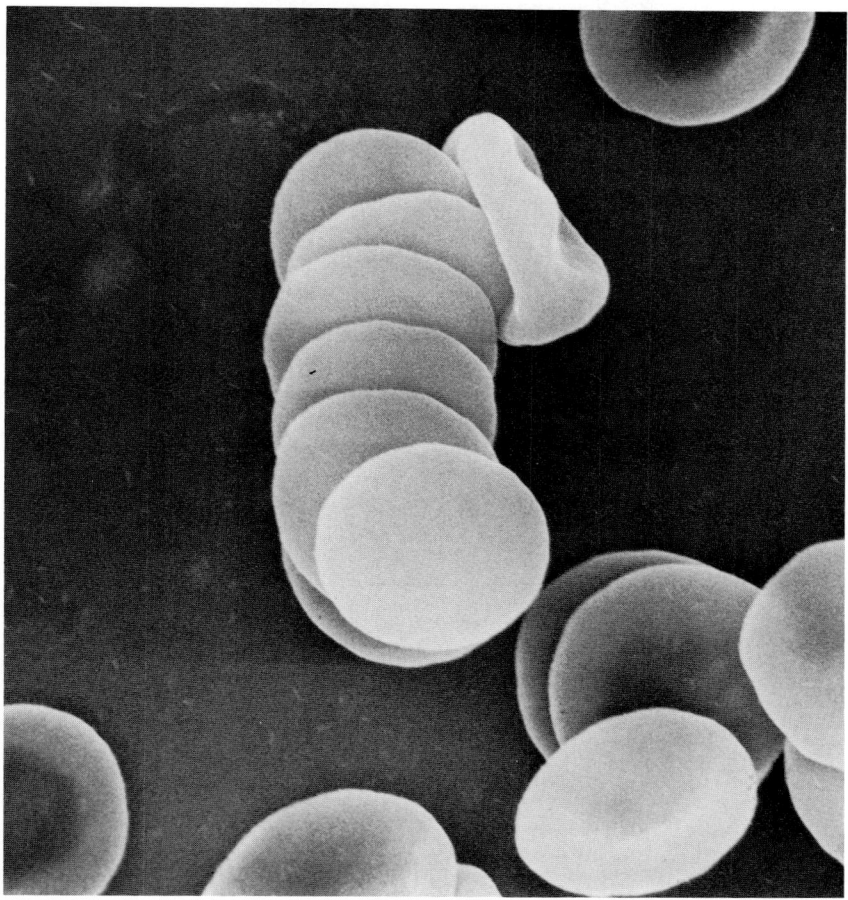

Fig. 5-5. Scanning electron micrograph of a group of erythrocytes displaying rouleaux formation. (× 7,900.) (Courtesy of F. G. Lightfoot.)

of the red cells are thus formed, called *hemocytoblasts* (see Fig. 5-6). The hemocytoblasts subsequently divide, producing *proerythroblasts*. These are large nucleated cells that possess no hemoglobin. Each proerythroblast now divides to form *basophilic erythroblasts*. These cells are slightly smaller than proerythroblasts, and their cytoplasm stains with basic dyes.

The basophilic erythroblasts now divide into *polychromatophilic erythroblasts* (see Fig. 5-6). These cells are smaller and have a small nucleus with condensed chromatin. The cytoplasm of these cells possesses hemoglobin, which is beginning to be synthesized at this stage. The polychromatophilic erythroblasts continue to divide, and the hemoglobin content of the cytoplasm increases. The nucleus becomes small and eccentric and stains deeply. The cell is now known as a *normoblast* (see Fig. 5-6). As the normoblast undergoes further development, the cytoplasm becomes filled with hemoglobin and the nucleus is extruded from the cell. This mature cell is known as the *red cell* or *erythrocyte*. The extruded nuclei are phagocytosed by the macrophages of the bone marrow. The newly formed erythrocytes pass between or through the endothelial cells of the marrow sinusoids and enter the blood circulation.

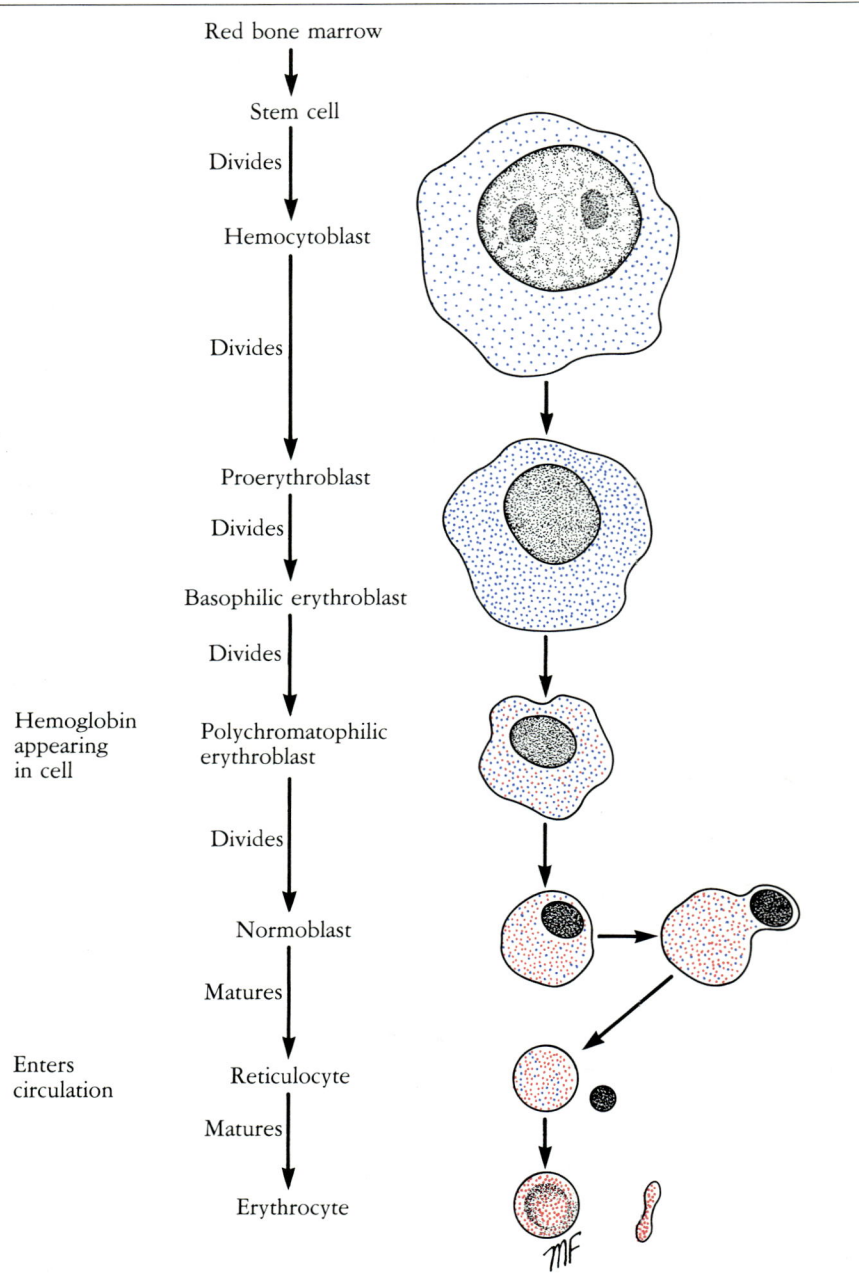

Fig. 5-6. *Formation of erythrocytes.*

Some of the new erythrocytes entering the blood contain small amounts of basophilic material interspersed with the hemoglobin in the cytoplasm. This material is the remains of the rough endoplasmic reticulum and may persist for 2 days. These reticulum-containing cells are known as *reticulocytes*. Normally, the total number of reticulocytes does not exceed one percent of the red cell series.

Control of Red Blood Cell Formation. The total number of red blood cells in the circulatory system is kept constant to provide adequte transport of oxygen from the lungs to the tissues. If a person has a decrease in the oxygen content of the blood, such as can occur following a severe hemorrhage or at a high altitude, where the concentration of oxygen in the air is greatly decreased, the hypoxia strongly stimulates the bone marrow to increase the red cell production. The substance responsible for stimulating the bone marrow is a glycoprotein called *erythropoietin*. Erythropoietin is thought to be synthesized in the kidney in response to hypoxia. It enters the blood and circulates for about 24 hours, during which it acts on the bone marrow and stimulates erythropoiesis. As would be expected, the transfusion of excess red cells leads to suppression of erythropoiesis. It is important to realize that the body possesses only a limited reserve of iron and that iron is necessary for the formation of hemoglobin. It is possible, therefore, that a lack of available iron in food or an inability to absorb it from the intestine will interfere with the response of the bone marrow to erythropoietin.

FATE OF RED BLOOD CELLS. The average life span of red cells is about 120 days. Although the cells possess no nuclei, active metabolic processes continue within the cytoplasm. It has been determined, however, that these processes become progressively reduced as the cells age. As the result of the stresses and strains that the cell is subjected to while it is whirled through the circulatory system, the red cell simply wears out. Once the plasma membrane ruptures, the cellular debris is removed from the blood circulation by reticuloendothelial macrophages, especially those of the spleen, liver, and bone marrow.

The hemoglobin within the red cells is released and digested and broken down into an iron-containing pigment called *hemosiderin,* a non-iron-containing pigment called *bilirubin,* and a protein called *globin.* The hemosiderin is either stored or taken to the bone marrow for the production of new hemoglobin in new red cells. The bilirubin is released into the blood and later secreted by the liver into the bile. The globin is metabolized in the liver.

White Blood Cells

Individual white cells, or leukocytes, are colorless, but when they are packed together, they are white. Unlike red cells, they possess a nucleus but have no hemoglobin. In the normal adult there are between *5,000 and 10,000 per cubic millimeter* of blood. In the bloodstream, they are spherical in shape and mobile. Whereas red cells perform their functions within the blood, white cells become active only when they leave the circulatory system and enter the tissues of the body.

White blood cells are of two main types: (1) those with granules in their cytoplasm, called *granulocytes,* and (2) those without granules in their cytoplasm, called *agranulocytes.* The granulocytes are of three types and are classified according to the staining of their granules into (1) *neutrophils,* (2) *eosinophils*, and (3) *basophils* (Fig. 5-7). The agranular leukocytes are of two types: (1) *lymphocytes,* so called because they are found in lymphoid tissue as well as in the bloodstream, and (2) *monocytes* (see Fig. 5-7). Because the nuclei of the granular leukocytes possess two or more lobes, they are frequently called *polymorphonuclear leukocytes.*

The approximate normal percentages of the different types of white blood cells in the adult are:

Neutrophils	55 to 60 percent
Eosinophils	1 to 3 percent
Basophils	0 to 0.7 percent
Lymphocytes	25 to 33 percent
Monocytes	3 to 7 percent

NEUTROPHILS. Neutrophils are the most numerous type of white cell, forming 55 to 60 percent of the

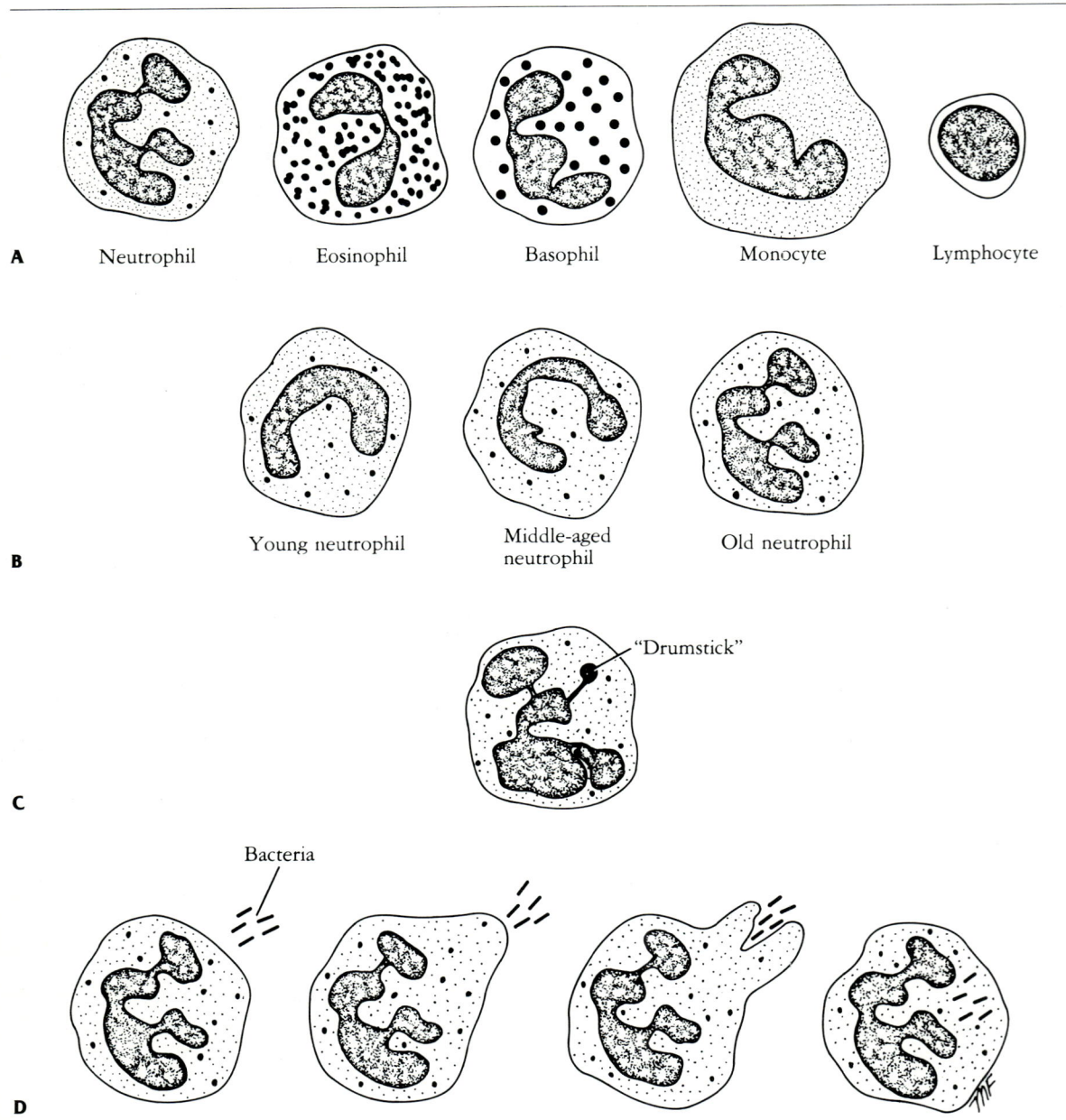

Fig. 5-7. (A) Structures of the different types of leukocytes; (B) age changes in a neutrophil; (C) neutrophil from a female, showing the X chromosome, which resembles a drumstick; (D) a neutrophil in the process of phagocytosing a group of bacteria.

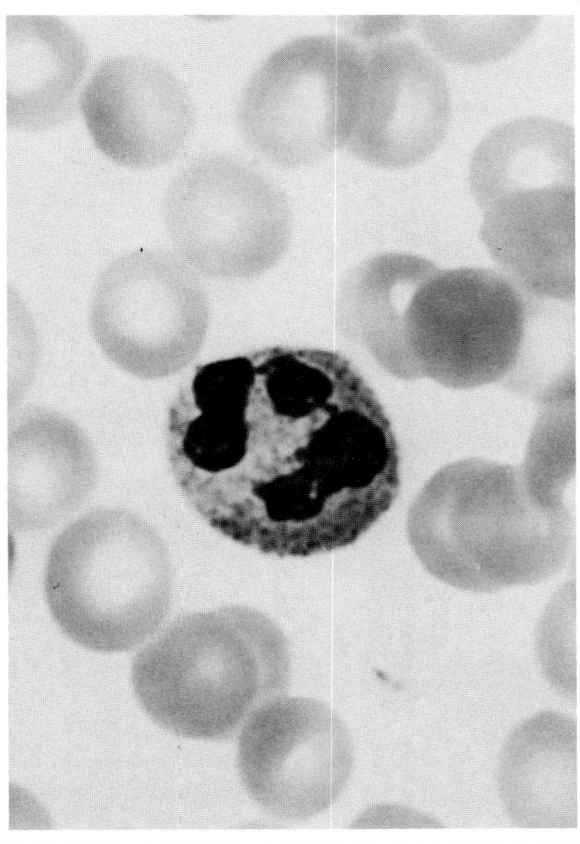

Fig. 5-8. Photomicrograph of a blood film, showing a mature neutrophil leukocyte surrounded by erythrocytes. Note that the neutrophil has a nucleus with three lobes connected by narrow strands. The cytoplasm contains large numbers of fine granules that are faintly stained; an occasional larger, more deeply stained granule is also visible. (Leishman stain; × 2,364.)

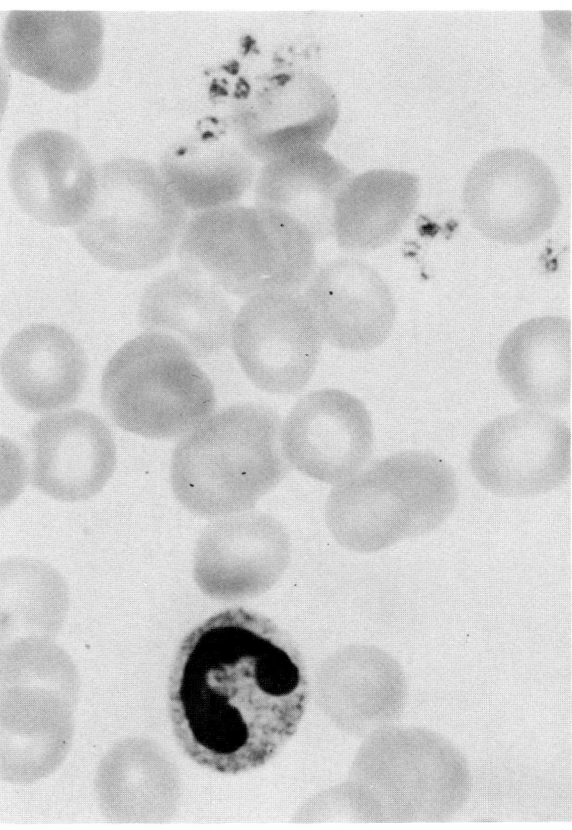

Fig. 5-9. Photomicrograph of a blood film, showing a young neutrophil leukocyte surrounded by erythrocytes. Note the shape of the nucleus of the neutrophil; compare with that in Figure 5-8. A number of platelets are seen as fine dots. (Leishman stain; × 1,700.)

white cell population. They measure about 10 to 12 μm in diameter, and their nuclei have two or more lobes connected by narrow strands (Figs. 5-8 and 5-9; see Fig. 5-7). A young neutrophil may show only slight lobulation of the nucleus, but as the cells age, the lobes increase in number. In a small percentage of neutrophils in women, the condensed chromatin of the X chromosome forms a small separate lobule of the nucleus that resembles a drumstick. It is thus possible to determine the sex of an individual by examining samples of neutrophils for the presence of the *sex* chromatin (see Figs. 5-7 and 2-5).

The cytoplasm of neutrophils contains large numbers of fine granules that stain faintly with neutral dyes. Scattered among the finer granules is an occasional larger granule that stains reddish-purple. The cytoplasmic granules are seen under the electron microscope to be lysosomes.

Neutrophils are actively mobile and phagocytic. They are attracted to bacteria by chemical substances liberated by the organisms, a process known as *chemotaxis*. The neutrophils send out pseudopodia

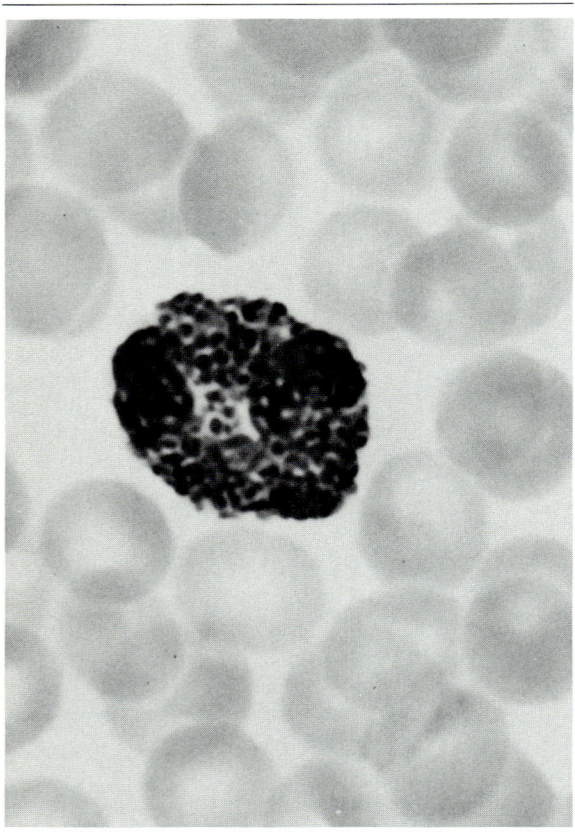

Fig. 5-10. Photomicrograph of a blood film, showing an eosinophil leukocyte surrounded by erythrocytes. The cytoplasm of the eosinophil is packed with coarse granules, and the dark-staining nucleus is just visible in the background. (Leishman stain; ×2,364.)

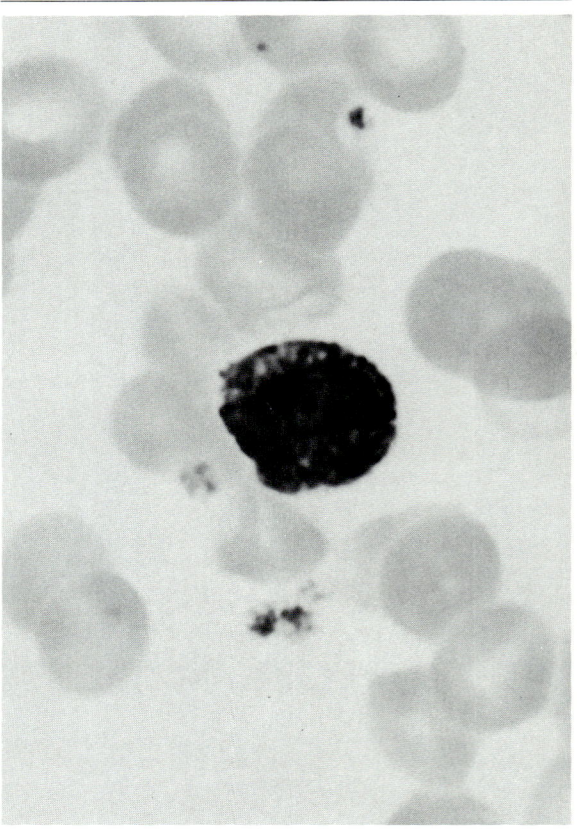

Fig. 5-11. Photomicrograph of a blood film, showing a basophil leukocyte surrounded by erythrocytes. The cytoplasm of the basophil is filled with deeply staining granules. A few platelets also can be seen in the film. (Leishman stain; ×2,364.)

that engulf the bacteria and other foreign matter. Once within the cytoplasm of the neutrophils, the bacteria are contained within membrane-bound vacuoles. Neutrophils contain large numbers of lysosomes that discharge their hydrolytic enzymes and bactericidal substances into the vacuoles, quickly destroying the bacteria. Neutrophils are thus one of our most important lines of defense against bacterial infection. Without neutrophils, an individual quickly dies of infection.

EOSINOPHILS. Eosinophils constitute about 1 to 3 percent of the white cell population. They measure about 10 to 12 μm in diameter (Fig. 5-10; see Fig. 5-7). The nucleus usually has two lobes, and the cytoplasm is packed with coarse, pink-staining granules. The granules are seen under the electron microscope to be lysosomes.

Eosinophils are motile but not as motile as neutrophils. They are phagocytic, but they ingest foreign protein rather than bacteria. They are found in the mucous membrane of the intestine, in the lungs, and in the dermis of the skin. Their function is in some manner related to the response of the body to foreign protein. They are found in increased numbers in tissues displaying allergic reactions and

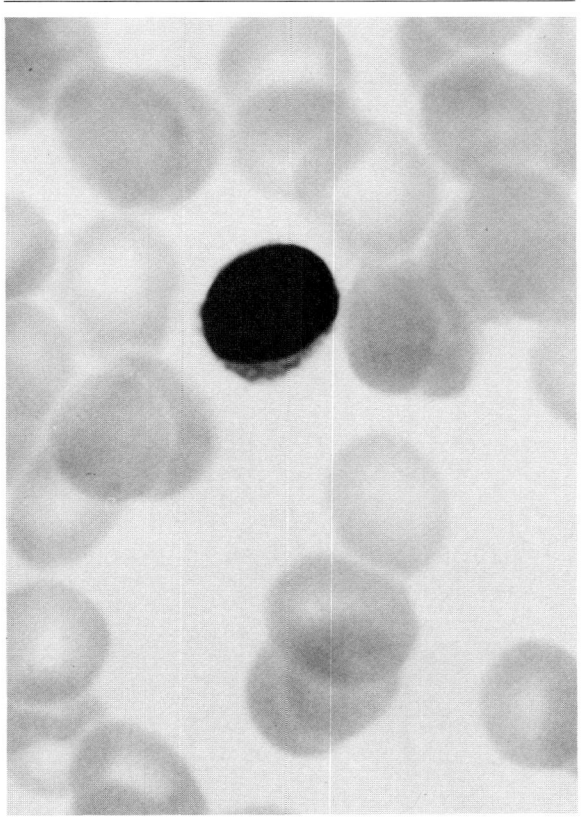

Fig. 5-12. Photomicrograph of a blood film, showing a small lymphocyte surrounded by erythrocytes. Note that the lymphocyte possesses a deeply stained, rounded nucleus surrounded by a thin rim of cytoplasm. (Leishman stain; ×2,364.)

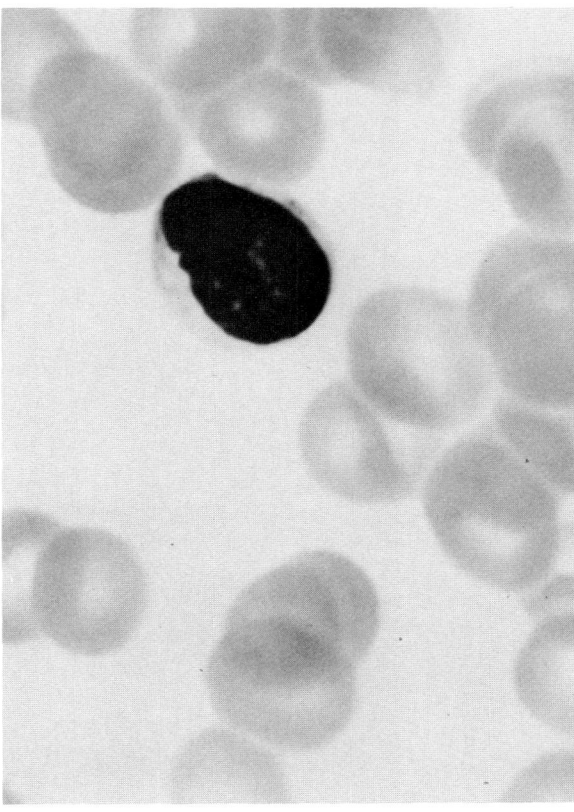

Fig. 5-13. Photomicrograph of a blood film, showing a large lymphocyte surrounded by erythrocytes. Compare with Figure 5-12. (Leishman stain; ×2,364.)

in the blood of individuals who experience allergic reactions. Eosinophils are believed to release substances that counteract the effects of histamine in allergic reactions. Hydrocortisone, a hormone that depresses allergic reactions, also lowers the numbers of eosinophils in the blood.

BASOPHILS. Basophils are few in number, forming only a maximum of 0.7 percent of the white cell population. A prolonged search may be required to find a basophil in a blood smear. These cells measure about 10 to 12 μm in diameter (Fig. 5-11; see Fig. 5-7). The nucleus is irregular in shape and may possess more than one lobe. The cytoplasm contains large, dark blue–staining granules that contain *heparin* and *histamine*. Examination with an electron microscope shows that the granules are bounded by a membrane.

Basophils are motile and phagocytic. Although their precise function is unknown, they are believed to release heparin into the bloodstream, where it probably serves as an anticoagulant. The release of histamine by basophils appears to be associated with allergic and inflammatory reactions (see p. 147).

LYMPHOCYTES. Lymphocytes constitute about 25 to 33 percent of the total white cell population. They vary in size from 7 to 12 μm in diameter (Figs. 5-12, 5-13, and 5-14). They have intensely staining, round

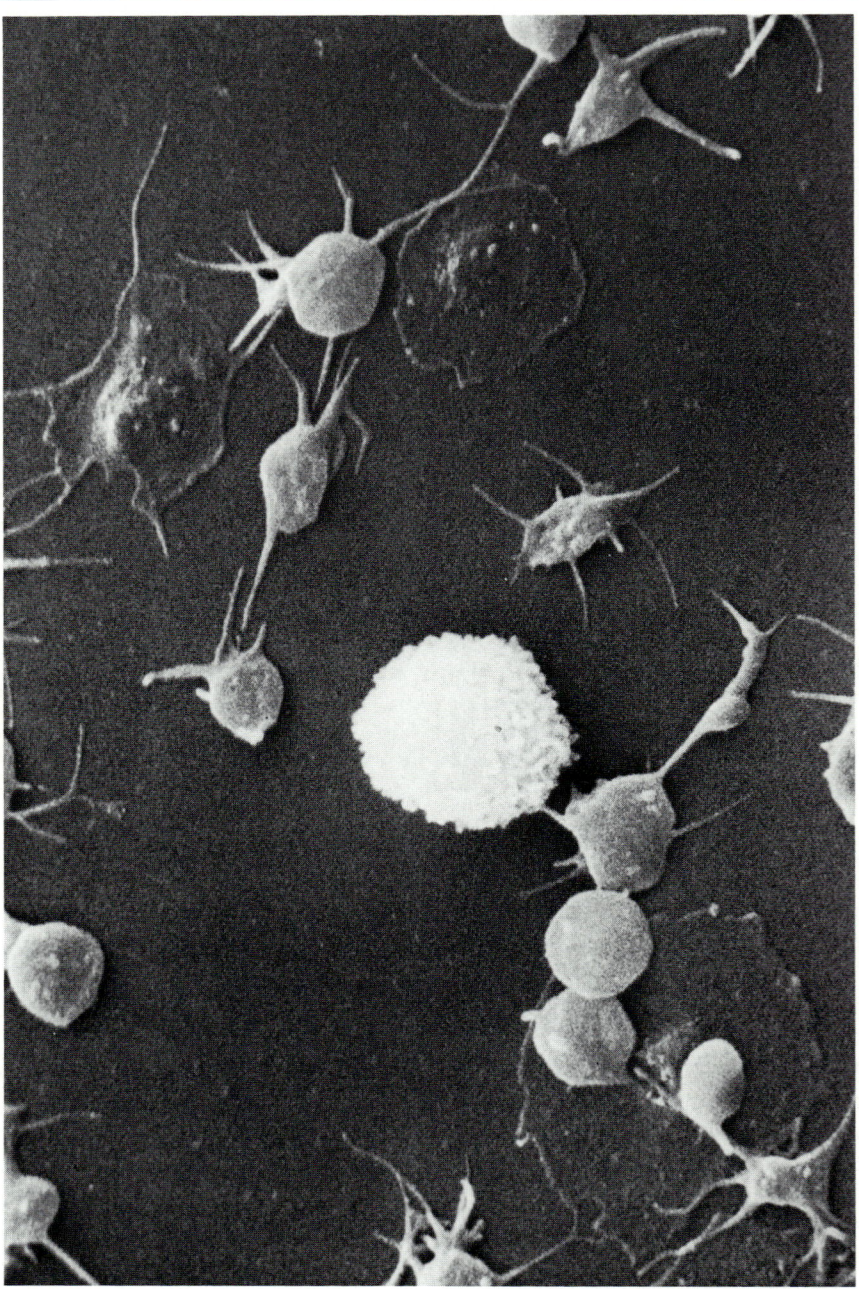

Fig. 5-14. Scanning electron micrograph of a blood film, showing a small lymphocyte (white in color, center) with multiple short processes projecting from its plasma membrane. Numerous platelets with branching processes also can be seen. Three flattened granular leukocytes are present as well. (×4,350.) (Courtesy of F. G. Lightfoot.)

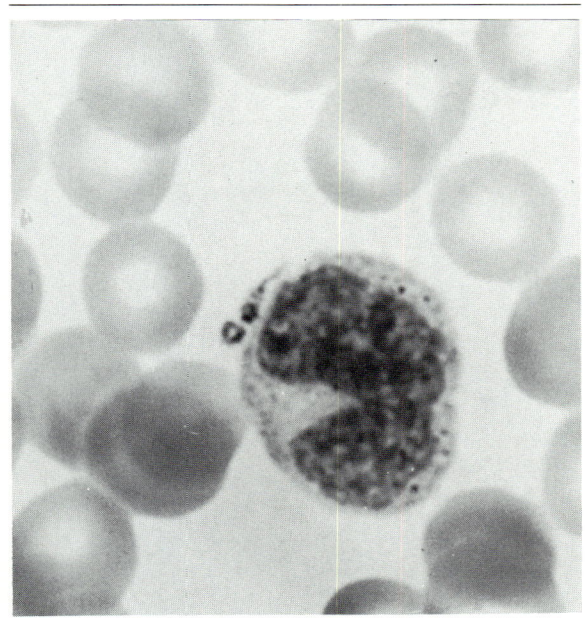

Fig. 5-15. Photomicrograph of a blood film, showing a monocyte surrounded by erythrocytes. Note that the monocyte possesses an indented nucleus that is less densely stained than that of a lymphocyte (see Figs. 5-12 and 5-13). Note also the presence of faintly stained granules in the cytoplasm. (Leishman stain; ×2,364.)

nuclei and a thin rim of clear cytoplasm. Lymphocytes are actively motile and are continually moving from the lymph nodes, spleen, and connective tissues, using the blood as their method of conveyance. The function of the lymphocytes is to provide the body with an immunological defense.

Lymphocytes have been classified into two main types, T and B lymphocytes. T lymphocytes have a long life span, probably years, and are formed in the bone marrow and later travel to the thymus. B lymphocytes live for shorter periods, probably weeks, and are also formed in the bone marrow. For further information concerning these important cells and their relation to plasma cells, see Chapter 9.

MONOCYTES. Monocytes constitute about 3 to 7 percent of the total white cell population. They are large cells and may measure as much as 17 μm in diameter (Figs. 5-15 and 5-16). The nucleus is ovoid and often indented and is less densely stained than that of the lymphocyte. The cytoplasm is abundant and stains blue-gray. Scattered throughout the cytoplasm are a number of azurophil granules that are lysosomes.

Monocytes are actively motile and leave the blood to enter the connective tissues, where they become tissue macrophages. They are phagocytic and devour invading microorganisms. They play an important role in the liberation of antigens prior to the activation of lymphocytes in the development of the immunological response.

FORMATION OF WHITE BLOOD CELLS. *Formation of Granulocytes.* Stem cells in the red bone marrow differentiate into *myeloblasts* (Fig. 5-17). These cells each have a large nucleus with three or more nucleoli. The cytoplasm is devoid of granules. These cells differentiate and acquire purple-staining cytoplasmic granules. Each cell is now called a *promyelocyte*. Further development takes place along three separate paths of differentiation to form the *neutrophil, eosinophil,* and *basophil* (see Fig. 5-17). These paths can be recognized by the appearance of specifically staining granules in the cytoplasm. One path leads to the development of the *neutrophil myelocyte,* the *neutrophil metamyelocyte,* and, finally, the *neutrophil.* In the same manner, eosinophil and basophil myelocytes and metamyelocytes are formed and ultimately differentiate into the mature cells. Just before the granulocytes are discharged from the bone marrow into the general circulation, the nuclei constrict and the development of lobes commences. Normally, it is only cells in the final stages of development that leave the bone marrow and enter the bloodstream.

Control of Granulocyte Formation. The numbers of granulocytes in the blood are kept remarkably constant. Physiological stress, such as severe exercise or bacterial infection, results in a rapid rise in the number of circulating neutrophils. Two populations of neutrophils exist: those circulating in the bloodstream and those that adhere to the endothelial lining of blood vessels. Should there be a sudden

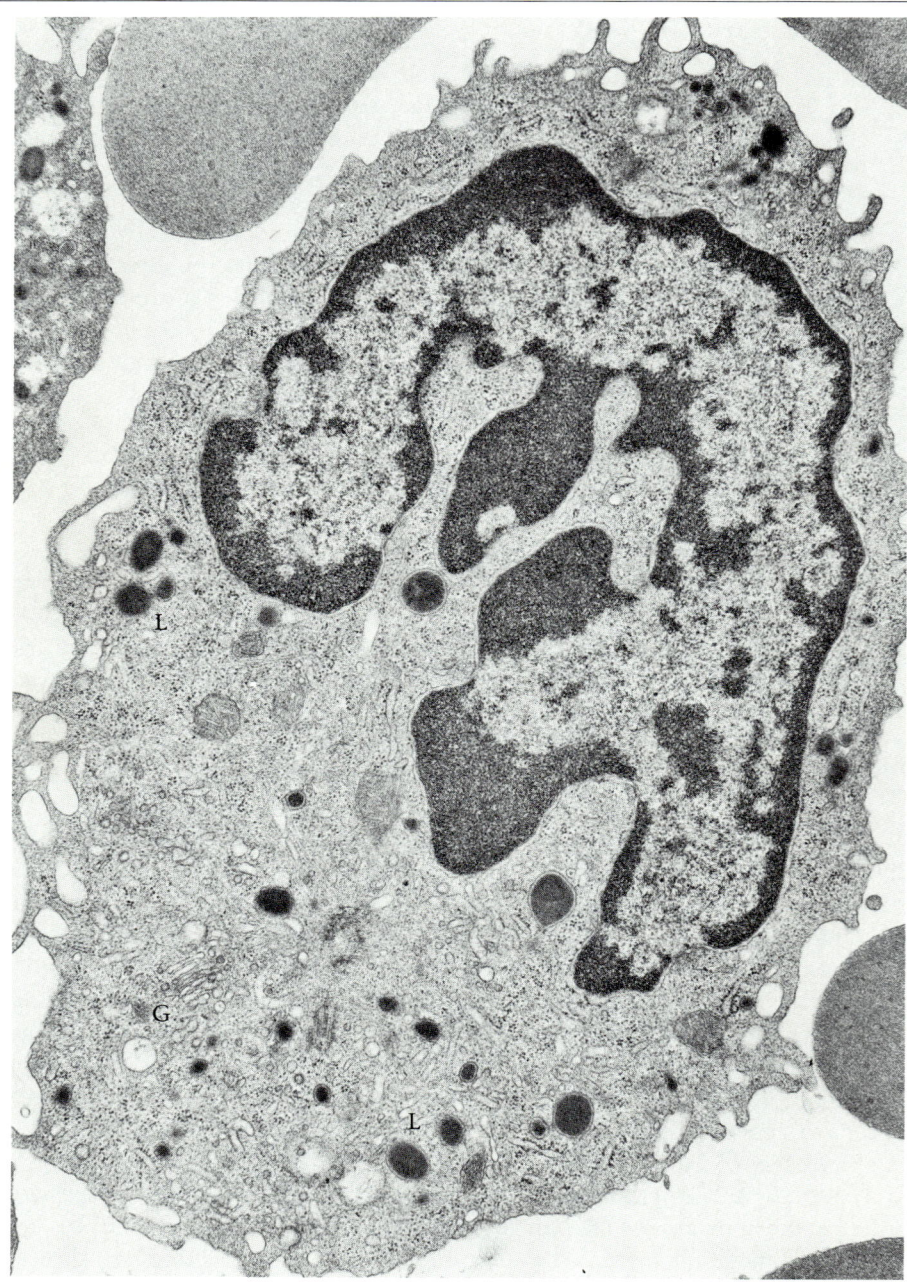

Fig. 5-16. Electron micrograph of a monocyte, showing an irregularly shaped nucleus, a Golgi complex (G), rough endoplasmic reticulum, free ribosomes, and several dark-staining lysosomes (L). (×16,000.) (Courtesy of Dr. B. Nichols.)

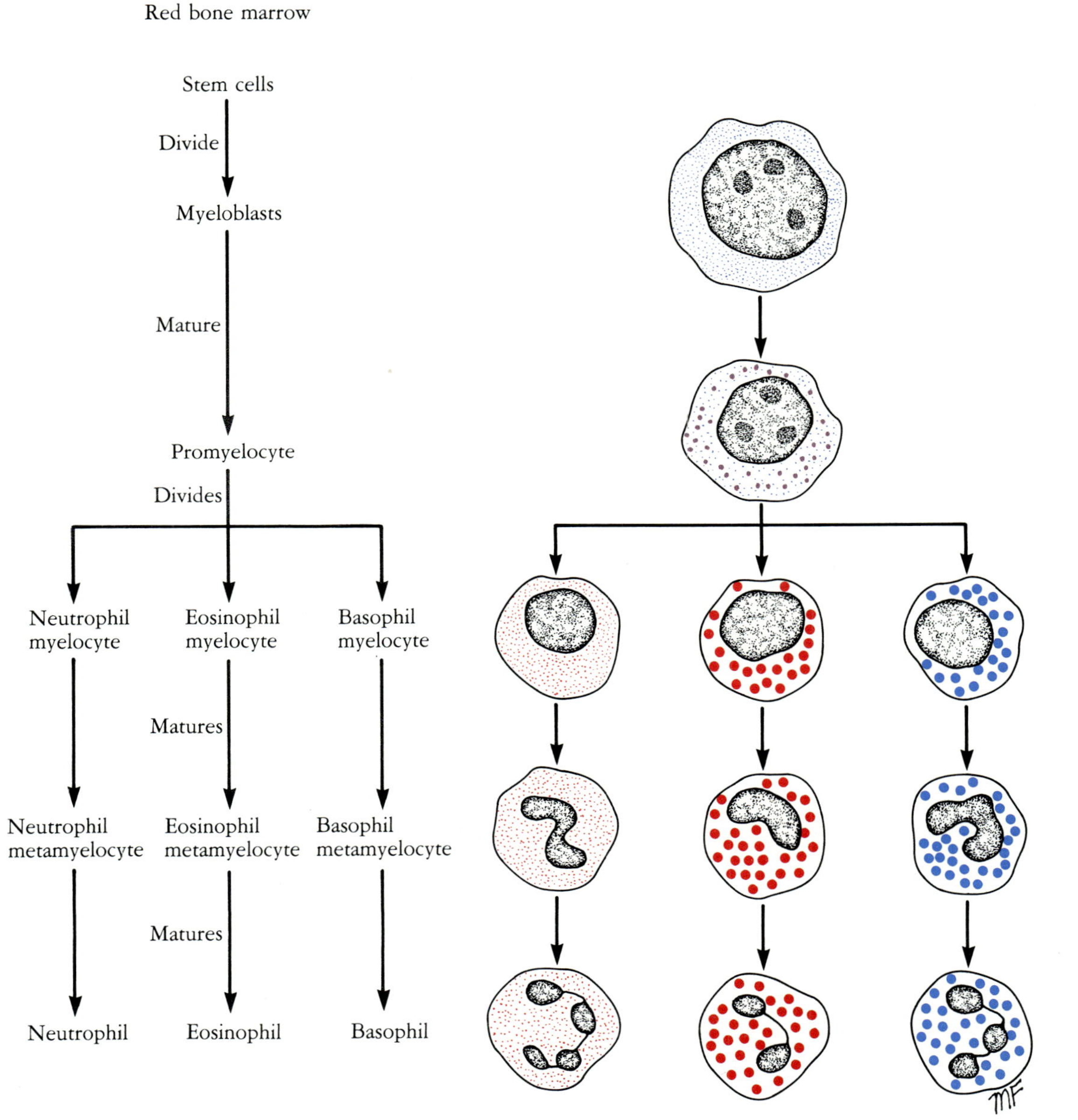

Red bone marrow

Stem cells

↓ Divide

Myeloblasts

↓ Mature

Promyelocyte

↓ Divides

| Neutrophil myelocyte | Eosinophil myelocyte | Basophil myelocyte |

↓ Matures

| Neutrophil metamyelocyte | Eosinophil metamyelocyte | Basophil metamyelocyte |

↓ Matures

| Neutrophil | Eosinophil | Basophil |

Fig. 5-17. Formation of granulocyte leukocytes.

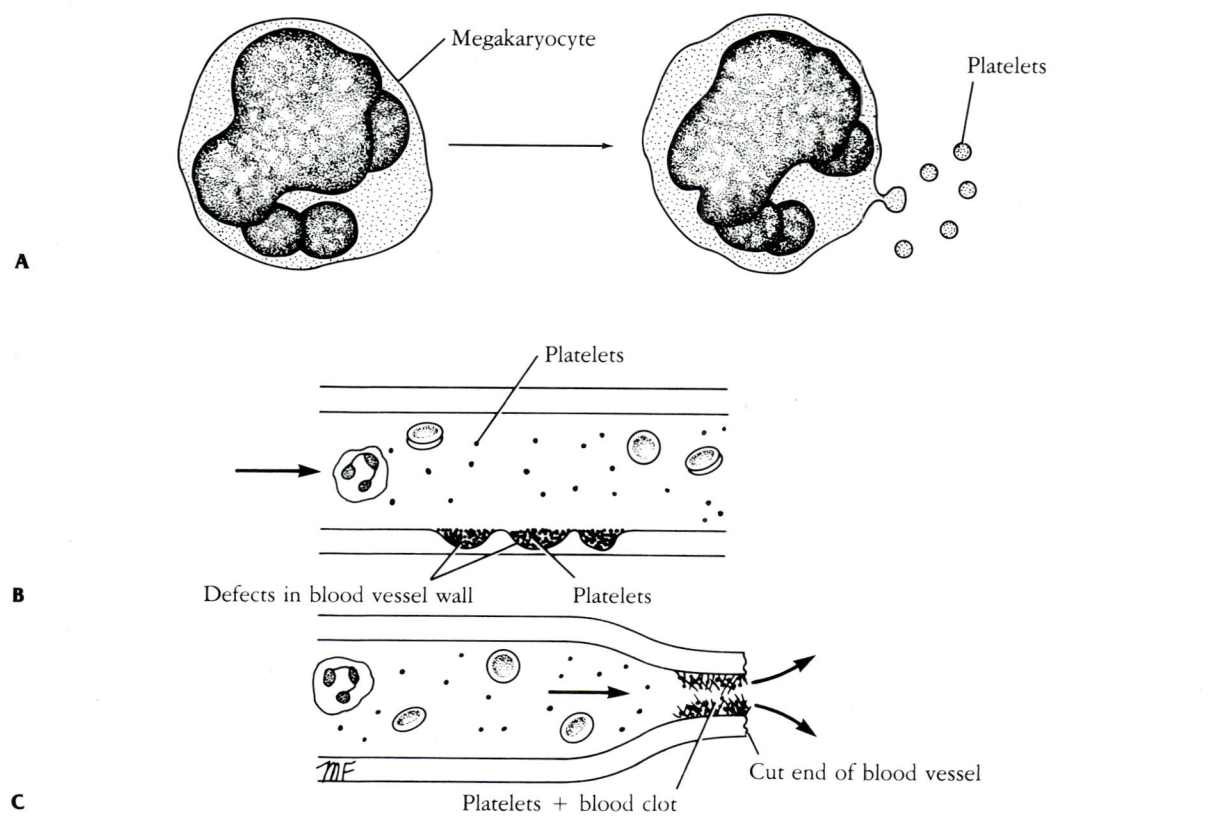

Fig. 5-18. (A) Formation of platelets from a megakaryocyte in bone marrow; (B) adherence of platelets to defects in the lining of a blood vessel wall; (C) platelets adhering to cut wall of blood vessel. Note that in (C), the blood vessel lumen has been narrowed by the contraction of the smooth muscle in its wall.

need to increase the numbers of circulating neutrophils, the latter group of cells is added to the circulating pool. In addition, the process of differentiation of the immature granulocytes in the bone marrow is hastened, so that many more new neutrophils appear in the blood. It is probable that a chemical agent similar to erythropoietin is responsible for controlling the production of new granulocytes in the bone marrow. In the presence of infection, some chemical substance is liberated from the invading organism that stimulates the increased production of neutrophils by the bone marrow.

Fate of Granulocytic White Cells. The normal life span of neutrophils is about 8 days. Most are believed to die combating invading organisms. Very little is known about the fate of eosinophils and basophils. They probably die after emigrating into tissues and are then phagocytosed by tissue macrophages.

Formation of Agranulocytes. The long-living T lymphocytes and the short-lived B lymphocytes are formed in the bone marrow; the T lymphocytes then enter the bloodstream and travel to the thymus. The two types of lymphocytes then populate the lymph nodes, the spleen, and connective tissues. Because these lymphocytes are programmed to react with specific antigens, when they meet those antigens, the T and B lymphocytes are stimulated to be changed into lymphoblasts and proliferate. Finally, specific antibodies are formed from plasma cells, as described on page 342. The lymphocytes are able to move freely throughout the body via the bloodstream and lymph.

The *monocytes* are also formed in the bone marrow. The primitive cells are known as *promonocytes*. After 1 to 3 days, the mature monocytes appear in the bloodstream. They remain in the bloodstream for about 3 days and then migrate into the tissues, where they die. The factors controlling monocyte formation are not known.

Platelets

Platelets, or thrombocytes, are small fragments of cytoplasm measuring about 2 to 5 μm in diameter. They possess no nuclei and are each completely surrounded by a plasma membrane (see Figs. 5-9, 5-11, and 5-14). There are normally *250,000 to 300,000 per cubic millimeter* of blood.

Platelets plug small defects in the endothelial lining of blood vessels and stop bleeding from severed small blood vessels by causing the blood to clot. When there is an endothelial defect, the lining of the blood vessel no longer has a smooth surface. As the blood flows along the lumen, platelets start to adhere to the floor and edges of the defect and accumulate until the defect no longer exists (Fig. 5-18). (See also the discussion of disease of arterial walls, page 328.)

When a blood vessel is cut, hemorrhage occurs. As the blood flows out of the opening in the wall of the vessel, platelets start to adhere to the damaged area (see Fig. 5-18). The continued accumulation of platelets at the site narrows and eventually closes the opening. The whole process is aided by contraction of the smooth muscle in the vessel wall, which constricts the blood vessel and narrows the opening. In addition, the blood in the area of platelet accumulation may clot.

COAGULATION OF BLOOD. Coagulation of blood occurs when blood is withdrawn from a patient and placed in a test tube, or when blood escapes from the cardiovascular system into connective tissue and stagnates. Coagulation of blood can also take place intravascularly when it comes into contact with a damaged or diseased area of the lining of a blood vessel. Essentially, the process consists in the formation of a network of *fibrin* fibers, in the meshes of which the blood cells become trapped. The jellylike red mass so formed is called a *blood clot*.

Mechanism of Blood Clotting. The mechanism of blood clotting is extremely complicated, and only a summary will be given here. There are two pathways by which the process is initiated: (1) the intrinsic pathway, which occurs within the blood itself, and (2) the extrinsic pathway, which occurs when blood escapes from the blood vessels and is exposed to damaged tissues.

In the *intrinsic pathway,* a series of reactions takes place (Fig. 5-19) involving several blood clotting factors. The process is commonly initiated when the blood comes into contact with a damaged or diseased part of the lining of a blood vessel. The reaction sequence finally activates factor X, and it, in the presence of phospholipids released from platelets and also in the presence of calcium, catalyzes the conversion of prothrombin to thrombin. Thrombin now catalyzes the conversion of fibrinogen to fibrin.

In the *extrinsic pathway,* a substance called *thromboplastin* is released from the damaged tissues (see Fig. 5-19). Thromboplastin, with the help of factor VII and calcium, activates factor X, which, in the presence of phospholipids from platelets and calcium, catalyzes the conversion of prothrombin to thrombin. Note that the last part of the mechanism is identical in the two pathways.

The fibrin appears in the blood as fine threads that quickly join one another to form a network. The blood cells become entangled in the network, and the plasma gels. A blood clot is red because of the trapped red cells. After a few minutes, the fibrin threads shorten, the platelets contract, and the blood clot shrinks. The yellow fluid expelled from the clot is called *serum*.

When blood is removed from the body and placed in a glass tube or bottle, it is the intrinsic mechanism that initiates the clotting, activated by the contact of factor XII and platelets with the glass wall. If the glass container is first siliconized and

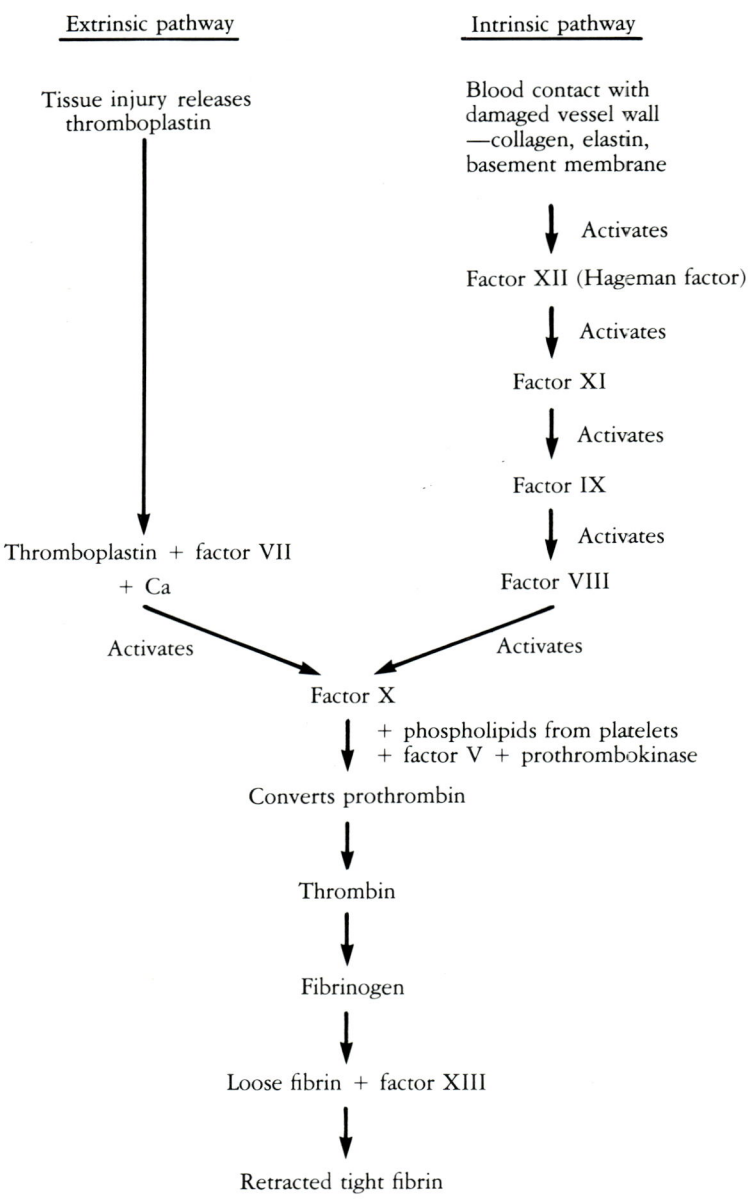

Fig. 5-19. Mechanisms for blood coagulation. Note the intrinsic and extrinsic pathways. The different clotting factors are numbered by order of discovery and not by sequence in the clotting reaction.

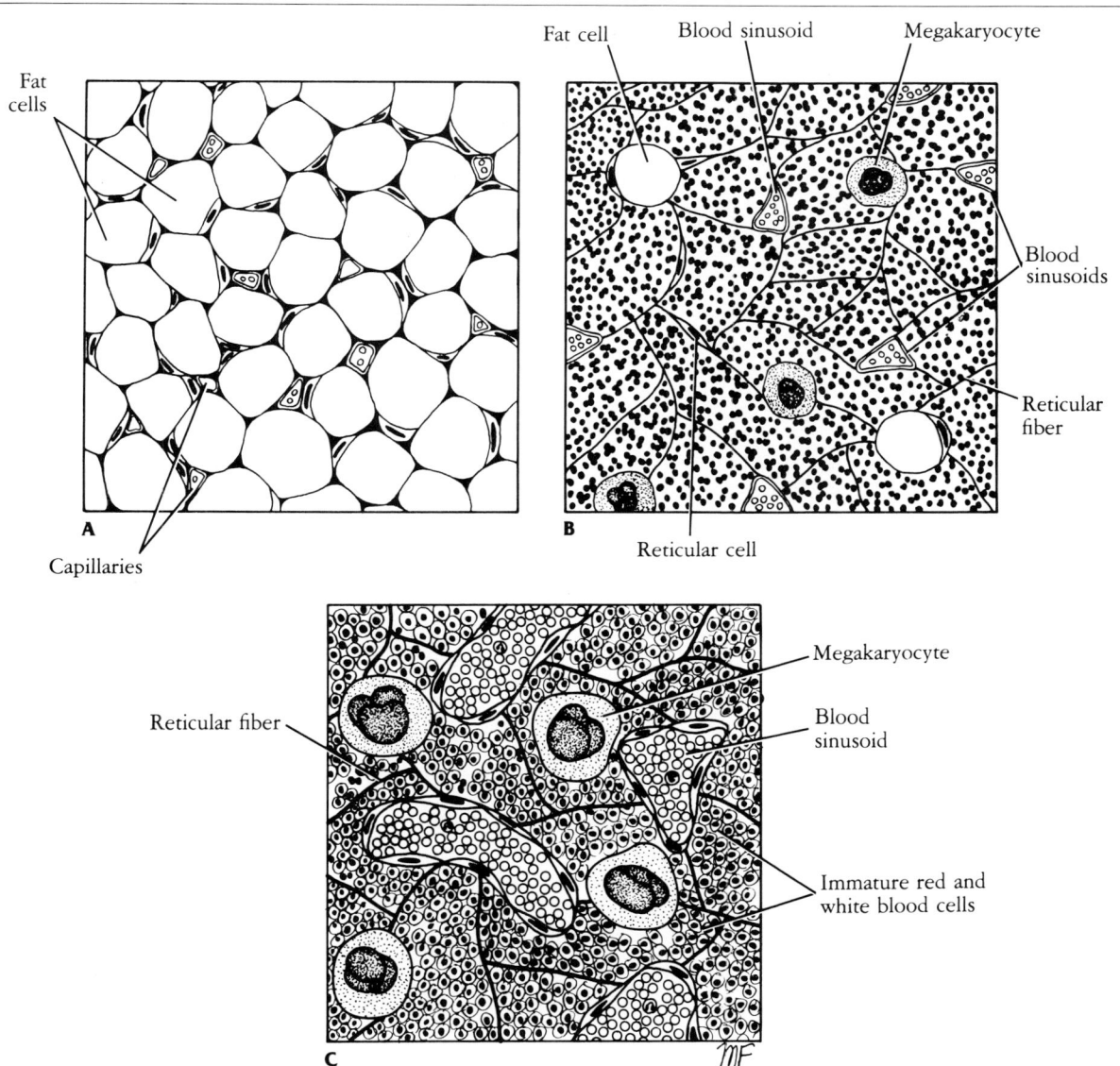

Fig. 5-20. Bone marrow. (A) Yellow marrow. Large numbers of fat cells filled with fat are visible. (B) Red marrow. Active blood cell formation is shown. Only two fat cells can be seen. (C) Magnified view of red marrow, showing numerous blood sinusoids. Between the sinusoids, the marrow network is filled with immature erythrocytes and leukocytes at different stages of development. Note the presence of four megakaryocytes.

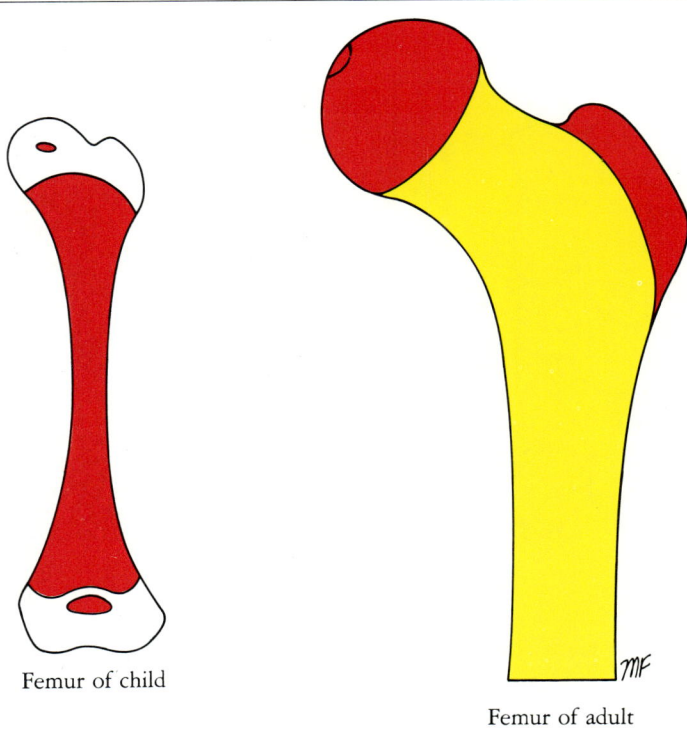

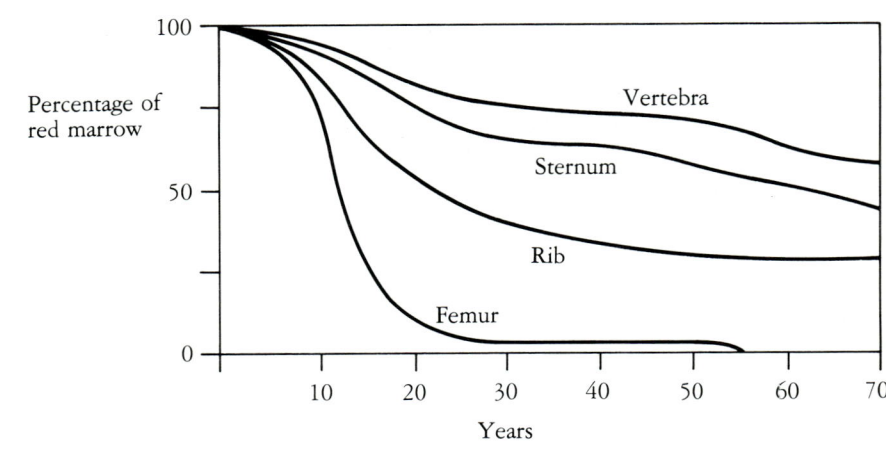

Fig. 5-21. (A) Distribution of red and yellow bone marrow in a young child and in an adult; (B) the changing percentage of red marrow with aging in a number of different bones.

made "nonwettable," the blood clotting mechanism can be delayed.

FORMATION OF PLATELETS. Platelets are formed from very large cells called *megakaryocytes* in the red bone marrow (see Figs. 5-18 and 5-23). The megakaryocytes send pseudopodia through the wall of the blood sinusoids of the marrow into the bloodstream. The pseudopodia then become detached, and the cytoplasmic fragments in the bloodstream form the platelets. Each cytoplasmic fragment or platelet is surrounded by a plasma membrane.

It is now believed that platelets contain *actin* and *myosin* filaments, similar to those seen in skeletal muscle, and these are responsible for the contraction of the platelets in a blood clot.

Control of Platelet Formation. A substance called *thrombopoietin* is present in the blood and increases the number of megakaryocytes in the bone marrow, thus stimulating the production of platelets. Experimental evidence suggests that, as the platelet numbers in the blood fall, the thrombopoietin concentration rises and platelet production is increased.

FATE OF BLOOD PLATELETS. Platelets have a life span of about 7 days. They are eventually phagocytosed by macrophages throughout the body.

Blood Plasma

Plasma is the fluid component of blood and is a light amber color. It forms about 55 percent of the total blood volume, of which 90 percent is water. One percent of plasma is inorganic substances such as potassium, sodium, chloride, and bicarbonate. Seven percent is plasma proteins, albumin, globulin, and fibrinogen. Another 1 percent is nonprotein organic substances. Plasma also contains dissolved gases, hormones, and pigments.

PLASMA PROTEINS. Because of the large size of the plasma protein molecules, under normal conditions, very little plasma protein is able to escape from the cardiovascular system. Plasma proteins serve several important functions: they (1) exert osmotic pressure in relation to tissue fluid formation (see p. 337), (2)

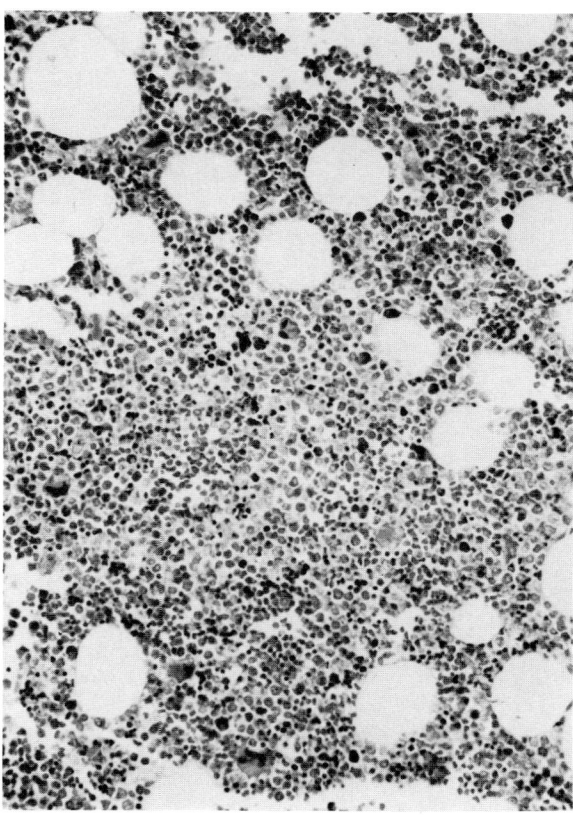

Fig. 5-22. Photomicrograph of a section of active red bone marrow, showing the reticular network and blood sinusoids to be packed with immature erythrocytes and leukocytes. The rounded, white empty spaces represent fat cells from which the fat has been dissolved during the preparation of the section. (H&E; ×200.)

play a part in blood clotting (see p. 171), (3) contribute to blood viscosity in relation to blood pressure (see p. 319), (4) serve as buffers in maintaining constant hydrogen ion concentration in the blood, (5) assist in the transport of iron and hormones by the formation of chemical complexes (see p. 632), and (6) assist in the development of immunity to infection and foreign proteins by the formation of gamma globulins (see p. 342).

Plasma proteins are formed in the liver by the hepatic cells and are synthesized from amino acids.

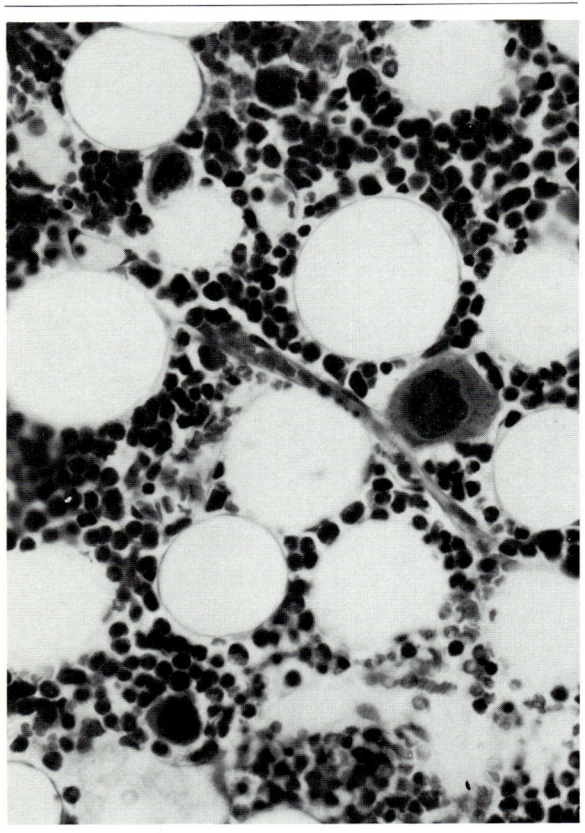

Fig. 5-23. *Photomicrograph of a high-power view of the section of red bone marrow seen in Figure 5-22, showing active blood cell formation and a number of empty fat cells. Three large megakaryocytes can also be seen. (H&E; ×400.)*

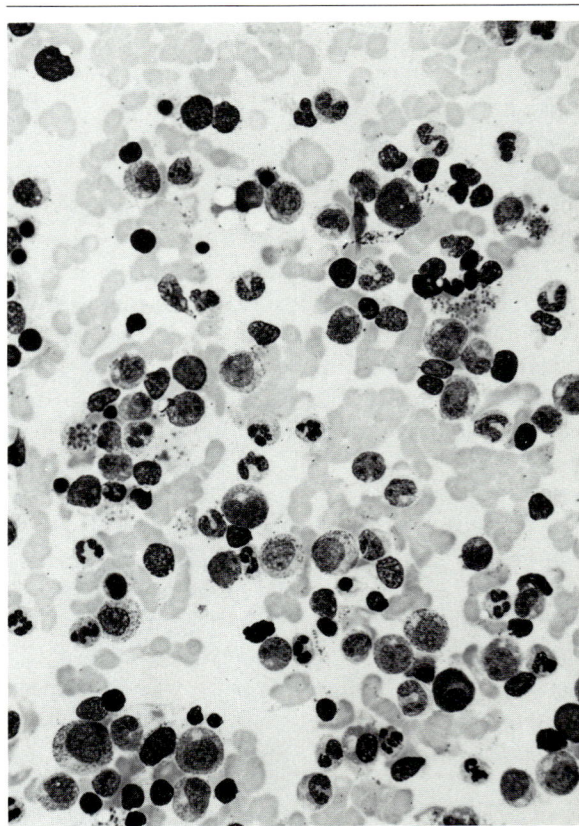

Fig. 5-24. *Photomicrograph of a smear taken from red bone marrow of the iliac crest, showing many immature and mature erythrocytes and leukocytes. Consult Figures 5-6 and 5-17. (Giemsa stain; ×400.)*

Gamma globulins, which form antibodies, are formed by plasma cells (see p. 342).

BONE MARROW

Bone marrow is found in the cavities of long bones and in the spaces of spongy bone. In the adult, there are two types of bone marrow, *red marrow* and *yellow marrow* (Fig. 5-20). Red marrow is red because of the hemoglobin in the large number of red cells it is producing. Yellow marrow is yellow because of the large number of fat cells it contains.

At birth, the bone marrow throughout the body is red and *hematopoietic* (blood forming). This blood-forming activity gradually lessens with age, and the red marrow is replaced by yellow marrow (Fig. 5-21). At 7 years of age, the child begins to develop yellow marrow in the distal bones of the limbs. This replacement of marrow gradually moves proximally, so that by adulthood, the red marrow is restricted to the bones of the skull, the vertebral column, the thoracic cage, the girdle bones, and the head of the humerus and the femur. Thus, in the adult only about half the bone marrow is red and hematopoietic. If there is a need for increased red cell production, the yellow marrow can be converted back into red marrow.

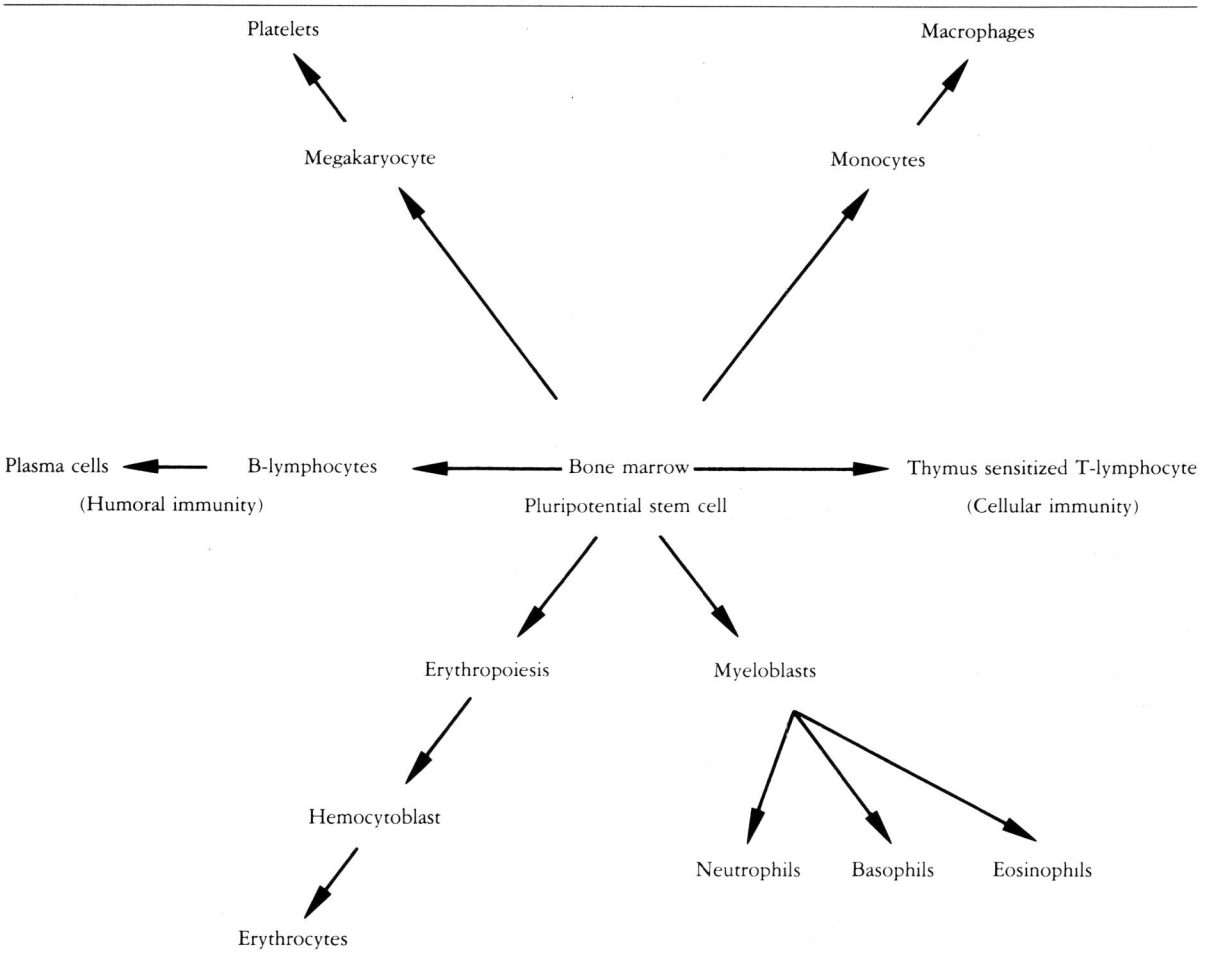

Fig. 5-25. Bone marrow pluripotential stem cell giving rise to the different types of blood cells, including the platelets.

Structure

Basically, bone marrow consists of a three-dimensional network of reticular fibers that support *reticular cells* (Figs. 5-22, 5-23, and 5-24; see Fig. 5-20). The nutrient artery supplying the marrow divides into arterioles and capillaries that in turn open into thin-walled blood sinusoids. The endothelium lining the sinusoids allows large numbers of newly formed blood cells that may arise outside the sinusoids to squeeze between the endothelial cells.

Structure of Red Marrow

In addition to the basic structure of a reticular network and blood sinusoids, there exist a large number of *pluripotential stem cells* (Fig. 5-25). These cells are called pluripotential cells because they are capable of giving rise to all the different types of blood cells. The offspring of the pluripotential cells are *unipotential cells* that undergo rapid mitotic division and develop in five different ways. In this way are formed (1) the red cells, (2) the granular white cells, (3) the lymphocytes, (4) the monocytes, and (5) the megakaryocytes and platelets. As the five lines of cells differentiate into mature cells, they fill up the cavities of the blood sinusoids. The entrance into the sinusoids is believed to open from time to time, and the newly formed cells are swept into the general circulation. Meanwhile, other sinusoids close, so that there is little blood flow, and they in turn start to accumulate new blood cells.

The details of development of each type of blood cell has been described (red cells, p. 158; white cells, p. 167; platelets, p. 175). *Megakaryocytes* are very large cells found in the bone marrow. They extend pseudopodia into the blood sinusoids to form platelets, as described on page 175.

CLINICAL NOTES

HEMORRHAGE

Hemorrhage is a loss of whole blood—cells and plasma—from the cardiovascular system. *External hemorrhage* occurs when the blood escapes from the body, as when an artery or vein is cut in a knife wound or when blood escapes from the vagina in uterine bleeding. *Internal hemorrhage* occurs when the blood escapes from the cardiovascular system but is retained within the body, as when the spleen is ruptured and the blood is retained within the peritoneal cavity. A large blood loss, whether external or internal, will have a consistent effect on the patient. The loss of red cells and hemoglobin immediately will affect the ability of the blood to transport oxygen, and the patient will become breathless. Because there is a reduction in circulating blood volume, the blood pressure will fall (Fig. 5-26).

Immediately, reflex mechanisms, such as vasoconstriction of the peripheral blood vessels, will be set in motion to counteract these changes. The patient will become pale, and the heart rate will increase. The contraction of blood vessels in the skin, intestines, and spleen partially will restore the blood volume and will ensure that the brain and heart receive an adequate blood supply. Recovery will take place, provided that the hemorrhage has not been massive and that the bleeding has been stopped. The described physiological responses are at best temporary, and it may take weeks or even months before the blood lost is replenished.

Almost immediately, an attempt is made to increase the blood volume. Water and electrolytes are withdrawn from the tissues and returned to the blood as a result of the fall in blood pressure at the venous end of the capillaries. Plasma proteins are replaced slowly from the diet, and several weeks may elapse before the blood cells are replaced. The red bone marrow becomes more active, but after a single large hemorrhage, it is rare for the inactive yellow marrow to become converted into active red marrow. It should be remembered that in an external hemorrhage, the red cells are lost outside the body, resulting in a depletion of the iron reserve, whereas in an internal hemorrhage into one of the cavities of the body, the iron is retained and can be reused by the bone marrow. For these reasons, a blood loss of any size is usually treated with a blood transfusion.

EXTRAMEDULLARY HEMATOPOIESIS

At birth, the red bone marrow is the source of all forms of blood cells. In a premature infant, the liver, spleen, and lymph nodes may retain their ability to form both red and white blood cells (Fig. 5-27), but this ability usually quickly disappears.

Loss of blood in the newborn may cause the liver and spleen to revert to their fetal blood-forming function. Here, again, this function should quickly disappear once the patient recovers from the blood loss.

In the adult, repeated hemorrhage or loss of red cells from disease can result in the conversion of the inactive yellow marrow in the bones of the limbs into active red marrow. If additional hematopoiesis is required, as in severe hemolytic disorders, the liver, spleen, and lymph nodes can revert to their fetal activities and become hematopoietic.

BLOOD REPLACEMENT: TRANSFUSION

A large hemorrhage may result in peripheral vascular failure or shock, because of the reduction in blood volume. The treatment is to try to stop the

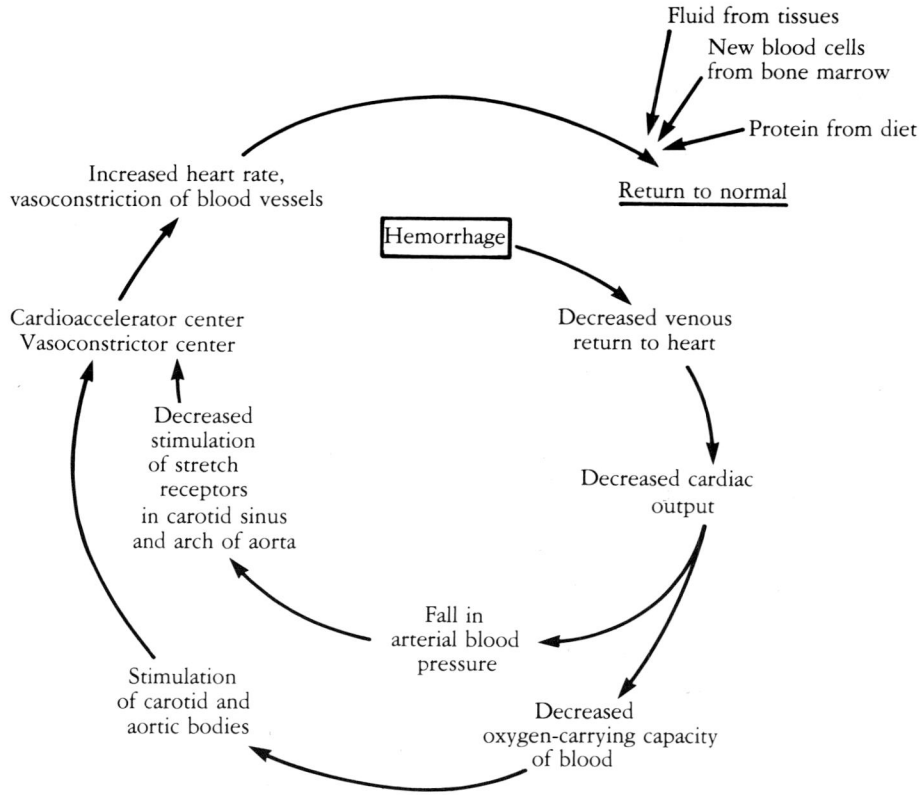

Fig. 5-26. The reaction of the body to hemorrhage, and the reflex mechanisms set in motion to counteract blood loss.

bleeding and to treat the peripheral vascular failure. The reduction in blood volume usually can be corrected by blood transfusion. If compatible blood is unavailable, plasma or a protein solution having the physical properties of blood can be given until there is a supply of compatible blood.

Blood Typing

When the blood of one individual (the donor) is transfused into the vein of another (the recipient) and the bloods are not carefully matched, the blood of the donor can cause a severe reaction and even the death of the recipient. This is because the red blood cells of different persons have different antigenic properties; as a result, the antibodies in the recipient's plasma react with the antigens of the red cells of the donor. The antibodies in the donor's plasma are so diluted by the recipient's plasma that they do not cause a reaction with the recipient's red cells. When mismatched blood is transfused, the donor's erythrocytes become clumped together—*agglutinate*—and block capillaries throughout the body. Later, the cells disintegrate and liberate their hemoglobin. The kidneys attempt to excrete the hemoglobin, resulting in an obstruction of the urinary tubules and renal failure. Bloods that react in this manner are said to be *incompatible*.

Two main groups of blood antigens present in the red cells are important in blood transfusion: the O-A-B groups and the Rh-HR groups.

O-A-B Blood Groups

Blood groups are named according to the antigens (agglutinogens) present on the plasma membranes

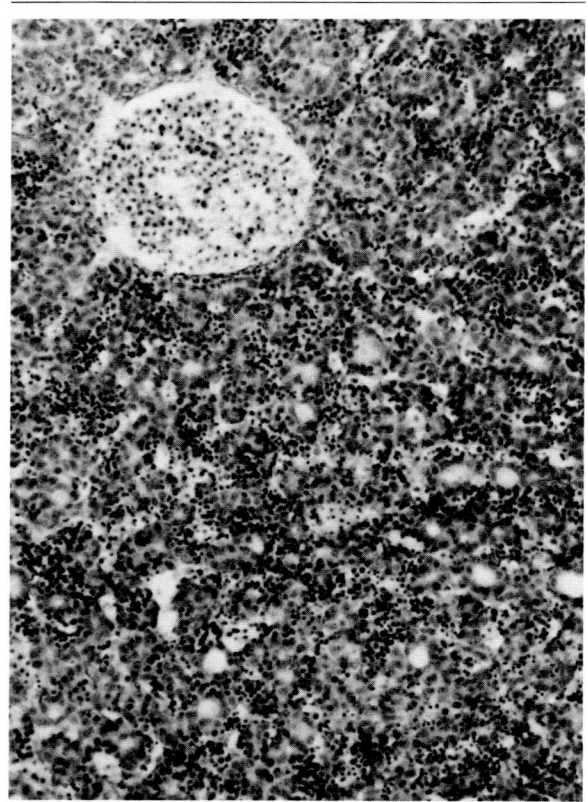

Fig. 5-27. Photomicrograph of section of a fetal liver, showing nucleated immature erythrocytes and leukocytes packed between the hepatocytes. Normally, the liver ceases to form blood cells before birth. (H&E; ×154.)

of the red cells. There are four O-A-B blood groups: group O blood has neither A nor B agglutinogens in the red cells; group A blood has only type A agglutinogens in the red cells; group B blood has only type B agglutinogens in the red cells; and group AB blood has both A and B agglutinogens in the red cells.

Persons with group O blood, although having no agglutinogens (antigens) in their red cells, have in their plasma anti-A and anti-B agglutinins (antibodies). Group A blood contains type A agglutinogens and anti-B agglutinins, and group B blood contains type B agglutinogens and anti-A agglutinins. In group AB blood, both A and B agglutinogens are present in the red cells but there are no agglutinins in the plasma.

A newborn has almost no agglutinins in the plasma. The titer for agglutinins reaches its maximum at about 10 years of age.

SLIDE TECHNIQUE OF BLOOD TYPING. In the slide technique, a drop of blood is removed from the person whose blood is to be typed. The blood is diluted about fifty times in isotonic saline to prevent clotting and to produce a suspension of red blood cells. Two drops of the red cell suspension are placed on a glass slide; a drop of anti-A agglutinin serum is mixed with one drop, and a drop of anti-B agglutinin serum is mixed with the second drop (Fig. 5-28). The slide is then examined under a microscope, and it is easy to see whether the red cells have agglutinized. The possible results of such a test are shown in Figure 5-28.

CROSS MATCHING. In an extreme emergency, when there is insufficient time to type the bloods of the donor and the recipient, one can test the bloods against each other. First, one prepares a saline suspension of red cells from the donor and tests it against the serum of the recipient. In a second test, a saline suspension of red cells from the recipient is tested against the serum of the donor. If agglutination of the red cells does not occur in either test, the bloods are compatible and a blood transfusion is safe.

Rh-HR Blood Groups

There are at least eight different Rh agglutinogens (named after the rhesus monkey that possesses the agglutinogen) and probably more than three HR agglutinogens. These blood groups are determined by taking a saline suspension of red cells and mixing it with specific antisera, as described previously. A person whose red cells react with anti-Rh antiserum is said to be Rh positive, and, conversely, Rh negative if the red cells do not react with anti-Rh antiserum. About 85 percent of whites are Rh positive, and about 15 percent are Rh negative.

When the blood of a person who is Rh positive is

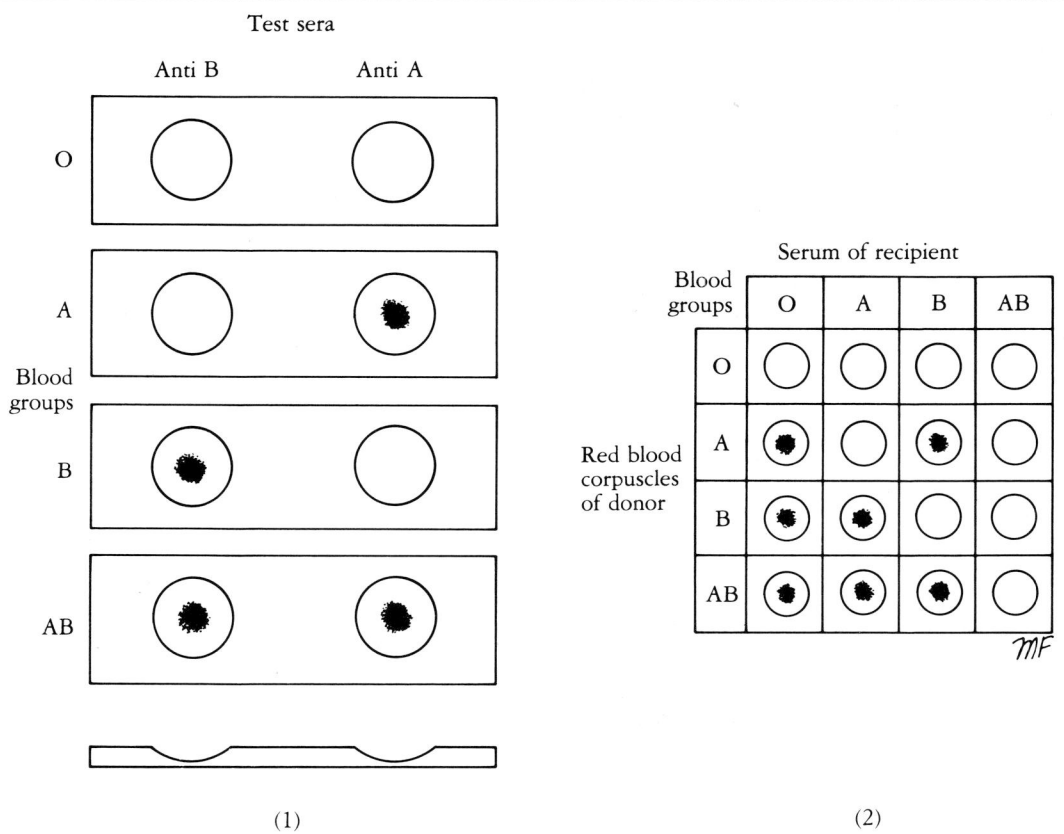

Fig. 5-28. Slide technique for blood typing. (1) shows the result of adding a drop of blood from different blood groups to anti-B and anti-A agglutinin test sera. (2) shows the results that can be predicted when a drop of blood from different blood groups is added to sera taken from different blood groups.

given intravenously to a recipient whose blood is Rh negative, the agglutinin (antibody) or anti-Rh factor is produced by the recipient. No agglutination follows. A later similar transfusion, however, will cause a severe reaction, because of the accumulation of the anti-Rh factor.

RH-NEGATIVE MOTHER. In an Rh-negative mother with an Rh-positive fetus (a trait the child inherited from an Rh-positive father), the mother will, during the course of the pregnancy, develop anti-Rh agglutinins. The anti-Rh agglutinins will diffuse across the placenta into the fetus, causing red cell agglutination. Provided that the mother has not been previously stimulated by a transfusion of Rh-positive blood, her first pregnancy with a Rh-positive fetus will not be adversely affected. The Rh-negative mother will have been sensitized, however, by the Rh-positive fetus. In a second or any subsequent pregnancy with an Rh-positive fetus, the anti-Rh factor of the mother will enter the fetal circulation and cause extensive hemolysis of the fetal red cells before and after birth. The blood disease is known as *erythroblastosis fetalis* and is fatal unless the child receives a large transfusion of Rh-negative blood at birth.

In Rh-negative women who have not been sensitized by receiving Rh-positive blood, the Rh sensitivity in pregnancy can be prevented by neutralizing the Rh-positive antigen by the administration of Rh-immune globulin.

BLOOD CLOTTING

The normal clotting mechanism has already been described (see p. 171). Blood does not clot in the normal vascular system because of the smoothness of the endothelial lining and the presence of a thin layer of protein on the inner surface of the endothelium that prevents the adherence of the platelets. In addition, the anticoagulant heparin, which is produced by connective tissue mast cells and the basophilic white cells of the blood, diffuses into the vascular system and inhibits the process of clotting.

Abnormalities

Liver Diseases

Hepatitis and cirrhosis may interfere with the normal formation of prothrombin by the liver. A lowered prothrombin level in the blood will cause excessive bleeding because of a delay in the clotting mechanism.

Vitamin K Deficiency

Vitamin K is fat-soluble. Any disorder that prevents adequate amounts of fat from being absorbed from the small intestine will result in vitamin K deficiency. For example, significant changes in the intestinal flora or obstruction of the common bile duct will cause vitamin K deficiency. Vitamin K is necessary for the formation of prothrombin (factor II) and other blood-clotting factors (factors VII, IX, and X) in the liver. All patients with liver disease or obstruction of the common bile duct should receive adequate amounts of vitamin K by injection.

Hemophilia

This disease is caused by a sex-linked recessive gene that results in an abnormal clotting mechanism; the clotting factor VIII is absent (see Fig. 5-19). In all cases, the disease is carried on the X chromosome and is thus handed down from the unaffected (carrier) females to affected sons. The signs and symptoms of the disease are caused by the failure of blood coagulation. Habitual hemorrhage from various parts of the body, either spontaneous or following slight trauma, is the main symptom of the disease. The treatment is directed toward protection of the child from wounds or abrasions and avoidance of unnecessary surgery. Transfusions of concentrated antihemophilic globulin may be given.

Thrombocytopenia

In this condition, the patient has a very low platelet count and has a tendency to bleed from the capillaries. In most patients, the cause is unknown, although the disease may be produced by the patient's developing immunity against his own platelets. Another cause is depression of the bone marrow by toxic drugs or radiation therapy. The treatment in acute cases is transfusion with whole blood. Splenectomy may be beneficial, because it normally removes large numbers of platelets from the blood.

Cardiovascular Thrombosis

The loss of smoothness of the endothelial lining of blood vessels or the heart caused by inflammation or degeneration is a common cause of intravascular thrombosis. At first, platelets adhere to the damaged area, forming an agglutinated mass that may interfere with blood flow (Fig. 5-29). Later, blood clotting may take place on the surface of the platelet mass and occlude the vessel lumen.

A coronary thrombosis is caused by the adherence of platelets to the diseased lining of the coronary arteries. The underlying degenerative disease of these arteries is called *atherosclerosis*.

Fig. 5-29. (A) Deposit of platelets on diseased area of lining of artery. (B, C) Development of intravascular thrombus. (D) Common sites of thrombosis in the cardiovascular system; a detached thrombus forms an embolus that may travel to the brain and lungs. (E) Cancer cells may travel from the primary site of the neoplasm as emboli and lodge in distant organs, forming metastases. (F) Disrupted fat cells in the yellow marrow of fractured long bones may enter the bloodstream and form emboli that terminate in the lungs, brain, or kidney.

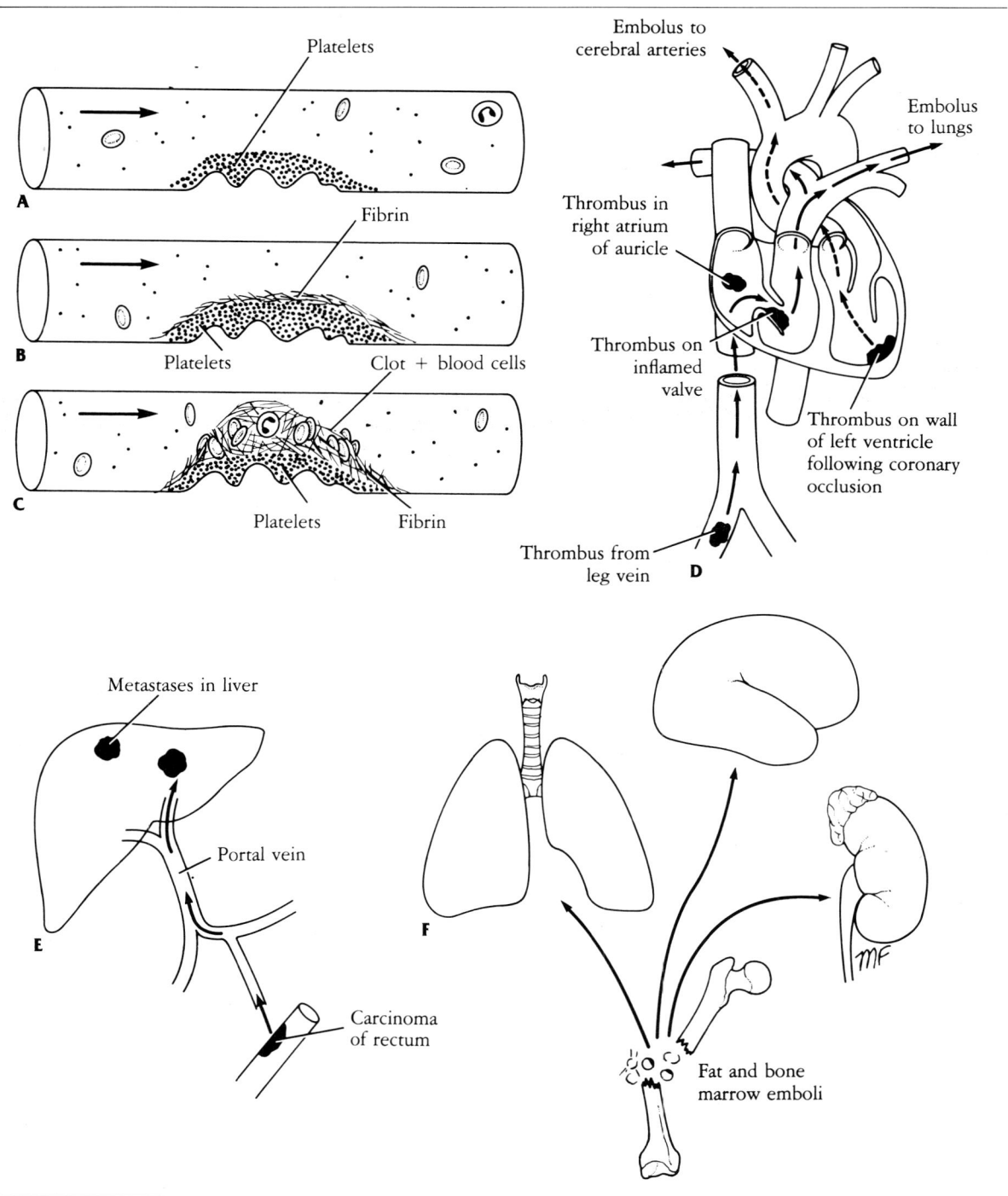

Embolus

An embolus is a foreign body traveling in the bloodstream. It can be composed of pieces of a thrombus, tissue cells, fat, or bubbles of gas. A thrombotic embolus, usually from a peripheral vein, may become detached from the vein wall and circulate through the cardiovascular system (see Fig. 5-29). It finally lodges in a vessel, such as the pulmonary artery, whose diameter is smaller than the embolus.

Anticoagulants

Anticoagulant drugs are used clinically to inhibit the clotting process, especially in patients in whom there is an increased risk of thrombosis.

Heparin, which is normally produced by the mast cells and the basophilic white cells in the body, also is produced commercially and can be given intravenously. Heparin acts by inhibiting the conversion of fibrinogen to fibrin. It also prevents the formation of prothrombin in the body. The small quantities of heparin normally present in the blood prevent blood coagulation in the normal circulation. When the drug is given intravenously, it acts quickly, but the effect is short lived.

Dicumarol, another anticoagulant, can be given orally but has no effect for 2 days. It acts by inhibiting the formation of prothrombin by competing with vitamin K in the liver. Its effect lasts several days, and it is commonly used in the treatment of phlebitis and coronary thrombosis. The dosage of the drug is determined by frequent estimations of the plasma prothrombin level.

Citrate and *oxalate* solutions are chemical agents that prevent blood coagulation by combining with the blood calcium, thus interfering with the clotting mechanism. Clinically, these substances are used in the preservation of blood either in blood samples or in blood transfusions.

RED AND WHITE CELL COUNTS

Types of Counts

It is now common practice for red and white cell counts to be performed by an *electronic counter.* A measured volume of diluted blood is passed through a small orifice guarded by an electric current passing between electrodes. The blood cells are poor electrical conductors, and as each one passes between the electrodes, the electrical current changes. The number of cells passing through the orifice can be expressed as changes in electrical current. The Coulter electronic counter works with an accuracy of about 2 percent.

A differential white cell count is carried out on a blood film on a glass slide that has been stained with Giemsa or Leishman stain. One hundred, two hundred, or five hundred stained white cells are counted and grouped according to the different cell types. The results for each group are expressed as a percentage of white cells—for example: lymphocytes, 30 percent.

Abnormalities

Anemia

Anemia is present if the hemoglobin concentration or red cell count in the peripheral blood is abnormally low. The cause of anemia may be an excessive loss of red cells from the circulation, as in a hemorrhage, or hemolysis of red cells. There may be a defective or deficient production of hemoglobin or red cells. A combination of excessive loss and deficient production resulting from disease may be the cause. Some examples of anemia follow.

ANEMIA CAUSED BY REPEATED HEMORRHAGE. A single large hemorrhage results in the mobilization of red cells stored in the bone marrow, and the hemoglobin and red cell counts initially may be little reduced. After 24 hours, however, the volume of blood has usually been restored by the passage of fluid from the tissues into the blood circulation, and the hemoglobin concentration and red cell counts drop. The red cells look normal in size and shape (*normocytic*) and in color (*normochromic*). The patient is said to have a normocytic, normochromic anemia.

If at this stage the patient has a low supply of iron stored in the body, because of repeated previous hemorrhages or lack of iron in the diet, the newly produced red cells will be smaller than normal (*microcytic*) and will contain less hemoglobin than normal (*hypochromic*).

APLASTIC ANEMIA. The red bone marrow may fail to produce sufficient numbers of red cells because of damage to the marrow cells by toxic chemicals or excessive irradiation. Such a condition is called aplastic anemia.

MEGALOBLASTIC ANEMIA. Vitamin B_{12} in small quantities is essential for the normal blood-forming function of the bone marrow (Fig. 5-30). In the mucus secreted by the fundus of the stomach is a chemical substance, called the *intrinsic factor,* that combines with vitamin B_{12} and allows it to be absorbed from the small intestine. Once the vitamin B_{12} is absorbed, it is stored in the liver and is slowly released to the bone marrow and other body tissues.

Pernicious anemia is a form of anemia in which the erythroblastic cells of the bone marrow become larger than normal. These cells are known as *megaloblasts*. The megaloblasts produce a larger-than-normal red cell called a *macrocyte.* The cell membranes of the macrocytes are excessively fragile, so that the cells have a short life. The resulting condition is a *macrocytic anemia.* The cause of pernicious anemia is an atrophic gastric mucosa that does not produce sufficient amounts of the intrinsic factor. This lack in turn leads to a failure of absorption of vitamin B_{12} and an abnormal development of large red cells.

HEMOLYTIC ANEMIA. In this form of anemia, the number of red cells produced by the bone marrow is normal but, because the cells are excessively fragile, their life span is short and the patient is anemic. Many forms of hemolytic anemia are inherited.

Sickle cell anemia occurs almost exclusively in blacks. The sickle shape of the red cell is caused by the presence of an abnormal form of hemoglobin. Such cells are very fragile, and the patient is seriously anemic.

POLYCYTHEMIA VERA. This disease is characterized by excessive production of red cells by the bone marrow. Because of the unregulated character of the red cell production, the disorder is regarded as neoplastic. The white cell counts and the platelet numbers may also be increased.

This condition must be distinguished from *secondary* or *physiological polycythemia,* which occurs in persons living at high altitudes, where the oxygen concentration is low.

LEUKOCYTOSIS. In this condition, the number of white cells in the blood becomes abnormally high. A differential white cell count will determine which type of white cell is responsible. An increase in the number of neutrophils is called *neutrophilia* and occurs in acute infections. An increase in the number of lymphocytes is called *lymphocytosis;* it occurs in whooping cough and many viral infections. An increase in the number of eosinophils is known as *eosinophilia* and tends to occur in allergic conditions, such as bronchial asthma, and in parasitic infections, such as intestinal worms.

LEUKEMIA. This condition is essentially an uncontrolled, neoplastic proliferation of white cells. The blood becomes populated with large numbers of immature white cells that are incapable of carrying out their normal functions. Both acute and chronic forms of the condition exist, and they are classified, according to the type of cell that is produced in excessive numbers, as granulocytic leukemia, lymphocytic leukemia, and monocytic leukemia.

LEUKOPENIA. In this condition, the number of white cells in the blood falls below the normal range. The reduction usually involves one type of cell, with the resulting condition called, for example, neutropenia or lymphopenia.

Neutropenia may occur in such conditions as typhoid fever, viral infections such as measles and mumps, and aplastic anemia secondary to exposure to toxic chemicals or excessive irradiation of the

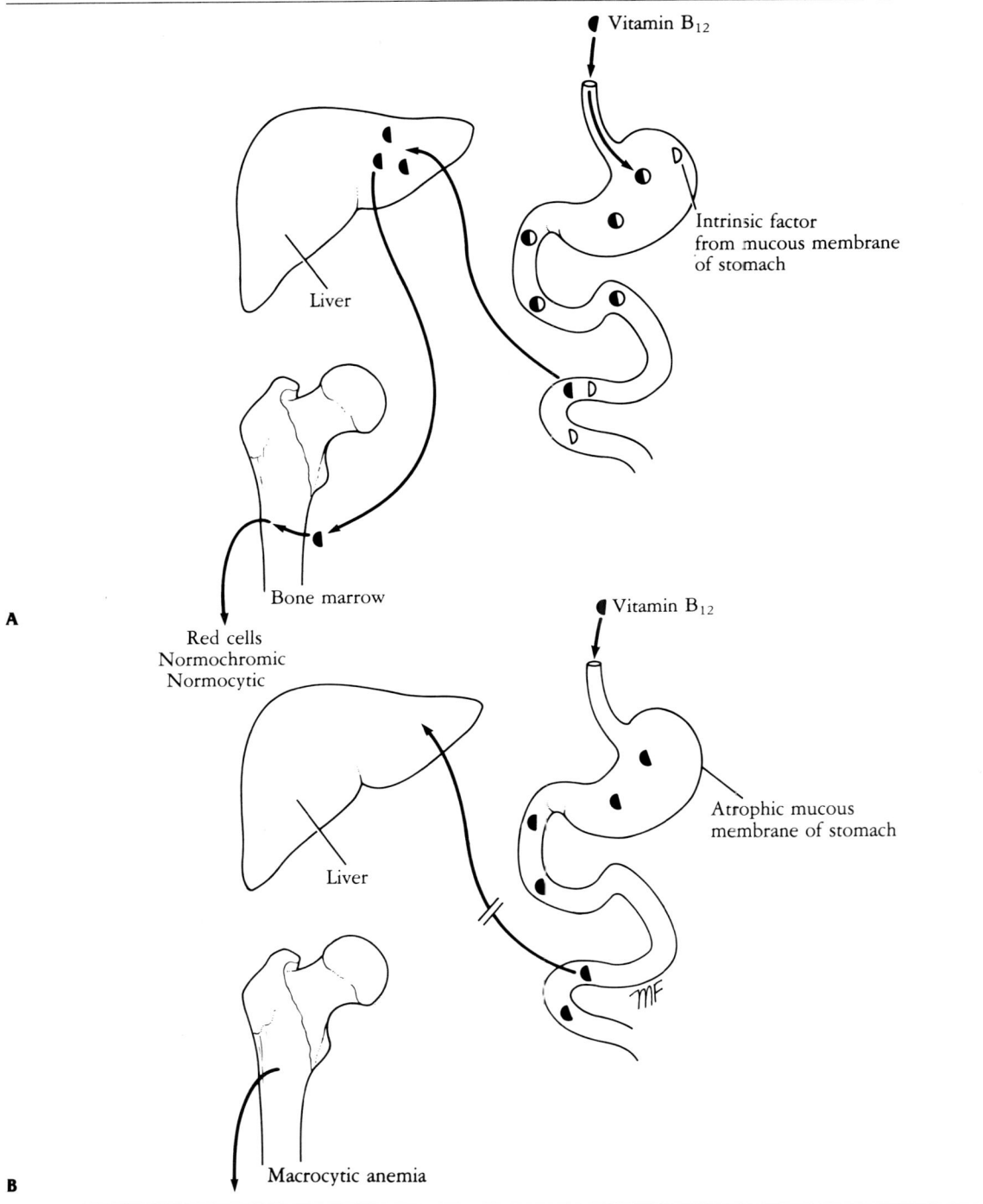

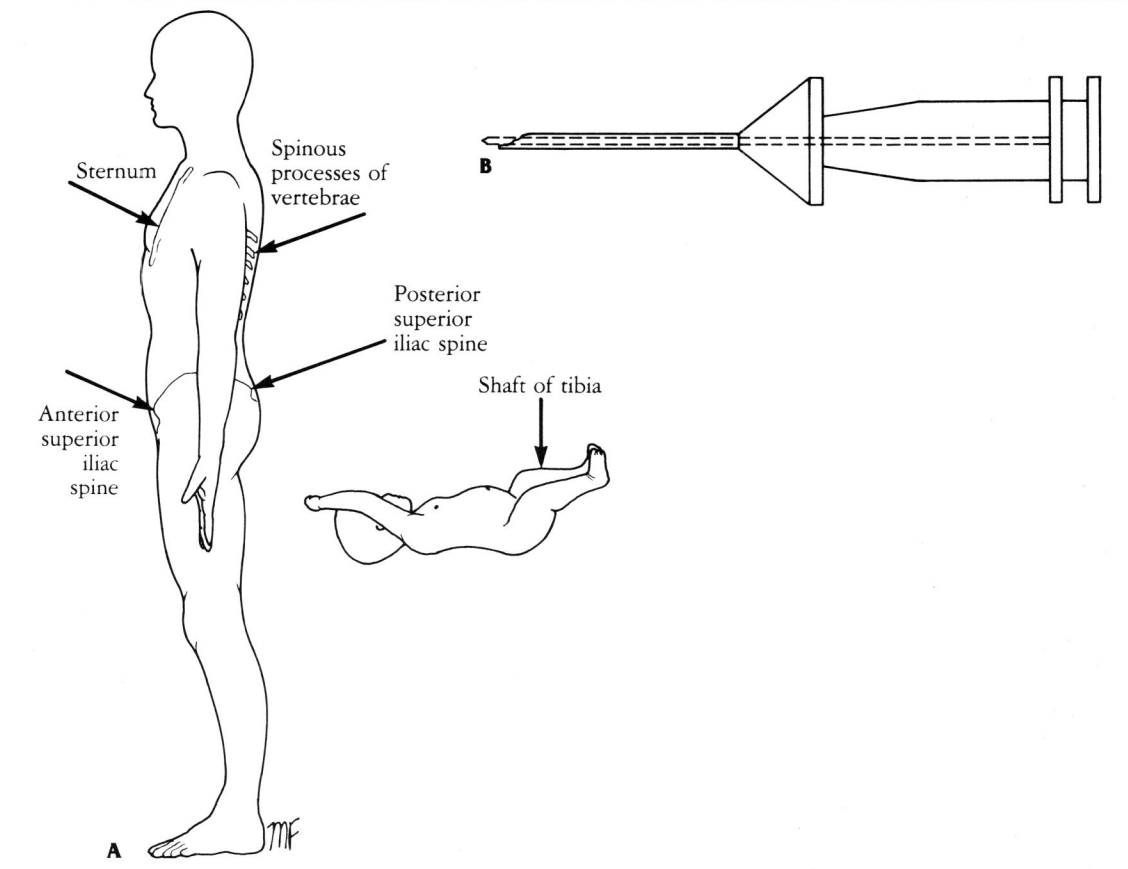

Fig. 5-31. (A) Common sites used for obtaining red bone marrow in adult and infant; (B) needle and stylet used for obtaining bone marrow biopsy specimen.

Fig. 5-30. (A) The path taken by vitamin B_{12} from the intestine to the red bone marrow. Note that the intrinsic factor allows the vitamin to be absorbed from the small intestine. (B) The underlying mechanism responsible for pernicious anemia. Note that the absence of the intrinsic factor prevents the absorption of vitamin B_{12}.

bone marrow. Examples of *lymphopenia* occur in Hodgkin's disease and following the administration of hormones, such as adrenocorticotropic hormone or cortisone.

BONE MARROW

Biopsy

Bone marrow biopsy may be useful in determining whether the production of red cells, granulocytic white cells, or platelets is normal (Fig. 5-31). It may also enable one to confirm the presence of other disease processes, such as metastatic carcinoma. When choosing a site for a biopsy, it is important to remember that as a person ages, the active red marrow in many bones is replaced by yellow marrow (see p. 176). The common sites at which to aspirate a bone marrow sample are the sternum, the iliac crest, and the posterior superior iliac spine. The aspirated material is smeared on a glass slide and stained. The specimen is then ready for study.

Bone Marrow Failure

In this condition, the bone marrow is unable to produce sufficient cells to replace those in the peripheral blood as they wear out. In about half the patients with marrow failure, the cause is unknown. There is, however, a large group of cases in which the cause can be found to be exposure to toxic chemicals or ionizing radiation.

Neoplasms

The leukemias and polycythemia vera may be regarded as neoplasms of the bone marrow. They have been described previously (p. 185).

BASIC PHYSIOLOGICAL AND MICROSCOPICAL FACTORS IN ACUTE INFLAMMATION

Inflammation may be defined as the series of changes that take place in response to injury or invasion by pathogenic organisms. In acute inflammation, the process is of short duration and may last from a few minutes to 1 or 2 days. The principal leukocytes involved are the neutrophils. In chronic inflammation, the process is of long duration and may last for months or years. The principal cells involved are the lymphocytes and the macrophages.

There are five cardinal clinical signs of acute inflammation: (1) swelling, (2) redness, (3) heat, (4) pain, and (5) loss of function. The cause may be trauma, exposure to chemicals, heat, cold, or infection. The first change is a transient vasoconstriction of the arterioles, which may last only a few seconds and is thought to be neurogenic or adrenergic in origin. This change is quickly followed by a dilatation of the arterioles and capillaries in response to the liberation of histamine and histaminelike substances locally by the tissues. The dilatation causes increased blood flow through the area and is responsible for the redness and heat. In this manner, the permeability of the blood vessel wall is increased, permitting large quantities of protein-rich fluid to escape into the tissues (Fig. 5-32). This localized inflammatory edema is responsible for the swelling of inflammation. The pain associated with these changes is caused by the pressure of the increased amounts of tissue fluid on the sensitive sensory nerve endings. The loss of function may be caused by the pain or by the accumulated tissue fluid's interfering with movements of the affected part. In many instances, this temporary loss of movement allows the injured part to rest and recover. The reduction in movement of the affected part also limits the spread of the infecting organisms. In addition, the local spread of organisms or toxic products is often retarded by the clotting of the protein-rich tissue fluid.

When tissues are damaged, chemical substances are liberated that enter the bloodstream. These then attract neutrophils to the damaged area. As a result of the vasodilatation of the capillaries and the outpouring of protein-rich tissue fluid, the circulation slows. The neutrophils start to stick to the walls of the capillaries in the damaged area; in other words, they migrate out of the axial stream and accumulate along the margins of the vessel wall. This phenomenon is known as *margination* (see Fig. 5-32). Chemotaxis now attracts the neutrophils through the vessel wall to the site of injury or infection. This movement of neutrophils is known as *diapedesis* (see Fig. 5-32).

Chemical substances liberated by invading organisms may stimulate the thermoregulation center of the body and cause the patient to experience a fever. Fever may have a beneficial effect on the chemical changes taking place at the site of injury. The same toxic chemical substances are believed to stimulate the release of mature neutrophils from the red bone marrow; thus, severe infections are associated with a mobilization of the first line of defense, namely, the neutrophils. Leukocytosis thus occurs.

On reaching the site of bacterial invasion, the neutrophils engulf the bacteria by phagocytosis. The bacteria now lie within a membranous sac within the cytoplasm of the neutrophil. Lysosomes fuse with the sac, and most of the bacteria are destroyed by

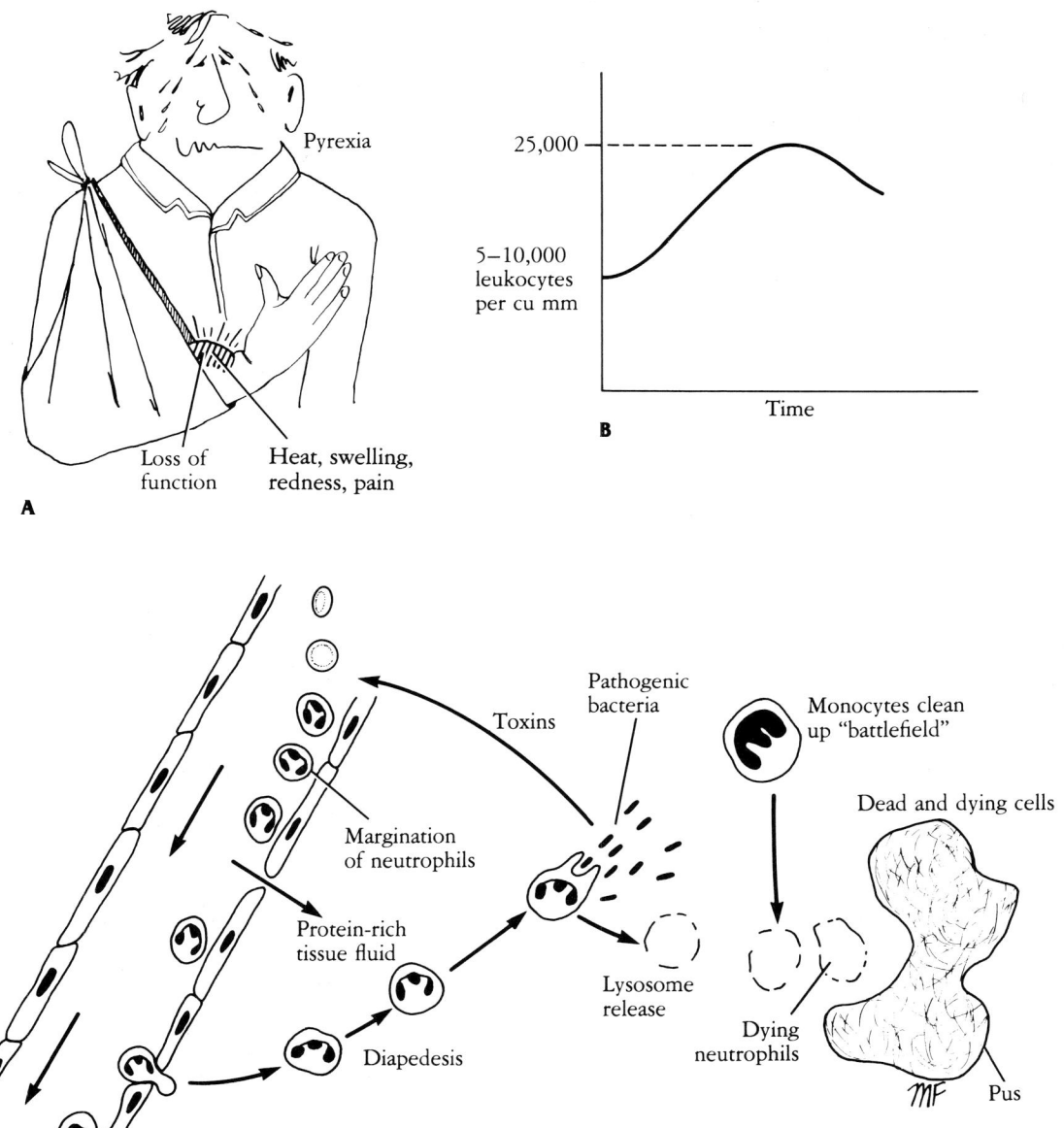

Fig. 5-32. (A) *Cardinal signs of acute inflammation;* (B) *example of increase in leukocyte count in a patient with a severe acute inflammatory lesion;* (C) *mobilization and deployment of neutrophils against invading pathogenic bacteria.*

the bactericidal substances and enzymes present within the lysosomes. Unfortunately, other bacteria, such as the tubercle bacillus, survive phagocytosis, and as long as they reside within the phagocyte, they are protected from antibacterial drugs. In many instances, the neutrophils release their lysosomes at the site of bacterial invasion, and the enzymes liberated not only destroy bacteria but bring about injury to tissues.

In most cases of acute inflammation caused by invading microorganisms, the organisms are repelled by the defending army of neutrophils and by the immune responses of the body. It must not be forgotten, however, that the battle takes a toll on both sides. The local accumulations of dead or dying neutrophils, the broken-down tissue cells, and the living and dead pathogenic organisms form a creamy yellow liquid known as *pus*. A local accumulation of pus is known as an abscess and must be drained surgically.

As the battle draws to a close, the neutrophils are gradually replaced by monocytes. These, on entering the area of conflict, quickly become macrophages. Initially, they assist the neutrophils in ridding the body of the invading organisms. Later, they dispose of the cellular debris as the inflammation subsides.

Almost immediately, the process of repair begins, and fibroblasts enter the area, accompanied by new capillary blood vessels. New connective tissue is formed, and in most areas of the body, epithelial cells regenerate.

CLINICAL PROBLEMS

For the answers to these problems, see page 788.

1. A 24-year-old woman is seen in the emergency room with severe vaginal bleeding. Her history reveals that she is 3 months pregnant, and a diagnosis of spontaneous abortion is made. The gynecologist is concerned about the volume of blood lost. What is the normal blood volume in a healthy adult? What type of transfusion would you give this patient? What tests would you perform before you started the transfusion?

2. List a number of clinical conditions in which a hematocrit determination would help the physician in making a diagnosis and monitoring the course of treatment.

3. A 56-year-old man complains to his physician of breathlessness on exertion. During the history taking, the patient mentions that he has suffered from severe hemorrhoids for a number of years. On questioning, he admits that on many occasions following defecation, he has noted his stools to be stained with bright red blood. Physical examination reveals nothing abnormal in the respiratory or cardiovascular systems. The patient's skin is sallow, and his nails are lusterless and concave. Examination of the conjunctiva shows excessive paleness in both eyes. The physician orders a red blood cell count and a hemoglobin estimation. Using your knowledge of the histology and physiology of the blood, can you explain this patient's symptoms and signs? Why did the physician request these blood examinations? What is the normal red blood cell count in the adult? What is the normal hemoglobin content of blood?

4. A 30-year-old college professor is granted sabbatical leave to continue his studies in astronomy. He selects an observatory high in the Swiss Alps and plans to stay there for a year. For the first few weeks following his arrival, he notices that he tends to be breathless on walking up steps and to tire very easily. After 2 months, the symptoms disappear. On returning to the United States a year later, he undergoes a medical checkup, and his physician reports that his red blood cell count is above normal. Can you explain this? Will the red cell count remain at this high level?

5. During a lecture to freshmen medical students, the professor asks if anyone can explain the connection between the blood and the pigments found in the bile. Can you answer this question?

6. A 5-year-old girl is found to have acute lymphocytic leukemia. The mother cannot understand

why infection can be a major complication when her child's white blood count is so high. Could you explain this to her?

7. How would you perform a differential white blood cell count? What is the approximate percentage of the different types of white blood cells in the adult? Name three common diseases in which each type of white blood cell separately may increase in number. Do you know of any disease in which the total number of white blood cells is diminished?

8. A red marrow biopsy specimen can be taken from the tibia in a young child, but in an adult, red marrow specimens are taken from the iliac crest or the sternum. Can you explain this phenomenon?

9. A 10-year-old boy falls while roller skating in the street. He receives a large abrasion of the right knee, which bleeds profusely. His parents roughly bandage the area and take him to the emergency room of a local hospital. Ten minutes later, he is examined by a doctor, and to the boy's amazement, the bleeding by this time has stopped. Describe the processes involved when a wound stops bleeding.

10. A 47-year-old man is admitted to the intensive care unit with a diagnosis of polycythemia vera and a pulmonary embolus. Why are patients with polycythemia vera prone to intravascular clotting of blood? What is an embolus? How does an embolus differ from a thrombus?

11. While making morning rounds with the attending physician, one of the house staff presents a patient suffering from dietary deprivation and impaired intestinal absorption caused by regional enteritis. One of the medications ordered is injection of vitamin K every other day. Why would dietary deprivation and impaired intestinal absorption cause a lack of vitamin K? What role does vitamin K play in blood physiology?

12. A 40-year-old woman is admitted to the hospital complaining of multiple small hemorrhagic spots in the skin, severe nose bleeding, and vaginal bleeding. While taking the patient's history, the physician asks her if she is taking any medicines. She replies that she had been having trouble getting to sleep at night and her doctor had prescribed some sleeping tablets. An examination of the prescription shows that the patient has been taking Sedormid (apronal) for the past 3 months. This drug is known to be toxic to bone marrow. Using your knowledge of histology and physiology, can you see any connection between the bleeding problems and the taking of Sedormid?

13. Neutrophils are said to be one of our most important lines of defense against pathogenic organisms. Can you explain this? Define the terms *margination, diapedesis,* and *pus.*

14. Using your knowledge of histology and physiology, explain the underlying mechanisms responsible for the cardinal signs of acute inflammation, namely, swelling, redness, heat, pain, and loss of function.

15. A 54-year-old man attends a clinic for weekly injections of vitamin B_{12}. His medical history includes a total gastrectomy for cancer of the stomach performed six months previously. Why is this patient receiving vitamin B_{12}? What is the function of vitamin B_{12}?

16. An expectant mother has a sample of her blood tested for A, B, O, and Rh groups. The woman is found to be Rh negative. It is decided to test the woman for the presence of Rh antibodies. Why? If the Rh antibodies are found in a mother's serum, the Rh genotype of the husband should be ascertained. Why? Is it important to know whether an Rh-negative mother has been transfused in the past with Rh-positive blood?

ADDITIONAL READING

Allison, A. C., et al. *Inflammation.* New York: Springer-Verlag, 1978.

Bainton, D. F., and Farquhar, M. G. Origin of granules in polymorphonuclear leucocytes: Two types derived from opposite faces of the Golgi apparatus in developing leucocytes. *J. Cell Biol.* 28:277, 1966.

Bainton, D. F., and Farquhar, M. G. Segregation and packaging of granules in eosinophilic leucocytes. *J. Cell Biol.* 45:54, 1970.

Bainton, D. F., Ullyot, J. L., and Farquhar, M. G. The development of neutrophilic polymorphonuclear leukocytes in human bone marrow. *J. Exp. Med.* 139:907, 1971.

Barr, R. D., Whang-Peng, J., and Perry, S. Hemopoietic stem cells in human peripheral blood. *Science* 190:284, 1975.

Becker, R. P., and De Bruyn, P. P. H. The transmural passage of blood cells into myeloid sinusoids and the entry of platelets into the sinusoidal circulation: A scanning electron microscopic investigation. *Am. J. Anat.* 145:183, 1976.

Bentfield-Barker, M. E., and Bainton, D. F. Ultrastructure of rat megakaryocytes after prolonged thrombocytopenia. *J. Ultrastruct. Res.* 61:201, 1977.

Bessis, M. *Living Blood Cells and Their Ultrastructure.* New York: Springer-Verlag, 1973.

Castle, W. B. Current concepts of pernicious anemia. *Am. J. Med.* 48:541, 1970.

Chao, F. C., Shepro, D., Tullis, J. L., Belamarich, F. A., and Curby, W. A. Similarities between platelet contraction and cellular motility during mitosis: Role of platelet microtubules in clot retraction. *J. Cell Sci.* 20:569, 1976.

Cline, M. J. *The White Cell.* Cambridge, Mass.: Harvard University Press, 1975.

Davidson, W. M., and Smith, D. R. A morphological sex difference in the polymorphonuclear neutrophil leucocytes. *Br. Med. J.* 2:6, 1954.

Escobar, M. R., and Friedman, H. (eds.). *Macrophages and Lymphocytes: Nature, Functions and Interaction.* New York: Plenum, 1979.

Everett, N. B., and Perkins, W. D. Hemopoietic stem cell migration. In Cairnie, A. B., Lala, P. K., and Osmond, D. G. (eds.), *Stem Cells of Renewing Cell Populations.* New York: Academic, 1976.

Goldwasser, E. K. Erythropoietin and the differentiation of red blood cells. *Fed. Proc.* 34:2285, 1975.

Gowans, J. L. Life span, recirculation, and transformation of lymphocytes. *Int. Rev. Path.* 5:1, 1966.

Gowans, J. L. Differentiation of the cells which synthesize the immunoglobulins. *Ann. Immunol. (Paris)* 125:201, 1974.

Gowans, J. L. *Blood Cells and Vessel Walls: Functional Interactions.* Princeton, N.J.: Excerpta Medica, 1980.

Gralnick, H. R. Intravascular coagulation. I. Differential diagnosis and conditioning mechanisms. *Postgrad. Med.* 62:68, 1977.

Gutman, G. A., and Weissman, I. L. Lymphoid tissue architecture: Experimental analysis of the origin and distribution of T-cells and B-cells. *Immunology* 23:465, 1972.

Handin, R. I., and Rosenberg, R. D. Hemorrhagic disorders. III. Disorders of primary and secondary hemostasis. In Beck, W. S. (ed.), *Hematology* (2nd ed.). Cambridge, Mass.: MIT Press, 1977, p. 547.

Hanifin, J. M., and Cline, M. J. Human monocytes and macrophages: Interaction with antigen and lymphocytes. *J. Cell Biol.* 46:97, 1970.

Kass, L. *Bone Marrow Interpretation.* Philadelphia: Lippincott, 1979.

Keleman, E., et al. *Atlas of Human Development.* New York: Springer-Verlag, 1979.

Klebanoff, S. J., and Clark, R. A. *The Neutrophil: Function and Clinical Disorders.* New York: Elsevier North-Holland, 1978.

Marchalonis, J. J. Lymphocyte surface immunoglobulins. *Science* 190:20, 1975.

Metcalf, D., and Moore, M. A. S. *Haemopoietic Cells.* Amsterdam: North-Holland, 1971.

Movat, H. Z. (ed.). *Inflammation, Immunity and Hypersensitivity: Molecular and Cellular Mechanisms* (2nd ed.). New York: Harper & Row, 1979.

Nichols, B. A., Bainton, D. F., and Farquhar, M. G. Differentiation of monocytes: Origin, nature and fate of their azurophil granules. *J. Cell Biol.* 50:498, 1971.

Osmond, D. G. Potentials of bone marrow lymphocytes. In Cairnie, A. B., Lala, P. K., and Osmond, D. G. (eds.), *Stem Cells of Renewing Cell Populations.* New York: Academic, 1976.

Polliack, A., et al. Identification of human B and T lymphocytes by scanning electron microscopy. *J. Exp. Med.* 138:607, 1973.

Raff, M. C. T and B lymphocytes and immune responses. *Nature* 242:19, 1973.

Ryan, G. B., and Majino, G. Acute inflammation. *Am. J. Pathol.* 86:183, 1977.

Spivak, J. L. (ed.). *Fundamentals of Clinical Hematology.* Hagerstown, Md.: Harper & Row, 1980.

Tanaka, Y., and Goodman, J. R. *Electron Microscopy of Human Blood Cells*. New York: Harper, 1972.

Travassoli, M., and Crosby, W. H. Fate of the nucleus of the marrow erythroblast. *Science* 179:912, 1973.

Till, J. E., et al. Regulation of blood cell differentiation. *Fed. Proc.* 34:2279, 1975.

Wall, R. T., et al. Human endothelial cell injury mechanism in vitro. *Thromb. Haemost.* 38:228, 1977.

Weiss, L. The hematopoietic microenvironment of the bone marrow: An ultrastructural study of the stroma in rats. *Anat. Rec.* 186:161, 1976.

Weiss, L., and Chen, L. T. The organization of hematopoietic cords and vascular sinuses in bone marrow. *Blood Cells* 1:617, 1975.

Whiteside, T. L., and Rowlands, D. T. T-cell and B-cell identification in the diagnosis of lymphoproliferative disease. *Am. J. Pathol.* 88:754, 1977.

Williams, W. W., Beutler, E., Erslev, A. J., and Rundles, R. W. *Hematology* (2nd ed.). New York: McGraw-Hill, 1977.

Wintrobe, M., et al. *Clinical Hematology* (7th ed.). Philadelphia: Lea & Febiger, 1974.

MUSCLE TISSUE

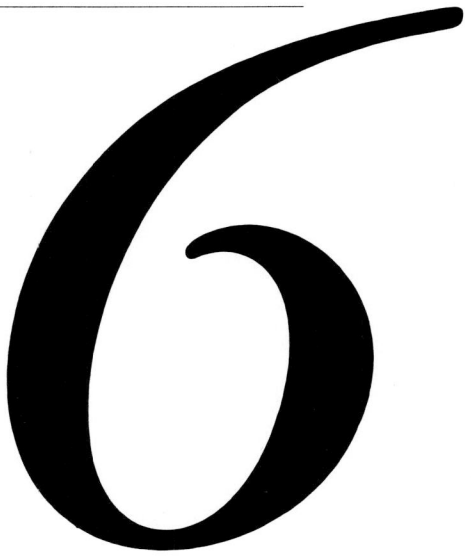

Muscle tissue is unique in that it can contract and perform mechanical work. This property results from the contractile properties of proteins contained in the cell cytoplasm. The muscle cells are commonly referred to as muscle fibers. There are three kinds of muscle tissue: skeletal, smooth, and cardiac. Skeletal and cardiac muscle is often called *striated muscle,* because the intracellular contractile proteins form an alternating series of transverse bands along the cell when viewed with the light microscope. Smooth muscle is so called because the contractile proteins are not arranged in the same orderly manner and the transverse bands are absent.

The muscle cells (fibers) are surrounded and supported by connective tissue that also supports their blood supply and nerve supply.

SKELETAL MUSCLE

Skeletal muscles are the muscles that produce the movements of the skeleton. They are under voluntary control and are sometimes called *voluntary muscles.* A skeletal muscle has two or more attachments. The attachment that moves the least is referred to as the *origin,* and that which moves the most, as the *insertion.* Under varying circumstances, the degree of mobility of the attachments may be reversed, and therefore the terms *origin* and *insertion* are interchangeable.

The fleshy part of a muscle is referred to as its *belly.* The ends of a muscle are attached to bones, cartilage, or ligaments by cords of fibrous tissue called *tendons.* Occasionally, flattened muscles are attached by a thin, strong sheet of fibrous tissue called an *aponeurosis.* The individual muscle fibers are either parallel or oblique to the long axis of the muscle. Because a muscle shortens by one-third or one-half its resting length when it contracts, it follows that muscles whose fibers run parallel to the line of pull will bring about a greater degree of movement than will those whose fibers run obliquely. The strength of a muscle depends not upon the length of its fibers but upon the total number of fibers present in the muscle. The increase in the size of a muscle that takes place as a result of repeated exercise is caused by an increase in the size of each muscle fiber and not by an increase in the number of fibers (that is, hypertrophy, not hyperplasia, takes place).

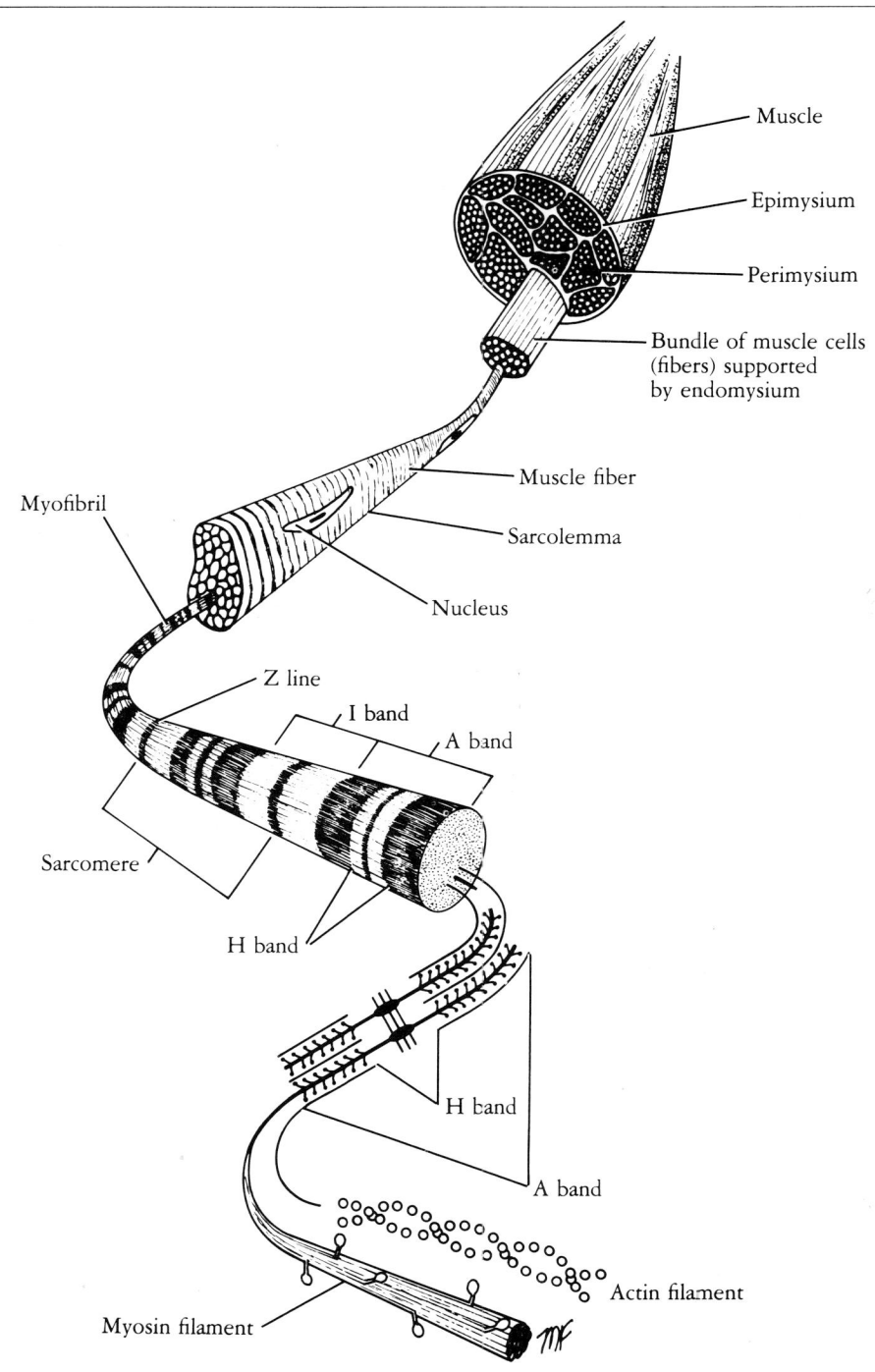

Light Microscopic Structure

Skeletal muscle fibers are extremely long, cylindrical, multinucleated cells measuring about 1 to 40 mm in length and from 10 to 100 μm in diameter. Each fiber is surrounded by an extracellular layer of polysaccharides that form a basal lamina. The fibers are bound together by connective tissue to form a muscle. A tough connective tissue sheath, the *epimysium,* surrounds the whole muscle (Fig. 6-1). From the epimysium, connective tissue septa pass into the muscle mass, binding together groups of muscle cells. This connective tissue is referred to as the *perimysium.* Each muscle fiber in turn is surrounded by a delicate connective tissue envelope, the *endomysium* (see Fig. 6-1).

The plasma membrane of skeletal muscle fibers (cells) is called *sarcolemma,* and the cytoplasm is referred to as *sarcoplasm.* The multiple nuclei of the muscle cells are found at the periphery of the cells, just beneath the plasma membrane (Figs. 6-2 and 6-3). Most of the sarcoplasm is occupied by longitudinally running *myofibrils,* which measure about 1 μm in diameter and give the fibers a longitudinally striated appearance. The myofibrils show a pattern of repeating crossbands (Fig. 6-4; see Fig. 6-2). Because these bands are in close register, they give rise to the cross striations of the whole muscle fiber.

When examined with the light microscope, each cross striation can be seen to be made up of a dark band called the *A band* and a light band called the *I band* (see Figs. 6-1 and 6-4). A transverse line, the *Z line,* bisects each I band. The *H bands* are the middle region of the A band. The area between two Z lines on a single myofibril is called a *sarcomere.*

Electron Microscopic Structure

The basic contractile unit of the muscle fiber is the sarcomere. With the electron microscope, the sarco-

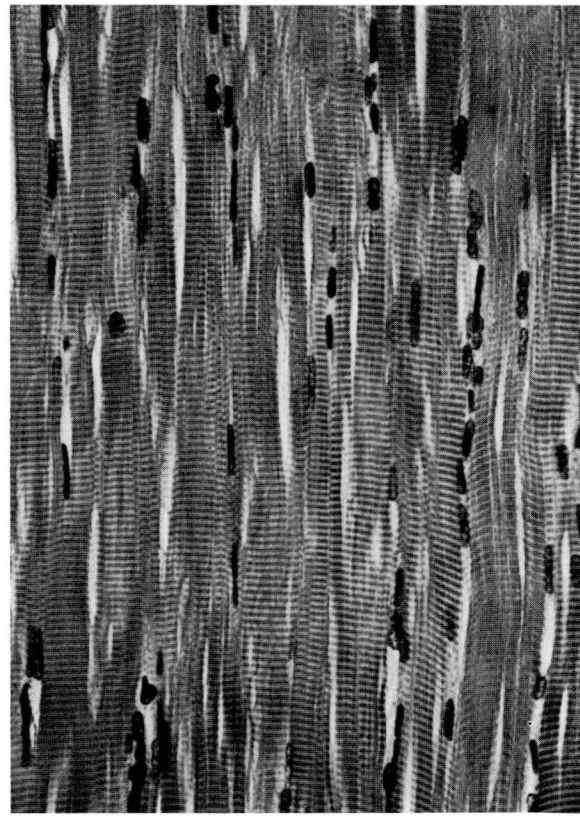

Fig. 6-2. Photomicrograph of longitudinal section of skeletal muscle, showing crossbanding and numerous peripherally located nuclei. (H&E; ×400.)

mere of each myofibril is seen to be made up of two types of longitudinally running filaments (Figs. 6-5 and 6-6). The thick filament (10 nm), composed of the protein *myosin,* occupies the A band. The thin filaments (5 nm), composed of the protein *actin,* are attached to the Z line and occupy the I band. The actin filaments also extend into the adjacent A bands, where they lie between the thick myosin filaments. When a muscle contracts, the thick and thin filaments slide past one another and pull the Z lines closer together, so that the myofibril and the muscle fibers shorten. The thick myosin filaments have lateral projections that attach to the thin actin

Fig. 6-1. Structure of skeletal muscle. Note the organization of the muscle fibers, the myofibrils, and the muscle filaments. Observe that a sarcomere, with its A, I, and H bands, extends between Z lines.

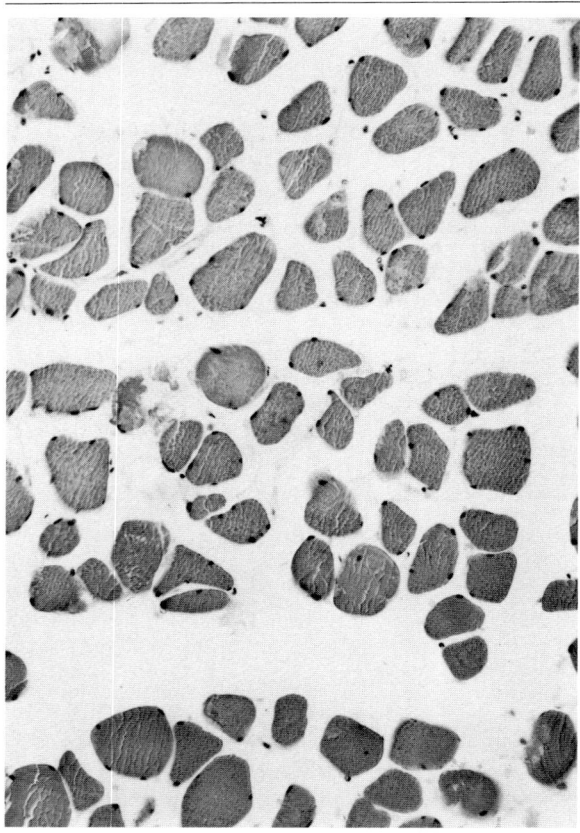

Fig. 6-3. Photomicrograph of transverse section of skeletal muscle, showing many muscle fibers with peripherally located nuclei. The muscle fibers are separated from one another by loose connective tissue, the endomysium. (H&E; ×200.)

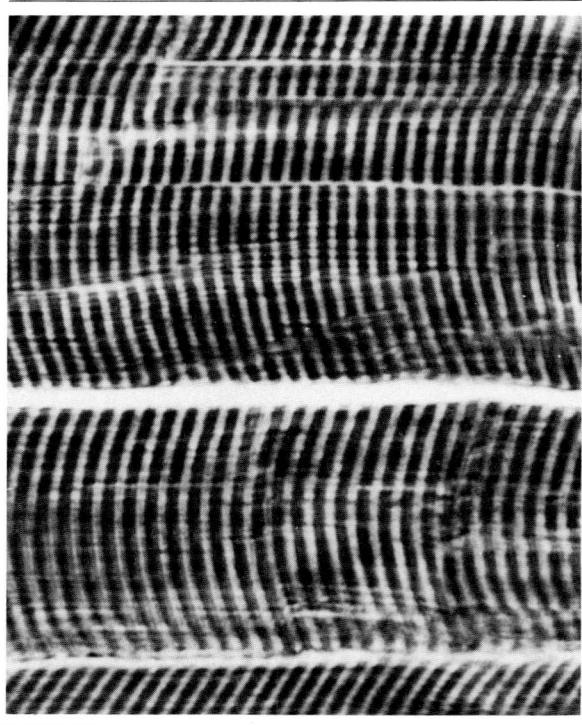

Fig. 6-4. Photomicrograph of longitudinal section of skeletal muscle, showing A and I bands. (Iron hematoxylin stain; ×1,200.)

filaments and bring about the movement of the actin filaments (see Fig. 6-1). The chemical reaction responsible for the movement of one set of filaments on the other is not known. The breakdown of adenosine triphosphate (ATP) by ATPase in the lateral projections is believed to provide the necessary energy (see p. 219).

The sarcolemma, which is the plasmolemma of muscle cells, is invaginated at the A-I junction to form the *T system* of tubules. Each T tubule extends transversely into the sarcoplasm, and the cavity of each tubule is continuous with the exterior (Fig. 6-7). Another system of tubules exists in the sarcoplasm and is known as the *sarcoplasmic reticulum*. These tubules, which are the smooth endoplasmic reticulum of muscle cells, run longitudinally and do not communicate with the exterior of the muscle cell (see Fig. 6-7). The T tubules and the sarcoplasmic reticulum play an important role in muscle contraction (see p. 218).

Skeletal muscle cells also contain the usual cell organelles and inclusions. Glycogen is found throughout the sarcoplasm, and the oxygen-binding protein *myoglobin* is also present.

Types of Skeletal Muscle Fibers

Skeletal muscles are made up of two main types of muscle fibers: (1) *red fibers,* which are of small diameter and possess large amounts of myoglobin in the sarcoplasm, and (2) *white fibers,* which are of large diameter and contain little myoglobin pigment. Red

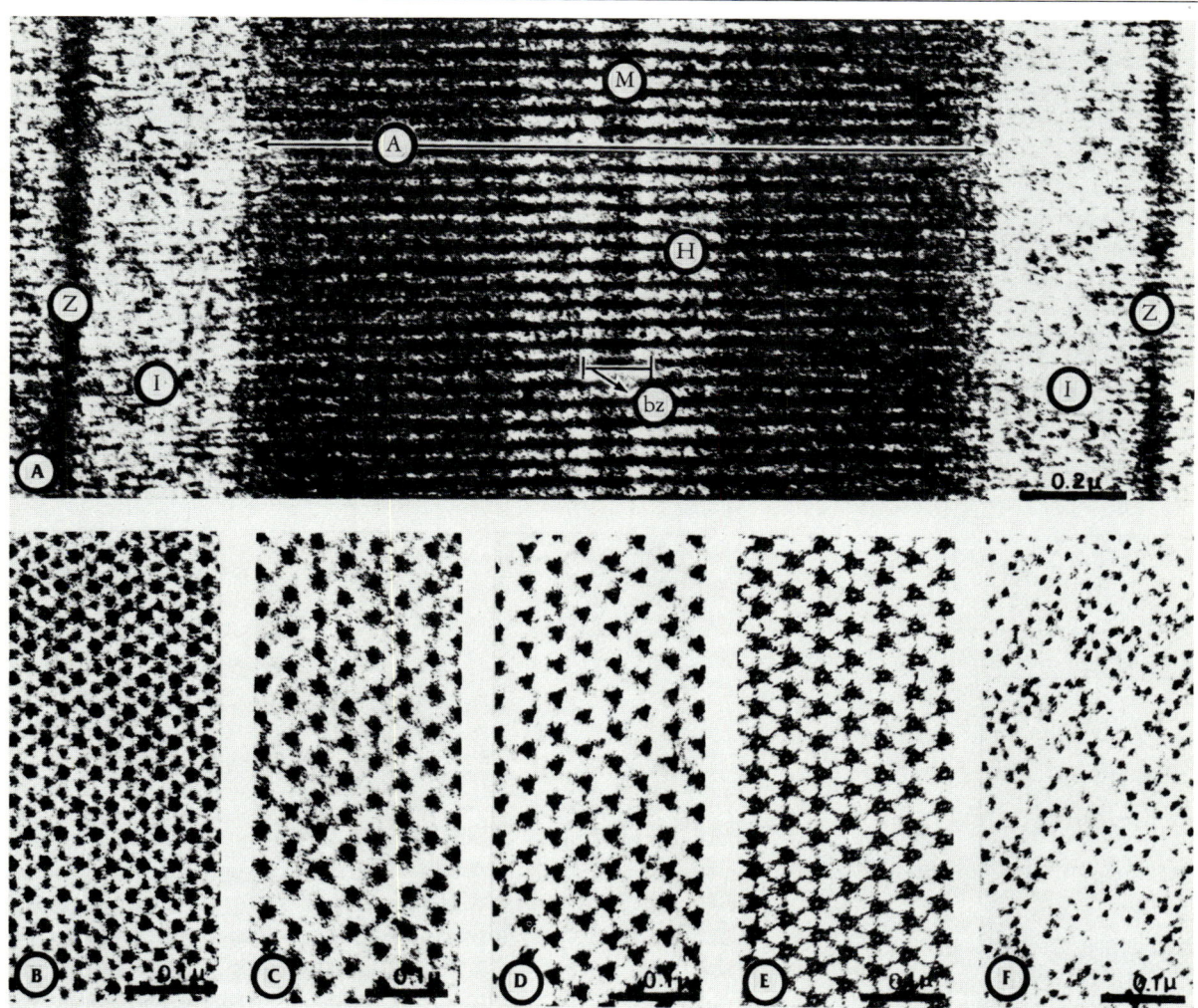

Fig. 6-5. Electron micrograph of a longitudinal section of skeletal muscle, showing a single sarcomere (A). Transverse sections of the different bands are shown below (B, C, D, E, F). The A band (←A→) consists of both thick and thin filaments (B). The H band (H) consists of thick filaments (C). The M band (M) consists of thick filaments with transverse extensions (E). The I band consists only of thin filaments (F). (Courtesy of Dr. F. A. Pepe.)

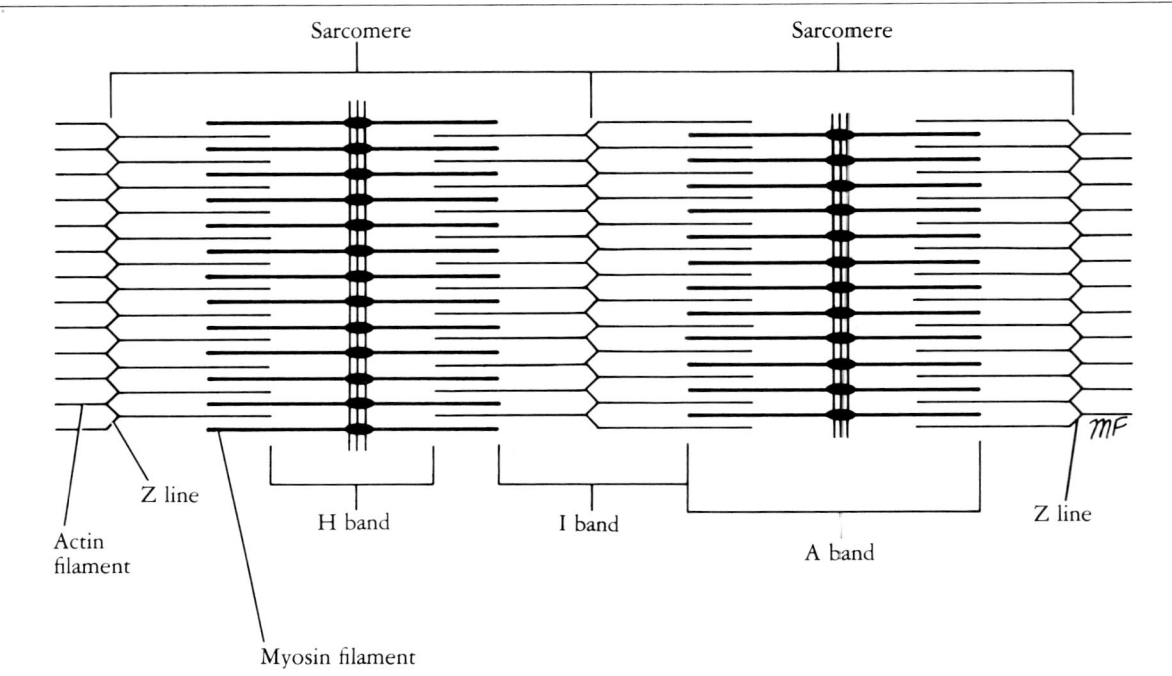

Fig. 6-6. Organization of sarcomeres in skeletal muscle.

fibers are capable of carrying out sustained activity over a prolonged period and are found in large numbers in postural muscles. White fibers are characterized by short bursts of activity. Most skeletal muscles are composed of a mixture of these two types of fibers.

SMOOTH MUSCLE

Smooth muscle is not under conscious control and is often called *involuntary muscle*. Depending on the organ, smooth muscle fiber may be made to contract by local stretching of the fibers, by nerve impulses from autonomic nerves, or by hormonal stimulation.

In the tubes of the body, smooth muscle provides the motive power for propelling the contents through the lumen. In the digestive system, it also causes the ingested food to be mixed thoroughly with the digestive juices. A wave of contraction of the circularly arranged fibers passes along the tube, milking the contents onward. By their contraction, the longitudinal fibers pull the wall of the tube proximally over the contents. This method of propulsion is called *peristalsis*.

In storage organs, such as the urinary bladder and the uterus, the fibers are irregularly arranged and interlaced. Their contraction is slow and sustained and causes the contents of the organs to be expelled. In the walls of the blood vessels, the smooth muscle fibers are arranged circularly, and they serve to modify the caliber of the lumen.

Light Microscopic Structure

Smooth muscle fibers consist of long, spindle-shaped cells measuring from 20 to 500 μm in length. The fibers are arranged in bundles or sheets and are offset relative to one another in such a way that the thick middle portion of one cell lies next to the thin ends of neighboring cells (Figs. 6-8 and 6-9). There is a single nucleus for each fiber, and it is centrally placed and ovoid (Fig. 6-10). The nucleus contains several nucleoli. In sections stained with

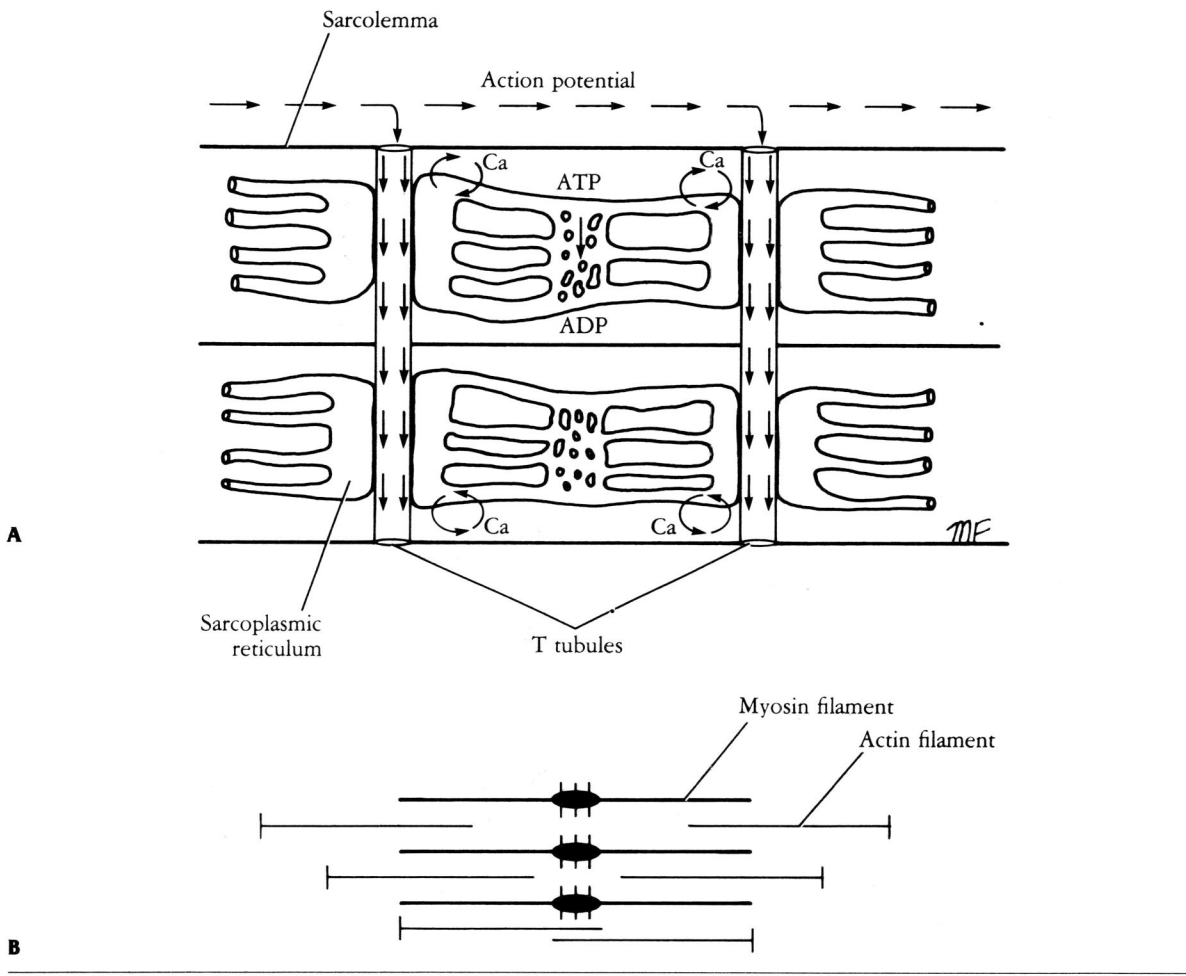

Fig. 6-7. (A) Longitudinal section of skeletal muscle, showing the pathway taken by an action potential that causes the release of calcium ions from the sarcoplasmic reticulum; the calcium ions are taken up again by the calcium pump. (B) Sliding movements of the actin filaments as a myofibril contracts.

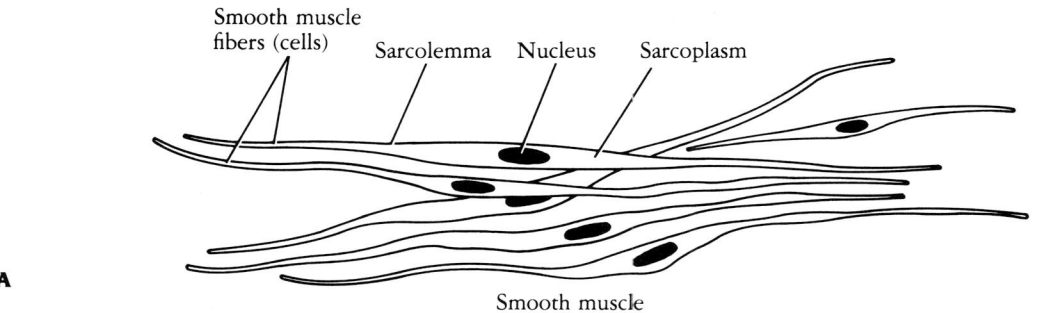

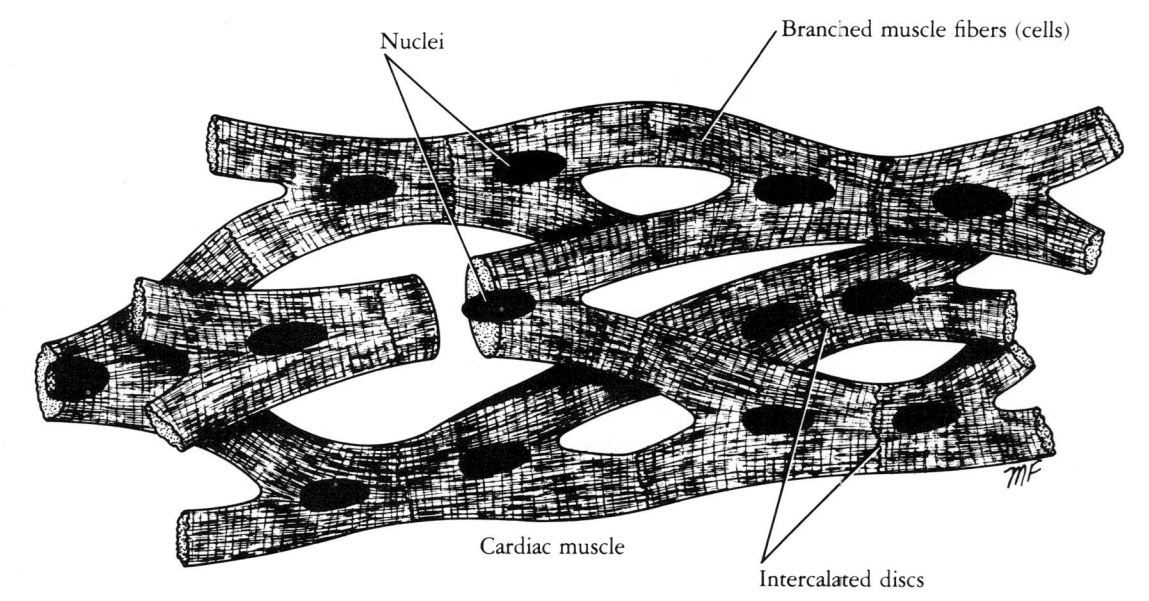

Fig. 6-8. Main features of the structure of (A) smooth muscle fibers and (B) cardiac muscle fibers. Note that an intercalated disc represents the coming together of the plasma membranes of two adjacent muscle cells; it is a site of junctional complexes.

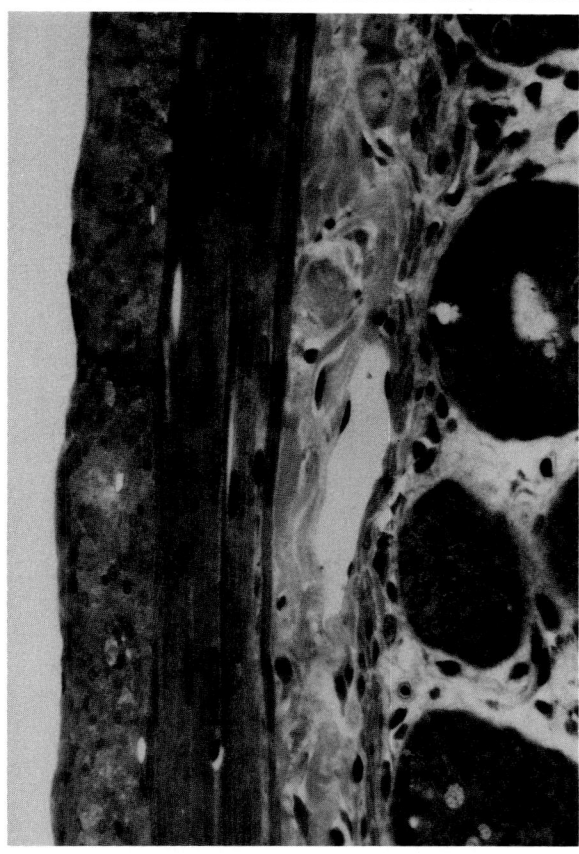

Fig. 6-9. Photomicrograph of transverse section of wall of small intestine. On the extreme left, the smooth muscle layer is cut transversely. Next to it is a layer of smooth muscle cut longitudinally; note the presence of fusiform nuclei in this layer. Plastic section. (H&E; ×400.)

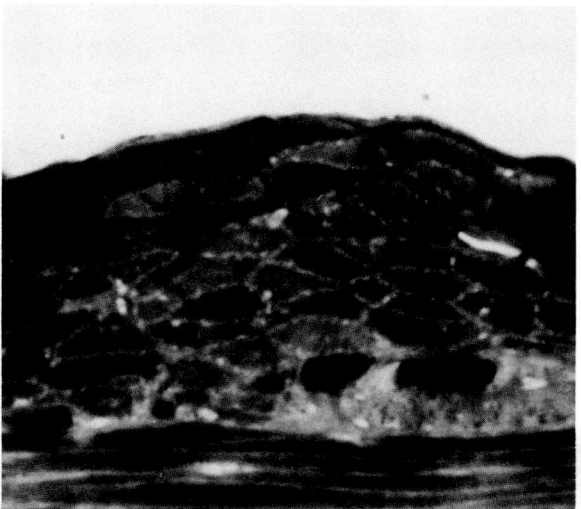

Fig. 6-10. Photomicrograph of transverse section of wall of small intestine, showing the outer layer of smooth muscle in cross section. Where the muscle fibers are cut in the region of the nucleus, note that the nucleus is centrally placed. Plastic section (H&E; ×1,000.)

hematoxylin and eosin (H&E), the sarcoplasm (cytoplasm of muscle cells) stains pink and is homogeneous, having no longitudinal or cross striations. With special stains, however, longitudinally running myofibrils can be recognized.

Electron Microscopic Structure

Electron micrographs show the usual structure, including nucleus, mitochondria, endoplasmic reticulum, free ribosomes, and a Golgi apparatus (Fig. 6-11). The greater part of the cytoplasm is filled with thin myofilaments that are collected into bundles to form the myofibrils. Although the myofibrils run longitudinally, there is no evidence of the crossbanding seen in skeletal muscle. Chemical analysis has demonstrated that smooth muscle contains both myosin and actin, and recently it has been shown that they form myofilaments, as in skeletal muscle, although the myofilaments are more difficult to demonstrate. It is thought that the sliding filament mechanism operates in the same manner as in skeletal muscle when smooth muscle contracts. Scattered throughout the sarcoplasm (see Fig. 6-11) and along the inner surface of the sarcolemma are ovoid dense areas in which myofilaments are embedded. It is believed that with contraction of the muscle fiber, the myofilaments pull on these dense areas, folding the sarcolemma. Gap junctions exist between adjacent smooth muscle fibers, permitting electrical excitation to pass from one cell to another.

CARDIAC MUSCLE

Cardiac muscle forms the greater part of the walls of the heart, forming the myocardium. It is arranged in

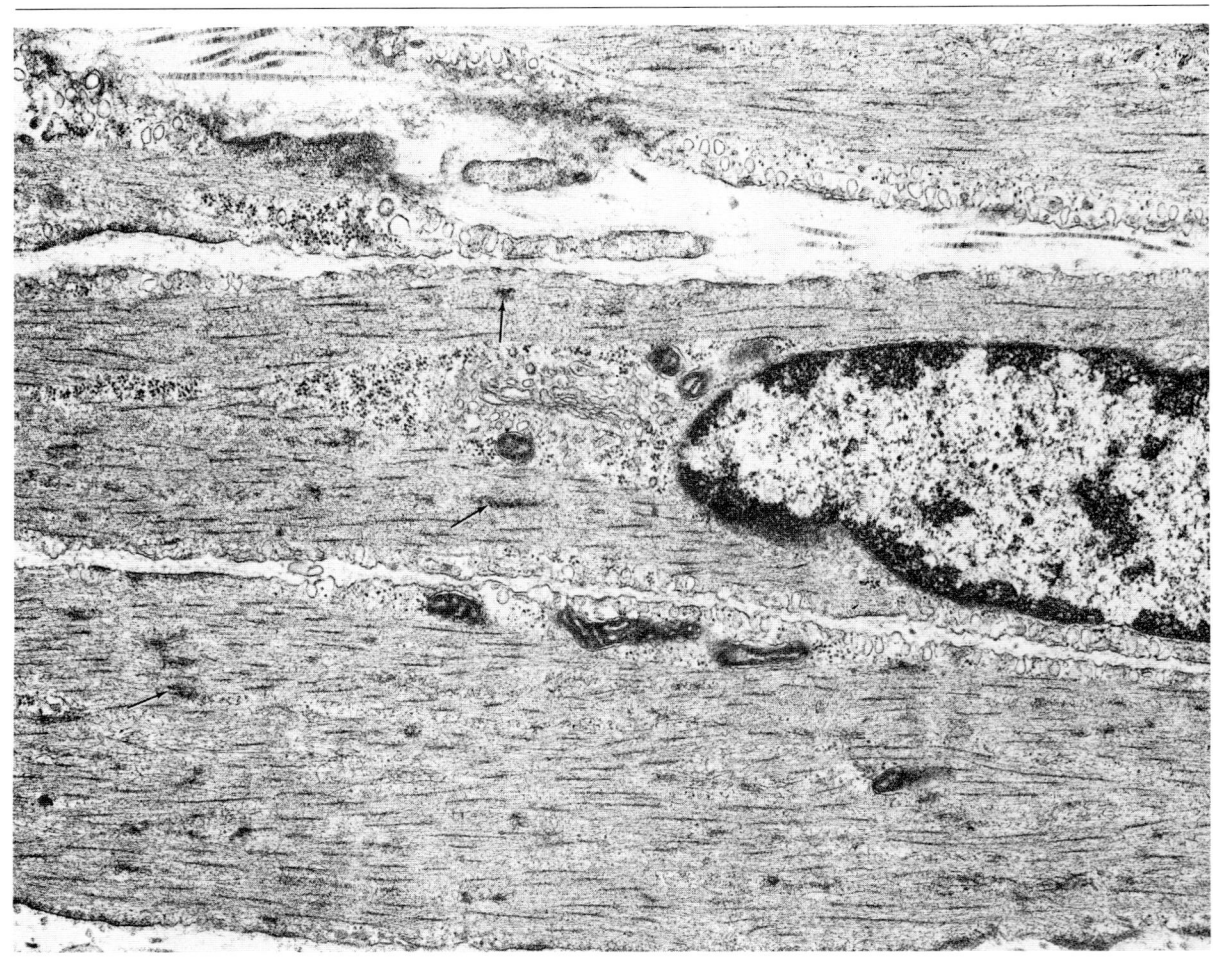

Fig. 6-11. Electron micrograph of longitudinal section of three smooth muscle fibers, showing a nucleus, Golgi apparatus, endoplasmic reticulum, and free ribosomes. Note the presence in the cytoplasm of numerous filaments and ovoid dense areas (arrows). ($\times 24,700$.) (Courtesy of Drs. A. P. Somlyo, C. E. Devine, A. V. Somlyo, and R. V. Rice.)

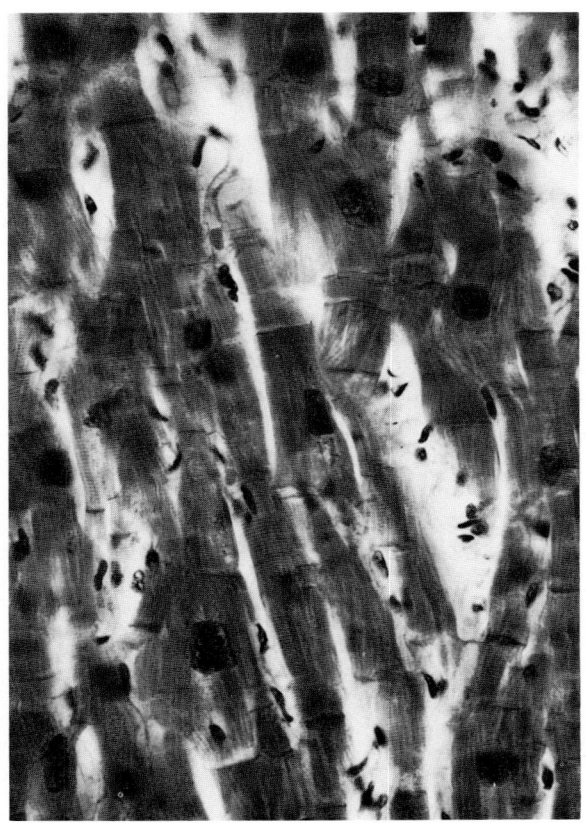

Fig. 6-12. Photomicrograph of longitudinal section of cardiac muscle, showing branching muscle fiber, crossbanding, centrally placed nuclei, and intercalated discs. (H&E; ×400.)

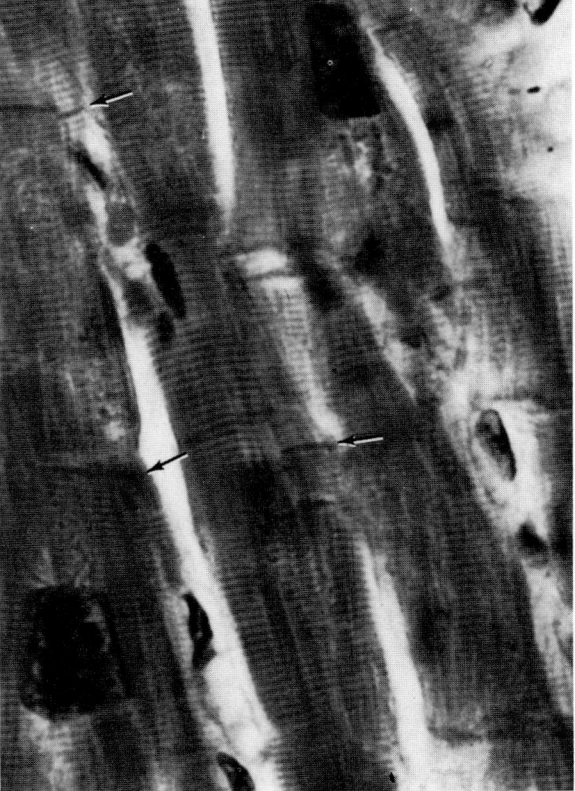

Fig. 6-13. Photomicrograph of high-power view of same longitudinal section of cardiac muscle as in Figure 6-12, showing detail of crossbands and intercalated discs (arrows). (H&E; ×1,000.)

layers that spiral around the heart. Cardiac muscle fibers (muscle cells) have the property of spontaneous and rhythmical contraction. Specialized cardiac muscle fibers form the *conducting system of the heart.* Cardiac muscle is involuntary and is supplied by the autonomic nervous system.

Light Microscopic Structure

Cardiac muscle cells are branched and possess centrally placed nuclei (Figs. 6-12–6-14; see Fig. 6-8). Each cell is about 80 μm long and 15 μm in diameter. The sarcoplasm contains myofibrils and shows cross striations similar to those of skeletal muscles.

Thus, we find A bands, I bands, H bands, and Z lines. Cardiac muscle cells differ from those of skeletal or smooth muscle in that the cells not only branch but are joined together by a special junctional complex known as the *intercalated disc* (see Fig. 6-13). The discs are seen as dark lines that run transversely in a step-wise manner across the fibers at the level of the Z lines.

Electron Microscopic Structure

The electron microscopic structure of cardiac muscle is very similar to that of skeletal muscle (Figs. 6-15 and 6-16). *Myosin* and *actin filaments* form the

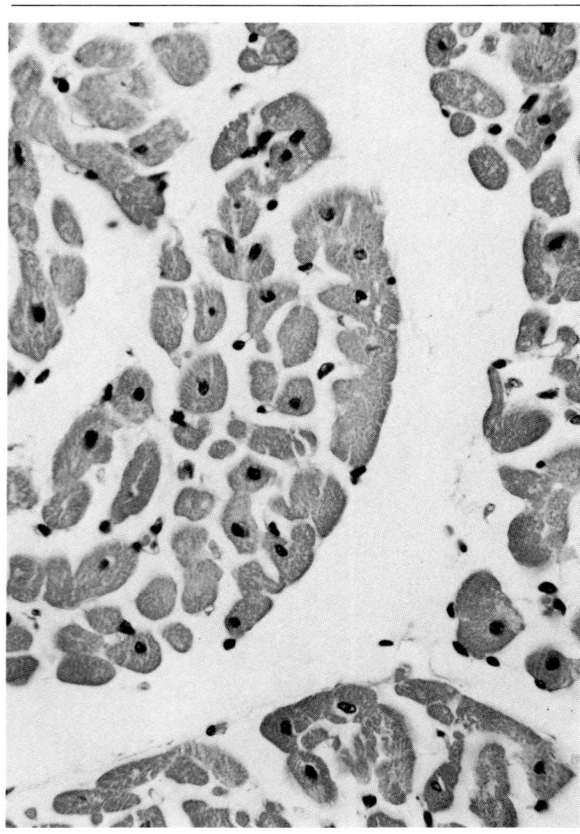

Fig. 6-14. Photomicrograph of transverse section of cardiac muscle, showing numerous muscle fibers with centrally placed nuclei. (H&E; ×400.)

myofibrils, but the latter are not arranged in such discrete groups as in skeletal muscle. The mitochondria are large and numerous, and the tubular invaginations of the sarcolemma that form the T system of cardiac muscle are less frequent, occurring at the Z lines of each sarcomere instead of at the A-I junction as in skeletal muscle. The sarcoplasmic reticulum is not as well developed as in skeletal muscle.

The intercalated discs (Fig. 6-17) consist of three regions: (1) the macula adherens (desmosome), (2) the fascia adherens, and (3) the gap junction. The macula adherens provides a spotlike attachment between adjacent muscle fibers. The fascia adherens attaches the actin filaments to the sarcolemma. The gap junctions, which are areas of low electrical resistance, allow the rapid spread of excitation from cell to cell.

Structure of the Conducting System of the Heart

The conducting system of the heart consists of specialized cardiac muscle present in the *sino-atrial node*, the *atrioventricular node*, the *atrioventricular bundle* and its right and left terminal branches, and the *subendocardial plexus*.

The *sino-atrial node* is the site where the contraction of the heart muscle is initiated and is often called the *pacemaker*. It forms the full thickness of the myocardium of the right atrium and is situated just to the right of the opening of the superior vena cava into the right atrium. Once initiated, the cardiac impulse spreads through the atrial myocardium to the atrioventricular node.

The *atrioventricular node* is situated beneath the endocardium on the right side of the lower part of the atrial septum just above the tricuspid valve. The cardiac impulse is conducted from this node to the ventricles by the *atrioventricular bundle*. The atrioventricular bundle is the only muscular connection between the myocardium of the atria and the myocardium of the ventricles.

The *atrioventricular bundle* descends on the right side of the membranous part of the ventricular septum. At the upper border of the muscular part of the septum, it divides into two branches, one for each ventricle. The branches become continuous with the *subendocardial plexus*. The sino-atrial and atrioventricular nodes consist of small cardiac muscle fibers embedded in vascular connective tissue. The nodes are innervated by postganglionic fibers of the autonomic nervous system.

The atrioventricular bundle, its right and left branches, and the subendocardial plexus are composed of cardiac muscle fibers that are usually larger than ordinary cardiac muscle fibers. These specialized fibers are sometimes called *Purkinje fibers*. The fibers have relatively few myofibrils; those that are

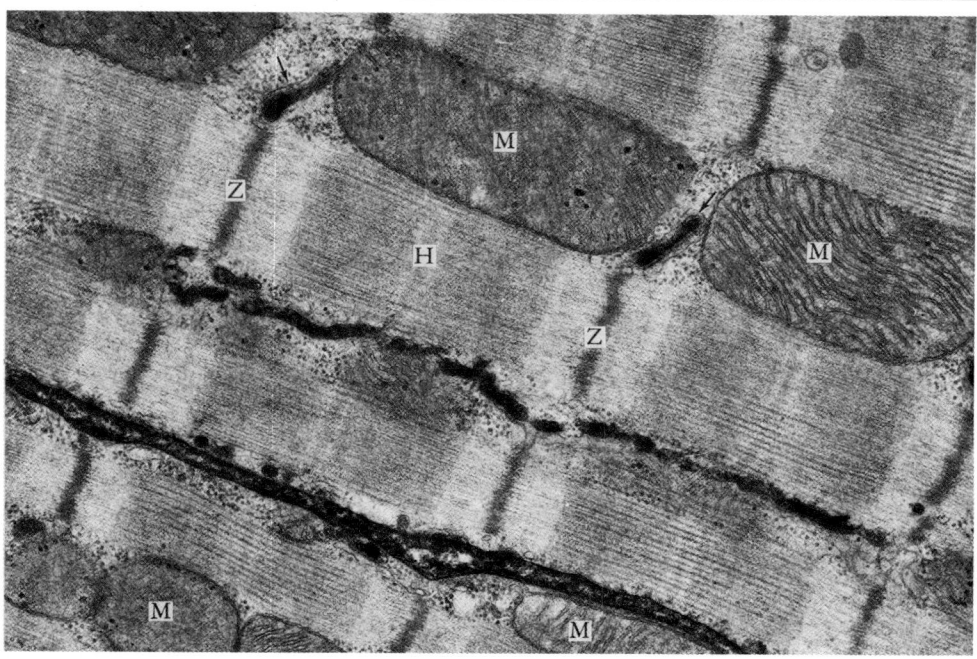

Fig. 6-15. Electron micrograph of longitudinal section of cardiac muscle, showing numerous mitochondria (M) between myofibrils and crossbanding. Note that the structure of the crossbands is similar to that in skeletal muscle. Note also the presence of two dark-staining T tubules (arrows). (Courtesy of Dr. W. G. Forssmann.)

present tend to be concentrated in the periphery of the cytoplasm. The center of the sarcoplasm is pale staining and contains large amounts of glycogen (Fig. 6-18). Electron microscopic examination reveals many mitochondria, a considerable amount of glycogen, poor development of the sarcoplasmic reticulum, and the absence of a T tubule system. The specialized cells are connected by numerous macula adherens and gap junctions.

The specialized cardiac muscle fibers of the sinoatrial and atrioventricular nodes have a higher rate of intrinsic rhythmical contraction and a slower speed of conduction than do ordinary cardiac muscle fibers. The specialized fibers of the atrioventricular bundle and its terminal branches, however, have a higher speed of conduction.

NERVE SUPPLY

Skeletal Muscle

The nerve trunk to a skeletal muscle is a mixed nerve, about 60 percent motor and 40 percent sensory; it also contains some sympathetic autonomic fibers. The nerve enters the muscle at about the midpoint on its deep surface, often near the margin; the place of entrance is known as the *motor point*. This arrangement allows the muscle to move with minimum interference with the nerve trunk. The motor nerve ends on entering the muscle by dividing into many branches, each of which terminates on a muscle fiber at the *motor end-plate* (Figs. 6-19 and 6-20). Each muscle fiber has at least one motor end-plate; the longer fibers possess more.

The sensory nerve fibers arise from specialized sensory endings lying within the muscle or tendons called *muscle spindles* and *tendon spindles*, respectively (Fig. 6-21). These endings are stimulated by tension in the muscle, which may occur during active con-

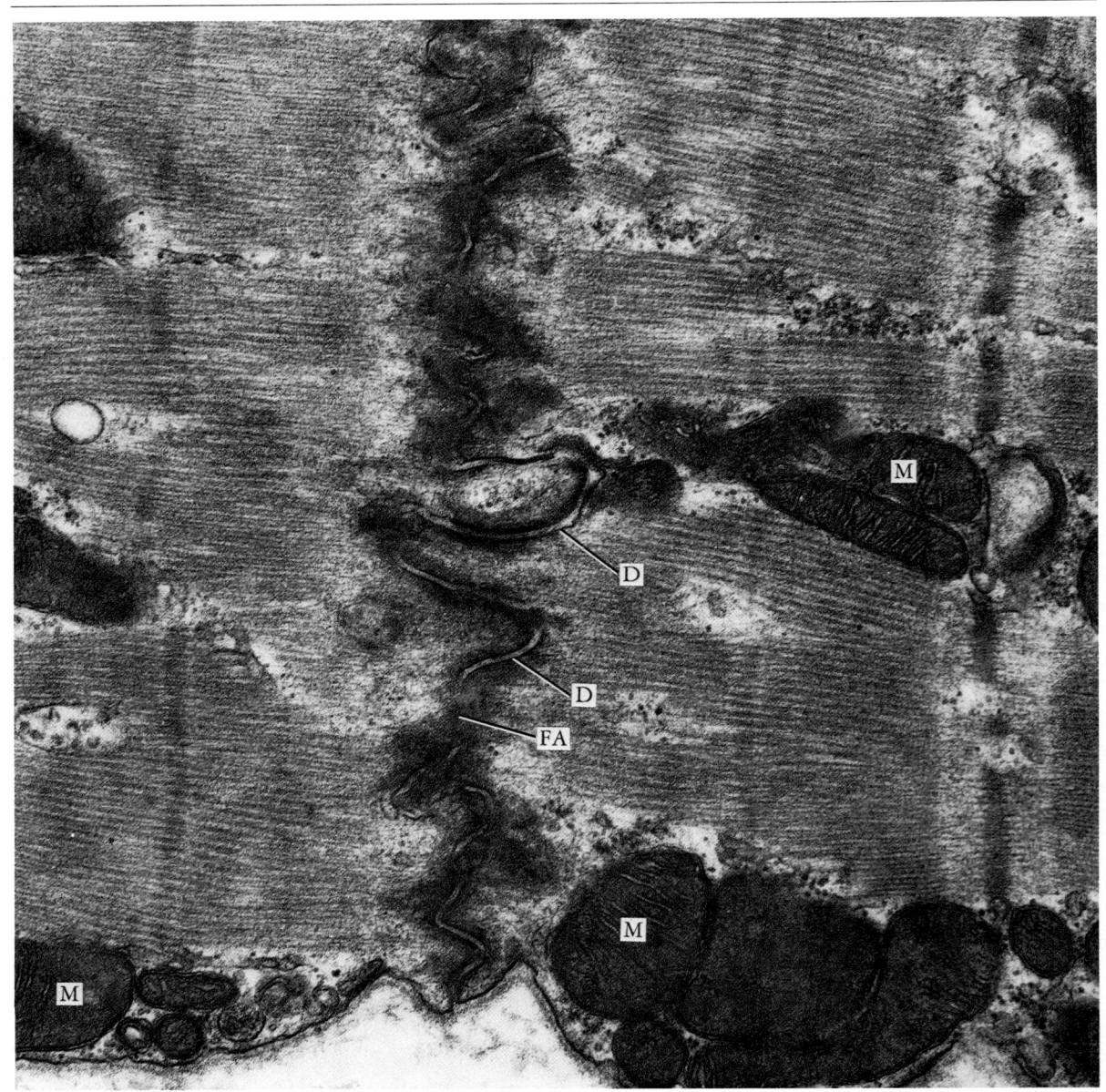

Fig. 6-16. Electron micrograph of longitudinal section of cardiac muscle, showing detailed structure of intercalated disc. Note the presence of desmosomes (D) and fascia adherens (FA). Numerous mitochondria (M) are present between the myofibrils. (×34,627.) (Courtesy of Dr. M. Koering.)

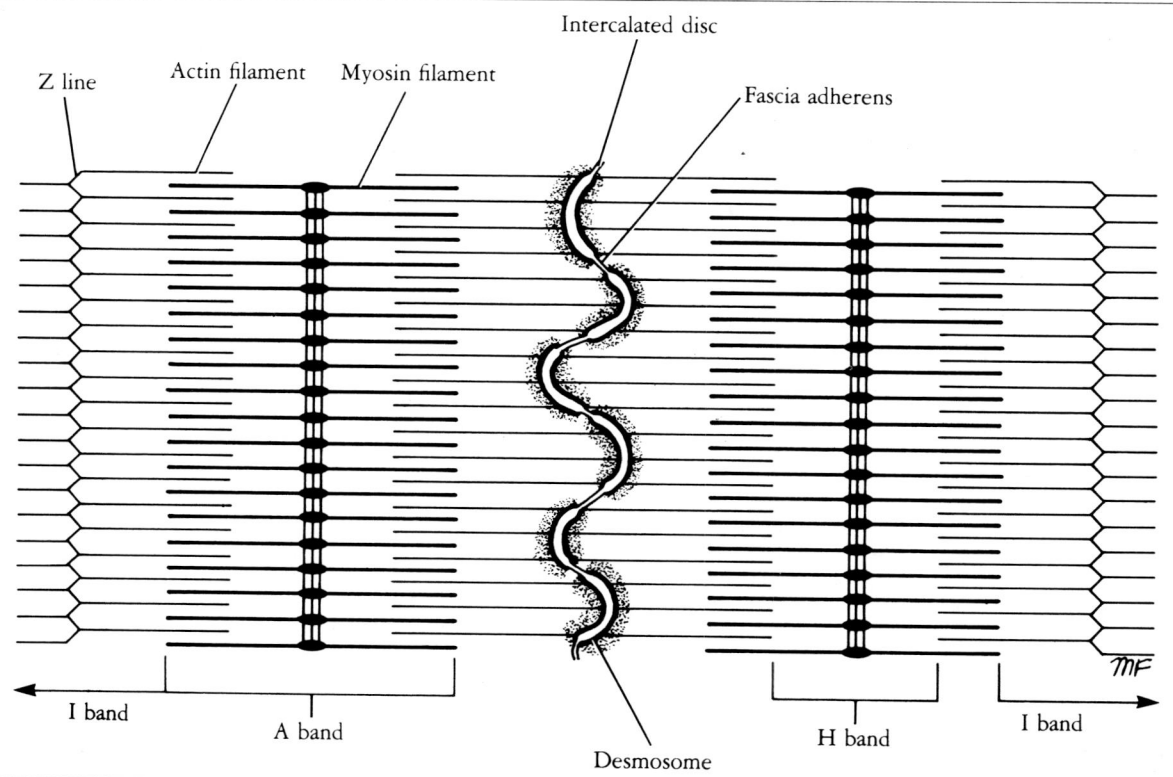

Fig. 6-17. Organization of actin and myosin filaments in a myofibril of cardiac muscle. Note the structure of an intercalated disc.

traction or by passive stretching. These sensory nerves convey information to the central nervous system regarding the degree of tension of the muscles. This information is essential for the maintenance of muscle tone and body posture and for coordinated voluntary movements.

The sympathetic fibers pass to the smooth muscle in the walls of blood vessels supplying the muscle. They serve to regulate the blood flow to the muscles.

Neuromuscular Junctions

As each motor nerve enters a skeletal muscle, it branches many times. A single branch then terminates on a muscle fiber at a site referred to as a *neuromuscular junction* or *motor end-plate* (see Fig. 6-21). The nerve fiber, or axon, now loses its myelin sheath and gives off a number of subsidiary branches. Each branch forms the *neural element* of the motor end-plate. It contains numerous mitochondria and vesicles. At the site of the motor end-plate, the surface of the muscle fiber is slightly raised and forms the *muscular element* of the plate, often known as the *sole plate* (Fig. 6-22). The elevation is caused by the local accumulation of numerous nuclei and mitochondria.

The terminal axon lies in a trough or groove of sarcolemma (see Fig. 6-22). The floor of the groove is formed into numerous folds called *junctional folds*, which serve to increase the surface area of the sarcolemma that lies close to the axon. The plasma membrane of the axon (the *axolemma* or *presynaptic*

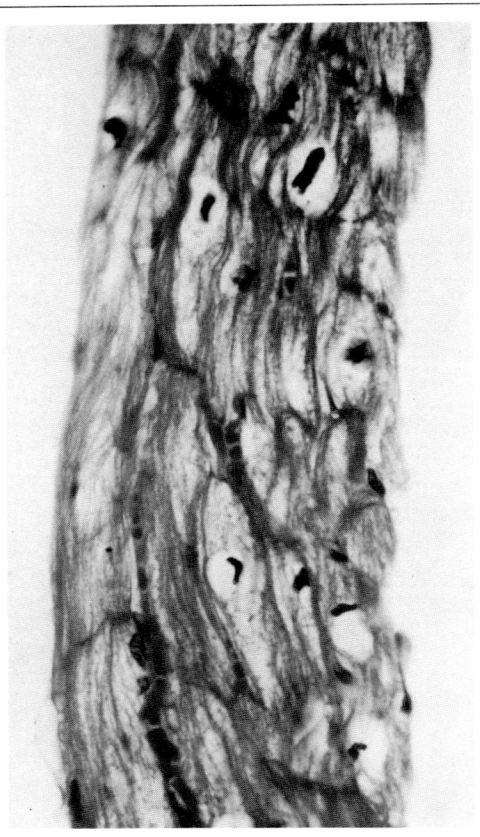

Fig. 6-18. Photomicrograph of section of Purkinje fibers of the heart. Note the peripheral distribution of the myofibrils. The central clear areas are rich in glycogen. (H&E; ×400.)

membrane) is separated from the plasma membrane of the muscle fiber (the sarcolemma or *postsynaptic membrane*) by a space about 20 to 50 nm wide. This space is known as the *synaptic cleft* (see Fig. 6-22). The synaptic cleft, which includes the depressions between adjacent junctional folds, is filled with the basement membranes of the axons and the muscle fiber and is composed largely of glycoprotein (see Fig. 6-22). The motor end-plate is strengthened by the connective tissue sheath of the nerve fiber, the endoneurium, which becomes continuous with the connective tissue sheath of the muscle fiber, the endomysium.

When a nerve impulse reaches a motor end-plate, it causes *acetylcholine* to be released from some of the axonal vesicles (Figs. 6-23 and 6-24). The vesicles discharge their acetylcholine into the synaptic cleft by a process of *exocytosis*. The acetylcholine now affects the sarcolemma (postsynaptic membrane), making it more permeable to sodium ions. By this means, a wave of depolarization passes over the surface of the sarcolemma (see Fig. 6-7) and is carried into the muscle fiber to the contractile myofibrils via the transverse T tubules.

The amount of acetylcholine released at the motor end-plate will depend on the number of nerve impulses arriving at the nerve terminal. Once the acetylcholine crosses the synaptic cleft, it immediately undergoes hydrolysis because of the presence of *acetylcholinesterase* in the sarcolemma. Skeletal muscle fiber contraction is thus controlled by the frequency of the nerve impulses arriving at the motor nerve terminal.

Neuromuscular Spindles

Neuromuscular spindles, or muscular spindles (Fig. 6-25), are found in skeletal muscle and are most numerous toward the tendinous insertion of the muscle. They provide sensory information used by the central nervous system in the control of muscle activity. Each spindle measures about 1 to 4 mm in length and is surrounded by a fusiform capsule of connective tissue. Within the capsule are six to fourteen slender *intrafusal muscle fibers;* the ordinary muscle fibers situated outside the spindles are referred to as *extrafusal fibers*. The intrafusal fibers of the spindles are of two types: the *nuclear bag* and *nuclear chain* fibers. The nuclear bag fibers are distinguished by the presence of numerous nuclei in the equatorial region, which consequently is expanded; also, cross striations are absent in this region. In the nuclear chain fibers, the nuclei form a single longitudinal row in the center of each fiber at the equatorial region. The nuclear bag fibers are larger in diameter than the nuclear chain fibers, and they extend beyond the capsule at each end to attach to the endomysium of the extrafusal fibers.

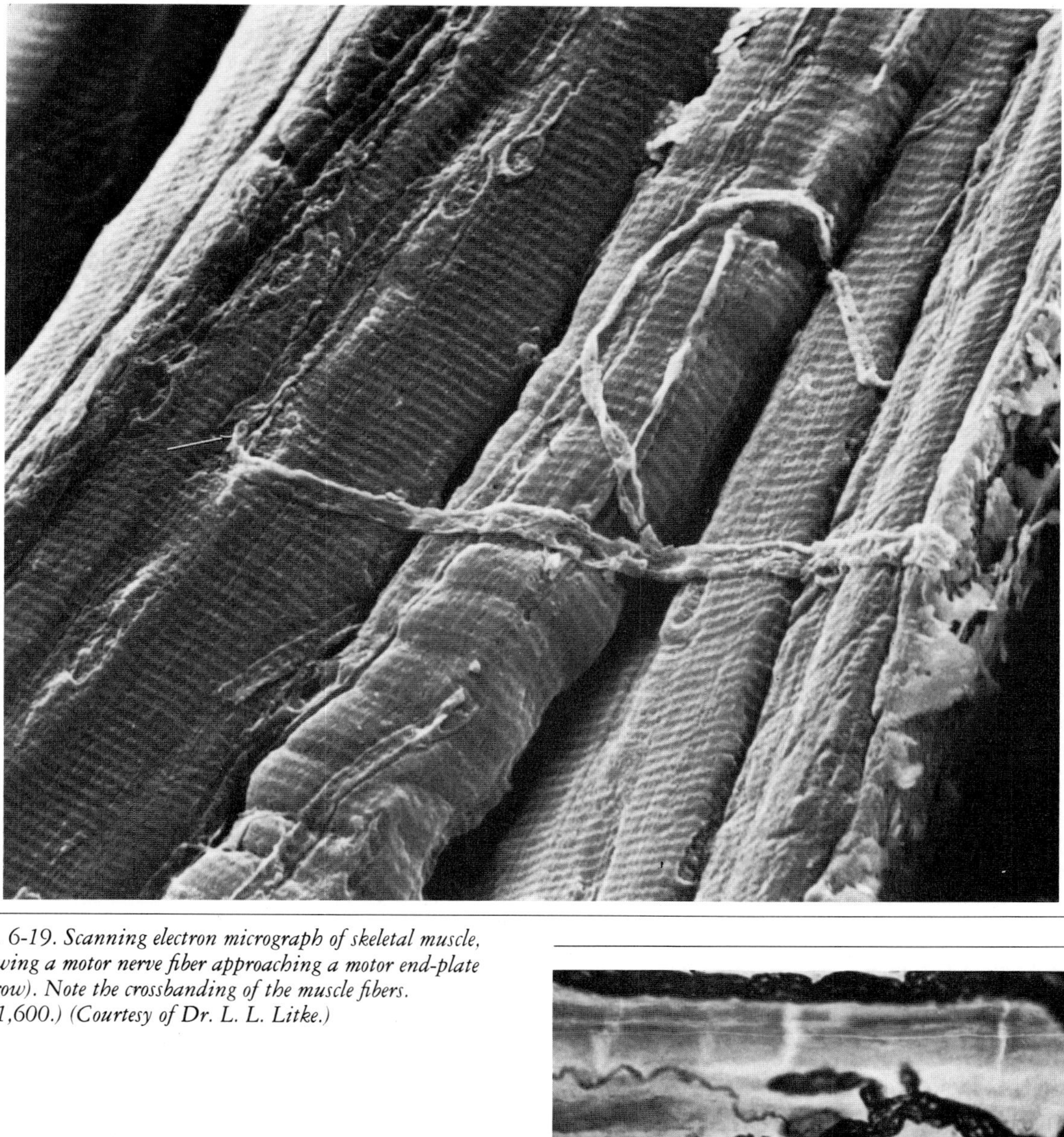

Fig. 6-19. Scanning electron micrograph of skeletal muscle, showing a motor nerve fiber approaching a motor end-plate (arrow). Note the crossbanding of the muscle fibers. (×1,600.) (Courtesy of Dr. L. L. Litke.)

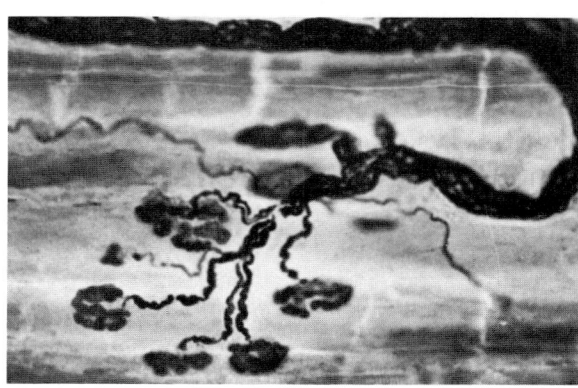

Fig. 6-20. Photomicrograph of preparation of skeletal muscle, showing a motor nerve branching prior to terminating on muscle fibers at motor end-plates. (Courtesy of Dr. M. J. T. Fitzgerald.)

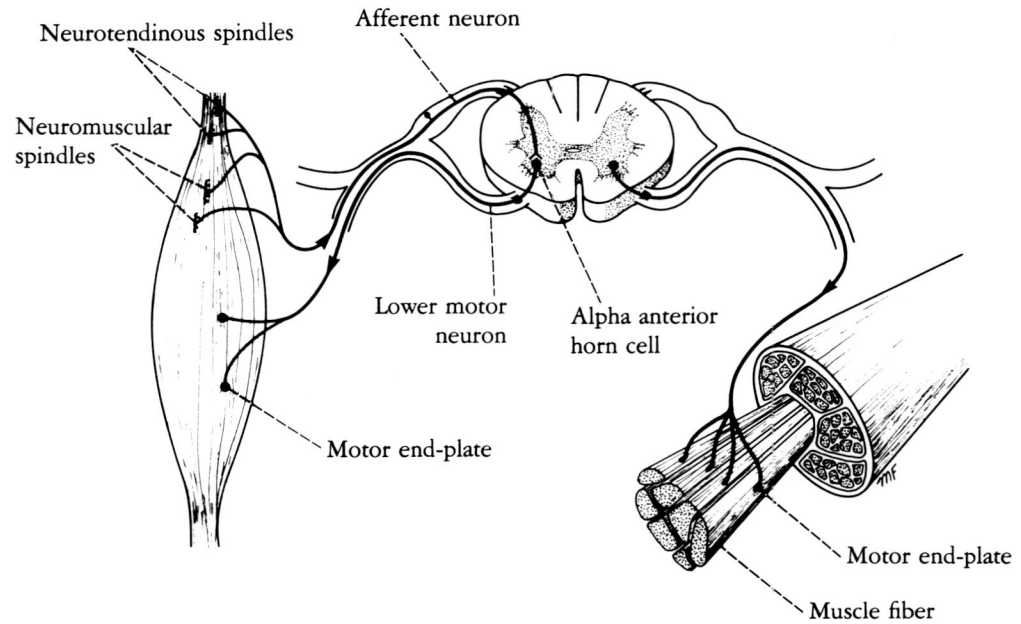

Fig. 6-21. Afferent neuron arising from neuromuscular spindles and neurotendinous spindles, and efferent lower motor neuron whose cell body is an alpha anterior horn cell within the spinal cord. Note that the efferent neuron terminates on a muscle fiber at a motor end-plate. A simple reflex arc, on which muscle tone depends, consists of an afferent and an efferent neuron that synapse together.

There are two types of sensory innervation of muscle spindles: the annulospiral and the flower spray. The *annulospiral endings* are situated at the equator of the intrafusal fibers (Fig. 6-26; see Fig. 6-25). As the large myelinated nerve fiber pierces the capsule, it loses its myelin sheath, and the naked axon winds spirally around the nuclear bag or chain portions of the intrafusal fibers.

The *flower spray endings* are situated mainly on the nuclear chain fibers some distance from the equatorial region. A myelinated nerve fiber slightly smaller than that of the annulospiral ending pierces the capsule and loses its myelin sheath, and the naked axon branches terminally and ends as varicosities.

Stretching of the intrafusal fibers results in stimulation of the annulospiral and flower spray endings, and nerve impulses pass to the spinal cord in the afferent neurons.

Motor innervation of the intrafusal fibers is provided by fine gamma motor fibers.

The neuromuscular spindle plays a very important role in controlling the activities of voluntary muscle. Slight stretching of a muscle results in stretching of the intrafusal fibers; the annulospiral and flower spray endings are stimulated, and impulses reach the spinal cord through the afferent neurons. The large alpha motor neurons in the anterior gray horns of the spinal cord are stimulated, nerve impulses reach the extrafusal fibers that form the main muscle mass, and the muscle contracts. This simple reflex action is based on the integrity of a two-neuron reflex arc involving an afferent neuron and an efferent neuron.

Neurotendinous Spindles

Neurotendinous spindles, or tendon spindles (Fig. 6-27), are most numerous near the junctions of tendons with muscles. They provide the central ner-

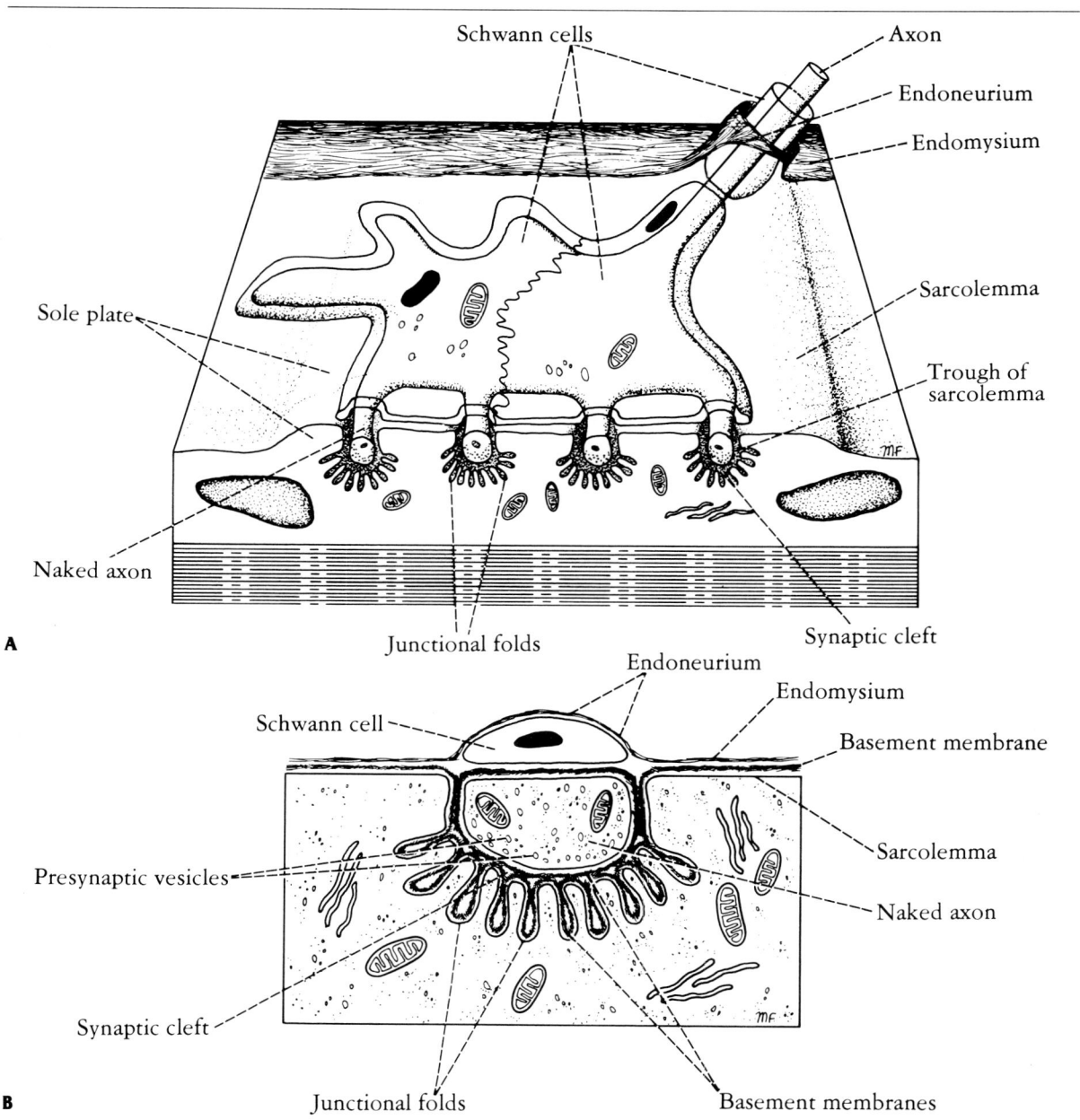

Fig. 6-22. (A) Skeletal neuromuscular junction; (B) enlarged view of a muscle fiber, showing a terminal naked axon lying in a surface groove of a muscle fiber.

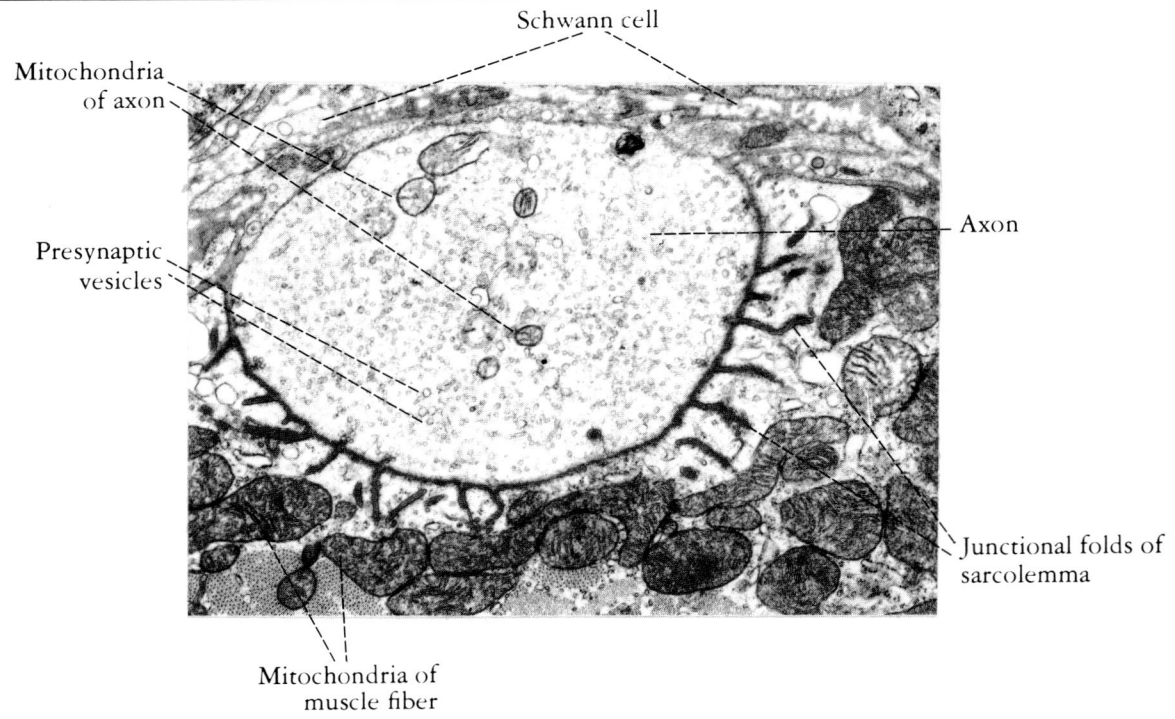

Fig. 6-23. Electron micrograph of cross section of axon at motor end-plate, showing axon lying in a trough of folded sarcolemma. (Courtesy of Dr. J. M. Kerns.)

vous system with information concerning tension within a tendon and are therefore associated with the control of muscle tone. Each spindle consists of a fibrous capsule that contains a small bundle of loosely arranged tendon fibers (intrafusal fibers). The tendon cells are larger and more numerous than those elsewhere in the tendon. One or more myelinated sensory nerve fibers pierce the capsule, lose their myelin sheaths, branch freely, and terminate in club-shaped endings.

Stretching of the tendon results in deformation of the nerve endings by the adjacent tendon fibers within the spindle.

Nerve Supply of Smooth Muscle

In smooth muscle where the action is slow and widespread, such as that within the wall of the intestine, the autonomic nerve fibers branch extensively, so that a single nerve fiber exerts control over a large number of muscle fibers. In some areas, for example, the longitudinal layer of smooth muscle in the intestine, only a few muscle fibers are associated with autonomic endings, and the wave of contraction passes from one muscle cell to another by means of gap junctions (Fig. 6-28).

In smooth muscle where the action is fast and where precision is required, such as occurs in the iris, the branching of the nerve fibers is less extensive, so that a single nerve fiber exerts control over only a few muscle fibers.

The autonomic nerve fibers, which are postganglionic, are nonmyelinated and terminate as a series of varicosed branches. An interval of from 10 to 100 nm may exist between the axon and the muscle fiber. At the site at which transmission is to occur, the Schwann cell is retracted and the axon lies within a shallow groove on its surface (see Fig. 6-

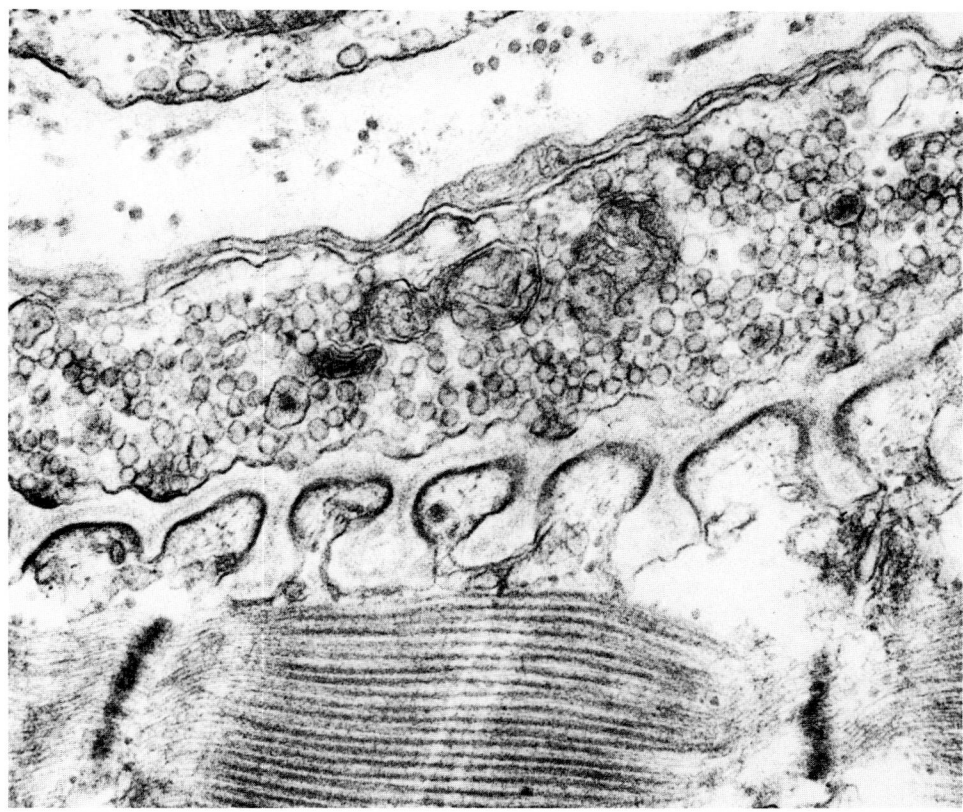

Fig. 6-24. Electron micrograph of a section of axon covered on its outer surface by a Schwann cell (top) and a much-folded sarcolemma (bottom). Note the presence of numerous vesicles within the axon. (×77,000.) (Courtesy of Dr. T. L. Lentz.)

28). Part of the axon thus is naked, permitting free diffusion of the transmitter substance from the axon to the muscle cell (see Fig. 6-28). Here the axoplasm contains numerous vesicles similar to those seen at the motor end-plates of skeletal muscle.

Smooth muscle is innervated by sympathetic and parasympathetic parts of the autonomic system. Those nerves that are cholinergic liberate acetylcholine at their endings by a process of exocytosis, the acetylcholine being present in the vesicles at the nerve ending. Those nerves that are noradrenergic liberate norepinephrine at their endings by a process of exocytosis. Both the acetylcholine and the norepinephrine bring about depolarization of the muscle fibers innervated, which then contract. The fate of these neurotransmitter substances differs. The acetylcholine is probably hydrolyzed in the presence of acetylcholinesterase in the sarcolemma of the muscle fiber. Experimental data of the past few years suggest that norepinephrine is taken up again by the nerve endings. In some areas of the body (such as bronchial muscle), the norepinephrine liberated from postganglionic sympathetic fibers causes smooth muscle to relax rather than to contract.

Cardiac Muscle

Nonmyelinated postganglionic autonomic nerves extend into the connective tissue between the ordinary cardiac muscle fibers and the specialized muscle fibers of the sino-atrial and atrioventricular

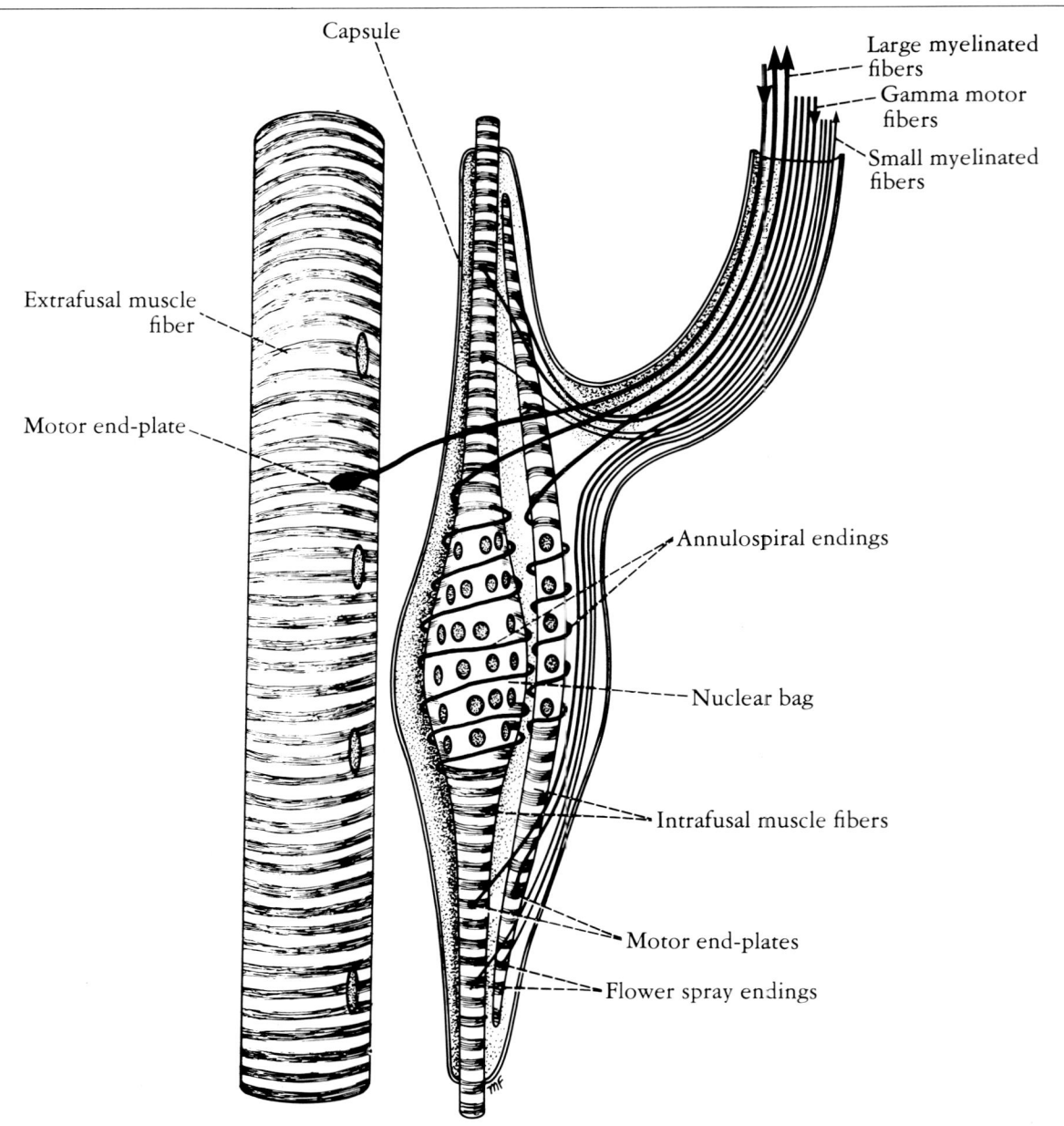

Fig. 6-25. Neuromuscular spindle. Two types of intrafusal fibers are visible: the nuclear bag and nuclear chain fibers.

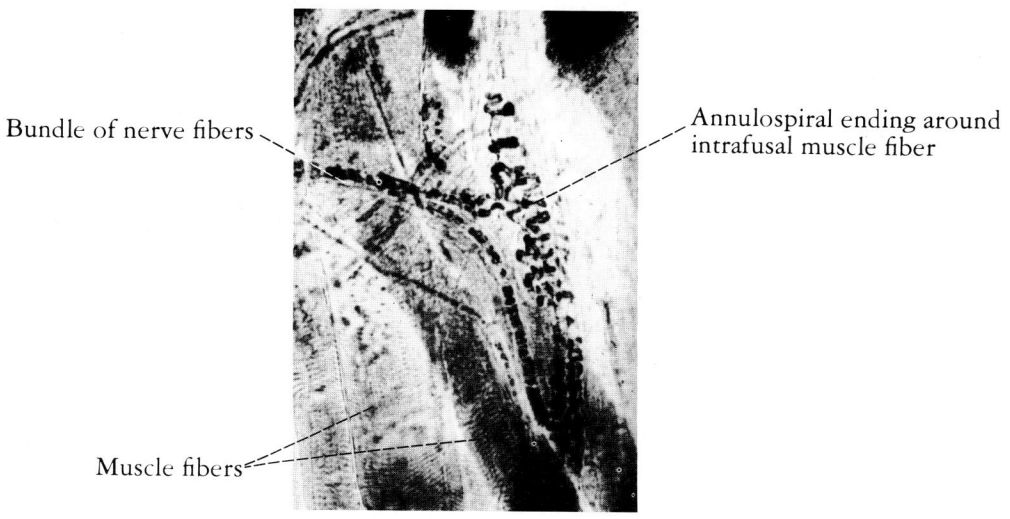

Fig. 6-26. Photomicrograph of a neuromuscular spindle. (Silver nitrate stain.)

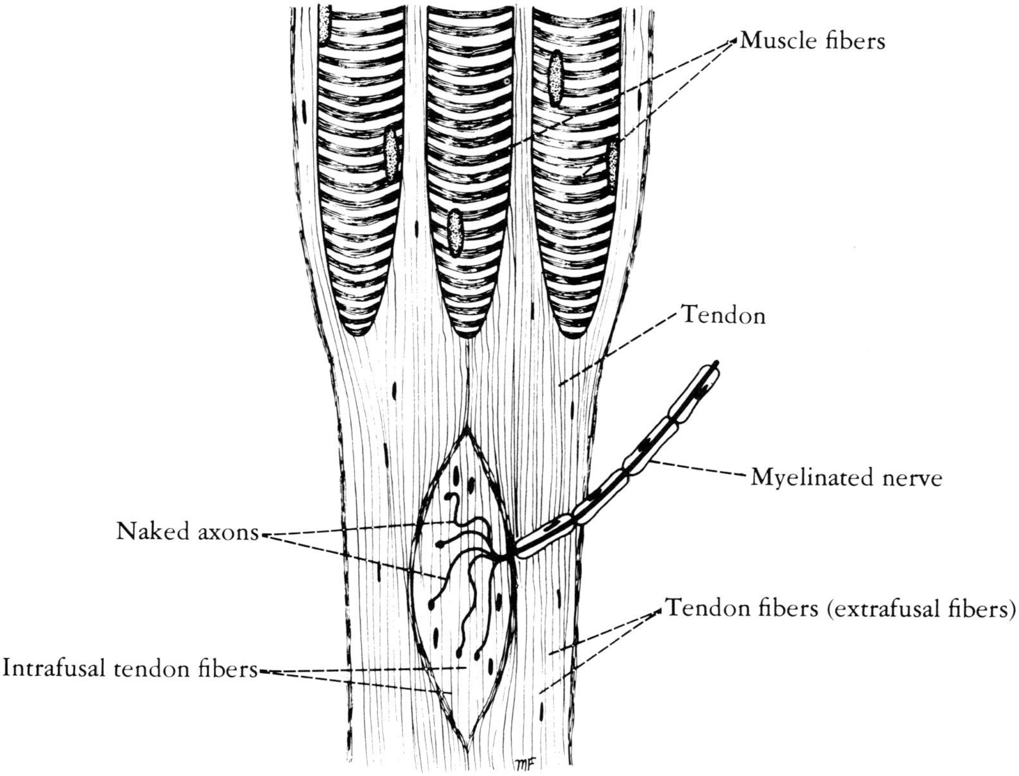

Fig. 6-27. Neurotendinous spindle.

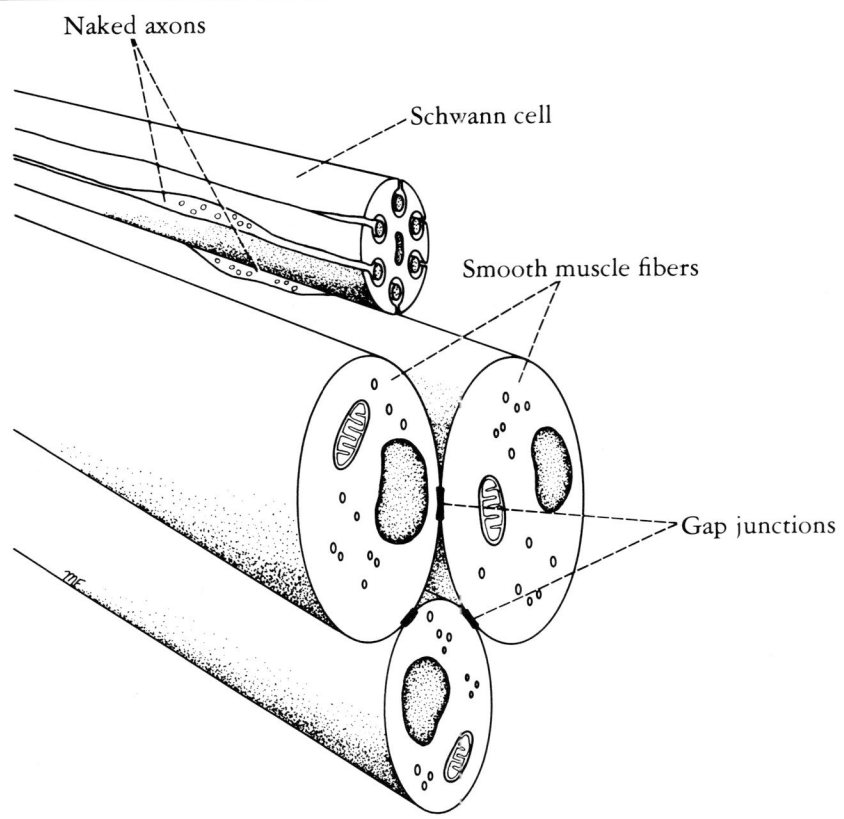

Fig. 6-28. Autonomic neuromuscular junction. Note the exposed axons close to the smooth muscle fibers.

nodes. They terminate close to the individual muscle fibers. Because of the gap junctions between abutting muscle fibers, excitation and contraction of one muscle fiber rapidly spreads to other fibers.

As is the case with smooth muscle, the axon at the site at which transmission is to occur rises to the surface of the Schwann cell and lies within a shallow groove. Part of the axon thus is naked, and free diffusion of the neurotransmitter substance from the axon to the muscle cell can occur.

MUSCLE CONTRACTION

Chemistry

In skeletal muscle, the nerve impulse on reaching the motor end-plate excites the sarcolemma (muscle plasma membrane). The action potential spreads along the sarcolemma and passes into the muscle cell via the tubular indentations, the T tubules (see Fig. 6-7). The sarcoplasmic reticulum in response releases calcium ions, which combine with the proteins *troponin* and *tropomyosin,* which are part of the actin filament. Bridge formation occurs between actin and myosin, and contraction takes place (see Fig. 6-7). Once the stimulus has ceased, the calcium ions are withdrawn from the sarcoplasmic matrix back into the sarcoplasmic reticulum, and the muscle begins to relax. Thus, the state of relaxation is thought to be caused by the troponin and tropomyosin, which are now free from the calcium ions and prevent the actin from interacting with myosin filaments. Troponin and tropomyosin are often referred to as the *regulator proteins* of muscle.

In smooth muscle and cardiac muscle, the chemistry of the contractile process is very similar to that in skeletal muscle. As noted previously, smooth muscle cells contain actin and myosin molecules, but they are not organized in the same way as in skeletal muscle or cardiac muscle.

Source of Energy

When a muscle contracts and work is performed, large amounts of ATP (adenosine triphosphate) are broken down by ATPase into adenosine diphosphate (ADP), with the liberation of energy. Additional energy is provided by the breakdown of phosphocreatine. The energy so produced in some way causes the actin filaments to move over the myosin filaments, so that the sarcomere length decreases. The whole chemical process is initiated by the spread of the action potential over the surface of the muscle cell and the release of calcium ions from the sarcoplasmic reticulum. After the muscle contraction is completed, the oxidation of glycogen provides energy for the resynthesis of phosphocreatine and ATP.

ACTION POTENTIAL OF MUSCLE

Skeletal Muscle

Skeletal muscle fibers are excited by the arrival of a nervous stimulus at the neuromuscular junction (motor end-plate). The neurotransmitter acetylcholine is released from the nerve ending and serves as a stimulus to the sarcolemma (plasma membrane) of the muscle fiber. The rapid depolarization of the sarcolemma creates a local reversed potential, called here the *end-plate potential*. If the end-plate potential is great enough, it will excite a spreading action potential in the surrounding sarcolemma of the muscle fiber.

As the action potential spreads over the surface of the muscle fibers, it enters the T tubules (see Fig. 6-7), causing depolarization to spread into the interior of the muscle fiber. Here the excitation activates the contractile process between the actin and myosin filaments. In some unknown way, the depolarization of the T tubules causes a release of calcium ions from the endoplasmic reticulum (see Fig. 6-7). The calcium now joins with the troponin and tropomyosin myofibrils, as discussed on page 218.

Smooth Muscle

Smooth muscle fibers have membrane potentials and action potentials and can be depolarized and repolarized in a manner similar to that of skeletal muscle fibers. They do not have a well-developed sarcoplasmic reticulum, however, and they lack a T tubule system.

Smooth muscle cells can be stimulated by autonomic nerve fibers or by hormones. Some smooth muscle cells, those closely packed together to form a single unit, undergo spontaneous rhythmic contractions and are not stimulated by nerves or hormones. In these cells, spontaneous depolarization of the plasma membranes occurs at regular intervals. The activities of separate single-unit cells in a group can be coordinated by gap junctions between adjacent cells that permit the active membrane potential to pass from cell to cell. One smooth muscle cell in a group becomes a kind of pacemaker and sets the pace; all the other cells follow in unison.

The contractile process in smooth muscle is similar to that in skeletal muscle but is much slower. The process of relaxation is prolonged and is also much slower than in skeletal muscle.

Cardiac Muscle

Cardiac muscle fibers have a well-developed sarcoplasmic reticulum and a T tubule system. Cardiac muscle fibers closely resemble single-unit smooth muscle fibers in that they can initiate spontaneous rhythmic contractions. There are also cell junctions between adjacent fibers that permit the muscle mass to contract as a whole.

The action potentials of the muscle fibers forming the conducting system of the heart and the myocardium of the ventricles possess a longer phase of depolarization (0.3 seconds) than do those cells that form the myocardium of the atrium (0.15 second). This means that the ventricles have adequate time to fill: the fibers will not contract during the refractory period, that is, while the cell membranes are depolarized.

CLINICAL NOTES

SKELETAL MUSCLE

Muscle Tone

Skeletal muscle tone, which can be appreciated by the recognition of a rubbery firmness of a muscle when it is palpated, is caused by the constant full contraction of a few muscle fibers within a muscle. To avoid fatigue, different groups of muscle fibers within a muscle are brought into action at different times. The muscle fibers contract in response to the asynchronous discharge of nervous impulses from the motor anterior gray column (horn) cells of the spinal cord or the motor nerve cells of the cranial nerve nuclei. Muscle tone is reflexly controlled from afferent nerve endings, the neuromuscular and neurotendinous spindles. It follows that any disease process that interferes with any part of the reflex arc will abolish the muscle tone; the muscle will be noncontractile and will feel doughlike on palpation. For example, syphilitic infection of the posterior root (tabes dorsales), destruction of the motor anterior gray column cells (as in poliomyelitis or syringomyelia), destruction of a segment of the spinal cord by trauma or pressure from a tumor, section of an anterior or posterior root of a spinal nerve, pressure on a spinal nerve by a prolapsed intervertebral disc, and section of a peripheral nerve (as in a stab wound) will all result in loss of muscle tone.

Although it has been emphasized that the basic mechanism underlying muscle tone is the integrity of a reflex arc, it must not be forgotten that this reflex activity is influenced by nervous impulses received by the motor nerve cells from all levels of the brain and spinal cord. Spinal shock, which follows injury to the spinal cord, will result in diminished muscle tone: the cerebellum facilitates the stretch reflex and in spinal shock is cut off from the spinal cord. The reticular formation normally increases muscle tone, but its activity is inhibited by higher cerebral centers. Therefore, if the higher cerebral control is interfered with by trauma or disease, the inhibition is lost and the muscle tone is exaggerated (*decerebrate rigidity*).

Motor Unit

A single motor unit of skeletal muscle consists of a motor nerve cell in the anterior gray column of the spinal cord (or its equivalent cell in a motor nucleus of a cranial nerve), its axon within a peripheral nerve, the myoneural junctions, and the muscle fibers supplied by the single motor nerve cell. In a large buttock muscle, such as the gluteus maximus, where fine control is unnecessary, a given motor neuron may supply as many as two hundred muscle fibers. In contrast, in the small muscles of the hand or the extrinsic muscles of the eyeball, where fine control is required, one nerve fiber supplies only a few muscle fibers. It follows that disease or injury to any part of a motor unit will affect the activity of the muscle concerned.

Muscle Fatigue

Muscle fatigue occurs after prolonged forceful contraction of a muscle. The motor nerve continues to function normally, the neuromuscular junction functions normally, and the muscle fibers show normal depolarization. The available ATP has been used up within the muscle fibers, however, and as a result, the contractions become weaker.

Muscle Atrophy

Muscle atrophy can result from a variety of conditions. These include disease of the motor nerve cell (e.g., poliomyelitis), section or disease of the peripheral nerve (e.g., polyneuritis), disorders of the myoneural junction (e.g., myasthenia gravis), and disease of the muscle itself (e.g., muscular dystrophy).

Muscle atrophy can also follow prolonged immobilization of joints, as occurs in the treatment of a fracture (e.g., atrophy of the quadriceps muscle, which occurs in knee joint immobilization). Atrophy of muscles occurs in the aged, in whom it is probably caused by diminished activity, chronic illness, and a diminished blood supply.

Microscopically, the nuclei become hyperchromatic and tend to assume a more central position within the muscle fibers. The muscle fibers become reduced in diameter, and there is a reduction in the mass of the myofibrils. The mitochondria start to break up and disappear. At first, the cross striations persist, but they later disappear as well. The amount of connective tissue in the endomysium and perimysium increases. Later still, the muscle fibers break up and the debris is phagocytosed by tissue macrophages. The muscle shrinks in size and becomes flabby.

Muscle Hypertrophy

Repeated exercise of muscles by athletes or those who "pump iron" results in the muscles' becoming stronger and larger. This development is caused by an increased number of myofibrils in each muscle fiber and is called *hypertrophy*. Once the training ceases and the workload diminishes, the muscles become smaller.

Muscle Regeneration

Destruction of a muscle fiber that includes its nuclei leads to a total breakdown of the fiber, which largely is replaced by proliferation of the connective tissue of the endomysium and perimysium. Should the nuclei survive, new sarcoplasm is formed and myofibrils reappear. In some situations, surviving sarcomeres send out buds in an attempt to re-form the fibers.

Effects of Neuromuscular Blocking Agents on Skeletal Muscle

D-Tubocurarine produces flaccid paralysis of skeletal muscle, affecting the extrinsic muscles of the eyeball first and then those of the face, the extremities, and, finally, the diaphragm.

This drug combines with the receptor sites at the sarcolemma normally used by acetylcholine and thus blocks the neurotransmitter action of acetylcholine. As the drug slowly is metabolized, the paralysis passes off. This drug is commonly used with light general anesthesia for abdominal surgery, when it is important to relax the abdominal muscles without depressing the vital centers of the central nervous system with deep general anesthesia.

Dimethyl tubocurarine, gallamine (Flaxedil), and *benzoquinonium* have similar effects.

Disease

Myasthenia Gravis

Myasthenia gravis is a disease characterized by drooping of the upper eyelids (ptosis), double vision (diplopia), difficulty in swallowing (dysphagia), difficulty in talking (dysarthria), and general muscular weakness and fatigue. The disease is caused by some abnormality at the neuromuscular junction. The following explanations have been suggested: (1) the muscle plasma membrane at the neuromuscular junction is less sensitive than normal to acetylcholine; (2) the amount of acetylcholine released from the motor nerve is less than normal; and (3) the condition is an example of an auto-immune disease, in which antibodies affect proteins in the neuromuscular junction, producing a curarelike blocking effect.

The condition is relieved by anticholinesterase drugs, such as *neostigmine*, that potentiate the action of acetylcholine.

Escape of Muscle Enzymes into the Blood during Muscle Disease

Skeletal muscle fiber sarcoplasm contains *creatine phosphokinase* and *aldolase*, and these escape into the bloodstream as the fibers are destroyed in muscle disease. Their levels are raised in, for example, muscular dystrophy, polymyositis, and traumatic injury to muscles. The same enzymes escape from cardiac muscle fibers in acute myocardial infarction.

Rigor Mortis

Following death, as a result of chemical changes in skeletal muscle, the muscle fibers of the body enter into sustained contraction. The process starts in the muscles of the face and then spreads to muscles of the trunk and the limbs. The contracture may last for several days, until the muscle fibers are destroyed by enzymes liberated from intracellular lysosomes.

SMOOTH MUSCLE

Hypertrophy and Hyperplasia

During pregnancy, in response to the increased production of estrogen, the smooth muscle cells of the uterus increase in size and undergo mitotic division in preparation for the expulsion of the fetus at the termination of the pregnancy. In pathological conditions, such as chronic obstruction of the intestinal or urinary tract, the smooth muscle in the intestinal or bladder walls undergoes hypertrophy and hyperplasia. A similar hypertrophy and hyperplasia of smooth muscle may occur in the walls of arterioles in patients with high blood pressure (hypertension) and in the walls of bronchi in patients with asthma.

Role of Smooth Muscle Fibers in Atherosclerosis

The smooth muscle fibers of the tunica media become distended with cholesterol in atherosclerosis. The cells form a plaque that protrudes into the lumen of the artery. The plaques enlarge as a result of the hypertrophy and hyperplasia of the smooth muscle cells that become filled with cholesterol. This overgrowth of smooth muscle tends to occur where an artery branches or bends sharply. It is at these sites that the arterial wall is subjected to the turbulent flow of blood and suffers from wear and tear. The plaques make the arterial wall rigid, so that it cannot dilate or contract in response to changing blood requirements. The plaque also roughens the tunica intima, so that blood may clot on its surface. The rigidity and narrowness of the artery may cause damage to or death of the tissue that it supplies with blood.

Regeneration of Smooth Muscle

Smooth muscle fibers show only a minimal ability to regenerate when injured. Dead smooth muscle fibers are usually replaced by connective tissue.

Ileus of the Gastrointestinal Tract

Ileus is a condition in which peristalsis ceases in the gastrointestinal tract; that is, the smooth muscle ceases to contract normally. *Adynamic ileus* is common and follows all abdominal operations. Essentially, it is caused by excessive sympathetic activity that inhibits the activity of the smooth muscle fibers. Function usually returns spontaneously in a few days.

Spastic ileus is caused by excessive uncoordinated contraction of the smooth muscle and occurs in heavy metal poisoning and uremia.

CARDIAC MUSCLE

Hypertrophy

When the workload of cardiac muscle is increased, the muscle fibers enlarge, but they do not increase in number. Such hypertrophy is commonly seen in systemic hypertension, when an increased force of left ventricular contraction is necessary to overcome the high blood pressure in the aorta. Similarly, right ventricular hypertrophy occurs in pulmonary hypertension.

Cardiac Muscle Ischemia

Ischemia occurs when the heart muscle receives an insufficient supply of oxygenated blood; the most common cause is atherosclerosis of the coronary arteries. In coronary occlusion, the glycogen content of the muscle fibers diminishes and muscle enzymes, such as creatinine phosphokinase, lactic dehydrogenase, and glutamic oxalacetic transaminase, escape from the fibers and increase in concentration in the blood serum. Laboratory tests can detect these changes in the serum enzymes and may assist in confirming the diagnosis of ischemic heart disease. The contractile ability of the muscle is reduced, and the irritability may be increased, often resulting in abnormal ventricular contractions and, in some cases, ventricular fibrillation.

Histologically, the regular arrangement of the myofibrils becomes lost. Later, the muscle fibers undergo degeneration and the area is invaded by leukocytes. The remains of the dead cardiac muscle fibers are phagocytosed by macrophages and are replaced by fibrous tissue laid down by proliferating fibroblasts.

When coronary occlusion affects the specialized

cardiac muscle found in the conducting system of the heart, the possible results range from the appearance of arrhythmias to complete heart block when the ventricles start to beat independently of the atria.

CLINICAL PROBLEMS

For the answers to these problems, see page 790.

1. During the closure of an abdominal wound, a surgeon approximates the cut edges of the muscle belly by inserting a series of interrupted sutures. He asks the student who is assisting him if he thinks that the sutures will tear through the delicate muscle cells when the patient coughs or strains postoperatively. He also asks if muscles possess tissue in addition to muscle fibers within their substance. How would you answer those questions?

2. A professor of histology states that all types of muscle, when appropriately stained, can be seen under the light microscope to possess longitudinal striations. If that is so, why are skeletal and cardiac muscles often called striated muscles, whereas the muscle found in the wall of the uterus or intestinal tract is referred to as smooth muscle?

3. Define muscle tone in skeletal muscle. Explain the basic physiological processes involved in the maintenance of muscle tone. Name three clinical conditions that can result in a loss of skeletal muscle tone.

4. What is meant by the terms *motor unit* and *motor end-plate?* Explain how a nervous impulse arriving at a motor end-plate can bring about the depolarization of the cell membrane of a muscle fiber. What is the name of the enzyme present at the motor end-plate that limits the stimulating process, and where is it located?

5. A 19-year-old student arrives at the university late for his lecture. Because the elevator is out of order, he is forced to run up six flights of stairs. On reaching the fourth floor, the student, who is in good physical condition, is forced to rest, because his leg muscles feel weak and he is out of breath. Explain why this healthy young adult is experiencing muscle weakness and breathlessness.

6. A 21-year-old man is concerned about his physical appearance. He decides to join the local gym and lift weights. After 3 months of training, he notices that his pectoralis major and biceps brachii muscles in both upper limbs have increased greatly in size. Using your knowledge of anatomy and physiology, explain the increase in the size of the muscles.

7. Define the following: (a) A band, (b) Z line, (c) sarcoplasmic reticulum, (d) T tubule, (e) white muscle fibers, (f) intercalated disc, (g) Purkinje fibers.

8. What are the essential functional and morphological differences between general cardiac muscle and that found in the conducting system of the heart?

9. Discuss the chemistry of muscle contraction. What is the source of energy for muscle contraction?

10. Describe the morphological changes that take place in skeletal muscle fibers when they undergo atrophy. Give clinical examples of skeletal muscle atrophy.

11. Give three examples of hypertrophy and hyperplasia of smooth muscle. What possible part can smooth muscle cells play in the development of atherosclerosis?

12. A 45-year-old man is found dead, with a bullet wound in his right temple. A revolver is tightly clenched in his right hand. The police decide that the man has committed suicide. The medical examiner has difficulty removing the gun from the victim's hand. Can you explain this difficulty? If the victim had been found 5 days later, would the same difficulty exist?

13. When the blood supply to cardiac muscle is cut off, as in coronary thrombosis, and the muscle fibers die, do they regenerate? If the fibers do not regenerate, what replaces the muscle?

14. How do autonomic nerve fibers terminate on smooth and cardiac muscle? What supplies the nervous control of the cardiac muscle in a heart that has been transplanted?

ADDITIONAL READING

Ashton, F. T., Somlyo, A. V., and Somlyo, A. P. The contractile apparatus of vascular smooth muscle: Intermediate high voltage stereo electron microscopy. *J. Mol. Biol.* 98:17, 1975.

Bourne, G. H. (ed.). *The Structure and Function of Muscle.* New York: Academic, 1972.

Buller, A. J. The physiology of skeletal muscle. In *MTP International Review of Science: Physiology.* Vol. 3. Baltimore, Md.: Baltimore University Park Press, 1975, p. 279.

Butler, R. A new grouping of intrafusal muscle fibers based on developmental studies of muscle spindles in the cat. *Am. J. Anat.* 156:115, 1979.

Challice, C. E., and Viragh, S. (eds.). *Ultrastructure of the Mammalian Heart.* New York: Academic, 1973.

Curtin, N. A., and Woledge, R. C. Energy changes in muscular contraction. *Physiol. Rev.* 58:690, 1978.

Daniel, E. E., and Sarna, S. The generation and conduction of activity in smooth muscle. *Annu. Rev. Pharmacol. Toxicol.* 18:145, 1978.

Devine, C. E., Somlyo, A. V., and Somlyo, A. P. Sarcoplasmic reticulum and mitochondria as calcium accumulation sites in smooth muscle. *Philos. Trans. R. Soc. Lond. {Biol.}* 265:17, 1973.

Drachman, D. B. Myasthenia gravis. *N. Engl. J. Med.* 298:136, 186, 1978.

Ebashi, S. Regulatory mechanism of muscle contraction with special reference to the Ca-troponin-tropomyosin system. *Essays Biochem.* 10:1, 1974.

Endo, M. Calcium release from the sarcoplasmic reticulum. *Physiol. Rev.* 57:71, 1977.

Forssmann, W. G., and Girardier, L. A study of the T system in rat heart. *J. Cell Biol.* 44:1, 1970.

Franzini-Armstrong, C. The structure of a simple Z line. *J. Cell Biol.* 58:630, 1973.

Gabella, G. I. Cellular structures and electrophysiological behavior: Fine structure of smooth muscle. *Philos. Trans. R. Soc. Lond. {Biol.}* 265:7, 1973.

Gabella, G. I., and Blundell, D. Nexuses between smooth muscle cells of the guinea-pig ileum. *J. Cell Biol.* 82:239, 1979.

Hughes, J. T. *Pathology of Muscle.* Philadelphia: Saunders, 1975.

Huxley, H. E. The contractile structure of cardiac and skeletal muscle. *Circulation* 24:328, 1961.

Huxley, H. E. The mechanism of muscular contraction. *Sci. Am.* 213(6):18, 1965.

Jones, P. A., Scott-Burden, T., and Gevers, W. Glycoprotein, elastin and collagen secretion by rat smooth muscle cells. *Proc. Natl. Acad. Sci. U.S.A.* 76:353, 1979.

Kaldor, G., and DiBattista, W. J. (eds.). *Aging in Muscle.* New York: Raven, 1978.

Mark, R. F. Synaptic repression at neuromuscular junctions. *Physiol. Rev.* 60:355, 1980.

Mauro, A., and Bischoff, R. (eds.). *Muscle Regeneration.* New York: Raven, 1979.

Nobel, D. *The Initiation of the Heartbeat.* New York: Oxford University Press, 1979.

Rayns, D. G. Myofilaments and cross bridges as demonstrated by freeze-fracturing and etching. *J. Ultrastruct. Res.* 40:103, 1972.

Schoenberg, G. F., and Needham, D. M. A study of the mechanism of contraction in vertebrate smooth muscle. *Biol. Rev.* 51:53, 1976.

Small, J. V. Studies on isolated smooth muscle cells: The contractile apparatus. *J. Cell Sci.* 24:327, 1977.

Somlyo, A. V. Bridging structures spanning the junctional gap at the triad of skeletal muscle. *J. Cell Biol.* 80:743, 1979.

Sommer, J. R., and Johnson, E. A. Cardiac muscle: A comparative study of Purkinje fibers and ventricular fibers. *J. Cell Biol.* 36:497, 1968.

Sommer, J. R., and Waugh, R. A. The ultrastructure of the mammalian cardiac muscle cell—with special emphasis on the tubular membrane systems. *Am. J. Pathol.* 82:192, 1976.

Tregear, R. T., and Marston, S. B. The cross-bridge theory. *Annu. Rev. Physiol.* 41:723, 1979.

Zubrzycha, E., and MacLennan, D. H. Assembly of the sarcoplasmic reticulum. *J. Biol. Chem.* 251:7733, 1977.

NERVE TISSUE 7

The nervous system is divided into two main parts, the *central nervous system*, consisting of the brain and spinal cord, and the *peripheral nervous system*, consisting of the cranial and spinal nerves and their associated ganglia. An important subdivision of the nervous system is the *autonomic nervous system*, which innervates involuntary structures, such as the heart, smooth muscle, and glands, throughout the body. The autonomic system is distributed throughout the central and peripheral nervous systems and consists of *sympathetic* and *parasympathetic* parts; in both, there are afferent and efferent nerve fibers.

STRUCTURE OF NERVE TISSUE

The basic units of the nevous system are the nerve cells. These cells are specialized to conduct nerve impulses over considerable distances at very great speeds. The *neuron* is the name given to the nerve cell and all its processes (Figs. 7-1 and 7-2). The long processes of a nerve cell are called *axons*, or *nerve fibers*; the short processes are *dendrites*.

The central nervous system is composed of large numbers of neurons supported by specialized tissue called *neuroglia*. The interior of the central nervous system is organized into *gray* and *white matter*. Gray matter consists of nerve cells and the proximal portions of their processes embedded in neuroglia. White matter consists of nerve fibers embedded in neuroglia.

The cranial and spinal nerves of the peripheral nervous system are grayish-white cords. They are made up of bundles of nerve fibers supported by delicate areolar tissue.

STAINING OF NERVE TISSUE

Before considering the detailed structure of nerve tissue, the student must be aware of the difficulties in staining nerve tissue for light microscopic examination.

The staining of nerve tissue with H&E is disappointing and shows very little structural detail. A variety of special neurological stains must be used for this purpose. For example, the Golgi and Cajal silver impregnation methods will reveal the cell body and its neurites. Cresyl violet will stain nuclei and Nissl granules. The myelin sheath of central and peripheral nerves can be stained with hematoxylin after mordanting with potassium bichromate. Osmium tetroxide also will stain myelin black when used with potassium bichromate. Methylene blue is

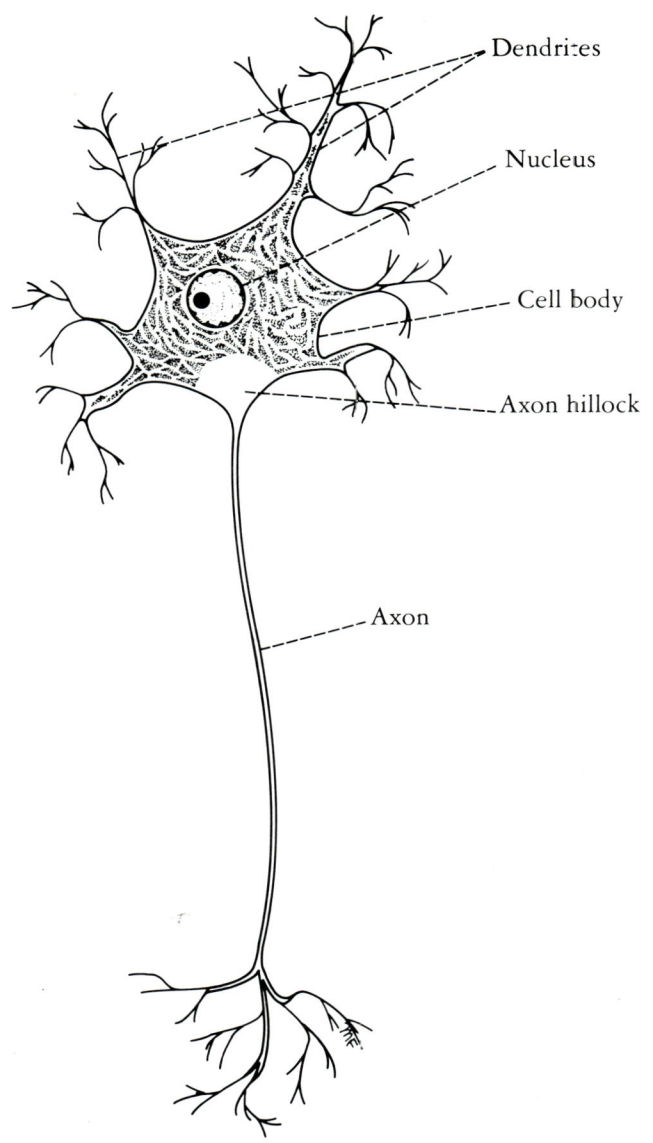

Fig. 7-1. *Neuron.*

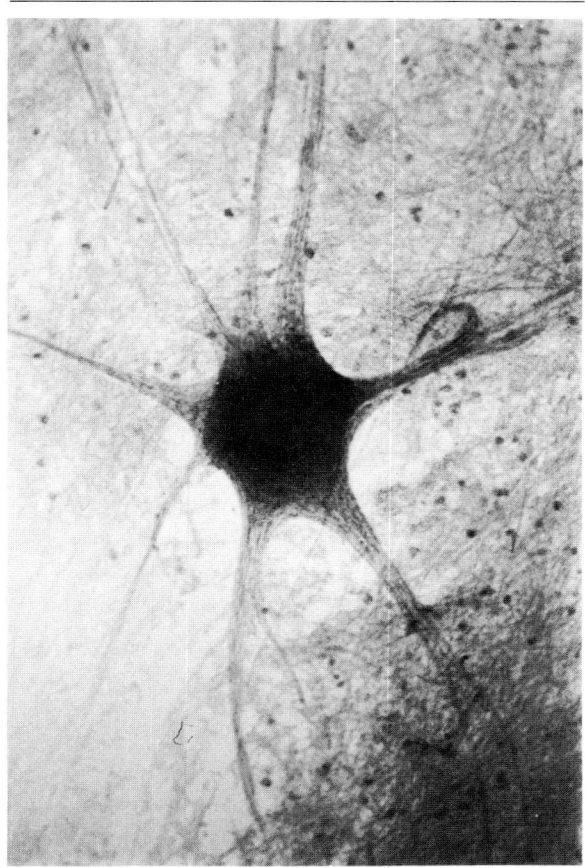

Fig. 7-2. Photomicrograph of a smear preparation of the spinal cord, showing a neuron with its cell body, or perikaryon, and its processes, or neurites. (×200.)

commonly used to stain nerve fibers and nerve endings. Only after studying a number of slides of nerve tissue that have been stained separately with many of these special stains is one able to understand the complete structure of nerve tissue.

THE NEURON

Classification

Although the cell body of a neuron may be as small as 5 μm or as large as 135 μm in diameter, the processes, or *neurites*, may extend over distances of more than 5 feet. The number, length, and mode of branching of the neurites provide a morphological method for classifying neurons.

Unipolar neurons are those in which the cell body has a single neurite that divides a short distance from the cell body into two branches, one proceeding to some peripheral structure and the other entering the central nervous system (Fig. 7-3). The branches of this single neurite have the structural and functional characteristics of an axon. In this type of neuron, the fine terminal branches found at the peripheral end of the axon, at the receptor site, are often referred to as the dendrites. Examples of this form of neuron are found in the posterior root ganglion.

Each *bipolar neuron* possesses an elongated cell body, from each end of which a single neurite emerges (see Fig. 7-3). Examples of this type of neuron are the retinal bipolar cells and the cells of the sensory cochlear and vestibular ganglia.

Multipolar neurons are those in which a number of neurites arise from the cell body (see Fig. 7-3). With the exception of the long process—the axon—the neurites are dendrites. Most neurons of the brain and spinal cord are of this type.

Neurons may also be classified according to size:

Golgi type I neurons have long axons that may be several feet in length in extreme cases (Figs. 7-4, 7-5, and 7-6). The axons of these neurons form the long fiber tracts of the brain and spinal cord and the nerve fibers of peripheral nerves. The pyramidal cells of the cerebral cortex, the Purkinje cells of the cerebellar cortex, and the motor cells of the spinal cord are Golgi type I neurons.

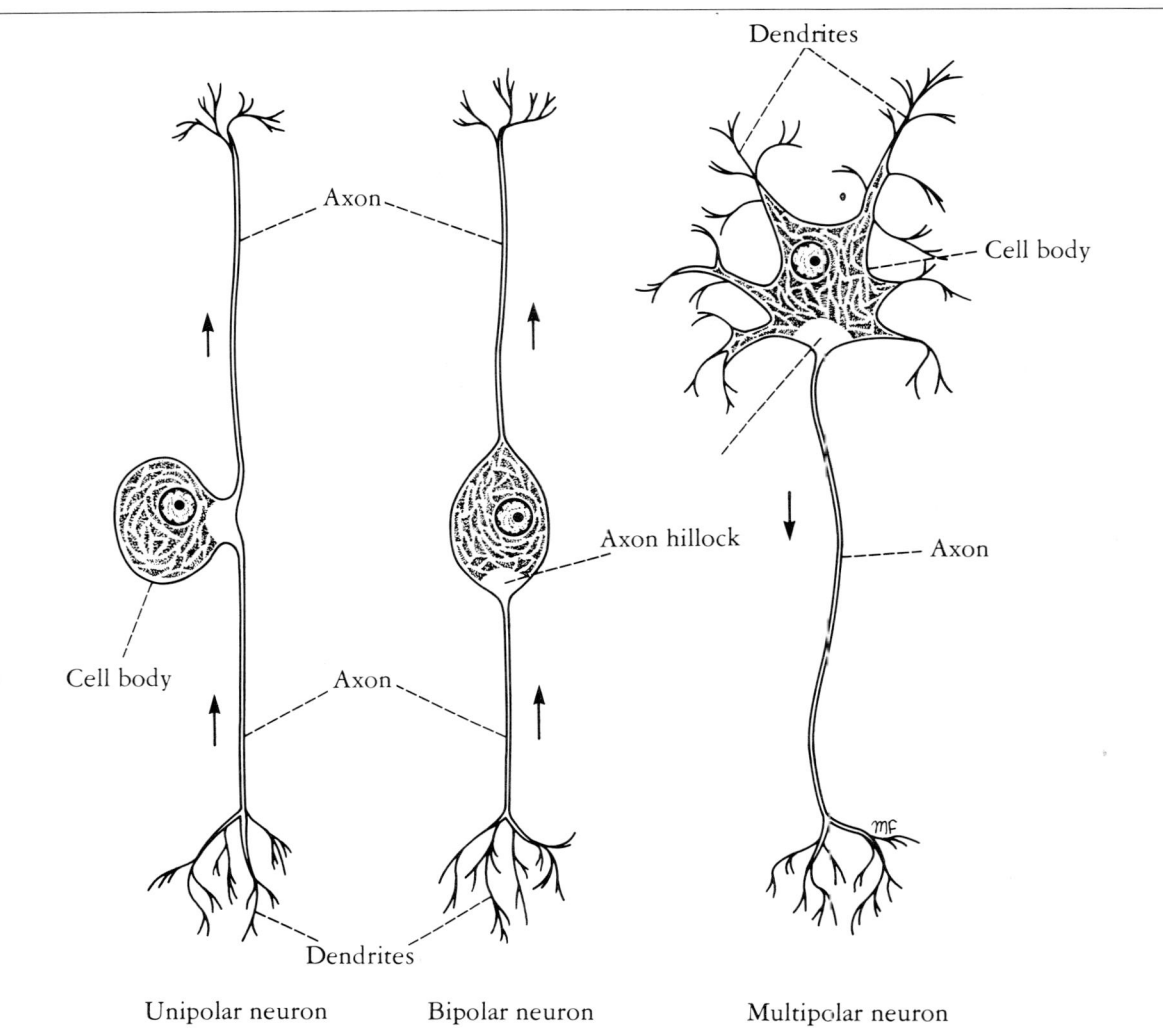

Fig. 7-3. Classification of neurons according to the number, length, and mode of branching of their processes (neurites).

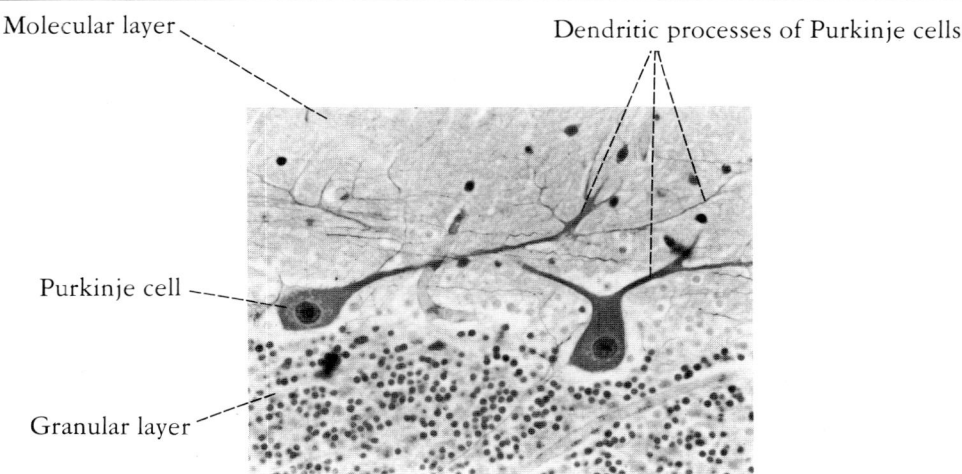

Fig. 7-4. *Photomicrograph of a section of the cerebellar cortex, showing two Purkinje cells. These are Golgi type I neurons. (Silver stain; ×260.)*

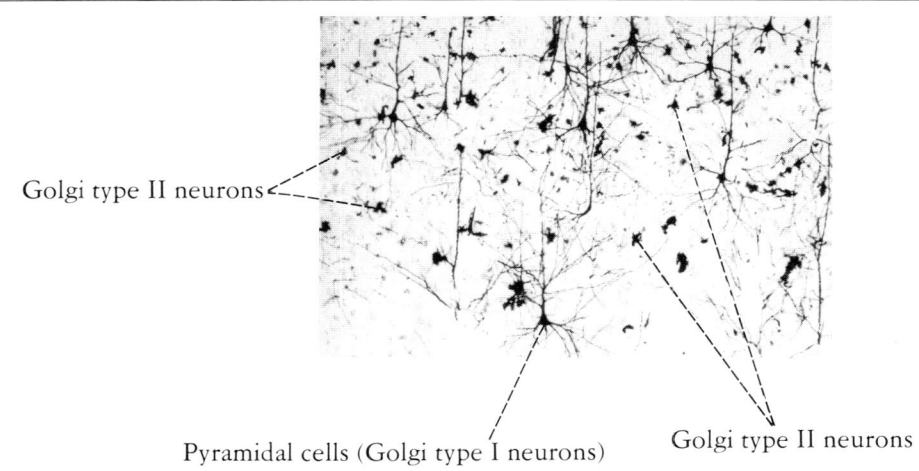

Fig. 7-5. *Photomicrograph of a section of the cerebral cortex. Note the presence of large pyramidal cells, which are Golgi type I neurons, and numerous Golgi type II neurons. (Silver stain; ×70.)*

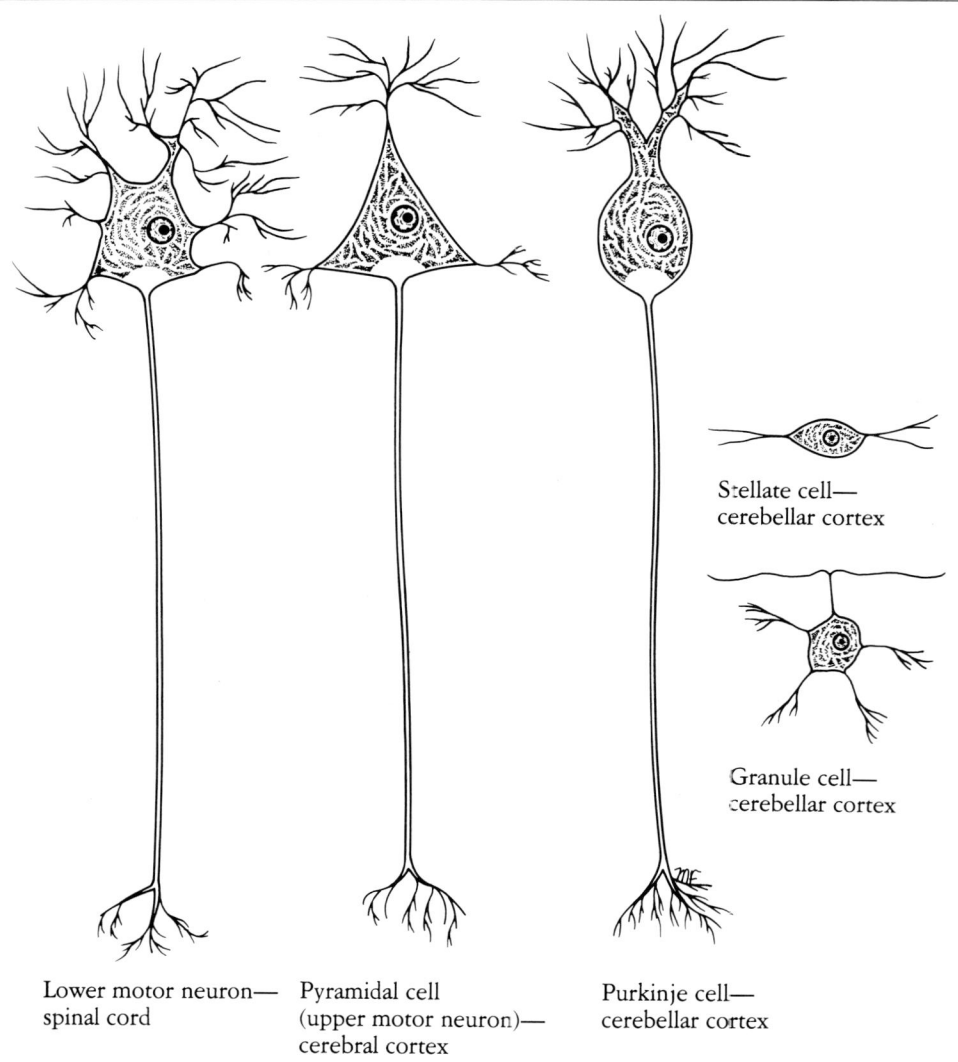

Fig. 7-6. *Different types of neurons.*

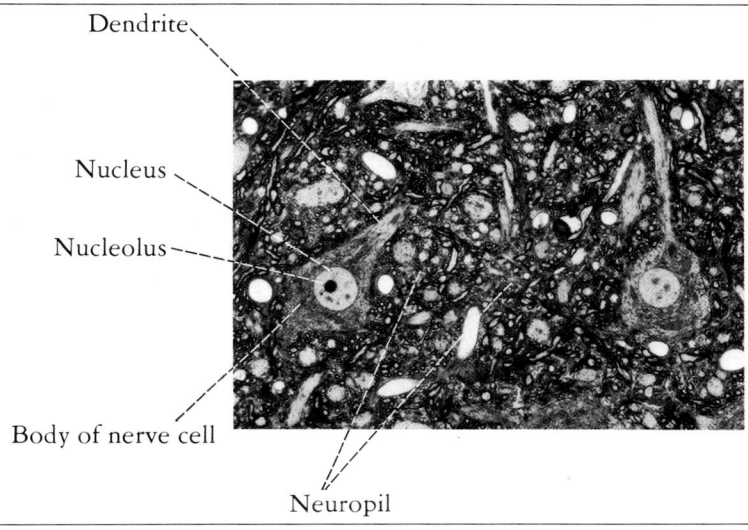

Fig. 7-7. Photomicrograph of section of anterior gray column of spinal cord, showing two large motor nerve cells. Note the prominent nucleolus in one of the nuclei. (Toluidine blue stain; ×300.)

A *Golgi type II neuron* has a short axon that terminates near the cell body or is entirely absent (see Figs. 7-5 and 7-6). These neurons greatly outnumber the Golgi type I neurons. The short dendrites that arise from these neurons give them a star-shaped appearance. These neurons are very numerous in the cerebral and cerebellar cortex and in the retina.

Structure

The *nerve cell body,* like the body of other cells, essentially consists of a mass of cytoplasm in which a nucleus is embedded (see Fig. 7-6); it is bounded externally by a plasma membrane. The volume of cytoplasm within the nerve cell body is often far less than the total volume of cytoplasm in the neurites. The cell bodies of the small granular cells of the cerebellar cortex measure about 5 μm in diameter, whereas those of the large anterior horn cells may measure as much as 135 μm in diameter.

The *nucleus* is typically large, rounded, and pale, and the fine chromatin granules are widely dispersed (Figs. 7-7 and 7-8; see Fig. 7-6). There is usually a single prominent nucleolus. The large size of the nucleolus probably is caused by the high rate of protein synthesis, which is necessary to maintain the protein level in the large cytoplasmic volume in the long neurites and in the cell body.

In the female, the compact X chromosome, or *Barr body,* is situated at the inner surface of the nuclear membrane (see p. 30).

Nerve cells possess a single nucleus, although those of the sympathetic and sensory ganglia are occasionally binucleate.

The *cytoplasm* is rich in granular and agranular endoplasmic reticulum (Fig. 7-9; see Fig. 7-12) and contains the following organelles and inclusions: (1) Nissl substance, (2) the Golgi apparatus, (3) mitochondria, (4) microfilaments, (5) microtubules, (6) lysosomes, (7) a centrosome, and (8) lipofuscin, melanin, glycogen, and lipid.

Nissl substance consists of granules distributed throughout the cytoplasm of the cell body except in the region close to the axon, called the *axon hillock* (Figs. 7-10 and 7-11). The granular material also extends into the proximal parts of the dendrites.

Electron micrographs show that the Nissl sub-

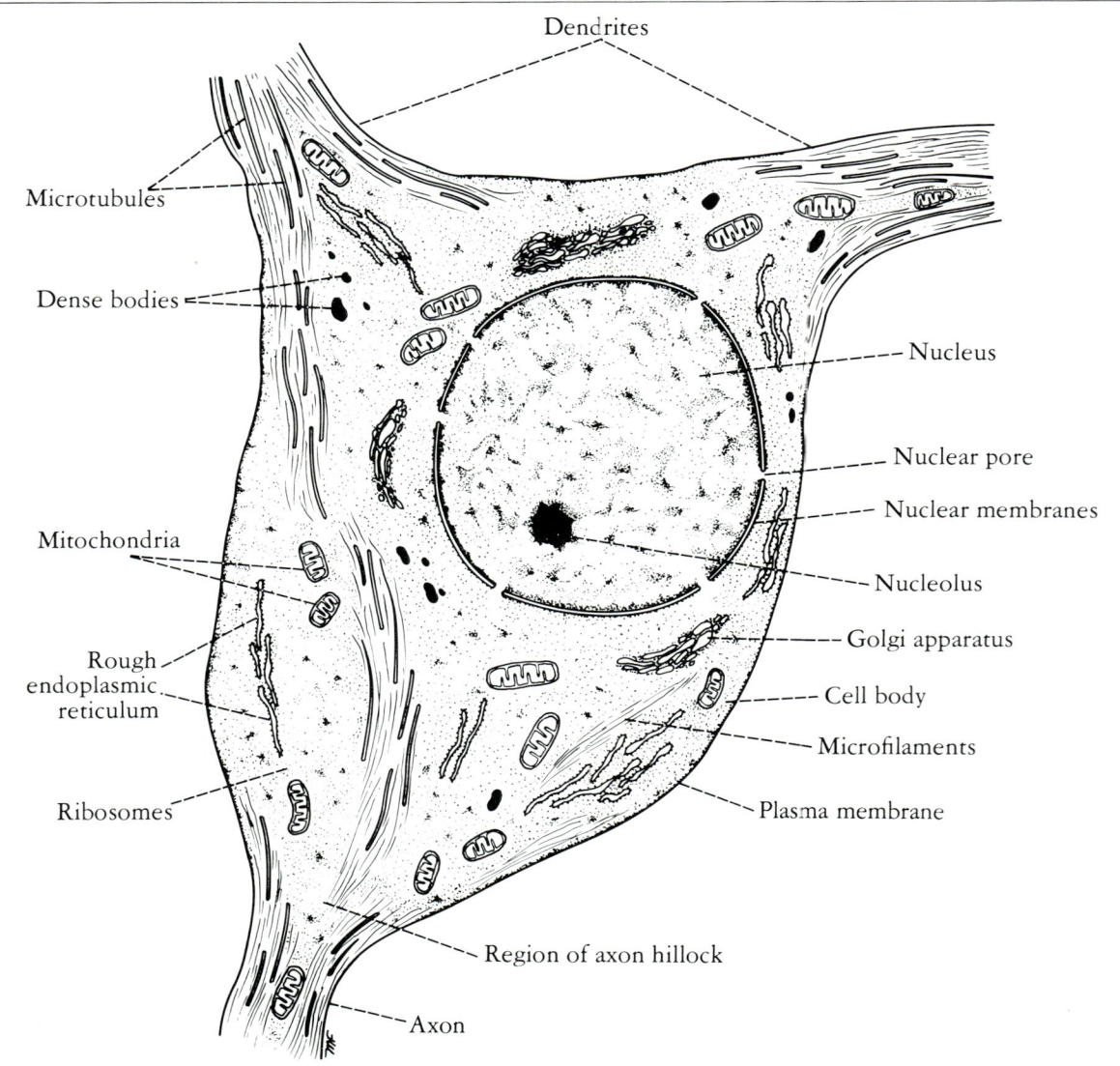

Fig. 7-8. Fine structure of a neuron.

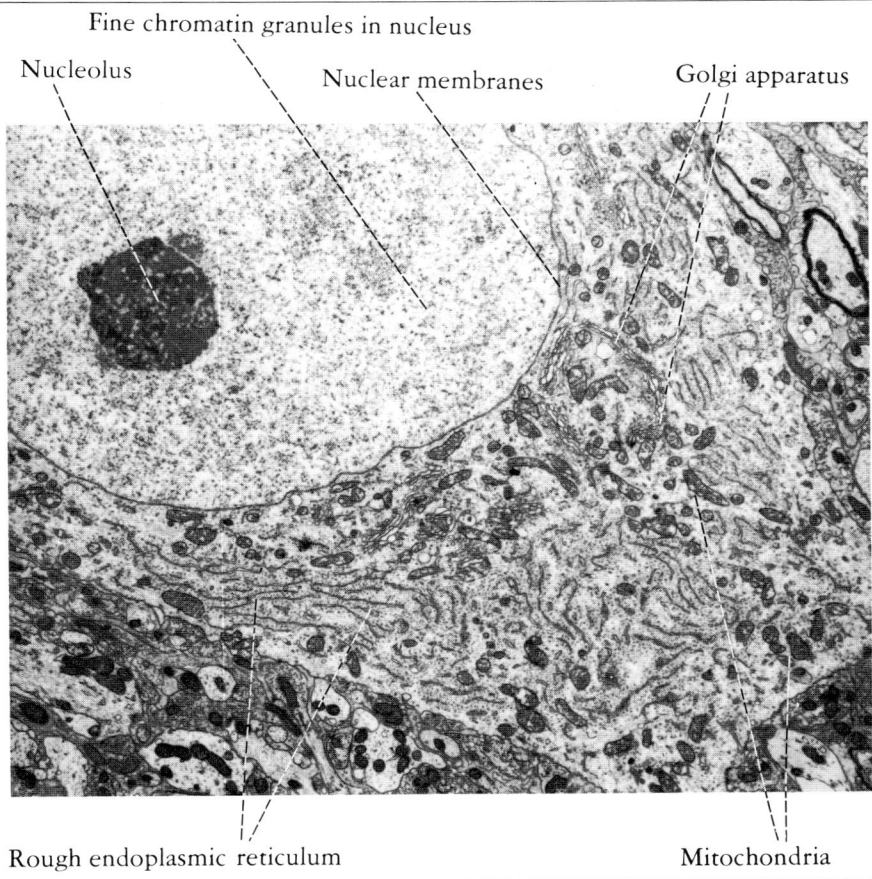

Fig. 7-9. Electron micrograph of a neuron, showing the structure of the nucleus and a number of cytoplasmic organelles. (Courtesy of Dr. J. M. Kerns.)

stance is composed of rough-surfaced endoplasmic reticulum (Fig. 7-12) and is arranged in the form of broad cisternae stacked on top of one another. Although many of the ribosomes are attached to the surface of the endoplasmic reticulum, many lie free in the intervals between the cisternae. Because the ribosomes contain ribonucleic acid (RNA), the Nissl substance is basophilic and can be well demonstrated under light microscope after staining with toluidine blue or other basic aniline dyes (Fig. 7-10).

The Nissl substance is responsible for synthesizing protein, which flows along the dendrites and the axon and replaces the proteins that are broken down during cellular activity. Fatigue or neuronal damage causes the Nissl substance to become concentrated at the periphery of the cytoplasm. This phenomenon, which gives the impression that the Nissl substance has disappeared, is known as *chromatolysis*.

The *Golgi apparatus,* when seen with the light microscope after staining with a silver-osmium method, appears as a network of irregular wavy threads around the nucleus. In electron micrographs it appears as clusters of flattened cisternae and small vesicles made up of smooth-surfaced endoplasmic reticulum (see Fig. 7-9). The function of the Golgi apparatus is discussed on page 45. *Mitochondria* are found scattered throughout the cell body, dendrites,

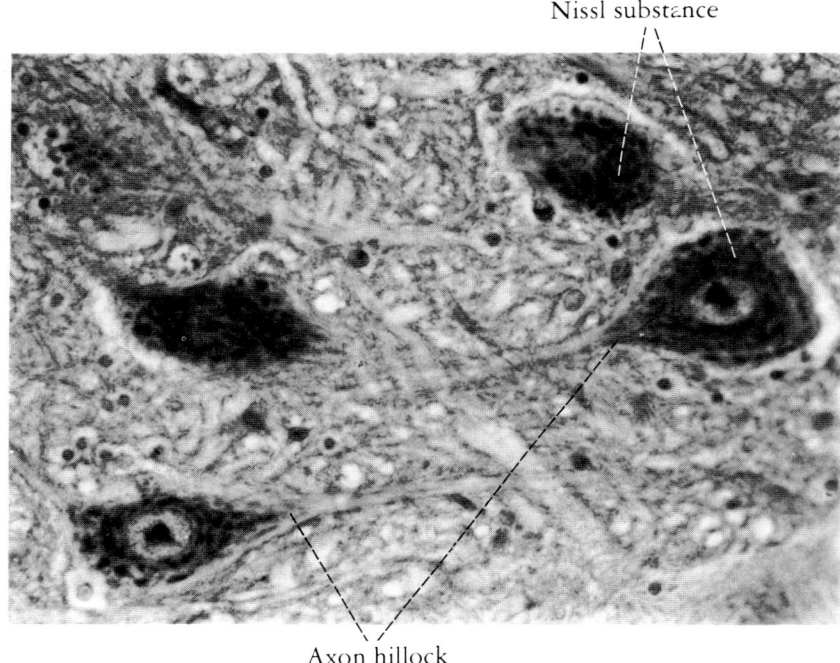

Fig. 7-10. Photomicrograph of section of anterior gray column of spinal cord, showing the presence of dark-staining Nissl substance in the cytoplasm of four neurons. (Toluidine blue stain; ×400.)

and axons (see Figs. 7-8 and 7-9). Their structure is similar to that seen in cells of other tissues.

Neurofibrils, visible with the light microscope when the cytoplasm is stained with silver, are numerous fibrils running parallel to one another through the cell body into the neurites (Fig. 7-13). With the electron microscope, the neurofibrils may be resolved into bundles of *microfilaments,* each filament measuring about 7 nm in diameter (Fig. 7-14). The function of these filaments is unknown.

Microtubules here are revealed with the electron microscope and are similar to those seen in other types of cells. They measure about 20 to 30 nm in diameter and are found interspersed among the microfilaments (see Fig. 7-14). They extend throughout the cell body and its processes. Microtubules are believed to transport substances from the cell body to the distal ends of the cell processes.

Lysosomes here are similar to those seen in other cell types.

Fig. 7-11. Electron micrograph of longitudinal section of a neuron from the cerebral cortex, showing the detailed structure of the region of the axon hillock and the initial segment of the axon. Note the absence of Nissl substance (rough endoplasmic reticulum) in the axon hillock and the presence of numerous microtubules in the axon. Note also the axon terminals (arrows) forming axo-axonal synapses with the initial segment of the axon. (×13,334.) (Courtesy of Dr. A. Peters.)

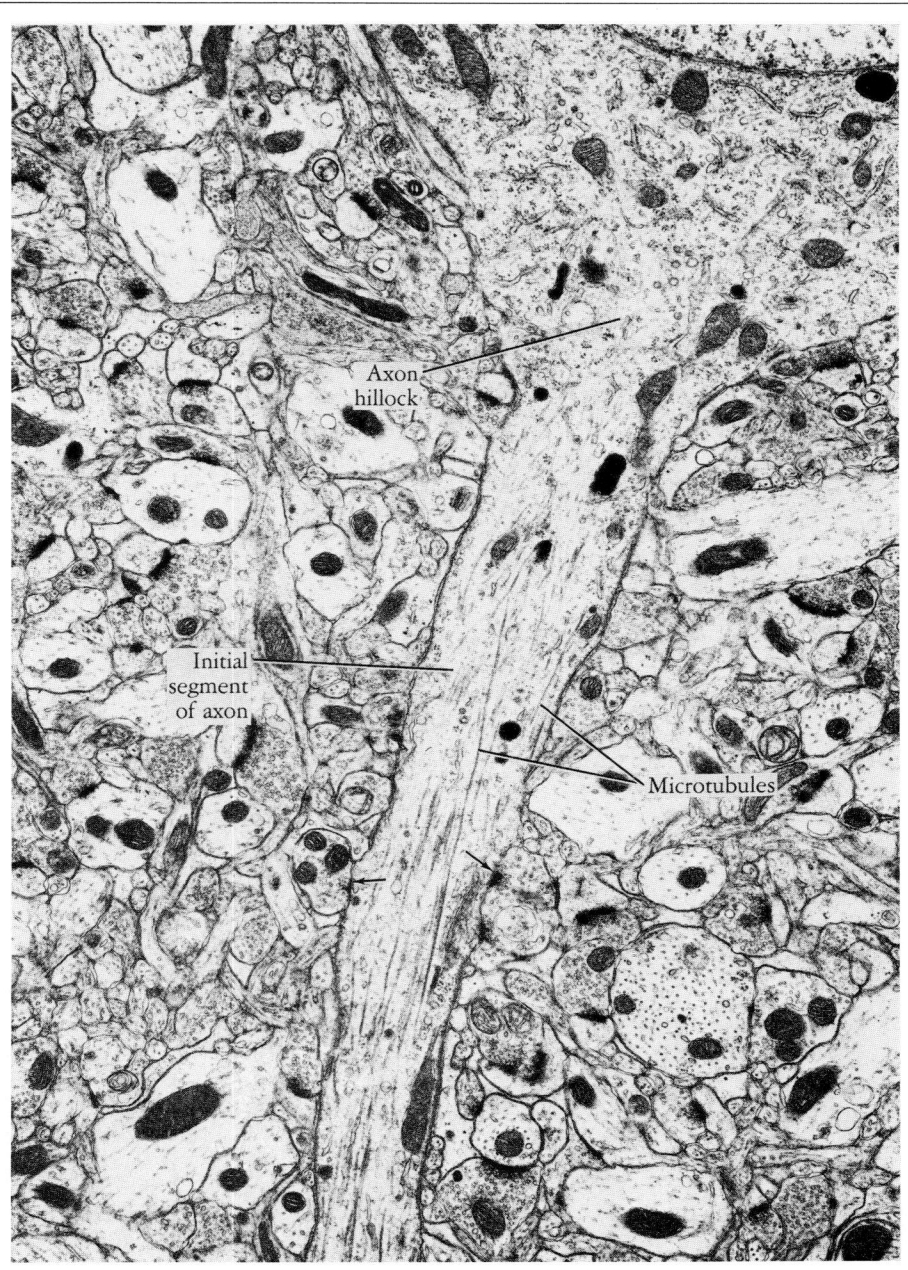

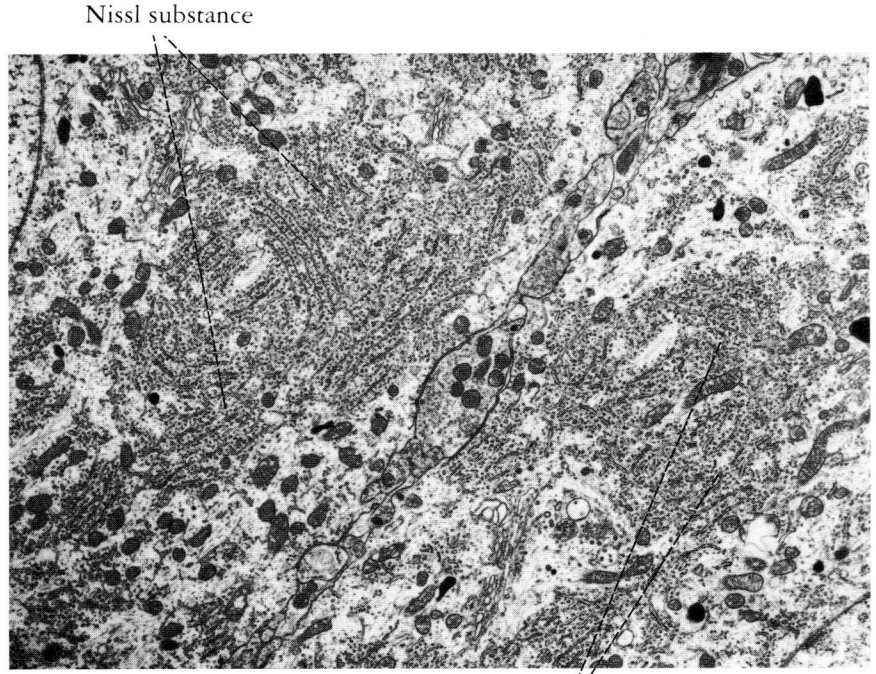

Nissl substance

Nissl substance

Fig. 7-12. Electron micrograph of cytoplasm of two neurons, showing the structure of Nissl substance. (Courtesy of Dr. J. M. Kerns.)

Fig. 7-13. Photomicrograph of a neuron, showing large numbers of neurofibrils in the cytoplasm of the cell body and the neurites. (Silver stain; ×868.)

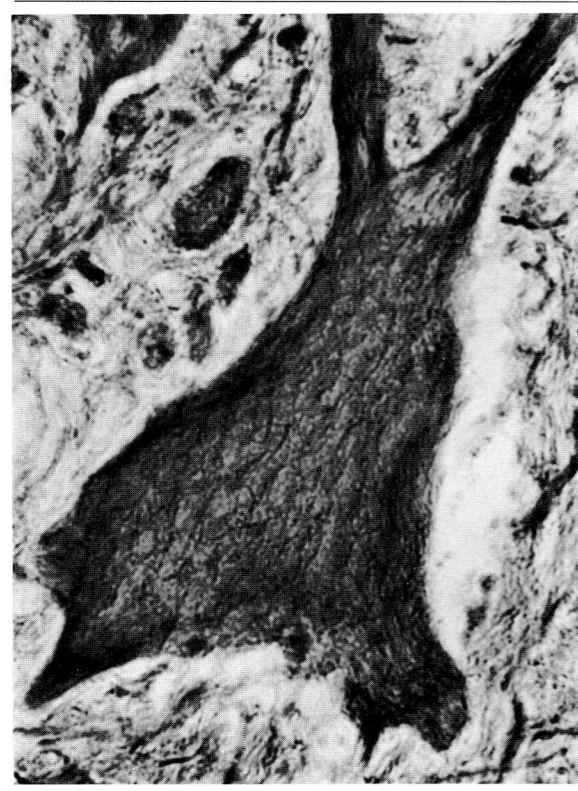

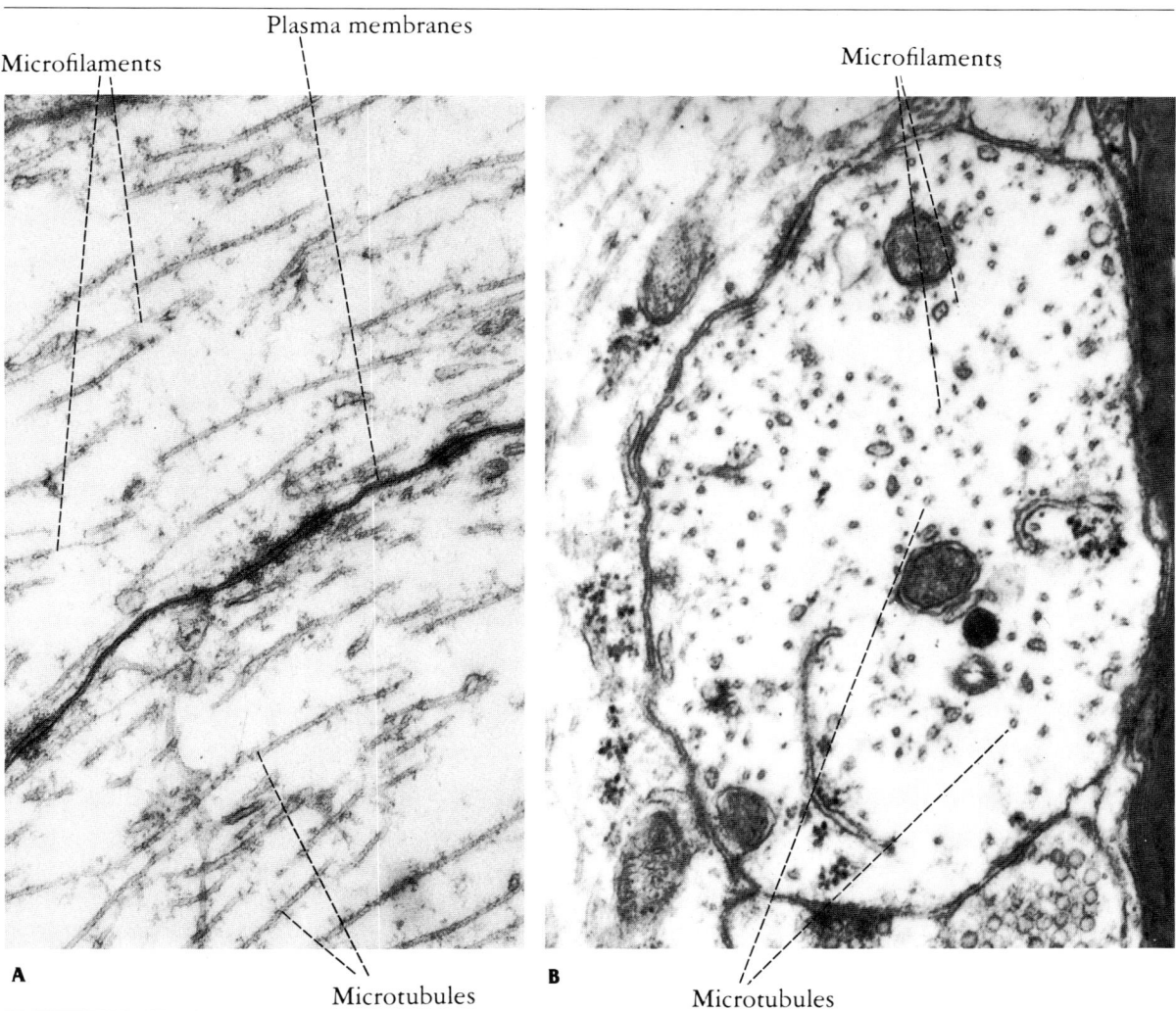

Fig. 7-14. Electron micrograph of dendrites, showing microfilaments and microtubules within their cytoplasm. (A) Longitudinal section of two adjacent dendrites; (B) transverse section of a dendrite. (Courtesy of Dr. J. M. Kerns.)

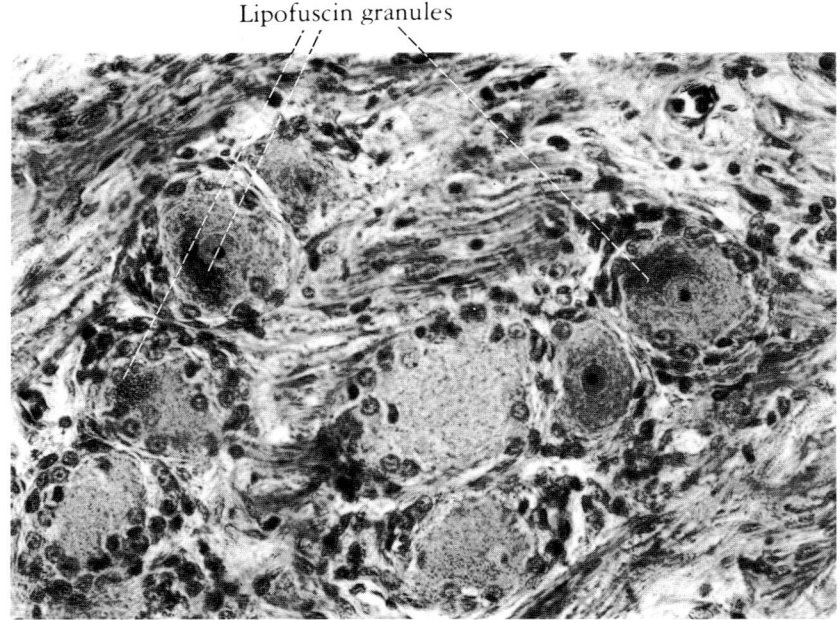

Fig. 7-15. Photomicrograph of longitudinal section of posterior root ganglion, showing lipofuscin granules within the cytoplasm of sensory neurons. (×400.)

The *centrosome* is seen in immature dividing nerve cells and occasionally in the mature neuron. This structure plays an important role in mitosis (see p. 34). Because mature neurons are incapable of dividing, the function of the centrosome in the mature neuron is unknown; it may be associated with the formation of microtubules.

Lipofuscin (pigment material) occurs as yellowish-brown granules within the cytoplasm (Fig. 7-15). It is believed to be formed as the result of lysosomal activity and represents a harmless metabolic by-product. Lipofuscin accumulates with age.

Melanin granules are found in the cytoplasm of cells in certain parts of the brain (for example, the substantia nigra of the midbrain). Their presence may be related to the catecholamine-synthesizing ability of these neurons.

Glycogen, which is a polymer of glucose, is seen in electron micrographs of nerve cells as electron-dense rosettes. It functions as a local source of energy.

Lipid occurs in the form of droplets and provides another local source of energy.

Plasma Membrane

The structure of the plasma membrane of a cell has been fully discussed in Chapter 2. It is sufficient to say here that the plasma membrane and the cell coat together form a semipermeable membrane that allows diffusion of certain ions but restricts others. In the resting (unstimulated state), a steady potential difference of about 80 mV is established that can be measured across the plasma membrane, the inside of the membrane being negative with respect to the outside (Fig. 7-16).

When the nerve cell is excited (stimulated), there is an increase in the permeability of the plasma membrane to Na^+ ions that diffuse through the plasma membrane into the cell cytoplasm from the tissue fluid (see Fig. 7-16). Because of such diffusion, the membrane becomes progressively *depolarized*. The sudden influx of sodium ions, followed by the altered polarity, produces the so-called *action potential*. This potential is, however, very brief

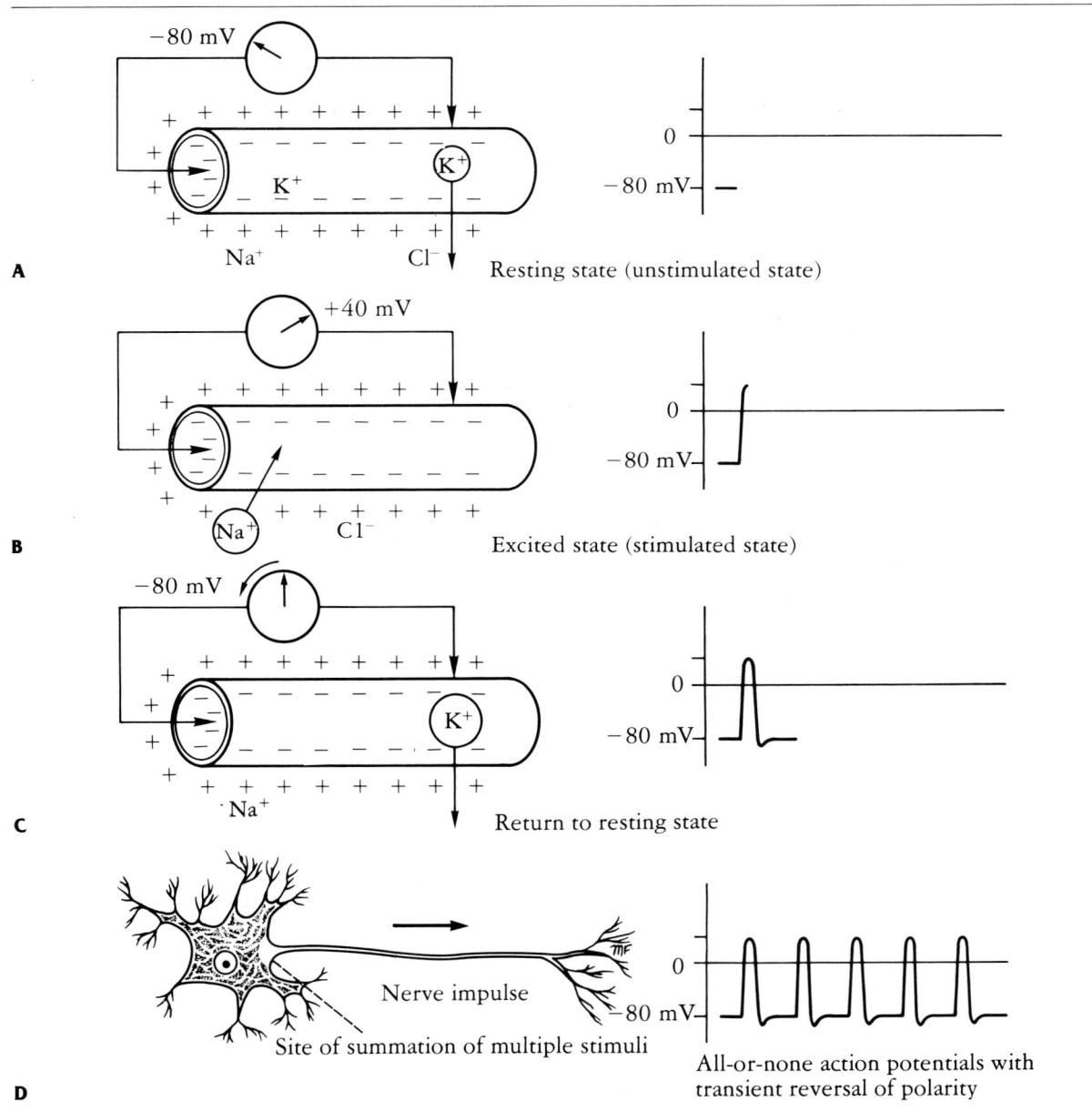

Fig. 7-16. Ionic and electrical changes that occur in a neuron when it is stimulated.

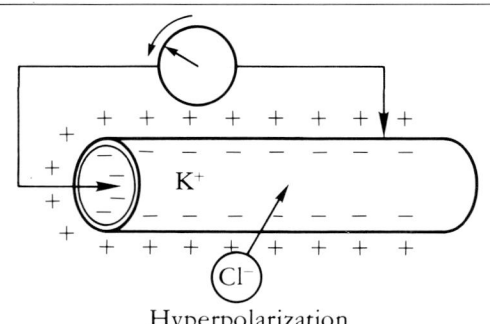

Fig. 7-17. Ionic and electrical changes that occur in a neuron during hyperpolarization.

Fig. 7-18. (A) Photomicrograph of a motor neuron in the anterior gray column on the spinal cord, showing the nerve cell body, two dendrites, and the surrounding neuropil. (Silver stain; ×700.) (B) Electron micrograph of a dendrite, showing axodendritic synapses. (Courtesy of Dr. J. M. Kerns.)

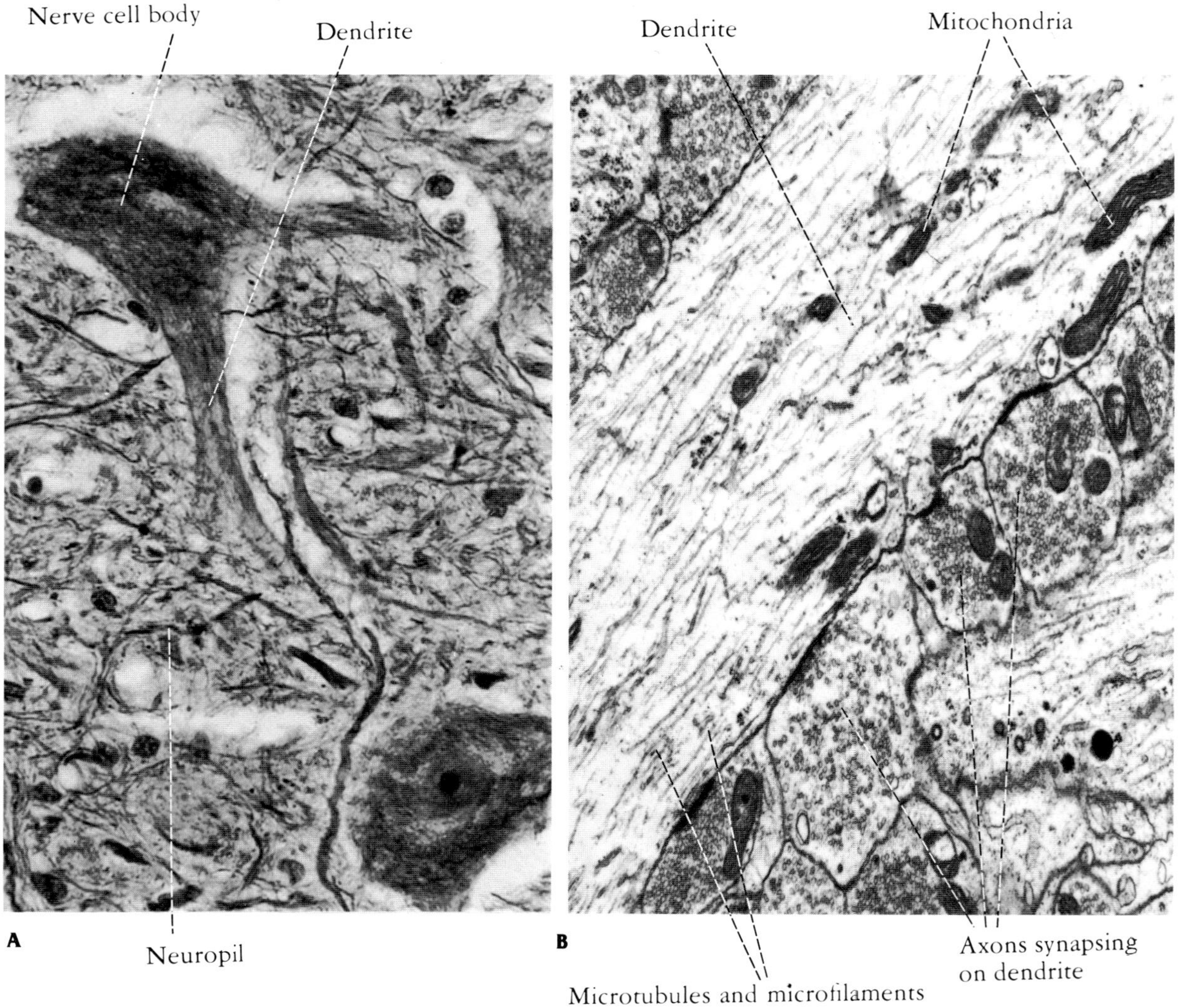

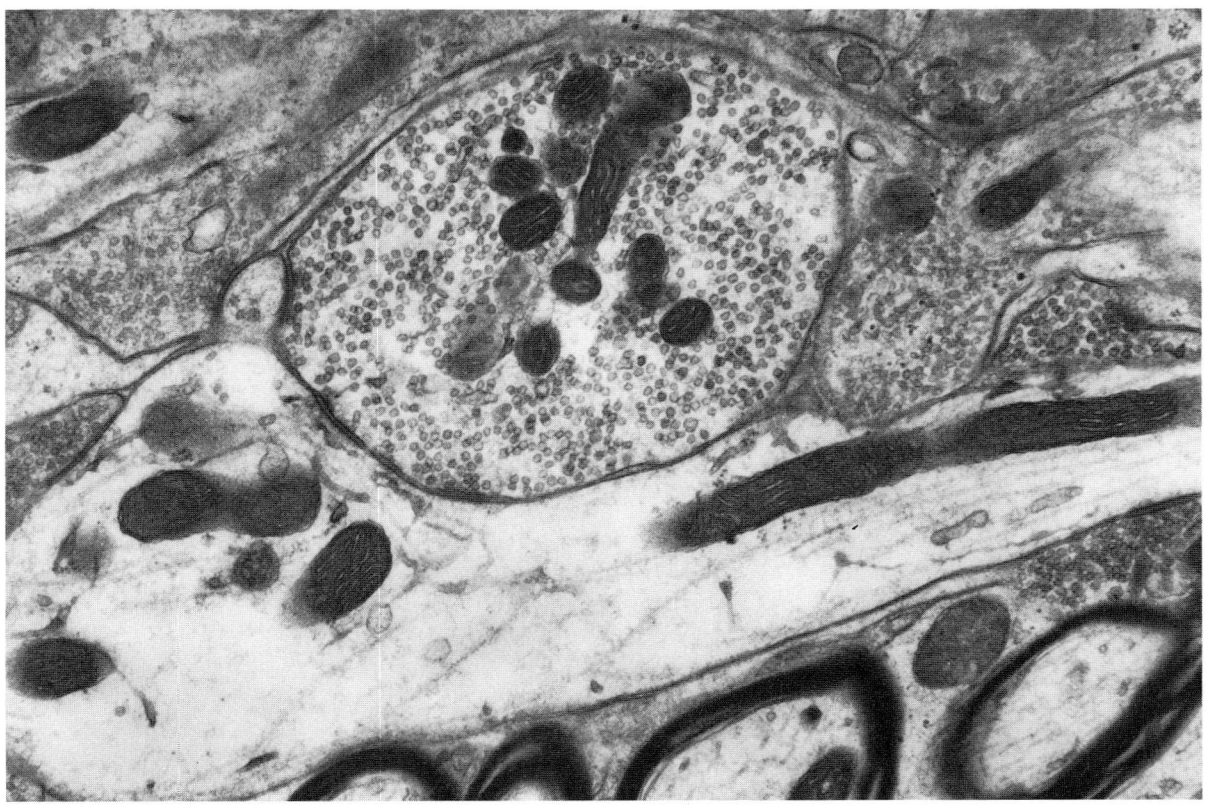

Fig. 7-19. Electron micrograph of an axon terminal contacting a dendrite. Note the large numbers of presynaptic vesicles and numerous mitochondria present in the axon terminal. (Courtesy of Dr. L. S. Ide.)

in duration, for very quickly, the K^+ ions start to flow from the cell cytoplasm and return the localized area of the cell to the resting state.

Once generated, the action potential spreads over the plasma membrane away from the site of initiation and is conducted along neurites as the *nerve impulse*. This impulse is self-propagated, and its size and frequency do not alter (see Fig. 7-16). Once the nerve impulse has spread over a given region of plasma membrane, another action potential cannot be elicited immediately. The duration of this nonexcitable state is referred to as the *refractory period*.

It is important to realize that the greater the strength of the initial stimulus, the larger will be the initial depolarization and the greater the spread into the surrounding areas of the plasma membrane. Should multiple excitatory stimuli be applied to the surface of a neuron, the effect can be *summated*. For example, subthreshold stimuli may pass over the surface of the cell body and be summated at the root of the axon, thereby initiating an action potential.

The inhibitory stimuli are believed to produce their effect by causing an influx of Cl^- ions through the plasma membrane into the neuron, thus producing hyperpolarization and reducing the excitatory state of the cell (Fig. 7-17).

Nerve Cell Processes

The processes of a nerve cell, often called neurites, may be divided into dendrites and an axon.

The *dendrites* are the short processes of the cell

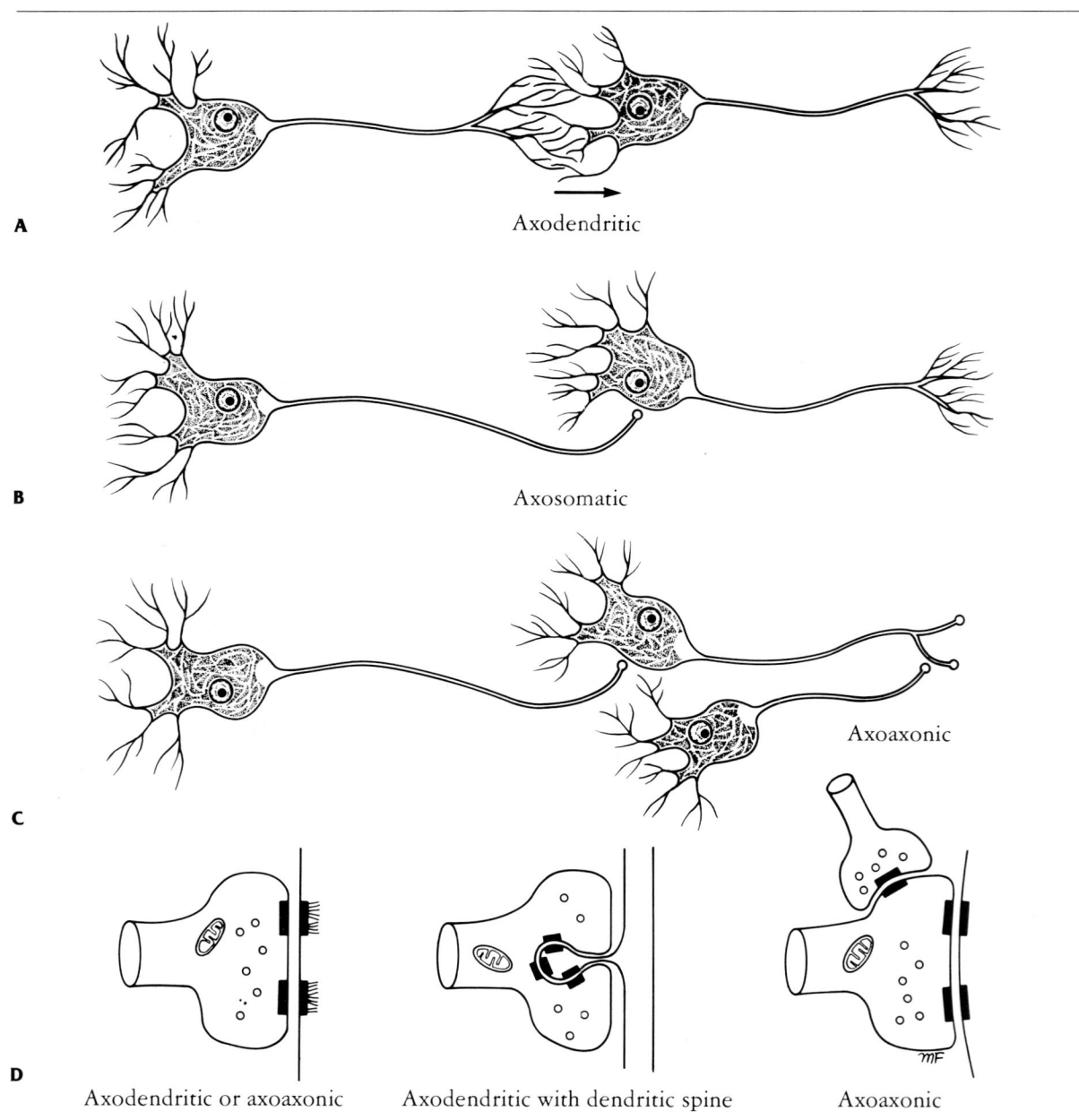

Fig. 7-20. The different types of synapses.

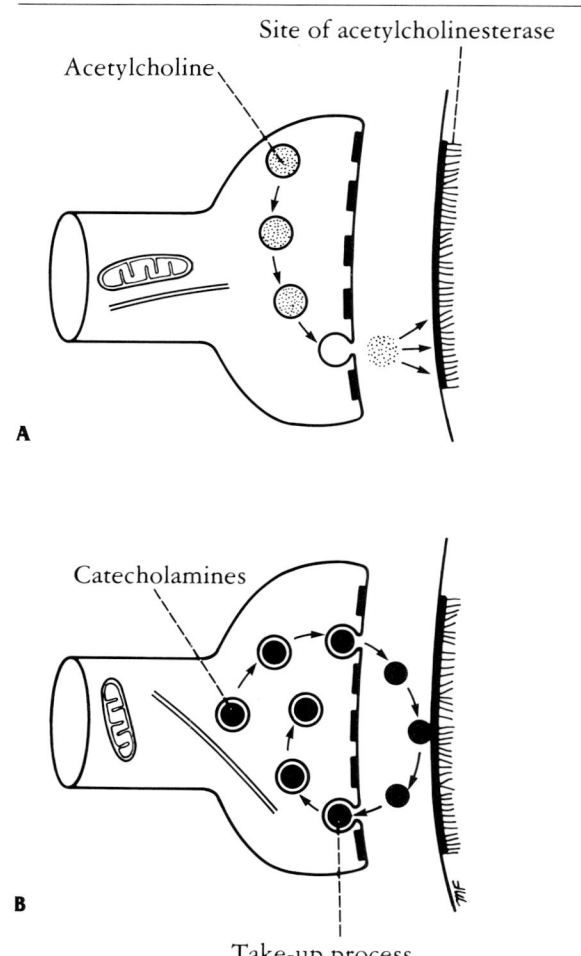

Fig. 7-21. Release of transmitters: (A) acetylcholine; (B) catecholamines.

body (Fig. 7-18). They taper as they extend from the cell body, and they often branch profusely. In many neurons, the finer branches bear large numbers of small projections called *dendritic spines*. The cytoplasm of the dendrites closely resembles that of the cell body and contains Nissl granules, mitochondria, microtubules, microfilaments, ribosomes, and agranular endoplasmic reticulum. Dendrites should be regarded merely as extensions of the cell body that serve to increase the surface area for the reception of axons from other neurons. Essentially, they conduct the nerve impulse toward the cell body.

Axon is the name given to the longest process of the cell body. It arises from a small, conical elevation on the cell body, devoid of Nissl granules, called the *axon hillock* (see Figs. 7-1 and 7-11). Occasionally, an axon arises from the proximal part of a dendrite. An axon tends to have a smooth contour and is uniform in diameter.

Axons tend not to branch close to the cell body; collateral branches may occur along their length. Shortly before their termination, axons commonly branch profusely. The distal ends of the terminal branches of the axons are often enlarged; they are called *terminals* or *boutons terminaux* (see Fig. 7-21).

Axons may be very short, as in many neurons of the central nervous system, or extremely long, as those that extend from a peripheral receptor in the skin of the toe to the spinal cord and from there to the brain.

The diameter of axons varies considerably with different neurons. Those of larger diameter conduct impulses rapidly, and those of smaller diameter conduct impulses very slowly.

The plasma membrane bounding the axon is called the *axolemma*. The cytoplasm of the axon is termed the *axoplasm*. Axoplasm differs from the cytoplasm of the cell body in possessing no Nissl granules or Golgi apparatus. The sites for the production of protein, namely RNA and ribosomes, are absent.

It is usually stated that an axon always conducts impulses away from the cell body. The axons of sensory posterior root ganglion cells are an exception; here the long neurite, which is indistinguishable from an axon, carries the impulse toward the cell body (see the discussion of unipolar neurons, p. 227).

AXOPLASMIC FLOW. Considerable experimental evidence shows that materials are transported along axons from the cell body to the terminals and, to a lesser extent, in the opposite direction. It has been noted previously that axons do not possess the ma-

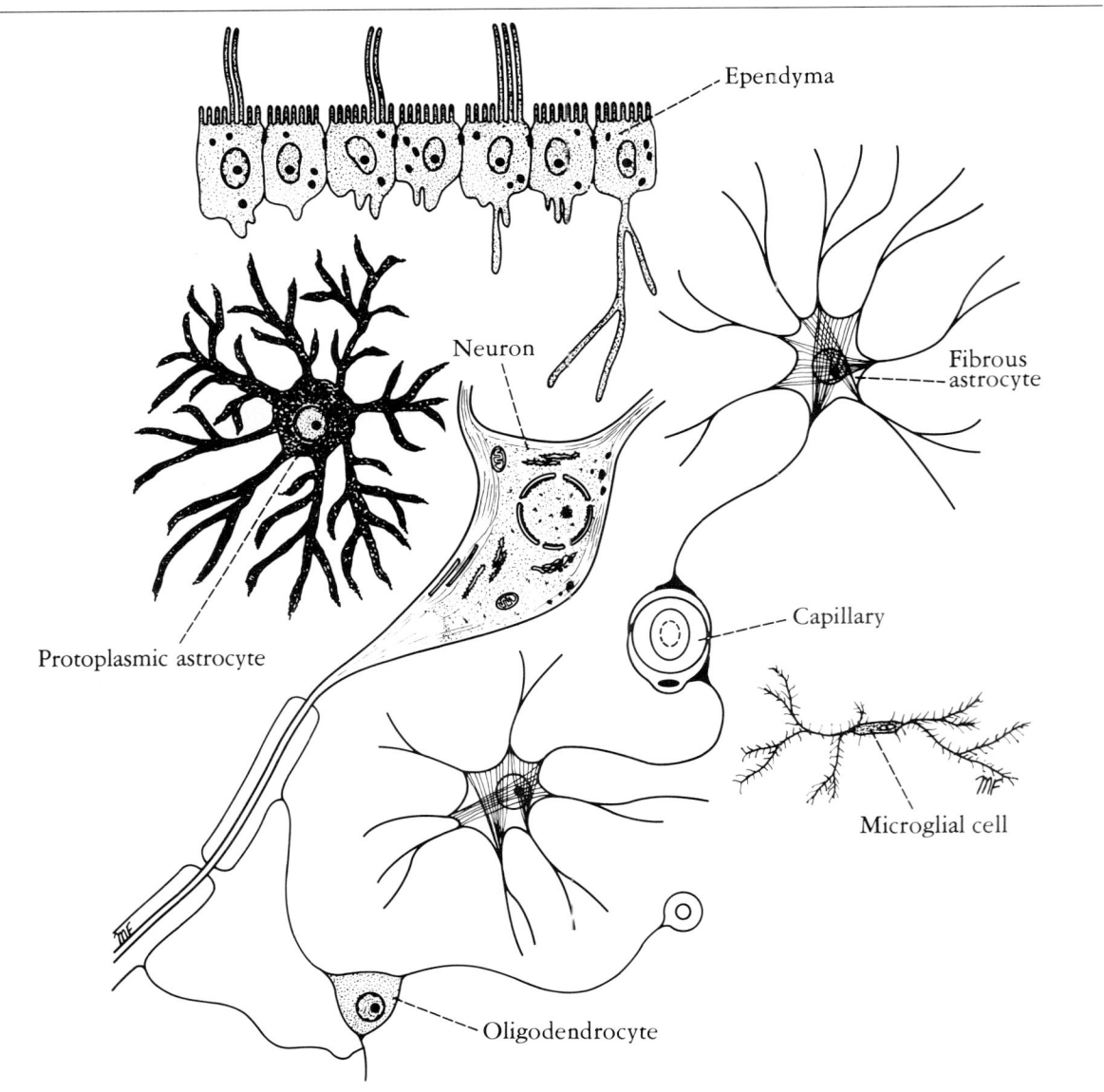

Fig. 7-22. Arrangement of different types of neuroglial cells.

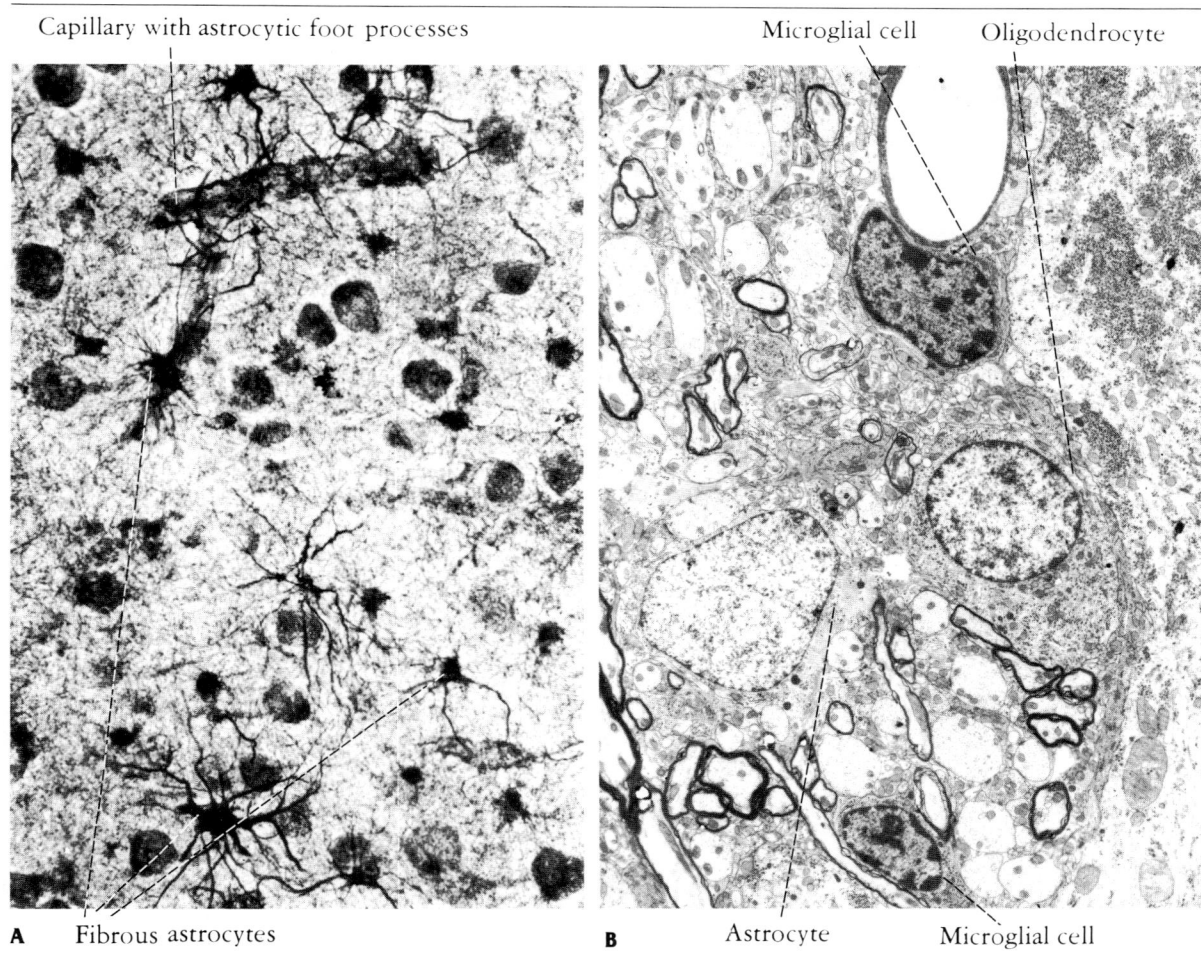

Fig. 7-23. (A) Photomicrograph of sections of gray matter of spinal cord, showing fibrous astrocytes. (×400.) (B) Electron micrograph, showing an astrocyte. (Courtesy of Dr. J. M. Kerns.)

chinery for manufacturing proteins; the cell body of the neuron is the site of such production. Proteins traveling distally along the axon are probably involved in protein replenishment of the axolemma following physiological activity. Axoplasmic flow is almost certainly involved in the build-up of materials at the axon terminals for the production of transmitter substances. The flow of the axoplasm in the opposite direction may explain how the cell bodies of nerve cells respond to changes in the distal ends of the axon.

The mechanism responsible for axoplasmic flow is not fully understood, although wavelike movements of the microtubules have been suggested as a cause of the streaming movements of the axoplasm.

Synapses

The nervous system consists of a large number of neurons that are linked together to form functional conducting pathways. Where two neurons come into close proximity and functional interneuronal

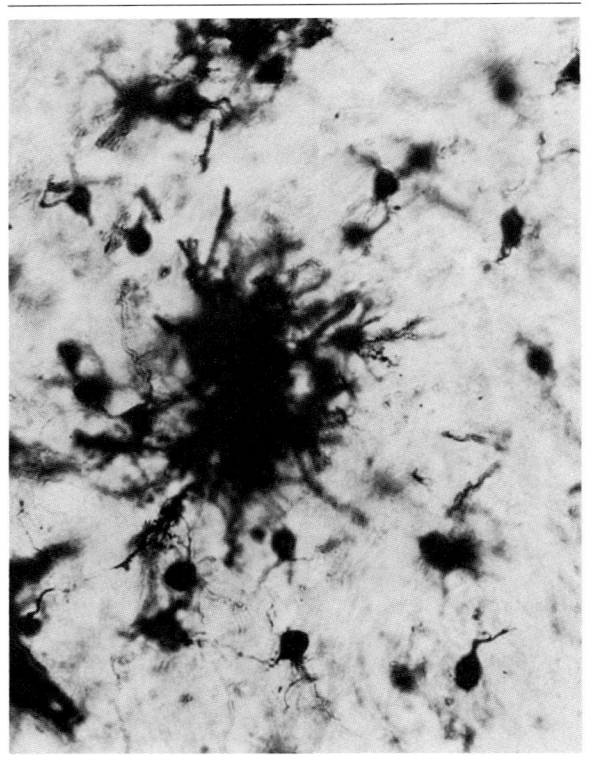

Fig. 7-24. Photomicrograph of a protoplasmic astrocyte in the cerebral cortex. (×400.)

communication occurs, the site of such communication is referred to as a *synapse* (Figs. 7-19 and 7-20). Communication at a synapse, under physiological conditions, takes place in one direction only. Synapses occur in a number of forms (see Figs. 7-19 and 7-20). The most common type is that which occurs between an axon of one neuron and the dendrite or cell body of a second neuron. As the axon approaches the synapse, it may have a terminal expansion (bouton terminal) or a series of expansions (bouton de passage), each of which makes synaptic contact. In other types of synapses, the axon synapses on the proximal segment of another axon, that is, proximal to the beginning of the myelin sheath, or there may be synapses between terminal expansions from different neurons. Depending on the site of the synapse, it is referred to as *axodendritic, axosomatic,* or *axoaxonic* (see Fig. 7-20).

Ultrastructure of Synapses

On examination with the electron microscope, synapses appear as areas of structural specialization (see Figs. 7-18B and 7-19). The apposed surfaces of the terminal axonal expansion and the neuron are called the *presynaptic* and *postsynaptic membranes,* respectively, and are separated by a *synaptic cleft* 20 nm wide. The presynaptic and postsynaptic membranes are thickened, and the adjacent underlying cytoplasm shows increased density. On the presynaptic side, the dense cytoplasm is broken up into groups, and on the postsynaptic side, the density often extends into a *subsynaptic web. Presynaptic vesicles,* mitochondria, and occasional lysosomes are present in the cytoplasm close to the presynaptic membrane (see Fig. 7-19). On the postsynaptic side, the cytoplasm often contains parallel cisternae. The synaptic cleft contains polysaccharides.

Transmission across a synapse is accomplished by the release of *neurotransmitters,* associated with the presynaptic vesicles, into the synaptic cleft. In the case of an excitatory synapse, the released transmitter causes a depolarization of the postsynaptic membrane; in the case of an inhibitory synapse, the transmitter causes hyperpolarization of the postsynaptic membrane. It is believed that the transmitter acetylcholine is stored in the clear presynaptic vesicles, whereas *catecholamines* are associated with the presence of dense-cored presynaptic vesicles (Fig. 7-21). The arrival of a nerve impulse at the presynaptic membrane results in the release of the transmitter substance into the synaptic gutter.

Neurotransmitters at Synapses

Acetylcholine and the catecholamines *norepinephrine, epinephrine,* and *dopamine* are the main neurotransmitters that have been researched extensively. Recent work on the central nervous system has suggested that synapses there may operate by means of other unknown chemical transmitters.

All neurotransmitters are released from their nerve endings by the arrival of the nerve impulse.

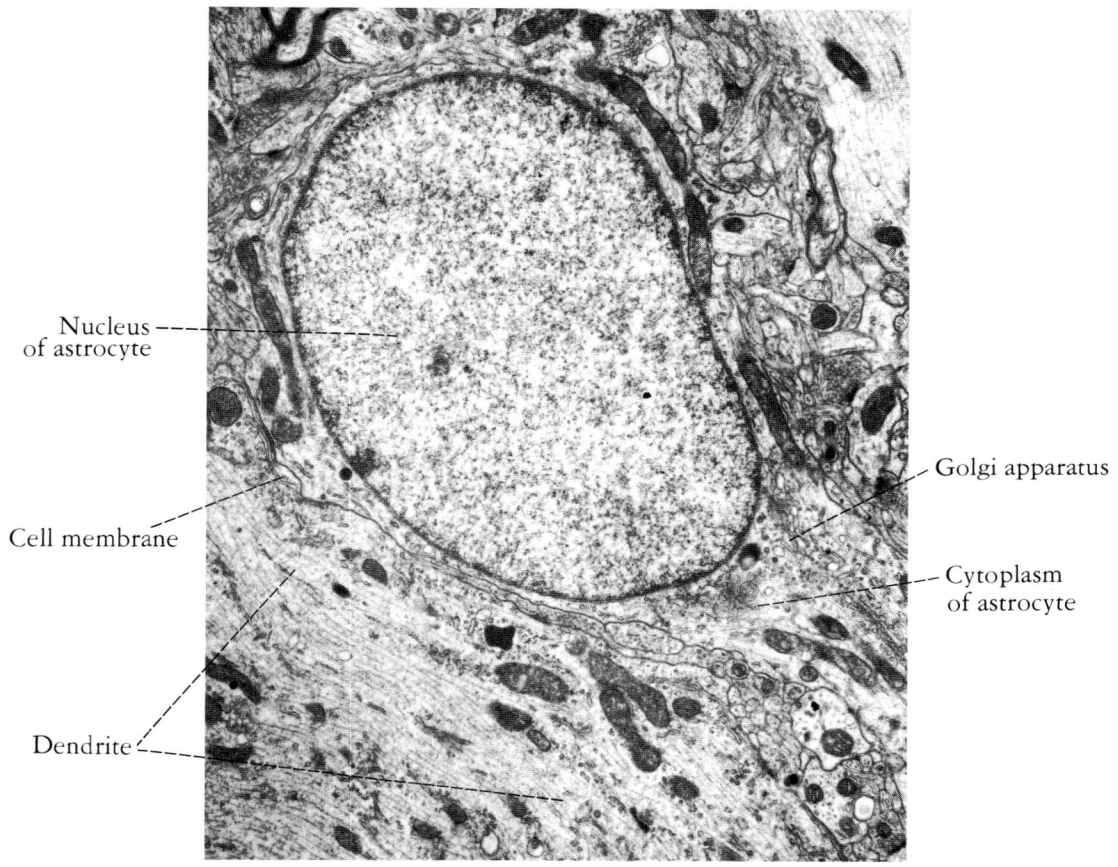

Fig. 7-25. Electron micrograph of a protoplasmic astrocyte in the cerebral cortex. (Courtesy of Dr. A. Peters.)

Once in the synaptic gutter, they achieve their objective by briefly raising or lowering the resting potential of the postsynaptic membrane. In the case of acetylcholine, the effect is limited by the destruction of the transmitter in the synaptic gutter by the enzyme *acetylcholinesterase* (see Fig. 7-21). In the case of the *cathecholamines,* the effect of the transmitter is limited by the return of the transmitter to the presynaptic nerve ending.

The distribution of the neurotransmitters varies in the different parts of the nervous system. *Acetylcholine* is found at the neuromuscular junction (see p. 209), in autonomic ganglia, and at parasympathetic nerve endings. In the hippocampus, the ascending reticular pathways, and the afferent fibers for the visual and auditory systems, the neurotransmitters are also cholinergic.

Norepinephrine is found at sympathetic nerve endings. In the central nervous system, it is found in high concentrations in the hypothalamus. *Dopamine* is found in high concentrations in different parts of the central nervous system, for example, in the basal ganglia.

Neuroglia

The neurons of the central nervous system are supported by special cells that are nonexcitable and do not conduct nerve impulses; together they are called

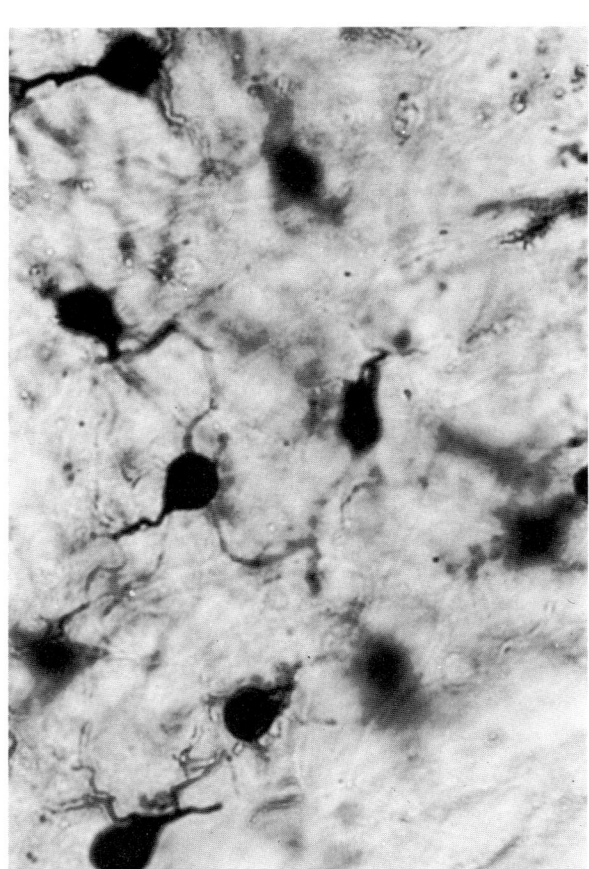
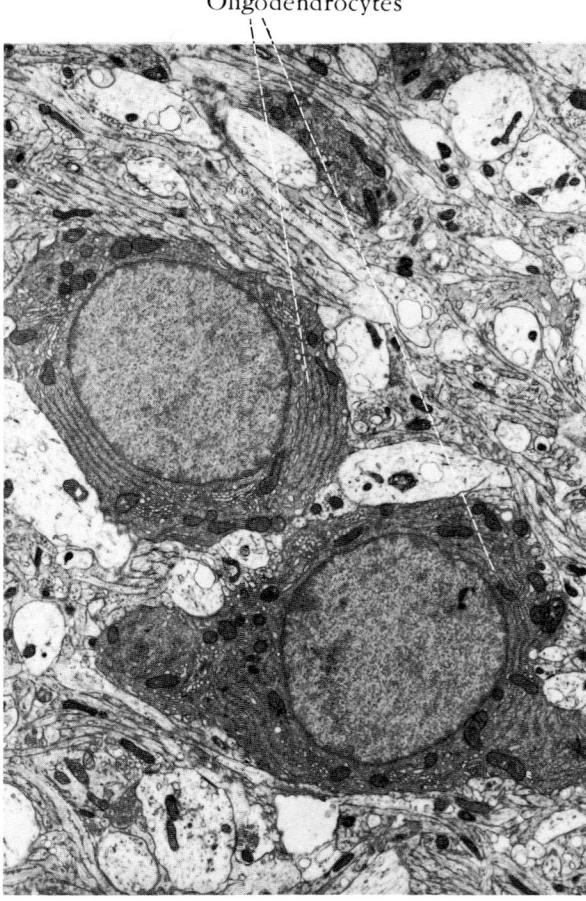

Fig. 7-26. (A) Photomicrograph of a group of oligodendrocytes. (×800.) (B) Electron micrograph of two oligodendrocytes. (Courtesy of Dr. J. M. Kerns.)

neuroglia (Fig. 7-22). Neuroglial cells are usually smaller than nerve cells and outnumber them five to ten times; they make up about half the total volume of the brain and spinal cord.

There are four types of neuroglial cells: astrocytes, oligodendrocytes, microglia, and ependyma (see Fig. 7-22).

Astrocytes

Astrocytes have small cell bodies with branching processes that extend in all directions. Many of the processes of these cells end in expansions on blood vessels (perivascular feet), on ependymal cells, and on the pia mater. There are two types of astrocytes, fibrous and protoplasmic.

Fibrous astrocytes are found mainly in the white matter, where their processes ramify among the nerve fibers (Fig. 7-23). Each process is long, slender, smooth, and not highly branched. The cell bodies and processes contain many filaments, which course through the cytoplasm.

Protoplasmic astrocytes are found mainly in the gray

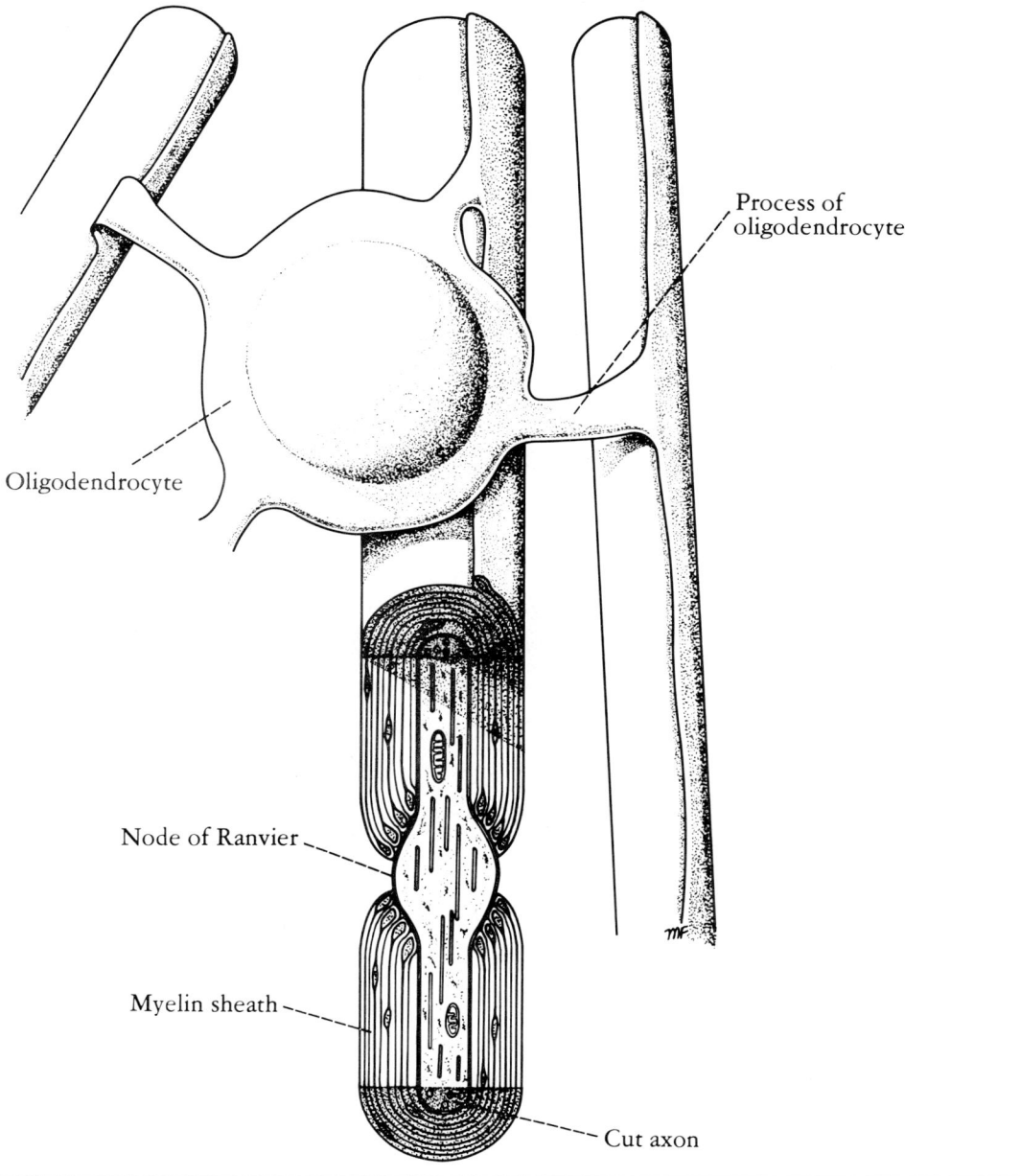

Fig. 7-27. Single oligodendrocyte with processes continuous with the myelin sheaths of four nerve fibers within the central nervous system.

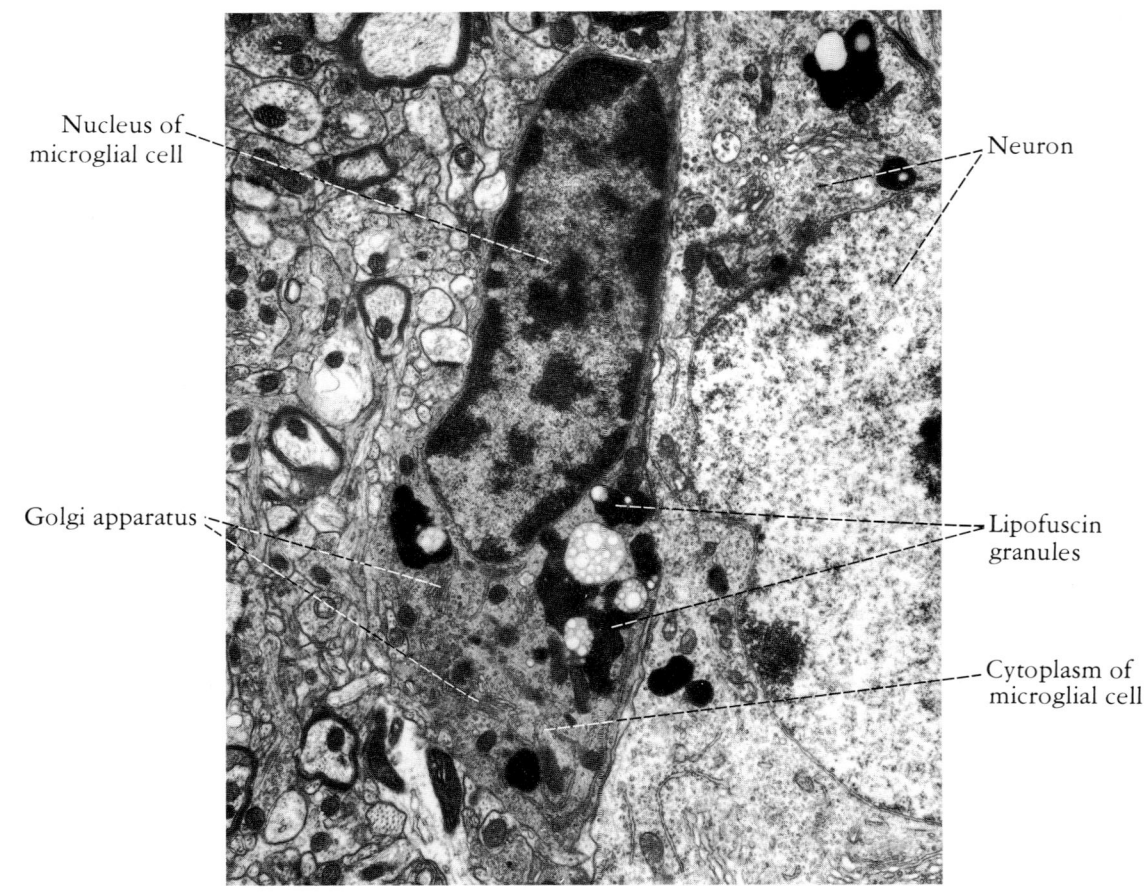

Fig. 7-28. Electron micrograph of a microglial cell in the cerebral cortex. (Courtesy of Dr. A. Peters.)

matter, where their processes ramify among the nerve cell bodies (Figs. 7-24 and 7-25). The processes are shorter, thicker, and more branched than those of the fibrous astrocytes. The cytoplasm of these cells contains fewer filaments than that of the fibrous astrocytes.

Oligodendrocytes

Oligodendrocytes have smaller cell bodies than do astrocytes and a few delicate processes. The filaments prominent in astrocytic cytoplasm are absent. Oligodendrocytes are frequently found in rows along nerve fibers or surrounding nerve cell bodies (Fig. 7-26). In electron micrographs, the processes of these cells are continuous with the myelin sheaths of the nerve fibers, and it is believed that the myelin of the central nervous system is formed by oligodendrocytes, much as the myelin of peripheral nerves is formed from Schwann cells (Fig. 7-27; see Fig. 7-30). The processes of a single oligodendrocyte may join the sheaths of more than one nerve fiber.

Microglia

The microglial cells are the smallest of the neuroglial cells and are found scattered throughout the central nervous system (Fig. 7-28). From their small cell bodies arise wavy, branching processes that give off

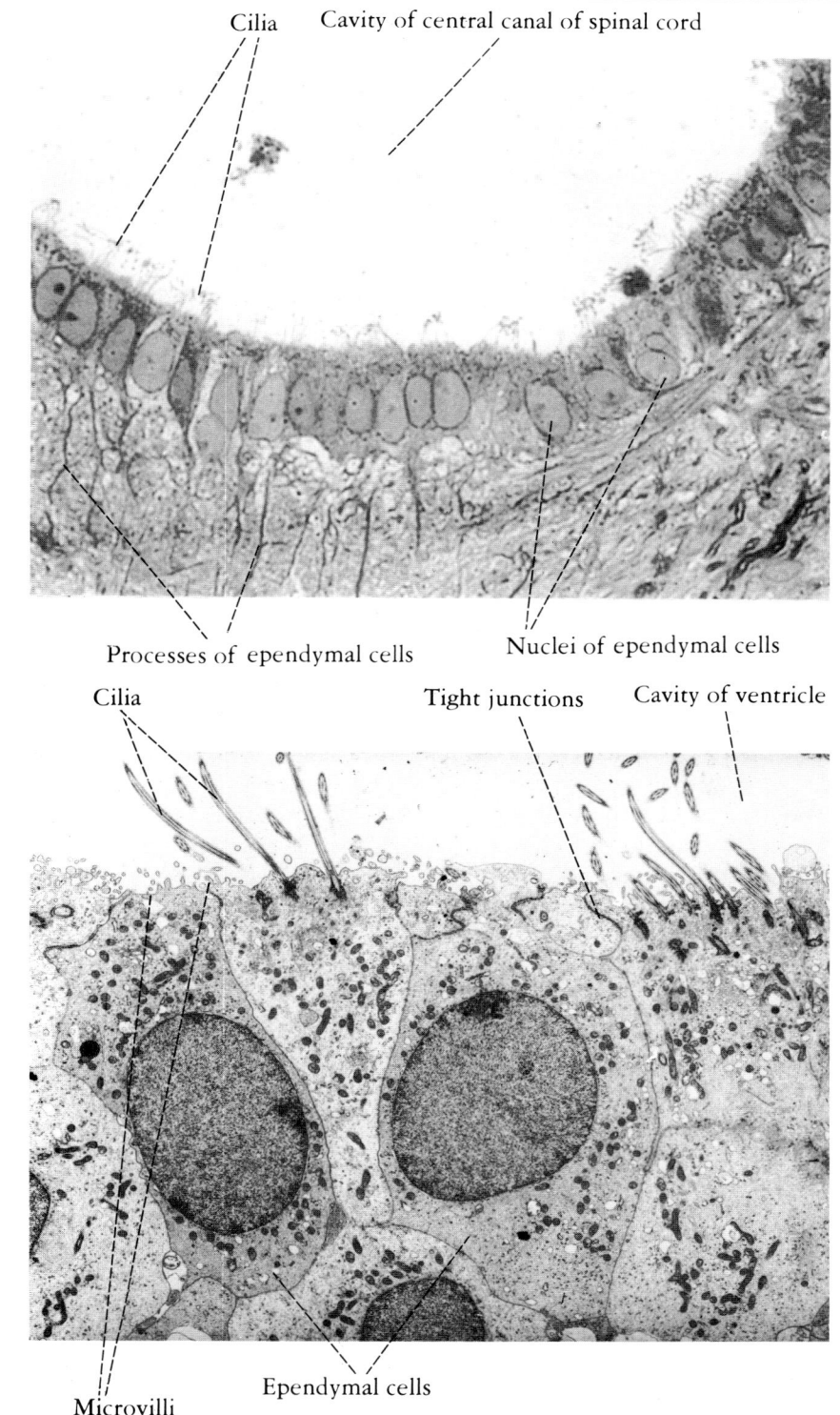

Fig. 7-29. A: Photomicrograph of ependymal cells lining the central canal of the spinal cord. B: Electron micrograph of ependymal cells lining the cavity of the third ventricle. (Courtesy of Dr. J. M. Kerns.)

numerous spinelike projections. Microglial cells are capable of ingesting vital dyes, such as trypan blue, and closely resemble connective tissue macrophages.

Ependyma

Ependymal cells line the cavities of the brain and spinal cord. They form a single layer of cells that are cuboidal and possess microvilli and cilia (Fig. 7-29). The cilia are often motile, and their movement contributes to the flow of the cerebrospinal fluid. The bases of the ependymal cells taper to long processes that branch and ramify among the other cells of the brain. Modified ependymal cells cover the blood vessels of the choroid plexuses.

Function of Neuroglia

Astrocytes, with their ramifying processes, form a supporting framework for nerve cells and nerve fibers within the central nervous system. The observations of Peters and Palay (1965) suggest that astrocytes act as insulators, separating neurons and their processes and preventing axon terminals from influencing neighboring and unrelated receptive neuronal surfaces. The processes may act as barriers to the diffusion of neurotransmitters. Some authors suggest that astrocytes take part in the metabolic activities of neurons. It is possible that metabolites are transported from the capillaries to the neurons through the perivascular feet, or that the byproducts of neuronal metabolism are transported along the same route to the capillary. Glia cells (astrocytes and oligodendrocytes) may interact metabolically with neurons. They may be responsible for absorbing excess K^+ ions and carbon dioxide in the extracellular fluid.

Oligodendrocytes are almost certainly involved in myelin formation, because connections have been demonstrated between myelin sheaths and oligodendrocytes in developing central nervous tissue. Oligodendrocytes are also believed to play a role in regulating the biochemical environment of neurons. This belief largely is based on the fact that these cells commonly are found clustered around neuronal cell bodies.

Microglial cells in the normal brain and spinal cord appear to be inactive. They resemble connective tissue macrophages and become actively phagocytic in disease.

Ependymal cells show branching processes in the basal border that extend radially and support the nervous tissue in the developing nervous system of the embryo. In later embryonic life, the basal processes in most areas are resorbed. The cells are ciliated, and the movements of the cilia help circulate the cerebrospinal fluid within the cavities of the central nervous system. Where the ependymal cells cover the blood vessels of the choroid plexuses, they are thought to have a secretory function and play an active part in the formation of cerebrospinal fluid. The presence of microvilli on the free surfaces of ependymal cells suggests that they also have an absorptive function.

NERVE FIBERS AND PERIPHERAL NERVES

Nerve Fibers

A nerve fiber is an axon (or a dendrite) of a nerve cell. The structure of axons and dendrites is described on pages 241 and 243. Bundles of nerve fibers found in the central nervous system are often referred to as *nerve tracts;* bundles of nerve fibers found in the peripheral nervous system are called peripheral nerves.

Two types of nerve fibers are present in the central and peripheral parts of the nervous system: myelinated and nonmyelinated fibers.

Myelinated Nerve Fibers

A myelinated nerve fiber is one that is surrounded by a myelin sheath. The myelin sheath is not part of the neuron but is formed by a supporting cell (Figs. 7-30 and 7-31). In the central nervous system, the supporting cell is called the oligodendrocyte; in the peripheral nervous system, it is called a Schwann cell.

The myelin sheath is a segmented, discontinuous layer interrupted at regular intervals by the nodes of Ranvier. Each segment of the myelin sheath is approximately 0.5 to 1 mm long. In the central nervous system, each oligodendrocyte may form and maintain myelin sheaths for as many as sixty nerve

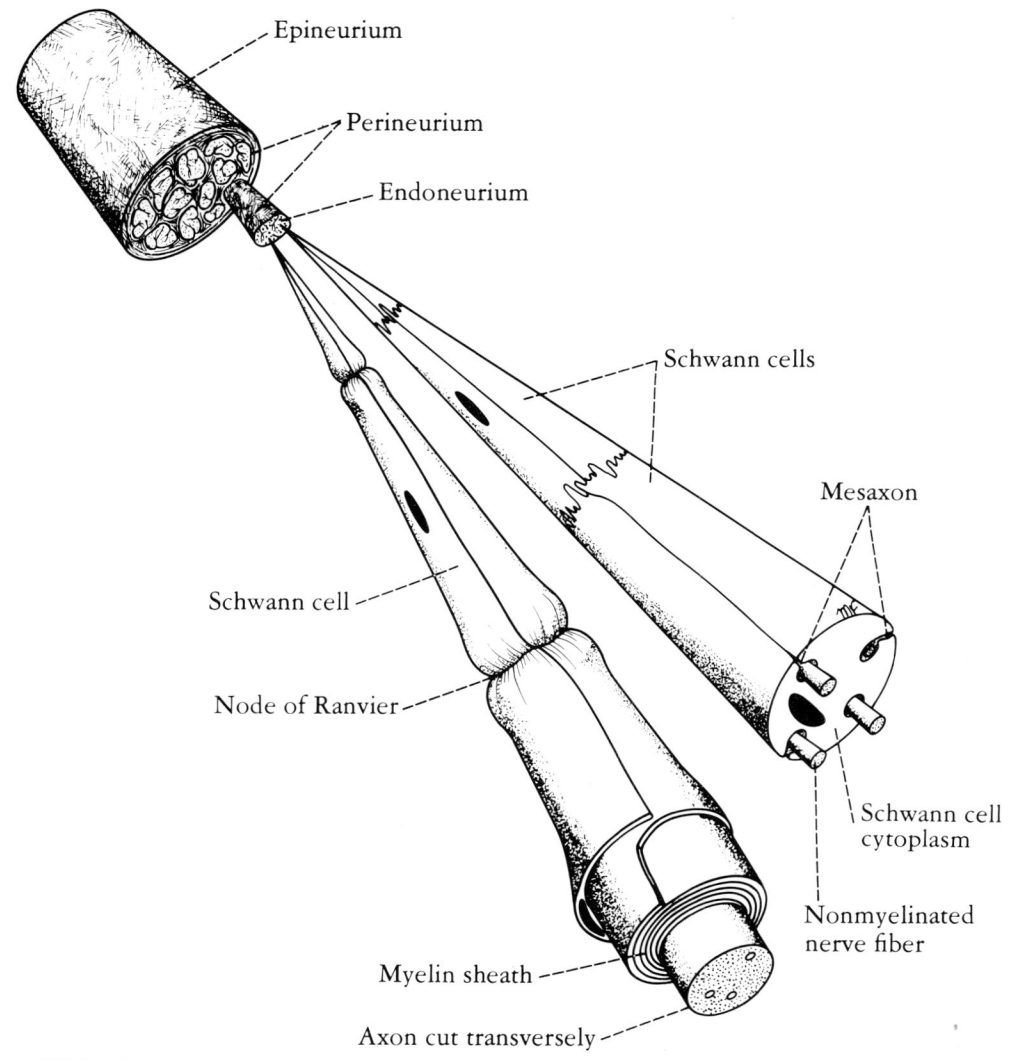

Fig. 7-30. Peripheral nerve. Note the connective tissue sheaths and the structure of myelinated and nonmyelinated nerve fibers.

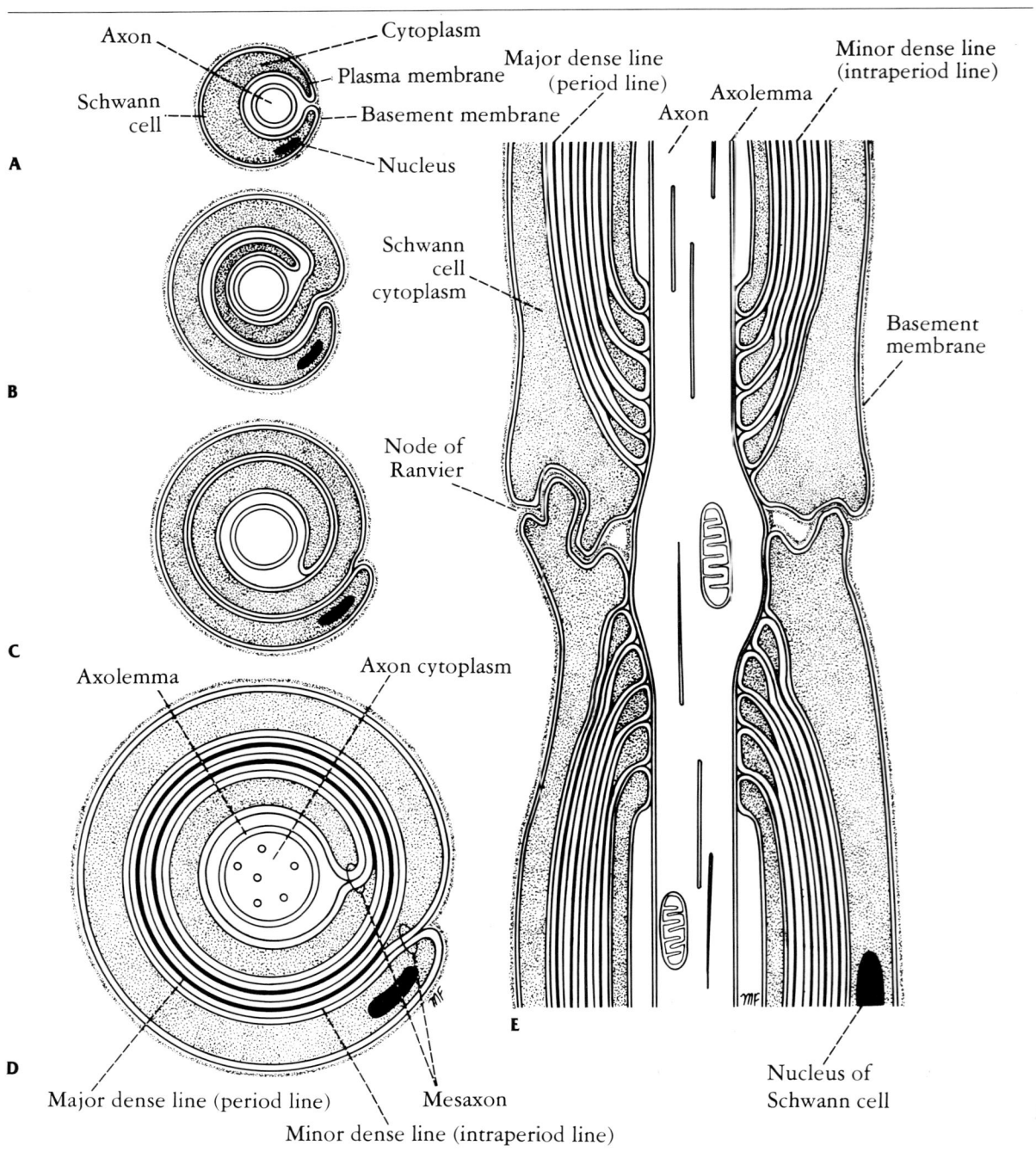

Fig. 7-31. Myelinated nerve fiber in a peripheral nerve. (A, B, C, D) Cross sections at different stages in the formation of the myelin sheath; (E) longitudinal section of a mature myelinated nerve fiber, showing a node of Ranvier.

fibers (axons). In the peripheral nervous system, there is usually only one Schwann cell for each segment of a single nerve fiber.

FORMATION OF MYELIN. Myelin sheaths begin to form during later fetal development and the first postnatal year. The process has been studied with the electron microscope.

In the *peripheral nervous system,* the nerve fiber or axon first indents the side of a Schwann cell (see Fig. 7-31). Later, as the axon sinks farther into the Schwann cell, the plasma membrane of the Schwann cell forms a *mesaxon,* which suspends the axon within the Schwann cell. Subsequently, it is thought, the Schwann cell rotates on the axon, so that the plasma membrane becomes wrapped repeatedly around the axon in a spiral. The spiral is clockwise in some segments and counterclockwise in others. At first, the wrappings are loose, but gradually the cytoplasm between the layers of the cell membrane disappears, leaving cytoplasm near the surface and in the region of the nucleus. The wrappings become tight with maturation of the nerve fiber. The thickness of the myelin depends on the number of spirals of Schwann cell membrane. Some nerve fibers are surrounded by only a few turns of the membrane; others have as many as fifty turns. In electron micrographs of cross sections of mature myelinated nerve fibers, the myelin is seen to be laminated (Figs. 7-32 and 7-33). Each lamella is 13 to 18 nm thick. The dark *major dense line,* about 2.5 nm thick, consists of two inner protein layers of the plasma membrane fused together. The lighter *minor dense line,* about 10 nm thick, is formed by the approximation of the outer surfaces of adjacent plasma membranes and is composed of lipid. The fused outer protein layers of the plasma membranes are very thin and form a thin intraperiod line situated in the center of the lighter lipid layer (Fig. 7-34; see Fig. 7-33).

The *incisures of Schmidt-Lanterman* are seen on longitudinal sections of myelinated nerve fibers (Fig. 7-35). They represent areas where the dark major dense line is not formed, as a result of the localized persistence of Schwann cell cytoplasm. This persistence of cytoplasm involves all the layers of the myelin, and thus there is a continuous spiral of cytoplasm from the outermost region of the Schwann cell to the region of the axon. This spiral of cytoplasm may provide a pathway for the conduction of metabolites from the surface region of the Schwann cell to the axon.

In the *central nervous system,* oligodendrocytes are believed to be responsible for the formation of the myelin sheaths. The plasma membrane of the oligodendrocyte becomes wrapped around the axon, and the number of layers will determine the thickness of the myelin sheath (see Fig. 7-27). The nodes of Ranvier are situated in the intervals between adjacent oligodendrocytes. A single oligodendrocyte may be connected to the myelin sheaths of as many as sixty nerve fibers. Moreover, a single oligodendrocyte may be associated with many nonmyelinated fibers (discussed later). For these reasons, the process of myelination in the central nervous system cannot take place by rotation of the oligodendrocyte on the axon, as the Schwann cell does in the peripheral nervous system. It is possible that myelination in the central nervous system occurs by the growth in length of the mesaxon of the oligodendrocyte, the mesaxon wrapping itself around the axon. There are incisures of Schmidt-Lanterman in nerve fibers of the central nervous system.

Nonmyelinated Nerve Fibers

The smaller axons of the central nervous system, the postganglionic axons of the autonomic part of the nervous system, and some fine sensory axons associated with the reception of pain are nonmyelinated.

In the *peripheral nervous system,* each axon, which is usually less than 1 μm in diameter, indents the surface of the Schwann cell so that the axon lies within a trough (Fig. 7-36; see Fig. 7-30). As many as fifteen or more axons may share a single Schwann cell, each lying within its own trough or sometimes sharing a trough. In some situations, the troughs are deep and the axons are deeply embedded in the Schwann cells, forming a mesaxon from the Schwann cell plasma membrane (see Fig. 7-30). The

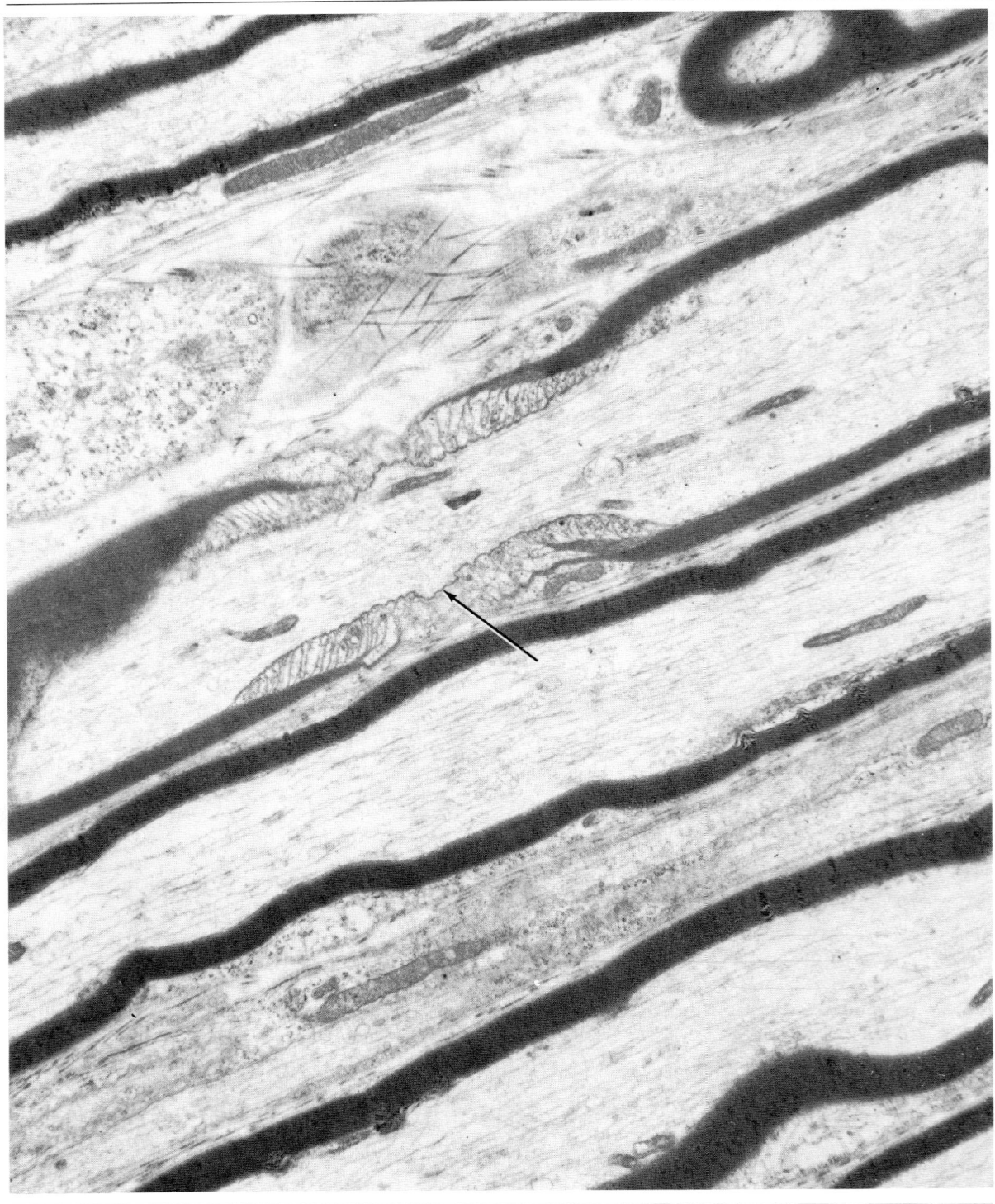

Fig. 7-32. Electron micrograph of a longitudinal section of several myelinated axons, showing the structure of a node of Ranvier (arrow). At the node, two adjacent Schwann cells terminate and the myelin sheaths become thinner by the turning off of the lamellae. Note the many microtubules and microfilaments within the axons. (×12,220.) (Courtesy of Dr. H. de F. Webster.)

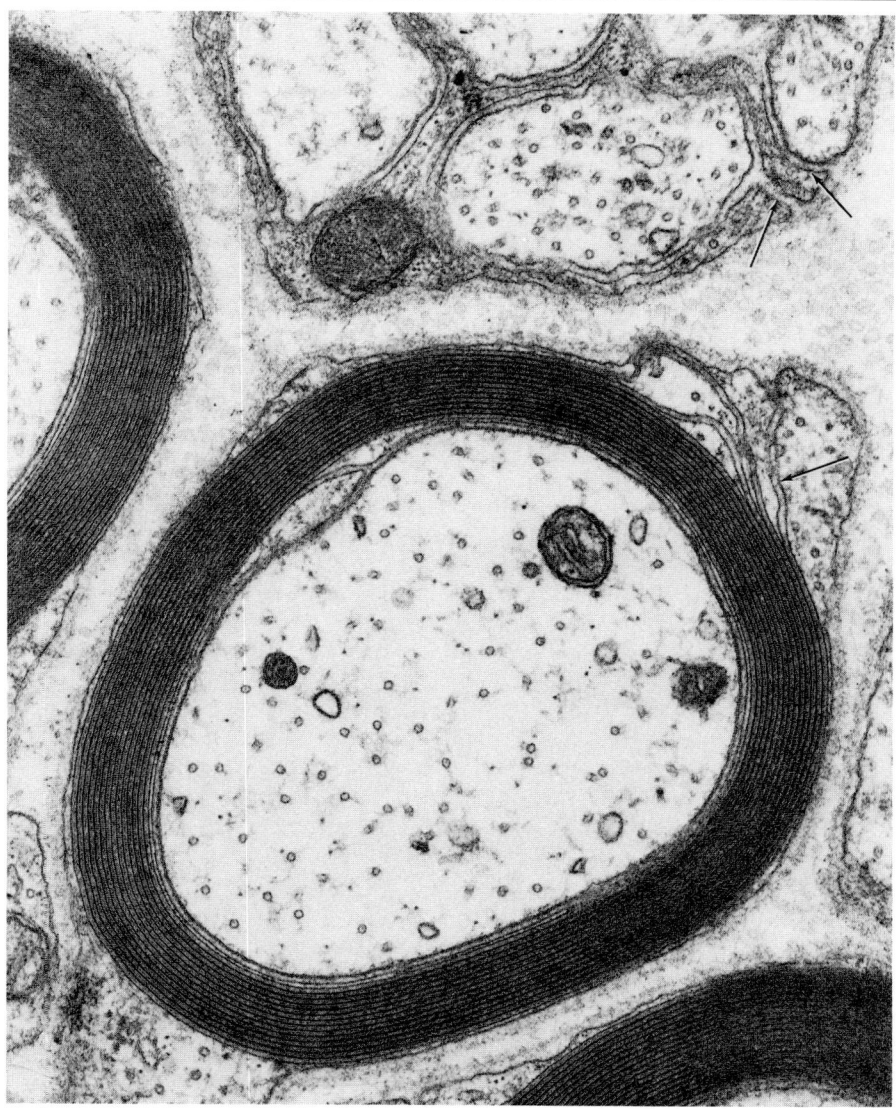

Fig. 7-33. *Electron micrograph of a transverse section of a peripheral nerve, showing a myelinated axon with spiral myelin lamellae (center). Note the mesaxon (arrow). Parts of two other myelinated fibers are also shown. A number of unmyelinated axons are enclosed in the peripheral cytoplasm of a Schwann cell (top). The mesaxons are indicated by arrows. (×28,000.) (Courtesy of Dr. H. de F. Webster.)*

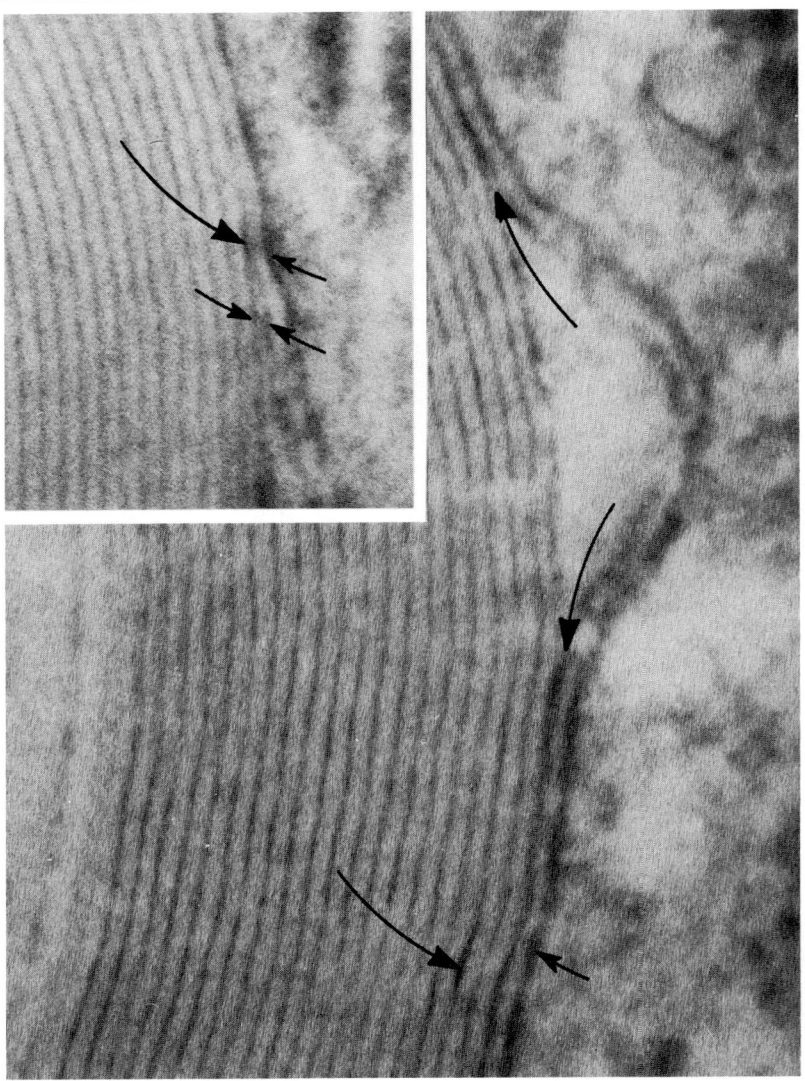

Fig. 7-34. Electron micrograph of a cross section of a myelinated peripheral nerve fiber, showing the immunocytochemical localization of myelin basic protein (small arrows). These immunostained cytoplasmic leaflets fuse to form the major dense lines (large arrows) of compact myelin. (×226,667.) (Courtesy of Dr. F. X. Omlin and colleagues.)

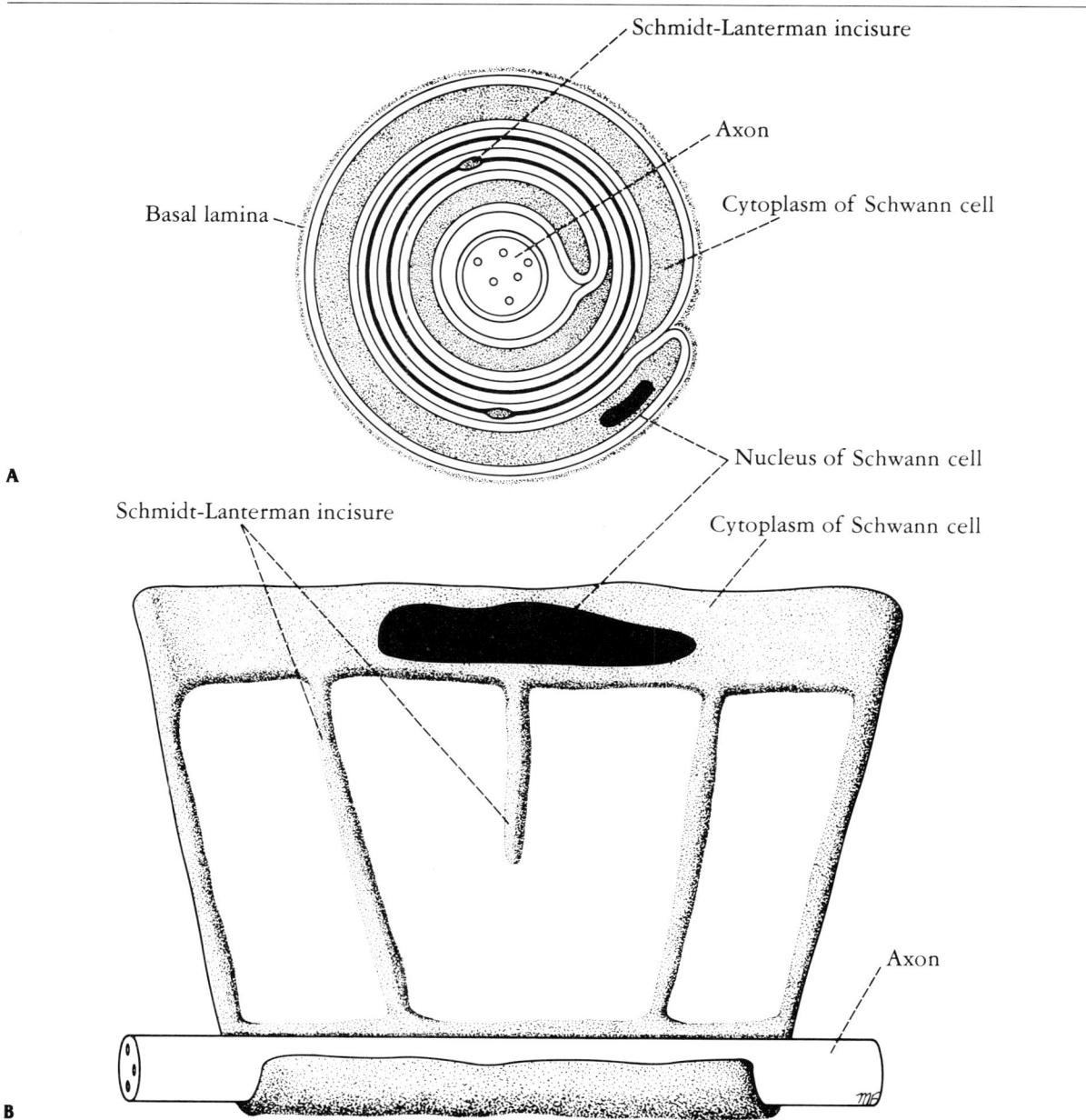

Fig. 7-35. Explanation of the Schmidt-Lanterman incisures in the myelin sheath of a peripheral nerve. (A) Transverse section of a myelinated nerve fiber; (B) myelinated nerve fiber in which the myelin sheath has been unrolled.

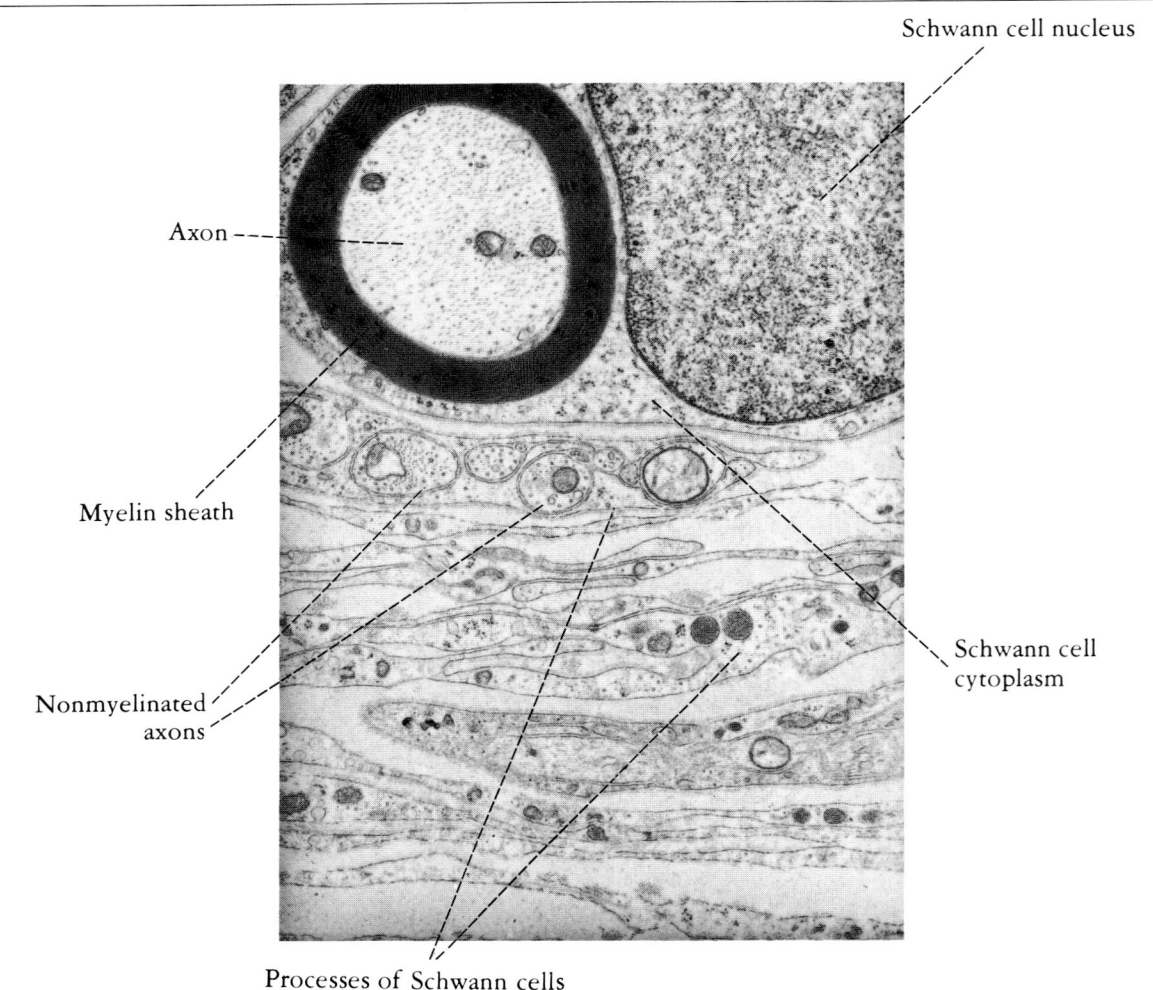

Fig. 7-36. *Electron micrograph of a transverse section of a myelinated nerve fiber and several nonmyelinated nerve fibers. (Courtesy of Dr. J. M. Kerns.)*

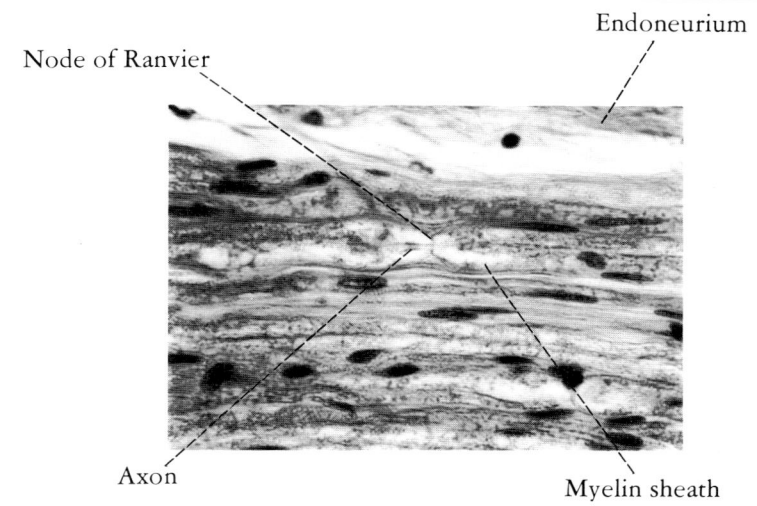

Fig. 7-37. Photomicrograph of a longitudinal section of a peripheral nerve, showing a node of Ranvier. (H&E; ×400.)

axons run from one Schwann cell to another, with a series of such cells occurring along the lengths of the axons. There are no nodes of Ranvier.

In areas where there are synapses or where motor transmission occurs, the axon emerges from the trough of the Schwann cell for a short distance, thus exposing the active region of the axon.

In the *central nervous system*, a single oligodendrocyte is related to one or several axons (see Fig. 7-27), and it is possible that they indent the plasma membrane.

Peripheral Nerves

The peripheral nerves are the cranial and spinal nerves. Each peripheral nerve consists of parallel bundles of nerve fibers that may be efferent or afferent axons, may be myelinated or nonmyelinated, and are surrounded by connective tissue sheaths (Figs. 7-37 and 7-38).

The nerve trunk is surrounded by a dense connective tissue sheath called the *epineurium* (see Fig. 7-30). Within the sheath are bundles of nerve fibers, each of which is surrounded by a connective tissue sheath called the *perineurium*. Between the individual nerve fibers is a loose, delicate connective tissue referred to as the *endoneurium*. The connective tissue sheaths support the nerve fibers and their associated blood vessels and lymphatic vessels.

Peripheral nerve fibers may be classified into three groups, depending on their site and speed of conduction:

Group A fibers are 1 to 22 μm in diameter and conduct at the rate of 5 to 120 m per second. They are myelinated, somatic, efferent or afferent fibers.

Group B fibers are 1 to 3 μm in diameter and conduct at 3 to 15 m per second. They are myelinated, efferent, preganglionic, autonomic fibers.

Group C fibers are 0.3 to 1.3 μm in diameter and conduct at 0.5 at 2 m per second. They are nonmyelinated, afferent or efferent, postganglionic, sympathetic fibers.

Spinal Nerves and Spinal Nerve Roots

There are thirty-one pairs of spinal nerves, which leave the spinal cord and pass through intervertebral foramina in the vertebral column. Each spinal nerve is connected to the spinal cord by two roots: the *anterior root* and the *posterior root* (Fig. 7-39). The anterior root consists of bundles of nerve fibers carrying nerve impulses away from the central nervous

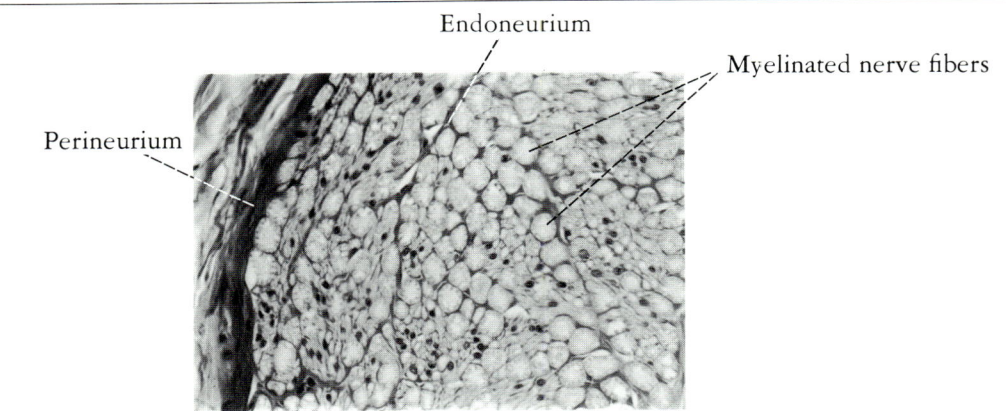

Fig. 7-38. Photomicrograph of a transverse section of a peripheral nerve, showing the perineurium, the endoneurium, and many myelinated nerve fibers. (H&E; ×275.)

system; these nerve fibers are called *efferent* fibers. The posterior root consists of bundles of nerve fibers carrying nerve impulses to the central nervous system; these nerve fibers are called *afferent* fibers. Because these afferent fibers are concerned with conveying information to the central nervous system, they are called *sensory* fibers. The cell bodies of these nerve fibers are situated in a swelling on the posterior root called the *posterior root ganglion*.

Cranial Nerves

There are twelve pairs of cranial nerves (see Fig. 7-39), which leave the brain and pass through foramina in the skull. Some of these nerves are composed entirely of afferent nerve fibers that bring sensations to the brain (olfactory, optic, and vestibulocochlear); others are composed entirely of efferent fibers (oculomotor, trochlear, abducent, accessory, and hypoglossal), and the remainder possess both afferent and efferent fibers (trigeminal, facial, glossopharyngeal, and vagus).

Ganglia

SENSORY GANGLIA. The sensory ganglia of the posterior spinal nerve roots and of the trunks of the trigeminal, facial, glossopharyngeal, and vagal cranial nerves have the same structure. Each ganglion is surrounded by a layer of connective tissue that is continuous with the epineurium and perineurium of the peripheral nerve. The neurons are unipolar, possessing cell bodies that are rounded or oval (Fig. 7-40). The cell bodies tend to be aggregated and separated by bundles of nerve fibers. A single non-myelinated process leaves each cell body and, after a convoluted course, bifurcates at a T junction into peripheral and central branches. The peripheral axon terminates in a series of dendrites in a peripheral sensory ending, and the central axon enters the central nervous system. On reaching the T junction, the nerve impulse passes directly from the peripheral axon to the central axon, thus bypassing the nerve cell body.

Each nerve cell body is closely surrounded by a layer of flattened cells called *capsular cells* or *satellite cells* (see Fig. 7-40). The capsular cells are similar in structure to Schwann cells and are continuous with these cells as they envelop the peripheral and central processes of each neuron.

AUTONOMIC GANGLIA. The autonomic ganglia are situated at a distance from the central nervous system. They are found in the sympathetic trunks, in prevertebral autonomic plexuses—for example, in the cardiac, celiac, and mesenteric plexuses—and as terminal ganglia in or close to viscera. Each ganglion

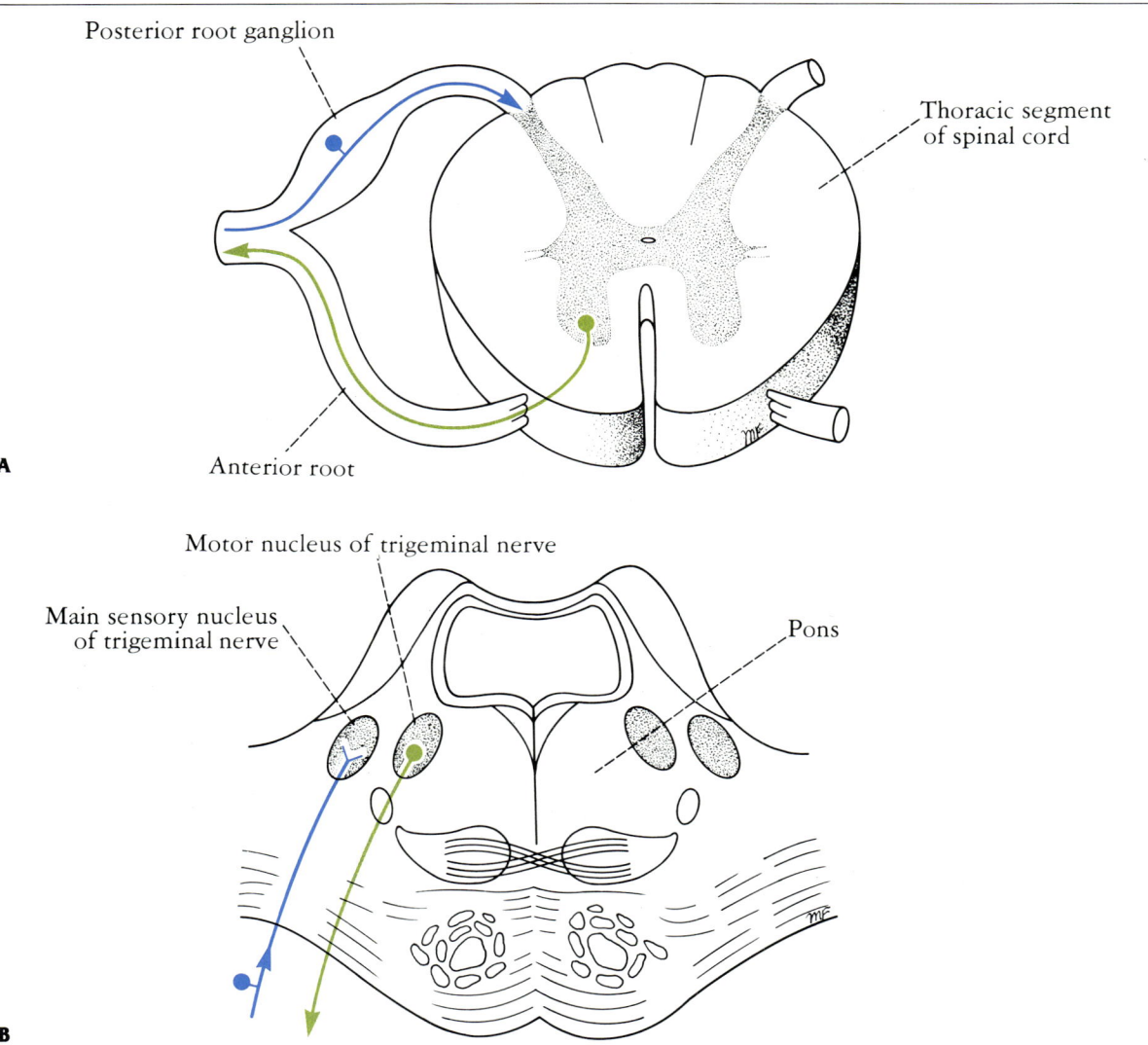

Fig. 7-39. (A) Transverse section of the thoracic region of the spinal cord, showing the formation of a spinal nerve from the union of an anterior and a posterior nerve root. (B) Transverse section of the pons of the hind brain showing the sensory and motor roots of the trigeminal nerve.

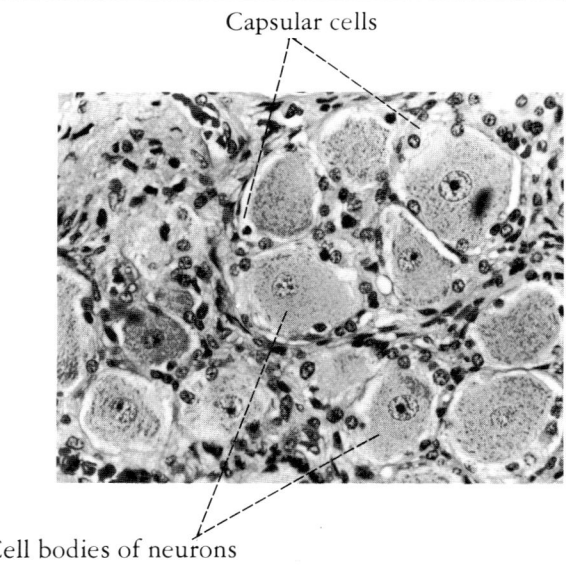

Cell bodies of neurons

Capsular cells

Fig. 7-40. Photomicrograph of longitudinal section of posterior root ganglion of spinal nerve. (H&E; ×400.)

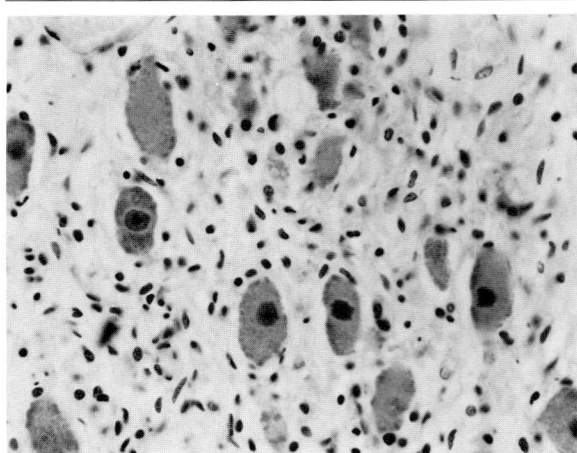

Fig. 7-41. Photomicrograph of longitudinal section of ganglion of the sympathetic trunk. (H&E; ×300.)

is surrounded by a layer of connective tissue that is continuous with the epineurium and perineurium of the peripheral nerve. The neurons are multipolar and possess irregularly shaped cell bodies (Fig. 7-41). The dendrites of the neurons make synaptic connections with the axons of preganglionic neurons. The axons of the neurons are of small diameter (C fibers) and nonmyelinated, and they pass to viscera, blood vessels, and sweat glands.

Each nerve cell body is closely surrounded by a layer of flattened cells called *capsular cells* or *satellite cells*. The capsular cells, like those of sensory ganglia, are similar in structure to Schwann cells and are continuous with them as they envelop the peripheral and central processes of each neuron.

Conduction in Peripheral Nerves

Normally, a resting nerve fiber is polarized so that the interior of the fiber is negative to the exterior; the potential difference across the axolemma is called the *resting membrane potential* (Fig. 7-42).

A nerve impulse is a self-propagating wave of electrical negativity that passes along the surface of the axolemma. To initiate this wave of electrical negativity, an adequate stimulus must be applied to the surface of the neuron. Such a stimulus alters the permeability of the membrane to Na^+ ions at the point of stimulation. Na^+ ions now rapidly enter the axon (see Fig. 7-42). The number of positive ions outside the axolemma quickly decreases to zero. The membrane potential therefore is reduced to zero and is said to be depolarized. A typical resting potential is 80 mV, with the outside of the membrane positive to the inside; the action potential is about 40 mV, with the outside of the membrane negative to the inside.

The negatively charged point on the outside of the axolemma now acts as a stimulus to the adjacent positively charged axolemma, and in less than 1 msec, the polarity of the adjacent resting potential is reversed (see Fig. 7-42). The action potential now has moved along the axolemma from the point originally stimulated to the adjacent point on the membrane. It is in this manner that the action potential travels along the full length of a nerve fiber.

As the action potential moves along the nerve fiber, the entry of the Na^+ ions into the axon ceases and the permeability of the axolemma to K^+ ions increases. Now K^+ ions rapidly diffuse out of the

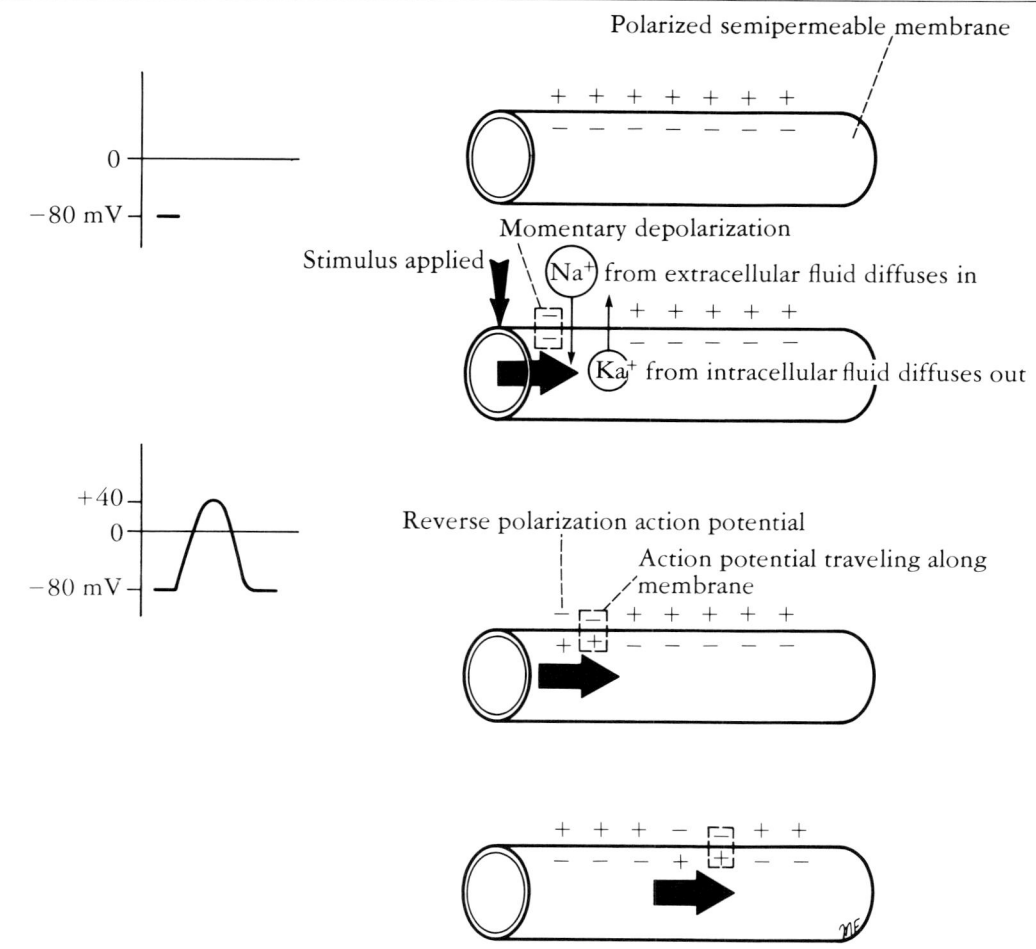

Fig. 7-42. Ionic and electrical changes that occur in a nerve fiber when it is conducting an impulse.

axon (because the concentration is much higher within the axon than outside), so that the original resting membrane potential is restored. The permeability of the axolemma now decreases, and the original state is restored by the active transport of Na^+ ions out of the axon and K^+ ions inward. The outer surface of the axolemma is again electrically positive compared to the inner surface.

For a short time after the passage of a nerve impulse along a nerve fiber, a second stimulus, however strong, cannot excite the nerve. This period of time is called the *absolute refractory period* and is followed by a further short interval during which the excitability of the nerve gradually returns to normal. This latter period is called the *relative refractory period*. Clearly, the refractory period makes a continuous excitatory state of the nerve impossible and limits the frequency of the impulses.

The *conduction velocity* of a nerve fiber is proportional to the cross-sectional area of the axon, the thicker fibers conducting more rapidly than those of smaller diameter. In the large motor fibers (alpha fibers), the rate is 80 to 120 m per second; the smaller sensory fibers have slower conduction rates.

In nonmyelinated fibers, the action potential passes continuously along the axolemma, progressively exciting neighboring areas of membrane (Fig. 7-43). In myelinated fibers, the presence of a myelin sheath serves as an insulator. Consequently, a myelinated nerve fiber can be stimulated only at the nodes of Ranvier. In these fibers, the action potential jumps from one node to the next (see Fig. 7-43). The action potential at one node sets up a current in the surrounding tissue fluid that quickly produces depolarization at the next node. This leaping of the action potential from one node to the next is referred to as *saltatory conduction*. It is a more rapid mechanism than is found in nonmyelinated fibers (see Fig. 7-43).

Sensory Nerve Endings

Receptors or sensory endings are found throughout the body in both somatic and visceral areas. It is fortunate that they are so widely distributed, because they enable the human subject to react to changes in the external and internal environment. Sensory endings may be classified by structure into nonencapsulated and encapsulated receptors.

NONENCAPSULATED RECEPTORS. *Free Nerve Endings*. Free nerve endings are widely distributed throughout the body (Fig. 7-44). They are found in the epithelia of the skin, cornea, and alimentary tract and in connective tissues, including the dermis, fascia, ligaments, joint capsules, tendons, periosteum, perichondrium, haversian systems of bone, tympanic membrane, and dental pulp. They are also present in muscle.

The afferent nerve fibers from free nerve endings are either myelinated or nonmyelinated and are always of small diameter. The terminal endings are devoid of a myelin sheath, and there are no Schwann cells covering their tips.

Although free nerve endings are commonly thought to be pain receptors because they are the only reception areas found in the cornea and the pulp of the teeth, areas of the body where pain is so often experienced, there is little scientific evidence to support this claim. Touch sensation also has been ascribed to these endings.

Merkel's Discs. Merkel's discs are found in hairless skin—for example, the fingertips (Figs. 7-45 and 7-46)—and in hair follicles. Essentially, they consist of free nerve endings derived from a dermal plexus of nerves that pass into the epidermis and terminate as disc-shaped expansions. Each expansion lies in contact with a single enlarged, dark-staining epithelial cell in the deeper part of the epidermis called the *tactile cell*. These corpuscles are presumed to be sensitive to touch.

Nerve Endings Related to Hair Follicles. All hair follicles are innervated from a plexus of nerves situated in the dermis, and myelinated nerve fibers reach the follicles from different directions (Fig. 7-47). The nerve fibers divide into branches below the duct of the sebaceous gland, and myelinated terminals wind around the follicle in its outer connective tissue sheath. Many naked axon filaments terminate among the cells of the outer root sheath. The hair acts as a lever, and any slight movement of the free end of the hair readily stimulates the axon filaments in the hair follicle. These nerve endings are extremely sensitive to touch, and they are therefore the main tactile organs in hairy skin.

ENCAPSULATED RECEPTORS. These receptors show wide variations in size and shape, but they have one common feature: the termination of the nerve is covered by a capsule.

Meissner's Corpuscles. Meissner's corpuscles, which are found in the dermal papillae of the skin (Figs. 7-48 and 7-49), are most numerous in the skin of the fingers, the palmar surface of the hand, and the plantar surface of the foot. Many also are present in the skin of the nipple and the external genitalia. The corpuscles are ovoid or cylindrical and are about 100 μm long and 50 μm wide. Each consists of a stack of flattened cells arranged transversely across the long axis of the corpuscle, enclosed by a capsule that is continuous with the endoneurium of the nerves that enter it. A few myelinated nerve fibers enter the deep end of the corpuscle; the majority lose their myelin sheaths, decrease in size, and

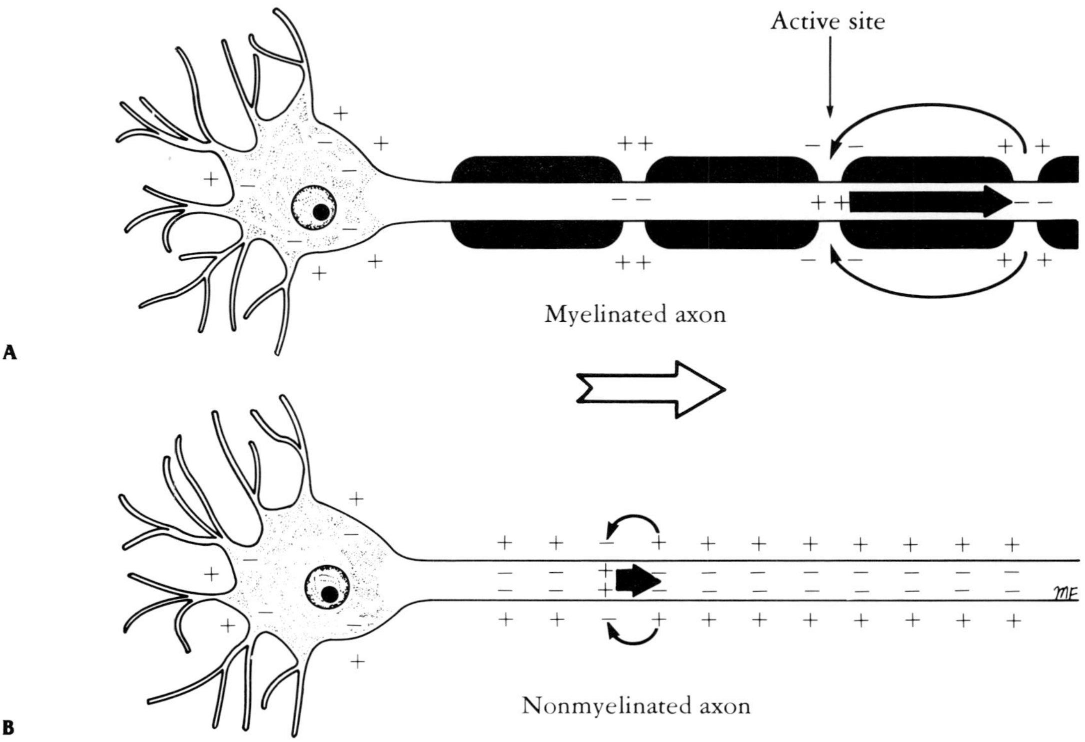

Fig. 7-43. Electrical changes that occur in (A) a stimulated myelinated axon and (B) a stimulated nonmyelinated axon.

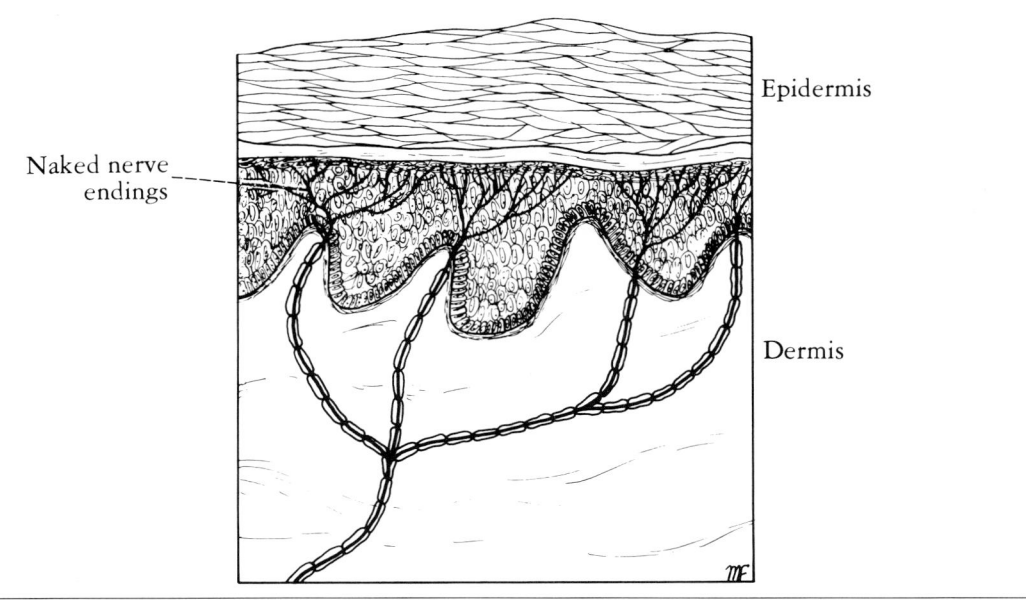

Fig. 7-44. Arrangement of free nerve endings in the skin. Note that the nerve fibers in the epidermis are naked.

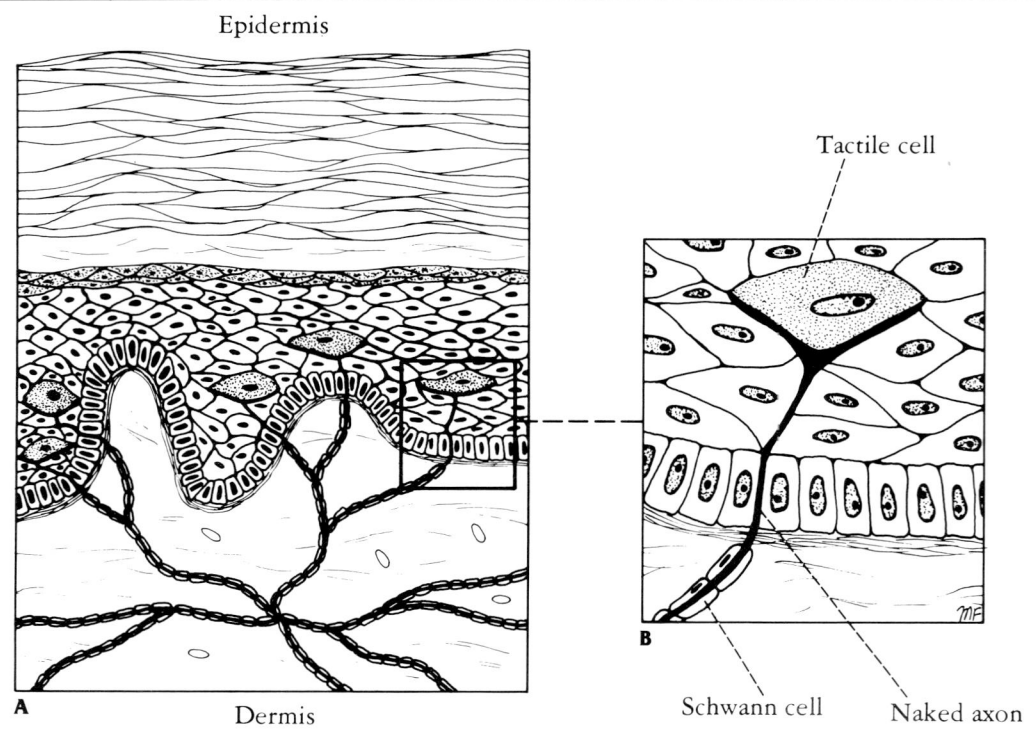

Fig. 7-45. *Merkel's discs in the skin.* (A) Low magnification. (B) Note expanded end of axon with stippled tactile cell.

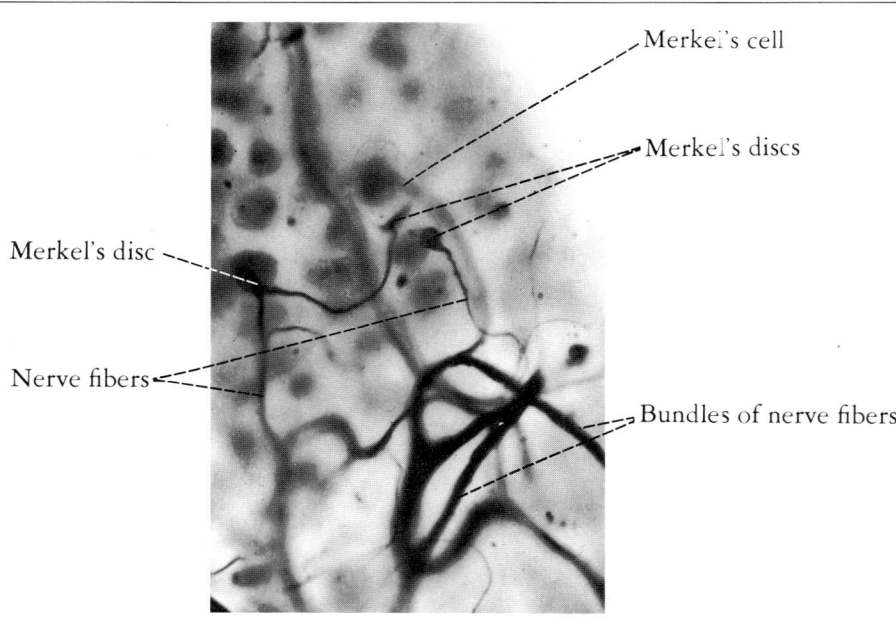

Fig. 7-46. *Photomicrograph of digital skin, showing nerve terminals ending in Merkel's discs.* (Silver stain.) (Courtesy of Dr. N. Cauna.)

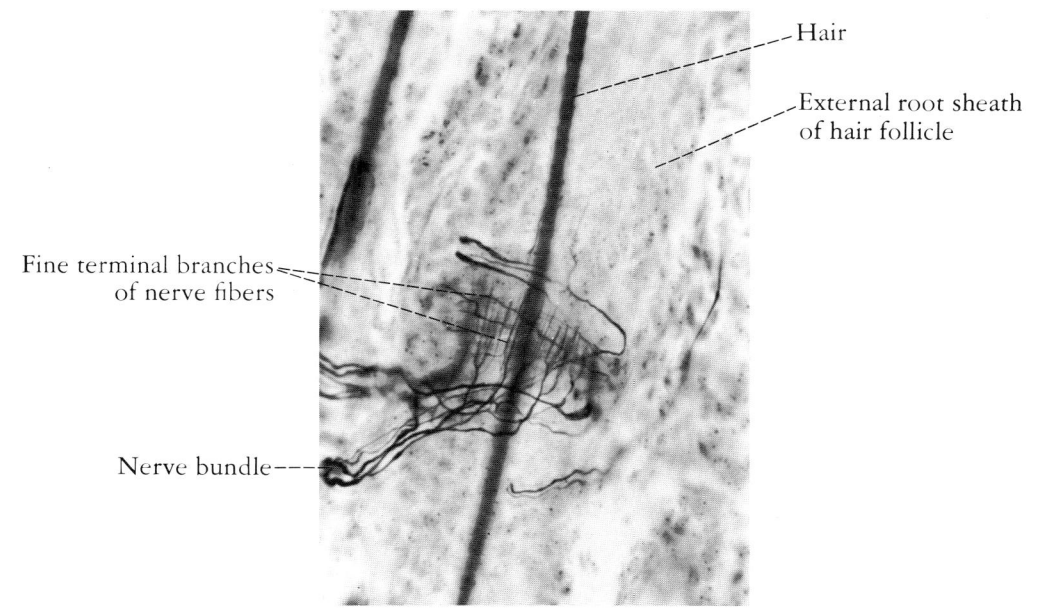

Fig. 7-47. Photomicrograph of nerve endings around hair follicle. (Silver stain.) (Courtesy of Dr. M. J. T. Fitzgerald.)

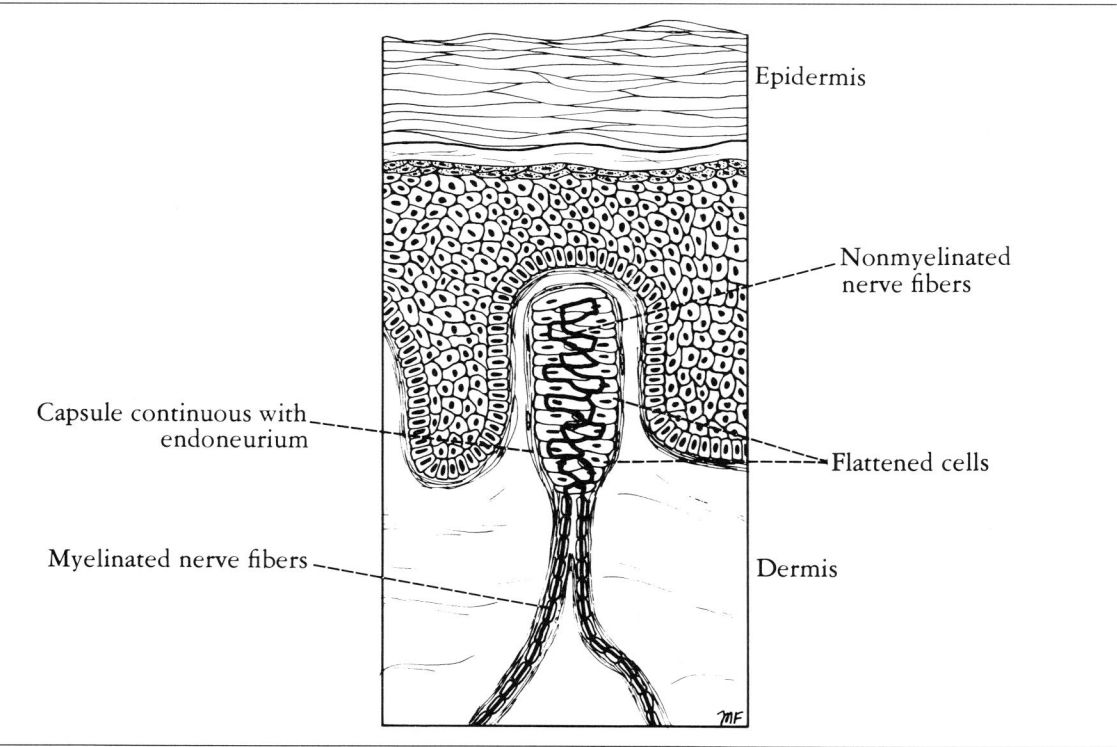

Fig. 7-48. Detailed structure of a Meissner's corpuscle in the skin.

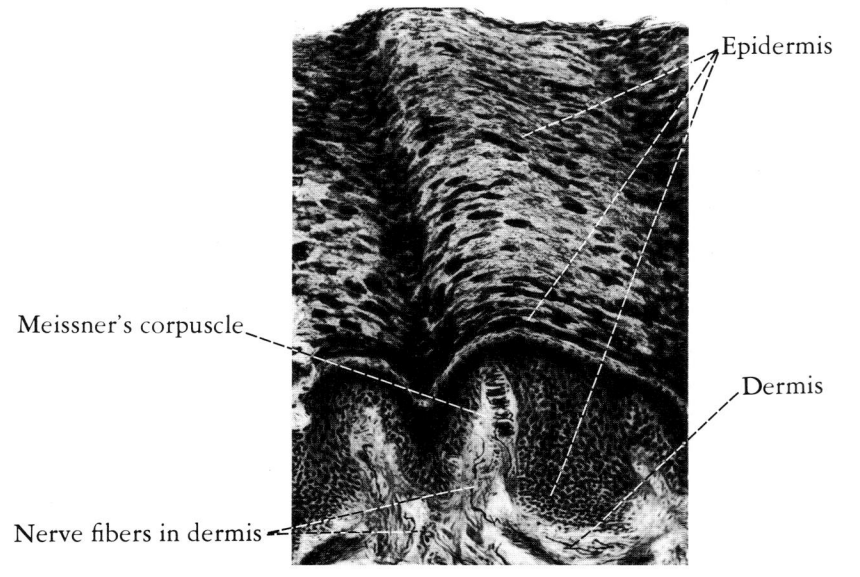

Fig. 7-49. Photomicrograph of a Meissner's corpuscle in the skin. (Silver stain.) (Courtesy of Dr. N. Cauna.)

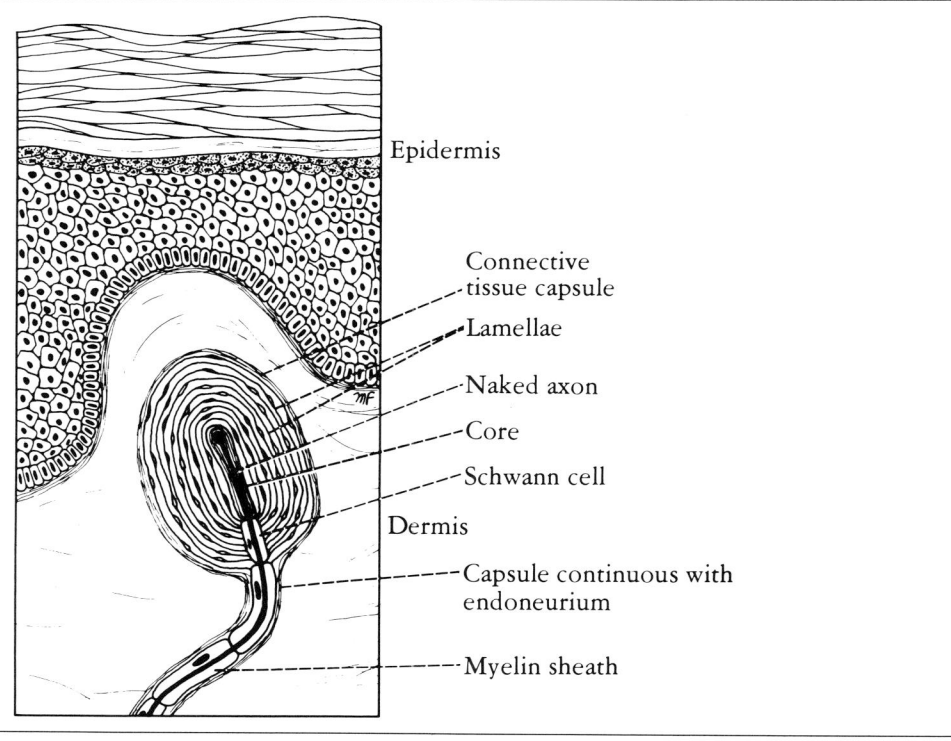

Fig. 7-50. Detailed structure of a Pacinian corpuscle in the skin.

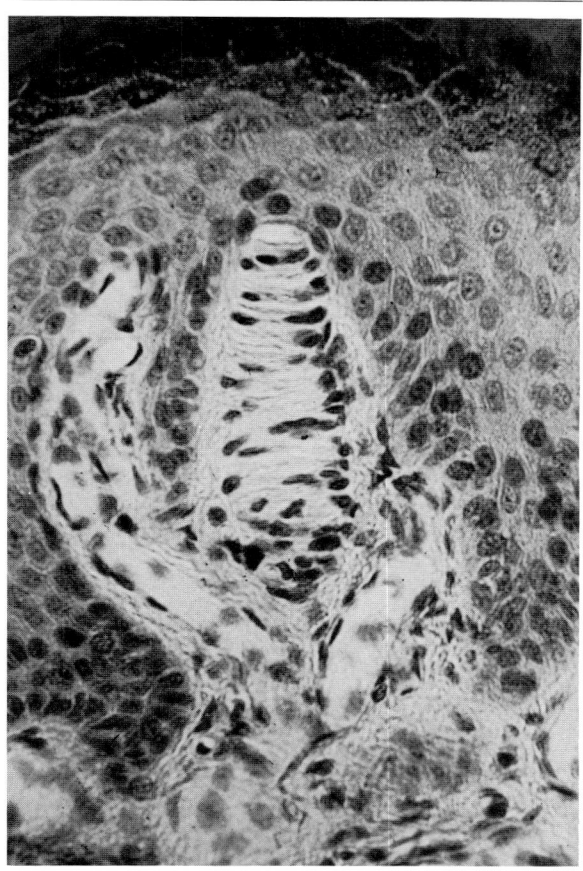

Fig. 7-51. Photomicrograph of a Pacinian corpuscle in the skin.

ramify among the epithelial cells. The nerve fibers never lose their covering of Schwann cells.

Meissner's corpuscles are believed to be extremely sensitive to touch and enable an individual to distinguish between two pointed structures when they are placed close together on the skin (two-point tactile discrimination). There is considerable reduction in their number with increasing age.

Pacinian Corpuscles. These corpuscles (Figs. 7-50 and 7-51) are widely distributed throughout the body and are abundant in the dermis, subcutaneous tissue, ligaments, joint capsules, pleura, peritoneum, nipples, and external genitalia. Each corpuscle is ovoid, measuring up to 4.5 mm long and 1 to 2 mm wide, and consists of a cylindrical core surrounded by numerous concentric lamellae. On section, the corpuscle resembles a sliced onion.

A large myelinated nerve fiber enters one pole of the corpuscle. First, it loses its myelin sheath and, shortly thereafter, its Schwann cell covering. The naked axon then passes through the center of the core and terminates in an expanded end. The naked axon contains numerous mitochondria. The nerve axon within the core is surrounded by about sixty closely packed lamellae formed of flattened cells. The core is surrounded by thirty or more concentric lamellae of flattened cells, which form the bulk of the corpuscle. Between adjacent lamellae are amorphous material and collagen fibers. On the outer surface of the corpuscle is a condensation of connective tissue forming the capsule, which is continuous with the endoneurium.

Pacinian corpuscles are sensitive to deformation and therefore respond to pressure or tension; they are probably also sensitive to vibration.

Bulbous Corpuscles of Krause. Bulbous corpuscles of Krause are found mainly in microcutaneous regions—for example, the lips and external genitalia (Fig. 7-52). The corpuscle is spheroidal and measures about 50 μm in diameter. It possesses a capsule that is continuous with the endoneurium. A single myelinated nerve fiber on entering the corpuscle loses its myelin and expands. Covered by its Schwann cells, the nerve fiber then branches, becomes coiled, or runs a straight course to terminate as an expanded end. The detailed structure of these corpuscles is subject to considerable variation. The precise function of these receptors is not known.

Neuromuscular Spindles and Neurotendinous Spindles

These structures have been fully described in Chapter 6 (see pp. 210 and 212).

Effector Endings

The motor nerve endings on skeletal, smooth, and cardiac muscle are described on pages 209, 214, and 215.

NERVE ENDINGS ON SECRETORY CELLS. Nonmyelinated postganglionic autonomic nerves extend in

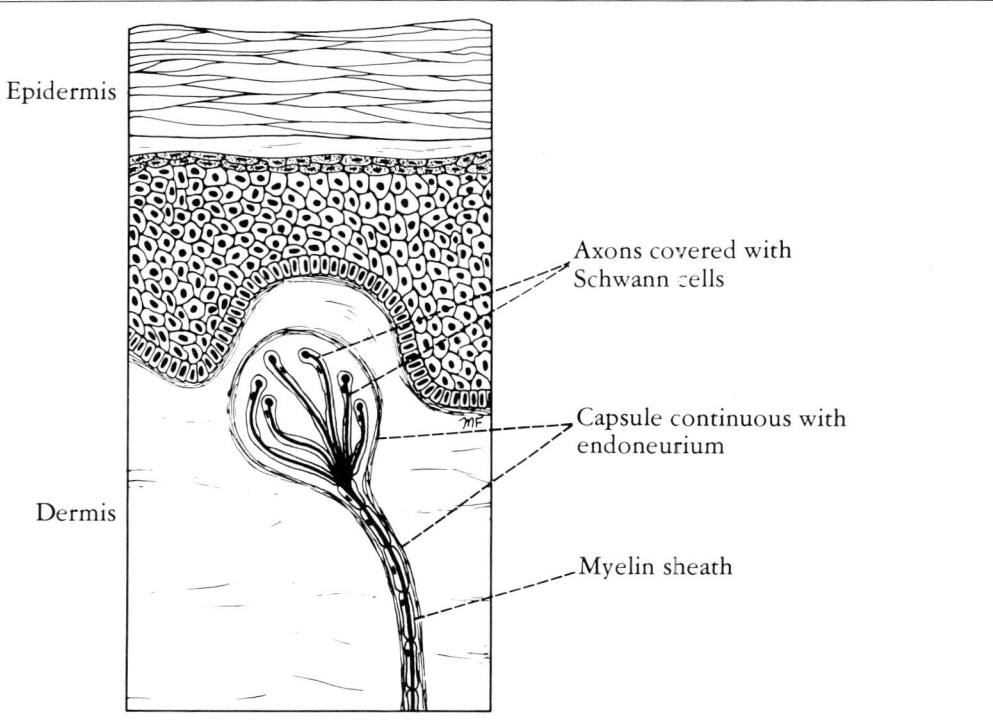

Fig. 7-52. Detailed structure of a bulbous corpuscle of Krause.

the connective tissue of glands and have been reported to ramify between adjacent secretory cells. In many glands, the nerve fibers have been found to innervate only the blood vessels.

NERVE TISSUE IN THE SPINAL CORD, CEREBELLUM, AND CEREBRUM

For a detailed description of the structure and function of these areas of the central nervous system, a textbook of neuroanatomy should be consulted. Only the main histological features will be described here.

Spinal Cord

The spinal cord is roughly cylindrical in shape and is composed of an inner core of gray matter surrounded by an outer covering of white matter (Figs. 7-53 and 7-54).

Gray Matter

Gray matter is seen on cross section as an H-shaped pillar with *anterior* and *posterior gray columns,* or *horns,* united by a thin *gray commissure* containing the small *central canal* (see Fig. 7-53). A small *lateral gray column* or *horn* is located in the thoracic and upper lumbar segments of the cord. The amount of gray matter at any given level of the spinal cord is related to the amount of muscle innervated at that level. Thus, the amount is greatest within the cervical and lumbrosacral enlargements of the cord, which innervate the muscles of the upper and lower limbs, respectively (see Fig. 7-53).

The nerve cells of the gray matter are multipolar, and the neuroglia forms an intricate network around the nerve cell bodies and their neurites. In the anterior gray columns, the majority of the nerve cells are

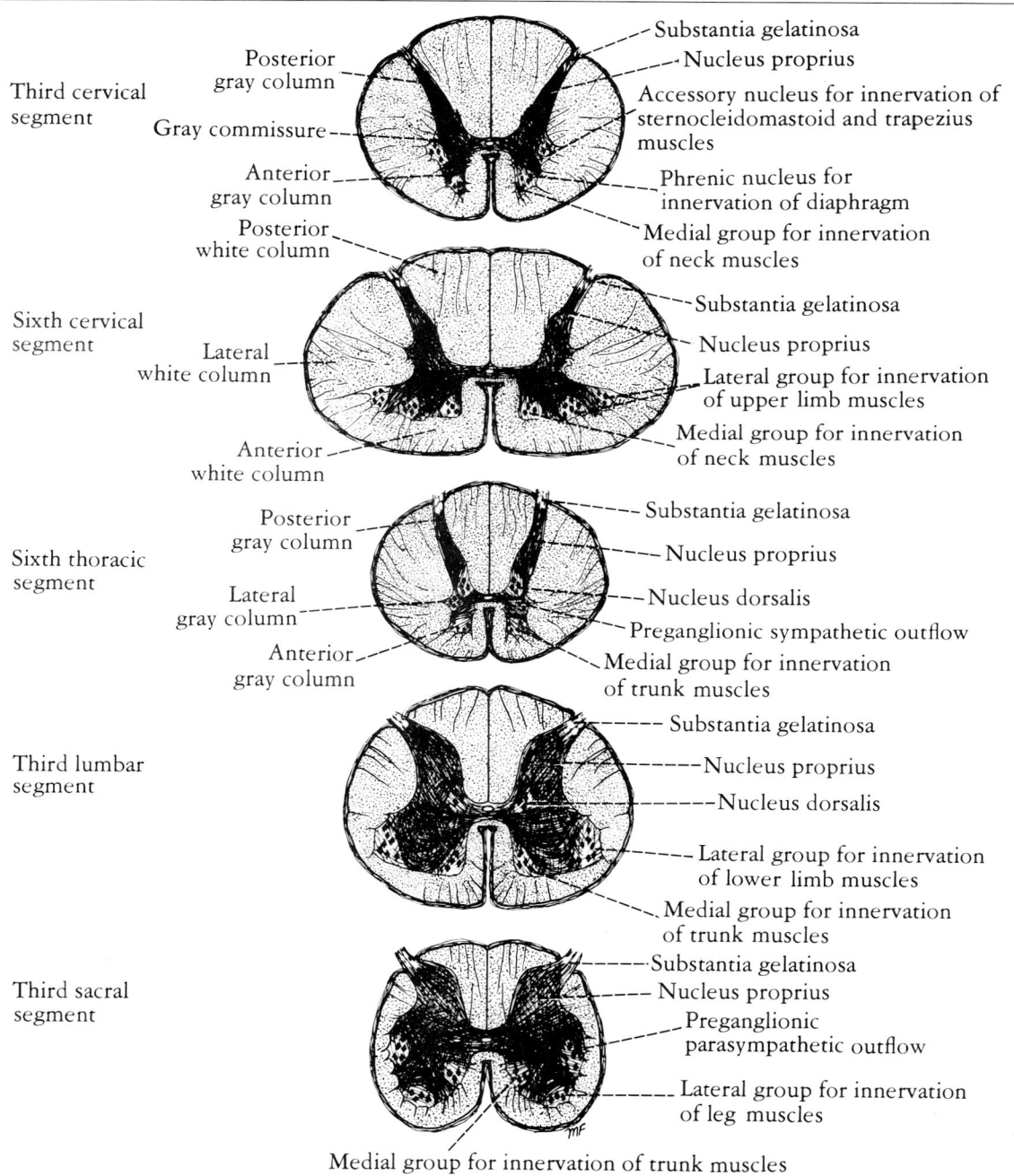

Fig. 7-53. Transverse sections of the spinal cord at different levels, showing the arrangement of the gray matter and white matter.

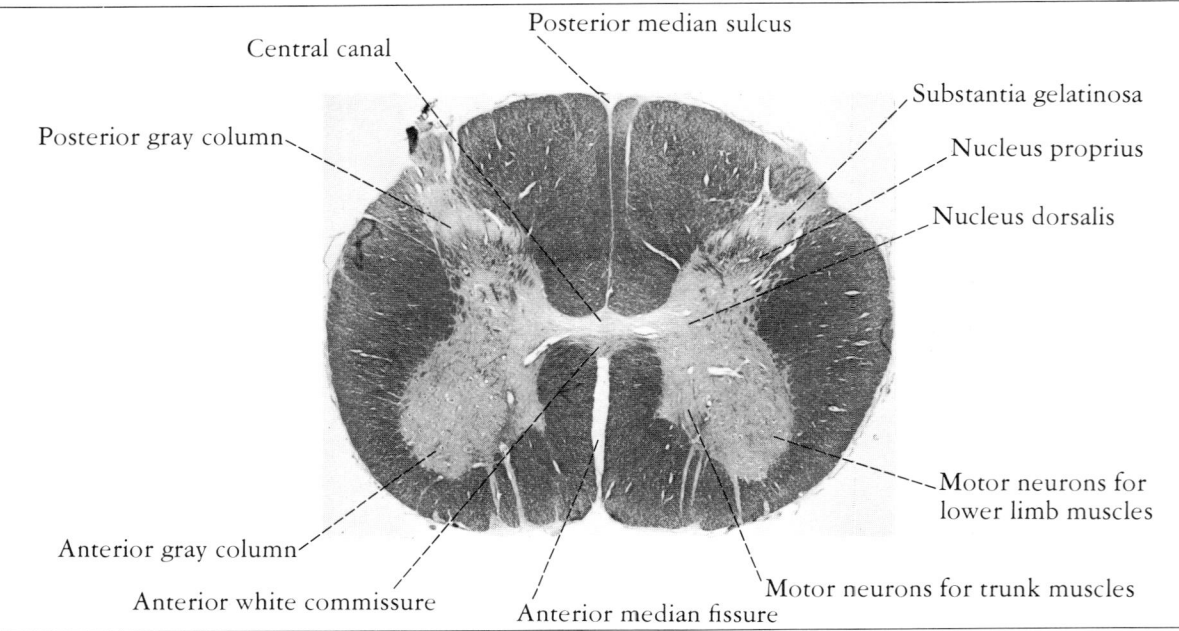

Fig. 7-54. *Photomicrograph of transverse section of the spinal cord at the level of the fourth lumbar segment. (Weigert stain.)*

large, and their axons pass out in the anterior roots of the spinal nerves to innervate skeletal muscles.

White Matter

As in other regions of the central nervous system, the white matter here consists of a mixture of nerve fibers, neuroglia, and blood vessels. It surrounds the gray matter, and its white color is caused by the high proportion of myelinated nerve fibers. The diameter of the nerve fibers varies from less than 1 μm to about 10 μm; fibers of 3 μm or less predominate.

For purposes of description, the white matter can be divided into anterior, lateral, and posterior white columns (see Fig. 7-53). The anterior column on each side lies between the midline and the point of emergence of the anterior nerve roots; the lateral column lies between the emergence of the anterior nerve roots and the entry of the posterior nerve roots; the posterior column lies between the entry of the posterior nerve roots and the midline.

Cerebellum

The cerebellum, the largest part of the hind brain, consists of two *cerebellar hemispheres* joined by a narrow median *vermis*.

The surface, or *cortex*, of the cerebellum contains many folds, separated by numerous transverse fissures. Each fold, or folium, contains a core of white matter covered superficially by gray matter (Fig. 7-55). The gray matter of the cortex can be divided into three layers: (1) an external layer, the *molecular layer*; (2) a middle layer, the *Purkinje cell layer*; and (3) an internal layer, the *granular layer* (see Figs. 7-4 and 7-55).

Molecular Layer

The molecular layer contains two types of neurons: the outer *stellate cell* and the inner *basket cell* (see Fig. 7-55). These neurons are scattered among dendritic arborizations and numerous thin axons that run par-

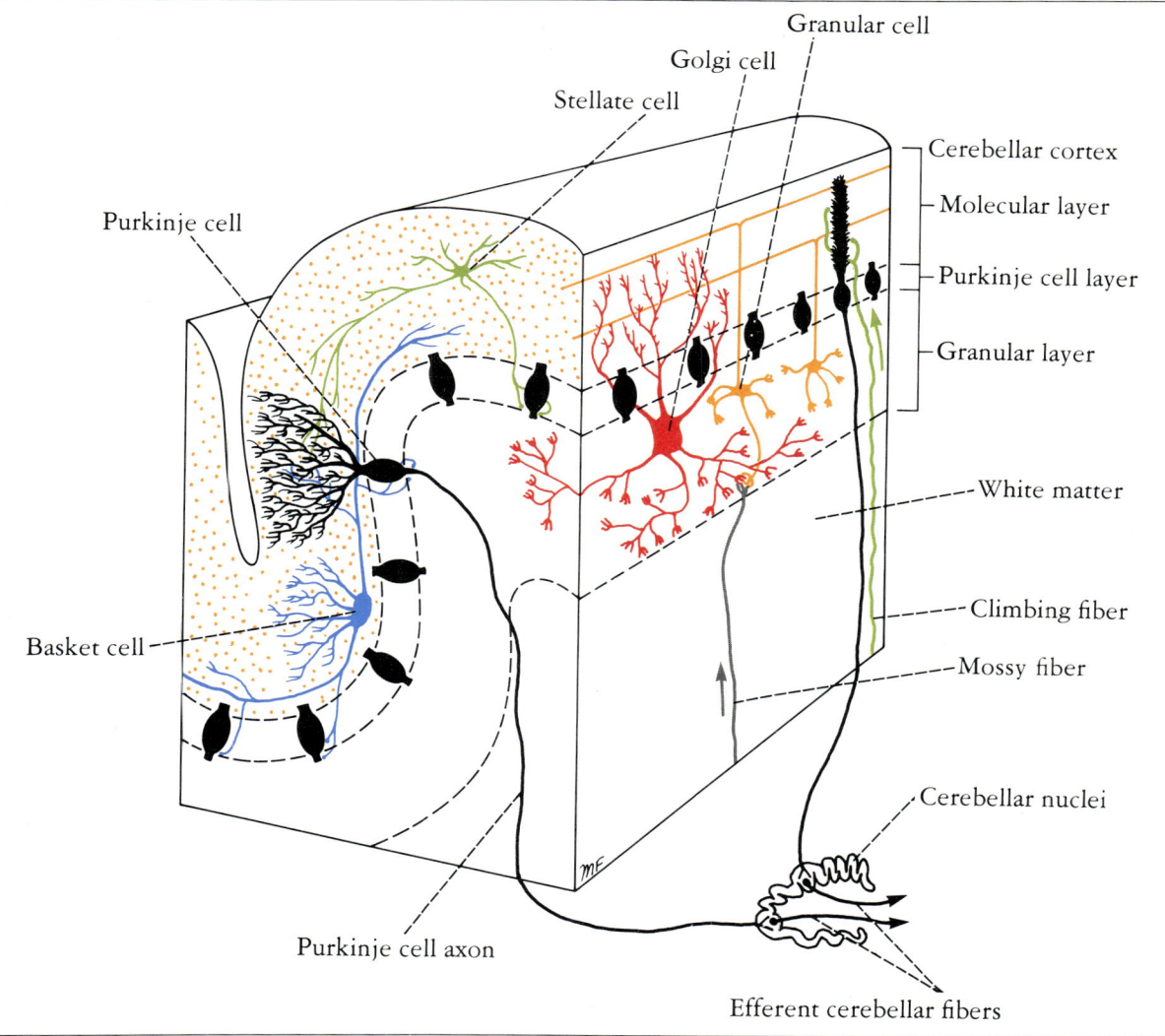

Fig. 7-55. Cellular organization of the cortex of the cerebellum. Note the afferent and efferent fibers.

allel to the long axis of the folia. Neuroglial cells are found between these structures.

Purkinje Cell Layer

The Purkinje cells are large Golgi type I neurons. They are flask-shaped and are arranged in a single layer (see Figs. 7-4 and 7-55). In a plane transverse to the folium, the dendrites of these cells pass into the molecular layer, where they undergo profuse branching (see Figs. 7-4 and 7-55). At the base of the Purkinje cell, the axon arises and passes through the granular layer to enter the white matter.

Granular Layer

The granular layer is packed with small cells with densely staining nuclei and scanty cytoplasm (see Figs. 7-4 and 7-55). Each cell gives rise to four or five dendrites, which make synaptic contact with the afferent mossy fibers. The axon of each granule cell passes into the molecular layer, where it bifurcates at a T junction, the branches running parallel to the long axis of the cerebellar folium (see Fig. 7-55). These fibers, known as *parallel fibers*, run at right angles to the dendritic processes of the Purkinje cells. The majority of the parallel fibers make synaptic contact with the dendrites of the Purkinje cells. Neuroglial cells are found throughout this layer. Scattered throughout the granular layer are Golgi cells (see Fig. 7-55). Their dendrites ramify in the molecular layer, and their axons terminate by splitting into branches that synapse with the dendrites of the granular cells (see Fig. 7-55).

The essential function of the cerebellum is to coordinate, by synergistic action, all reflex and voluntary muscular activity. It permits voluntary movements to take place with precision and economy of effort.

Cerebrum

The cerebral hemispheres are covered with a layer of gray matter, the *cerebral cortex*. Located in the interior of the cerebral hemispheres are the *lateral ventricles*, masses of gray matter, the *basal nuclei*, and nerve fibers. The nerve fibers are embedded in neuroglia and constitute the white matter.

Structure of the Cerebral Cortex

The surface area of the cortex is increased by its *convolutions*, or *gyri*, which are separated by *fissures*, or *sulci*. The cerebral cortex, like gray matter elsewhere in the central nervous system, consists of a mixture of nerve cells, nerve fibers, neuroglia, and blood vessels. The following types of nerve cells are present in the cerebral cortex: (1) pyramidal cells, (2) stellate cells, (3) fusiform cells, (4) horizontal cells of Cajal, and (5) cells of Martinotti (Fig. 7-56).

The *pyramidal cells* take their name from the shape of their cell bodies (see Fig. 7-56). The majority of the cell bodies measure 10 to 50 μm long. There are, however, giant pyramidal cells, also known as *Betz cells*, whose cell bodies measure as much as 120 μm; these are found in the motor precentral gyrus of the frontal lobe.

The apices of the pyramidal cells are oriented toward the surface of the cortex. From the apex of each cell, a thick apical dendrite extends upward toward the surface, giving off collateral branches. From the basal angles, several dendrites pass laterally into the surrounding nervous tissue. The axon arises from the base of the cell body and either terminates in the deeper cortical layers or, more commonly, enters the white matter of the cerebral hemisphere as a projection, association, or commissural fiber.

The *stellate cells*, sometimes called granule cells because of their small size, are polygonal. Their cell bodies measure about 8 μm in diameter (see Fig. 7-56). These cells have multiple branching dendrites and a relatively short axon that terminates on a nearby neuron.

The *fusiform cells* have their long axis perpendicular to the surface and are concentrated mainly in the deepest cortical layers (see Fig. 7-56). Dendrites arise from each pole of the cell body. The inferior dendrite branches within the same cellular layer, whereas the superficial dendrite ascends toward the surface of the cortex and branches in the superficial

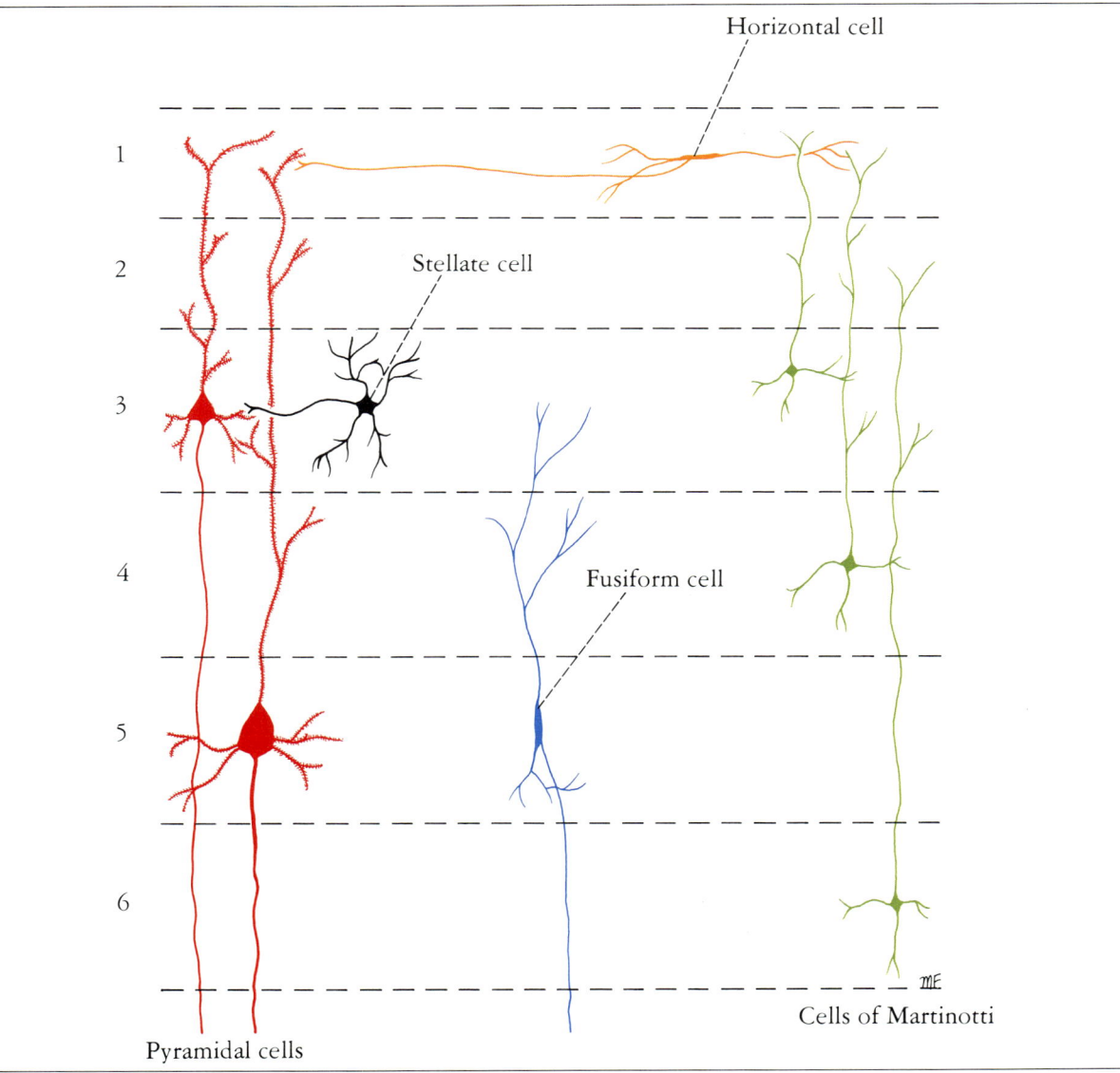

Fig. 7-56. Main types of neurons found in the cerebral cortex.

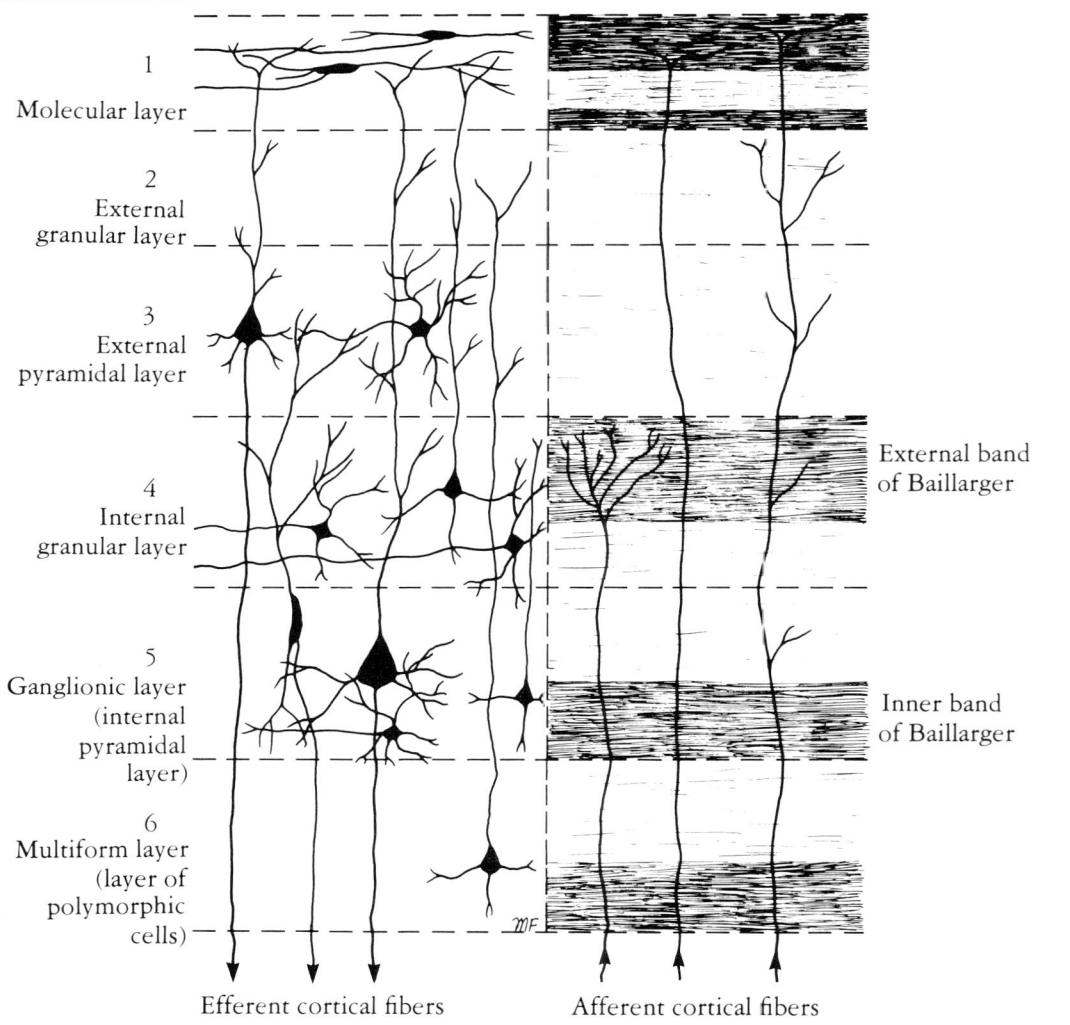

Fig. 7-57. Layers of the cerebral cortex; the neurons are shown on the left and the nerve fibers on the right.

layers. The axon arises from the inferior part of the cell body and enters the white matter as a projection, association, or commisural fiber.

The *horizontal cells of Cajal* are small, fusiform, horizontally oriented cells found in the most superficial layers of the cortex (see Fig. 7-56). A dendrite emerges from each end of the cell, and an axon runs parallel to the surface of the cortex, making contact with the dendrites of pyramidal cells.

The *cells of Martinotti* are small multipolar cells present throughout the levels of the cortex (see Fig. 7-56). The cell has short dendrites, but the axon is directed toward the surface of the cortex, where it ends in a more superficial layer.

For descriptive purposes, the cerebral cortex can be divided into six layers distinguished by the types, density, and arrangement of their cells (Fig. 7-57; see Fig. 7-56). Areas of specialization occur, as, for example, in the motor cortex in the precentral gyrus, where there is a relative absence of granular cells in the second and fourth layers, and in the sensory cortex in the postcentral gyrus, where there is a relative absence of pyramidal cells in the third and fifth layers.

Nerve Fibers of the Cerebral Cortex

The nerve fibers of the cerebral cortex are arranged both radially and tangentially (see Fig. 7-57). The *radial fibers* run at right angles to the cortical surface. They include the afferent entering projection, association, and commissural fibers that terminate within the cortex, and the axons of pyramidal, stellate, and fusiform cells, which leave the cortex to become projection, association, and commissural fibers of the white matter of the cerebral hemisphere.

The *tangential fibers* run parallel to the cortical surface and are for the most part collateral and terminal branches of afferent fibers. They include also the axons of horizontal and stellate cells and collateral branches of pyramidal and fusiform cells. The tangential fibers are most highly concentrated in layer 4 and layer 5, where they are referred to as the outer and inner *bands of Baillarger*, respectively (see Fig. 7-57).

For the mechanisms and functions of the cerebral cortex, the student is referred to a textbook of neuroanatomy.

CLINICAL NOTES

REACTION OF A NEURON TO INJURY

The first reaction of a nerve cell to injury is loss of function. Whether the cell recovers or dies will depend on the severity and duration of exposure to the damaging agent.

Injury to the Nerve Cell Body

If death occurs quickly—for example, in a few minutes from lack of oxygen—no morphological changes will be apparent immediately. Morphological evidence of cell injury requires a minimum of 6 to 12 hours of survival (Robbins and Angell, 1971). The nerve cell becomes swollen and rounded, the nucleus swells and is displaced toward the periphery of the cell, and the Nissl granules become dispersed toward the periphery of the cytoplasm. This phenomenon, which gives the impression that the Nissl substance has disappeared, is known as *chromatolysis* (Fig. 7-58). At this stage, the neuron can recover. If the neuronal injury is not so severe as to cause death, the reparative changes can start. The cell resumes its former size and shape, the nucleus returns to the center of the cell body, and the Nissl granules take up their normal position.

When cell death is imminent or has just occurred, the cell cytoplasm stains dark with basic dyes (hyperchromatism) and the nuclear structure becomes unclear. The final stage occurs after cell death. The cytoplasm becomes vacuolated, and the nucleus and cytoplasmic organelles disintegrate. The neuron now is dissolved and removed by phagocytes. In the central nervous system, this function is performed by the microglial cells; later, the neighboring astrocytes proliferate and replace the neuron with scar tissue. In the peripheral nervous system, the tissue macrophages remove the debris and the local fibroblasts replace the neuron with scar tissue.

Injury to the Nerve Cell Processes

The cytoplasm of a neuron is dependent for its survival on being connected, however indirectly, with the nucleus. The nucleus plays a key role in the synthesis of proteins, which pass into the cell processes and replace proteins that have been metabolized by the cell activity. Thus, the cytoplasm of axons and dendrites will quickly undergo degeneration if these processes are separated from the nerve cell body.

If the axon of the nerve cell is divided, degenerative changes will take place in the distal segment that

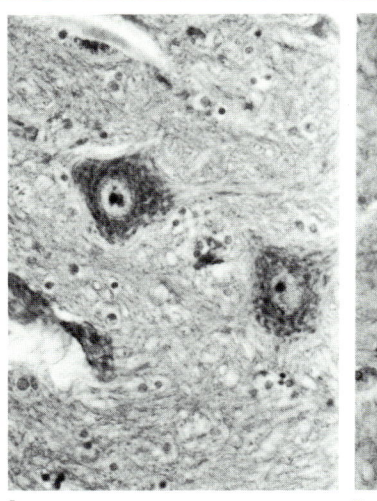 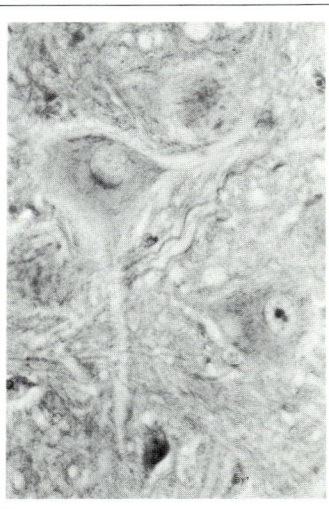

Fig. 7-58. Photomicrographs of motor neurons of the anterior gray column of the spinal cord. (A) shows Nissl substance in normal neurons; (B) shows chromatolysis in motor neurons following section of anterior roots of spinal nerve. (Toluidine blue stain; ×400.)

is separated from the cell body and in a portion of the axon proximal to the injury. Changes may also occur in the cell body from which the axon arises.

Changes in the Distal Segment of the Axon

Changes spread distally from the site of the lesion (Fig. 7-59) and include its terminations; the process is referred to as *wallerian degeneration*. By the third or fourth day, the axon is broken into fragments (see Fig. 7-59), and the debris is digested by the surrounding Schwann cells and tissue macrophages. The entire axon is destroyed within a week.

Meanwhile, the myelin sheath slowly breaks down and lipid droplets appear within the Schwann cell cytoplasm (see Fig. 7-59). Later, the droplets are extruded from the Schwann cell and subsequently are phagocytosed by tissue macrophages. The Schwann cells now begin to proliferate rapidly and become arranged in parallel cords within the persistent basement membrane. The endoneurial sheath and the contained cords of Schwann cells are sometimes referred to as a *band fiber*.

In the central nervous system, degeneration of the axons and myelin sheaths follows a similar course, and the debris is removed by the phagocytic activity of the microglial cells. Little is known about the role of oligodendrocytes in this process.

Changes in the Proximal Segment of the Axon

The changes in the proximal segment of the axon are similar to those that take place in the distal segment (see Fig. 7-59) but extend proximally above the lesion only as far as the first node of Ranvier. The proliferating cords of Schwann cells in the peripheral nerves bulge from the cut surfaces of the endoneurial tubes.

Changes in the Nerve Cell Body from Which the Axon Arises

The changes that can occur in the cell body following injury to its axon are often referred to as *retrograde degeneration*; the changes that take place in the proximal segment of the axon commonly are included under this heading.

The most characteristic change occurs in the cell body within the first 2 days following injury and

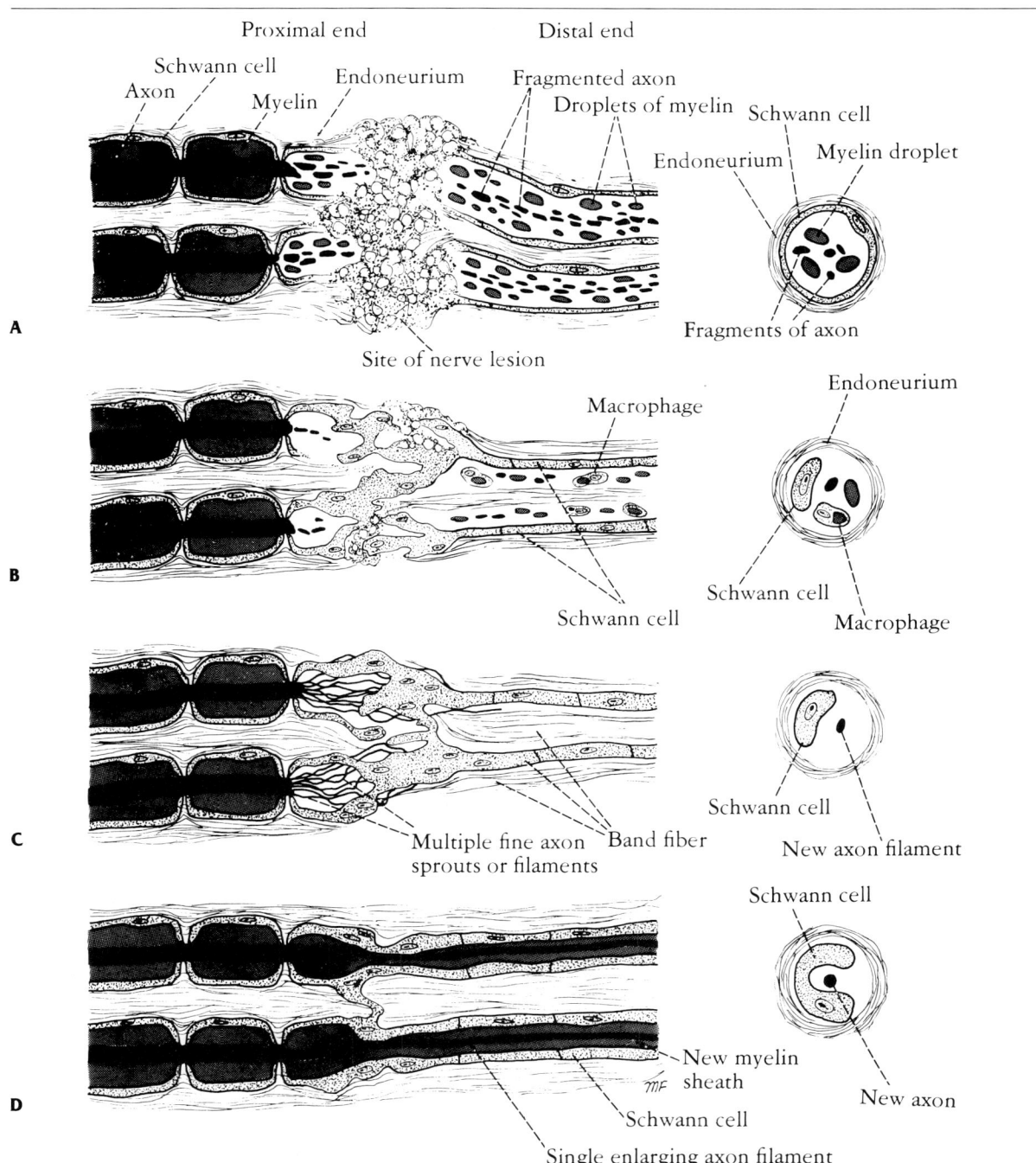

Fig. 7-59. *The main changes during degeneration and regeneration in a divided peripheral nerve.*

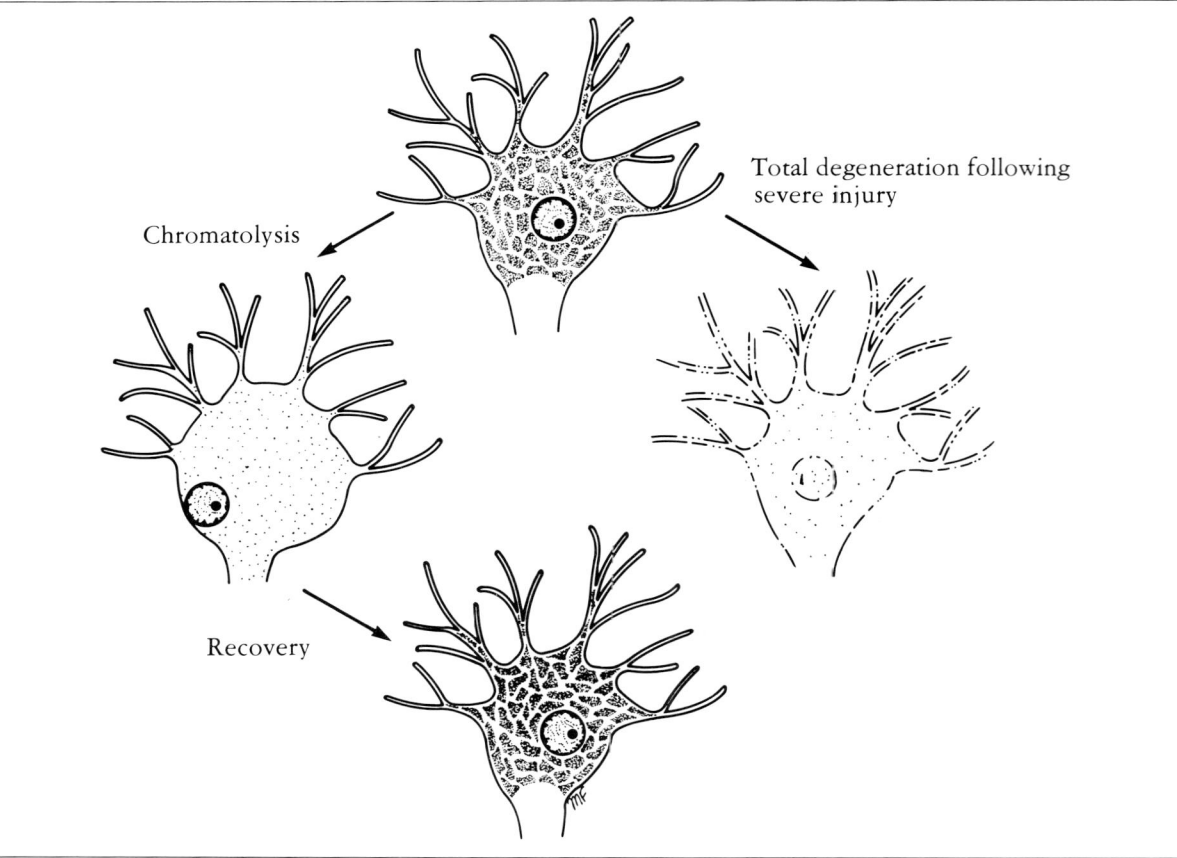

Fig. 7-60. *The changes that can take place in a nerve cell body following division of one of its processes.*

reaches its maximum within 2 weeks. The Nissl material becomes fine, granular (Fig. 7-60; see Fig. 7-58), and dispersed thoughout the cytoplasm (as described previously with injury to the cell body), a process known as chromatolysis. Chromatolysis begins near the axon hillock and spreads to all parts of the cell body. In addition, the nucleus moves from its central location toward the periphery of the cell, and the cell body becomes swollen and rounded (see Fig. 7-60). The degree of chromatolysis and of cell swelling is greatest when the injury to the axon is close to the cell body. In some neurons, very severe damage to the axon close to the cell body may lead to death of the neuron. Damage to the most distal process, in contrast, may lead to little or no detectable change in the cell body. The dispersal of the Nissl material, that is, the cytoplasmic RNA, and the swelling of the cell are caused by cellular edema. The loss of staining affinity of the Nissl material occurs because of a destruction of cytoplasmic RNA. The cause of the movement of the nucleus away from the center of the cell is not known.

Recovery of a Neuron following Injury

In contrast to the rapid onset of retrograde degeneration, the recovery of the nerve cell body and regeneration of its processes may take several months.

Recovery of the Nerve Cell Body

In recovery, the nucleolus moves to the periphery of the nucleus and polysome clusters reappear in the cytoplasm. These changes indicate that RNA and protein synthesis is being accelerated in preparation for the re-formation of the axon. Thus, there is a reconstitution of the original Nissl structure, a decrease in the swelling of the cell body, and a return of the nucleus to its characteristic central position (see Fig. 7-60).

Regeneration of the Axon

Regrowth of the axon is possible in peripheral nerves and appears to depend on the presence of endoneurial tubes and the special qualities possessed by Schwann cells. In the central nervous system, there is an attempt to regenerate the axons, evidenced by sprouting of the axons, but there is no indication that restoration of function takes place. The regeneration process is aborted by the absence of endoneurial tubes (which are necessary to guide the regenerating axons), the failure of oligodendrocytes to serve in the same manner as Schwann cells, and the laying down of scar tissue by the active astrocytes.

REGENERATION OF AXONS IN PERIPHERAL NERVES. The satisfactory regeneration of axons and the return of normal function will depend on the following factors:

1. In crushed nerve injuries, where the axon is divided or its blood supply has been interfered with but the endoneurial sheaths remain intact, the regenerative process may be very satisfactory.
2. In nerves that have been completely severed, there is much less chance of recovery, because the regenerating fibers from the proximal stump may be directed to an incorrect destination in the distal stump. For example, cutaneous fibers may enter incorrect nerve endings or motor nerves may supply incorrect muscles.
3. If the distance between the proximal and distal stumps of the completely severed nerve is greater than a few millimeters or the gap becomes filled with proliferating fibrous tissue or simply is filled by adjacent muscles that bulge into the gap, the chances of recovery are very poor. The outgrowing axonal sprouts escape into the surrounding connective tissue and form a tangled mass, or *neuroma*. In these cases, early close surgical approximation of the severed ends, if possible, greatly improves the chances of recovery.
4. If mixed nerves (those containing sensory, motor, and autonomic fibers) are completely severed, the chances of a good recovery are very much less than if the nerve is purely sensory or purely motor. The reason for this is that the regenerating fibers from the proximal stump may be guided to an incorrect destination in the distal stump; for example, cutaneous fibers may enter motor endoneurial tubes, and vice versa.
5. Inadequate physiotherapy for the paralyzed muscles will result in their degenerating before the regenerating motor axons have reached them.
6. Infection at the site of the wound will seriously interfere with regeneration.

If one assumes that the proximal and distal stumps of the severed nerve are in close apposition, the following regenerative processes take place (see Fig. 7-59): The Schwann cells, having undergone mitotic division, fill the space within the basal lamina of the endoneurial tubes of the proximal stump as far proximally as the next node of Ranvier, and in the distal stump as far distally as the end-organs. Where a small gap exists between the proximal and distal stumps, the multiplying Schwann cells form a number of cords to bridge the gap.

Each proximal axon end now gives rise to multiple fine sprouts, or filaments, with bulbous tips. As they grow, these filaments advance along the clefts between the Schwann cells and thus cross the interval between the proximal and distal nerve stumps. Many such filaments enter the proximal end of each

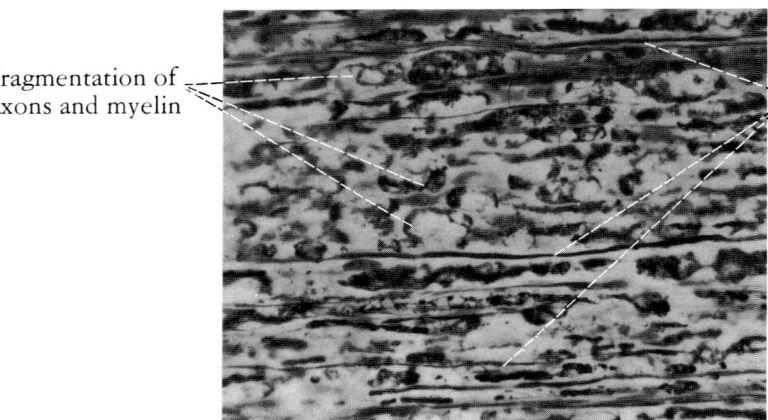

Fig. 7-61. Photomicrograph of longitudinal section of distal stump of an injured sciatic nerve, showing evidence of degeneration and axon regeneration. (Courtesy of Dr. M. J. T. Fitzgerald.)

endoneurial tube and grow distally in contact with the Schwann cells (Fig. 7-61). It is clear that the filaments from many different axons may enter a single endoneurial tube. Only one filament persists, however, the remainder degenerating, and that one filament grows distally to reinnervate a motor or sensory end-organ. Although they cross the gap between the severed nerve ends, many filaments fail to enter an endoneurial tube and instead grow out into the surrounding connective tissue. The formation of multiple sprouts or filaments from a single proximal axon greatly increases the likelihood that a neuron will become connected to a sensory or motor ending. It is not known why one filament within a single endoneurial tube should be selected to persist while the remainder degenerate.

Once the axon has reached the end-organ, the adjacent Schwann cells start to lay down a myelin sheath. This process begins at the site of the original lesion and extends distally. By this means, the nodes of Ranvier and the Schmidt-Lanterman incisures are formed.

Many months may elapse before the axon reaches its appropriate end-organ, depending on the site of the nerve injury. The rate of growth has been estimated to be about 2 to 4 mm daily. If, however, one takes into consideration the almost certain delay incurred by the axons as they cross the site of the injury, an overall regeneration rate of 1.5 mm daily is a useful figure for clinical use. Even if all the difficulties outlined are overcome and a given neuron reaches the original end-organ, the enlarging axonal filament within the endoneurial tube reaches only about 80 percent of its original diameter. For this reason, the conduction velocity will not be as great as in the original axon. Moreover, a given motor axon tends to innervate more muscle fibers than it did formerly, so that the control of muscle is less precise.

DEGENERATION

Transneuronal Degeneration

The responses of a single neuron to injury have been considered in the previous section. In the central nervous system, it is recognized that if one group of neurons is injured, a second group farther along the pathway that serves the same function may also show degenerative changes. This phenomenon is referred to as *anterograde transneuronal degeneration*. For example, if the axons of the ganglion cells of the retina are severed, not only do the distal ends of the axons that go to the lateral geniculate bodies undergo degeneration, but the neurons in the lateral geniculate bodies with which these axons form synapses also undergo degeneration. In fact, a further set of neurons may be involved in the degenerative process in the visual cortex.

Neuronal Degeneration Associated with Senescence

Many neurons degenerate and disappear during fetal development. This process is believed to be caused by their failure to establish adequate functional connections. During postnatal life, gradual neuronal degeneration continues. It has been estimated that by old age, an individual may have lost up to 20 percent of the original number of neurons. This loss may account to some extent for the loss of efficiency of the nervous system associated with senescence.

ACTION OF LOCAL ANESTHETICS ON NERVE CONDUCTION

Local anesthetics are drugs that block nerve conduction when applied locally to a nerve fiber in suitable concentrations. Their site of action is the axolemma, and they interfere with the transient increase in permeability of the axolemma to Na^+ ions. They also reduce the permeability of the axolemma of the resting axon to Na^+, K^+, and other ions. The sensitivity of nerve fibers to local anesthetics is related to the size of the nerve fibers. Small nerve fibers are more susceptible than are large fibers; small fibers are also slower to recover.

Cocaine has been used clinically to block nerve conduction. Unfortunately, it is a strong stimulant of the cerebral cortex and readily causes addiction. *Procaine* is a synthetic compound widely used as a local anesthetic agent.

TUMORS OF NEURONS AND PERIPHERAL NERVES

It is important to remember that the nervous system is made up of many different types of tissues. In the central nervous system, there are neurons, neuroglia, blood vessels, and meninges; in the peripheral nervous system, one finds neurons, Schwann cells, connective tissue, and blood vessels. Tumors of neurons in the central nervous system are rare, but tumors of peripheral neurons are not uncommon (Florey, 1970).

The *neuroblastoma* occurs in association with the suprarenal gland; it is highly malignant and occurs in infants and children. The *ganglioneuroma* occurs in the suprarenal medulla or sympathetic ganglia; it is benign and occurs in children and adults. The *pheochromocytoma* occurs in the suprarenal medulla; it is usually benign and gives rise to hypertension, because it secretes norepinephrine and epinephrine.

A *benign fibroma* or a *malignant sarcoma* may arise in the connective tissue of a peripheral nerve and does not differ from similar tumors elsewhere. *Neurolemmomas* are believed to arise from Schwann cells. They arise from any nerve trunk, cranial or spinal, and in any part of its course. Primary tumors of the axons are very rare.

SYNAPTIC BLOCKING AGENTS

Transmission of a nervous impulse across a synapse is accomplished by the release of neurotransmitters into the synaptic gutter. The released transmitter then exerts its effect on the postsynaptic membrane.

The synapse is a region in which transmission is easily blocked. As a general rule, long chains of neurons with multiple synapses are more easily blocked than shorter, simpler chains of neurons. General anesthetic agents are effective because they have the ability to block synaptic transmission.

Preganglionic fibers enter autonomic ganglia and synapse with the postganglionic sympathetic or parasympathetic neurons. On reaching the termination of the preganglionic nerve, the nerve impulse brings about the release of acetylcholine, which excites a nervous impulse in the postganglionic neuron.

Ganglionic blocking agents can be divided into three groups, according to their mechanisms of action. Those of the first group, which includes the *hexamethonium* and *tetraethylammonium salts*, resemble acetylcholine and compete with it at the postsynaptic membrane; they thus inhibit transmission across a synapse. Those of the second group, which includes *nicotine*, have the same action as acetylcholine on the postsynaptic membrane but are not destroyed by cholinesterase. The result is a prolonged depolarization of the postsynaptic membrane, during which it is insensitive to further stimulation by acetylcholine. Unfortunately, this depolarization block is associated with initial stimulation, and these drugs therefore are not suitable for clinical use. Agents of the third group, which includes procaine, inhibit the release of acetylcholine from the preganglionic fibers.

Many of the cholinergic blocking agents used in the peripheral nervous system have little or no effect on the cholinergic synapses of the central nervous system, because they are unable to cross the blood-brain barrier in significant concentrations. *Atropine, scopolamine,* and *diisopropylphosphorofluoridate* (DPF) can cross the barrier effectively, and their effects on human behavior have been studied extensively. Similarly, it is believed that many psychotropic drugs bring about changes in the activities of the central nervous system by influencing the release of catecholamines at synaptic sites. The *phenothiazines*, for example, are thought to block dopamine receptors on postsynaptic neurons.

NEUROGLIA

Reactions to Injury

The reaction of neuroglial cells to injury, whether caused by physical trauma or by vascular occlusion, is characterized by hyperplasia and hypertrophy of the astrocytes, which become fibrous irrespective of their antecedent structure; in addition, hypertrophy and hyperplasia of the microglial cells occur. The proliferation of the astrocytes is referred to as *astrocytosis* or *gliosis*. The loss of neuronal tissue is not compensated for in volume by the glial hypertrophy. The cytoplasm of the enlarged astrocytes contains large numbers of fibrils and glycogen granules. The dense feltwork of astrocytic processes that is found in the areas of neuronal degeneration produces the so-called *gliotic scar*. The degree of gliosis is much greater in the presence of residual damaged neuronal tissue than following a clean surgical excision in which no traumatized brain tissue remains. This is why, in patients with focal epilepsy caused by a large gliotic scar, the scar is excised surgically, leaving a minimal glial reaction.

Oligodendrocytes respond to injury by expanding and showing vacuolation of their cytoplasm; the nuclei also tend to become pyknotic. Severe damage to oligodendrocytes probably would result in demyelination.

Microglial cells in inflammatory and degenerative lesions of the central nervous system retract their processes and migrate to the site of the lesion. Here they proliferate and are actively phagocytic, and their cytoplasm becomes filled with lipids and cell remnants. They are joined in their scavenger activity by histiocytes that migrate from the meninges and neighboring blood vessels.

Neoplasms

According to Walton (1977), tumors of neuroglia account for 40 to 45 percent of intracranial tumors. Such tumors are referred to as *gliomas*. Tumors of astrocytes are those most commonly encountered and include *astrocytomas, glioblastomas*, and *medulloblastomas*. Except for the ependymomas, tumors of the neuroglia are highly invasive. Thus, it is difficult to achieve complete surgical removal, and there is a great possibility of recurrence after operation. These tumors often infiltrate without interfering with the function of neighboring neurons. As a result, the tumor is often very much larger than the symptoms and physical signs indicate.

CLINICAL PROBLEMS

For the answers to these problems, see page 791.

1. During an operation for repair of the radial nerve, which had been sectioned by a stab wound, the surgeon asks a medical student if the nerve fibers contained within the radial nerve are axons or dendrites. How would you answer this question? What is the structure of a peripheral nerve?

2. In a histological section of nervous tissue, one of the characteristic features noted is the large size of the nucleoli. What is the function of a nucleolus, and why do you think it is large in nerve cells?

3. An 18-year-old man is examined by a neurosur-

geon 12 months after an injury to the right forearm in which the median nerve was severed. At the initial operation, shortly after the injury had occurred, debridement was performed and the separated nerve ends were tagged with radiopaque sutures. Unfortunately, the wound was infected, and surgical repair of the nerve was deferred. Is it practical to consider repairing a peripheral nerve after a delay of 12 months?

4. During the examination of the cell body of a neuron in an electron micrograph, a student is puzzled by the number and varied appearance of membrane-bound vesicles seen within the cytoplasm. How would you classify the different types of vesicles found in the cytoplasm?

5. When a nerve cell is stimulated, the permeability of the plasma membrane changes, permitting certain ionic movements to take place across the membrane. What is the structure of the plasma membrane? Is the permeability of the plasma membrane increased or decreased when the nerve cell is stimulated? What is the action of local analgesics on the plasma membrane?

6. The synapse is a region where nervous transmission is easily blocked. Clinically, the ganglion-blocking drugs used act by competing with acetylcholine released from the nerve endings in the ganglia. Name two groups of drugs that have been used for this purpose, and indicate the site at which they act.

7. Axoplasmic flow is believed to be involved in the buildup of materials at the axon terminals for the production of transmitter substances. Such flow is sometimes referred to as anterograde flow. Retrograde axoplasmic flow is also thought to occur. What structures present in the cytoplasm of the neuron may be involved in these processes?

8. A 20-year-old man is seen in the emergency room following an automobile accident. A diagnosis of fracture dislocation of the fourth thoracic vertebra is made, with injury to the spinal cord as a complication. It is decided to perform a laminectomy, because it is believed that the spinal cord should be decompressed to avoid permanent injury to the tracts of the cord. What is a nerve tract in the spinal cord? How does it differ in structure from a peripheral nerve?

9. Define the following: (a) myelin sheath, (b) node of Ranvier, (c) Schmidt-Lanterman incisure, (d) satellite cells in sensory and autonomic ganglia.

10. Multiple sclerosis is a demyelinating disease of the central nervous system. There are many other diseases of the nervous system that have the common pathological feature of destruction of the myelin sheaths of nerve fibers. How does myelination normally take place in (a) peripheral nerves and (b) central nervous system tracts? When does myelination of nerves normally take place?

11. During a neurobiology lecture, the professor repeatedly refers to the terms *type A and B nerve fibers, resting membrane potential, absolute refractory period, conduction velocity,* and *saltatory conduction.* Can you define each of these terms?

12. What is meant by the following: (a) wallerian degeneration, (b) band fiber, (c) transneuronal degeneration?

13. A well-known politician is attending a rally when a youth suddenly steps forward and shoots him in the back. The patient cannot feel anything in either leg and is paralyzed from the waist down. At operation, the bullet is removed and considerable damage to the spinal cord is noted. What changes take place in the spinal cord when the nerve fibers are damaged? Does regeneration take place in the central nervous system?

14. A 35-year-old woman, while walking past some workers digging a hole in the road, suddenly becomes aware of a foreign body in her left eye. Because the cornea is extremely sensitive, she suffers considerable discomfort. What sensory endings are present in the cornea? Is the cornea sensitive to stimuli other than pain?

15. A 60-year-old man visits his physician because

for the past 3 months, he has been experiencing an agonizing stabbing pain over the middle part of the right side of his face. The pains last a few seconds but may be repeated several times. "The pain is the worst I have ever experienced," he tells his physician. He has noticed particularly that a draft of cold air on his face or the touching of a few scalp hairs in the temporal region triggers the pain. Physical examination reveals no sensory or motor loss of the trigeminal nerve. A diagnosis of trigeminal neuralgia is made. Using your knowledge of histology, can you explain why hairs are so sensitive to touch?

16. During a practical class in pathology, a student is shown a slide illustrating a particular form of cerebral tumor. At the edge of the section, there is a small area of the cerebral cortex. The instructor asks the student whether the tissue has been removed from a motor or a sensory area of the cortex. What are the main differences in structure between the motor and sensory areas of the cerebral cortex?

17. When looking at a histological slide of the cerebellar cortex, one is struck by the uniformity of the cellular arrangement. What different types of neurons are found in the cerebellar cortex?

18. At a postmortem examination, a third-year medical student is handed a slice of the cerebrum and asked what proportion of the central nervous system is composed of neuroglia. How would you answer that question? Which cells are more numerous, neurons or neuroglial cells?

19. While discussing the different types of intracranial tumors, a neurologist repeatedly uses the terms *microglia* and *neuroglia*. What are these structures?

20. At the end of a seminar entitled "The Neuroglia," a physiologist, a pathologist, and an anatomist take part in an intense discussion on the possible functions of neuroglia in the central nervous system. What do you know about the functions of neuroglial cells?

ADDITIONAL READING

Asbury, A. K., and Johnson, P. C. *Pathology of Peripheral Nerves*. Philadelphia: Saunders, 1978.

Axelrod, J. Neurotransmitters. *Sci. Am.* 230(6):58, 1974.

Bodian, D. Neuron junctions: A revolutionary decade. *Anat. Rec.* 174:73, 1972.

Bradley, W. G. *Disorders of Peripheral Nerves*. New York and London: Oxford University Press, 1974.

Brightman, M. W., and Reese, T. S. Junctions between intimately apposed cell membranes in the vertebrate brain. *J. Cell Biol.* 40:648, 1969.

Bunge, R. P., Bunge, M. B., and Cochran, M. Some factors influencing the proliferation and differentiation of myelin-forming cells. *Neurology* (N.Y.) 28:59, 1978.

Ceccarelli, B., and Clementi, F. (eds.). *Neurotoxins: Tools in Neurobiology*. New York: Raven, 1979.

Ceccarelli, B., and Hurlbut, W. P. Vesicle hypothesis of the release of quanta of acetylcholine. *Physiol. Rev.* 60:396, 1980.

Chouchkov, C. V. Cutaneous receptors. In *Advances in Anatomy, Embryology and Cell Biology*. Vol. 54. Vienna and New York: Springer-Verlag, 1978.

Dyck, P. J., and Hopkins, A. P. Electron microscopic observations on degeneration and regeneration of unmyelinated fibers. *Brain* 95:223, 1972.

Friede, R. L., and Samorajski, T. The clefts of Schmidt-Lanterman: A quantitative electron microscopic study of their structure in developing and adult sciatic nerves of the rat. *Anat. Rec.* 165:89, 1969.

Heuser, J. E., and Reese, T. S. Evidence for recycling of synaptic vesicle membrane during transmitter release of the frog neuromuscular junction. *J. Cell Biol.* 57:315, 1973.

Iggo, W. E. Cutaneous and subcutaneous sense organs. *Br. Med. Bull.* 33:97, 1977.

Jacobson, M., and Hunt, R. K. The origins of nerve-cell specificity. *Sci. Am.* 228(2):26, 1973.

Kaeser, H. E. Nerve conduction velocity measurements. In Vinken, P. J., and Bruyn, G. W. (eds.), *Handbook of Clinical Neurology*. Vol. 2. Amsterdam: Elsevier, 1970.

Katz, B. Elementary components of synaptic transmission. *Naturwissenschaften* 66:606, 1979.

Krstić, R. V. Observations on the nodes of Ranvier of

rat sciatic nerve fibers under the scanning and transmission electron microscope. *Period. Biol.* 76:105, 1974.

Landon, D. N. (ed.). *The Peripheral Nerve.* Chapman and Hall, 1976.

Lewis, A. J. *Mechanism of Neurological Disease.* Boston: Little, Brown, 1976.

Lowenstein, W. R. (ed.). Principles of receptor physiology. In *Handbook of Sensory Physiology.* Vol. 1. New York: Springer-Verlag, 1971.

Morales, R., and Duncan, D. Specialized contacts of astrocytes with astrocytes and other cell types in the spinal cord of the cat. *Anat. Rec.* 182:255, 1975.

Nicoll, R. A., et al. Substance P as a transmitter candidate. *Annu. Rev. Neurosci.* 3:227, 1980.

Nishi, K., Oura, C., and Pallie, W. Fine structure of pacinian corpuscles in the mesentary of the cat. *J. Cell Biol.* 43:539, 1969.

Palay, S. L., and Chan-Palay, V. *Cerebellar cortex: Cytology and Organization.* Vienna and New York: Springer-Verlag, 1974.

Peters, A., Palay, S. L., and Webster, H. F. *The Fine Structure of the Nervous System: The Neurons and Supportive Cells.* Philadelphia: Saunders, 1976.

Seddon, H. J. *Surgical Disorders of Peripheral Nerves.* Edinburgh and London: Longman, 1972.

Snell, R. S. Changes in the histochemical appearances of cholinesterase in a mixed peripheral nerve following nerve section and compression injury. *Br. J. Exp. Pathol.* 38:34, 1957.

Trojaborg, W. Rate of recovery in motor and sensory fibers of the radial nerve: Clinical and electrophysiological aspects. *J. Neurol. Neurosurg. Psychiatry* 33:625, 1970.

Walton, J. N. *Brain's Diseases of the Nervous System* (8th ed.). New York and London: Oxford University Press, 1977.

Wuerker, R. B., and Kirkpatrick, J. B. Neuronal microtubules, neurofilaments, and microfilaments. *Int. Rev. Cytol.* 33:45, 1972.

CARDIOVASCULAR SYSTEM

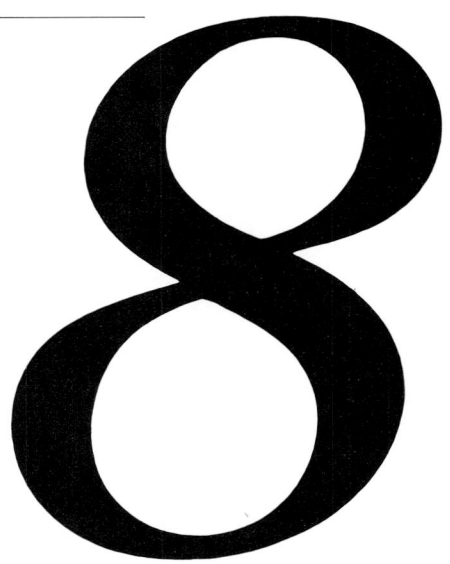

The cardiovascular system consists of the heart (the pump), a closed system of blood vessels, and the blood. It is the body's transportation system. The blood picks up oxygen and the products of digestion from the respiratory and digestive systems and delivers them to the cells of the body. From the cells the blood picks up the products of metabolism, such as carbon dioxide and lactic acid, and delivers them to the excretory organs. In addition, blood transports hormones from the endocrine glands to their target organs. It also delivers white blood cells and antibodies to sites of infection and helps regulate body temperature. The cardiovascular system thus plays a vital role in maintaining the constancy of the internal environment (homeostasis).

The blood leaves the heart through tubes called *arteries*, which branch repeatedly until fine arteries, or *arterioles*, measuring about 0.1 mm in diameter are formed. The arterioles lead the blood into extremely small tubes called *capillaries*. The blood starts its return journey to the heart by passing through small veins called *venules*. The venules join together to form *veins*. The larger veins finally return the blood to the heart.

THE HEART

The heart is a cone-shaped, hollow, muscular organ that is divided by septa into four chambers, the *right* and *left atria* and the *right* and *left ventricles* (Fig. 8-1). Each atrium has an earlike appendage called the *auricle*.

Blood returns to the right atrium through the *superior* and *inferior venae cavae* (see Fig. 8-1). It passes into the right ventricle through the *right atrioventricular valve*, or *triscupid valve*. When the right ventricle contracts, the blood is pumped through the pulmonary valve into the pulmonary arteries to the lungs. After passing through the lung capillaries, where it absorbs oxygen and gives up carbon dioxide, the blood is conveyed to the left atrium by the four pulmonary veins (two from each lung). The blood then flows through the left atrium and the *left atrioventricular valve*, or *mitral valve*, into the left ventricle. Finally, the blood is pumped from the left ventricle through the *aortic valve* into the aorta and its branches and flows to all parts of the body, only to return eventually to the right atrium to repeat the cardiac cycle.

The shorter course taken by the blood from the

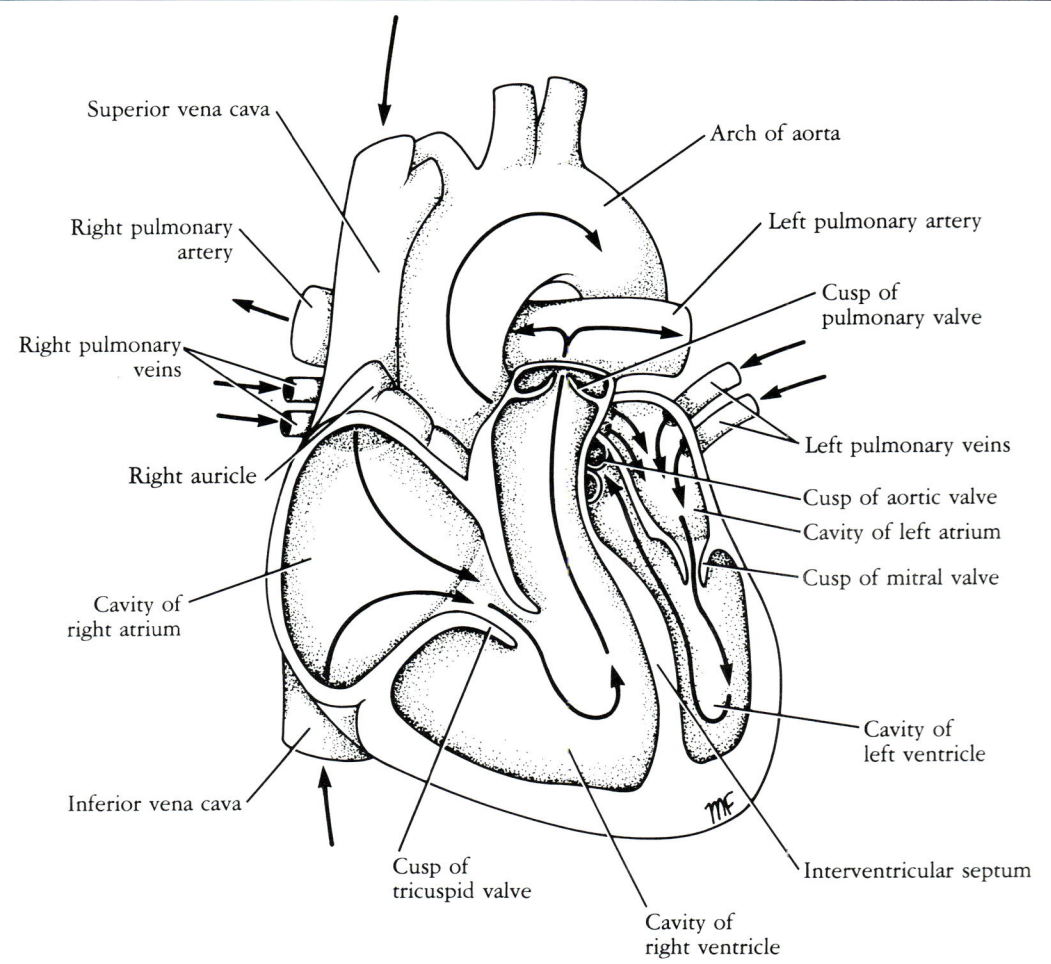

Fig. 8-1. The heart. The pathway taken by the blood as it circulates through the various chambers during the cardiac cycle is shown.

right side of the heart to the lungs and back to the left side of the heart is called the *pulmonary circulation*. The much longer course taken by the blood from the left side of the heart through the rest of the body and back to the right side of the heart is called the *systemic circulation*.

Microscopic Structure
Wall of the Heart
The heart wall consists of three layers: the inner layer, or endocardium; the middle layer, or myocardium; and the outer layer, or epicardium (Fig. 8-2).

ENDOCARDIUM. The endocardium lines all the internal surfaces of the heart and is continuous with the tunica intima of the blood vessels entering and leaving the heart. It is the layer of the heart wall that lies in contact with the blood (see Fig. 8-2). The endocardium consists of an *endothelium* and a *subendothelial layer*. The endothelium consists of polygonal squamous cells. The subendothelium is thin and consists of delicate connective tissue that contains numerous elastic fibers and some bundles of

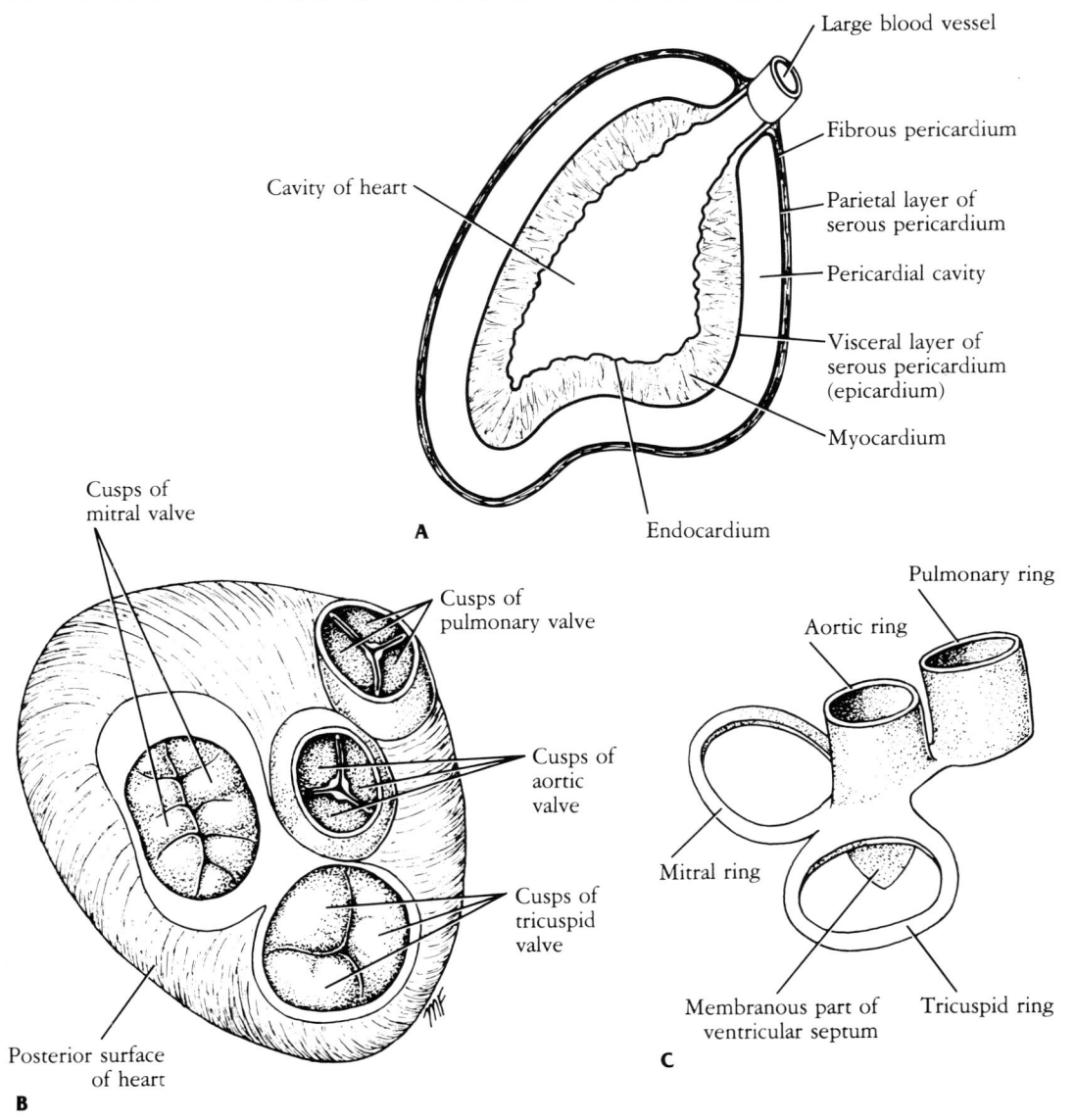

Fig. 8-2. A: The different layers of the heart and its coverings; note that the pericardial cavity is normally a very small space containing pericardial fluid. B: The valves of the heart, superior view; the atria and the great vessels have been removed. C: The fibrous skeleton of the heart.

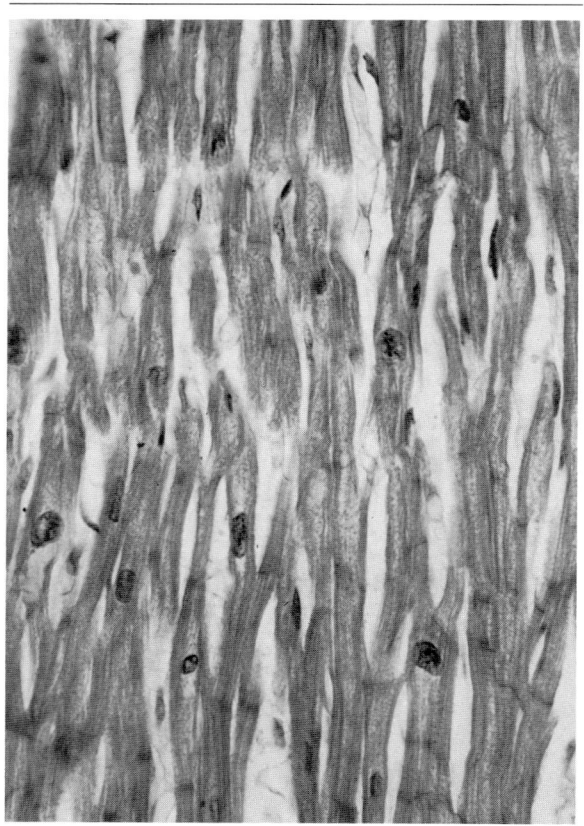

Fig. 8-3. Photomicrograph of a section of cardiac muscle, showing branched fibers, centrally placed nuclei, cross striations, and intercalated discs. (H&E; ×400.)

smooth muscle. Connecting the endocardium to the myocardium is loose connective tissue containing blood vessels, nerves, and terminal branches of the conducting system.

MYOCARDIUM. The myocardium forms the main mass of the heart and is composed of cardiac muscle (Fig. 8-3). The structure of cardiac muscle is fully considered on page 203. In the atria, the myocardium is relatively thin, because the pressure within the atria rises by only about 6 mm Hg when the atria contract to force the blood into the ventricles. In the ventricles, the myocardium is thick, and, because the systolic blood pressure in the systemic circulation is about six times higher than in the pulmonary circulation, it is not surprising to find that the myocardium of the left ventricle is about three times as thick as that of the right ventricle.

The cardiac muscle fibers are attached to the fibrous skeleton of the heart and are separated from one another by connective tissue. The arrangement of the muscle fibers is extremely complicated. The superficial fibers are common to the two atria, whereas the deeper fibers are confined to each atrium. In the ventricles, the fibers are arranged in a spiral, and most of them end in the papillary muscles (see p. 296). The cardiac muscles of the atria and ventricles are completely separated by the fibrous skeleton of the heart, the only connection being the conducting system of the heart.

EPICARDIUM. The epicardium, the outermost covering of the heart, forms the visceral layer of the *serous pericardium* (see Fig. 8-2). The serous pericardium forms the wall of the *pericardial cavity* and is protected on the outside by a tough fibrous coat called the *fibrous pericardium*.

The epicardium consists of an outer layer of flattened mesothelial cells resting on a layer of connective tissue. The connective tissue contains nerves and the coronary arteries and veins. Adipose tissue is sometimes found in large amounts around the coronary blood vessels. A small amount of *pericardial fluid* is produced by the mesothelial cells of the serous pericardium and passes into the pericardial cavity. The normal volume of pericardial fluid is about 50 ml. This fluid lubricates the apposing surfaces of the serous pericardium and allows the heart to move freely during contraction and relaxation.

Skeleton of the Heart

The skeleton of the heart consists of fibrous rings that surround the atrioventricular and arterial orifices (see Fig. 8-2). It is composed of dense fibrous tissue and provides attachment for the cardiac muscle fibers of the atria and ventricles and for the cusps of the atrioventricular valves. Its function is to limit

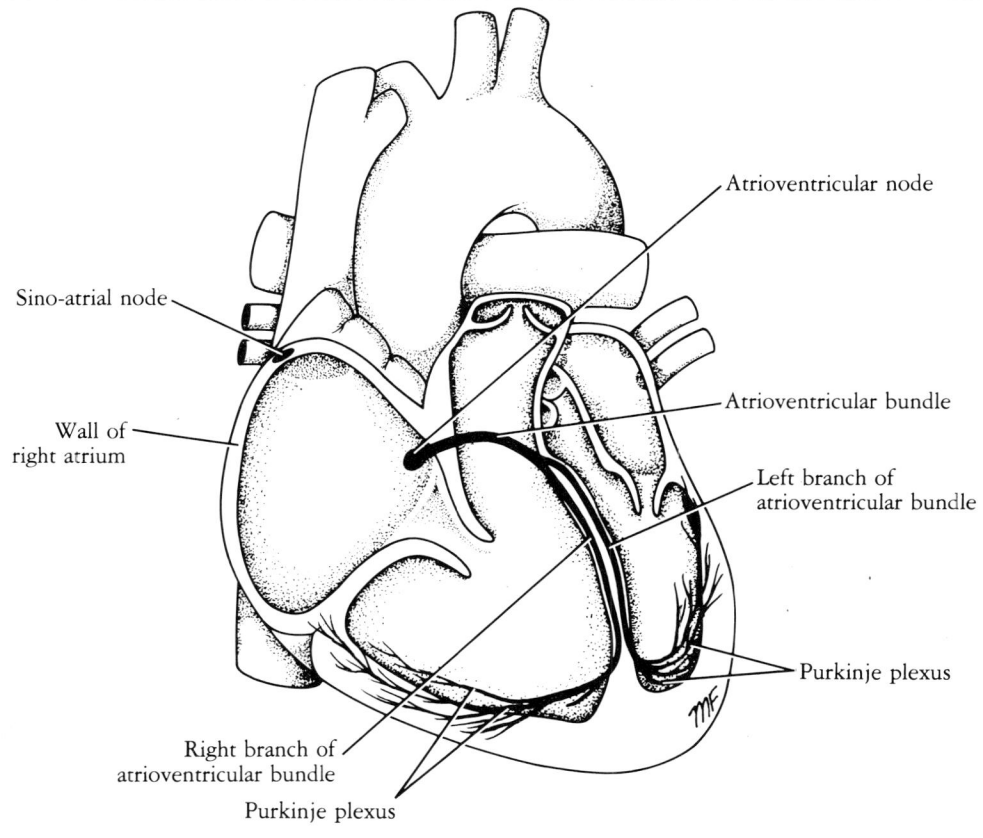

Fig. 8-4. The heart. The arrangement and position of the different parts of the conducting system are indicated.

the diameter of the atrioventricular and arterial orifices and to provide a solid foundation for the valves of the heart during the different phases of the cardiac cycle.

Conducting System of the Heart

The conducting system of the heart consists of (1) the sino-atrial node, (2) the atrioventricular node, (3) the atrioventricular bundle, and (4) the Purkinje plexus. The histological characteristics of the conducting system are described on page 206.

SINO-ATRIAL NODE. The sino-atrial node, located in the wall of the right atrium at the root of the superior vena cava (Fig. 8-4), spontaneously gives origin to rhythmical impulses that spread in all directions through the cardiac muscle of the atria and cause the muscle to contract. The sino-atrial node is sometimes called the *pacemaker,* because it controls the rate of contraction of the entire heart.

The action potential originating in the specialized cardiac muscle fibers of the sino-atrial node spreads to the surrounding muscle fibers and reaches the atrioventricular node in about 0.04 second.

ATRIOVENTRICULAR NODE. The atrioventricular node is strategically placed in the lower part of the atrial septum (see Fig. 8-4), just above the fibrous skeleton of the heart, which separates the myocardium of the atria from that of the ventricles. It can be likened to a radio receiver that picks up the excitation wave as it passes through the atrial myocardium.

The speed of conduction of the cardiac impulse through the atrioventricular node (about 0.11 second) is such that sufficient time is allowed for the atria to empty their blood into the ventricles before the ventricles start to contract. From the atrioventricular node, the cardiac impulse is conducted to the ventricles by the atrioventricular bundle (see Fig. 8-4).

ATRIOVENTRICULAR BUNDLE. The atrioventricular bundle (bundle of His) is the only pathway of cardiac muscle that connects the myocardium of the atria and the myocardium of the ventricles; it is thus the only route along which the cardiac impulse can travel from the atria to the ventricles (see Fig. 8-4). The specialized cardiac muscle fibers, which are fast-conducting and make up the atrioventricular bundle, are commonly referred to as *Purkinje fibers*. The atrioventricular bundle divides into right and left terminal branches, which lie on either side of the ventricular septum and extend toward the apex of the heart.

PURKINJE PLEXUS. The right and left terminal branches of the atrioventricular bundle become continuous with small branches that spread around each ventricular chamber and back toward the base of the heart. These fine terminal branches are referred to as the *Purkinje plexus* (Fig. 8-5; see Fig. 8-4). The cardiac impulse travels from the beginning of the atrioventricular bundle to the terminal branches of the Purkinje plexus in about 0.03 second. This rapid spread of the cardiac impulse ensures that the entire myocardium of the ventricles is stimulated to contract at almost exactly the same time.

It can thus be seen that the conducting system of the heart is responsible not only for generating rhythmical cardiac impulses but also for conducting these impulses throughout the myocardium of the heart.

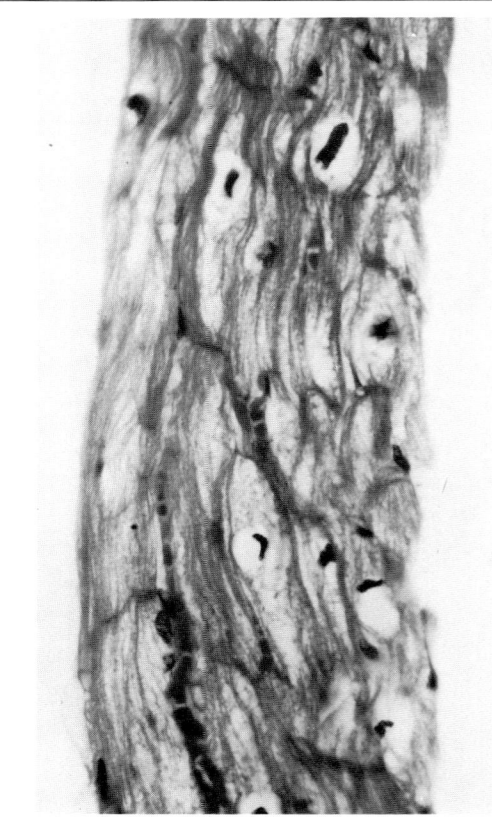

Fig. 8-5. *Photomicrograph of a section of Purkinje fibers of the heart, showing the peripheral distribution of myofibrils. The central clear areas are rich in glycogen. (H&E; ×400.)*

Valves of the Heart

TRICUSPID VALVE. The tricuspid valve guards the right atrioventricular orifice (see Figs. 8-1 and 8-2). It has three cusps, which are attached by their bases to the fibrous atrioventricular ring of the skeleton of the heart. Each cusp consists of a double layer of endocardium, with a small amount of connective tissue forming the core. The endocardium on the atrial surface is thicker than that on the ventricular surface.

The margins and ventricular surfaces of the cusps are connected to small muscular projections on the ventricular walls, the *papillary muscles*, by a number of tendinous cords, the *chordae tendineae* (Fig. 8-6).

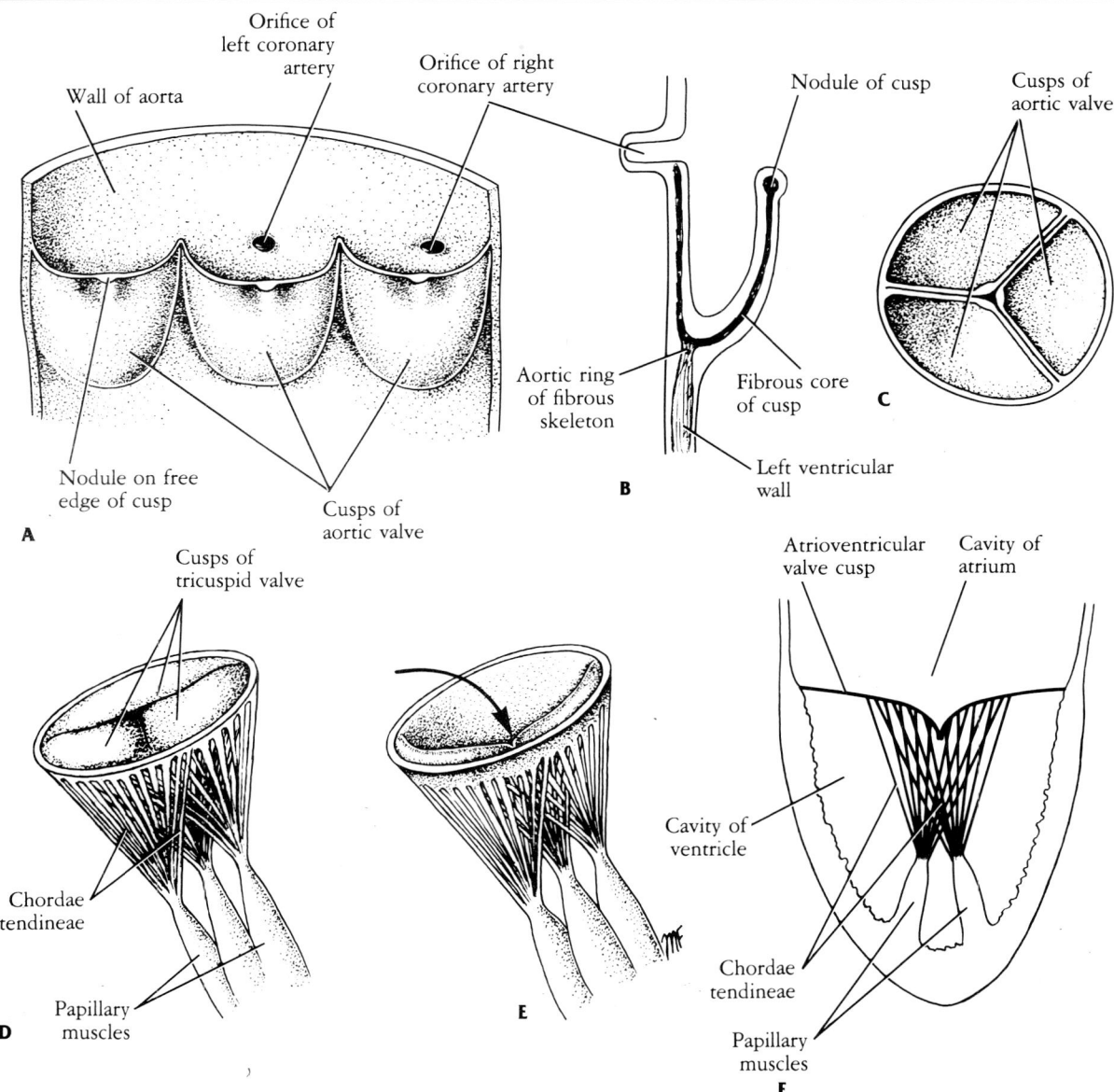

Fig. 8-6. A: Attachment of the cusps of the aortic valve to the wall of the aorta; B: section of a cusp of the aortic valve; C: superior view of the cusps of the aortic valve with the valve in the closed position; D: cusps of the tricuspid valve in the closed position; E: cusps of the tricuspid valve in the open position; F: section of atrioventricular valve, showing the attachment of the chordae tendineae to the cusps.

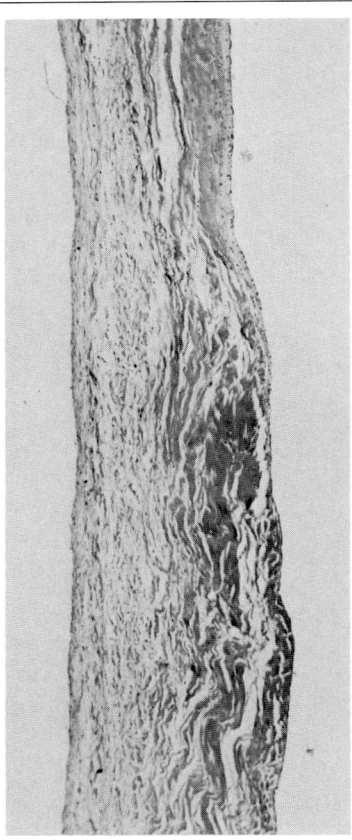

Fig. 8-7. Photomicrograph of section of cusp of mitral valve, showing the core of connective tissue and the covering of endothelial cells on both surfaces. (H&E; ×40.)

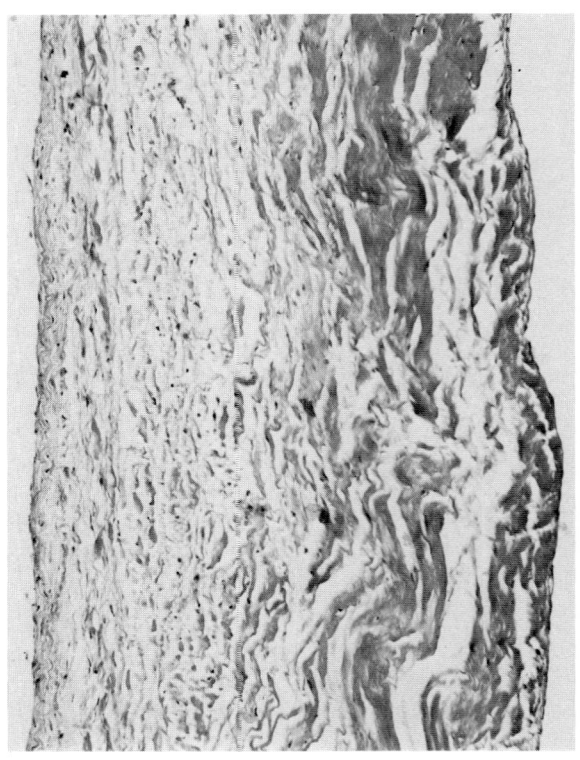

Fig. 8-8. Photomicrograph of high-power view of section of cusp of mitral valve shown in Figure 8-7, showing the loose connective tissue core of the cusp and the flattened endothelial cells covering its surfaces. (H&E; ×90.)

The chordae tendineae are composed of dense fibrous tissue and are covered with endocardium. When the ventricle contracts, the papillary muscles contract and prevent the cusps from being forced into the atrium and turning inside out as the intraventricular pressure rises.

MITRAL VALVE. The mitral valve guards the left atrioventricular orifice (see Figs. 8-1 and 8-2). It consists of two cusps, one anterior and one posterior, that have a structure similar to that of the cusps of the tricuspid valve (Figs. 8-7 and 8-8). The attachment of the chordae tendineae and the function of the valve cusps are also similar to those of the cusps of the tricuspid valve.

PULMONARY VALVE. The pulmonary valve guards the pulmonary orifice (see Fig. 8-1). It consists of three semilunar cusps, one posterior and two anterior. Each cusp consists of a double layer of endocardium, with a small amount of connective tissue forming the core. At the base of each cusp, the connective tissue is continuous with the fibrous skeleton of the heart. At the center of the free edge, the connective tissue is thickened to form a fibrous nodule (see Fig. 8-2).

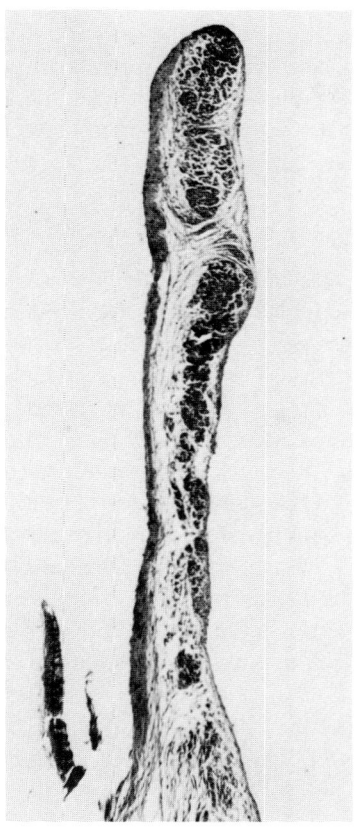

Fig. 8-9. Photomicrograph of section of cusp of aortic valve; the free edge of the cusp lies above. (H&E; ×40.)

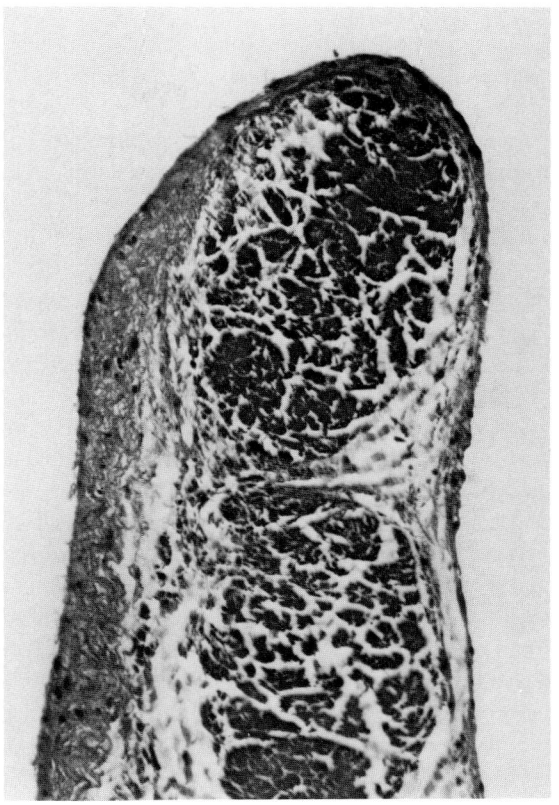

Fig. 8-10. Photomicrograph of high-power view of section of cusp of aortic valve shown in Figure 8-9, showing the core of connective tissue and the covering of endothelial cells on its surfaces. (H&E; ×100.)

The curved lower margin of each cusp is continuous with the arterial wall. The open mouths of the cusps are directed upward. During ventricular systole, the cusps of the valve are pressed against the wall of the pulmonary trunk by the outrushing blood. During ventricular diastole (relaxation), blood flows back toward the heart and enters the open mouths of the cusps, which promptly fill, come into apposition in the center of the lumen, and close the pulmonary orifice.

AORTIC VALVE. The aortic valve guards the aortic orifice (see Figs. 8-1, 8-2, and 8-6) and is almost identical in structure and function to the pulmonary valve (Figs. 8-9 and 8-10). One cusp is situated on the anterior wall, and two are located on the posterior wall. The aortic valve prevents the regurgitation of blood from the aorta into the left ventricle.

Blood Supply of the Heart

The blood supply of the heart comes from the right and left coronary arteries. The blood is collected by the cardiac veins, most of which join the coronary sinus and drain into the right atrium. The structure of the important coronary arteries is described on page 308.

Physiology of Cardiac Muscle

The resting potential of general cardiac muscle is about -85 mV. The action potential of cardiac muscle rises to about $+20$ mV and differs from that of skeletal muscle in that it is very prolonged. This prolonged action potential is accompanied by an increased period of contraction. The reason for this prolonged action potential is not known, but it may be caused by a decrease in the permeability of the cell membrane to potassium ions over this period. At the end of the action potential, the permeability of the membrane to potassium suddenly increases and rapid repolarization takes place.

Cardiac muscle fibers are crossed by *intercalated discs,* which are the cell membranes that separate adjacent cardiac muscle cells (see p. 205). The electrical resistance across these discs is very small, allowing action potentials to travel from one cardiac muscle cell to another with minimal delay. Therefore, if one muscle cell is stimulated, the action potential spreads to all the muscle cells very rapidly. Bear in mind, however, that although all the muscle fibers of both atria and all the muscle fibers of both ventricles are closely interconnected, the muscle of the atria is separated from that of the ventricles by the fibrous skeleton of the heart, and the only connection between the two functional units is the atrioventricular bundle.

Cardiac muscle has three important properties: excitability and contractility, rhythmicity, and conductivity.

Excitability and Contractility

Cardiac muscle responds to stimuli by contracting. If the stimulus is strong enough to cause a response, the muscle will contract to its maximum; that is, it obeys the *all-or-none law.* Thus, if the stimulus is too weak, the muscle will not contract, and if the stimulus is greater than is necessary to produce a contraction (the threshold strength), the force of contraction will not be increased.

Cardiac muscle will not respond to a stimulus during the action potential—that is, while it is contracting—thus differing from skeletal muscle. The time during which cardiac muscle is unresponsive to an adequate stimulus is called the *absolute refractory period.* When cardiac muscle starts to repolarize, its excitability gradually recovers. The period of depressed but gradually increasing excitability is called the *relative refractory period.*

Rhythmicity

Cardiac muscle has the power to generate its own contractile impulse and does not need an external stimulus. Not only is the impulse spontaneous, but it occurs rhythmically. Because of the absolute refractory period, summation of contractions and tetanus cannot occur as they do in skeletal muscle. For the heart to perform satisfactorily as a pump, the cardiac muscle must contract and then there must be a pause to allow the chambers to fill with blood. Then contraction can take place again.

Should the cardiac muscle be stimulated by some unusual agent while relaxing and the stimulus is strong enough, the muscle will contract, producing a premature beat or *extrasystole.* Following the extra systole is an especially long rest pause called a *compensatory pause.* This pause occurs because the normal cardiac impulse reaches the cardiac muscle at regular intervals from the sino-atrial node. When an extra systole of, say, the ventricle occurs, the next normal impulse to arrive from the node will reach the ventricle during the absolute refractory period of the ventricular muscle. The cardiac muscle will not respond; hence, the long pause.

Conductivity

As was stated earlier, because the intercalated discs provide little hindrance to the spread of the action potential between individual muscle cells, the excitability process spreads rapidly from one area of cardiac muscle to another. The speed of conduction is especially well developed in the Purkinje fibers of the atrioventricular bundle and the Purkinje plexus. For example, the rate of conduction in Purkinje fibers is 4 m per second, and in the ordinary cardiac muscle of the ventricular wall it is 0.4 m per second.

The Cardiac Cycle

The heart is a muscular pump. The series of changes that takes place within it as it fills with blood and empties is referred to as the *cardiac cycle*. The normal heart beats about 70 times per minute in the resting adult and about 130 times per minute in the newborn.

Deoxygenated or venous blood is continuously being returned to the right atrium by two large veins, the *superior* and *inferior venae cavae* (see Fig. 8-1). The superior vena cava drains the upper part of the body; the inferior vena cava, the lower part of the body. When the right atrioventricular valve is closed, the venous blood is temporarily accommodated in the right atrium. Once ventricular diastole (relaxation) occurs, the right atrioventricular valve opens and the blood passively flows from the right atrium into the right ventricle. When the right ventricle is nearly full, atrial systole (contraction) occurs and forces the remainder of the blood in the right atrium into the right ventricle. The sino-atrial node initiates the wave of contraction in the right atrium (see Fig. 8-4), which commences around the openings of the large veins and milks the blood toward the right ventricle. This prevents any reflux of blood into the veins.

The cardiac impulse, having reached the atrioventricular node, is conducted to the papillary muscles by the atrioventricular bundle and its branches (see Fig. 8-4). The papillary muscles now begin to contract and take up the slack of the chordae tendineae. Meanwhile, the right ventricle starts contracting and the right atrioventricular valve closes. The spread of the cardiac impulse along the atrioventricular bundle and its terminal branches, including the Purkinje plexus, ensures that myocardial contraction occurs at almost the same time throughout the ventricles.

Once the right intraventricular blood pressure exceeds that in the pulmonary trunk, the semilunar cusps of the pulmonary valve are pushed aside and the blood is ejected from the heart. On conclusion of ventricular systole, blood begins to move back toward the right ventricle and immediately fills the pockets of the semilunar cusps of the pulmonary valve. The cusps move into apposition and completely close the pulmonary orifice into the right ventricle.

The blood now flows through the pulmonary arteries to the lungs (see Fig. 8-1). After passing through the lung capillaries, where it absorbs oxygen and gives up carbon dioxide, the blood is conveyed to the left atrium by the four pulmonary veins (two from each lung). The blood then flows through the left atrium, the left atrioventricular orifice, and the left ventricle in exactly the same manner that it traversed the right side of the heart, as described previously. Finally, blood is pumped from the left ventricle into the aorta and then flows to all parts of the body, only to return eventually to the right atrium to repeat the cardiac cycle.

Although the two ventricles contract at the same time, it must be understood that the right ventricle is the pump for the pulmonary circulation and the left ventricle is the pump for the systemic circulation. Because the systolic blood pressure in the systemic circulation is about six times that in the pulmonary circulation, it is not surprising that the myocardium of the left ventricle is about three times the thickness of that of the right ventricle.

Measures of Cardiac Activity

Cardiac Output

Cardiac output is the quantity of blood pumped out of each ventricle per minute. In the young male, it averages about *5.6 liters per minute* under ordinary conditions of mental and physical rest. Cardiac output is greatly increased during muscular exercise and may reach *20 liters per minute.* Cardiac output is also increased during emotional excitement, digestion, and the later months of pregnancy.

The left and right ventricles must have equal cardiac outputs, so that equal volumes of blood pass through the systemic and pulmonary circulations.

Stroke Volume

Stroke volume is the volume of blood pumped out of one ventricle at each beat of the heart. Under resting condition this equals *60 to 70 ml.* The cardiac output thus equals the stroke volume multiplied by the heart rate. In other words, any change in the heart rate or stroke volume will alter cardiac output.

Venous Return and the Frank-Starling Law

The blood flow into the right atrium of the heart is called the *venous return*. Within physiological limits, the heart is capable of pumping out into the arteries all the blood that comes to it without permitting excessive damming of blood in the veins. The heart has this ability to adapt to the changing venous return because the force of contraction of cardiac muscle depends on the degree to which it is stretched. Thus, if the venous return increases during diastole, an extra volume of blood will enter the chambers of the heart and the muscle will be stretched to a greater extent; the muscle will contract with an increased force, so that the extra blood is pumped out of the heart into the arteries. Simply stated, the Frank-Starling law says that the greater the volume of blood that enters the heart during diastole, the greater will be the volume of blood ejected into the aorta.

Heart Rate

The heart rate in the young adult male at rest is about *70 beats per minute.* At birth, the heart rate is about *130 per minute,* and it diminishes progressively until adolescence. The heart rate is accelerated by such factors as emotional excitement, muscular exercise, high environmental temperatures, and digestion. Athletes have slower resting heart rates than do persons leading sedentary lives.

The term used to describe an increase in heart rate is *tachycardia. Bradycardia* is used to describe a heart rate of less than 60 beats per minute.

CONTROL OF HEART RATE. One of the outstanding characteristics of cardiac muscle is its ability to contract spontaneously and rhythmically. This quality is especially well developed in the cardiac muscle fibers of the conducting system of the heart. The sino-atrial node is the source of the *cardiac impulse,* which causes the heart to beat independently of all external influences. This inherent rhythmic rate of contraction can be modified, however, by the activity of the vagus and sympathetic nerves and by chemical agents. Thus, the efficiency of the pump can be adjusted to meet the demands of daily living (Fig. 8-11).

Nervous Control. Vagus Nerve. The activity of the vagus nerve slows the heart rate and diminishes the force of contraction. The nerve cells in the dorsal motor nucleus of the vagus are sometimes referred to as the *cardioinhibitory center* (see Fig. 8-11).

Cardiac Sympathetic Nerves. The activity of the cardiac sympathetic nerves increases the heart rate and increases the force of contraction. These nerves have little influence on the heart rate at rest. The sympathetic nerve cells in the spinal cord are sometimes referred to as the *cardioaccelerator center* (see Fig. 8-11).

Higher Nervous Centers. Emotions such as anger, fear, and excitement can increase the heart rate greatly (see Fig. 8-11). Impulses in such situations are conducted by nerve fibers from the cerebral cortex and the hypothalamus to the cardioinhibitory center and the cardioaccelerator center.

Respiration and Heart Rate. In children, quiet inspiration and expiration are associated with cardiac acceleration and slowing, respectively. This phenomenon is called *sinus arrhythmia.* It is caused by nervous connections between the respiratory center and the cardioinhibitory center and between the cardioinhibitory and cardioaccelerator centers (see Fig. 8-11); it is also caused by changes in the venous return during different phases of respiration. In adults, sinus arrhythmia occurs only when breathing is deepened voluntarily.

Cardiac Reflexes. The Bainbridge Reflex. An increase in atrial pressure causes an increase in heart rate (see Fig. 8-11). Stretch receptors situated in the atrial wall are stimulated, and nervous impulses pass along the vagus nerves to the medulla oblongata, where they inhibit the cardioinhibitory center and increase the heart rate. This phenomenon is called the *Bainbridge reflex.*

The Baroreceptor Afferent Reflexes. The common carotid artery near its bifurcation, or the internal carotid artery at its commencement in the neck,

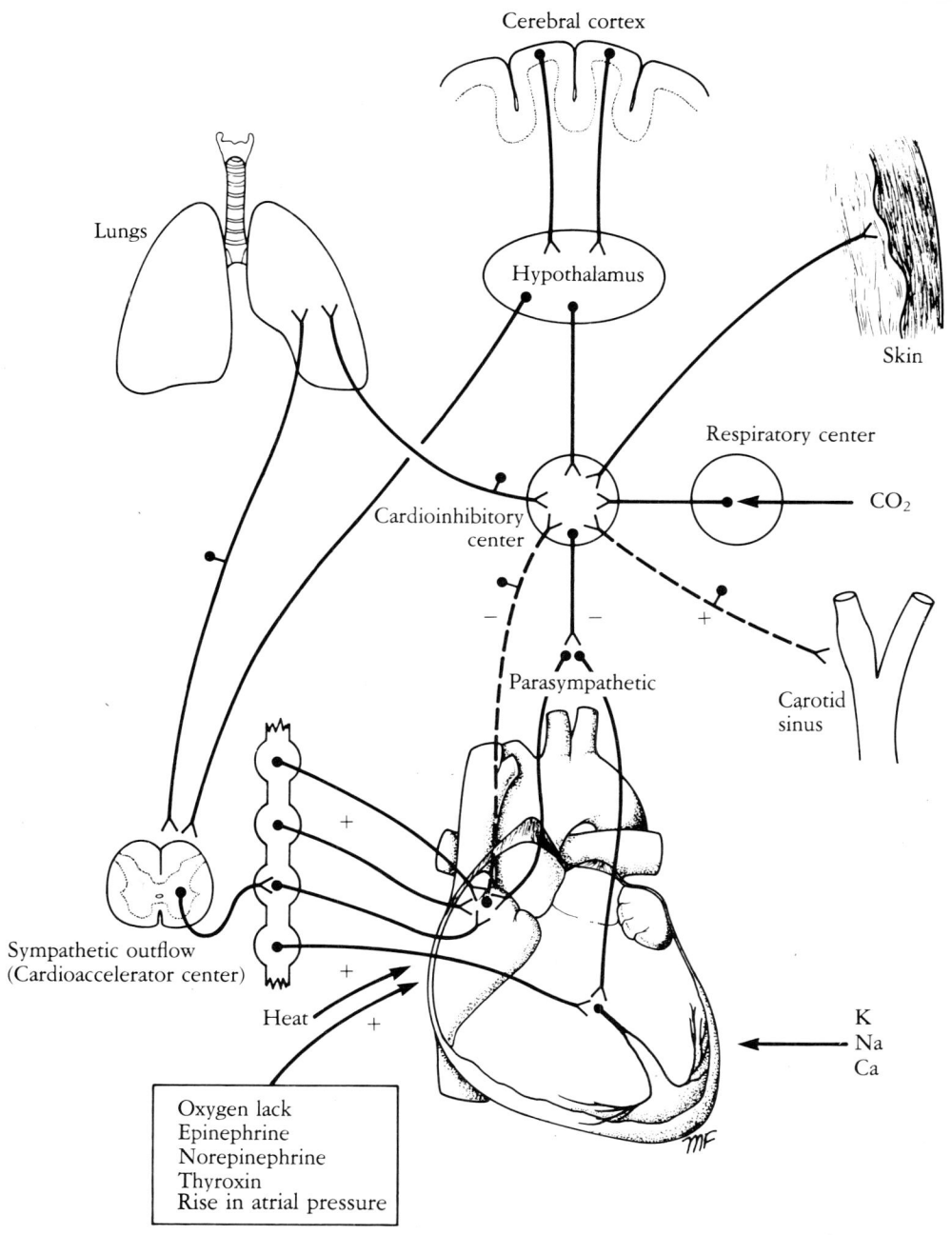

Fig. 8-11. The various factors that can influence the heart rate.

shows a slight enlargement called the *carotid sinus* (see Fig. 8-11). Stretch receptors in the wall of the sinus are stimulated by a rise in blood pressure. Nervous impulses ascend in the glossopharyngeal nerve and stimulate the cardioinhibitory center (and the vasodilator center) and cause reflex slowing of the heart. A similar set of stretch receptors is situated in the wall of the aortic arch. Nervous impulses ascend in the vagus nerve and stimulate the cardioinhibitory center (and the vasodilator center) and cause reflex slowing of the heart. Other baroreceptors are located in the walls of many large arteries in the neck and thorax.

General Afferents. The stimulation of almost any sensory nerve in the body will cause a change in the heart rate (see Fig. 8-11). For example, painful stimulation of the trigeminal nerve, which is the sensory nerve supply to the skin of the face, will cause slowing of the heart rate.

Chemical Control. Oxygen Lack. Anoxia causes cardiac acceleration, probably by direct action of oxygen lack on the sino-atrial node (see Fig. 8-11). If oxygen lack is severe or prolonged, cardiac slowing occurs and, finally, the heart ceases to contract.

Excess Carbon Dioxide. Inhalation of excess carbon dioxide causes cardiac acceleration (see Fig. 8-11). This result is probably caused by the spread of nervous impulses from the respiratory center to the cardiac centers. Prolonged exposure to excess carbon dioxide slows the heart rate.

Hormones. Norepinephrine and Epinephrine. The sympathetic postganglionic nerves increase the rate and force of heart contraction by liberating norepinephrine at their endings. When activated by stimulation of its sympathetic nerve supply, the suprarenal medulla liberates epinephrine and norepinephrine into the bloodstream. The two hormones have similar effects on the heart, although that of epinephrine is greater (see Fig. 8-11).

Acetylcholine. The parasympathetic postganglionic nerves decrease the rate and force of contraction of the heart by liberating acetylcholine at their endings (see Fig. 8-11). The effect of this hormone on the heart is limited by its rapid destruction by cholinesterase.

Thyroxin and Tri-iodothyronine. These hormones, produced by the thyroid gland, greatly increase the heart rate (see Fig. 8-11). They have a direct effect on the excitability of heart muscle.

Body Temperature. A rise in body temperature greatly increases the heart rate (see Fig. 8-11) by a direct stimulating effect on the sino-atrial node.

Muscular Exercise. Muscular exercise also greatly increases the heart rate. The various mechanisms of this increase are shown in Figure 8-11.

Electrical Changes in the Heart: The Electrocardiogram

Contracting cardiac muscle is relatively electrically negative compared with resting muscle. The spread of the wave of depolarization (the cardiac impulse) through the heart causes electrical currents to spread into tissues around the heart. The placement of electrodes on the body surface on opposite sides of the heart enables one to detect those electrical changes produced by the heart. The recording of these electrical changes is called an *electrocardiogram* (Fig. 8-12).

The normal electrocardiogram is made up of five waves known by the letters *P, Q, R, S,* and *T*. The P, R, and T waves are positive—that is, above the baseline of the record—whereas the Q and S waves are negative (see Fig. 8-12).

The P wave is caused by the spread of the cardiac impulse over the atria and represents atrial depolarization prior to contraction. The Q, R, and S waves are caused by the spread of the cardiac impulse over the ventricles prior to contraction and represent ventricular depolarization. The T wave is caused by currents produced by the ventricles as they recover from the state of depolarization (i.e., ventricular repolarization).

The P-Q interval or the P-R interval (the Q wave is often absent) is the interval between the beginning of the P wave and the beginning of the Q or R

Fig. 8-12. A: Position of the electrodes for recording the standard electrocardiographic leads; B: normal electrocardiograms with three standard leads; C: enlarged view of a normal electrocardiogram, showing the P, Q, R, S, and T waves.

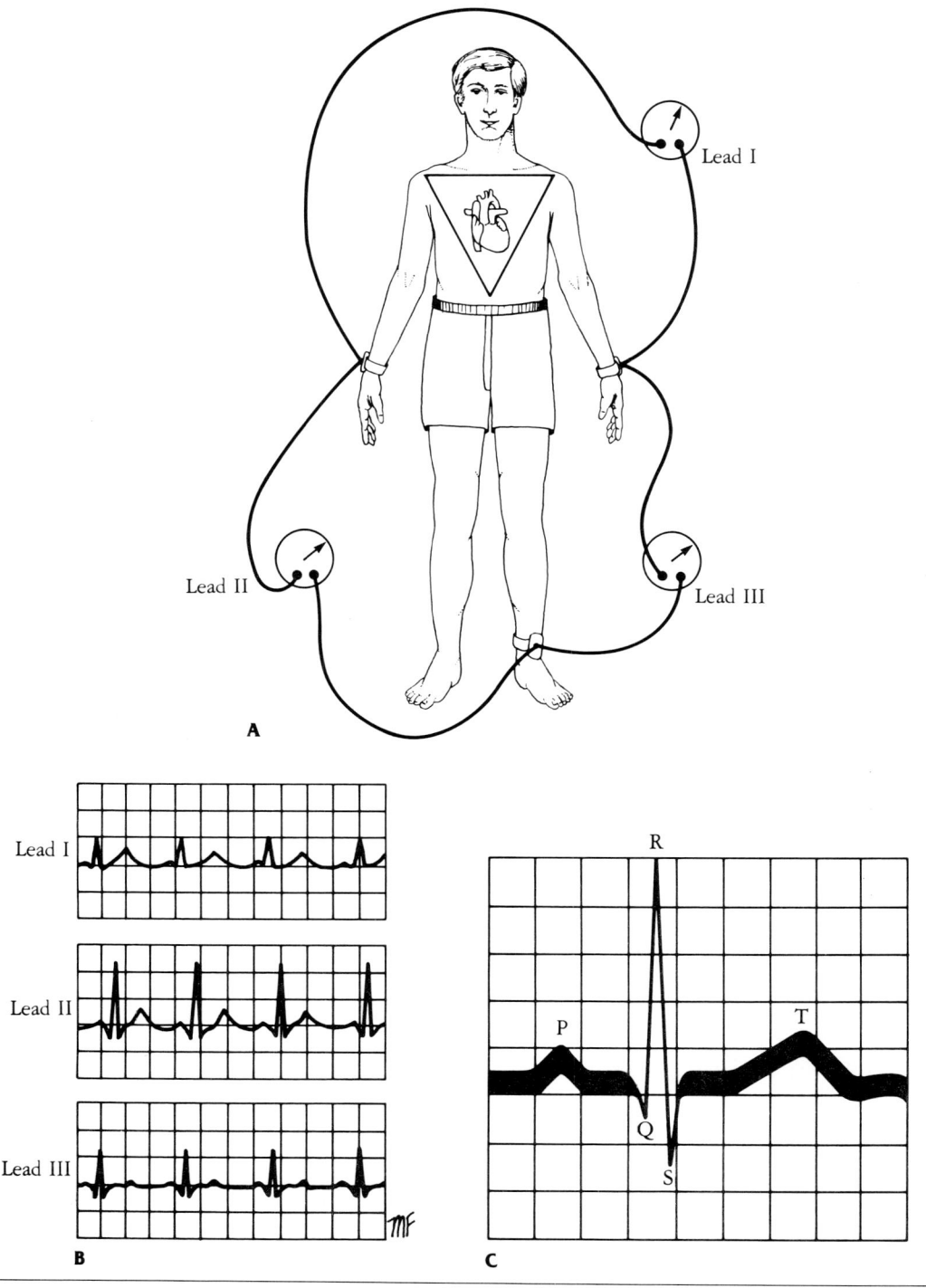

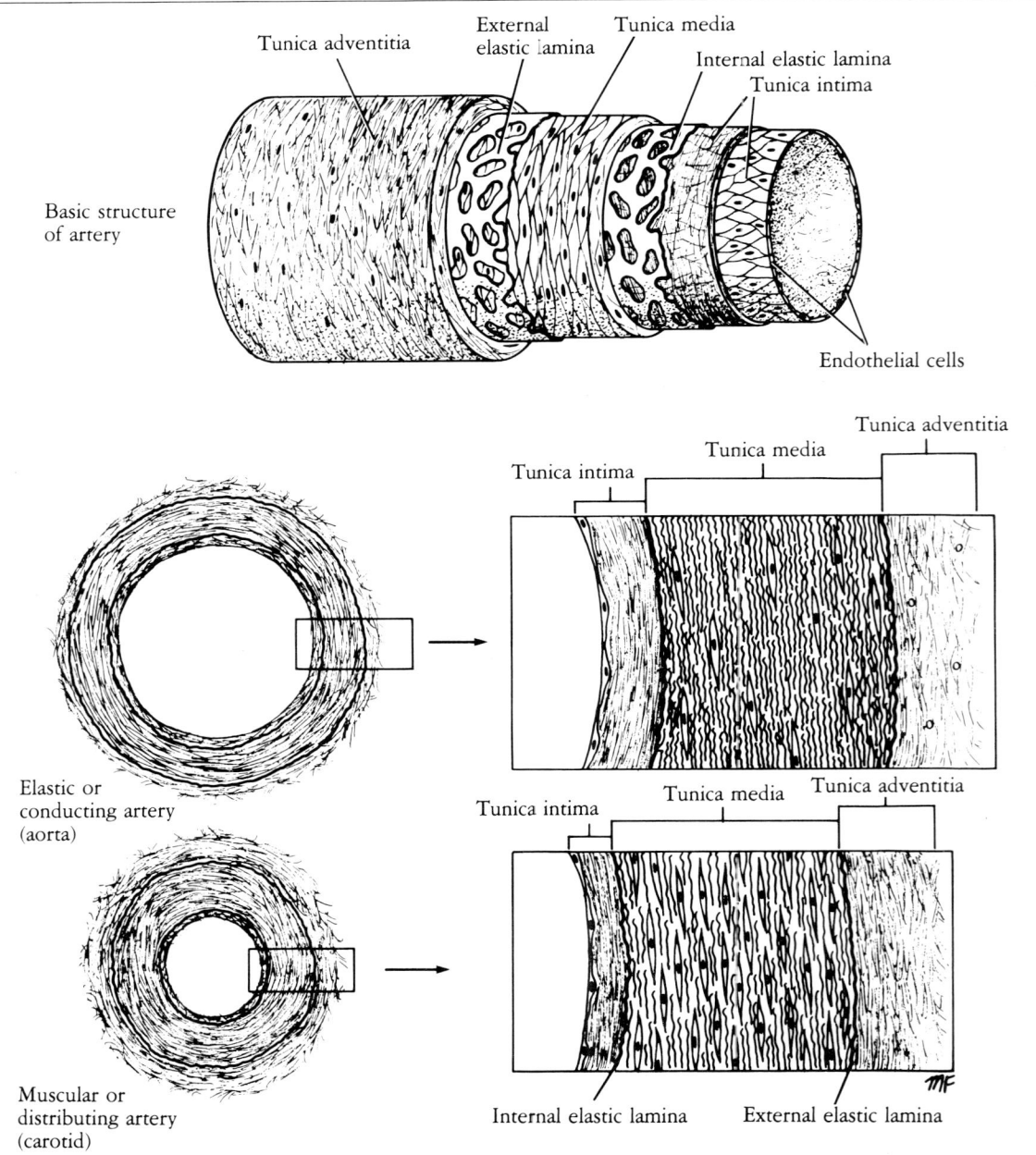

Fig. 8-13. Basic structure of an artery and sections of an elastic or conducting artery and a muscular or distributing artery. Note that the tunica media of the aorta contains numerous elastic fibers and only a few smooth muscle fibers, whereas the tunica media of the carotid artery contains many smooth muscle fibers as well as elastic fibers.

wave. It represents the time that has elapsed between the beginning of the contraction of the atria and the beginning of the contraction of the ventricles and is normally about 0.16 second.

The Q-T interval is the interval between the beginning of the Q wave and the end of the T wave. It represents the time taken for the ventricular contraction and is about 0.3 second.

Electrocardiograms are recorded by using three standard leads that are connected to the arms and legs:

Right arm and left arm is called *lead I.*
Right arm and left leg is called *lead II.*
Left arm and left leg is called *lead III.*

The electrocardiograms for leads I, II, and III are recorded simultaneously (see Fig. 8-12). On inspection, they are similar to one another. The sum of the potentials of leads I and III, however, equals the potential of lead II. Damage to atrial or ventricular muscle may alter the pattern of the electrocardiograms in some leads and not change other leads.

Precordial Chest Leads

Because the anterior surface of the heart is situated close to the anterior chest wall, it is common clinical practice to use a chest lead that records mainly the electrical potential in the cardiac muscle that lies close to the electrode. This practice may be important in detecting pathological changes in the cardiac muscle of the right and left ventricles. The chest electrode is usually placed at six separate sites over the anterior surface of the heart.

BLOOD VESSELS

Main Vessels

There are five main types of blood vessels: arteries, arterioles, capillaries, venules, and veins.

Arteries

The arteries are the blood vessels that conduct blood away from the heart to the organs and tissues. They branch repeatedly along their course, forming arteries of progressively smaller diameter. It is cus-

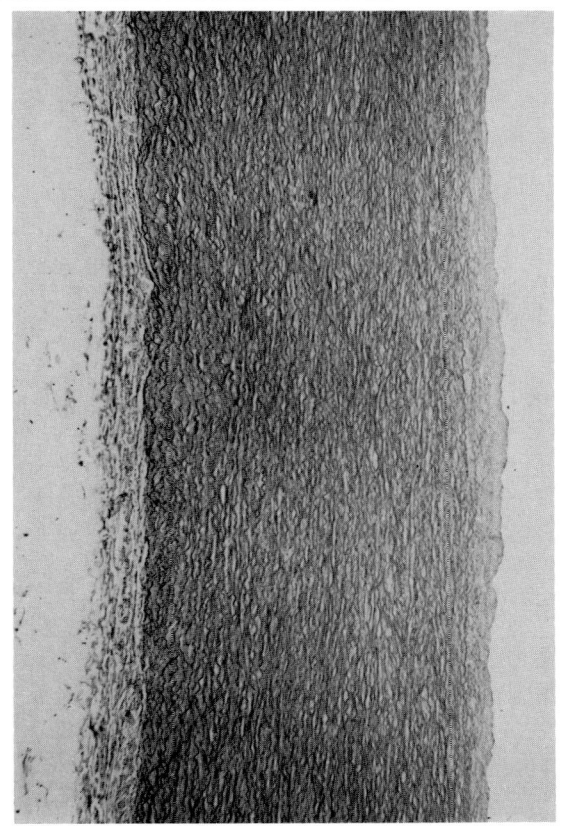

Fig. 8-14. Photomicrograph of transverse section of the aorta, showing the loose connective tissue of the tunica adventitia on the left and the thick tunica media and the tunica intima on the right. (H&E; × 40.)

tomary to classify arteries into elastic, or conducting, arteries and muscular, or distributing, arteries. The walls of arteries are thick and strong and consist of three coats: (1) the tunica intima (internal coat), (2) the tunica media (middle coat), and (3) the tunica adventitia (outer coat). These three coats are seen most distinctly in the muscular arteries.

ELASTIC OR CONDUCTING ARTERIES. Elastic, or conducting, arteries are the large arteries, such as the aorta and pulmonary, brachiocephalic, common carotid, and iliac arteries. These arteries have the following basic structure (Figs. 8-13 and 8-14).

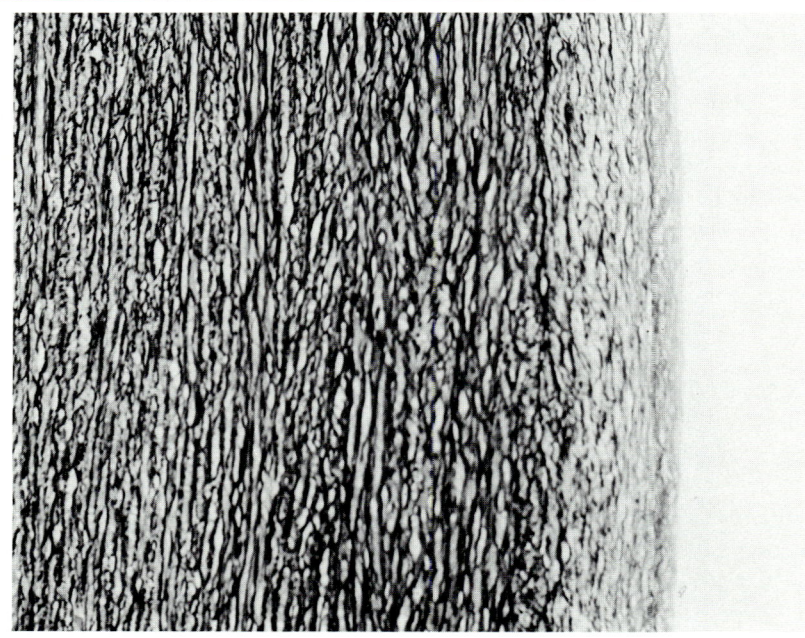

Fig. 8-15. Photomicrograph of transverse section of the aorta, showing part of the tunica media on the left and the thin tunica intima and the lumen on the right. Large numbers of black-stained elastic fibers can be seen in the tunica media. (Resorcin fuchsin stain; × 100.)

Tunica Intima. This layer consists of a lining of epithelial cells resting on a layer of connective tissue. The tunica intima is bounded externally by a lamina of fenestrated elastic tissue known as the *internal elastic lamina* (see Fig. 8-13). This lamina may be difficult to recognize, because it merges with the elastic laminae of the tunica media.

Tunica Media. This layer consists largely of successive layers of fenestrated elastic laminae, between which are bundles of collagen fibers and smooth muscle cells (Fig. 8-15; see Fig. 8-13). The outermost elastic lamina corresponds to the *external elastic lamina* found in other kinds of arteries.

The large amount of elastic tissue present in the tunica media of elastic arteries (see Fig. 8-15) allows the arterial wall to become distended by the blood ejected from the heart during ventricular systole. The elastic recoil of these arteries that occurs when the ventricles are relaxing is largely responsible for maintaining the arterial blood pressure during diastole of the heart.

Tunica Intima. This layer consists of a lining of endothelial cells resting on a layer of connective tissue. The tunica intima is bounded externally by a lamina of fenestrated elastic tissue known as the *internal elastic lamina* (see Fig. 8-13). This lamina may be difficult to recognize, because it merges with the elastic laminae of the tunica media.

MUSCULAR OR DISTRIBUTING ARTERIES. Muscular, or distributing, arteries are the medium-sized arteries, such as the brachial, radial, ulnar, femoral, and tibial arteries. The coronary arteries are also muscular. These arteries have the following basic structure (Figs. 8-16, 8-17, and 8-18; see Fig. 8-13).

Tunica Intima. This layer consists of a lining of endothelial cells resting on a layer of connective tissue. The tunica intima is bounded externally by a

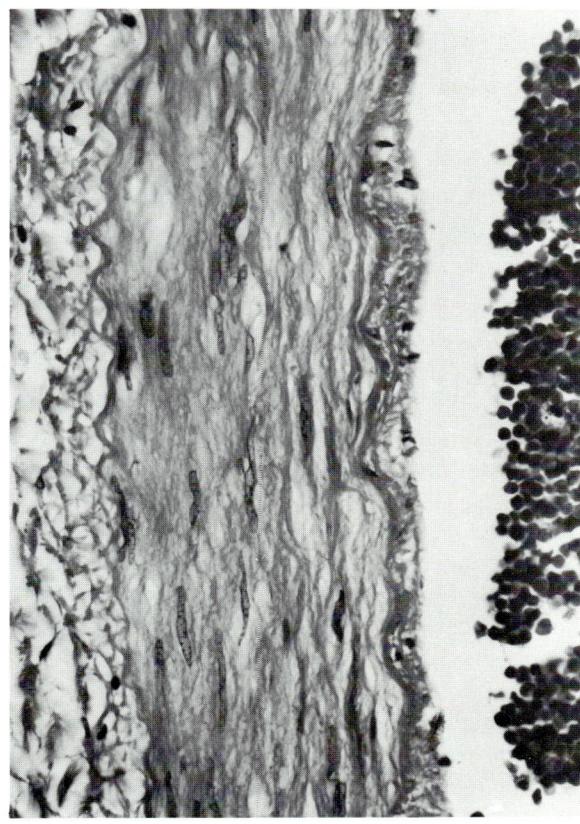

Fig. 8-16. Photomicrograph of transverse section of a small muscular artery, showing the tunica adventitia on the left and the lumen containing blood cells on the right. Note the presence of large numbers of smooth muscle fibers with fusiform nuclei in the tunica media. (H&E; × 400.)

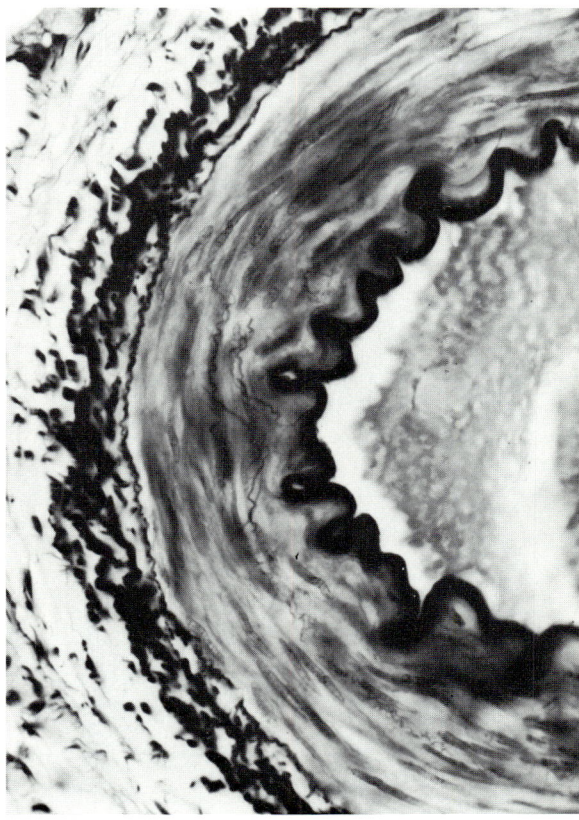

Fig. 8-17. Photomicrograph of transverse section of a small muscular artery, showing the tunica adventitia on the left and the lumen containing blood on the right. Note the concentration of wavy, black-staining elastic fibers forming the internal and external elastic laminae. (Resorcin fuchsin stain; × 400.)

distinct lamina of fenestrated elastic tissue known as the *internal elastic lamina* (see Fig. 8-17).

Tunica Media. This layer consists largely of concentric layers of smooth muscle cells mixed with a few bundles of collagen fibers and occasional elastic fibers. The tunica media is bounded externally by a distinct layer of elastic tissue known as the *external elastic lamina* (see Fig. 8-17). The large number of circularly arranged smooth muscle cells in the tunica media of muscular arteries permits the autonomic nervous system to control the flow of blood through these vessels and thus regulate the blood supply to different organs of the body.

Tunica Adventitia. This layer is composed of a thick layer of connective tissue (see Figs. 8-16 and 8-17) that merges with the surrounding connective tissues. Numerous nonmyelinated axons, which are postganglionic sympathetic nerve fibers, are found in the tunica adventitia. These nerve fibers stimulate the contraction of the smooth muscle cells in the tunica media and thus regulate the diameter of the lumina of these arteries.

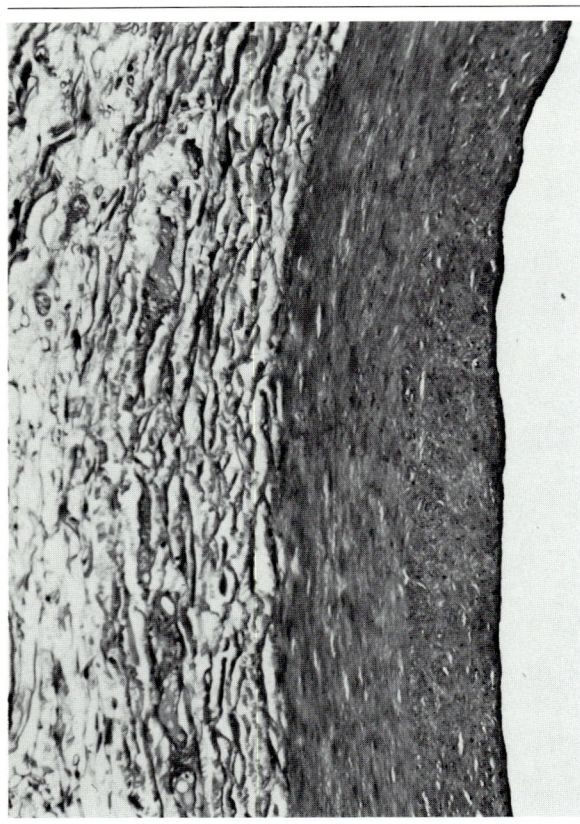

Fig. 8-18. Photomicrograph of transverse section of a coronary artery (muscular type of artery), showing the tunica adventitia on the left and the lumen on the right. Note the tunica media, composed of numerous concentric layers of smooth muscle fibers. (H&E; × 100.)

Arterioles

An arteriole is an artery having a diameter of less than 0.1 mm; an arteriole characteristically has a very thick wall relative to the size of its lumen (Fig. 8-19). Arterioles possess the usual three coats, but the tunica media is made up almost entirely of circularly arranged smooth muscle cells. The tunica adventitia possesses autonomic nerve fibers that bring about contraction of the smooth muscle and thus control the size of the lumen of the vessel.

The terminal branch of many arterioles, sometimes called a *metarteriole,* has a small lumen and only a few smooth muscle cells in its tunica media (see Fig. 8-25). At the junction of the metarteriole with the capillary, however, there is a band of smooth muscle called the *precapillary sphincter.* The precapillary sphincter intermittently contracts, opening and closing the arteriolar-capillary junction.

Capillaries

When traced peripherally, arterioles break up into small blood vessels called capillaries. The lumen of a typical capillary is about 7 to 9 μm wide, that is, slightly wider than a red blood cell. The wall of a capillary is composed of a single layer of endothelial cells resting on a basement membrane (Fig. 8-20; see Fig. 8-19). The endothelial cells can be seen under the electron microscope to be held together by tight junctions (maculae occludens) (Figs. 8-21 and 8-22). Numerous pinocytotic vesicles are seen; they are involved in transporting materials across the endothelial cells in either direction.

There are two types of capillaries, as demonstrated under the electron microscope: continuous and fenestrated (see Figs. 8-19, 8-21, and 8-22). In both types, the endothelial cells form a continuous lining of the capillary, but in the fenestrated capillaries, the cells show tiny holes less than 100 nm in diameter. It is believed that these so-called holes are in fact closed by a diaphragm that is thinner than a cell membrane and that allows dissolved substances to pass through easily.

Occasional cells called *pericytes* are found within the basement membrane of the endothelial cells (see Fig. 8-19). These cells are noncontracting, and their function is not known.

Venules

Venules receive the blood from the capillaries and are of a larger diameter than capillaries. The structure of a small venule is identical to that of a continuous capillary (Fig. 8-23). Some smooth muscle fibers are situated in the connective tissue surrounding the endothelial cells in large venules.

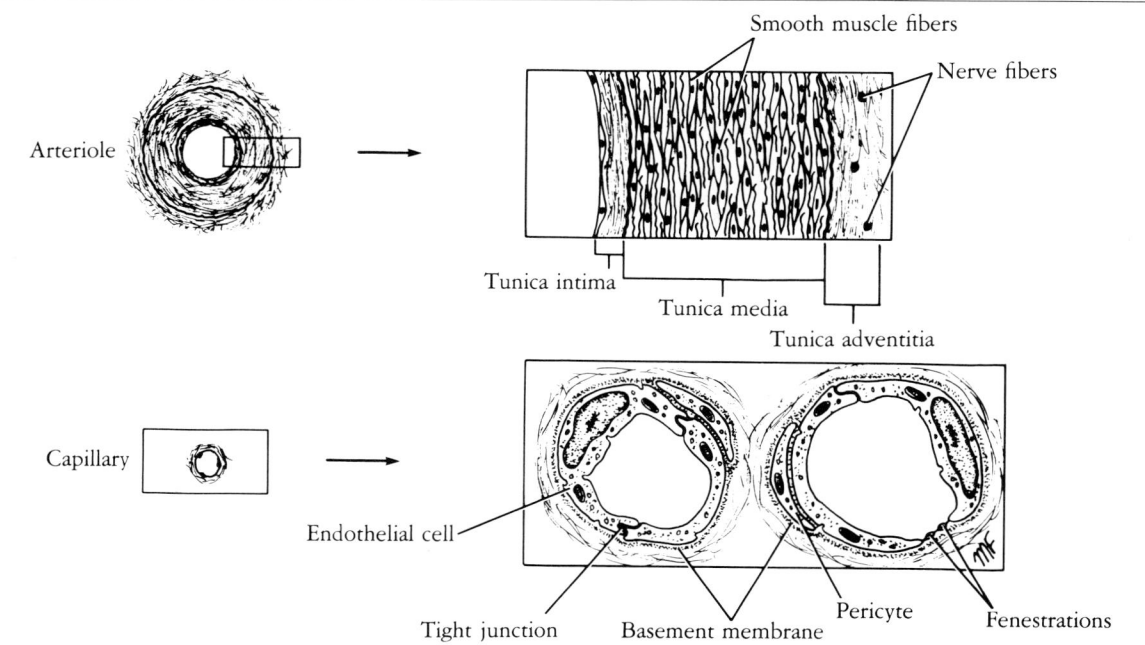

Fig. 8-19. Basic structure of an arteriole and a capillary. Note the two types of capillaries, continuous and fenestrated.

It is at the capillaries and the small venules that oxygen and nutritive materials pass from the blood into the tissue fluid and the carbon dioxide and the waste products of tissue metabolism pass into the bloodstream. The walls of blood vessels larger than capillaries and venules are impervious to gases and liquids.

Veins

Veins are the blood vessels that conduct blood back to the heart from the capillaries of the organs and tissues. The smallest veins, the venules, closely resemble capillaries and were discussed in the previous paragraphs. The diameters of veins tend to be larger than those of the corresponding arteries. As the venous tributaries unite to form larger veins, their walls become thicker.

The walls of veins, like those of arteries, consist of three coats: the tunica intima, the tunica media, and the tunica adventitia (see Fig. 8-23).

MEDIUM-SIZED VEINS. These veins include the distal veins of the limbs and the veins of the viscera.

Tunica Intima. This consists of a lining of endothelial cells resting on a thin layer of connective tissue.

Tunica Media. This layer is thinner than that found in arteries and consists of circularly arranged smooth muscle fibers mixed with connective tissue.

Tunica Adventitia. This is a thick layer, thicker than the tunica media. It is composed of loose connective tissue containing bundles of collagen fibers and elastic networks. Longitudinally arranged bundles of smooth muscle cells are also frequently found in this layer. Many vasa vasorum are present.

Valves. Many veins are provided with valves that allow the blood to flow toward the heart but not in the opposite direction (see Fig. 8-23). Most of the valves have two leaflets (are bicuspid), and each leaflet is composed of a fold of tunica intima. The

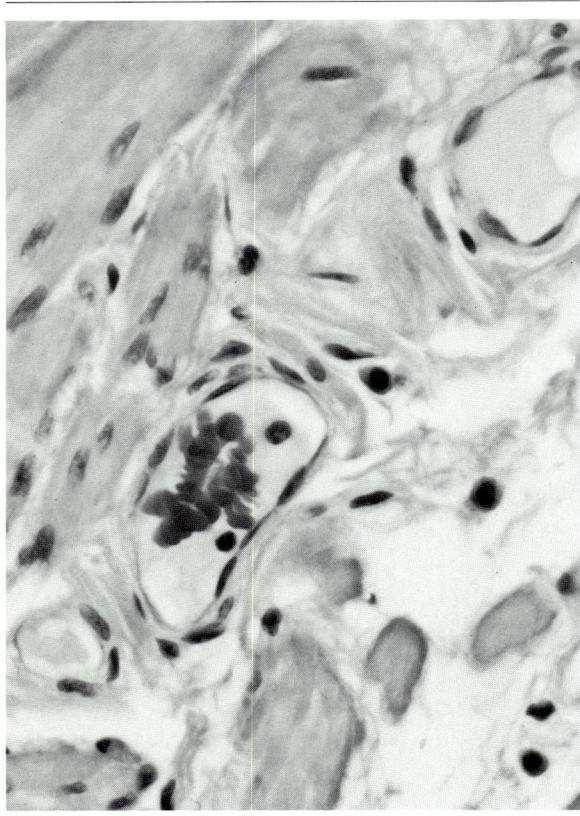

Fig. 8-20. Photomicrograph of a transverse section of a blood capillary and two lymph capillaries. Note that the blood capillary is lined with flattened endothelial cells. (H&E; ×373.)

valves within veins that pass between muscles allow the veins to serve as pumps and aid the return of venous blood to the heart.

LARGE VEINS. These veins include the superior and inferior venae cavae, the portal vein, and the iliac veins; the renal and mesenteric veins have a similar structure (Fig. 8-24; see Fig. 8-23).

Tunica Intima. This consists of a lining of endothelial cells resting on a thick layer of connective tissue.

Tunica Media. This is a thin layer and consists of circularly arranged smooth muscle fibers mixed with connective tissue (see Fig. 8-23).

Tunica Adventitia. This is the thickest layer of the wall. It is composed of loose connective tissue containing bundles of longitudinally running collagen fibers and smooth muscle cells. Elastic networks are also present (see Fig. 8-24). Situated within the tunica adventitia are many small blood vessels, the vasa vasorum; lymphatic vessels and nerves are also present.

Other Structures

Sinusoids

Sinusoids are found in the bone marrow, spleen, liver, and some endocrine glands. They are very thin-walled blood vessels having an irregular cross diameter. The sinusoids are lined by endothelium supported by a minimum of connective tissue. In the bone marrow and spleen, there are gaps between the endothelial cells that permit the passage of blood cells. In the liver, the sinusoids are lined by endothelial cells, some of which are phagocytic and are members of the reticuloendothelial system. These are known as *Kupffer cells.* In the suprarenal cortex and the islets of Langerhans in the pancreas, the endothelial cells are fenestrated, as in fenestrated capillaries.

Arteriovenous Anastomoses

In certain areas of the body, notably the skin, the blood is shunted from the arterioles directly into the venules without having to circulate through a capillary network. Such a bypass is referred to as an *arteriovenous anastomosis* or *AV shunt* (Fig. 8-25). The walls of the shunt are thick and muscular and are well supplied with vasomotor nerve fibers.

In the nail beds of the fingers and toes and the auricle of the ear, the arteriovenous anastomoses are branched and tortuous and form a specialized organ called the *glomus* (see Fig. 8-25).

Arteriovenous anastomoses control blood flow and assist in temperature regulation of the body. In

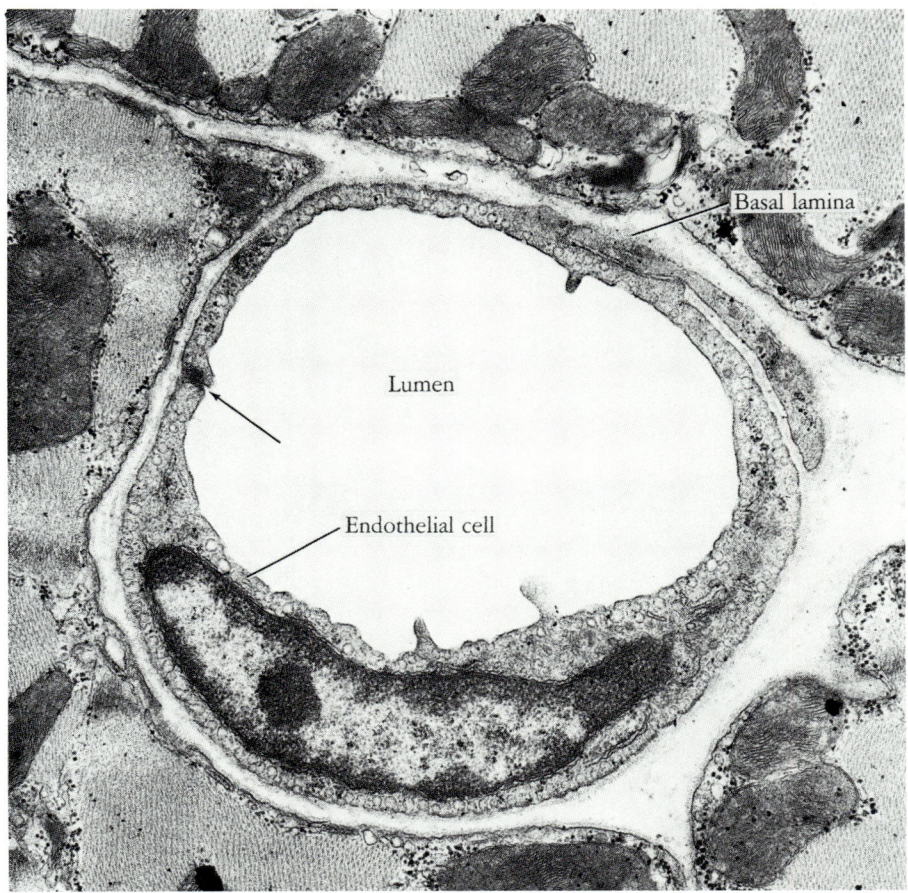

Fig. 8-21. Electron micrograph of a transverse section of a continuous capillary, showing the endothelial cells forming a continuous lining of the capillary. Note that the endothelial cells are held together by tight junctions (arrow). ($\times 21,000$.) (Courtesy of Dr. J. Rhodin.)

the skin, for example, the constriction or dilatation of an AV shunt will control the blood flow through the capillaries and thus conserve heat or increase heat loss in the body.

Anatomical End Arteries and Functional End Arteries

Anatomical end arteries are vessels whose terminal branches do not anastomose with branches or arteries supplying adjacent areas. Functional end arteries are vessels whose terminal branches *do* anastomose with those of adjacent arteries, but the caliber of the anastomosis is insufficient to keep the tissue alive if one of the arteries becomes occluded. Coronary arteries are examples of functional end arteries.

Carotid Sinus

The carotid sinus is a slight dilatation of the terminal part of the common carotid artery or the beginning of the internal carotid artery (see Fig. 8-25). The carotid arteries are muscular arteries and serve to distribute blood to the head and neck. In the carotid sinus, the tunica media is thinner than elsewhere

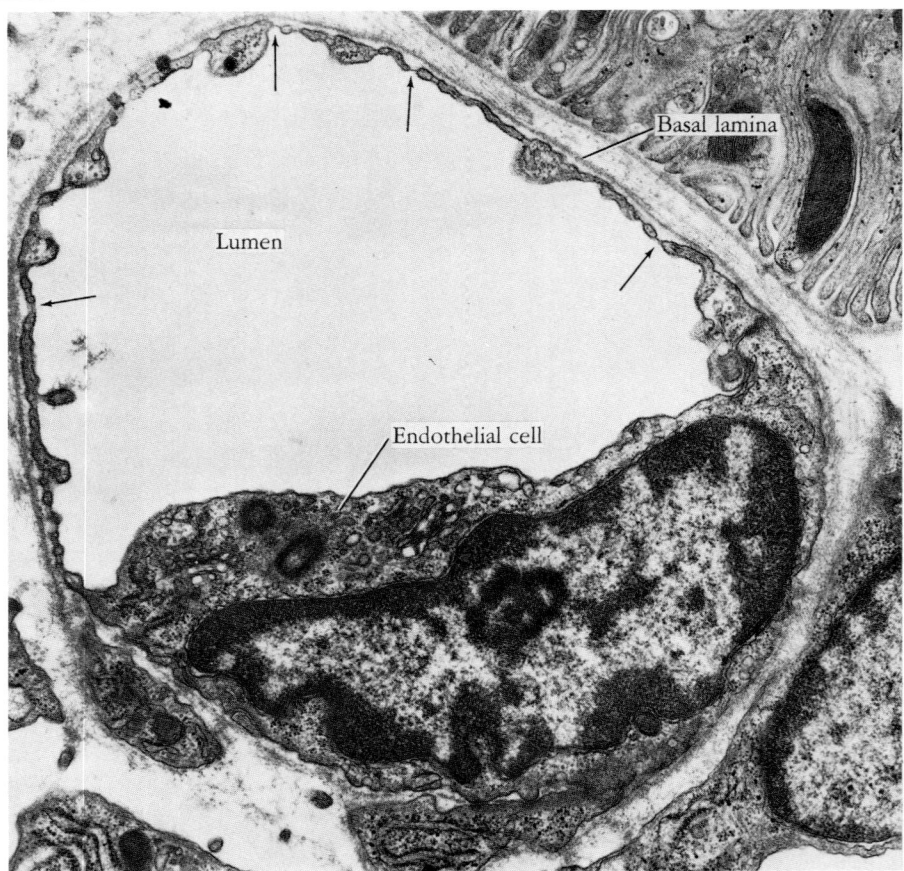

Fig. 8-22. Electron micrograph of a transverse section of a fenestrated capillary. Note that the so-called holes in the endothelial cells (arrows) are in fact closed by a thin diaphragm. (× 18,000.) (Courtesy of Dr. J. Rhodin.)

and contains many nerve endings of the glossopharyngeal nerve. The thinness of the tunica media permits pressure changes within the lumen of the sinus to be transmitted readily to the sensory endings in the tunica adventitia. For example, a rise in arterial blood pressure will cause an increased number of impulses to ascend the glossopharyngeal nerve, resulting in the slowing of the heart rate and vasodilatation of peripheral blood vessels.

Similar stretch receptors are found in the wall of the aortic arch.

Carotid Body

The carotid body is a highly vascular structure measuring a few millimeters in diameter. It is situated close to the bifurcation of the common carotid artery. Similar structures, known as aortic bodies, are located near the arch of the aorta.

The carotid body consists of groups of cells between which lie sinusoidlike capillaries (Fig. 8-26). Numerous nerve fibers that are branches of the glossopharyngeal nerve end on the cells. The cells are chemoreceptors sensitive to excess carbon dioxide and reduced oxygen tensions in the blood circulating through the capillaries of the organ; they are also sensitive to changes in blood pH. When the chemoreceptors are stimulated, more afferent nerve

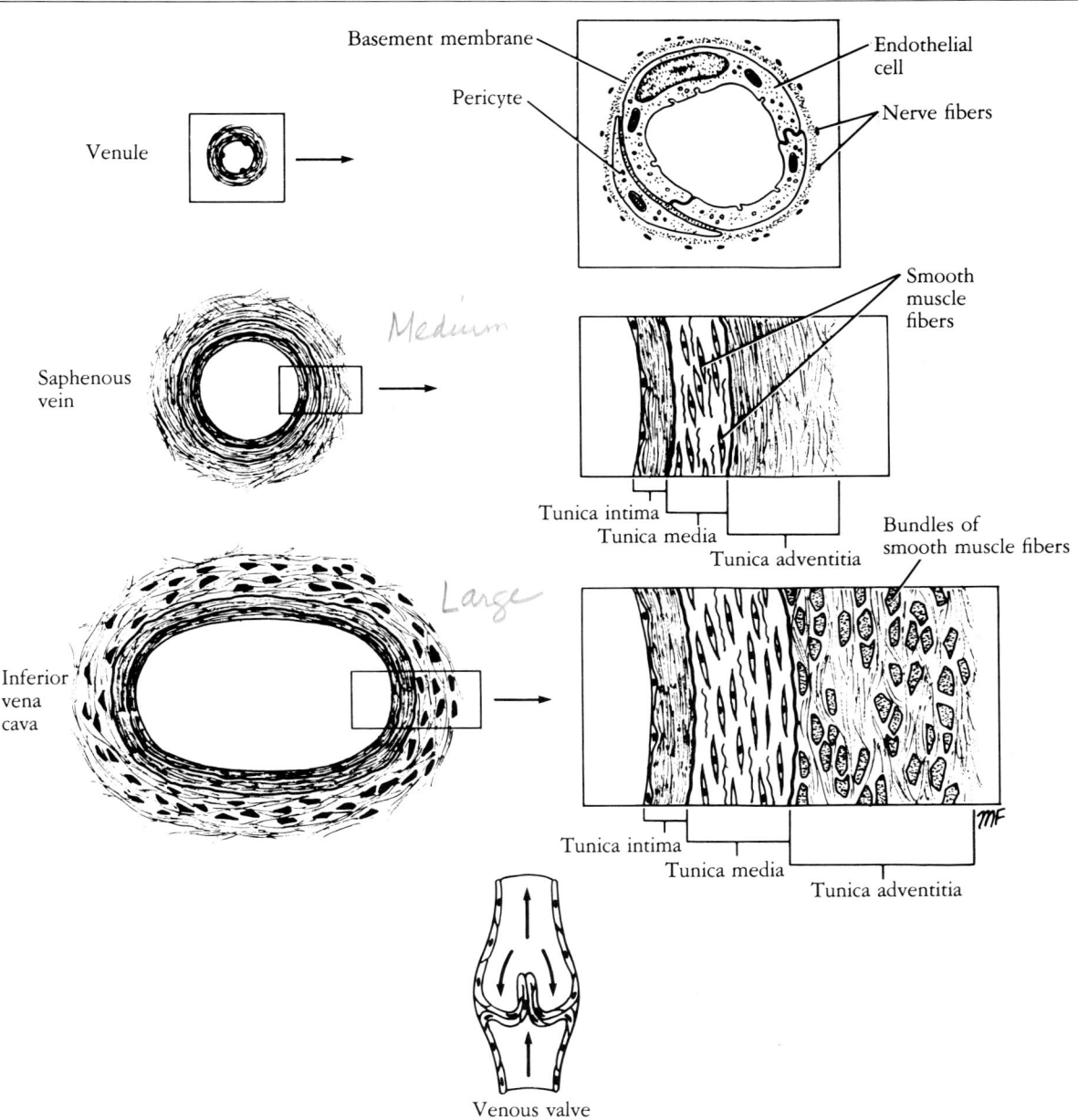

Fig. 8-23. Basic structure of a venule, a medium-sized vein, the saphenous vein, and a large vein, the inferior vena cava.

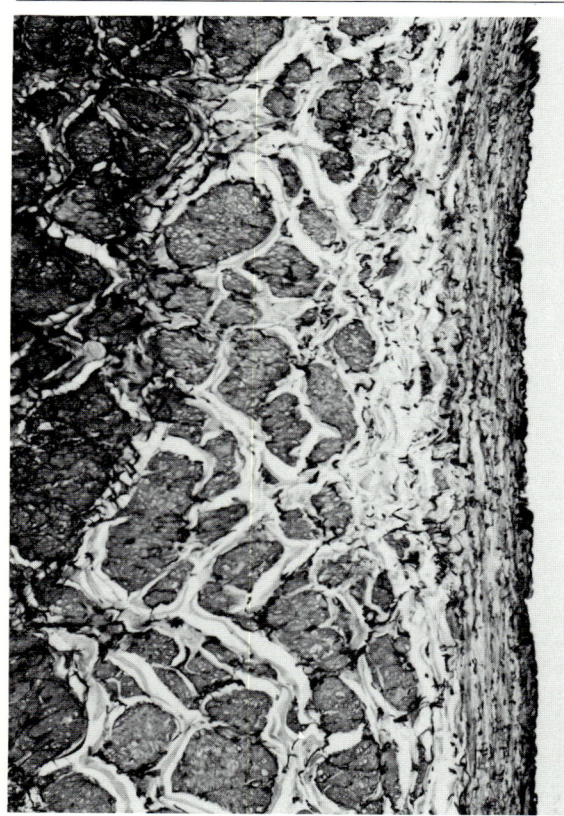

Fig. 8-24. Photomicrograph of a transverse section of the inferior vena cava. The lumen is on the right side. Note the tunica adventitia containing large bundles of smooth muscle fibers that run longitudinally. Note also the black-staining elastic fibers. (Resorcin fuchsin stain; × 100.)

impulses ascend the glossopharyngeal nerve and increase the heart and respiration rates.

Blood Pressure

Arterial Blood Pressure

The blood in arteries is under a relatively high pressure that rises and falls with each beat of the heart (Fig. 8-27). The highest pressure attained in the aorta and peripheral arteries occurs during the contraction of the left ventricle (systole), when blood is pumped into the arteries. The lowest pressure occurs when the left ventricle is relaxed (diastole). Under ordinary resting conditions, the *systolic pres-* *sure* in a young male is about 120 mm Hg (± 10 mm Hg). The minimum or *diastolic pressure* is about 80 mm Hg.* The pulsation in the arteries is caused by the difference between the systolic and diastolic pressures and is called the *pulse pressure* (120 − 80 = 40 mm Hg).

MAINTENANCE OF NORMAL ARTERIAL BLOOD PRESSURE. The following factors are responsible for the maintenance of normal blood pressure:

(1) Cardiac output
(2) Blood volume
(3) Blood viscosity
(4) Elasticity of blood vessels
(5) Peripheral resistance

Cardiac Output. Cardiac output is the volume of blood pumped out of each ventricle per minute. An increase in the cardiac output will result in an increase in the mean arterial blood pressure. The increased output may be caused by an increase in the heart rate or in the stroke volume. The stroke volume may rise as a result of an increase in the force of contraction of the heart or in the venous return to the heart. It follows that a decrease in cardiac output will cause a fall in the mean arterial blood pressure.

Blood Volume. The arterial blood pressure is produced by the ejection from the heart into the arteries of a volume of blood that cannot immediately escape through the small peripheral vessels, the ar-

---

*The upper limit of normal in a young male at rest is 140 mm Hg systolic pressure and 90 mm Hg diastolic pressure.

Fig. 8-25. General structure of (A) a microcirculatory network, with the blood being fed into the capillary plexus through an arteriole and drained away by a venule; note the distribution of the smooth muscle fibers and the presence of precapillary sphincters; (B) an arteriovenous anastomosis with large numbers of rounded smooth muscle fibers; (C) a glomus, in which the vascular channels are surrounded by rounded smooth muscle fibers called glomus cells; (D) the carotid sinus, emphasizing the thin tunica media and the thick tunica adventitia containing nerve endings.

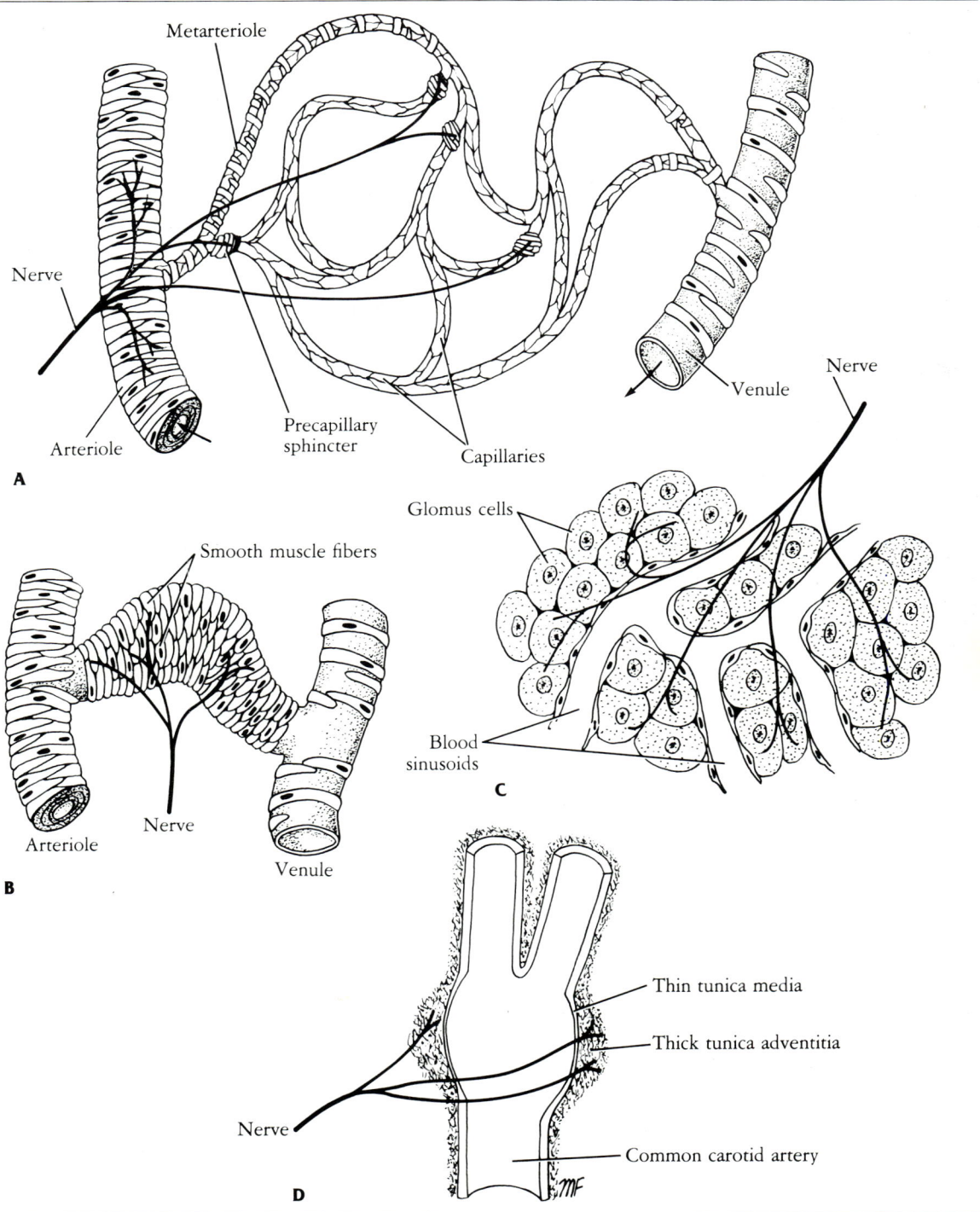

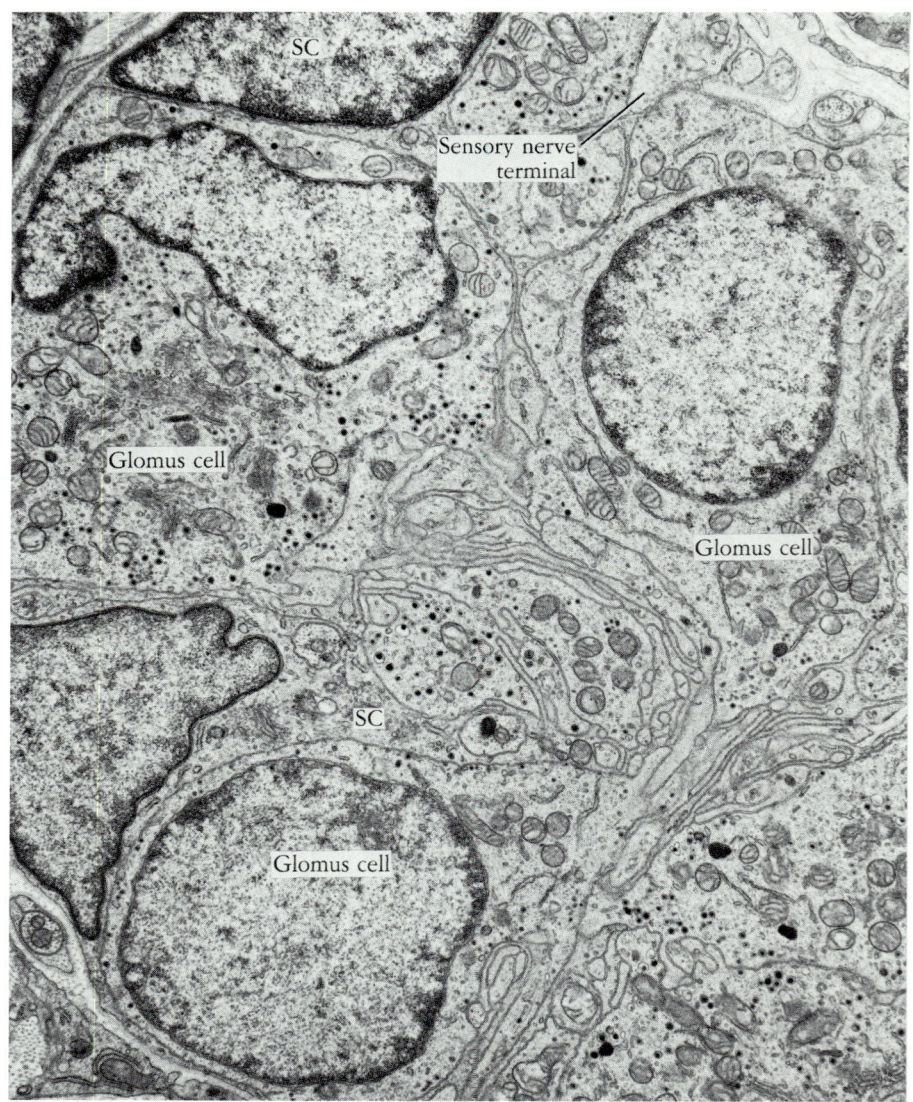

Fig. 8-26. Electron micrograph of section of the carotid body, showing numerous epithelioid (glomus) cells and two supporting cells (SC). A sensory nerve terminal is seen at the top of the picture (pointer). No blood capillaries are seen in this section. (×13,500.) (Courtesy of Dr. J. T. Hansen.)

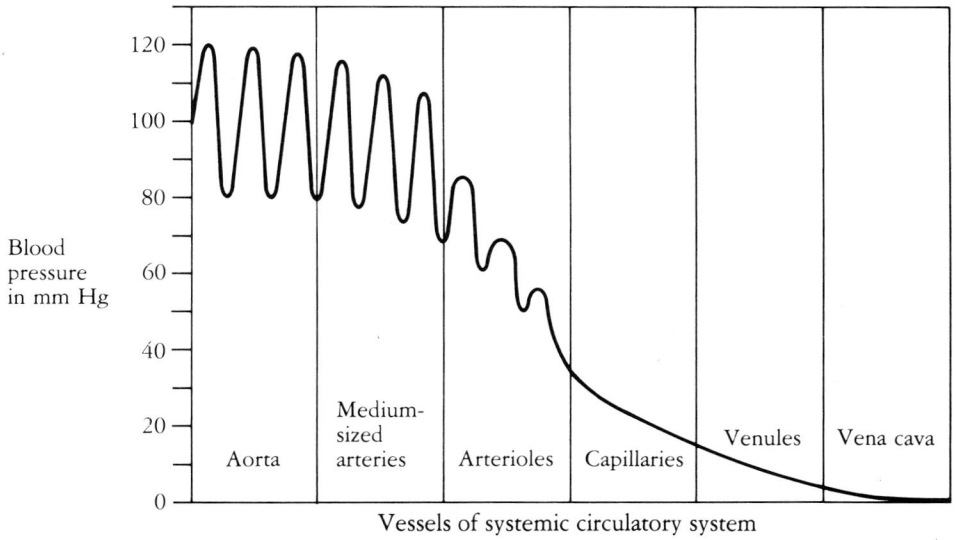

Fig. 8-27. Blood pressure in different blood vessels of the circulatory system.

terioles, into the venous system. If the volume of blood is not large enough to overfill the arteries, the blood pressure will fall.

Blood Viscosity. The presence of proteins and cells within the blood makes it thicker than water and less able to pass through small tubes, such as arterioles. It is the resistance to the passage of this viscous liquid through the arterioles that helps maintain the blood pressure.

Elasticity of Blood Vessels. If, during the ejection phase of the heart, the blood were discharged into rigid arteries (Fig. 8-28), the systolic blood pressure would be high but there would be no diastolic pressure. The walls of the large arteries, however, contain elastic tissue, so when the blood is ejected from the heart, the large arteries are distended by the force of the ventricular contraction. Thus, during ventricular diastole, when no further blood is leaving the heart, the elastic walls of the blood vessels recoil, driving the blood onward under pressure. Diastolic blood pressure therefore largely depends on the elasticity of the blood vessels.

For the elasticity of blood vessels to contribute to the maintenance of blood pressure, the blood cannot escape freely (see Fig. 8-28) from the peripheral arteries; there must be some peripheral resistance provided by the blood viscosity and the arterioles to cause the large elastic arteries to distend during ventricular systole.

Peripheral Resistance. The small diameter of the lumen of the arteriole, which is controlled by the smooth muscle in its wall, effectively provides resistance at the periphery of the arterial system to the passage of blood into the veins. If the arterioles are constricted, the blood is held back in the arterial system and the systolic blood pressure rises. The elastic arterial walls are stretched further, and consequently the diastolic blood pressure rises also. Should the arterioles become dilated, the opposite effect is produced and the blood pressure falls.

The diameters of the arterioles of the abdominal viscera can be changed easily by modifying the activity of the sympathetic nerves supplying the smooth muscle in the arteriolar walls. Should vasodilatation occur following an emotional experience, the blood capacity of the dilated arterioles and capillaries becomes enormous and nearly equal to the total blood volume. Under these circumstances, the venous re-

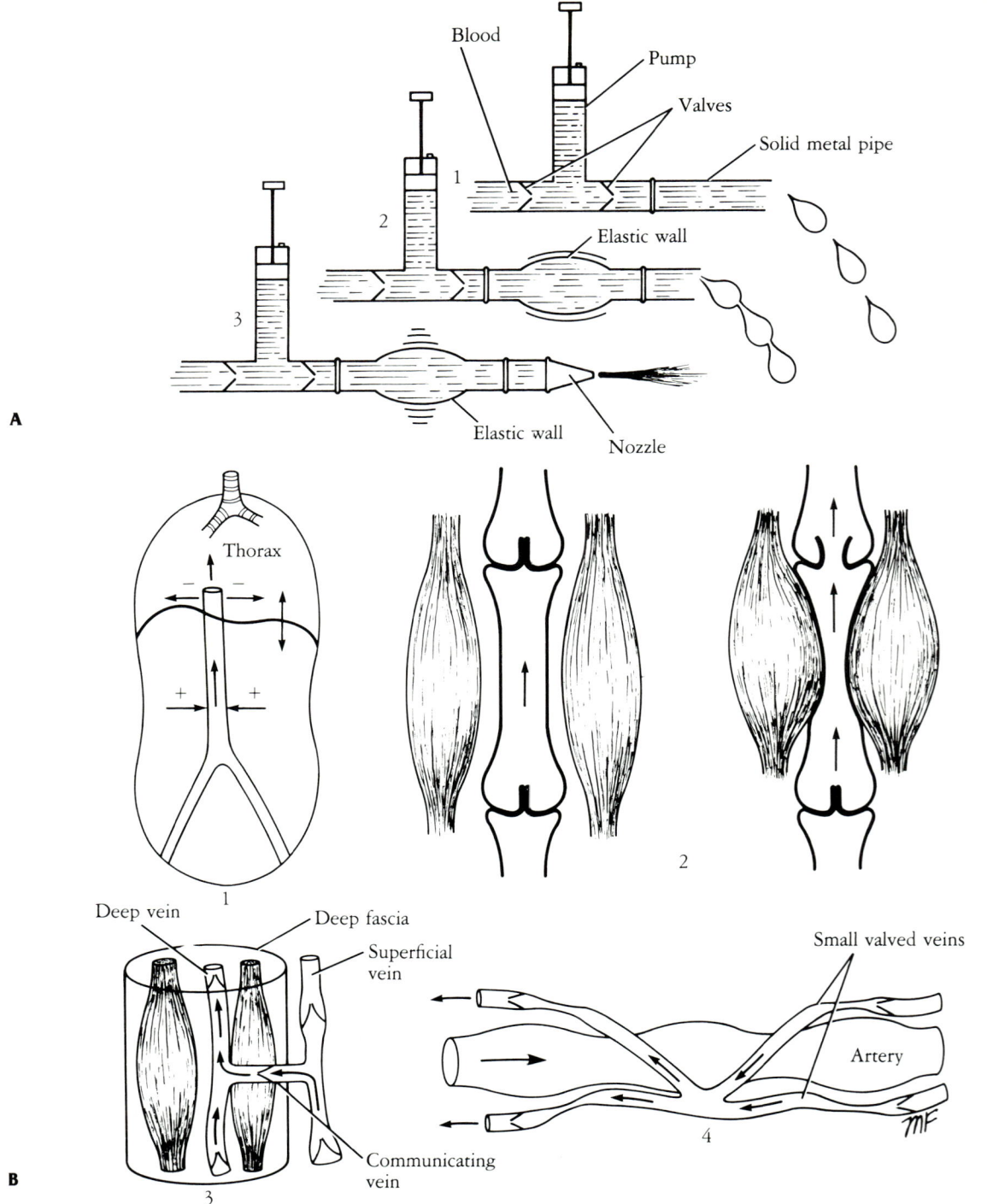

Fig. 8-28. (A) Factors responsible for maintaining normal arterial blood pressure. (B) Mechanisms that aid venous return: 1, abdominothoracic pump; 2 and 3, skeletal muscle pump; 4, arterial pump.

turn falls drastically, the cardiac output falls, the arterial blood pressure falls, and the patient may faint.

In a normal healthy individual, all the five factors discussed contribute to keeping the mean arterial blood pressure within normal limits under varying physiological conditions.

Capillary and Venous Pressures

Once the blood passes through the arterioles, the blood pressure falls sharply. The pressure is about *25 mm Hg* at the arterial end of the capillary and about *10 mm Hg* at the venous end. The pressure of blood in the large veins is low and in the inferior vena cava may be only about *5 mm H$_2$0*.

Mechanisms Aiding Venous Return to the Heart
Abdominothoracic Pump

During inspiration, the decrease in intrathoracic pressure and the increase in intra-abdominal pressure following the descent of the diaphragm result in venous blood being sucked up into the right atrium. At the same time, the blood is forced up from below by pressure on the inferior vena cava within the abdomen. This cyclical change in the intrathoracic and intra-abdominal pressure is very effective and is known as the abdominothoracic pump (see Fig. 8-28).

Skeletal Muscle Pump

Valved veins running between layers of active skeletal muscles milk the blood toward the right atrium (see Fig. 8-28). Suitably placed valves in the communicating vein connecting these deeply placed veins and the superficial veins prevent the venous blood from escaping into the superficial veins.

Arterial Pump

Valved venae comitantes, which closely accompany many of the limb arteries, cause the pulsation of the arterial walls pressing on the veins, thus aiding the passage of venous blood toward the heart (see Fig. 8-28).

Control of Blood Vessels
Vasoconstrictor and Vasodilator Centers

The *vasoconstrictor center* consists of groups of neurons in the medulla oblongata of the brain (Fig. 8-29). The center is connected by nerve fibers to sympathetic nerve cells lying in the lateral gray horn of the thoracic and upper lumbar parts of the spinal cord. Nerve impulses are constantly descending from the center to these nerve cells in the spinal cord. The sympathetic cells give origin to the *vasoconstrictor fibers,* which are distributed to the smooth muscle in the arteries, arterioles, venules, and small veins. An increase in the discharge of nerve impulses from the vasoconstrictor center is followed by a decrease in the size of the lumina of these vessels. Superimposed on the activity of the vasoconstrictor center is the control exerted by the hypothalamus and even the cerebral cortex.

The *vasodilator center* consists of groups of neurons associated with the dorsal nucleus of the vagus (see Fig. 8-29). The discharge of nerve impulses from this center inhibits the activity of the vasoconstrictor center in a direct action of one center upon the other. Thus, the vasodilator center reduces the degree of sympathetic vasoconstriction, allowing the dilatation of the small blood vessels.

Sympathetic Vasodilator Nerve Fibers

Most blood vessels of the body are constricted by the activity of the sympathetic nerve fibers. The sympathetic fibers to skeletal muscle blood vessels and cardiac muscle vessels, however, inhibit the smooth muscle in their walls and thus produce moderate vasodilatation. The vasodilator effect is minimal on the general circulation and does not affect the blood pressure.

Sympathetic Nerve Fibers to the Suprarenal Medulla

Preganglionic sympathetic nerve fibers travel to the suprarenal medulla, where the cells are stimulated to secrete norepinephrine and epinephrine into the bloodstream. These two hormones then act directly on the peripheral blood vessels, causing vasoconstriction, except in the blood vessels of skeletal and cardiac muscle, which dilate.

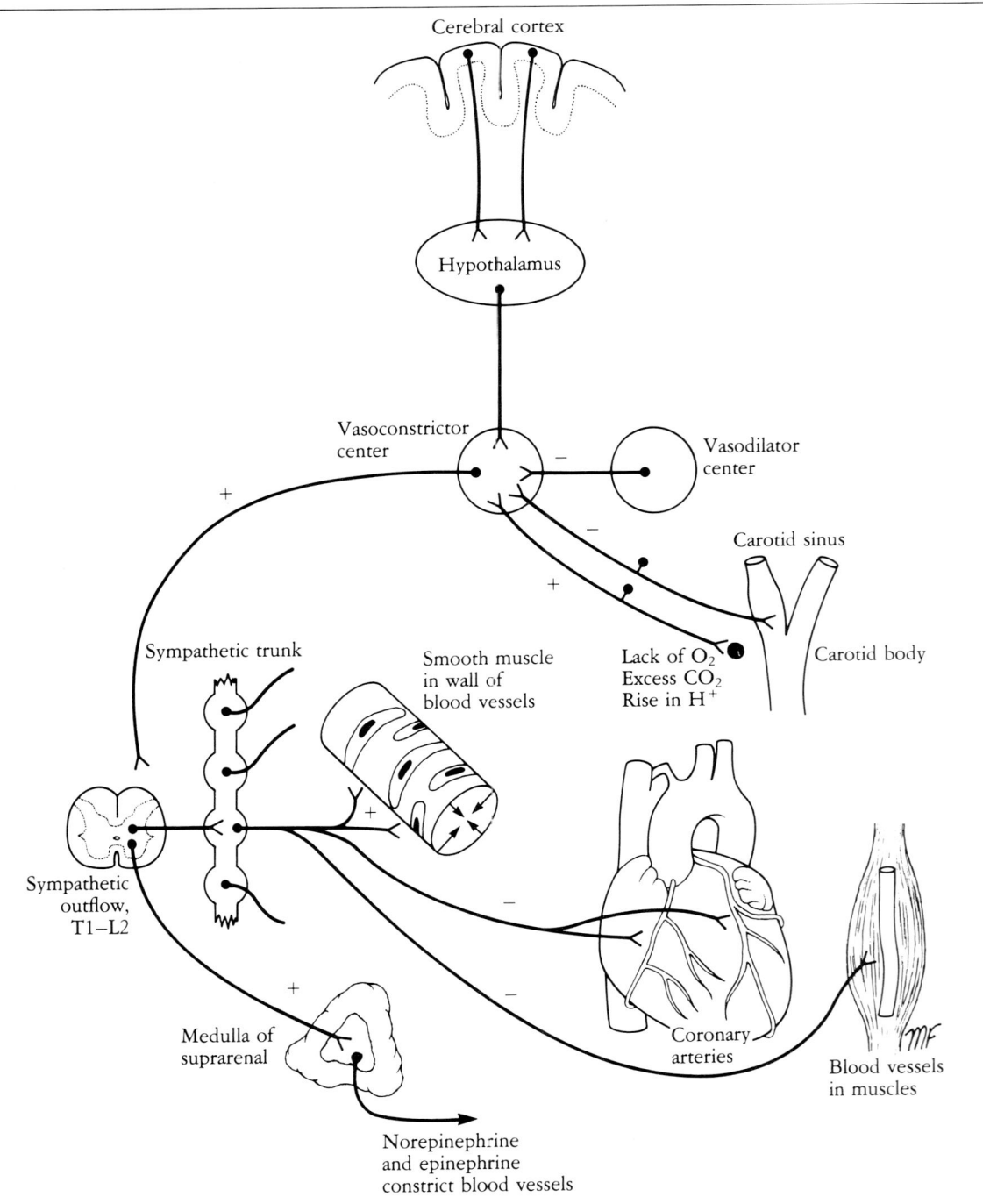

Fig. 8-29. Factors that control the diameter of the blood vessels of the circulatory system.

Vascular Reflexes

PERIPHERAL NERVE STIMULATION. A strong stimulus applied to any peripheral nerve will increase the activity of the vasoconstrictor center and raise blood pressure.

CAROTID AND AORTIC PRESSOR RECEPTORS. Nerve endings that are stimulated by stretching are situated in the walls of the *carotid sinus* and the *aortic arch* (see Fig. 8-29). When the blood pressure rises in these vessels and stretches their walls, nerve impulses ascend in the glossopharyngeal nerve (from the carotid sinus) and the vagus (from the aorta) to the vasoconstrictor center in the medulla oblongata and inhibit the activity of the center. This inhibition results in a reduced vasoconstriction of the small blood vessels; the peripheral resistance thereby is reduced, causing the blood pressure to fall. A fall in blood pressure in these large blood vessels is followed by a reduction in the inhibitory impulses passing to the vasoconstrictor center, and the resulting increased vasoconstriction raises the blood pressure once again. The pressor receptors thus serve as a governor and assist the body in the fine tuning of the blood pressure to suit the body's needs.

CAROTID AND AORTIC BODY REFLEXES. Chemoreceptors in the vascular *carotid body* and *aortic body*, situated near the carotid sinus and arch of the aorta, respectively, are stimulated by a decrease in the oxygen tension, an increase in the carbon dioxide tension, and an increase in the hydrogen ion concentration within the blood. Nerve impulses ascend to the brain from the carotid body in the glossopharyngeal nerve and from the aortic body in the vagus nerve (see Fig. 8-29). As a result, the vasoconstrictor center and the inspiratory center are stimulated, raising the blood pressure and increasing pulmonary ventilation.

Local Control of Blood Flow in Tissues

The walls of the arterioles leading into a capillary plexus and the larger venules leading out of the plexus have a well-defined smooth muscle coat. In contrast, the small branches of the arterioles, the *metarterioles*, have little smooth muscle in their walls. At the site at which a metarteriole joins a capillary, there is a band of smooth muscle forming a *precapillary sphincter* (see Fig. 8-25).

Two main forms of control of blood flow in tissues exist: local chemical control and nervous control.

LOCAL CHEMICAL CONTROL. Low concentrations of oxygen and high concentrations of carbon dioxide, hydrogen ions, and other tissue metabolites exert a direct inhibitory action on the smooth muscle of the metarterioles and the precapillary sphincter, increasing the blood flow to the tissue (see Fig. 8-25).

NERVOUS CONTROL. Sympathetic vasoconstrictor nerve fibers pass to the smooth muscle of the arterioles and large venules but not to the metarterioles. Activation of these sympathetic fibers causes the general body blood pressure to rise but reduces the local blood flow.

It is important to realize that in a tissue undergoing a high rate of metabolic activity, the local chemical control can overcome the general nervous control.

SPECIAL BLOOD CIRCULATIONS

Coronary Circulation

The right and left coronary arteries supply the cardiac muscle with blood that is drained back into the right atrium through (1) the coronary sinus, (2) the anterior cardiac vein, and (3) small veins that drain directly from the walls of the heart into the heart chambers.

The flow of blood through the coronary arteries is greatest during ventricular diastole, because during systole, the contracting ventricular walls compress the coronary vessels. The coronary arteries are made to dilate via the sympathetic nerve fibers and by the hormones norepinephrine and epinephrine. The vagus does not affect blood flow.

Pulmonary Circulation

Pulmonary circulation consists of the passage of blood from the right ventricle through the lungs to the left atrium. The volume of blood flowing through the lungs is equal to that flowing through the systemic circulation. The systolic pulmonary arterial pressure is about *22 mm Hg,* and the diastolic pressure is about *8 mm Hg.*

The pulmonary blood vessels are innervated by the sympathetic nerves and the vagus. The former are vasoconstrictors; the latter is a vasodilator. These nerves play a minor role in the control of the pulmonary circulation.

Hepatic Circulation

Blood originating in the gastrointestinal tract, from the lower one-third of the esophagus to halfway down the anal canal, and from the spleen, pancreas, and gallbladder, is conveyed to the liver by the portal vein. This vein is unique in that it begins as a capillary network and ends in the liver by dividing into capillaries and sinusoids. All the liver sinusoids converge on the central vein of each liver lobule, and these veins ultimately join to form the hepatic veins, which drain into the inferior vena cava.

The portal vein conveys the products of digestion from the gastrointestinal tract to the liver cells. The portal blood has a relatively low oxygen content. The liver cells receive their oxygen via the blood in the hepatic artery, which joins the portal blood in the liver sinusoids.

CLINICAL NOTES

PERICARDIUM

The pericardium is a fibrous sac lined by a serous membrane. A small amount of fluid (50 ml) is normally present within the pericardial cavity to prevent friction between the visceral and parietal layers of the serous pericardium. The pericardium holds the heart in position, prevents sudden dilatation of its chambers, and aids venous filling of the atria during ventricular systole. The last of these functions occurs as a result of the negative intrapericardial pressure developed by the sudden emptying of the ventricles.

Pericarditis

Inflammation of the pericardium is usually caused by spread of disease from the myocardium or surrounding structures. The condition is accompanied by an excessive accumulation of pericardial fluid, which may be clear or serous, as in rheumatic disease, or purulent, as in bacterial infections. Excess fluids in the pericardial cavity may impede the filling of the heart during diastole. Later, fibrous adhesions within the pericardial cavity may impair cardiac function by constricting the chambers of the heart and the venae cavae.

MYOCARDIAL ISCHEMIA

Inadequate blood supply to the myocardium results in the patient's experiencing severe pain over the middle of the sternum that often spreads to one or both arms, the root of the neck, and even the jaw. The pain is assumed to be caused by the accumulation of metabolites and by oxygen deficiency, which stimulate the sensory nerve endings in the myocardium.

The myocardium receives its blood supply through the right and left coronary arteries. Although the coronary arteries have numerous anastomoses at the arteriolar level, they are essentially functional end arteries. A sudden block of one of the large branches of either coronary artery will inevitably lead to necrosis of the cardiac muscle (myocardial infarction) in that vascular area and often to the death of the patient. The great majority of cases of blockage of the coronary arteries are caused by atherosclerotic narrowing of the lumen, sometimes accompanied by thrombosis of the blood.

Arteriosclerotic disease of the coronary arteries may present itself in three ways, depending on the rate of narrowing of the lumina of the arteries: (1) a general degeneration and fibrosis of the myocardium, which occurs over a period of many years and is caused by a gradual narrowing of the coronary arteries; (2) angina pectoris, cardiac pain that occurs on exertion and is relieved by rest; in this condition, the coronary vessels are so narrowed that myocardial ischemia occurs on exertion but not at rest; and (3) myocardial infarction, in which coronary flow is suddenly reduced or stopped and the cardiac muscle undergoes necrosis. Myocardial infarction is the major cause of death in industrialized nations.

VALVULAR DISEASE OF THE HEART

Rheumatic fever is the most common cause of acquired valvular disease. Rheumatic fever is a hypersensitivity reaction to β-hemolytic group A streptococci, which have produced attacks of pharyngitis. The heart and the joints are the main affected areas.

Although the initial inflammatory response may be minimal, it may cause the edges of the heart valve cusps to stick together. Later (possibly many years later), fibrous thickening and deposits of calcium occur, followed by loss of flexibility and shrinkage. Narrowing (stenosis) and valvular incompetence (regurgitation) result, and the heart ceases to function as an efficient pump.

In rheumatic disease of the mitral valve, not only do the cusps undergo fibrosis and shrink, but the chordae tendineae shorten, preventing closure of the cusps during ventricular systole. The tricuspid valve is less commonly affected by disease, but the changes produced are similar.

Valvular Heart Murmurs

Apart from the sounds of the valves closing, lūb–dūp, the blood passes through the normal heart silently. Should the valve orifices become narrowed or the valve cusps distorted and shrunken by disease, however, a rippling effect is set up that leads to turbulence and vibrations that are heard as heart murmurs.

CONGESTIVE HEART FAILURE

This condition stems from the inability of the heart to perform efficiently as a mechanical pump. *Left-sided congestive heart failure* is caused by overload of or damage to the left ventricle, such as hypertension (high blood pressure) or coronary arteriosclerosis. Left-sided congestive heart failure results in a backup of blood in the pulmonary circulation, with pulmonary edema; shortness of breath is the common symptom. *Right-sided congestive heart failure* can be a result of defective pulmonary circulation caused by lung disease or disease of the tricuspid or pulmonary valve. In these conditions, there is a backup of venous blood in the right atrium and the superior and inferior venae cavae. The right atrium consequently often becomes enlarged, and there is often congestion of the veins of the neck.

DISEASES OF THE CONDUCTING SYSTEM OF THE HEART

The sino-atrial node is the spontaneous source of the cardiac impulse. The atrioventricular node is responsible for picking up the cardiac impulse from the atria. The atrioventricular bundle is the only route by which the cardiac impulse can spread from the atria to the ventricles. Failure of the bundle to conduct the normal impulses will result in alterations in the rhythmic contraction of the ventricles (arrhythmias) or, if there is complete bundle block, complete dissociation between the atrial and ventricular rates of contraction. The common cause of defective conduction through the bundle is atherosclerosis of the coronary arteries, which results in a diminished blood supply to the bundle.

Extrasystoles

The cardiac impulse, instead of arising normally in the sino-atrial node, may arise in the atrial wall, the atrioventricular node, or the atrioventricular bundle. When the additional impulse arises in the atrium, it is picked up by the atrioventricular node and bundle and the ventricles contract. The ventricular muscle now enters a complete (absolute) refractory period, so that when the normal cardiac impulse arrives, the ventricles do not contract. A compensatory pause follows.

When the cardiac impulse arises in the atrioventricular node, it travels both upward into the atria and downward into the ventricles, so that the atria and the ventricles contract at about the same time.

When the impulse arises in the atrioventricular bundle, the ventricles immediately contract, and this contraction is followed by a compensatory pause.

Atrial Flutter

In this condition, it is believed that the cardiac impulse, originating from the sino-atrial node, travels in a circle of cardiac muscle that extends around the right atrium, joining the entrances of the superior and inferior venae cavae. Such a rapid circus movement of the cardiac impulse causes the wave of the conduction to be spread repeatedly over the atria at a very rapid rate completely independent of the sino-atrial node. The rate of atrial contraction in atrial flutter is between 200 and 350 times per minute. The atrioventricular bundle is unable to conduct impulses at such a high rate, so the ventricles contract at a slower rate than the atria.

Atrial Fibrillation

In this condition, the atrial wall does not contract as a whole but simply twitches at a rate of 450 to 600 times per minute. The cardiac impulse is not a single impulse; instead, there are many impulses traveling in different directions at the same time. The rhythm of the ventricles is very irregular.

Atrial flutter and fibrillation are commonly associated with coronary arteriosclerosis, hyperthyroidism, and mitral stenosis.

Ventricular Fibrillation

This condition is similar to atrial fibrillation in that the ventricles contract in a completely disorganized manner instead of contracting as a whole; that is, the muscle merely quivers. Consequently, the ventricles cease to be an effective mechanical pump, and the cardiac output is totally inadequate to meet bodily needs. Unless the condition is corrected immediately, death quickly follows.

Diagnosis and Treatment

Electrocardiogram

Clinically, the electrocardiogram (ECG) is referred to as the EKG. This abbreviation is used to avoid confusion with other similar-sounding abbreviations, such as EEG (electroencephalogram). A great deal of important information can be obtained by studying electrocardiograms in patients with cardiac disease; for example, changes in wave form or disturbances of wave order can be discovered. Any change in the conduction of the cardiac impulse from the sino-atrial node to the Purkinje plexus will be reflected in abnormal electrical currents around the heart, which in turn will cause an alteration in the shape and timing of the waves in the electrocardiogram. Any serious disease of cardiac muscle can be detected by studying the electrocardiograms obtained from different leads.

In addition to the more obvious problems of cardiac arrhythmias and heart block, ventricular hypertrophy and dilatation and effects of coronary ischemia can all be detected by this method.

Pacemaker

In patients whose sino-atrial node is not functioning normally or who show a pathological block of the conducting system of the heart, an electronic apparatus called a pacemaker can be used to initiate the heart beat; it may be used temporarily or permanently.

Defibrillation

In cases of life-threatening arrhythmias, a high-voltage electric current is delivered to the patient for a short time, causing the entire myocardium to be depolarized. This treatment terminates the arrhythmia, and in successful cases the sino-atrial node once again becomes the natural pacemaker of the heart.

ARTERIES

When discussing the structure of arteries in this chapter, we emphasized that all arteries possess a tunica intima, a tunica media, and a tunica adventitia, and that these coats are seen most clearly in the muscular (distributing) arteries.

Age Changes in Arteries

In the young, the tunica intima is thin. With advancing years, the connective tissue of this coat becomes thicker because of the accumulation of mucopolysaccharides and the appearance of *myointimal cells,* which synthesize collagen and elastic fibers.

The elastic fibers in the tunica media of the larger blood vessels degenerate with age and are replaced by bundles of collagen fibers, causing the vessels to become more rigid. The loss of elastic tissue causes the vessels to elongate and become tortuous.

Congenital Defects in Arteries

Developmental Aneurysm

About 1 percent of adults show a poor development of the tunica media in the cerebral arteries of the circulus arteriosus. The condition is localized and occurs at the site of branching of the cerebral arteries. With time, the weakened blood vessel wall gradually gives way and balloons outward under the influence of the arterial blood pressure. Sudden rupture of the simple aneurysm into the subarachnoid space may lead to sudden death.

Coarctation of the Aorta

This condition consists of a congenital narrowing of the aorta just distal to the origin of the left subclavian artery. The narrowing lies very close to the site of attachment of the ligamentum arteriosum. It is a condition that arises after birth and is believed to occur because an unusual quantity of ductus arteriosus muscle is incorporated in the wall of the aorta. As a result, when the ductus arteriosus contracts, the ductal muscle in the aortic wall also contracts and the aortic lumen becomes narrowed. Later, when fibrosis takes place, the aortic wall is also involved, and permanent narrowing occurs.

Arteriosclerosis

Arteriosclerosis is the name given to a group of arterial disorders characterized by thickening of the walls and loss of elasticity. The most important disorder is *atherosclerosis,* in which there are fibrofatty plaques in the tunica intima. The next most important is a condition in which there is calcification of the tunica media. Last in importance is *arteriolosclerosis,* in which there is thickening of the walls of the small arteries. Only atherosclerosis will be considered here.

Atherosclerosis

Atherosclerosis most commonly involves the aorta and the coronary and cerebral arteries and leads to myocardial ischemia or infarction and cerebral ischemia or infarction. Atherosclerosis is a killing disease, myocardial infarction being responsible for at least 20 percent of all deaths in the United States. It is a very common disease in affluent countries like Great Britain and the Scandinavian countries; the incidence is much lower in Asia. The disease is much more common in men. Diet and life-style greatly influence the incidence, although genetic factors, high blood pressure, cigarette smoking, and diabetes are very important factors.

The atheromatous plaque is the most important lesion of the disorder. It arises in the tunica intima, and as it enlarges, it protrudes into the lumen of the artery, reducing the blood flow through it. Microscopically, the plaque may have a superficial portion composed of collagen bundles and smooth muscle cells. Beneath this layer is a mixture of lipid material and cellular debris, the lipid being cholesterol and cholesteryl ester. Many of the smooth muscle cells show lipid inclusions. Other cells, thought to be macrophages, also contain many lipid globules.

As the atheromatous plaque enlarges over years, it may become calcified or undergo ulceration on its luminal surface, or thrombosis of blood may occur on its roughened luminal surface. In the larger arteries, such as the aorta, the danger lies in the possibility that a thrombus will be dislodged from the plaque and form an embolus, which then will quickly circulate with the arterial blood until it reaches a vessel whose diameter is too small to let it pass. Severe peripheral arterial occlusion then occurs. Although the plaque clearly develops in the tunica intima, the underlying tunica media also undergoes atrophy with loss of elastic tissue. The weakened wall may then undergo stretching and form an aneurysm.

In the coronary and cerebral arteries, the important complication is the gradual narrowing of the arterial lumen, which may lead to arterial insufficiency with myocardial infarction or stroke.

DEVELOPMENT OF ATHEROSCLEROSIS. It is inappropriate to discuss in detail here the theories concerning the pathogenesis of atherosclerosis, but the following comments will be made. It is possible that the endothelial cells of the tunica intima are damaged by stress, leading to leakage of plasma lipids into the underlying connective tissue. Platelets may then adhere to the damaged intimal surface. The smooth muscle cells of the tunica media may then migrate into the tunica intima in response to the initial intimal injury, or secondary to the accumulation of plasma lipids in the connective tissue of the intima. Moreover, experimental evidence indicates that the accumulated platelets may liberate a growth factor that stimulates the proliferation of smooth muscle cells. The newly formed smooth muscle cells then phagocytose the lipoproteins. They are also responsible for laying down new collagen and elastic fibers and for the accumulation of proteoglycans.

This sequence of events appears to explain the development of atherosclerosis, but the cause of this condition has not been determined with certainty.

Arterial Blood Pressure

Clinically, arterial blood pressure is measured indirectly by an instrument known as a sphygmomanometer, which may be of the mercury or aneroid type. The blood pressure is measured with the patient lying or sitting comfortably with the arm relaxed. The patient's arm is bared, and a blood pressure cuff, consisting of a flat rubber bag enclosed in a cloth, is wrapped snugly around the arm above the elbow. The cloth prevents the rubber bag from stretching under pressure. The rubber bag is then inflated with air by means of a small hand pump, and the pressure of the air within the bag is measured by means of a mercury manometer connected to the bag. The air pressure within the bag is raised until the lumen of the brachial artery is obliterated and the radial pulse disappears. The air pressure is then gradually released through a valve until the blood begins to pass through the brachial artery once again. If the examiner listens with a stethoscope placed over the brachial artery just below the cuff, a faint tapping sound will be heard in time with the heart beat as the blood starts to pass through the compressed artery. At the moment at which this sound is first heard, the air pressure within the bag should be read, and this will indicate the *systolic pressure*. As more air is released from the rubber bag, more blood is able to pass through the brachial artery and the tapping sounds become louder. Finally, the sounds suddenly acquire a muffled quality and then disappear. The reading of the air pressure when the sounds become muffled is the *diastolic pressure*. To measure it, air has to be pumped back into the bag once the sound has disappeared, and the air again slowly released until the muffled sounds reappear.

The systolic blood pressure in a normal healthy young adult at rest is approximately 120 mm Hg; the diastolic pressure is approximately 80 mm Hg.

Other methods, such as arterial catheterization, can be used to monitor and record a patient's blood pressure.

Hypertension

An abnormally high blood pressure is accompanied by an abnormally high peripheral resistance; therefore, the diagnosis depends on recording a high diastolic arterial pressure. A patient who is resting quietly and has a systolic blood pressure in excess of 140 mm Hg and 90 mm Hg diastolic pressure is considered to have hypertension. Hypertensive patients may be divided into two main groups: (1) those with essential hypertension, in which the cause is unknown, and (2) those with secondary hypertension, in which the cause may be renal, endocrine, or mechanical, such as congenital narrowing (coarctation) of the aorta.

DISEASES OF VEINS

Veins are characteristically thin-walled, and the tunica intima, tunica media, and tunica adventitia are not well defined. Bacterial organisms and tumor cells easily can penetrate their walls and spread to distant parts of the body via the bloodstream.

Varicose Veins

A vein is said to be varicosed when its diameter is greater than normal and it is elongated and tortuous. Prolonged increased venous pressure is responsible for the stretching of the thin walls of the veins. Varicose veins occur at three sites: (1) superficial veins of the lower limbs; (2) veins at the lower end of the esophagus, where they are called *esophageal varices;* and (3) veins of the anal canal, where they are called *hemorrhoids.*

Varicosed superficial veins of the lower limbs are responsible for considerable discomfort, pain, and suffering in innumerable persons. There are many predisposing causes, including hereditary weakness of the vein walls, incompetent valves, and elevated intra-abdominal pressure as a result of multiple pregnancies or abdominal tumors. Microscopically, the vein wall usually shows some thickening, because of increased amounts of connective tissue in the tunica intima and additional smooth muscle cells in the tunica media.

In severe cases, there is a stasis of venous blood in the tissue and an excessive accumulation of tissue fluid (edema). The poor circulatory flow with inadequate oxygen transport, and the local accumulation of tissue metabolites, leads to dermatitis and ulcer formation.

Thrombophlebitis

This condition is most commonly seen in the superficial veins of the leg, where the blood undergoes thrombosis (see p. 182). It is accompanied by an inflammatory reaction in the wall of the vein that gives rise to pain, swelling, and redness along the course of the vein. It is a common complication of varicose veins. Fortunately, the thrombus adheres strongly to the wall of the vein and it is rare for the thrombus to break away to form an embolus.

Phlebothrombosis

Thrombosis of blood within a vein may occur in patients immobilized in bed, especially after surgery. It occurs during pregnancy, in patients with advanced malignant disease, and in those with a slow venous return, as found in heart failure. Oral contraceptives containing estrogen predispose women to phlebothrombosis. In all these conditions, the blood is likely to clot and form a thrombus. The thrombus forms most commonly in the deep veins of the leg, especially those of the calf, possibly because the calf veins of a patient lying in bed are subject to unusual outside pressures as a result of the weight of the limb.

Phlebothrombosis occurs spontaneously without symptoms or signs. The thrombus dams the venous blood and alters the circulation. More important, the thrombus usually does not adhere strongly to the vein wall and may break free, forming an *embolus.* The embolus rapidly travels through the right side of the heart and finally lodges in the lungs, a very serious and often fatal complication known as *pulmonary embolism.*

Vein Grafts

Saphenous vein autografts can be used to revascularize the myocardium in severe atherosclerosis of the coronary arteries. An end-to-side venocoronary anastomosis may be made with very fine sutures. Occluded arteries of the lower limbs may also be bypassed by bridging the defect with a vein. After a time, the grafted vein wall thickens in response to the raised intraluminal pressure.

CLINICAL PROBLEMS

For the answers to these problems, see page 794.

1. A 40-year-old man is admitted to the hospital with severe substernal pain. On physical examination, a pericardial friction rub is heard with the stethoscope during forced expiration with the pa-

tient leaning forward. A diagnosis of acute pericarditis is made and confirmed by the finding of electrocardiographic changes. Using your knowledge of histology, describe the structure and function of the different parts of the pericardium. Is the pericardial fluid normally produced as a secretion or by transudation from the capillaries? Can fibrous contraction of the pericardium or excessive production of pericardial fluid embarrass cardiac function?

2. An 8-year-old girl is examined by a pediatrician because of complaints of pains in her joints. The pains had started a week previously and first involved her left elbow and right shoulder joints. She has had a sore throat for 3 weeks. On examination, her left elbow and right shoulder joints appear normal, but her right knee and left wrist and ankle joints are painful on movement and tender to touch. On the pediatrician's listening to the heart, the mitral and aortic valves exhibit soft blowing systolic murmurs, indicating mitral and aortic regurgitation. A diagnosis of rheumatic fever is made based on the joint problems and heart findings. Although the heart lesions in this condition involve all three layers of the heart wall, the most serious are those of the endocardium. The cusps of the mitral and aortic valves are often thickened and distorted by the inflammatory process. Describe the normal microscopic structures of the mitral and aortic valves. Indicate how they function. Using your knowledge of histology and physiology, explain how rheumatic heart disease interferes with the function of the valves.

3. The myocardium forms the main mass of the heart. Describe the structure of cardiac muscle and indicate how its fibers are ideally suited to their function. What are the microscopic and physiological differences between ordinary cardiac muscle and that of the conducting system of the heart? Define the following: all-or-none law; absolute refractory period; compensatory pause.

4. A 65-year-old man is examined by his physician and found to have right-sided heart failure. As the patient lies propped up on pillows in bed, his physician notices that the blood in the external jugular veins can be seen easily, rising nearly as high as the angle on the mandible. What is the significance of the blood level in the external jugular vein? Define venous return and explain the Frank-Starling law.

5. A 45-year-old man is admitted to the coronary care unit with a diagnosis of left ventricular failure and cardiogenic shock resulting from a severe myocardial infarction. He had awakened at 3 A.M. with agonizing pain over the front of his chest. His skin is pale and cold, and sweating is evident. His radial pulse is weak, rapid, and irregular, and his blood pressure is 100/70 mm Hg. Both external jugular veins are engorged with blood, and moist sounds are heard with a stethoscope in the lower lobes of both lungs. Can you explain how left ventricular failure can cause these symptoms and signs? Define cardiac output and stroke volume.

6. Describe the electrical changes that take place in cardiac muscle when it contracts. What is an electrocardiogram? What is peculiar about the structure of cardiac muscle that permits the action potentials to spread rapidly across the heart?

7. Describe the microscopic structure of large elastic arteries, medium-sized muscular arteries, and arterioles. How is the structure of these different types of arteries related to their function?

8. Define the terms *capillary, metarteriole,* and *precapillary sphincter.* What factors locally control blood flow in tissues?

9. Describe the structures of a coronary artery. What factors control the coronary circulation? What is a functional end artery?

10. What age changes normally take place in the structure of arteries? How do these changes affect the efficiency of the circulatory system?

11. Compare the structures of a venule, a medium-sized vein, and a large vein. Describe how the structure of these vessels assists in the return of venous blood to the heart.

12. The structure of arteries is well adapted to con-

veying blood under high pressure from the heart to the tissues of the body. What factors normally control the arterial blood pressure? Is the pressure within the pulmonary arteries the same as in the systemic arteries? What is the structure of a blood sinusoid? What is an arteriovenous anastomosis?

13. Atherosclerosis is a killer disease involving arteries. What cells and tissues of an artery are involved in the disease process?

14. A 47-year-old woman visits her physician complaining of a dull, aching pain in the lower part of both legs. She states that the pain has been getting progressively worse since the birth of her sixth child and is particularly bad at the end of a long day of standing. She has also noticed that the skin along the medial side of her legs has started to show irritation. On examination, the patient is seen to have widespread varicosities involving both the great and small saphenous veins. What is the normal microscopic structure of a saphenous vein? What changes take place when such a vein becomes varicosed?

ADDITIONAL READING

Alpert, N. R., et al. Heart muscle mechanics. *Annu. Rev. Physiol.* 41:521, 1979.

Baez, S. Microcirculation. *Annu. Rev. Physiol.* 39:391, 1977.

Bennett, H. S., Luft, J. H., and Hampton, J. C. Morphological classification of vertebrate blood capillaries. *Am. J. Physiol.* 196:381, 1959.

Bishop, V. S., et al. Factors influencing cardiac performance. *Int. Rev. Physiol.* 9:239, 1976.

Casley-Smith, J. R. The functioning and interrelationships of blood capillaries and lymphatics. *Experientia* 32:1, 1976.

Chou, T. *Electrocardiography in Clinical Practice.* New York: Grune & Stratton, 1979.

Durrer, D., et al. Human cardiac electrophysiology. In Dickinson, C. J., and Marks, J. (eds.), *Development in Cardiovascular Medicine.* Lancaster, England: MTP Press, 1978, p. 53.

Edanaga, M. Scanning electron microscope study of the endothelium of the vessels. *Arch. Histol. Jpn.* 37:1, 1974.

Fawcett, D. W. The fine structure of capillaries, arterioles, and small arteries. In Reynolds, S. R. M., and Zweifach, B. W. (eds.), *The Microcirculation: A Symposium on Factors Influencing Exchange of Substances across Capillary Wall.* Urbana: University of Illinois Press, 1959, p. 1.

Fernando, N. V. P., and Movat, H. Z. The smallest arterial vessels: Terminal arterioles and metarterioles. *Exp. Mol. Pathol.* 3:1, 1964.

Guyton, A. C. *Arterial Pressure and Hypertension.* Philadelphia: Saunders, 1980.

Guyton, A. C., et al. *Circulatory Physiology: Cardiac Output and Its Regulation* (2nd ed.). Philadelphia: Saunders, 1973.

Hans, J. (ed.). *Cardiac Arrhythmias.* Springfield, Ill.: Thomas, 1972.

James, D. G. (ed.). *Circulation of the Blood.* Pitman Books, England, 1978.

Johnson, P. C. *Peripheral Circulation.* New York: Wiley, 1978.

Karnovsky, M. J. The ultrastructural basis of capillary permeability studied with peroxidase as a tracer. *J. Cell Biol.* 35:213, 1967.

Karnovsky, M. J. The ultrastructural basis of transcapillary exchanges. *J. Gen. Physiol.* 52:643, 1968.

Keatinge, W. R., and Harman, M. C. Local mechanisms controlling blood vessels. New York: Academic, 1979.

Maul, G. G. Structure and formation of pores in fenestrated capillaries. *J. Ultrastruct. Res.* 36:768, 1971.

Muir, A. R. Observations on the fine structure of the Purkinje fibers in the ventricles of the sheep's heart. *J. Anat.* 91:251, 1957.

Parmley, W. W., and Talbot, W. Heart as a pump. In Berne, R. M., et al. (eds.), *Handbook of Physiology.* Sec. 2, Vol. 1. Baltimore: Williams & Wilkins, 1979, p. 429.

Rhodin, J. A. G. Ultrastructure of mammalian venous capillaries, venules and small collecting veins. *J. Ultrastruct. Res.* 25:452, 1968.

Scott, M. N., and Fawcett, D. W. Myocardial ultrastructure. In Langer, G. A., and Brady, T. W. (eds.), *The Mammalian Myocardium.* New York: Wiley, 1974.

Shepherd, J. T., and Vanhoutte, P. M. *The Human Car-*

diovascular System: Facts and Concepts. New York: Raven, 1979.

Simionescu, N., Simionescu, M., and Palade, G. E. Recent studies on vascular endothelium. *Ann. N.Y. Acad. Sci.* 275:64, 1976.

Sperelakis, N. Propagation mechanisms in heart. *Annu. Rev. Physiol.* 41:441, 1979.

Thaemert, J. C. Fine structure of the atrioventricular node as viewed in serial sections. *Am. J. Anat.* 136:43, 1973.

Trautwein, W. Membrane currents in cardiac muscle fibers. *Physiol. Rev.* 53:793, 1973.

Wolf, S., et al. (eds.). *Structure and Function of the Circulation.* New York: Plenum, 1979.

Wolff, J. R. Ultrastructure of the terminal vascular bed as related to function. In Kaley, G., and Altura, B. M. (eds.), *Microcirculation.* Vol. 1. Baltimore: University Park Press, 1977, p. 95.

LYMPHATIC SYSTEM

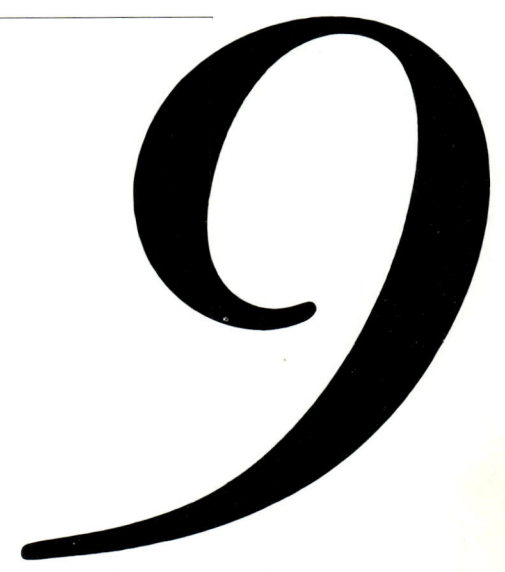

The lymphatic system consists of lymphatic vessels and lymphatic tissues. The lymphatic vessels are tubes that assist the cardiovascular system in the removal of tissue fluid from the interstitial spaces of the body; the vessels then return the fluid to the blood. The lymphatic system is essentially a drainage system, and there is no circulation. Lymphatic vessels are found in most tissues and organs in the body but are absent from the central nervous system, the eyeball, the internal ear, the epidermis, cartilage, and bone.

The smallest lymphatic vessels, the lymphatic capillaries, begin as blind-ended tubes. They differ markedly from blood capillaries in that they can absorb proteins and large particulate matter from the tissue spaces, whereas the fluid absorbed by the blood capillaries is an aqueous solution of inorganic salts and sugar. *Lymph* is the name given to tissue fluid once it has entered a lymphatic vessel.

The lymphatic tissue is not one of the primary tissues of the body but is a type of connective tissue that contains large numbers of lymphocytes. The lymphatic tissue is organized into the following organs or structures: (1) the thymus, (2) the lymph nodes, (3) the spleen, and (4) the lymphatic nodules.

The lymphatic tissue is essential for the immunological defenses of the body against bacteria and viruses.

LYMPHATIC VESSELS

Structure

The lymphatic vessels (lymph vessels) may be divided into lymphatic capillaries, medium-sized lymphatic vessels, and lymphatic ducts.

Lymphatic Capillaries

Lymphatic capillaries are small, thin-walled, endothelium-lined tubes surrounded by a thin layer of delicate connective tissue (Figs. 9-1 and 9-2). They vary in shape and size, and they anastomose freely to form networks. The endothelial cells overlap one another, but there is a distinct gap between adjacent cells. Unlike blood capillaries, lymphatic capillaries possess no pericytes, and a continuous basal lamina is absent. Attached to the outer surfaces of the endothelial cells are bundles of filaments that extend outward into the surrounding connective tissue. These filaments are called *lymphatic anchoring filaments*. Under the light microscope, lymphatic capillaries appear as small, empty tubes running in com-

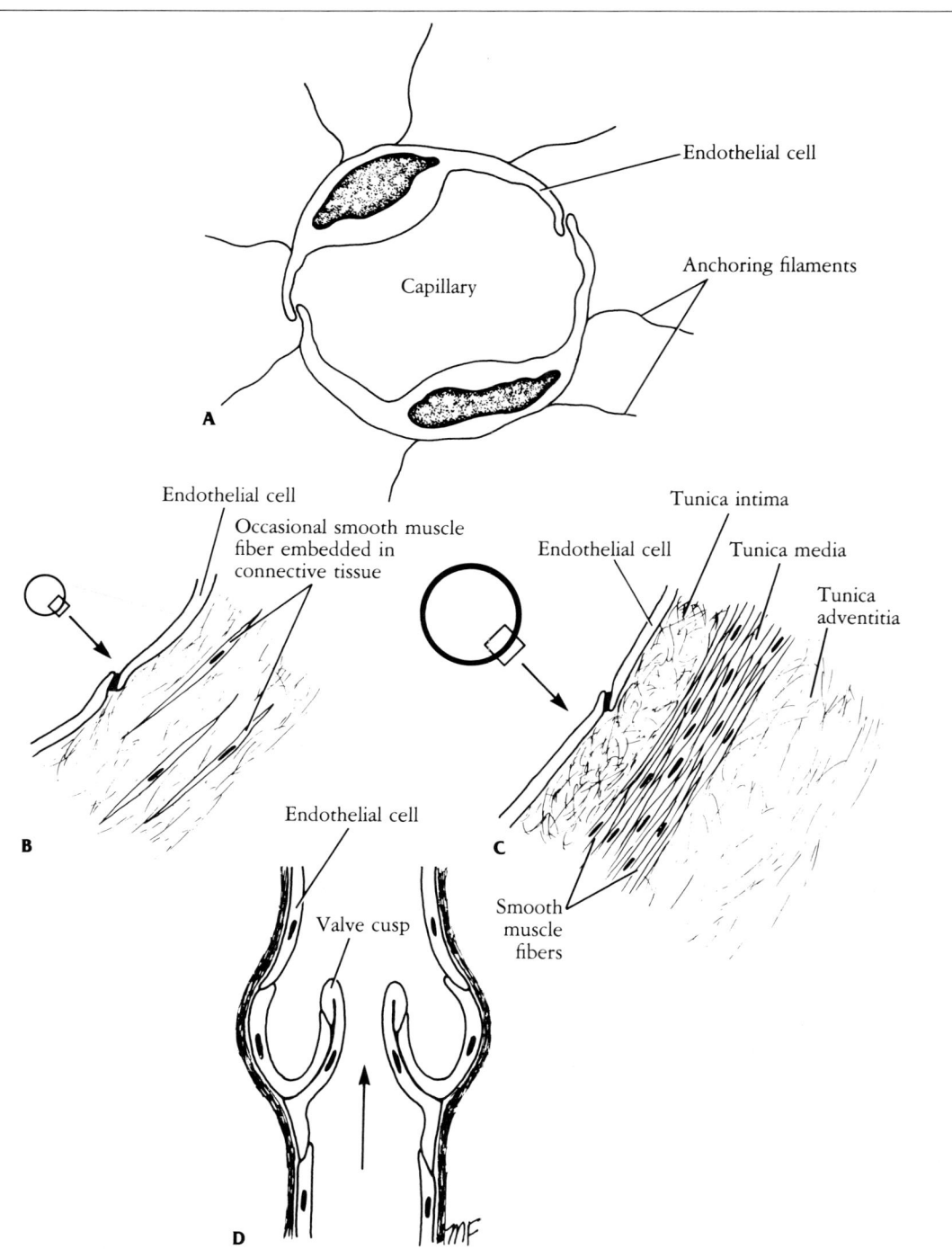

Fig. 9-1. Cross-sectional structure of (A) lymphatic capillary, (B) medium-sized lymphatic vessel, and (C) the thoracic duct. (D) shows a longitudinal section of a large lymphatic vessel at the site of a bicuspid valve.

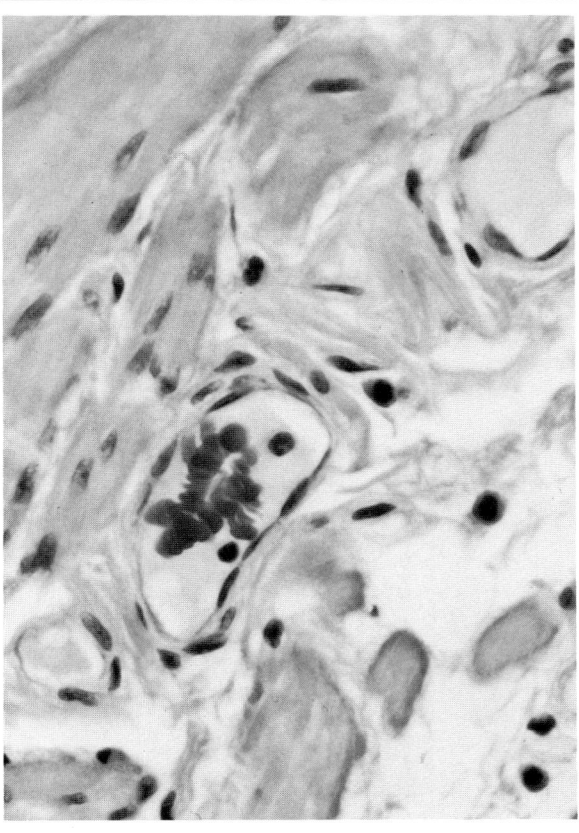

Fig. 9-2. Photomicrograph showing cross sections of a blood and two lymphatic capillaries. Note that the vessels are lined with flattened endothelial cells. (H&E; ×373.)

pany with blood capillaries. As stated previously, lymphatic capillaries are absent from the central nervous system, the eyeball, the internal ear, the epidermis, cartilage, and bone.

Medium-Sized Lymphatic Vessels

The lymphatic capillaries are drained by large, thicker-walled vessels. Outside the endothelial cells are a layer of connective tissue and an occasional smooth muscle fiber (see Fig. 9-1). These vessels join together to form successively larger vessels with even thicker walls. The amount of connective tissue increases, and the smooth muscle fibers form a distinct layer. Simple *bicuspid valves* (see Fig. 9-1), consisting of two layers of endothelial cells supported by a core of connective tissue, now appear. The free edges of the cusps point in the direction of lymph flow. Just proximal to the valve, the lymphatic vessel dilates slightly. The valves on lymphatic vessels are more numerous than those on veins.

Lymphatic Ducts

The medium-sized lymphatic vessels successively join one another to form even larger vessels (see Fig. 9-1). Finally, these converge and join to form two ducts, the *thoracic duct* and the *right lymphatic duct*. These ducts possess three recognizable but indistinct layers: the tunica intima, the tunica media, and the tunica adventitia (see Fig. 9-1). The walls of these large ducts thus resemble those of veins but are thinner.

The *tunica intima* consists of a layer of endothelial cells lying on a thin layer of connective tissue, the *tunica media* is composed largely of smooth muscle, and the *tunica adventitia* comprises connective tissue and bundles of longitudinally running smooth muscle fibers.

The large lymphatic ducts, like the medium-sized vessels, possess numerous biscuspid valves. They also have autonomic nerve fibers and small blood vessels in the tunica adventitia.

The thoracic duct opens into the venous system at the root of the neck on the left side by joining the junction of the left internal jugular vein and the subclavian vein or either one of these vessels. The right lymphatic duct opens into the venous system at the root of the neck on the right side by joining the junction of the right internal jugular vein and the subclavian vein or either one of these vessels.

Arrangement of Lymphatic Vessels of the Body

The lymphatic vessels differ from the blood vessels in that they are part of a drainage system, and they drain their contents in one direction only. As mentioned previously, the lymphatic vessels commence at the periphery as a network of small capillaries. These are widely distributed in the dermis, in the subcutaneous tissues, in muscles, and in the connective tissues of the thoracic and abdominal viscera. In

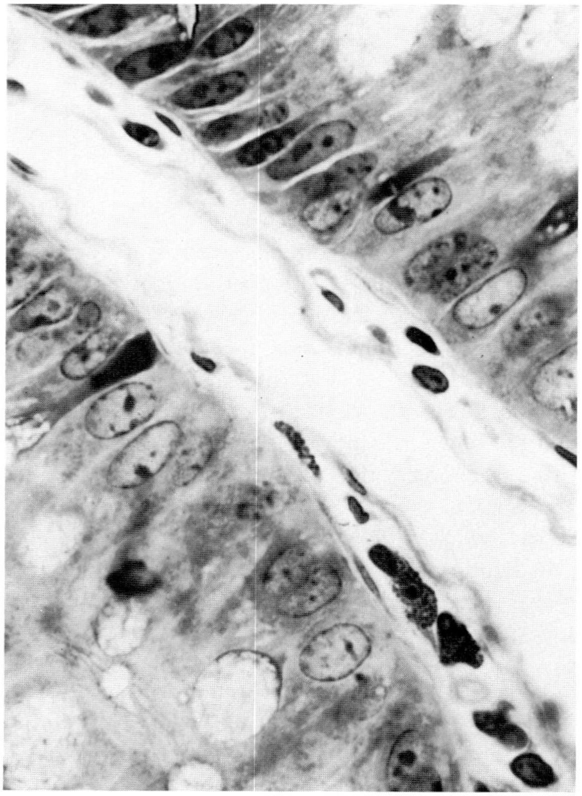

Fig. 9-3. Photomicrograph of a longitudinal plastic section of a central lacteal lying within a villus of the small intestine. In this section, the lumen of the lacteal is empty. (H&E; ×1,000.)

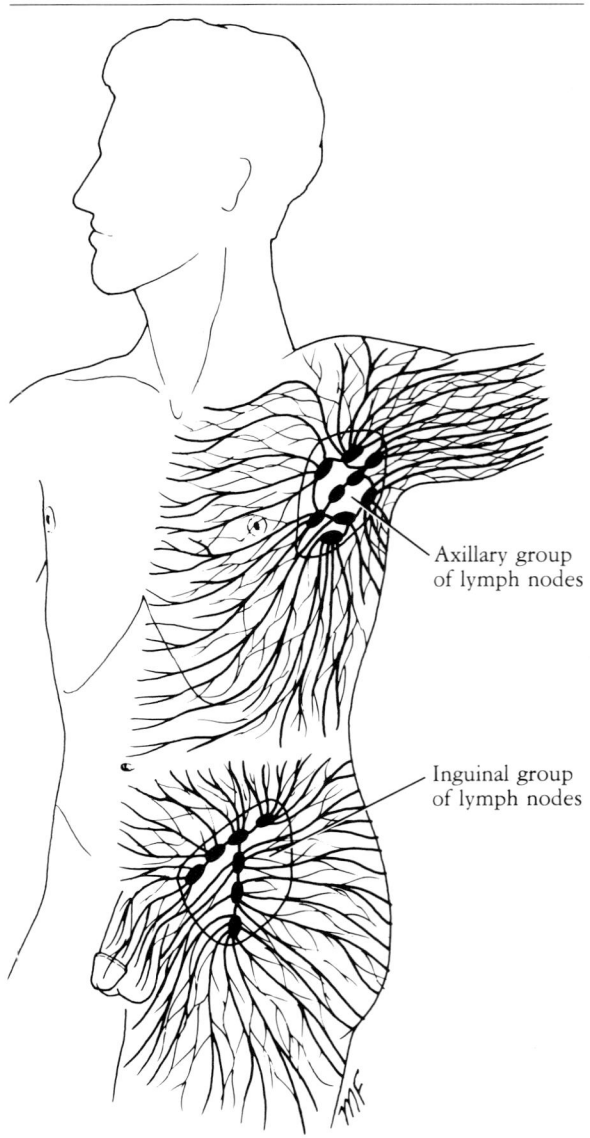

Fig. 9-4. Lymphatic vessels from the upper and lower limbs converging on lymph nodes situated at the roots of the limbs.

the mucous membrane of the small intestine, a single lymphatic capillary lies in the center of each villus, ending blindly near its tip. This capillary is called a *lacteal* (Fig. 9-3), because of its milky appearance after a fatty meal. A large proportion of the fat in food is absorbed into the lacteals in the form of droplets called *chylomicrons* (see Fig. 11-60).

The lymph from the peripheral plexuses passes into larger collecting vessels. At strategic points along the course of these vessels are small, ovoid masses of lymphatic tissue called *lymph nodes* (Fig. 9-4). For example, at the root of the upper limb are the *axillary lymph nodes,* and the *inguinal lymph nodes* are found at the root of the lower limb. During its passage from the tissue spaces to the blood, all lymph has to pass through at least one lymph node.

The direction of the flow of lymph is determined by the valves of the lymphatic vessels (see Fig. 9-1). The local dilatations of the vessels in the regions of the valves give the lymphatic vessels a beaded appearance.

Lymphatic vessels tend to run in the loose connective tissue alongside blood vessels. In the limbs, the superficial lymphatic vessels of the skin and subcutaneous tissue tend to follow the superficial veins; the deeper lymphatic vessels follow the deep arteries and veins. The deep fascia (e.g., the fascia lata of the thigh) separates the superficial vessels from the deep vessels, and these vessels unite only at the roots of the limbs, where they join the main collecting vessels.

The lymph from the greater part of the body reaches the blood via the thoracic duct. The lymph from the right side of the head and neck, the right upper limb, and the right side of the thorax, however, reaches the blood via the right lymphatic duct.

TISSUE FLUID AND LYMPH

An understanding of the formation and reabsorption of tissue fluid in a blood capillary is basic to the understanding of the physiology of lymph formation.

Formation and Reabsorption of Tissue Fluid

The flow of fluid from the blood through the blood capillary wall into the tissue spaces is dependent on (1) the capillary blood pressure, (2) the interstitial fluid pressure, (3) the osmotic pressure of the plasma proteins, and (4) the osmotic pressure of the colloid of the interstitial fluid. According to Guyton (1981),* the capillary blood pressure at the arterial end is about 25 mm Hg (Fig. 9-5) and at the venous end about 10 mm Hg. The interstitial fluid pressure is less than atmospheric pressure and measures about 6.3 mm Hg. The osmotic pressure of the plasma proteins is about 28 mm Hg. The osmotic pressure of the colloid of the interstitial fluid is about 5 mm Hg.

At the arterial end of the capillary, the total force trying to move fluid out of the lumen of the capillary into the tissue space is 36.3 mm Hg, which is calculated as follows:

Capillary blood pressure	25	mm Hg
Interstitial fluid pressure	6.3	mm Hg
Interstitial fluid colloid pressure	5	mm Hg
Total force	36.3	mm Hg

The plasma protein osmotic pressure of about 28 mm Hg is opposing this force. Therefore, the total effective outward force is 36.3 less 28, or 8.3 mm Hg.

At the venous end of the capillary, the total force trying to move fluid from the tissue space into the lumen of the capillary is 28 mm Hg and is produced by the osmotic pressure of the plasma proteins (see Fig. 9-5). Opposing this inward force is an outward force of 21.3 mm Hg, which is calculated as follows:

Capillary blood pressure	10	mm Hg
Interstitial fluid pressure	6.3	mm Hg
Interstitial fluid colloid pressure	5	mm Hg
Total force	21.3	mm Hg

Therefore, the total effective inward force into the capillary lumen is 28 less 21.3, or 6.7 mm Hg.

It is clear that at the arterial end of the capillary, tissue fluid is being actively formed, and at the venous end, tissue fluid is being absorbed back into the capillaries and small venules. The movement of reabsorption apparently accounts for only 90 percent of the drainage of tissue fluid, the remaining 10 percent being drained into the lymphatic capillaries. Only substances of low molecular weight, such as water, sodium chloride, glucose, and urea, can pass rapidly through a blood capillary wall. Substances of large molecular weight, such as proteins, are removed from the tissue spaces via the lymphatic capillaries.

---

*Guyton, A. C. *Textbook of Medical Physiology* (6th ed.). Philadelphia: Saunders, 1981.

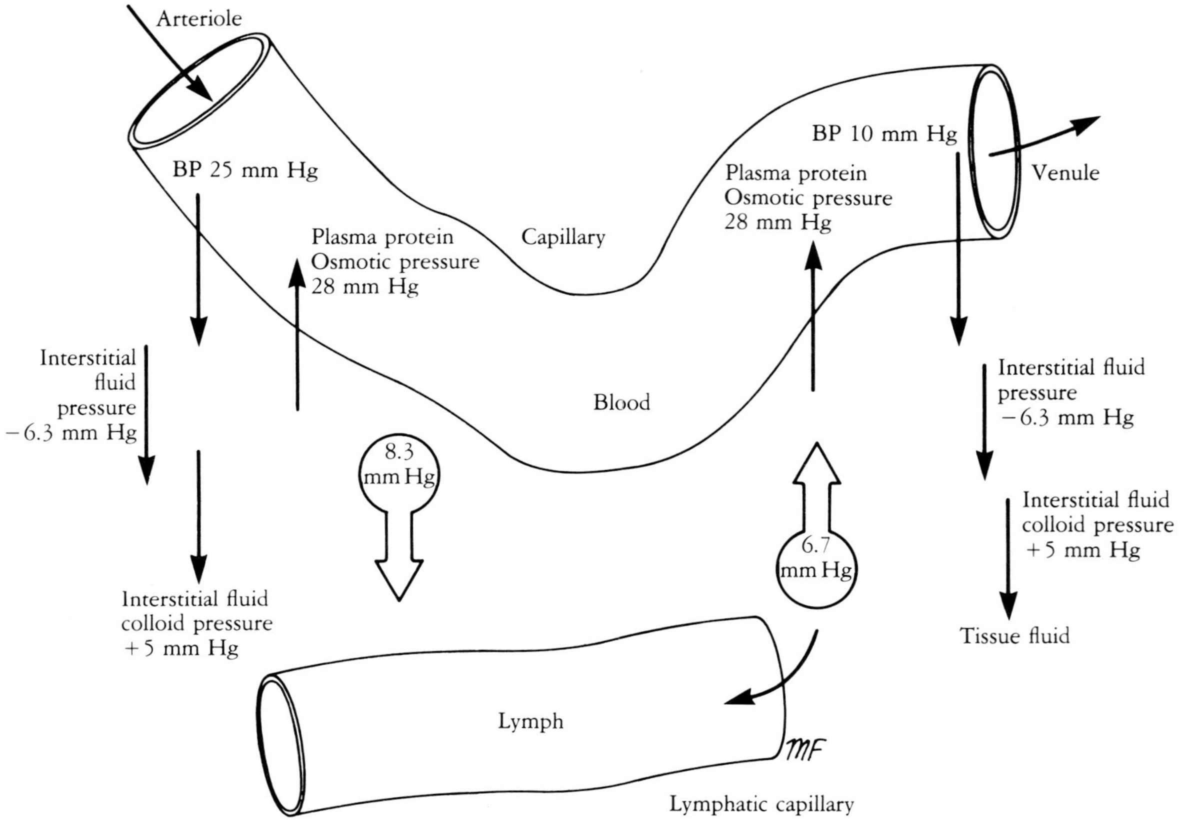

Fig. 9-5. Pressures involved in the production and reabsorption of tissue fluid in a blood capillary. Note that about 10 percent of the tissue fluid is absorbed into lymphatic capillaries, where it is known as lymph.

Formation of Lymph

Lymph has been defined as tissue fluid after it has entered a lymphatic vessel. In the previous paragraph, it was pointed out that about 10 percent of tissue fluid leaves the intercellular spaces via the lymphatic capillaries. It was also explained that substances of high molecular weight in tissue fluid leave the tissue spaces through the lymphatic vessels. The lymphatic capillaries are constantly siphoning off tissue fluid that enters their lumina and becomes lymph.

The passage of substances of large molecular weight, such as proteins, into a lymphatic capillary is easily accomplished because of the gaps between the endothelial cells and the absence of a continuous basal lamina (see Fig. 9-1). The overlap of adjacent edges of the endothelial cells provides a flap valve, so that once the substances have passed through the intercellular gaps, they are trapped within the lymphatic lumen.

Factors Controlling Lymph Flow

The following factors influence the flow of lymph from the lymphatic capillary to the bloodstream: (1) the pressure of tissue fluids, (2) the lymphatic capillary pump and the valves of lymphatic vessels, (3) the contraction of smooth muscle in the walls of lymphatic vessels, (4) the pressure on thin-walled lymphatic vessels by surrounding skeletal muscles and the pulsations of adjacent arteries, and (5) the thoraco-abdominal pump.

The more tissue fluid formed—whether by a raised arterial blood pressure, an increase in the permeability of the blood capillary wall, or a fall in plasma protein concentration—the higher the pressure of tissue fluid. This rise in pressure in turn will increase the flow of tissue fluid into the lymphatic capillaries. It is thought that the endothelial cells of capillaries contain contractile fibers (although these have not been demonstrated) that can cause the cells to contract. The effect of this so-called *lymphatic capillary pump* is to force lymph onward through the bicuspid valves, which prevent the backflow of lymph.

The squeezing effect of the smooth muscle cells in the walls of the lymphatic vessels and the pressure exerted by neighboring pulsating arteries and active skeletal muscles will have a similar effect, forcing the lymph onward while the lymphatic valves prevent the backflow of lymph.

During respiration, the alternating positive pressure exerted on the lymphatic vessels within the abdomen and the simultaneous negative pressure exerted on the thin-walled thoracic duct in the thorax, both caused by the descent of the diaphragm, assist the flow of lymph along the valved thoracic duct. This mechanism is known as the abdomino-thoracic pump. It will be remembered that the same mechanism greatly aids the return of venous blood to the right atrium of the heart (see p. 321).

LYMPHATIC TISSUE

Lymphatic or lymphoid tissue has a basic network of reticular fibers and reticular cells (Fig. 9-6). The majority of the reticular cells serve to form the reticular fibers; some, however, are fixed macrophages and belong to the reticuloendothelial system. Lying within the spaces of the reticular network are large numbers of lymphocytes, which may or may not be associated with plasma cells (Figs. 9-7, 9-8, and 9-9; see Fig. 9-6).

T and B Lymphocytes

Two kind of lymphocytes are present in peripheral lymphatic tissues, T and B lymphocytes. They are morphologically indistinguishable.

T Lymphocytes

The so-called thymus-dependent or T lymphocytes originate in the bone marrow and migrate to the cortex of the thymus, where they proliferate and undergo differentiation. Many die, but the remainder leave the thymus via the blood and migrate between the bloodstream and the peripheral lymphatic organs. T lymphocytes can be identified because they possess a specific surface antigen. They may survive for many years, and are responsible for *cellular immunity*. They constitute about 70 percent of the blood lymphocytes.

The mechanism of cellular immunity takes place as follows. The specific antigen combines with the receptor on the surface of the T lymphocyte. This process may take place at the site of entrance of the antigen into the body or in any lymphatic tissue in the body to which the antigen has been taken. The lymphocyte now enlarges and becomes a *lymphoblast* (see Fig. 9-6). The lymphoblast starts to multiply and produces a group, or clone, of new T lymphocytes that are genetically programmed to respond to this one specific antigen. These new lymphocytes circulate throughout the body and release chemical substances called *lymphokines*. The lymphokines act locally in the area of the antigen and are cytotoxic to the cells producing the antigen; they also stimulate the activity of the macrophages and prevent them from leaving the area. It must be emphasized that lymphokines act only over short distances, so the T lymphocyte must be very close to the source of the antigen. Moreover, the production of this form of immunity is a much slower process than the development of humoral immunity. The possible control of T lymphocytes by the thymic hormone thymosine is discussed on page 343.

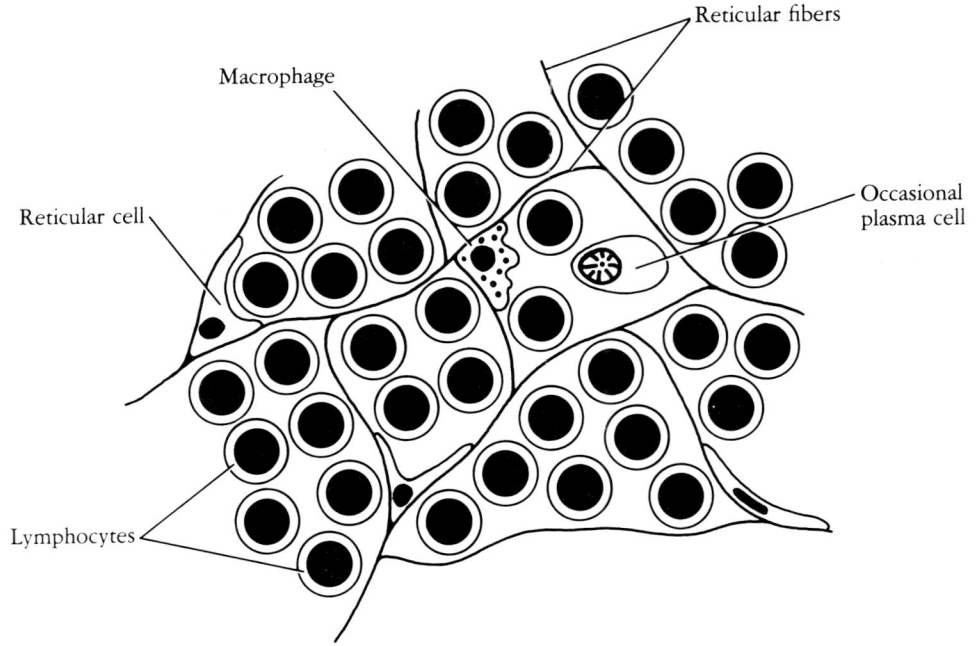
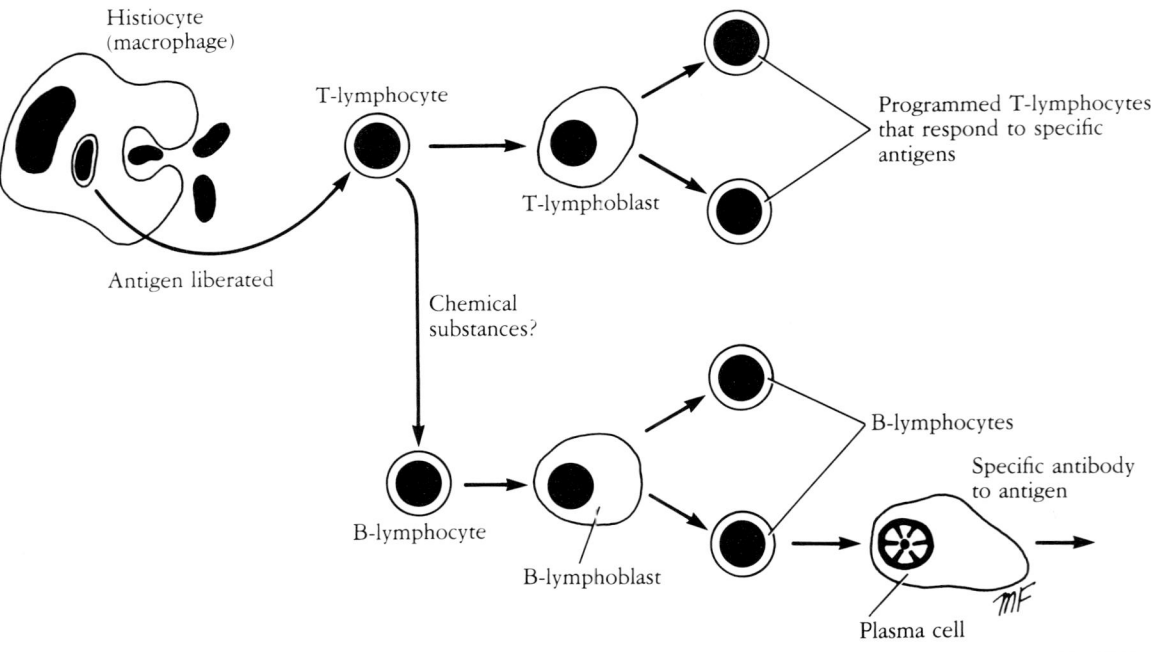

Fig. 9-6. (A) *General basic structure of lymphatic tissue.* (B) *Stages in the formation of specific antibodies from the time the antigens are liberated by macrophages. Note that the plasma cell is mainly responsible for the last stage in the formation of specific antibodies.*

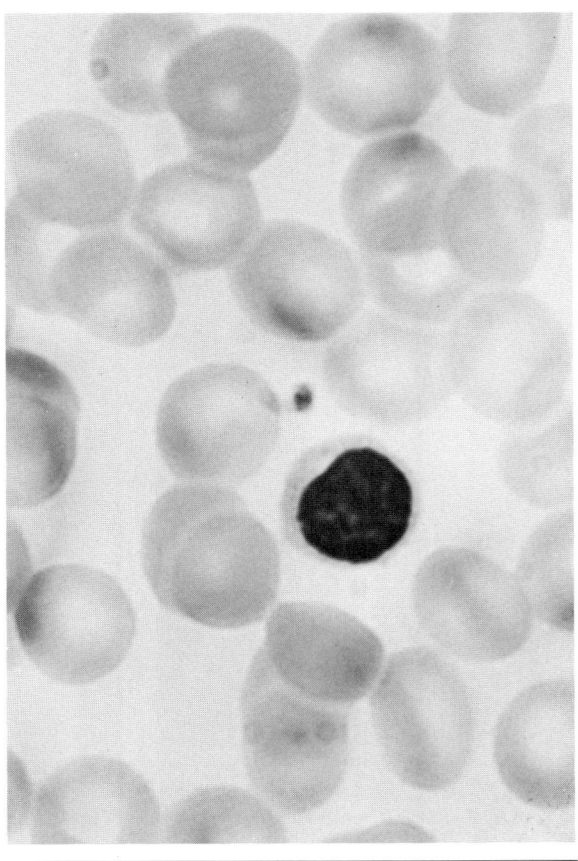

Fig. 9-7. Photomicrograph of a blood smear, showing a lymphocyte surrounded by numerous erythrocytes. Note that it is impossible morphologically to distinguish between T and B lymphocytes. (Wright's stain; ×2,364.)

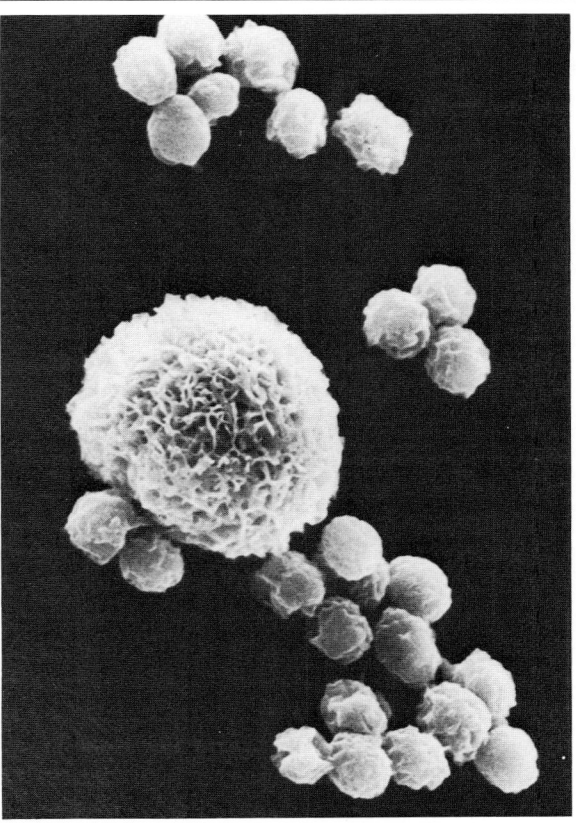

Fig. 9-8. Scanning electron micrograph of peripheral blood, showing numerous lymphocytes and a monocyte (center). (×1,952.) (Courtesy of F. G. Lightfoot.)

T LYMPHOCYTES AND TISSUE GRAFTING. If skin, for example, is transplanted from one patient to another and the two individuals are genetically not closely related, a homograft reaction takes place in the host at the site of contact with the graft. The area becomes infiltrated with *graft rejection cells*. These cells are activated T lymphocytes that have become stimulated by the antigens produced by the foreign graft. The T lymphocytes produce a cytotoxic lymphokine in response to the antigen, which causes lysis and death of the cells of the graft, resulting in rejection of the graft. In this situation, the T lymphocytes are often referred to as *killer cells*. Note that in grafting between identical twins the grafts are not rejected.

B Lymphocytes

B lymphocytes originate from the stem cells of bone marrow and possibly also from stem cells in the lymphatic tissue of the gastrointestinal tract. They circulate through the blood and lymphatic tissues throughout the body and constitute about 30 percent of the blood lymphocytes. They have a shorter life span than T lymphocytes, probably lasting only a few weeks. B lymphocytes are responsible for the development of *humoral immunity*.

The development of humoral immunity takes

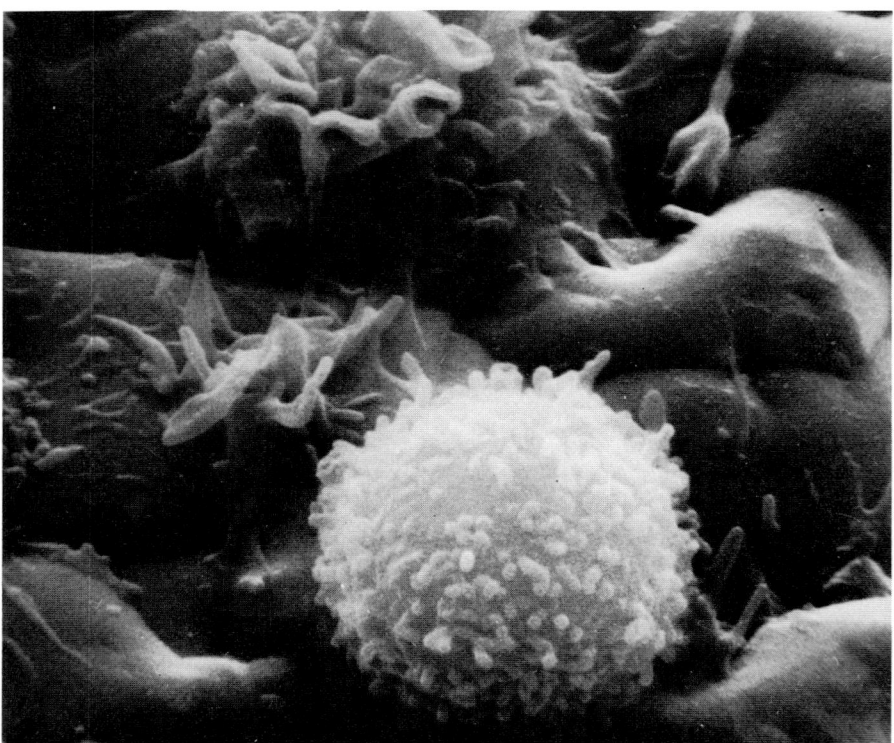

Fig. 9-9. Scanning electron micrograph of peripheral blood, showing a lymphocyte under high magnification. Note that the cell surface shows numerous microvilli. (×8,800.) (Courtesy of Dr. A. Polliack.)

place as follows. On entering the body, the antigen combines with a specific antibody present on the surface of the B lymphocyte. This process stimulates the B lymphocyte to enlarge and differentiate into a *lymphoblast,* which in turn multiplies, producing a series of new B lymphocytes. The B lymphocytes then undergo differentiation and form *plasma cells* (see Fig. 9-6). The plasma cells now form antibodies that react specifically with the original antigen.

B lymphocytes can themselves secrete specific antibodies to antigens in addition to differentiating into plasma cells. The amount of antibody produced by B lymphocytes is smaller than that produced by plasma cells, but it is known to be released at an earlier stage in the immunological response.

The antibodies thus produced are largely in the form of gamma globulins that are quickly distributed throughout the body in the bloodstream; hence, the name *humoral immunity.*

The T lymphocyte probably plays a key role in the production of humoral immunity in the majority of antibody-antigen reactions. It is believed that the T cell reacts first with the antigen and in some manner, probably by liberating chemical substances, stimulates the appropriate B lymphocyte. This cell then enlarges to form the lymphoblast, which multiplies to form more B lymphocytes; these in turn form plasma cells, which form antibodies. It has been shown as well that the T lymphocyte can inhibit the production of humoral immunity by the B lymphocyte in certain circumstances. Also, the tissue macrophage may assist in the development of humoral immunity by liberating the antigen from the invading cell.

The complicated relationship that exists between the T and B lymphocytes, the plasma cells, and the tissue macrophages is summarized in Figure 9-6.

Types of Lymphatic Tissue

Lymphatic tissue is found in the following forms: the thymus, the lymph nodes, the spleen, and the lymphatic nodules.

Thymus

The thymus is a flattened, bilobed structure lying in the thorax between the sternum and the pericardium. In the newborn, it is at its greatest size relative to the size of the body. It continues to grow until puberty, but thereafter undergoes involution, the organ being replaced by fibrofatty tissue. The thymus is a unique lymphatic tissue in that lymphatic vessels do not drain into it; lymphatic vessels do, however, leave it.

STRUCTURE. The thymus is surrounded by a delicate connective tissue capsule (Fig. 9-10) from the inner surface of which connective tissue partitions, or trabeculae, extend into the organ, partially subdividing it into *lobules*. Unlike other lymphatic organs, the thymus has a framework of branching reticular cells, the reticular fibers being practically absent. Lying within the meshwork of reticular cells are lymphocytes.

At the periphery of each lobule, the lymphocytes are small and densely packed. This area is known as the cortex (Fig. 9-11; see Fig. 9-10). In the center of the lobule, the lymphocytes are fewer; this area is known as the *medulla*. Also present in the medulla are characteristic structures known as *Hassall's corpuscles*. These are rounded structures that stain pink with eosin and measure about 50 μm in diameter. Each corpuscle consists of flattened reticular cells concentrically wrapped around one another (Fig. 9-12; see Fig. 9-10). Their function is unknown.

The majority of the lymphocytes of the thymus are nonfunctional. They become immunocompetent only when they move into the blood or other lymphatic organs.

LYMPHOCYTES OF THE THYMUS. The cortex of the thymus is made up of large numbers of lymphocytes. In the medulla, the lymphocytes are present in smaller numbers. Lymphocytes are continuously being produced in the cortex by the division of existing lymphocytes or lymphoblasts. Many of these cells die while they are in the thymus and are phagocytosed by macrophages. The remainder migrate toward the medulla and enter the bloodstream through the capillary walls.

In the embryo, the thymus is the first lymphatic organ to receive lymphocytes. These arise from cells in the yolk sac and later form the bone marrow and migrate to the thymus in the bloodstream. Descendants of these thymus lymphocytes (T lymphocytes) reenter the bloodstream and migrate to other peripheral lymphatic organs, which they populate. While these T lymphocytes reside within the thymus, they are specially antigen-sensitized. It is these T lymphocytes that are seeded out to the peripheral lymphatic organs. They are responsible for *cellular immunity*. This special processing of the lymphocytes in the thymus and their release and entrance into other lymphatic organs takes place mainly just before birth and for a few months thereafter. It follows that the removal of the thymus toward the end of the first year of life or at any time thereafter will not impair cellular immunity.

T lymphocytes cooperate with B lymphocytes (see p. 342) and assist them in the formation of antibodies.

THYMIC HORMONE. There is considerable evidence that the thymus secretes a hormone, called *thymosin*, that stimulates the activities of the T lymphocytes throughout the body. It is thought that the hormone causes the proliferation of these lymphocytes and increases their cellular immunity activity. Thymosin is produced by the reticular cells of the organ. Other peptide hormones produced by the thymus have recently been shown to have similar effects.

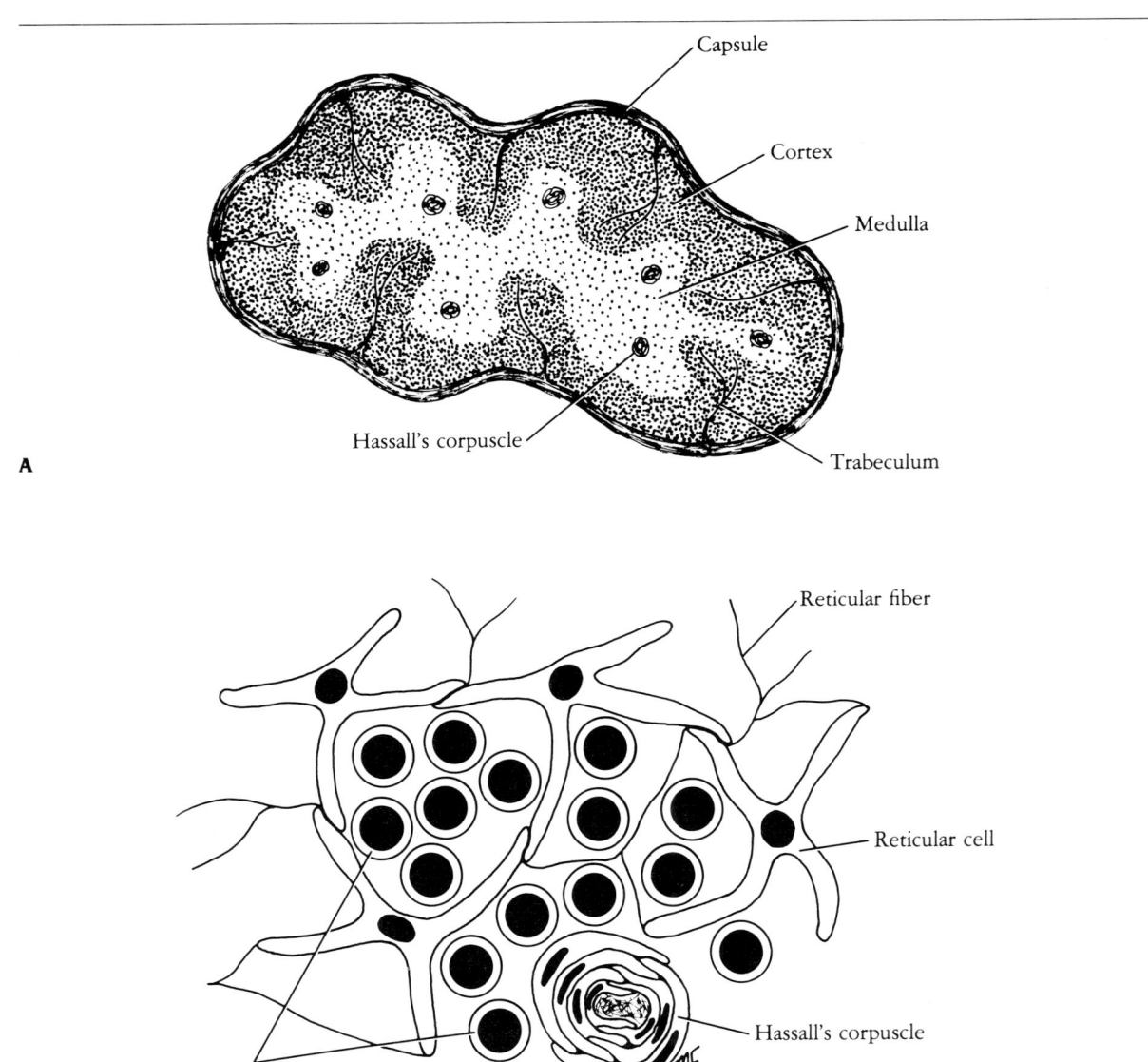

Fig. 9-10. (A) General structure of the thymus. (B) Detailed structure of the medulla of the thymus. Note that the stellate reticular cells form a three-dimensional net filled with lymphocytes.

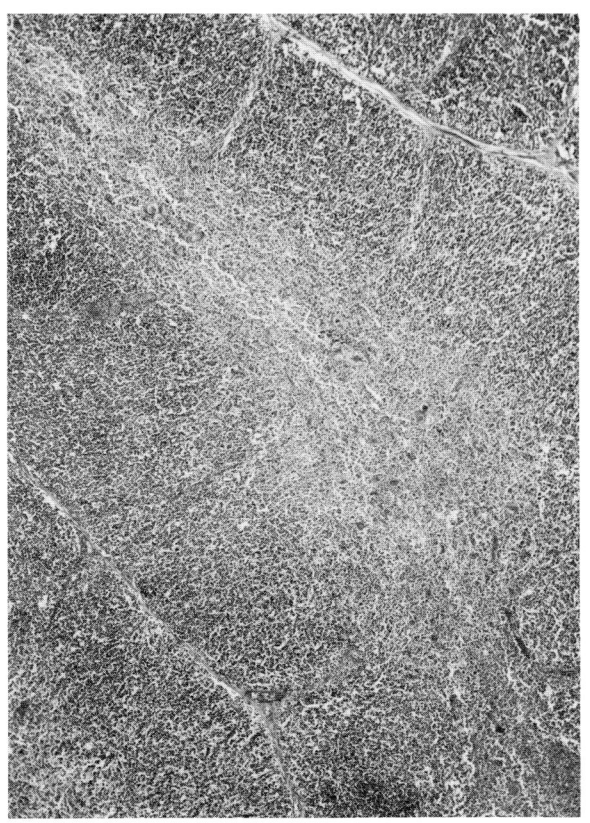

Fig. 9-11. Photomicrograph of a section of the thymus, showing parts of several lobules. Note that each lobule has a densely staining cortex and a lighter-staining central portion, the medulla. (H&E; ×40.)

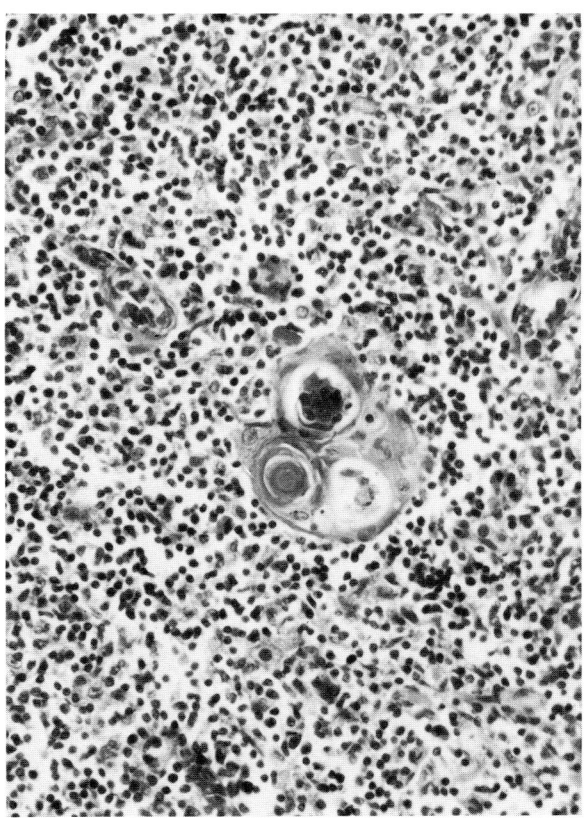

Fig. 9-12. Photomicrograph of a section of the medulla of a lobule of the thymus, showing a Hassall's corpuscle (center) consisting of concentric rings of flattened cells. Note that the central cells of the corpuscle are undergoing degeneration. (H&E; ×266.)

FUNCTION OF THE THYMUS. The thymus populates peripheral lymphatic organs, such as the lymph nodes and spleen, with immunocompetent T lymphocytes that are responsible for cellular immunity. It is thus one of the most important organs concerned with defense against infection. The activity of the T lymphocytes appears to be controlled to some extent by the thymic hormone. After puberty, when immunocompetence has been established, the thymus is of less importance and begins to atrophy.

Lymph Nodes

Lymph nodes are widely distributed throughout the body and lie along the course of lymphatic vessels (Fig. 9-13). They are ovoid or kidney-shaped and vary in size from a few millimeters to as much as 2 cm in length. Lymph nodes are usually found in groups that are associated with the lymphatic drainage of a particular region or organ.

Each lymph node is surrounded by a tough fibrous capsule that sends into the node a number of fibrous partitions called *trabeculae*. Suspended from the trabeculae is a three-dimensional network of re-

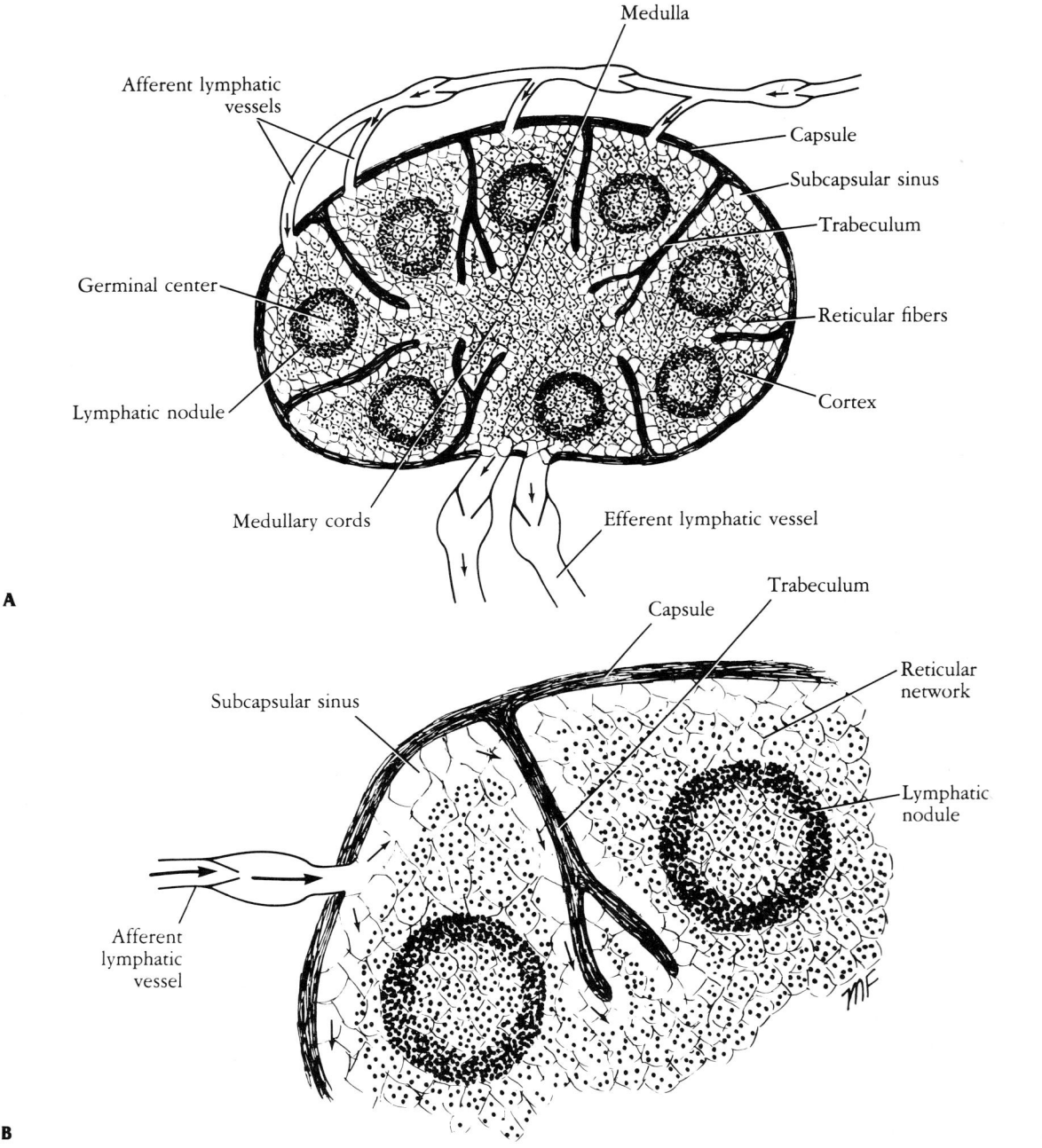

Fig. 9-13. (A) General structure of a lymph node. (B) Structure of the cortex under high magnification. Note the pathway taken by the lymph through the subcapsular sinus and along the trabeculae to the medulla.

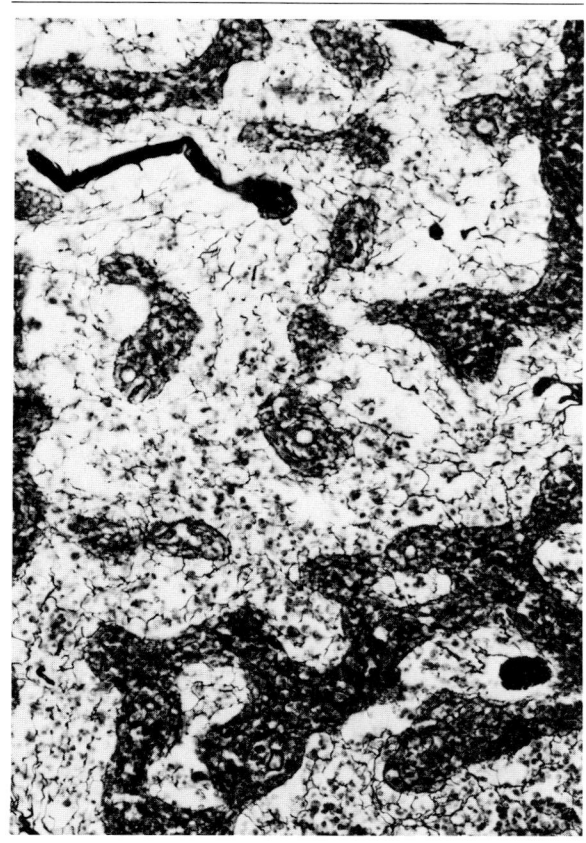

Fig. 9-14. Photomicrograph of a section of a lymph node, showing parts of trabeculae and the reticular network. The reticular fibers are seen as fine black lines. (Silver stain; ×200.)

ticular fibers and reticular cells (Fig. 9-14). The meshes of the network are filled with lymphocytes. There are also plasma cells and macrophages.

The lymphatic tissue is organized into an outer cortex and an inner medulla (Fig. 9-15). The cortex is made up of *lymphatic nodules* possessing *germinal centers* (see p. 354). The medulla is formed of strands, or cords, of lymphatic tissue called *medullary cords*. Macrophages are present in greater numbers in the medulla than in the cortex. B lymphocytes, which are concerned with the production of humoral immunity, are found mainly in the lymphatic nodules, whereas T lymphocytes, which are concerned with cellular immunity, are found mainly in the deeper cortex and the medulla.

Lymph enters a lymph node by a number of valved *afferent lymphatic vessels* that pierce the capsule on its convex surface (see Fig. 9-13). Once inside the capsule, the lymph enters the *subcapsular sinus*, an area of the reticular network devoid of lymphocytes (Fig. 9-16). The lymph moves through the subcapsular sinus until it reaches a fibrous trabeculum. Here, it is forced to turn into the interior of the node and percolates between adjacent lymphatic nodules. It then enters the medulla and finally leaves the node by one or two *efferent lymphatic vessels* that emerge from the hilus. The arrangement of the valves in the afferent and efferent lymphatic vessels permits the lymph to flow in one direction through the lymph node.

BLOOD SUPPLY AND NERVE SUPPLY. Blood vessels and sympathetic nerves pass into a lymph node at the hilum. The arteries enter the trabeculae and are distributed to the medulla and cortex. Capillary plexuses are formed in the medullary cords and the lymphatic nodules. The plexuses drain into venules that ultimately join veins that leave the node at the hilum. Lymphocytes circulating in the bloodstream enter the lymphatic tissue by passing between the cells lining the venules. Having passed through the lymphatic tissue, lymphocytes leave the node in the efferent lymphatic vessels, only to reenter the bloodstream through the thoracic duct or the right lymphatic duct.

The sympathetic nerves are vasomotor in function.

FUNCTION. Essentially, a lymph node serves as a filter. Any foreign particles in the lymph, whether bacteria or inert material, are trapped in the nodes as the lymph slowly diffuses through the meshwork of reticular fibers. A good example of this process is seen on examination of a bronchial lymph node. Inhaled carbon particles pass in the lymph from the alveolae and are trapped in the bronchial lymph nodes (Fig. 9-17). The macrophages attached to the reticular fibers phagocytose the particles as they pass by.

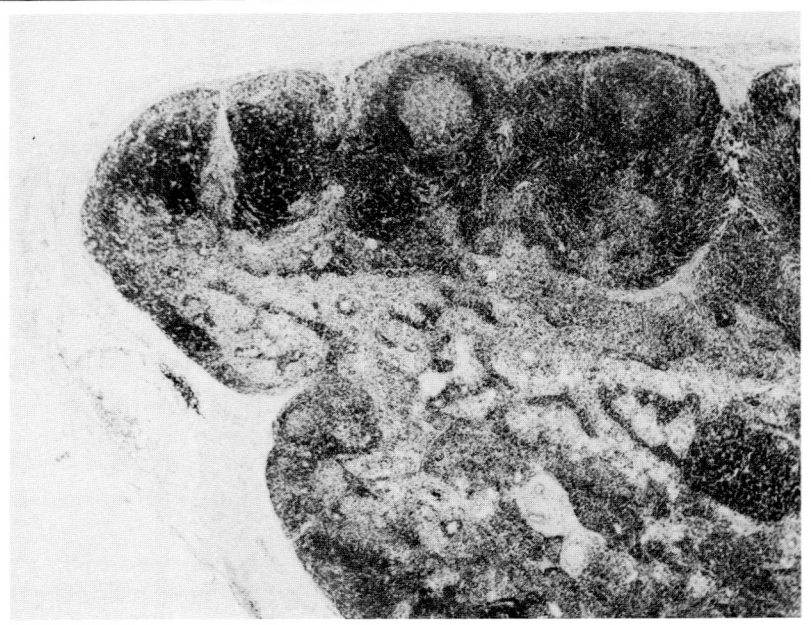

Fig. 9-15. Photomicrograph of a section of a portion of a lymph node, showing the fibrous capsule, several cortical lymph nodules, and part of the medulla. (H&E; ×40.)

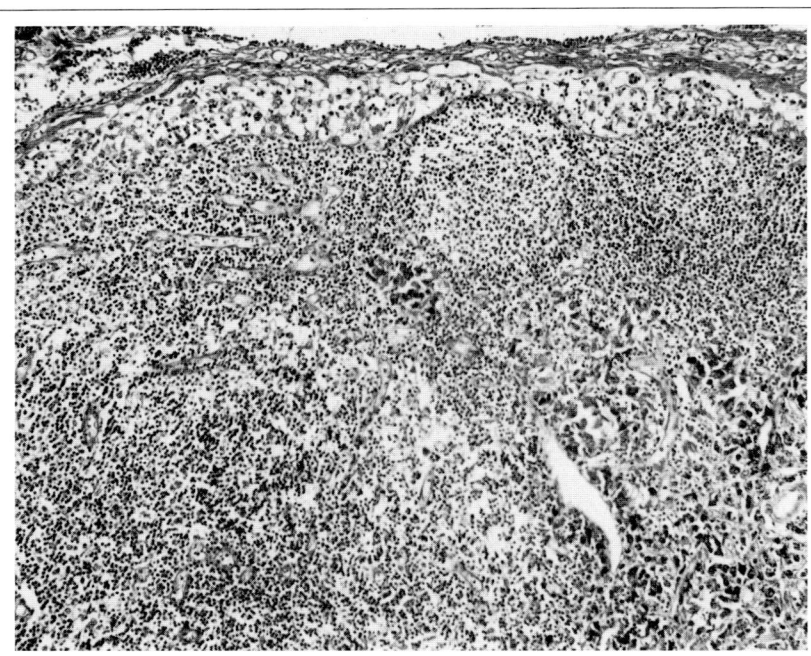

Fig. 9-16. Photomicrograph of part of the cortex of a lymph node, showing the fibrous capsule and the subcapsular sinus. Portions of several lymph nodules are also present. (H&E; ×100.)

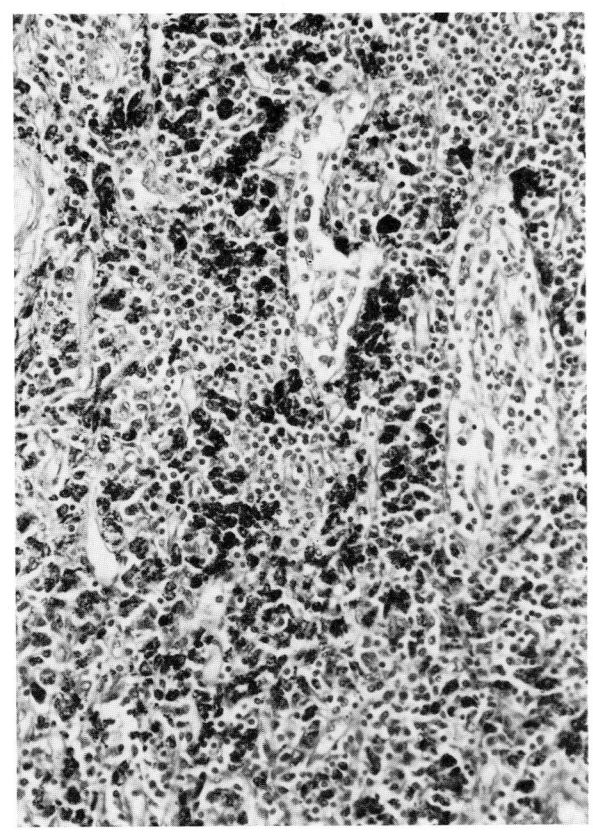

Fig. 9-17. Photomicrograph of part of the medulla of a bronchial lymph node, showing the accumulation of carbon particles in the macrophages. The carbon particles were inhaled into the lungs and passed to the lymph node, where they were phagocytosed by the macrophages. The medullary cords are packed with lymphocytes. (H&E; ×200.)

Toxins in the entering lymph initiate an immune response from the lymphocytes (see p. 339). The B lymphocytes proliferate and differentiate into plasma cells. The plasma cells then produce specific antibodies (gamma globulins) to the antigen, which are released into the lymph leaving the node. The lymph carries the antibodies to the blood in the neck via the thoracic duct and the right lymphatic duct, and they are widely disseminated throughout the body.

The T lymphocytes respond in a similar fashion by proliferating and differentiating as a result of stimulation by a specific antigen. They do not form plasma cells and antibodies, however. They develop a group of cytotoxic lymphocytes that are disseminated throughout the body.

The efferent lymph is therefore cleaner; it is richer in antibodies and contains more lymphocytes than the afferent lymph.

Spleen

The spleen is the largest single mass of lymphatic tissue in the body. It is situated in the abdomen just beneath the left half of the diaphragm. The spleen is generally ovoid and has a notched anterior border. Unlike lymph nodes, it does not lie along the course of lymphatic vessels but along the course of the systemic circulation, having a large splenic artery and a splenic vein.

The spleen is surrounded by peritoneum. Beneath the peritoneum is a fibrous *capsule* containing some smooth muscle cells. From the interior of the capsule, fibrous *trabeculae* extend into the organ (Fig. 9-18). Suspended from the capsule and trabeculae is a three-dimensional network of reticular fibers (Fig. 9-19), attached to which are reticular cells and macrophages. The interior of the spleen is filled with *splenic pulp*. On section, the spleen is seen to possess two types of pulp, white and red (Figs. 9-20 and 9-21). The white pulp forms small grayish islands less than a millimeter in diameter that are scattered throughout the remainder of the pulp, which is the red pulp.

The *white pulp* consists of nothing more than cuffs or sheaths of lymphoid tissue around the small branches of the splenic artery after the branches have left the trabeculae (Fig. 9-22; see Fig. 9-21). The lymphoid sheaths in structure resemble the cortex of lymph nodes. The meshes of the reticular network are filled with lymphocytes. Scattered along the course of each sheath are *lymph nodules* that project from its surface. The lymphocytes of the periarterial sheath are predominantly T lymphocytes; those of the lymph nodules are mainly B lymphocytes.

The *red pulp* consists of blood that is circulating

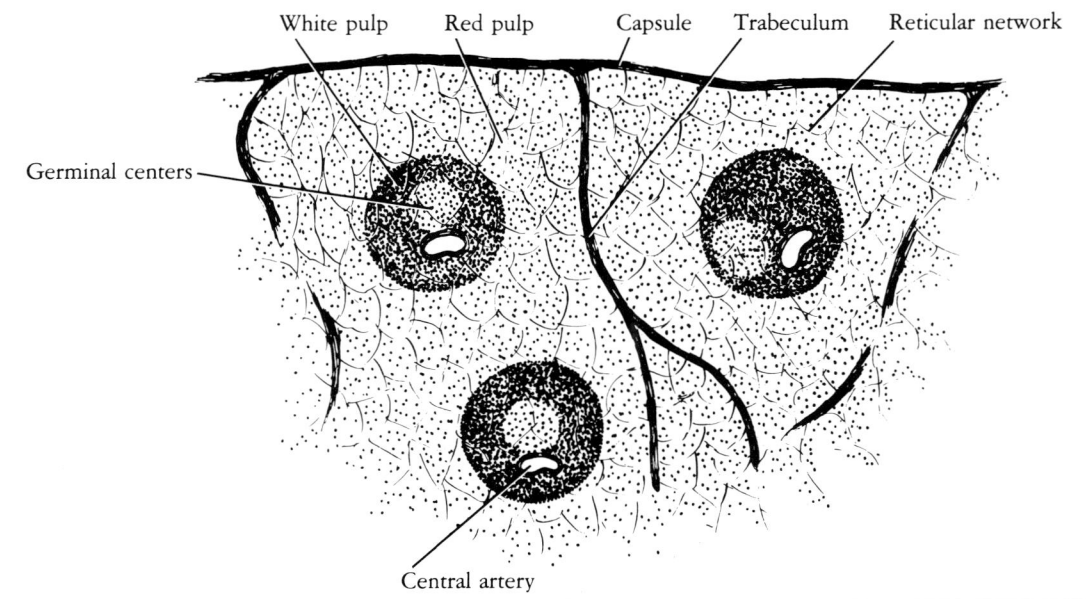

Fig. 9-18. Basic structure of the spleen. Note the red pulp and white pulp. Understand that the white pulp consists of nothing more than cuffs of lymphoid tissue around small branches of the splenic artery.

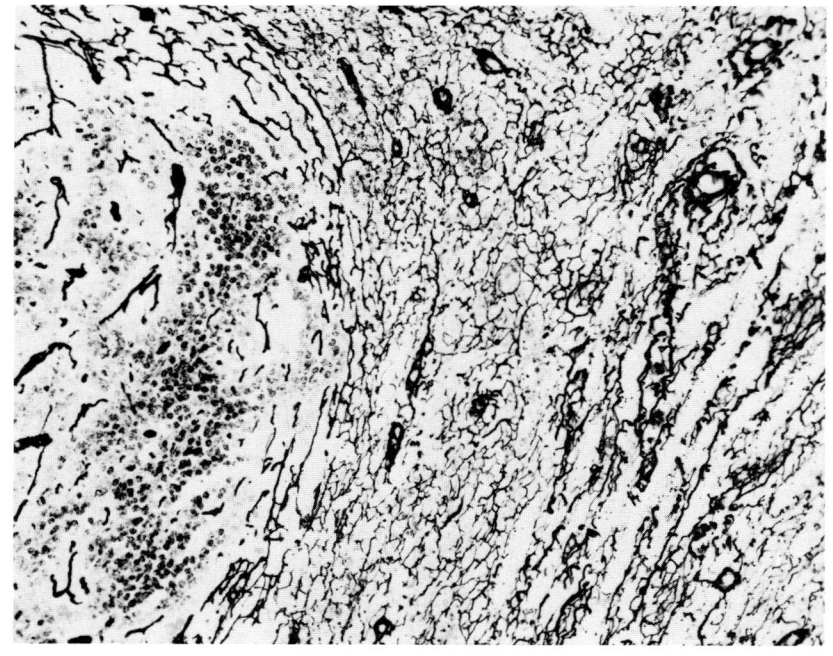

Fig. 9-19. Photomicrograph of a section through the red pulp and white pulp of the spleen, showing the black-stained reticular fibers that form a three-dimensional supporting network. (Silver stain; ×200.)

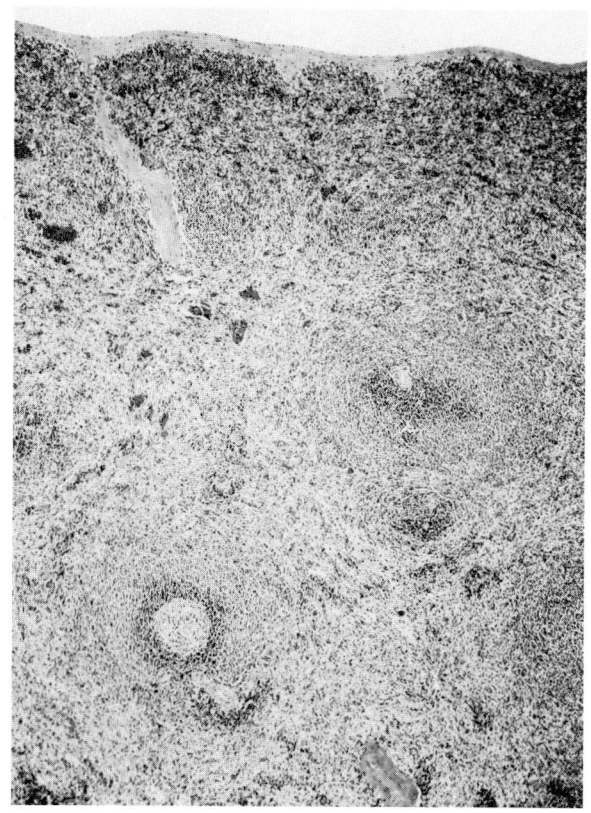

Fig. 9-20. Photomicrograph of a section of the spleen, showing the capsule and one trabeculum (top). Note the several nodules of white pulp surrounding branches of the splenic artery. The remainder of the section is made up of red pulp. (H&E; ×40.)

through the meshwork of reticular fibers (Fig. 9-23). The red color is caused by the large numbers of red cells in the blood. Attached to the reticular fibers are reticulocytes and large numbers of macrophages. Coursing through the red pulp are numerous venous sinuses and sinusoids.

BLOOD SUPPLY. The structure and organization of the spleen can be understood if the branches of the splenic artery are followed into the hilum of the spleen (see Fig. 9-21). Each branch enters a trabeculum in which it branches repeatedly. The smallest branches of the artery then leave the trabeculae and are supported by the reticular network. The outer coat of the small arteries is infiltrated with lymphocytes to form the sheaths or *white pulp*. The arteries in the center of each sheath not surprisingly are referred to as *central arteries*. Each central artery finally terminates by branching into small straight vessels (penicilliary arterioles), which in turn become capillaries in the red pulp. The central artery gives off a branch which supplies the white pulp.

In the red pulp are numerous wide and irregular passageways within the reticular network known as *venous sinusoids*. The walls of the sinusoids are formed of longitudinally arranged fusiform endothelial cells. Numerous gaps or slits exist between adjacent endothelial cells and provide a pathway for blood to enter the venous sinusoids from the red marrow (see Fig. 9-21). The outer surface of the venous sinusoids is supported by the reticular network. The venous sinusoids join one another and are drained by the red pulp veins that enter the trabeculae. The trabecular veins finally join one another at the hilum of the spleen to form the splenic vein.

BLOOD CIRCULATION THROUGH THE SPLEEN. We have seen that arterial blood passes through the white pulp within the central arteries. We also have noted that each central artery terminates by branching into small, straight vessels. The question now arises of whether the blood passes into capillaries and then into the venous sinusoids (*the closed theory*), or whether it pours from the open ends of the straight vessels directly into the open spaces of the red pulp (*the open theory*), later returning to the venous system by passing through the gaps between the endothelial cells forming the walls of the venous sinusoids. It is probable that in the human spleen both pathways are used.

FUNCTIONS. *Filter.* One of the main functions of the spleen is to filter from the blood damaged and worn-out blood cells and platelets. As the blood diffuses through the reticular meshwork in the red pulp, macrophages engulf these cells by phagocytosis.

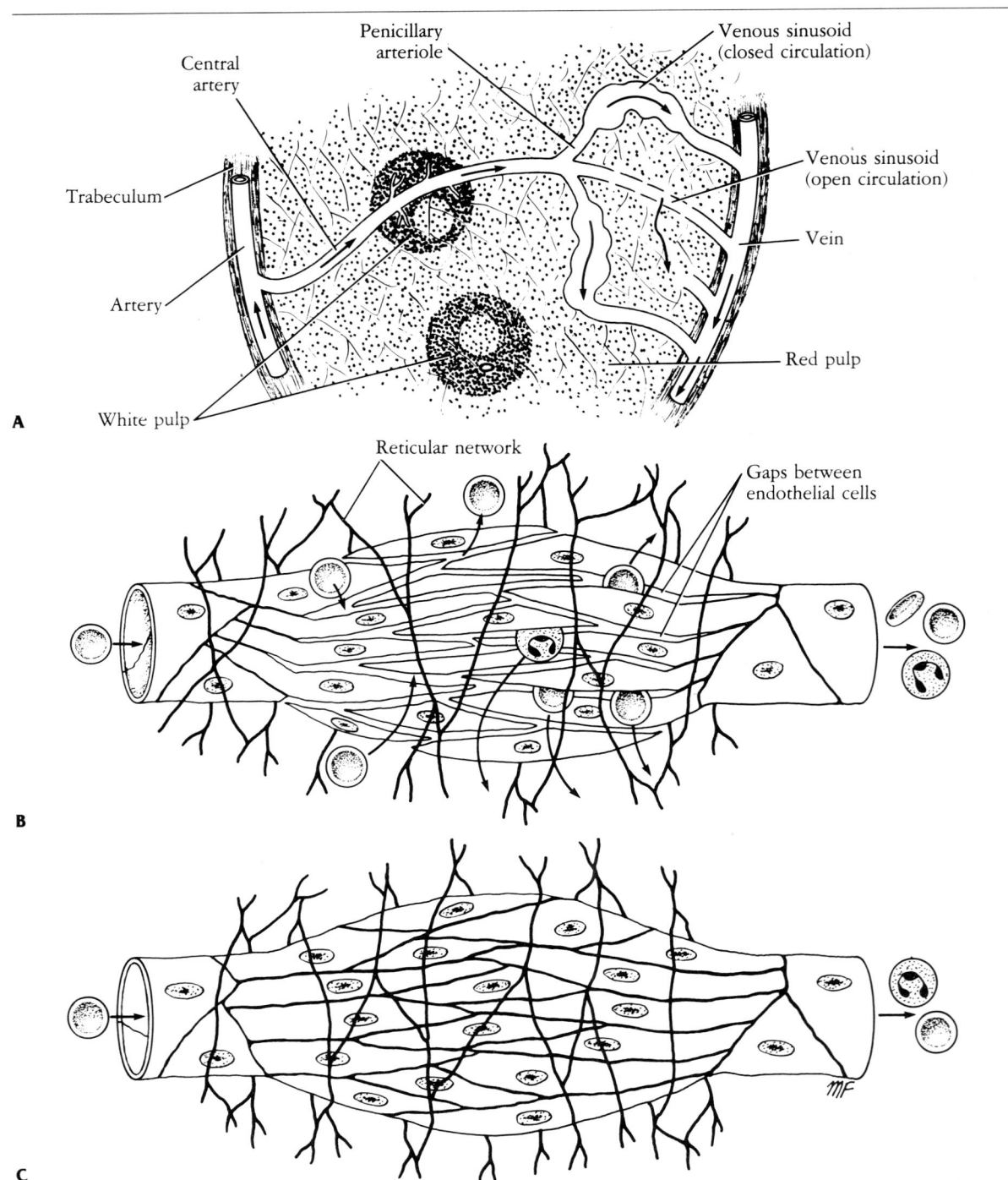

Fig. 9-21. Closed and open blood circulations through the spleen. A: The passage of blood from an artery in a trabeculum through the splenic pulp to a vein in a trabeculum. Note the two alternative routes. B: A venous sinusoid with gaps between the tapering endothelial cells. Blood cells enter or leave the sinusoid by passing through its wall and are forced to squeeze through the slitlike gaps between the endothelial cells. The venous sinusoid is supported by a network of reticular fibers. C: A venous sinusoid in which the tapering endothelial cells are in close apposition, preventing the blood cells from passing through its wall.

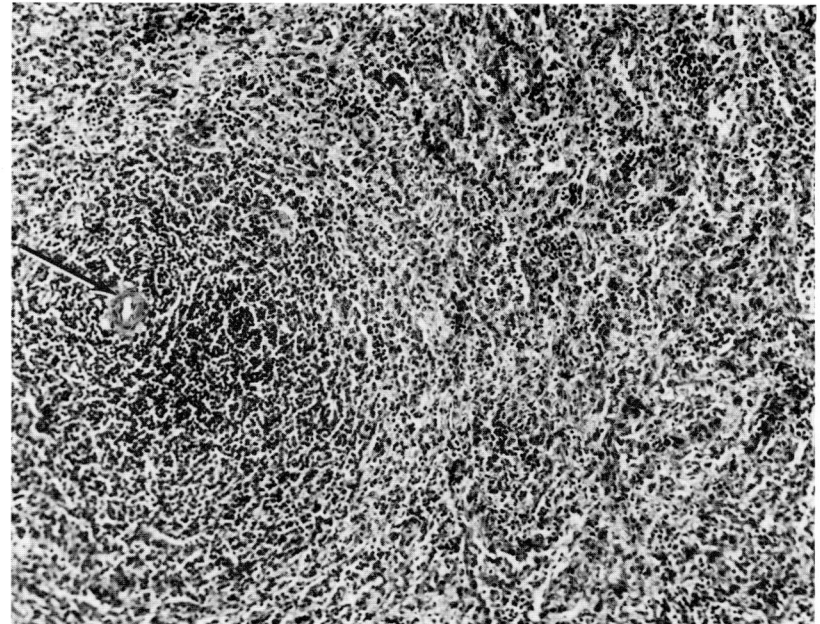

Fig. 9-22. Photomicrograph of a section of part of the spleen, showing a lymphatic nodule (white pulp) with a central artery (arrow). The red pulp is seen around the white pulp. (H&E; ×100.)

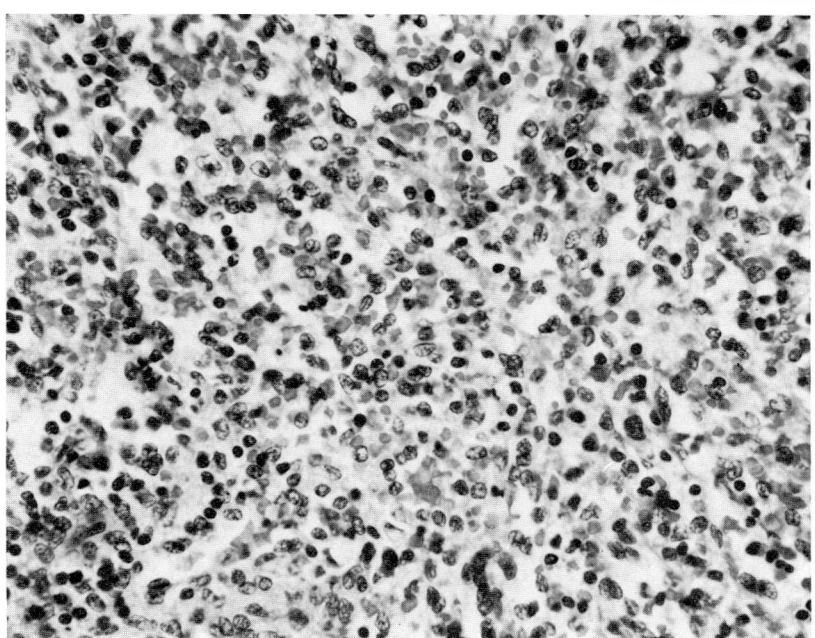

Fig. 9-23. Photomicrograph of a section of part of the spleen, showing the red pulp. The red pulp contains many venous sinusoids filled with blood; the hemoglobin in the erythrocytes is responsible for the red color of the pulp. (H&E; ×400.)

Associated with the destruction of erythrocytes is the breakdown of hemoglobin by lysosomal enzymes. The iron of the hemoglobin is temporarily stored in the macrophages as ferritin or hemosiderin and is available for the formation of new erythrocytes in the red bone marrow (see p. 158). The spleen is therefore a major organ for the storage of iron. The *heme* fraction of the hemoglobin is broken down within the macrophages to bilirubin. This then passes via the bloodstream, bound to albumin, to the liver, where it is secreted in the bile.

Immune Defense and the Formation of New Lymphocytes. Foreign particles, including bacteria and viruses, that are circulating in the blood may stimulate a strong immune response in the spleen (compare with the function of a lymph node). The reticular network of the red and white pulp traps the antigen, allowing it to come into contact with the T and B lymphocytes. The T lymphocytes, concerned with providing cellular immunity, are situated close to the central artery of the lymphatic sheaths. The B lymphocytes, concerned with humoral immunity, are located in the periphery of the white pulp. In this manner, the spleen contributes to both cellular and humoral immunity.

Blood-forming Function. Lymphocytes and macrophages are formed in the spleen throughout life. In the fetus, the spleen forms blood cells in the same manner as does the red bone marrow. Just before birth, the spleen loses the function of forming erythrocytes and granular leukocytes; this function is taken over entirely by the red bone marrow. In certain pathological conditions in which there is destruction of bone marrow, this function may be resumed by the spleen in postnatal life.

Blood Reservoir. The reticular network filters off and separates blood cells from the plasma and may store them for varying periods of time. The stored red cells and platelets form a reserve pool that can be drawn upon in an emergency.

Lymphatic Nodules

Lymphatic nodules are circumscribed collections of lymphatic tissue found in the cortex of lymph nodes, at the periphery of the lymphatic sheaths (white pulp) of the spleen, and in the connective tissue of the mucous membrane of the respiratory and intestinal tracts (Figs. 9-24 and 9-25).

Each nodule has a basic three-dimensional network of reticular fibers and reticular cells; within the meshes of the network are T and B lymphocytes. A nodule usually possesses a lighter-staining central area, called the *germinal center*, that is the active site of lymphocyte production. Germinal centers are absent from lymphatic nodules before birth; they appear only following the exposure of the nodule to a foreign antigen.

Most lymphatic nodules occur singly in loose connective tissue and are nonencapsulated. Others—for example, in the tonsil or ileum—become fused. In the lower part of the ileum, the fused nodules are called *Peyer's patches* (Fig. 9-26). Remember that the lymph nodes and spleen are lymphatic organs that contain lymphatic nodules but that the thymus does not contain lymphatic nodules.

FUNCTIONS OF LYMPHATIC NODULES. Antigens may penetrate the mucous membrane lining the respiratory and alimentary tracts and even the genitourinary tract and gain entrance to the connective tissue. It is not surprising, therefore, to find collections of lymphocytes in the form of nonencapsulated nodules just beneath the epithelium lining these tubular tracts. T and B lymphocytes provide an important line of defense against bacterial, viral, and other sources of antigens.

TONSILS. The tonsils form a discontinuous ring of lymphatic tissue around the entrance of the mouth and nose into the pharynx (Fig. 9-27). They consist of paired palatine tonsils, paired tubal tonsils, a lingual tonsil, and a nasopharyngeal tonsil. The tonsils are strategically placed at the entrance to the respiratory and digestive systems and respond immunologically to foreign antigens entering these systems.

The *palatine tonsils* are located in the lateral walls of the oral pharynx between the palatoglossal and palatopharyngeal arches (Figs. 9-28 and 9-29). The

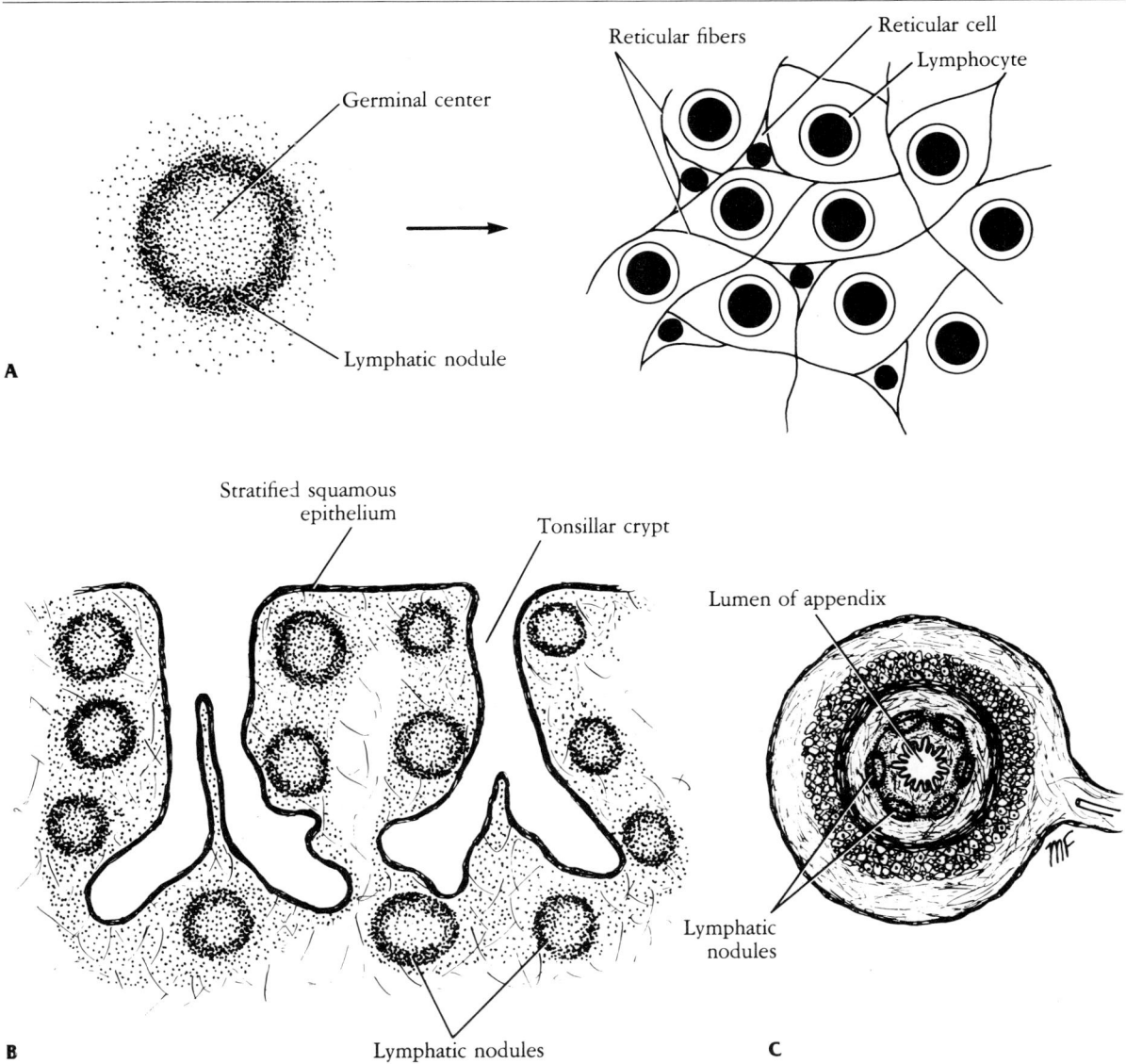

Fig. 9-24. A: The basic structure of a lymphatic nodule; B: the arrangement of the lymphatic nodules in the tonsil; C: the position of the lymphatic nodules in a cross section of the appendix.

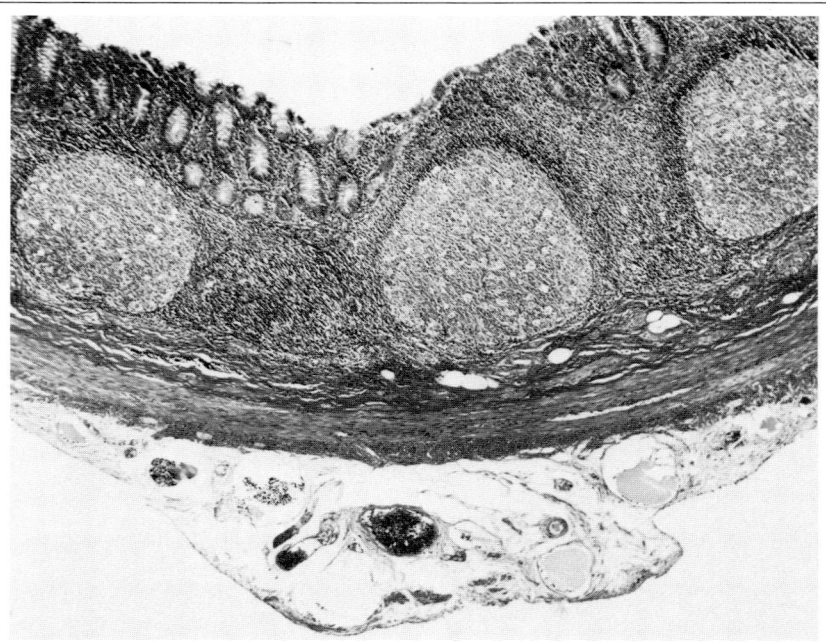

Fig. 9-25. Photomicrograph of a cross section of part of the appendix, showing the large lymphatic nodules in the submucosa. (H&E; ×40.)

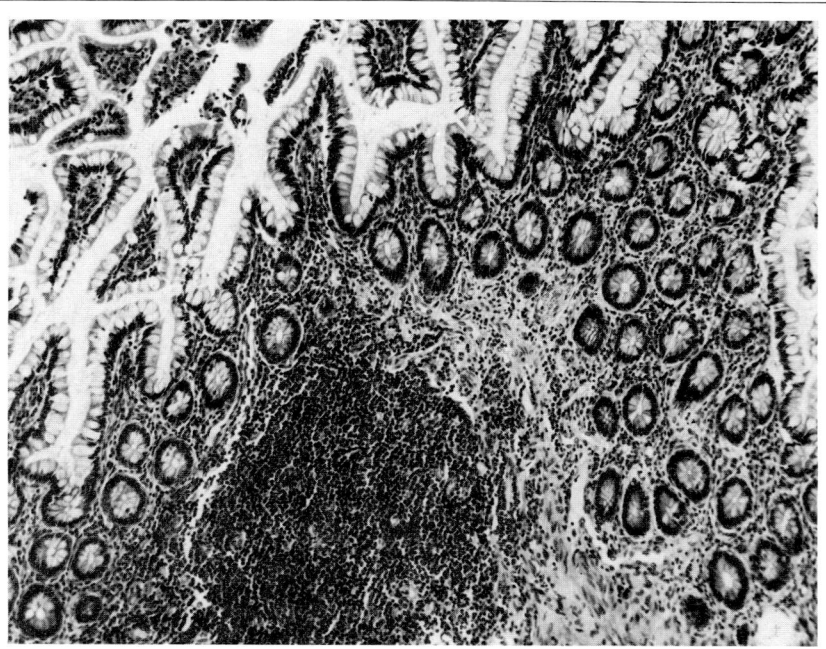

Fig. 9-26. Photomicrograph of section of the mucous membrane and submucosa of the lower part of the ileum, showing part of a lymphatic nodule in a Peyer's patch. (H&E; ×100.)

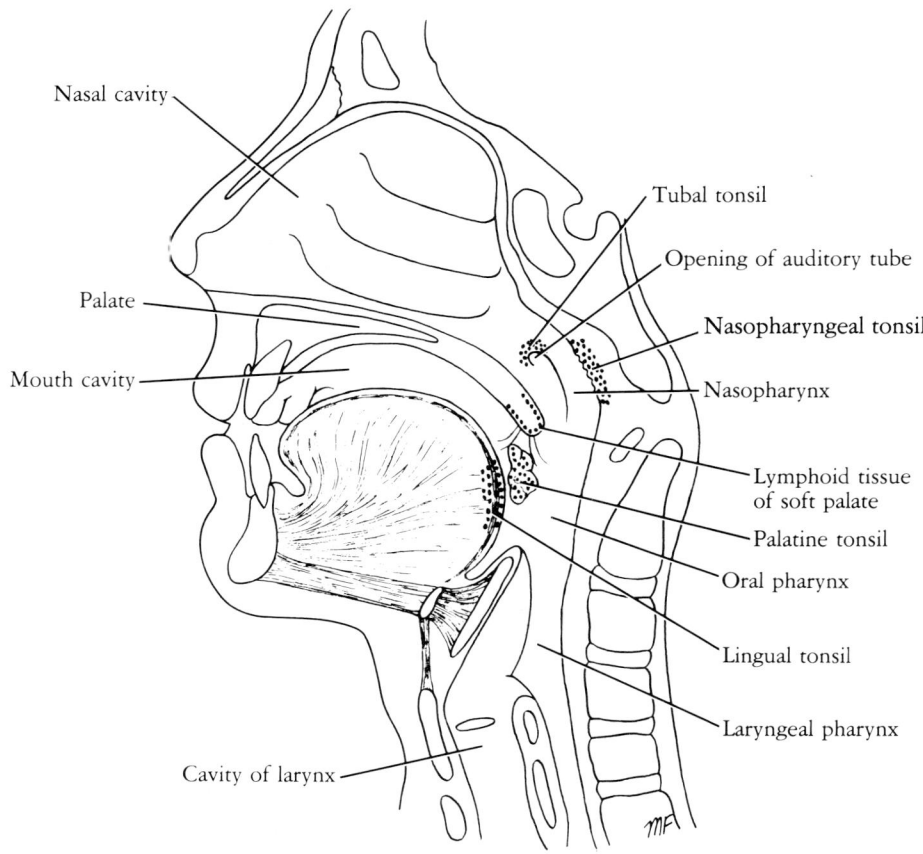

Fig. 9-27. Distribution of lymphatic tissue around the entrance of the mouth and nose into the pharynx.

tubal tonsils are located in the lateral wall of the nasopharynx around the opening of the auditory tube. The *lingual tonsil* is situated on the posterior third of the tongue, and the *nasopharyngeal tonsil* (Fig. 9-30) is located in the roof of the nasopharynx. Because all the tonsils have a basically similar structure, only the structure of the palatine tonsil will be described here.

Palatine Tonsils. Each tonsil has a free medial surface that projects into the cavity of the pharynx. The surface is pitted by numerous small openings leading into the *tonsillar crypts* (see Figs. 9-28 and 9-29).

The tonsils consist of masses of lymphatic tissue lying within the connective tissue of the mucous membrane. The mucous membrane is covered with stratified squamous epithelium continuous with that of the mucosa of the pharynx. Occasionally, the epithelium dips down into the lymphatic tissue, forming the tonsillar crypts (see Fig. 9-29).

The lymphatic tissue of the tonsils contains numerous lymphatic nodules with germinal centers. Many of the lymphocytes formed in the nodules migrate through the epithelial lining of the tonsillar crypts. From there, they pass into the cavity of the pharynx, where they degenerate in the saliva.

The tonsil is covered on its lateral surface by a layer of dense connective tissue called the *capsule*.

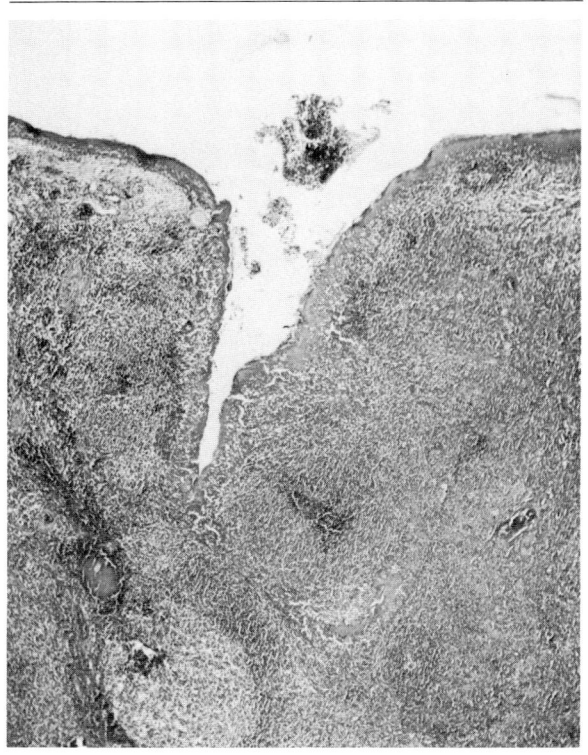

Fig. 9-28. Photomicrograph of section of the palatine tonsil, showing a tonsillar crypt surrounded by lymphatic nodules. (H&E; ×40.)

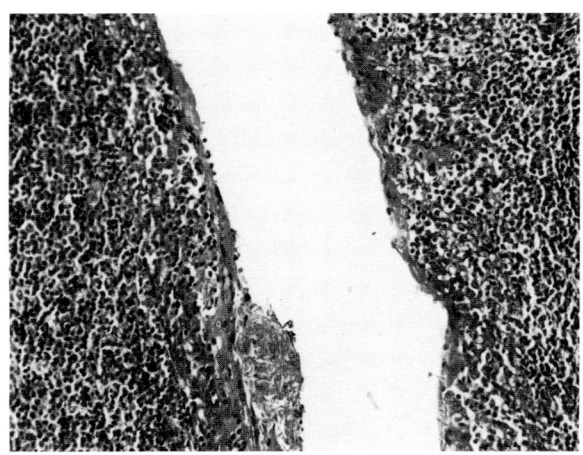

Fig. 9-29. Photomicrograph of a longitudinal section of a tonsillar crypt, showing the crypt to be bounded on each side by a dense accumulation of lymphatic tissue. Note that the stratified squamous epithelium lining the crypt is being invaded by lymphocytes, which pass into the lumen of the crypt and out into the cavity of the pharynx. (H&E; ×140.)

THE RETICULOENDOTHELIAL SYSTEM (MONONUCLEAR PHAGOCYTE SYSTEM)

In 1892 Metchnikoff recognized a group of cells that are widely scattered throughout the body and have the common function of being able to phagocytose actively and store vital dyes, such as trypan blue, when they are introduced into the body of an animal. Aschoff in 1924 proposed the collective name of *reticuloendothelial system* for these cells, because many of them are associated with reticular

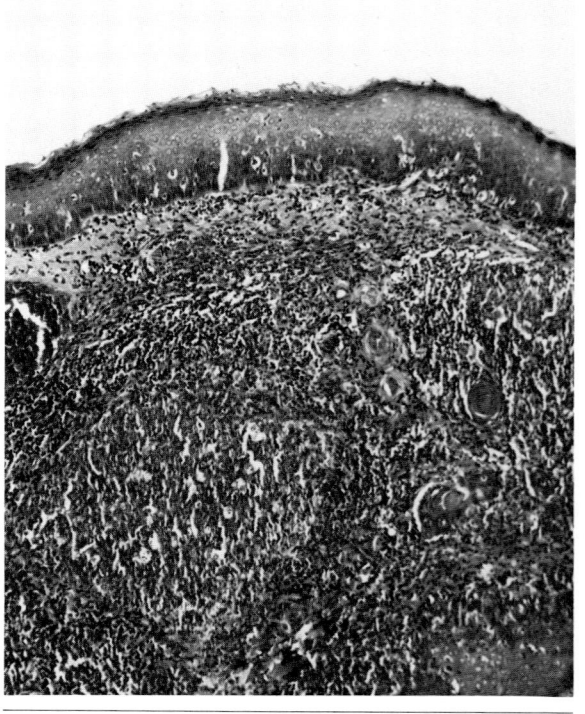

Fig. 9-30. Photomicrograph of a section through the nasopharyngeal tonsil, showing the stratified squamous epithelium lining the pharyngeal wall (top) and large amounts of lymphatic tissue in the mucous membrane and submucosa. (H&E; ×92.)

Table 9-1. The cell components of the reticuloendothelial system

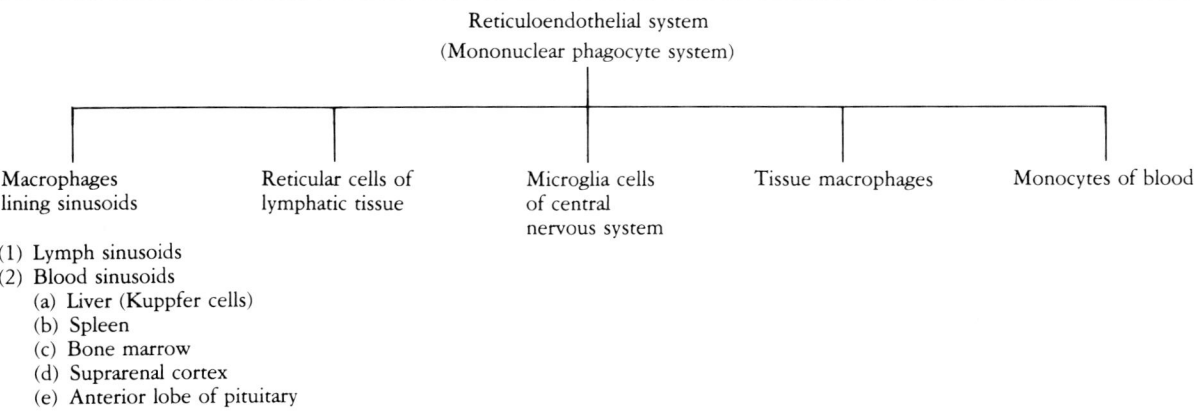

fibers in tissues or are endothelial cells that line the blood sinusoids in the liver, spleen, bone marrow, and suprarenal and pituitary glands. The different cells of the reticuloendothelial system are shown in Table 9-1.

It is now generally accepted that not all the cells of this system are reticular cells or endothelial cells, and the term *reticuloendothelial system* has been replaced by *mononuclear phagocyte system;* this term includes all phagocytic cells within the body except the polymorphonuclear leukocytes.

Mononuclear phagocyte cells are thought to arise from the bone marrow as monocytes. The monocytes circulate around the body in the blood and take up temporary or permanent residence in tissues such as the Kupffer cells of the liver (Fig. 9-31), the macrophages of connective tissue, and lymphatic tissue. When stimulated by foreign particulate matter, the cells proliferate, detach themselves, and move back into the circulation.

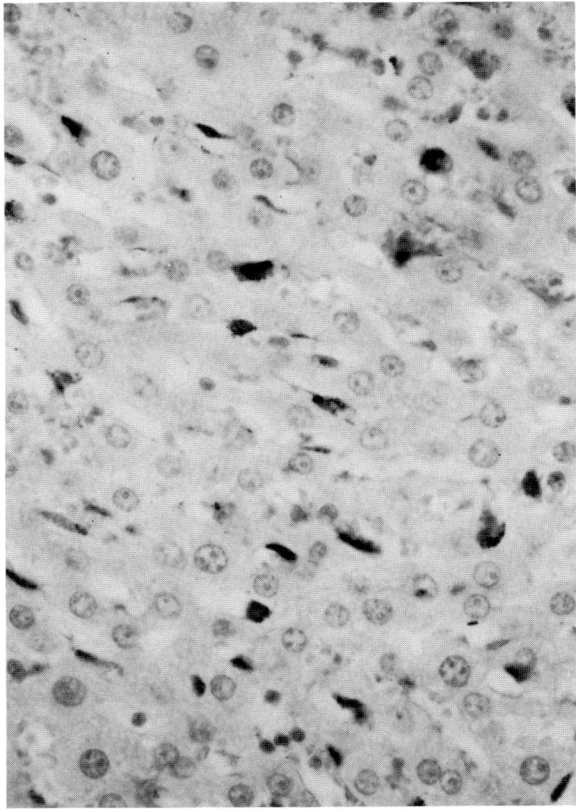

Fig. 9-31. Photomicrograph of a section of a guinea pig liver following the subcutaneous injection of trypan blue three days previously. The accumulation of dye granules is visible within the cytoplasm of Kupffer cells lining the blood sinusoids. (H&E; ×400.)

The ameboid and phagocytic activities of these mononuclear cells provide the body with a strong defense against microorganisms. Not only do these cells phagocytose and destroy many microorganisms, but they assist the lymphocytes in establishing immune responses by liberating the antigen from the invading organisms.

CLINICAL NOTES

EDEMA

Edema is an abnormal accumulation of tissue fluid within the intercellular spaces. As a result of gravity, edema tends to appear first in the dependent parts, such as the ankles and feet. The ease with which edema fluid collects is related to the density of the tissues. For example, excess tissue fluid collects readily in the loose connective tissues of the eyelids, scrotum, or vulva.

Basically, edema is a result of an upset in the dynamics of the formation and absorption of tissue fluid in the region of the blood and lymphatic capillaries. The common causes of edema are as follows:

Increased Blood Capillary Pressure

Increase in blood capillary pressure can be caused by venous obstruction stemming from such conditions as (1) pressure of the pregnant uterus on the inferior vena cava, (2) heart failure, and (3) venous thrombosis in which the blood clot obstructs the vein.

Increased capillary pressure can also be caused by arteriolar dilatation from such conditions as (1) infection, such as the common boil, in which the edema is worsened by the escape of plasma proteins into the tissues, which osmotically attract fluid outside the capillary; and (2) hives, or urticaria, an allergic condition resulting in the release of histamine into the tissues, thereby causing arteriolar dilatation.

Hypoproteinemia

This condition may be caused by (1) a leakage of plasma proteins from the blood into the urine, as in the disease of the kidney known as nephrosis, in which large quantities of albumin are lost from the plasma each day; and (2) diets deficient in protein.

Lymphatic Obstruction

An inability to absorb protein from the tissue fluid into the lymphatic capillary will result in an accumulation of protein in the tissue fluid outside the capillary and cause edema. This occurs in several conditions: (1) Congenital lymphatic obstruction (Milroy's disease), which occurs when the lymphatic vessels, especially those of the lower limbs, fail to develop. (2) Surgical removal of lymph nodes and associated lymphatic vessels in an attempt to remove completely cancer cells that may have spread from their primary locus. This form of edema commonly occurs in the upper limbs following a radical mastectomy for carcinoma of the breast. In this operation, the axillary group of lymph nodes is removed along with the diseased breast. (3) Filariasis. This is a mosquito-spread disease, common in the tropics, in which the worm larvae enter the lymphatic vessels and progressively block the lymph nodes. After a number of years, the lymphatic drainage of the leg may become totally obstructed and the grossly edematous lower limb may resemble that of an elephant; hence, the name *elephantiasis*. (4) Malignant metastases in lymph nodes and lymphatic vessels; these may cause edema of the skin of the breast or arm in advanced carcinoma of the breast.

Retention of Fluid in the Body

Failure of the kidneys to excrete adequate quantities of water in an individual who continues to consume normal quantities of water and electrolytes will invariably lead to accumulation of fluid in the tissue spaces.

LYMPHATIC VESSELS

Infection

Infection of the lymphatic vessels, *lymphangitis*, is a common occurrence. Red streaks along the course of the lymphatic vessels are characteristic of the condition. For example, a severe infection of the thumb may be followed by the spread of the bacteria into the lymphatic vessels draining the area. Red streaks may be seen on the anterior aspect of the forearm, following the course of the cephalic vein.

Once the infection reaches the lymph nodes, the nodes become enlarged and tender, a condition known as *lymphadenitis*.

Lymph Flow in Lymphatic Vessels

The factors responsible for normal lymph flow in lymphatic vessels have been discussed (see p. 338). There are clinical situations in which it is important to diminish the speed of lymph flow. For example, a patient who has a severe bacterial infection of the hand may have the arm immobilized in a sling as an important part of the treatment. This procedure reduces the muscular activity of the limb and, consequently, the lymph flow, lessening the possibility of bacterial spread via the lymphatic vessels and diminishing the rate of entry of toxins into the bloodstream via the lymph. In some conditions, it may be appropriate to have the patient rest in bed in order to reduce lymph flow.

Other clinical conditions may warrant treatment that increases the lymph flow in lymphatic vessels. In postural edema, an individual who has been standing in one position for hours may experience swelling of the ankles and feet. Increasing lymph flow also may be important in someone who has had a limb immobilized for a long period in a cast. Suitable muscular exercises, raising the limb to use the force of gravity, or massage applied to the area will aid the flow of lymph along valved lymphatic vessels.

SPREAD OF MALIGNANT DISEASE

Lymphatic vessels provide a pathway for the spread of certain types of malignant tumors from their site of origin. When the cancer cells reach a lymph node, they may be stopped temporarily by the meshwork of reticular fibers. If the environment is suitable, however, the cancer cells may continue to multiply in situ, leading to the formation of a secondary growth, or metastasis. Therefore, a surgeon treating a cancer patient is not content merely to remove the primary growth but must also remove the lymphatic vessels and lymph nodes that drain the area of the growth. This treatment is the only rational way of excising the cancer cells totally and preventing the possible appearance of secondary growth.

Lymph Node Neoplasms

Neoplasms that have spread to regional lymph nodes and caused a metastasis there far outnumber primary tumors of lymph nodes. Tumors arising primarily from lymph nodes include lymphomas, Hodgkin's disease, and lymphocytic leukemia. A lymphoma is a tumor composed mainly of lymphocytes and, sometimes, histiocytes. Hodgkin's disease is a condition that arises in lymph nodes and exhibits a characteristic giant cell known as the Reed-Sternberg cell; lymphocytes and histiocytes are also present. Although Hodgkin's disease tends to spread from one lymph node to another, it is purposely referred to as a disease rather than a neoplasm, because whether it is a tumor or an inflammatory response to an unknown organism has not been determined. Lymphatic leukemia is a malignant neoplasm of lymphocytes. Acute lymphocytic leukemia is a common form of cancer in children.

LYMPHATIC TISSUES

Lymph Node Infections

Lymph nodes may be involved in acute or chronic infections. A general enlargement of lymph nodes is suggestive of a general infection such as *German measles (rubella), syphilis, tuberculosis,* or *brucellosis.* An enlargement restricted to a group of nodes, however, suggests a local infection.

Thymus

The role of the thymus in the sensitization of lymphocytes and the formation of T lymphocytes is described on page 343. The part that T lymphocytes play in cellular immunity also has been fully discussed.

Allograft Rejection

At about the time of birth, T lymphocytes leave the thymus and populate the peripheral lymphatic tissue; it is these cells that will bring about rejection of an allograft. Grafts between identical twins or from a individual to himself will survive indefinitely, because there is no antigenic response. Although the thymus in the adult continues to influence the activities of the T lymphocytes, possibly by means of thymosin, thymectomy has been unsuccessful in preventing the rejection of allografts.

Attempts to suppress the immunocompetent lymphocytes with drugs have been moderately successful. Allograft survival can now be prolonged by the combined use of adrenal steroids (direct action on lymphocytes), azathioprine (inhibits deoxyribonucleic acid and ribonucleic acid synthesis by lymphocytes), and antilymphocyte serum.

Congenital Absence of the Thymus

As a consequence of congenital absence of the thymus, the patient lacks T lymphocytes and, therefore, cellular immunity. This rare disease has been treated successfully by the transplantation of the thymus from an embryo.

Tumors of the Thymus

Thymomas are tumors of the thymus and are some of the most common tumors found in the anterior mediastinum. Many of the tumors are associated with myasthenia gravis and aplasia of blood cells. It is thought that these diseases are autoimmune in origin and may develop as a result of the formation of T lymphocytes that react to the individual's own tissues. Myasthenia gravis, as discussed earlier, is a disease in which there is a possible reduction of acetylcholine receptors at the motor end-plates of skeletal muscle. Thymomas are neoplasms of the reticular cells that form the framework of the interior of the thymus. The reticular cells resemble epithelial cells in that they possess desmosomes and many organelles commonly seen in epithelial cells. Thymomas may be benign or malignant.

Spleen

Hypersplenism

In this condition, the normal destructive capabilities of the spleen in relation to the blood have been increased abnormally, producing *anemia, leukopenia,* or *thrombocytopenia.* Many patients with these conditions are cured by splenectomy.

Idiopathic Thrombocytopenic Purpura

In this condition, there is a slow, continuous bleeding from the mucous membranes, the nose, and other parts of the body because of a lack of platelets in the blood. The cause is unknown. Splenectomy is advised in patients in whom spontaneous remission does not occur after 6 months. The rationale of this treatment is that it removes the main center in the body where the platelets are normally extracted from the circulation.

CLINICAL PROBLEMS

For the answers to these problems, see page 797.

1. A 23-year-old woman is treated in the emergency room for an infected right index finger. Three days previously, she had got a rose thorn in her finger while gardening. On examination, the finger is red, tender, and very swollen. After removing the thorn and applying a dressing, the physician prescribes a course of antibiotics. He asks the nurse to put the patient's right arm in a sling, and warns the patient not to move the arm excessively. Explain why the patient's arm has been placed in a sling.

2. A 54-year-old man visits a dermatologist because of a skin infection of the auricle of the right ear. The patient explains that he had scratched the ear accidentally while putting on his glasses 4 days previously. Since that time, his ear has become greatly swollen, and his wife has noted that the right side of his neck is also swollen. A diagnosis of impetigo is made, and the patient is given an antibiotic to take orally. The dermatologist advises the patient to place a warm compress over the ear twice daily to

reduce the auricular swelling. Using your knowledge of anatomy and physiology, explain the following: (a) Why is the ear swollen? (b) Why is the right side of the neck swollen? (c) Why will the application of a warm compress to the ear reduce the swelling?

3. Define the following terms used to describe the lymphatic system: (a) lymph, (b) reticulocyte, (c) subcapsular sinus of a lymph node, (d) Hassall's corpuscle, (e) red pulp of spleen, (f) T lymphocyte.

4. A 58-year-old woman following a right radical mastectomy (which involves removal of the right breast and the right axillary lymph nodes) has lymphatic edema of the right arm because of obstruction of the normal lymph flow. Describe the main factors responsible for lymph flow.

5. Describe the structure of (a) a lymphatic capillary, (b) a medium-sized lymphatic vessel, and (c) a large lymphatic duct, and indicate where possible the functional significance of the structures mentioned.

6. The lymphatic system is the center for the immunological defenses of the body. Explain cellular and humoral immunity. Do you think that the lymphatic vessels and lymph nodes help us in limiting the spread of carcinoma?

7. Typhoid fever is an acute infection of the body resulting from the ingestion of food contaminated with typhoid bacilli. There is a generalized enlargement of the lymphatic tissues of the body, including the spleen and lymph nodes and the lymphatic tissue of the intestinal tract. Where is lymphatic tissue found in the intestinal tract? What is the special name given to the aggregations of lymphatic tissue found in the distal part of the ileum?

8. Define the following: (a) lacteal, (b) chylomicron, (c) lymphokine, (d) lymphatic germinal center, (e) lymphangitis.

9. Compare and contrast the functions of a lymph node and the spleen. Discuss the open and closed theories of blood circulation through the spleen.

10. Explain the mechanism of allograft rejection. What form of immunity is lacking in a patient who has a congenital absence of the thymus?

ADDITIONAL READING

Aurameas, S., and Leduc, E. H. Detection of simultaneous antibody synthesis in plasma cells and specialized lymphocytes in rabbit lymph nodes. *J. Exp. Med.* 131:1137, 1970.

Bellanti, J. A. *Immunology II*. Philadelphia: Saunders, 1979.

Boyse, E. A., and Cantor, H. Surface characteristics of T-lymphocyte subpopulations. *Hosp. Pract.* 12:81, 1977.

Burke, J. S., and Simon, G. T. Electron microscopy of the spleen. I. Anatomy and microcirculation. *Am. J. Pathol.* 58:127, 1970.

Cato, L. V. Some endocrine aspects of the thymus gland. *Jpn. J. Med. Sci. Biol.* 28:289, 1976.

Chen, L. T. Microcirculation of the spleen: An open or closed circulation? *Science* 201:157, 1978.

Chen, L. T., and Weiss, L. Electron microscope study of the red pulp of human spleen. *Am. J. Anat.* 134:425, 1972.

Clodius, L. (ed.). *Lymphedema*. Stuttgart: Thieme, 1977.

Enriquez, P., and Neiman, R. S. *The Pathology of the Spleen: A Functional Approach*. Chicago: American Society of Clinical Pathologists, 1976, p. II.

Fujita, T. A scanning electron microscope study of the human spleen. *Arch. Histol. Jpn.* 37:187, 1974.

Gowans, J. L., and Knight, E. J. The route of recirculation of lymphocytes in the rat. *Proc. R. Soc. Lond.* [*Biol.*] 159:257, 1964.

Guyton, A. C., et al. *Dynamics and Control of the Body Fluids*. Philadelphia: Saunders, 1975.

Hirasawa, Y., and Tokuhiro, H. Electron microscopic studies of the normal human spleen, especially on the red pulp and the reticuloendothelial cells. *Blood* 35:201, 1970.

Katz, D. H. *Lymphocyte Differentiation, Recognition and Regulation*. New York: Academic, 1977.

Leak, L. V., and Burke, J. F. Ultrastructural studies on

the lymphatic anchoring of filaments. *J. Cell Biol.* 36:129, 1968.

Luk, S. C., Nopajaroonsri, C., and Simon, G. T. The architecture of the normal lymph node and hemolymph node: A scanning and transmission electron microscope study. *Lab. Invest.* 29:258, 1973.

Nelson, D. S. (ed.). *Immunobiology of the Macrophage.* New York: Academic, 1976.

Nicoll, P. A., and Taylor, A. E. Lymph formation and flow. *Annu. Rev. Physiol.* 39:73, 1977.

Paul, W. E., and Benacerraf, B. Functional specificity of thymus-dependent lymphocytes. *Science* 195:1293, 1977.

Raff, M. C. T and B lymphocytes and immune responses. *Nature* 242:19, 1973.

Raviola, E., and Karnovsky, M. J. Evidence for a blood-thymus barrier using electron opaque tracers. *J. Exp. Med.* 136:466, 1972.

Salmon, S. E., and Seligmann, M. B-cell neoplasia in man. *Lancet* 2:1230, 1974.

Sprent, J. Circulating T and B lymphocytes of the mouse. I. Migrating properties. *Cell Immunol.* 7:10, 1973.

Weiss, L. *The Cells and Tissues of the Immune System.* Englewood Cliffs, N.J.: Prentice-Hall, 1972.

Weiss, L. A scanning electron microscopic study of the spleen. *Blood* 43:665, 1974.

Yoffey, J. M., and Courtice, F. C. (eds.). *Lymphatics, Lymph and Lymphomyeloid Complex.* New York: Academic, 1970.

RESPIRATORY SYSTEM

10

The exchange of oxygen and carbon dioxide between the body and its environment is called respiration. Respiration can be divided into two phases. Phase I is the exchange of gases between the inspired air and the blood and is called *external respiration*. Phase II occurs at the cellular level and is the exchange of gases between the blood and the tissues; it is called *internal respiration*.

The organs of the respiratory system can be divided into those that conduct air from outside the body to the interior of the lungs and form the *conducting portion* of the system, and those that are sites of gaseous exchange and are known as the *respiratory portion*. The conducting portion consists of the nose, pharynx, larynx, trachea, and bronchi. The respiratory portion consists of the small respiratory bronchioles, the alveolar ducts, the alveolar sacs, and the alveoli.

CONDUCTING PORTION

Nose

The nose consists of the external nose and the nasal cavity.

The external nose has a free tip and is attached to the forehead by the *root*, or *bridge*, of the nose. The external orifices of the nose are the two *nostrils*, or *nares* (Fig. 10-1). Each nostril is bounded laterally by the *ala* and medially by the *nasal septum*. The framework of the external nose is composed of bones above and plates of hyaline cartilage below. The skin over the dorsum and sides of the nose is thin and contains many sebaceous glands.

The *nasal cavity* extends from the nostrils, or nares, in front to the choanae behind. It is divided into right and left halves by the *nasal septum*. The posterior part of the septum is made up of bone, and the anterior part is made up of plates of hyaline cartilage.

The lateral wall of the nasal cavity is marked by three projections called the *superior, middle,* and *inferior nasal conchae*. The area below each concha is referred to as a *meatus* (Fig. 10-2; see Fig. 10-1).

The wider portion of the nasal cavity just behind the anterior nares is called the *vestibule*. The skin covering the outer surface of the nose enters the nose through the anterior nares and lines the anterior part of the vestibule. Here the skin has many hair follicles and sebaceous and sweat glands (Fig.

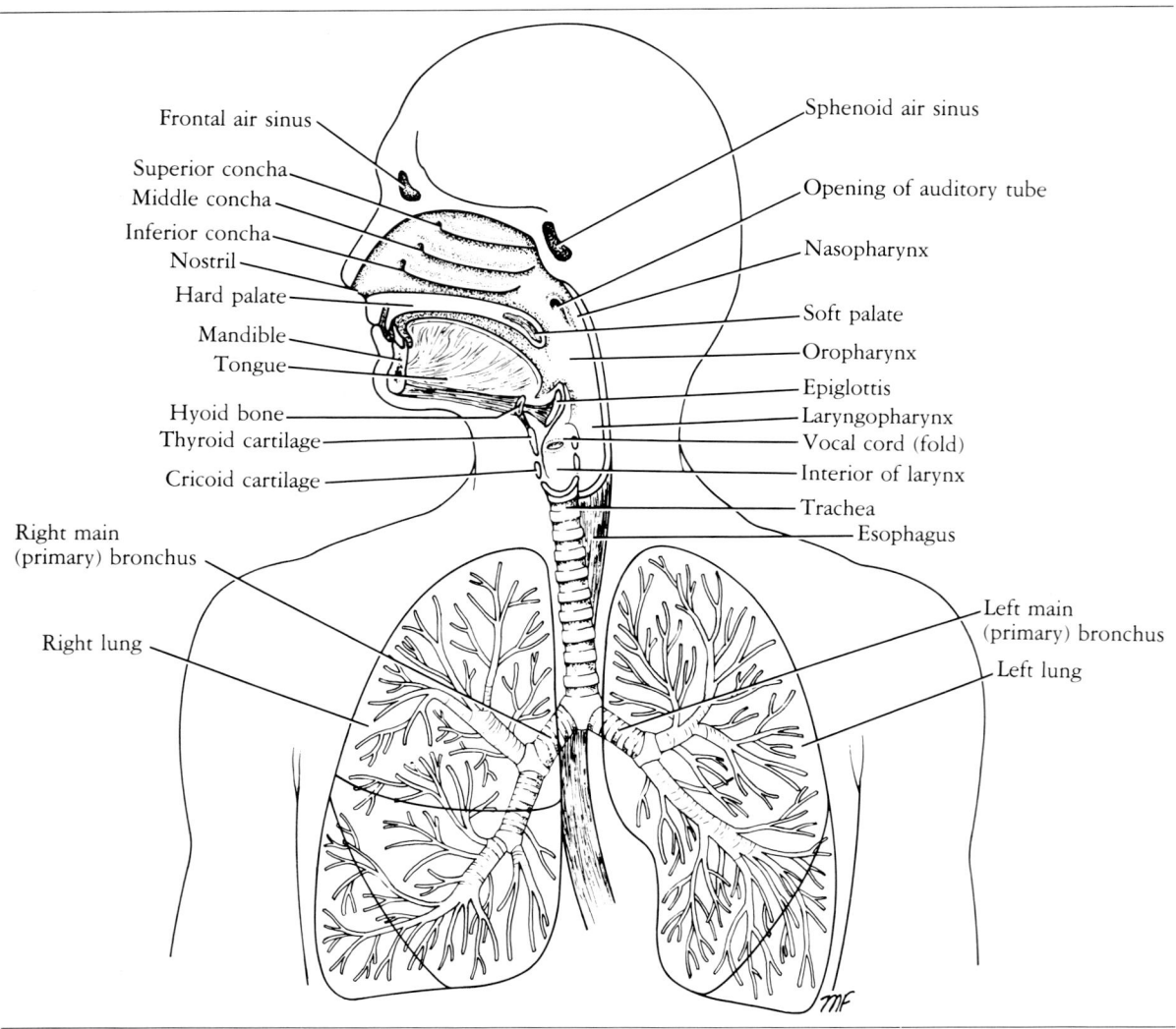

Fig. 10-1. General arrangement of the different parts of the respiratory system. Those organs that conduct air to the interior of the lungs form the conducting portion, and those that are sites of gaseous exchange form the respiratory portion.

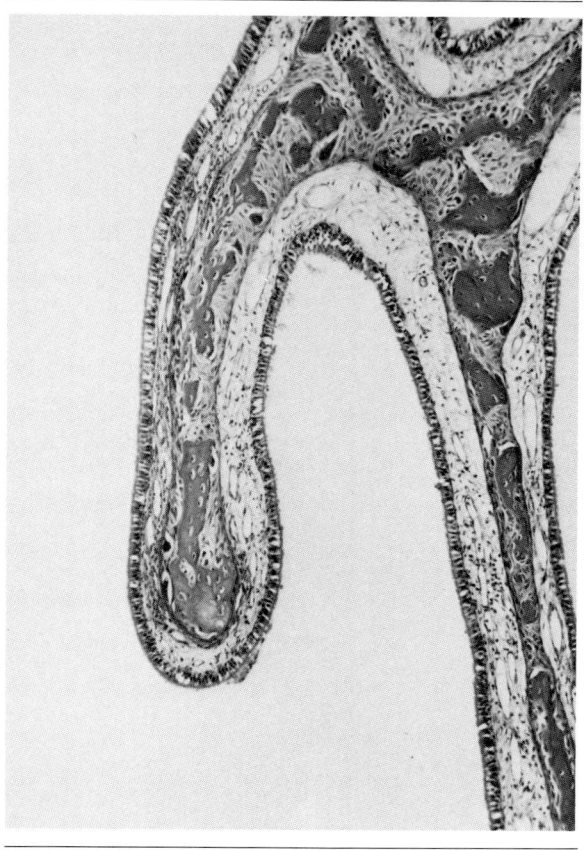

Fig. 10-2. Photomicrograph of section through the inferior concha of the nose. The bony projection is covered by mucous membrane that is connected to the periosteum by the lamina propria. (H&E; ×100.)

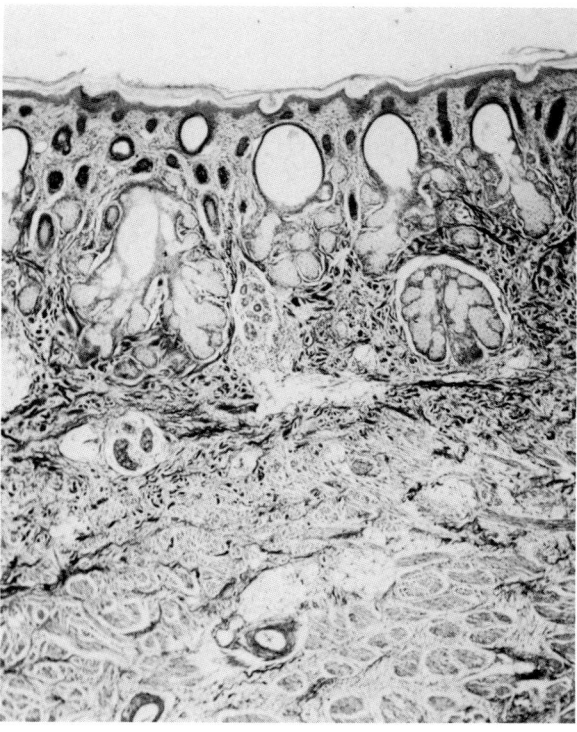

Fig. 10-3. Photomicrograph of section of the vestibule of the nose, showing many large sebaceous and sweat glands. (H&E; ×40.)

10-3). The hairs serve as a filter and strain large particles from the inspired air. The posterior part of the vestibule is lined with nonkeratinized stratified squamous epithelium, continuous posteriorly with pseudostratified ciliated columnar epithelium and goblet cells.

The remaining portion of the nasal cavities is lined with mucous membrane. The mucous membrane is of two types, olfactory and respiratory.

The *olfactory mucous membrane* lines the upper surface of the superior concha and the area of the lateral wall above it (spheno-ethmoidal recess). It also lines a corresponding area on the nasal septum and lines the roof. Its function is the reception of olfactory stimuli, and for this purpose it possesses specialized olfactory nerve cells. The central axons of these cells (the olfactory nerve fibers) pass through the openings in the cribriform plate of the ethmoid and end in the olfactory bulbs. There are also supporting and basal cells in the mucous membrane (for details, see p. 769). The surface of the mucous membrane is kept moist by the secretions of numerous serous glands (Fig. 10-4).

The *respiratory mucous membrane* lines the lower part of the nasal cavities (Fig. 10-5). Its function is to warm, moisten, and clean the inspired air. The mucous membrane consists of a layer of pseudostratified ciliated columnar epithelium with goblet cells,

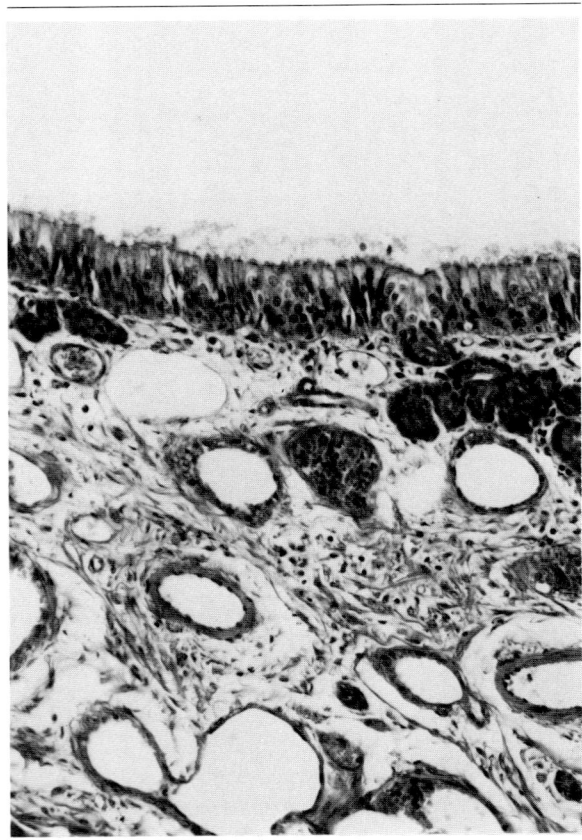

Fig. 10-4. Photomicrograph of section of the olfactory mucous membrane covering the upper surface of the superior concha. The thick epithelium consists of specialized olfactory cells and supportive and basal cells; glands and venous plexuses are present in the lamina propria. (H&E; ×200.)

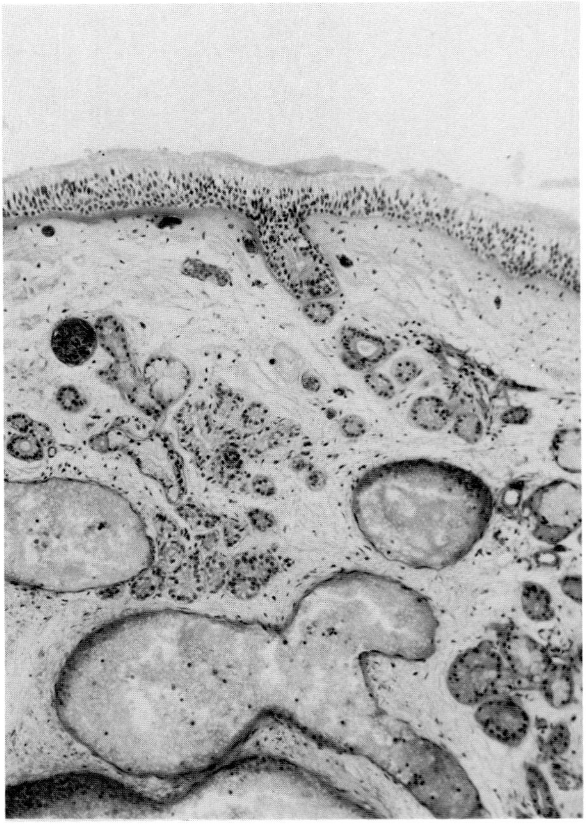

Fig. 10-5. Photomicrograph of section of the respiratory mucous membrane, showing the mucous membrane and numerous glands and venous plexuses in the lamina propria. (H&E; ×100.)

resting on a basal lamina (Fig. 10-6). Beneath the basal lamina is the lamina propria, consisting of fibroconnective tissue containing numerous mucous and serous glands. The lamina propria is attached to the periosteum or perichondrium forming the walls of the nasal cavity.

The inspired air is warmed by a plexus of veins in the lamina propria of the mucous membrane (see Fig. 10-5). Moisture is added to the inspired air by evaporation of the secretions poured onto the surface of the mucous membrane by the glands and goblet cells. Inspired dust particles are removed from the air by the moist, sticky surface of the mucous membrane. The contaminated mucus is moved backward continuously by the ciliary action of the columnar ciliated epithelium that covers the surface. On reaching the pharynx, the mucus is swallowed.

Paranasal Sinuses

The paranasal sinuses are air-filled cavities found in the bones around the nasal cavities. They are present in the maxilla, frontal, sphenoid, and ethmoid

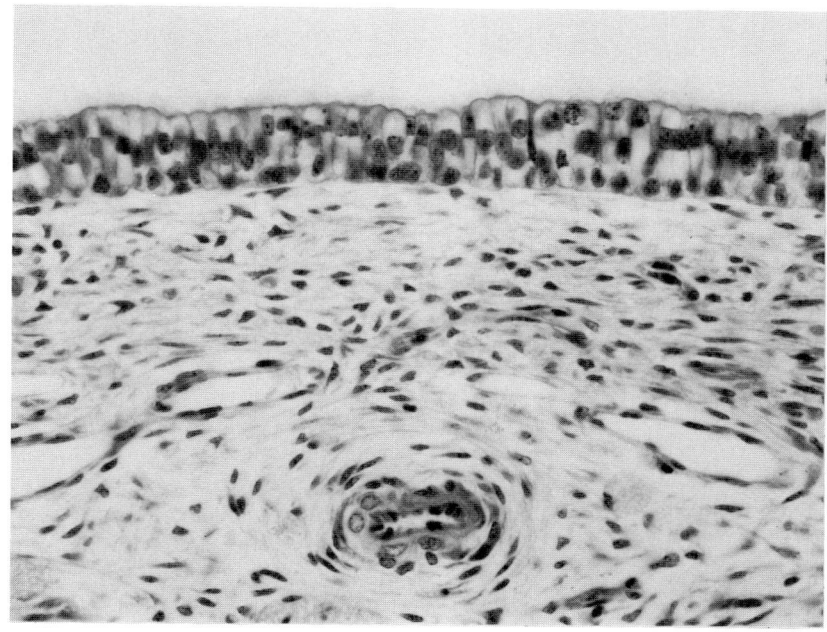

Fig. 10-6. Photomicrograph of section of the respiratory mucous membrane, showing the lining of pseudostratified ciliated columnar epithelium with goblet cells. The lamina propria contains a duct of a mucous gland and several small veins. (H&E; ×400.)

bones (see Fig. 10-1). The maxillary and frontal sinuses open into the middle meatus of the nose; the sphenoid sinus opens into the spheno-ethmoidal recess above the superior concha. There are three ethmoidal sinuses; the anterior and middle ethmoidal sinuses open into the middle meatus, and the posterior ethmoidal sinus opens into the superior meatus.

The paranasal sinuses are lined with mucous membrane that is continuous with that lining the nasal cavity. The mucous membrane is attached to the underlying periosteum by a thin layer of connective tissue; the membrane is covered with pseudostratified ciliated columnar epithelium and contains goblet cells. The mucous formed in the sinuses is moved to the nasal cavities by the action of the cilia. Drainage of the mucus is also achieved by the siphon action created during blowing of the nose.

The function of the sinuses is to act as resonators to the voice. When the apertures of the sinuses are blocked or the sinuses become filled with fluid, the quality of the voice is changed markedly.

Pharynx

The nasal cavities open posteriorly into the pharynx, or throat, which serves as a common passage for air and food (see Fig. 10-1). The pharynx is a musculomembranous tube extending from the base of the skull to the level of the sixth cervical vertebra, where it becomes continuous with the esophagus. The part of the pharynx behind the nose is called the *nasopharynx,* the part behind the mouth the *oropharynx,* and the part behind the larynx the *laryngopharynx.* During swallowing, the food has the right of way and the passage of air temporarily is arrested.

The wall of the pharynx is composed of four layers: (1) mucous membrane, (2) submucosa, (3) muscular coat, and (4) connective tissue coat. The mucous membrane of the nasopharynx is lined with

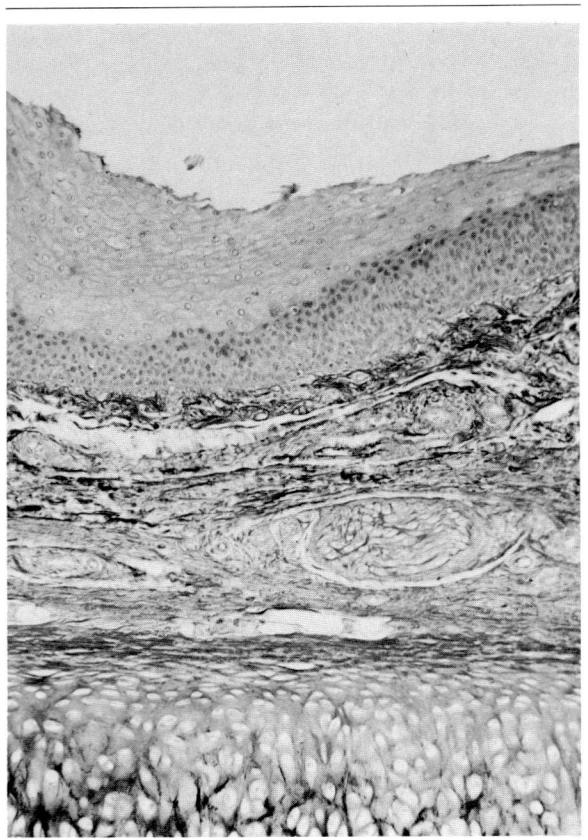

Fig. 10-7. Photomicrograph of section of the epiglottis. The mucous membrane covering the anterior surface (top) is lined with stratified squamous nonkeratinized epithelium. Note the elastic cartilage in the lower part of the photograph. (H&E; ×100.)

pseudostratified ciliated columnar epithelium. Where the surface is subject to trauma from food, as in the oral pharynx and laryngopharynx, the mucous membrane is lined with stratified squamous epithelium. The submucosa is made up of loose connective tissue that binds the mucous membrane to the muscle layer. The muscular coat is formed of striated voluntary muscle and comprises the superior, middle, and inferior constrictor muscles and the stylopharyngeus and salpingopharyngeus muscles. The connective tissue coat covers the outside of the pharyngeal wall and is sometimes called the *buccopharyngeal membrane.* It blends with the connective tissue of neighboring structures.

Lymphatic tissue is present in large amounts in the mucous membrane of the pharynx in the form of the tonsils (for details, see p. 354).

Larynx

The larynx is a specialized organ that provides a protective sphincter at the inlet of the air passages and is responsible for voice production. Above, it opens into the laryngeal part of the pharynx; below, it is continuous with the trachea.

The framework of the larynx is made up of cartilages, including the *thyroid cartilage,* the *cricoid cartilage,* the *arytenoid cartilages,* and the *epiglottis* (see Fig. 10-1). The thyroid, cricoid, and arytenoid cartilages are composed of hyaline cartilage; the epiglottis is composed of elastic cartilage (Fig. 10-7). The cartilages are connected by membranes and ligaments and moved by skeletal muscles.

The larynx is lined with mucous membrane. Under the mucous membrane on each side of the larynx are the *vocal ligaments,* which connect the arytenoid cartilages to the thyroid cartilage. The ligaments are composed of bundles of elastic fibers, with a few collagen fibers, and produce ridges, or folds, of mucous membrane called *vocal folds,* or *vocal cords* (Fig. 10-8; see Fig. 10-1). The gap between the vocal folds is called the *rima glottidis.* The vocal folds can be moved by skeletal muscles acting on the arytenoid cartilages. These muscles are often referred to as the intrinsic muscles of the larynx to distinguish them from the extrinsic laryngeal muscles, which move the larynx as a whole.

Voice sounds are produced by causing a strong stream of air to pass up through the rima glottidis from the trachea and bronchi.

An additional pair of folds of mucous membrane, sometimes called the false vocal cords, are present above the vocal folds. These are known as *vestibular folds* (see Fig. 10-8). They are fixed and have no known function.

The mucous membrane lining the larynx is cov-

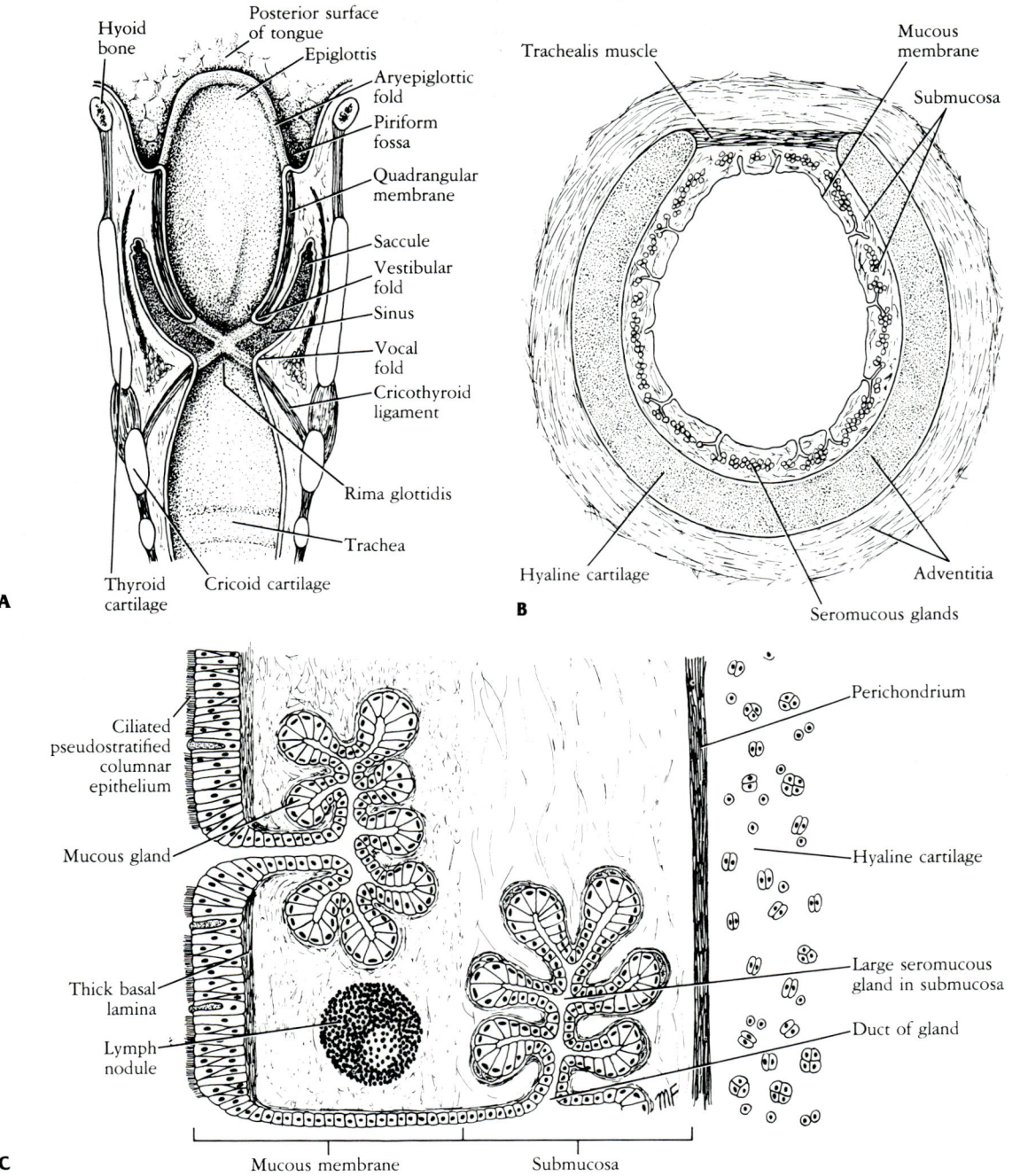

Fig. 10-8. General structure of (A) the larynx as seen in coronal section and (B) the trachea as seen in cross section. (C) shows the detailed structure of the mucous membrane and submucosa of the trachea.

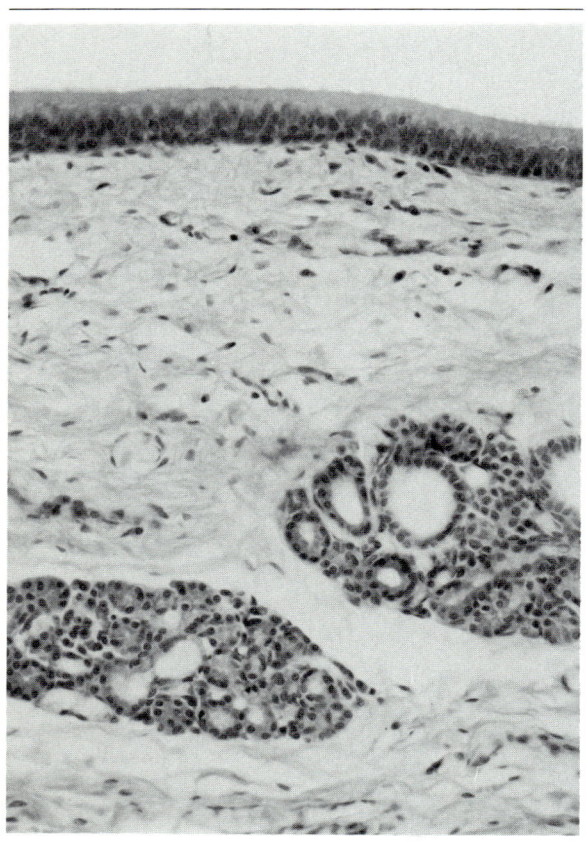

Fig. 10-9. Photomicrograph of mucous membrane and submucosa lining the larynx. The surface is covered with pseudostratified ciliated columnar cells. Note the presence of glands in the submucosa. (H&E; ×200.)

ered with pseudostratified ciliated columnar epithelium with goblet cells (Fig. 10-9). The cilia beat upward toward the pharynx, moving the mucus and adherent particles to the laryngeal part of the pharynx, where they are swallowed. The lamina propria contains many serous and mucous glands that pour their secretions onto the free surface. Lymph nodules are scattered throughout the lamina propria of the mucous membrane.

Over the vocal folds, where there is a considerable amount of wear and tear because of vibration, the surfaces are covered with stratified squamous nonkeratinized epithelium (Fig. 10-10). The mucous membrane covering the anterior surfaces of the epiglottis is also subject to wear and tear from the passage of food and friction against the tongue; this area is also covered with stratified squamous nonkeratinized epithelium.

Above the vocal folds, the lumen of the larynx expands to form the *sinus of the larynx* (see Fig. 10-8). Extending superiorly from the sinus on each side is the *laryngeal saccule,* a blind-ended tube lined with mucous membrane containing many goblet cells. The mucus from these cells runs inferiorly and lubricates the vibrating vocal folds.

Sphincteric Function

There are two sphincters in the larynx, at the inlet and at the rima glottidis.

The sphincter at the inlet is used only during swallowing. As the bolus of food passes backward between the tongue and the hard palate, the larynx is pulled up beneath the back of the tongue. The epiglottis is pushed backward by the tongue and serves as a cap over the laryngeal inlet. The bolus of food (or fluid) now enters the esophagus by passing over the epiglottis or moving down the grooves on either side of the laryngeal inlet, called the *piriform fossae* (see Fig. 10-8).

In coughing or sneezing, the rima glottidis serves as a sphincter. After inspiration, the vocal folds are adducted and the muscles of expiration are made to contract strongly. As a result, the intrathoracic pressure rises, whereupon the vocal folds suddenly are abducted. The sudden release of the compressed air often will dislodge foreign particles or mucus from the respiratory tract and carry the material up into the pharynx. Here, the material is either swallowed or expectorated.

In abdominal straining associated with micturition, defecation, or parturition, the air often is held temporarily in the respiratory tract by closure of the rima glottidis after deep inspiration. The muscles of the anterior abdominal wall then contract, and the upward movement of the diaphragm is prevented by the presence of compressed air within the respira-

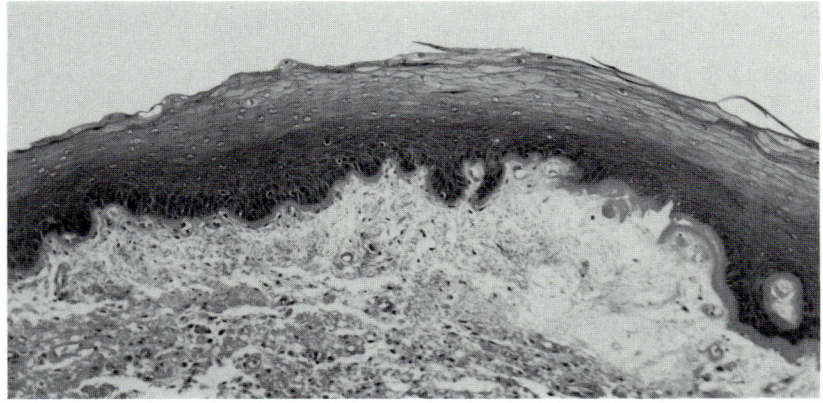

Fig. 10-10. Photomicrograph of section of the vocal folds (cords), showing the surface covered with stratified squamous nonkeratinized epithelium. (H&E; ×100.)

tory tract. After a prolonged effort, the person often releases some of the air by opening the rima glottidis momentarily, producing a grunting sound.

Voice Production

The intermittent release of expired air between the adducted vocal folds results in their vibration and in the production of sound. The *frequency,* or *pitch,* of the voice is determined by changes in the length of and tension in the vocal ligaments. The *quality* of the voice depends on the resonators above the larynx, namely, the pharynx, mouth, and paranasal sinuses. The quality is controlled by the muscles of the soft palate, tongue, floor of the mouth, cheeks, lips, and jaws. *Normal speech* depends on the modification of the sound into recognizable consonants and vowels by the use of the tongue, teeth, and lips. Vowel sounds are usually purely oral and are produced with the soft palate raised; that is to say, the air is channeled through the mouth rather than the nose.

Speech involves the intermittent release of the expired air between the adducted vocal folds. *Singing* requires a more prolonged release of the expired air between the adducted vocal folds. In *whispering,* the vocal folds are adducted but the arytenoid cartilages are separated; the vibrations are given to a constant stream of expired air that passes through the posterior part of the rima glottidis.

Trachea

The trachea is a mobile, fibroelastic tube situated in the lower part of the neck and the upper part of the thorax. It is continuous with the inferior end of the larynx above; below, at the level of the sternal angle, it divides into two branches, the *right* and *left main (primary) bronchi* (Fig. 10-11). Embedded in the wall of the trachea are a series of U-shaped bars of hyaline cartilage that keep the lumen patent (see Fig. 10-8). Located posteriorly, between the ends of each horseshoe cartilage, are bundles of smooth muscle fibers, the *trachealis muscle* (see Fig. 10-15).

The wall of the trachea has three coats, the mucous membrane, the submucosa, and the adventitia. The *mucous membrane* is lined with pseudostratified ciliated columnar epithelium with numerous goblet cells (Figs. 10-12 and 10-13; see Fig. 10-8). The epithelium rests on a thick basal lamina. The lamina propria is composed of loose connective tissue and contains many scattered lymphoid nodules. Some seromucous glands are also present.

The *submucosa* is composed of loose connective tissue in which are embedded numerous seromu-

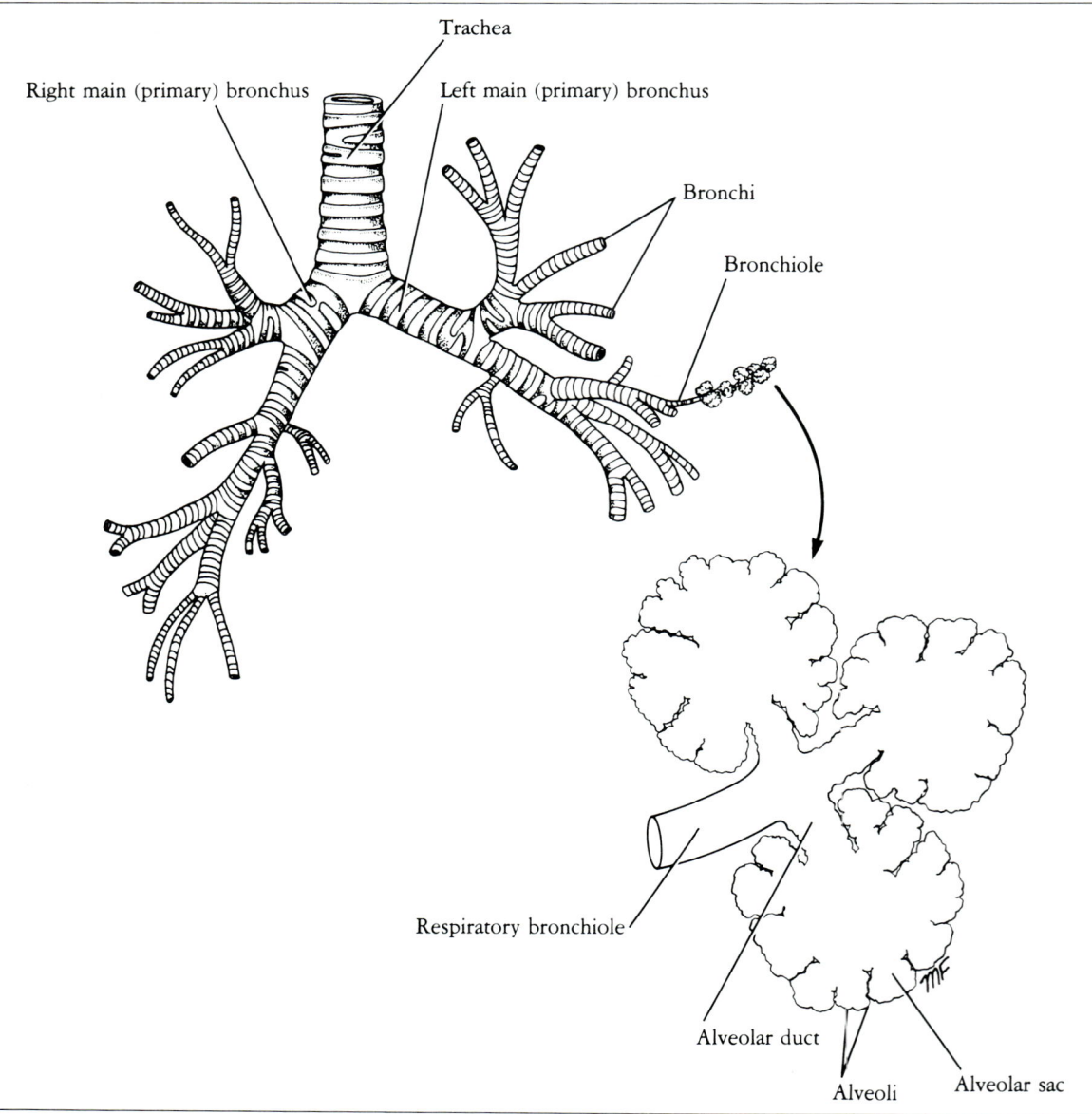

Fig. 10-11. Relationship among the bronchi, the bronchioles, the respiratory bronchioles, the alveolar ducts, the alveolar sacs, and the alveoli. Note the path taken by the inspired air from the trachea to the alveoli.

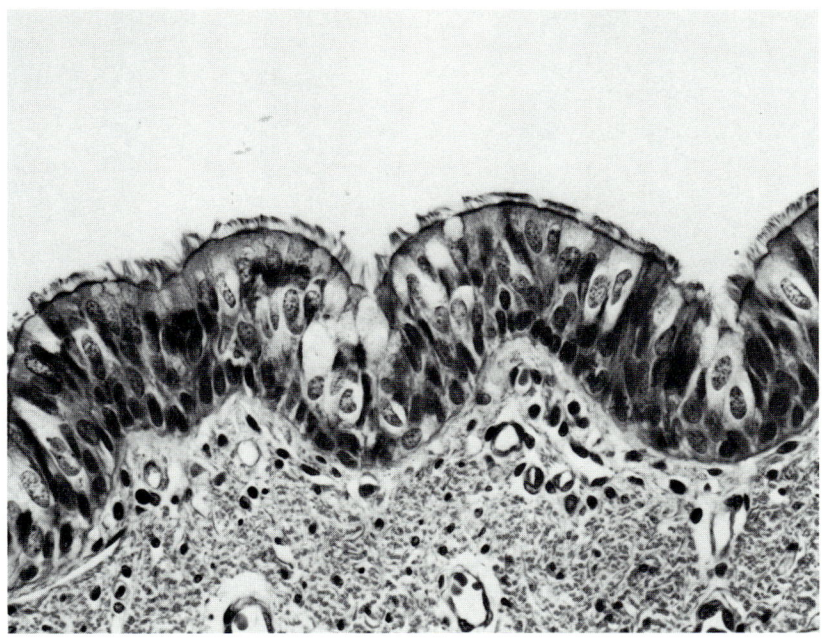

Fig. 10-12. Photomicrograph of a section of the mucous membrane lining the trachea, showing the surface covering of pseudostratified ciliated columnar epithelium with goblet cells. Note that the epithelium rests on a basal lamina. (H&E; ×400.)

cous glands (Figs. 10-14 and 10-15). The glands open by ducts into the lumen of the trachea.

The *adventitia,* the outer layer, contains the horseshoe bars of hyaline cartilage, the trachealis muscle, and fibroelastic tissue (see Fig. 10-8). It also contains blood vessels, lymphatic vessels, and nerves and blends with the surrounding connective tissue.

The trachea conducts air from the larynx to the bronchi of the lungs. The lumen of the trachea can be narrowed by the contraction of the trachealis muscle that occurs in response to parasympathetic stimulation. The sympathetic fibers cause relaxation of the trachealis muscle.

Mediastinum and Pleurae

The thoracic cavity contains a median partition, called the *mediastinum,* and the laterally placed pleurae and lungs (Fig. 10-16). The mediastinum extends superiorly to the thoracic inlet and inferiorly to the diaphragm; it extends anteriorly to the sternum and posteriorly to the vertebral column. The mediastinum contains the heart and major blood vessels, the trachea and esophagus, and the remains of the thymus. The mediastinum is covered on its lateral surface by the *parietal pleura,* which also lines the thoracic wall and covers the upper surface of the diaphragm. At the hilum, or root, of the lung, the pleura is reflected from the mediastinum over the lung as the *visceral pleura* (see Fig. 10-16). The visceral pleura completely covers the outer surfaces of the lungs and extends into the depths of the interlobar fissures (see Fig. 10-16).

The parietal and visceral layers of pleura are separated from each other by a slitlike space, the *pleural cavity* (see Fig. 10-16). This cavity normally contains a small amount of tissue fluid, the *pleural fluid,* which covers the surfaces of the pleura in a thin film and permits the two layers to move against each other with minimal friction.

The parietal and visceral layers of pleura each

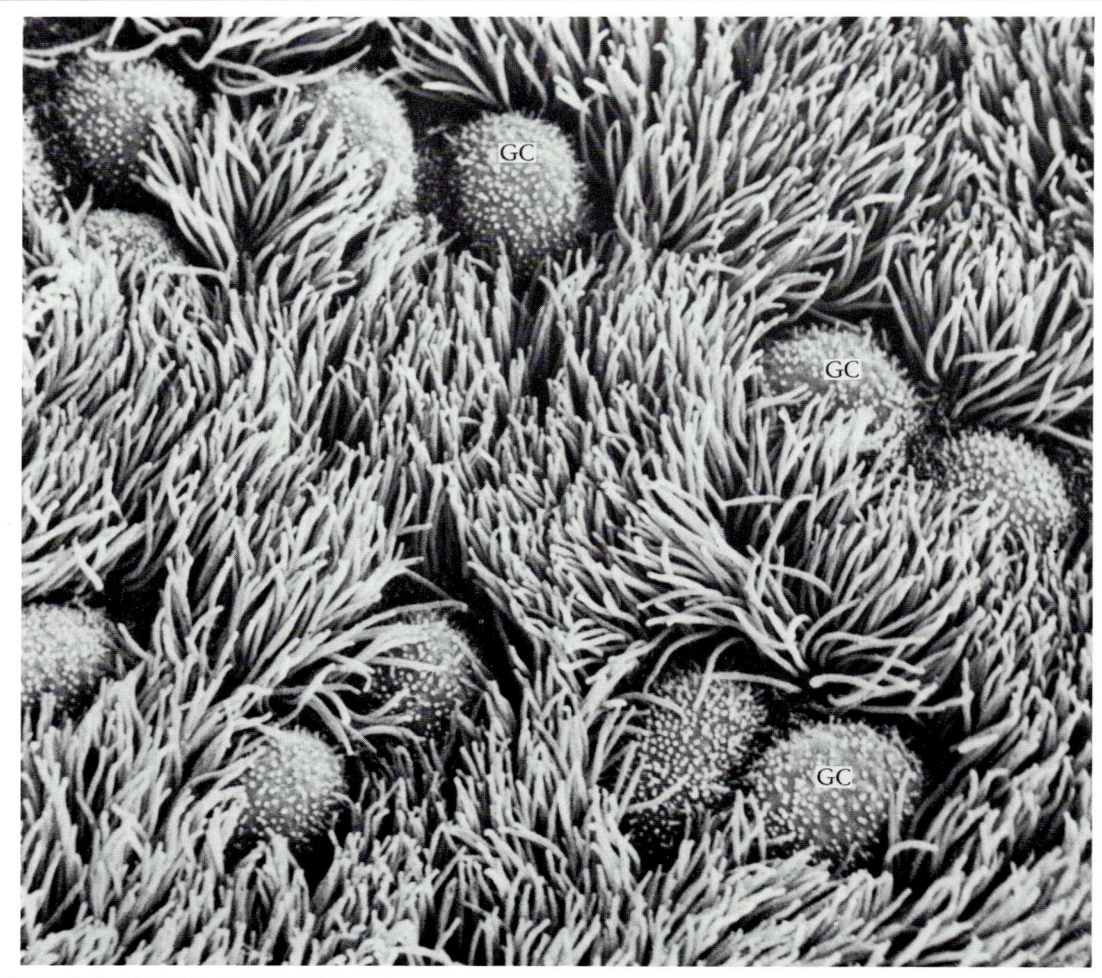

Fig. 10-13. Scanning electron micrograph of surface epithelial cells of the mucous membrane of the trachea, showing ciliated columnar cells and goblet cells (GC). ($\times 3,300$.) (Courtesy of Dr. P. M. Andrews.)

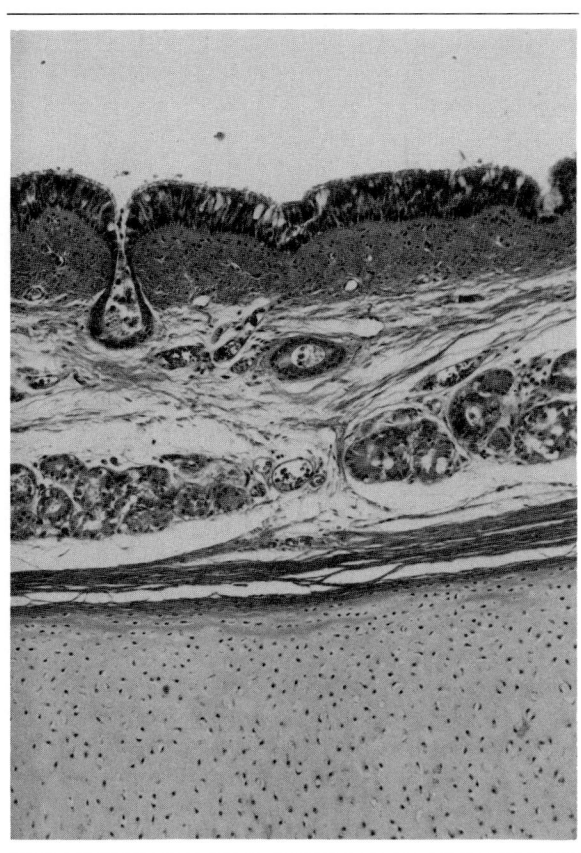

Fig. 10-14. Photomicrograph of a cross section of a portion of the trachea, showing mucous membrane, submucosa with serous and mucous glands, and part of a hyaline cartilaginous bar. (H&E; ×100.)

Fig. 10-15. Photomicrograph of a cross section of the posterior part of the trachea, showing a small part of a hyaline cartilaginous bar. Note the bundles of smooth muscle fibers forming the trachealis muscle (arrows). Note also the serous and mucous glands embedded in the muscle. (H&E; ×100.)

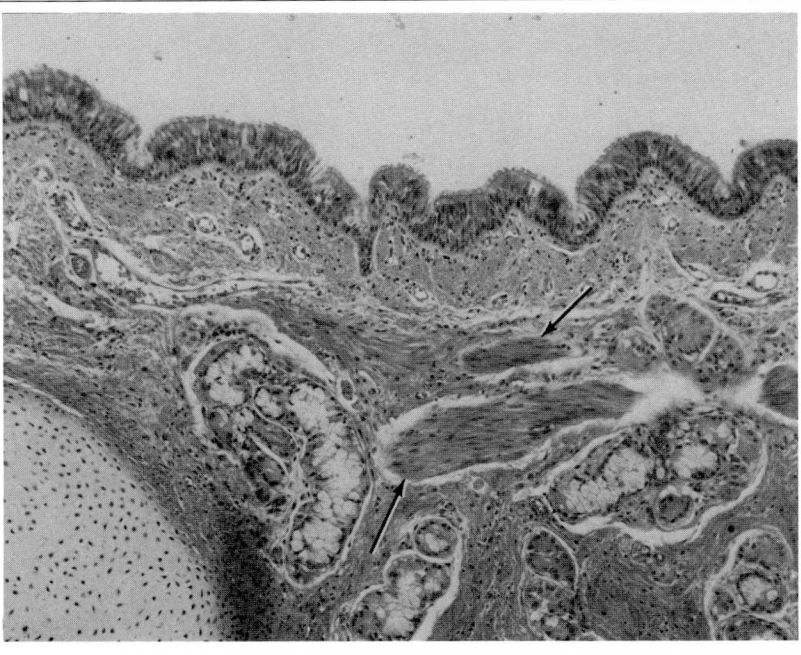

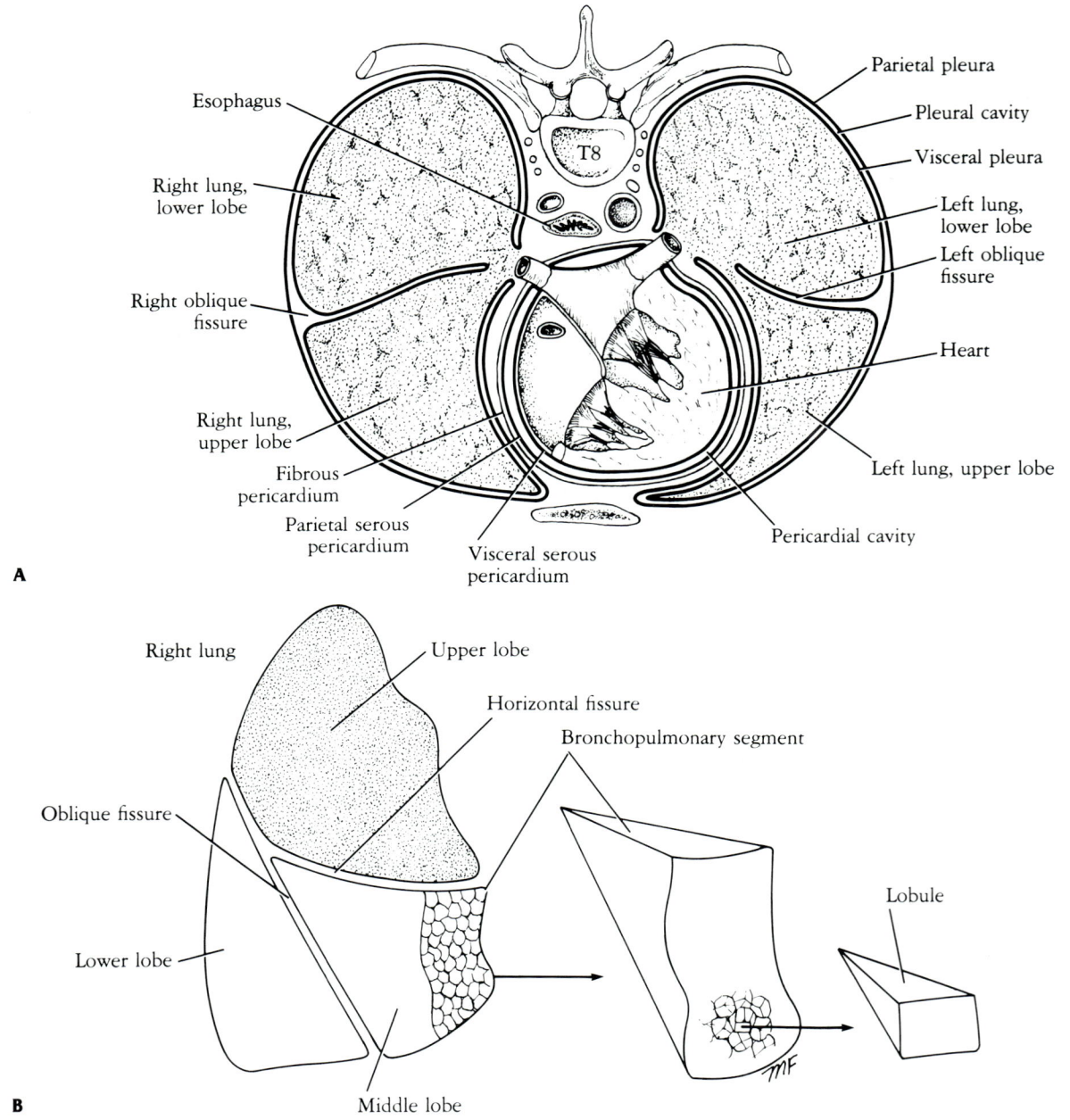

Fig. 10-16. A: Cross section of the thorax. Note the detailed arrangement of the pleura and pleural cavity and the fibrous and serous pericardia. B: Subdivisions of the right lung, passing from the three lobes to a bronchopulmonary segment to a lobule.

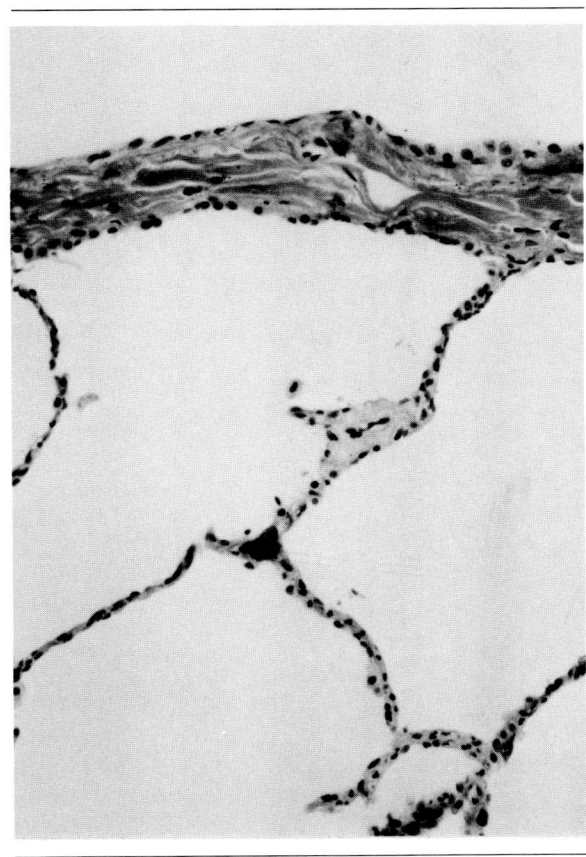

Fig. 10-17. Photomicrograph of a section through the surface of the lung, showing the visceral layer of pleura to consist of flattened mesothelial cells resting on connective tissue. Portions of numerous alveolar walls are also visible. (H&E; ×200.)

consist of a layer of flattened mesothelial cells resting on a thin layer of connective tissue (Fig. 10-17).

Lungs

The lungs are paired organs connected to the mediastinum by a cuff of pleura. The cuff is attached to the lung at the hilum, or root, and it is here that structures enter and leave the lung. The right lung has three lobes, known as the *upper, middle,* and *lower lobes.* The left lung has two lobes, called the *upper* and *lower lobes.*

The right main bronchus is wider, shorter, and more vertical than the left (see Fig. 10-11). It enters the right lung at the hilus, where it divides into secondary bronchi that pass to the upper, middle, and lower lobes. The left main bronchus passes to the left and downward and enters the left lung at the hilus, where it divides into secondary bronchi that pass to the upper and lower lobes. Each secondary bronchus divides to form tertiary bronchi. A tertiary bronchus enters a segment of a lobe of the lung called a *bronchopulmonary segment.* In addition, each bronchopulmonary segment receives an artery, a branch of the pulmonary artery, and a vein, a tributary of the pulmonary vein. Each bronchopulmonary segment is pyramid shaped, with its apex pointing toward the root of the lung and its base facing the lung surface (Fig. 10-16).

On entering a bronchopulmonary segment, each tertiary bronchus divides repeatedly into smaller and smaller bronchi. As the bronchi become smaller, the U-shaped bars of hyaline cartilage found in the trachea are gradually replaced by irregular plates of cartilage, which become smaller and fewer in number. The mucous membrane is thinner, and the pseudostratified ciliated columnar epithelium (Fig. 10-19) is replaced by ciliated columnar cells with many goblet cells. Smooth muscle is present within the submucosa and, in the smaller bronchi, forms a single complete layer of circularly arranged fibers.

The smallest bronchi divide and give rise to *bronchioles,* which are less than 1 mm in diameter. It is the bronchioles that enter the small units of the lungs known as the *lung lobules* (see Fig. 10-18). Bronchioles possess no cartilage in their walls and are lined with ciliated columnar cells. The submucosa possesses a complete layer of circularly arranged smooth muscle fibers. The seromucous glands found in the submucosa of the larger bronchi disappear.

The bronchioles then divide and give rise to *terminal bronchioles.* These are lined with nonciliated columnar or cuboidal cells (Fig. 10-18).

RESPIRATORY PORTION

The terminal bronchioles divide and give rise to *respiratory bronchioles,* which show delicate, air-con-

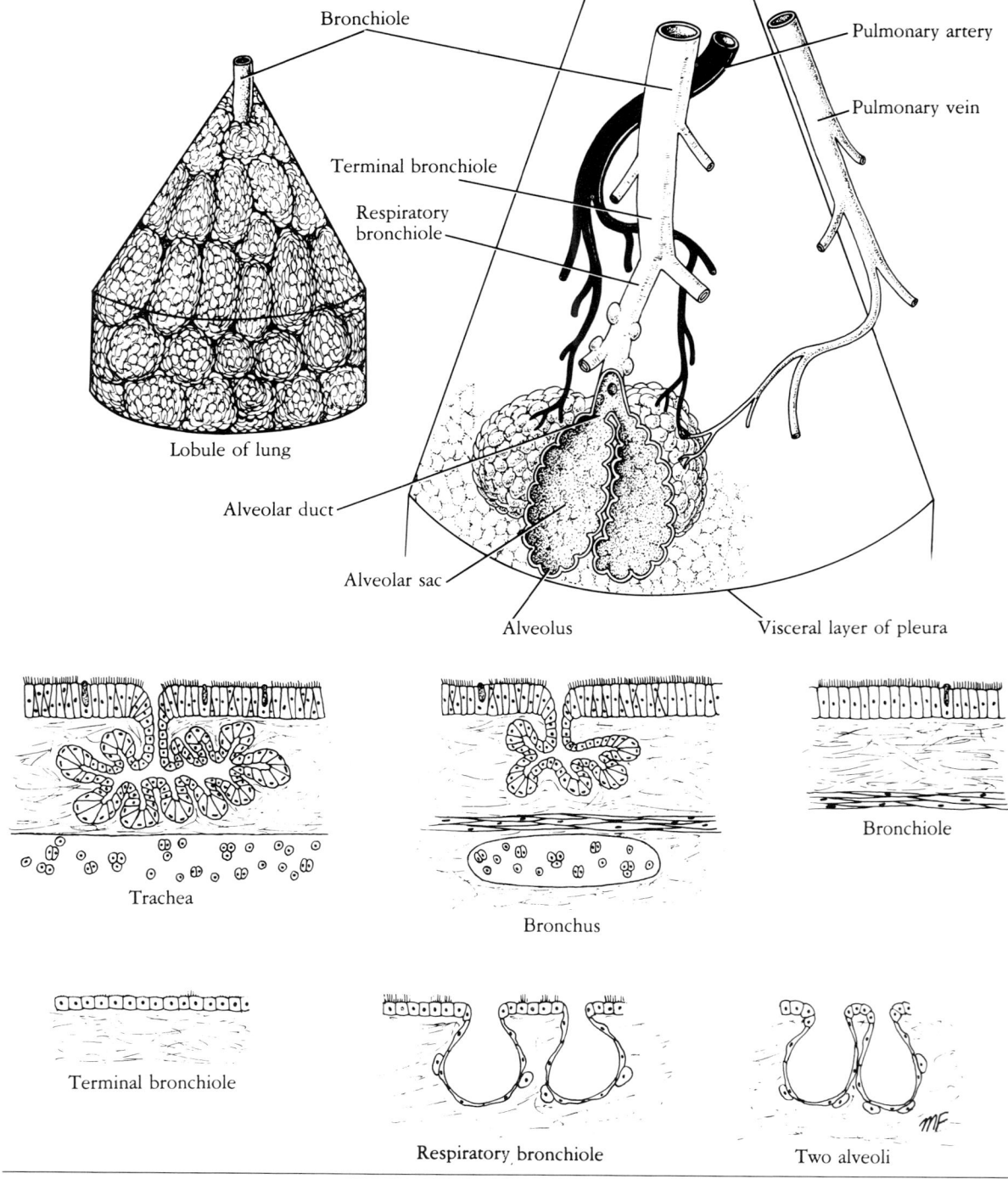

Fig. 10-18. Detailed structure of the lobule of the lung. The main structural changes that take place in the mucous membrane of the respiratory system as one passes from the trachea through the bronchi of diminishing size to the alveoli are summarized at the bottom of the figure.

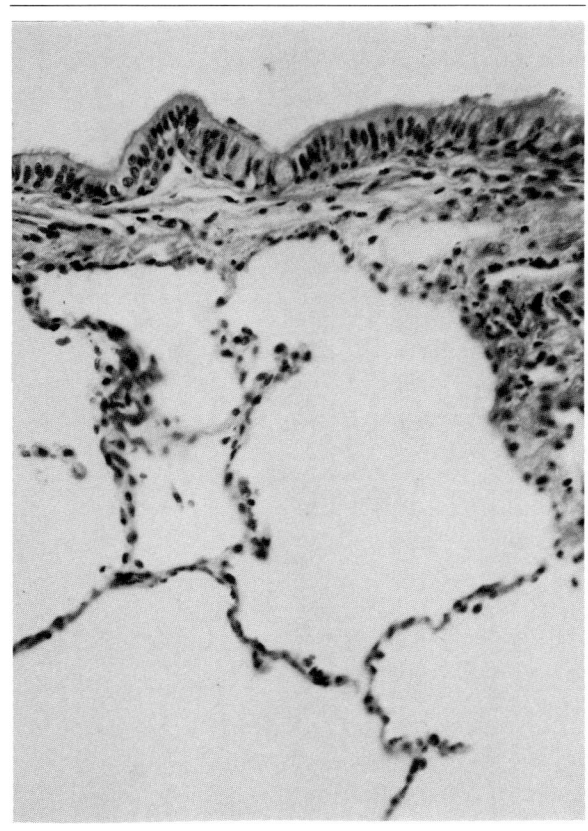

Fig. 10-19. Photomicrograph of a section of part of the wall of a medium-sized bronchus (top) and adjacent alveoli. Note that the mucous membrane is lined with pseudostratified ciliated columnar epithelium. Many smooth muscle fibers are present in the submucosa. (H&E; ×200.)

taining outpouchings from their walls (Fig. 10-20). Gaseous exchange between the blood and the air takes place in the walls of these outpouchings; hence, the name *respiratory bronchiole*. The diameter of a respiratory bronchiole is about 0.5 mm. The wall of a respiratory bronchiole is lined with cuboidal epithelium (see Fig. 10-18). The epithelium rests on connective tissue containing interlacing smooth muscle fibers and elastic fibers.

The respiratory bronchioles end by branching into *alveolar ducts* (see Figs. 10-18 and 10-20), tubular passages with numerous thin-walled outpouchings called *alveolar sacs* (Fig. 10-21). The wall of the alveolar duct is lined with cuboidal epithelium supported by connective tissue containing elastic fibers and a few smooth muscle fibers.

The alveolar sacs consist of several *alveoli* opening into a single chamber (Figs. 10-23 and 10-24; see Figs. 10-18 and 10-22). The walls of the alveoli (interalveolar septa) are composed of very thin flattened cells supported by delicate connective tissue containing elastic fibers (Fig. 10-25; see Fig. 10-22). Each alveolus is surrounded by a rich network of blood capillaries. Examination of the wall of an alveolus with the electron microscope (Figs. 10-26, 10-27, and 10-28) shows that the alveoli are in fact lined with simple squamous cells (type I), but there is an occasional cuboidal cell (type II) responsible for secreting *surfactant* into the lumen. The surfactant reduces the surface tension on the lining cells and permits the alveolar walls to separate from one another as air enters during inspiration. Surfactant is a lipoprotein material and appears in the lungs at about the thirtieth week of intra-uterine life.

Another type of cell seen bulging into the alveolus or residing in the space between adjacent alveoli is the *alveolar phagocyte* (Fig. 10-29; see Fig. 10-26). Such cells are believed to be derived from the monocytes of the blood. They migrate through the capillary wall to enter the tissue spaces and then pass through the epithelial lining of the alveolus to lie free in the lumen of the alveolus. These cells serve as phagocytes and remove debris, such as carbon particles, from the lumen of the alveolus (Fig. 10-30). They migrate up the bronchial tree and are ultimately swallowed with the mucus.

Respiratory Membrane

Electron microscopic study of the alveolar walls (see Figs. 10-26 and 10-27) shows that the lumen of the alveolus is separated from the lumen of the blood capillary by the following: (1) surfactant-containing fluid produced by the type II alveolar cells, (2) the alveolar squamous epithelium or type I cell, (3) the epithelial basement membrane, (4) a minute tissue space, (5) the blood capillary basement membrane, which fuses with the epithelial basement membrane

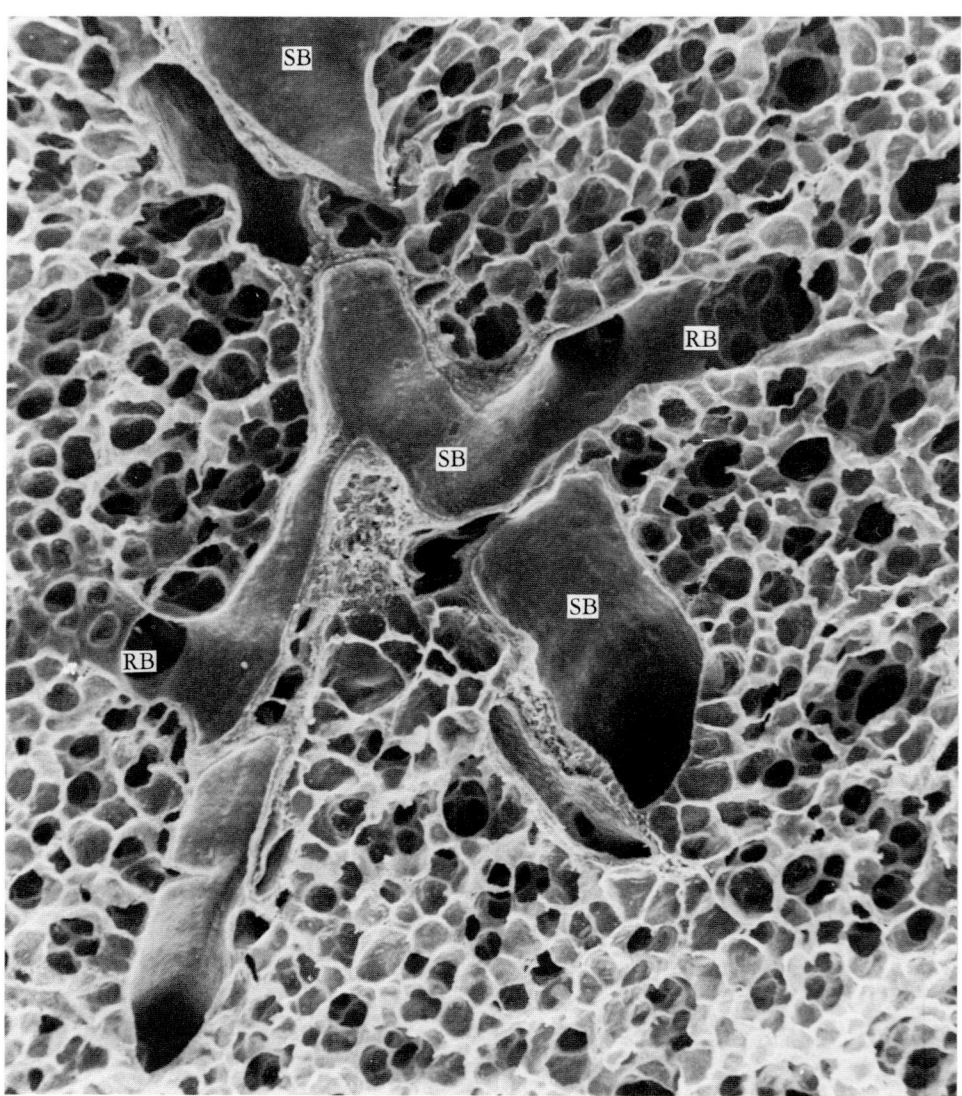

Fig. 10-20. Scanning electron micrograph of the lung, showing a small bronchiole (SB) and a respiratory bronchiole (RB) with many alveoli opening from its walls. Numerous alveolar sacs also can be seen. (×80.) (Courtesy of Dr. P. M. Andrews.)

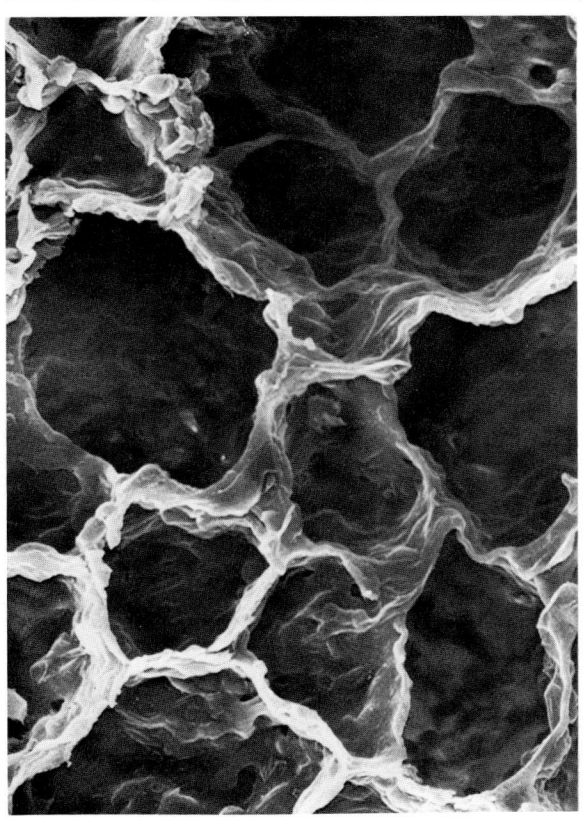

Fig. 10-21. Scanning electron micrograph of the lung, showing numerous alveolar sacs. The alveoli are the depressions, or alcoves, along the walls of the alveolar sac. (×430.) (Courtesy of Dr. M. Koering.)

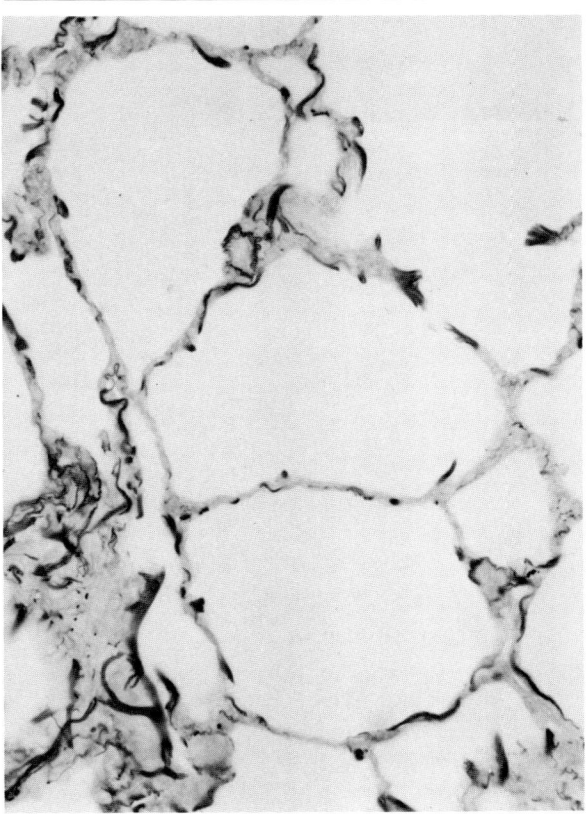

Fig. 10-22. Photomicrograph of a section of the lung stained to show the elastic fibers in the walls of the alveolar sacs and the alveoli. (Resorcin fuchsin stain; ×200.)

in many places, and (6) the capillary squamous endothelium.

The combination of these layers is known as the *respiratory membrane* and averages about 0.5 μm in thickness. It is at the respiratory membrane that gaseous exchange takes place between the air in the alveolar lumen and the blood within the capillary (see Fig. 10-32).

The bronchi, the terminal bronchioles, the respiratory bronchioles, the alveolar ducts, the alveolar sacs, the alveoli, and the blood and lymphatic vessels and nerves are all held together by connective tissue to form the lung. Recall that a pulmonary artery enters the hilus of each lung, carrying oxygen-poor and carbon dioxide–rich blood to the lungs for gaseous exchange. Having passed through the network of capillaries that surrounds the alveoli, the blood leaves the lungs oxygen rich and carbon dioxide poor via the pulmonary veins.

It should be remembered that the lungs receive a double blood supply, from the pulmonary and bronchial arteries. The bronchial arteries are able to supply the lungs adequately and keep the lung tissue alive should the pulmonary artery suddenly be blocked, as in pulmonary embolism.

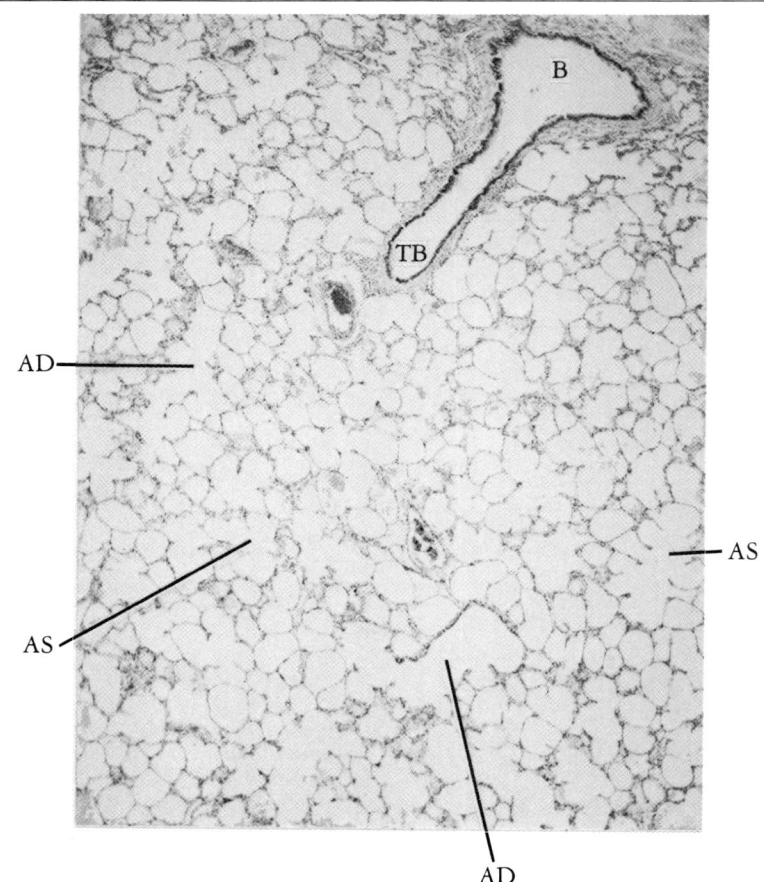

Fig. 10-23. Photomicrograph of a section of the lung, showing a bronchiole (B) giving rise to a terminal bronchiole (TB). Note the alveolar duct (AD), alveolar sacs (AS), and many alveoli. (H&E; ×40.)

MECHANICS OF RESPIRATION

Respiration consists of two phases, *inspiration,* or breathing in, and *expiration,* or breathing out. These processes are accomplished by the alternating increase and decrease in the capacity of the thoracic cavity. The rate of respiration varies from sixteen to twenty per minute in normal resting subjects and is faster in children and slower in the elderly.

Inspiration

Quiet Inspiration

The thoracic cavity can be compared to a box with a single entrance at the top, which is a tube, the trachea (Fig. 10-31). The volume of the box can be increased by elongating all its diameters, thereby reducing the pressure of the air within it; this will result in air under atmospheric pressure (760 mm Hg) entering the box through the tube.

Consider now the three diameters of the thoracic cavity and how they can be increased (see Fig. 10-31).

VERTICAL DIAMETER. Theoretically, the roof could be raised and the floor lowered. The roof is formed by the suprapleural membrane and is fixed. The floor, however, is formed by the mobile diaphragm. When the diaphragm contracts, the domes become

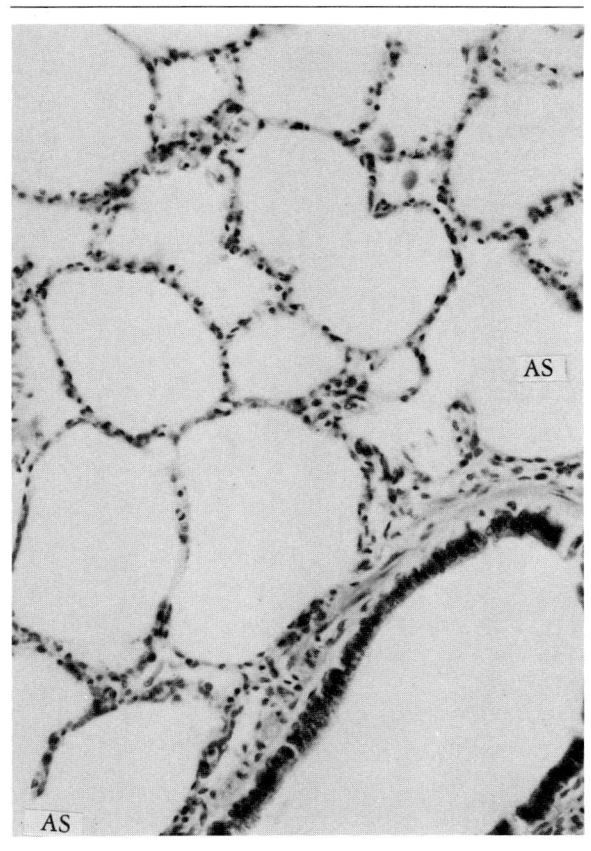

flattened and the level of the diaphragm is lowered (see Fig. 10-31).

ANTEROPOSTERIOR DIAMETER. If the downward-sloping ribs are raised at their sternal ends, the anteroposterior diameter of the thoracic cavity will be increased and the lower end of the sternum will be thrust forward (see Fig. 10-31). These changes can be brought about by fixing the first rib by the contraction of the scaleni muscles of the neck and contracting the intercostal muscles (see Fig. 10-31). By this means, all the ribs are drawn together and raised toward the first rib.

TRANSVERSE DIAMETER. The ribs articulate in front with the sternum via their costal cartilages and behind with the vertebral column. The ribs curve downward as well as forward around the chest wall; they therefore resemble bucket handles (see Fig.

Fig. 10-24. Photomicrograph of a section of the lung, showing a portion of a bronchiole lined with ciliated columnar epithelium. Adjacent to this structure are two alveolar sacs (AS) and numerous alveoli. (H&E; ×200.)

Fig. 10-25. Photomicrograph of a section of parts of the walls of four alveoli. Note that the walls of the alveoli are composed of flattened cells supported by delicate connective tissue. Each alveolus is surrounded by a rich network of blood capillaries (not shown). (H&E; ×400.)

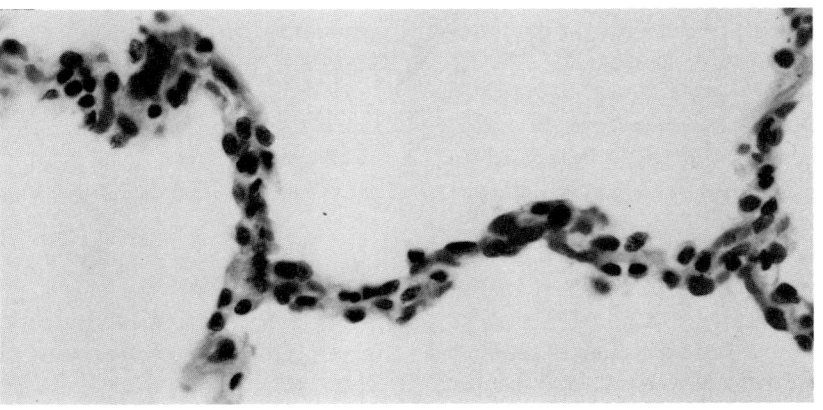

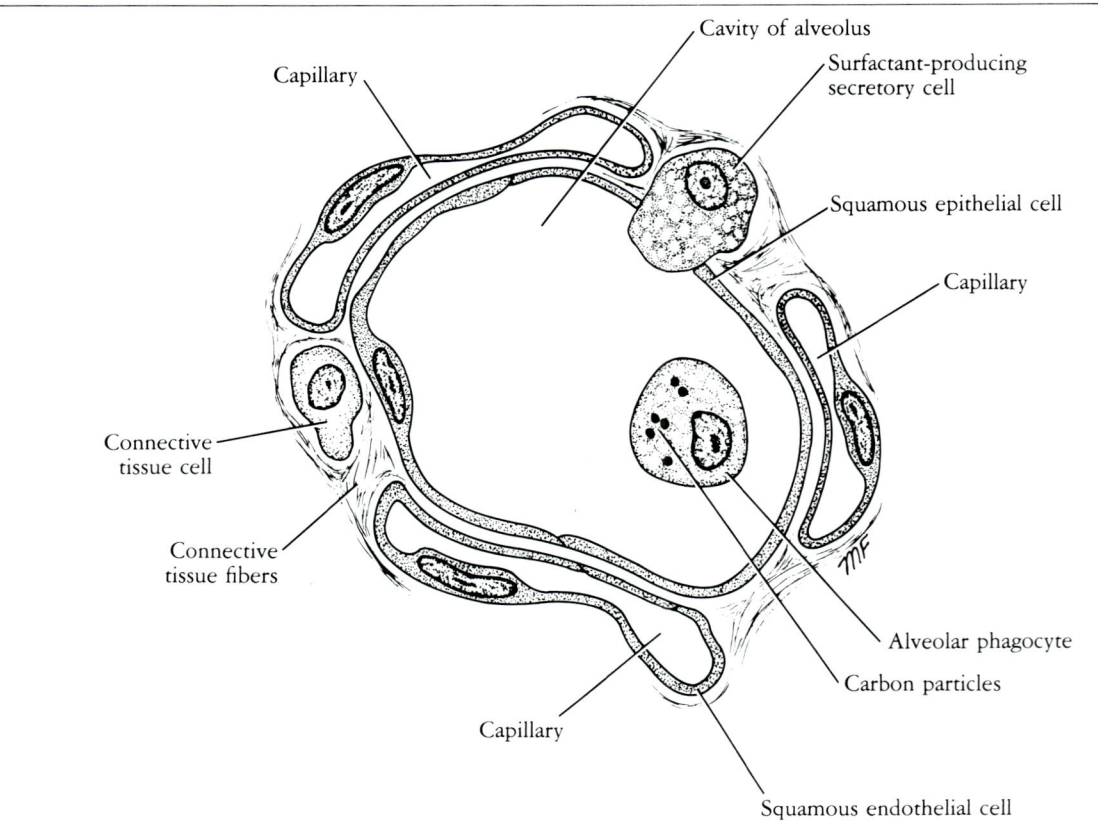

Fig. 10-26. *Detailed structure of the respiratory membrane.*

10-31). It follows that if the ribs are raised (like bucket handles), the transverse diameter of the thoracic cavity will be increased. As described previously, this change can be accomplished by fixing the first rib and raising the other ribs to it by contracting the intercostal muscles (see Fig. 10-31).

An additional factor is the effect of the descent of the diaphragm on the abdominal viscera and the tone of the muscles of the anterior abdominal wall. As the diaphragm descends on inspiration, the intra-abdominal pressure rises. This rise in pressure is accommodated by the reciprocal relaxation of the abdominal wall musculature. A point is reached, however, when no further abdominal relaxation is possible, and the liver and other upper abdominal viscera act as a platform that resists further diaphrag-

matic descent. On further contraction of the diaphragm, its central tendon will be supported from below, and its shortening muscle fibers will assist the intercostal muscles in raising the lower ribs (see Fig. 10-31).

In addition to the diaphragm and the intercostals, other, less important muscles also contract on inspiration and assist in elevating the ribs: the *levatores costarum muscles* and the *serratus posterior superior muscles*.

Forced Inspiration

Deep forced inspiration is accompanied by a maximal increase in the capacity of the thoracic cavity. Every muscle that can raise the ribs is brought into

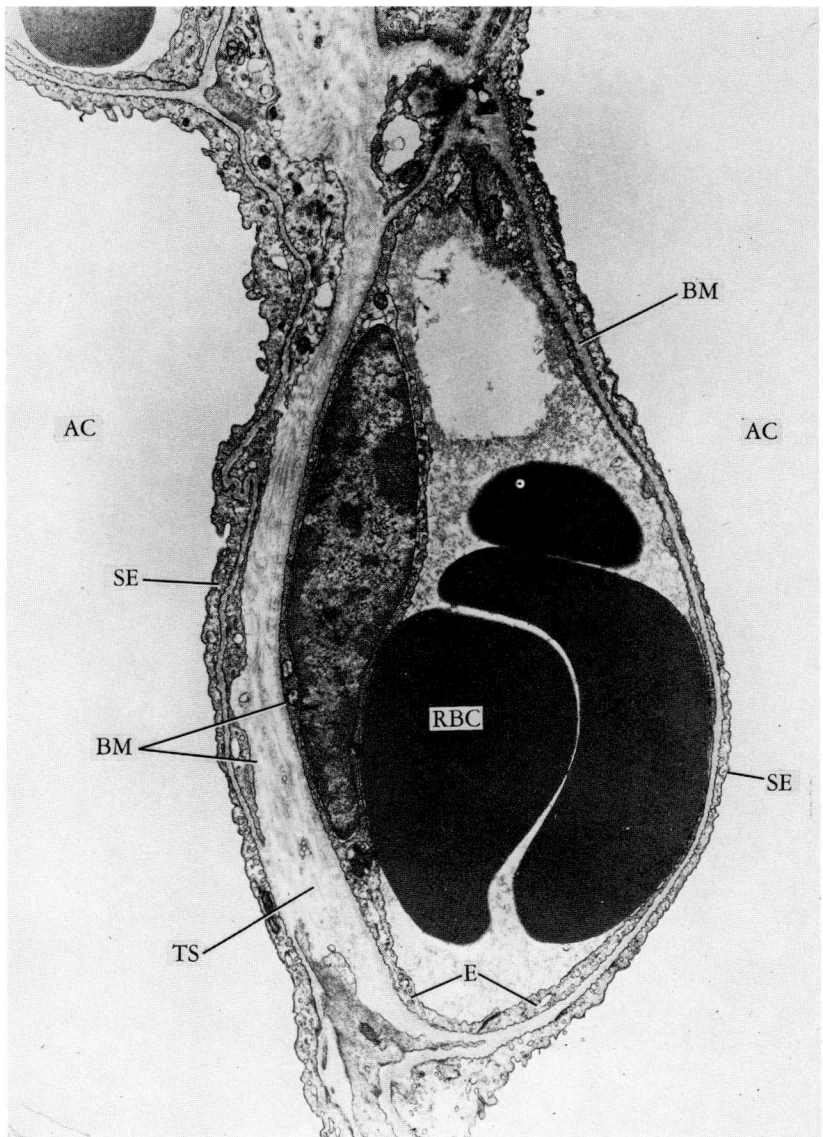

Fig. 10-27. Electron micrograph through a capillary in the alveolar wall (interalveolar septum). The alveolar cavity (AC) is lined with squamous epithelium (SE) (type I cells). The capillary containing erythrocytes (RBC) is lined with endothelium (E). The two layers of cells are separated from each other by a basement membrane (BM); the small tissue space (TS) is also visible. (×9,400.) (Courtesy of Dr. E. R. Weibel.)

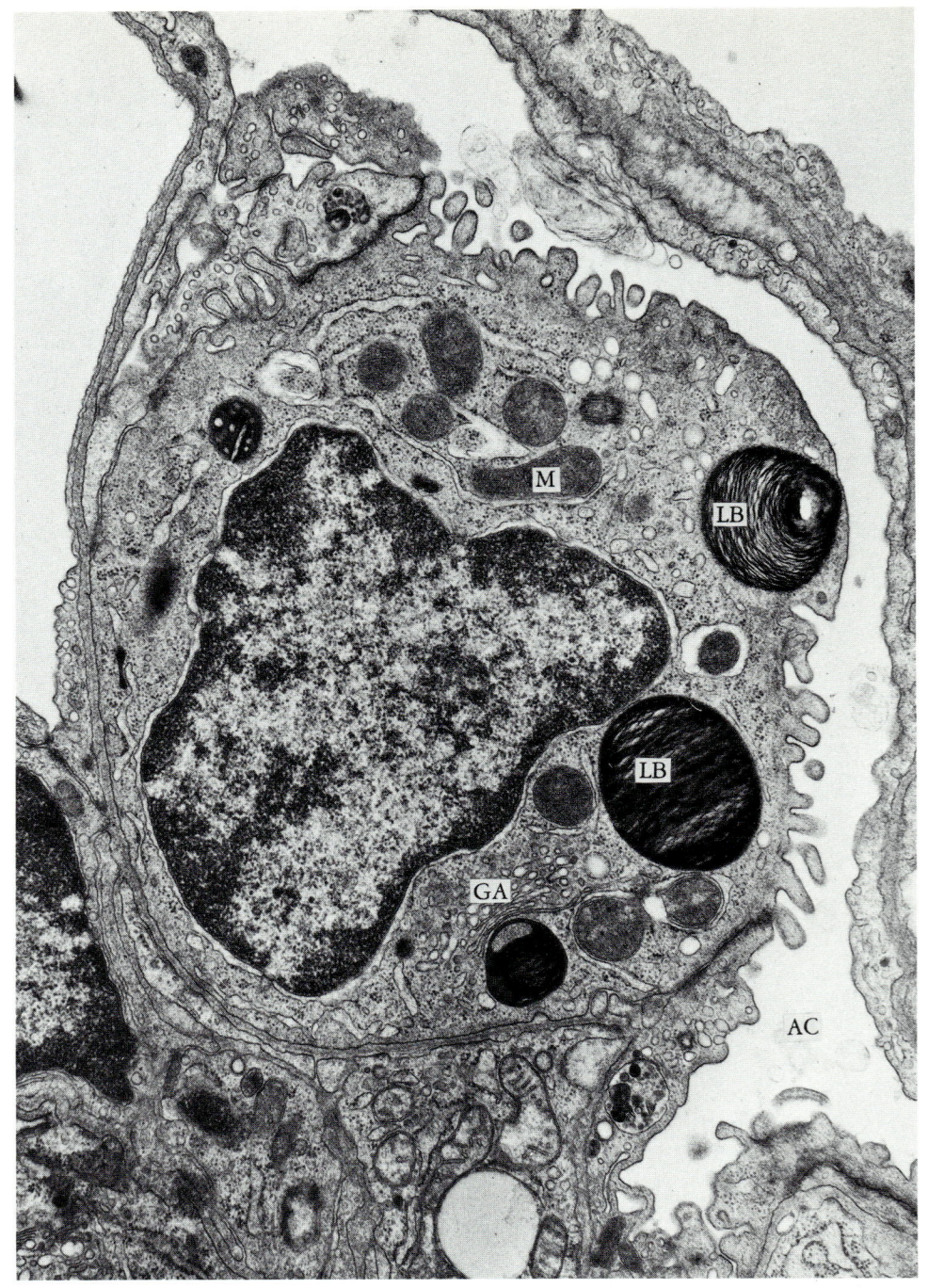

Fig. 10-28. Electron micrograph through two alveolar walls (interalveolar septa) showing a cuboidal (type II) epithelial cell responsible for secreting surfactant. Note the lamellar bodies (LB), mitochondria (M), and Golgi apparatus (GA) within the cytoplasm. The alveolar cavity (AC) is clearly visible (×19,000.) (Courtesy of Dr. M. C. Williams.)

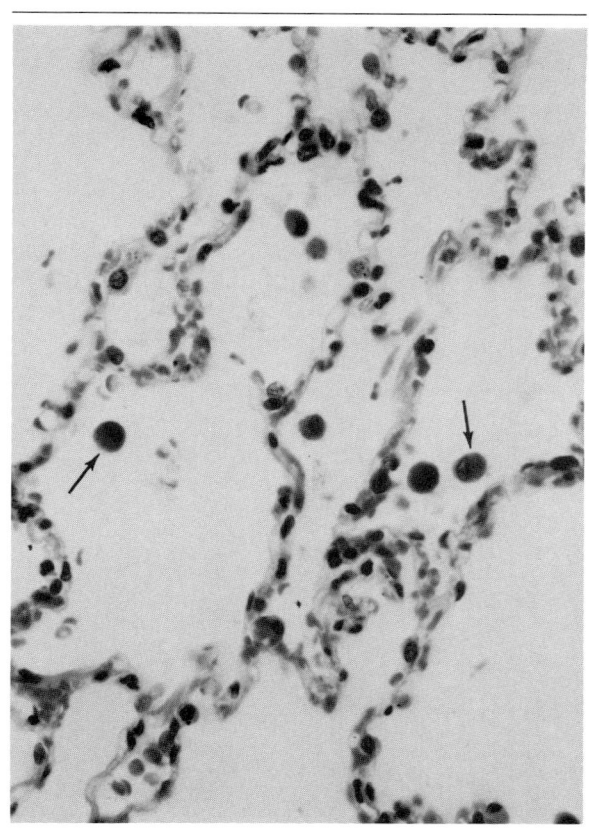

Fig. 10-29. Photomicrograph of a section of the lung, showing "heart failure cells" (arrows) in alveoli from a patient who died of left-sided heart failure. (H&E; ×400.)

Fig. 10-30. Photomicrograph of a section of the lung, showing numerous carbon particles in phagocytes that are lying free in the connective tissue between an artery and a small bronchus. These phagocytes have absorbed the inhaled carbon particles in the lumen of an alveolus and then migrated through the alveolar wall. The individual from whom this specimen was taken lived in a city. (H&E; ×200.)

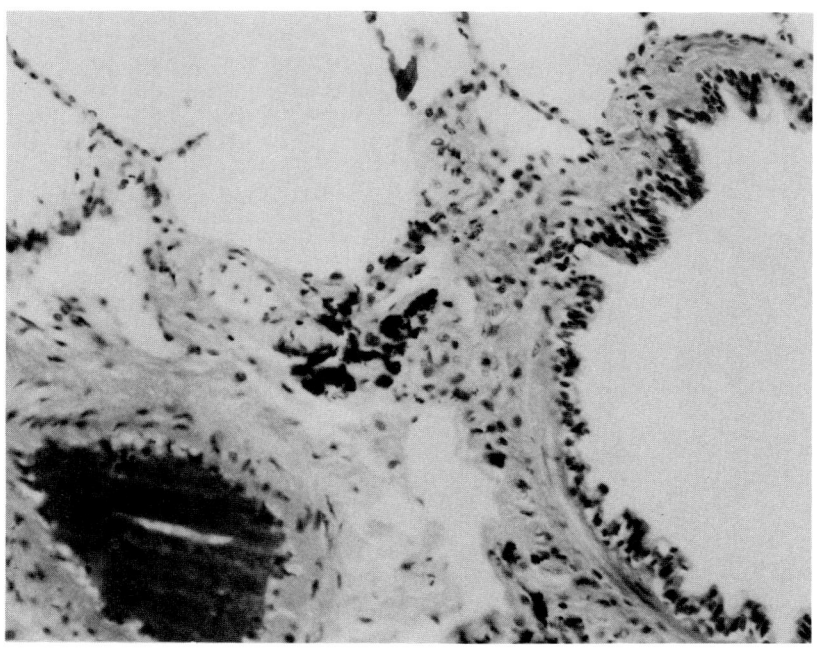

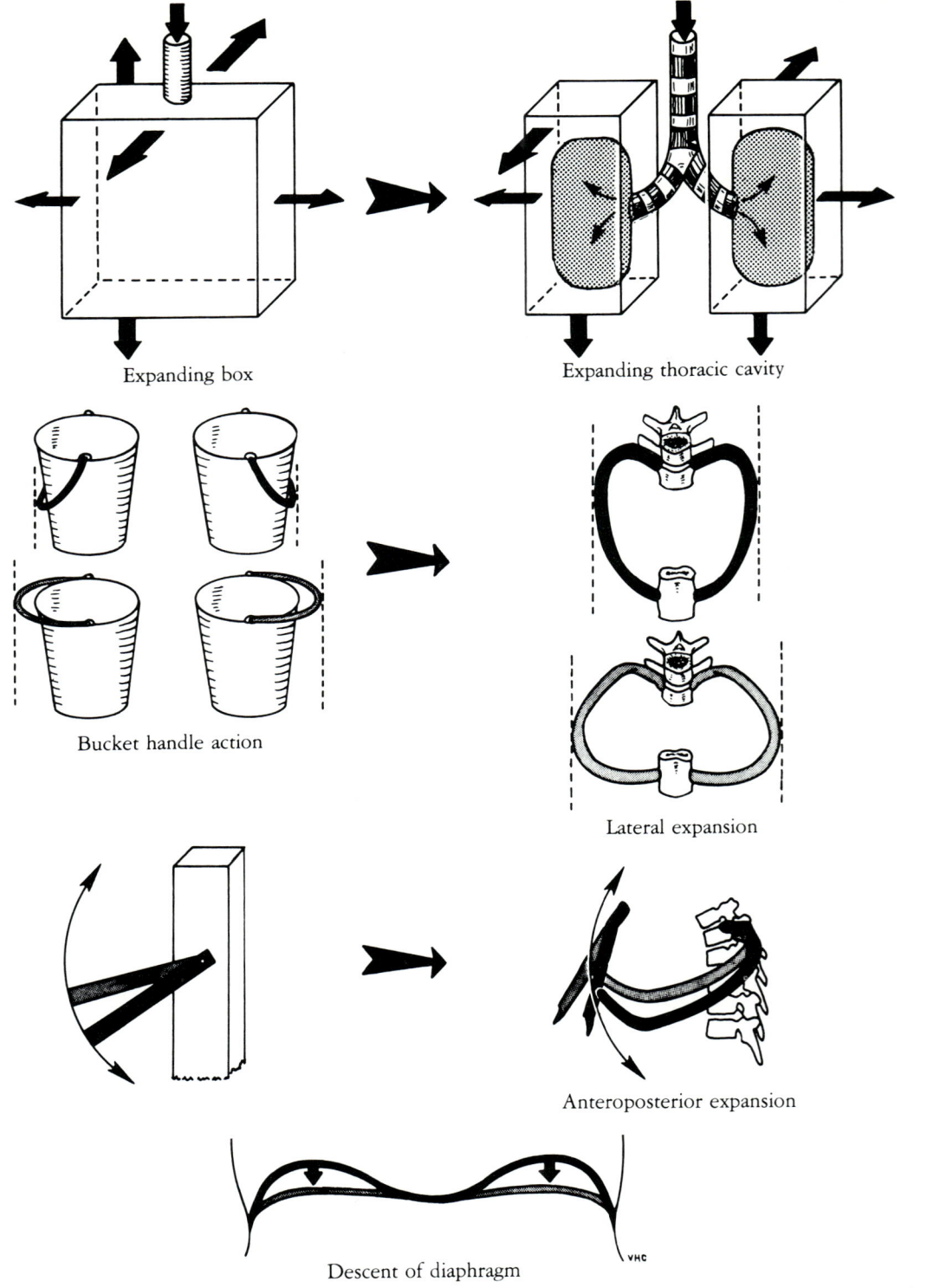

Fig. 10-31. Ways in which the capacity of the thoracic cavity is increased during inspiration.

action, including the scalenus anterior and medius and the sternocleidomastoid muscles of the neck. In respiratory distress, the action of all the muscles already engaged becomes more violent and the scapulae are fixed by the trapezius, levator scapulae, and rhomboid muscles, enabling the serratus anterior and pectoralis minor muscles to raise the ribs. If the individual supports the upper limbs by grasping a chair back or table, the sternal origin of the pectoralis major muscles can also assist the process.

Lung Changes on Inspiration

On inspiration, the root of the lung descends and the level of the bifurcation of the trachea may be lowered by as much as two vertebrae. The bronchi elongate and dilate and the alveolar capillaries dilate, assisting the pulmonary circulation. Air is drawn into the bronchial tree as a result of the positive atmospheric pressure exerted through the upper part of the respiratory tract and the negative pressure on the outer surface of the lungs brought about by the increased capacity of the thoracic cavity. With the expansion of the lungs, the elastic tissue in the bronchial walls and connective tissue is stretched. As the diaphragm descends, the costodiaphragmatic recess of the pleural cavity opens and the expanding sharp lower edges of the lungs descend.

Expiration

Quiet Expiration

Quiet expiration is largely a passive phenomenon and is brought about by the elastic recoil of the lungs, the relaxation of the intercostal muscles and diaphragm, and an increase in the tone of the muscles of the anterior abdominal wall, which forces the relaxing diaphragm upward. The *serratus posterior inferior muscles* play a minor role in pulling down the lower ribs.

Forced Expiration

Forced expiration is an active process brought about by the forcible contraction of the musculature of the anterior abdominal wall. The quadratus lumborum muscle also contracts, and pulls down the twelfth ribs. It is conceivable that under these circumstances, some of the intercostal muscles contract and pull the ribs together, depressing them to the lowered twelfth rib. The serratus posterior inferior and the latissimus dorsi muscles may also play a minor role.

Lung Changes on Expiration

On expiration, the roots of the lungs ascend, along with the bifurcation of the trachea. The bronchi shorten and contract. The elastic tissue of the lungs recoils, and the lungs become smaller. With the upward movement of the diaphragm, increasing areas of the diaphragmatic and costal parietal pleura come into apposition and the costodiaphragmatic recess is reduced in size. The lower margins of the lungs shrink and rise.

Types of Respiration

In babies and young children, the ribs are nearly horizontal. Thus, infants must rely mainly on the descent of the diaphragm to increase their thoracic capacity on inspiration. Because this diaphragmatic descent is accompanied by a marked and easily visible inward and outward excursion of the anterior abdominal wall, respiration at this age is referred to as the *abdominal type of respiration.*

After the second year, the ribs become more oblique, and the adult form of respiration is established.

In the adult, there is a sexual difference in the type of respiratory movements. The female relies mainly on the movements of the ribs rather than the descent of the diaphragm on inspiration. This is referred to as the *thoracic type of respiration.* The male uses both the thoracic and abdominal forms of respiration but mainly the abdominal form.

PULMONARY PRESSURES

Intra-alveolar Pressure

With each inspiration and expiration, when the capacity of the thoracic cavity increases and decreases, the pressure in the alveoli rises and falls. With inspiration, the intra-alveolar pressure becomes *less* than the atmospheric pressure, so air moves into the alveolar lumina. Conversely, with expiration, the intra-alveolar pressure becomes *greater* than the atmospheric pressure, so air moves out of the alveolar lumina.

Pleural Cavity Pressure (Intrapleural Pressure)

Any gas or fluid within the pleural cavity (i.e., the space between the visceral and parietal layers of pleura) is absorbed into the capillaries supplying the visceral and parietal layers. This absorption produces a partial vacuum and causes the visceral layer of pleura covering the lung to adhere to the parietal layer of pleura lining the chest wall. Thus, the pressure within the pleural cavity is negative. When the thoracic walls move away from the lungs, the thoracic walls apply suction to the lungs, and the lungs enlarge. The reverse effect occurs on expiration. A small amount of *pleural fluid* always remains within the pleural cavity to serve as a lubricant and allow the visceral pleura to slide over the parietal pleura.

Two further factors should be remembered. As the lungs are made to expand, the elastic fibers within the lung substance are stretched and the tension within these fibers rises. Also, the surface tension of the fluid within the alveolar lumina attempts to force the alveoli to collapse, explaining why the expanded lung is always ready to collapse away from the thoracic wall.

Compliance

Compliance is the ease with which a hollow viscus may be distended. In the lungs, compliance may be assessed by measuring the volume increase resulting from an increase in intra-alveolar pressure. Thus, the compliance of the lungs will be reduced if they are involved in fibrotic disease or if the bronchi become blocked. Deformities of the thoracic cage, disease of the rib joints, and paralysis of the intercostal muscles will all reduce the compliance of the lungs, because they decrease the expansibility of the thoracic cage.

VOLUMES OF AIR

Air in the Lungs

Tidal volume is the volume of air inspired and expired with each normal breath during quiet breathing. It amounts to about 500 ml. *Inspiratory reserve volume* is the additional volume of air that can be inspired above and beyond the normal tidal volume when the individual makes the maximum inspiratory effort. It amounts to about 3,000 ml in the young male adult. *Expiratory reserve volume* is the additional volume of air that can be expired above and beyond the normal tidal volume when the individual makes the maximum expiratory effort. It amounts to about 1,100 ml in the young male adult. *Residual volume* is the volume of air that remains within the lungs after the individual has made the maximum expiratory effort. It amounts to about 1,200 ml in the young male adult. *Vital capacity* is the sum of total tidal volume (500 ml), the inspiratory reserve volume (3,000 ml), and the expiratory reserve volume (1,100 ml) and equals about 4,600 ml in the young male adult.

Alveolar Air and Dead Space Air

The alveolar air is the air within the alveolar lumen. The air within the conducting tubes of the respiratory system—namely, that within the nasal cavities, the pharynx, the larynx, the trachea, and the bronchi—is called anatomical *dead space air* and amounts to about 150 ml. The volume of air that enters the alveoli with each inspiration is thus equal to the tidal volume minus the dead space volume.

GASEOUS EXCHANGE WITHIN THE LUNGS (EXTERNAL RESPIRATION)

When fresh air has entered the lumina of the alveoli, an exchange of respiratory gases (oxygen and carbon dioxide) takes place between the alveolar air and the blood (Fig. 10-32) because of pressure gradients of the respiratory gases.

The pulmonary artery blood that enters the lungs contains oxygen at a relatively low pressure (37 mm Hg) and carbon dioxide at a relatively high pressure (46 mm Hg); it is in fact the mixed venous blood from all parts of the body (see Fig. 10-32). The pulmonary blood then traverses the capillaries covering the alveoli. Here, the blood is separated from the air in the alveolar lumina only by the *respiratory membrane*. At the end of inspiration, the alveolar air

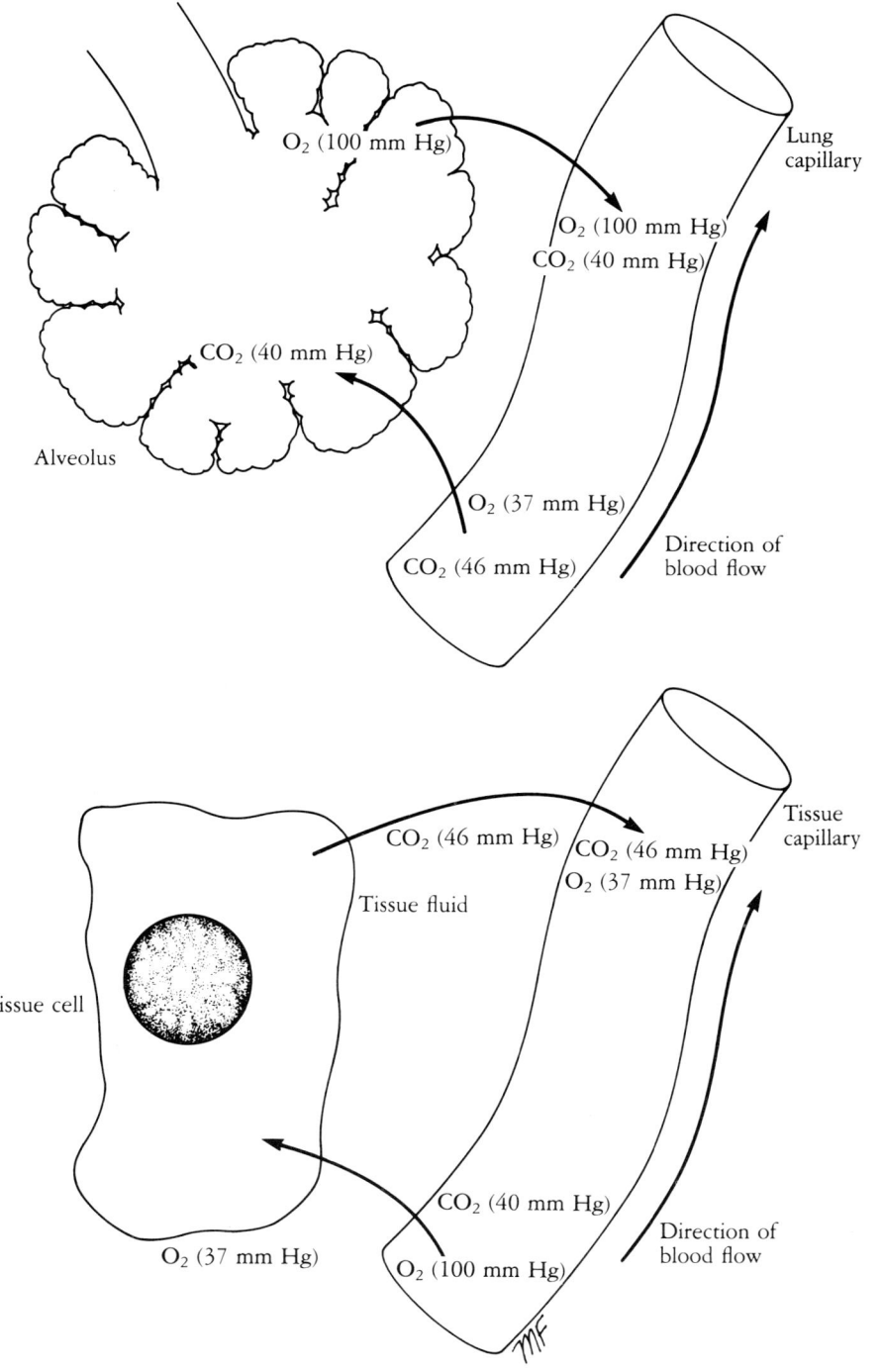

Fig. 10-32. Gaseous exchanges that take place because of pressure gradients: (A) exchange between the alveolar air and the blood in the lungs; (B) exchange between the blood and the tissue fluid and tissue cells.

contains oxygen at a relatively high pressure (100 mm Hg) and carbon dioxide at a relatively low pressure (40 mm Hg). Because of the existing pressure gradients, gaseous equilibrium quickly is established by the diffusion of oxygen into the blood and the diffusion of carbon dioxide from the blood into the alveolar air (see Fig. 10-32). The blood leaving the lungs by the pulmonary veins thus contains oxygen at a higher pressure (100 mm Hg) and carbon dioxide at a lower pressure (40 mm Hg) than does the blood entering the lungs (see Fig. 10-32).*

GASEOUS TRANSPORT WITHIN THE BLOOD

Oxygen Transport

About 97 percent of the oxygen transported from the lungs to the tissue is carried in chemical combination with the hemoglobin in the red blood cells; the remaining 3 percent is dissolved in the plasma. The combination of oxygen with hemoglobin forms the chemical *oxyhemoglobin*. This is a loose combination and easily reversible. When the blood in the pulmonary capillaries is exposed to relatively high oxygen pressure in the alveolar air, oxygen binds with the hemoglobin, but when the blood in the capillaries of the general body tissues is exposed to tissue fluid that has relatively low pressures of oxygen, the oxygen is quickly released from the hemoglobin.

An examination of the oxygen-hemoglobin dissociation curve (Fig. 10-33) shows the progressive rise in the percent of the hemoglobin that has combined with oxygen to form oxyhemoglobin as the pressure of oxygen increases. In the blood leaving the lungs in the pulmonary veins, the oxygen saturation is about 97 percent. Here, the pressure of oxygen is about 100 mm Hg. In the tissues, however, the oxygen saturation may be as low as 70 percent and the pressure of oxygen is only about 40 mm Hg.

A number of different factors are known to displace the hemoglobin dissociation curve to the right or the left. For example, an increased blood acidity, an increased carbon dioxide concentration within the blood, or an increased blood temperature will displace the curve to the right (see Fig. 10-33). A decreased acidity of the blood will shift the curve to the left. The significance of these facts is apparent when one considers the effects of increased tissue activity, such as severe muscular exercise, on oxygen transport: an increase in local temperature within the muscles because of increased metabolic activity, and an increased production of carbon dioxide and lactic acid. As a result, the capillary blood in the muscles readily will unload its oxygen, so that a greater volume of oxygen is delivered to the active tissue.

Carbon Dioxide Transport

Carbon dioxide is transported from the tissues to the lungs in several ways: as bicarbonate, in physical solution, and in combination with hemoglobin and plasma proteins.

Most carbon dioxide (70 percent) is transported in the form of bicarbonate ions. On diffusing from the tissue fluid into the water of the blood plasma (Fig. 10-34), carbon dioxide enters the red cells and rapidly combines with water to form *carbonic acid* (H_2CO_3). This reaction is catalyzed by the enzyme *carbonic anhydrase* within the red cell. The carbonic acid then rapidly dissociates into hydrogen and bicarbonate ions. The hydrogen ions quickly combine with the hemoglobin, which effectively removes the hydrogen ions from the fluid within the red cells (i.e., it acts as a chemical buffer). The excess bicarbonate ions within the red cells now diffuse into the plasma (see Fig. 10-34). To maintain electrical neutrality within the red cells, chloride ions rapidly diffuse from the plasma into the red blood cells, a phenomenon referred to as the *chloride shift*.

About 7 percent of all carbon dioxide is transported in physical solution in the blood to the lungs. About 15 to 25 percent of all carbon dioxide is transported in the blood to the lungs in *loose, easily reversible combination* with hemoglobin and plasma proteins (see Fig. 10-34).

It should be emphasized that the amount of car-

---

*Actually, the oxygen pressure in the pulmonary veins leaving the lungs is usually slightly less than 100 mm Hg, because not all the alveoli are equally ventilated, and venous shunts may exist, causing blood to bypass some of the alveoli.

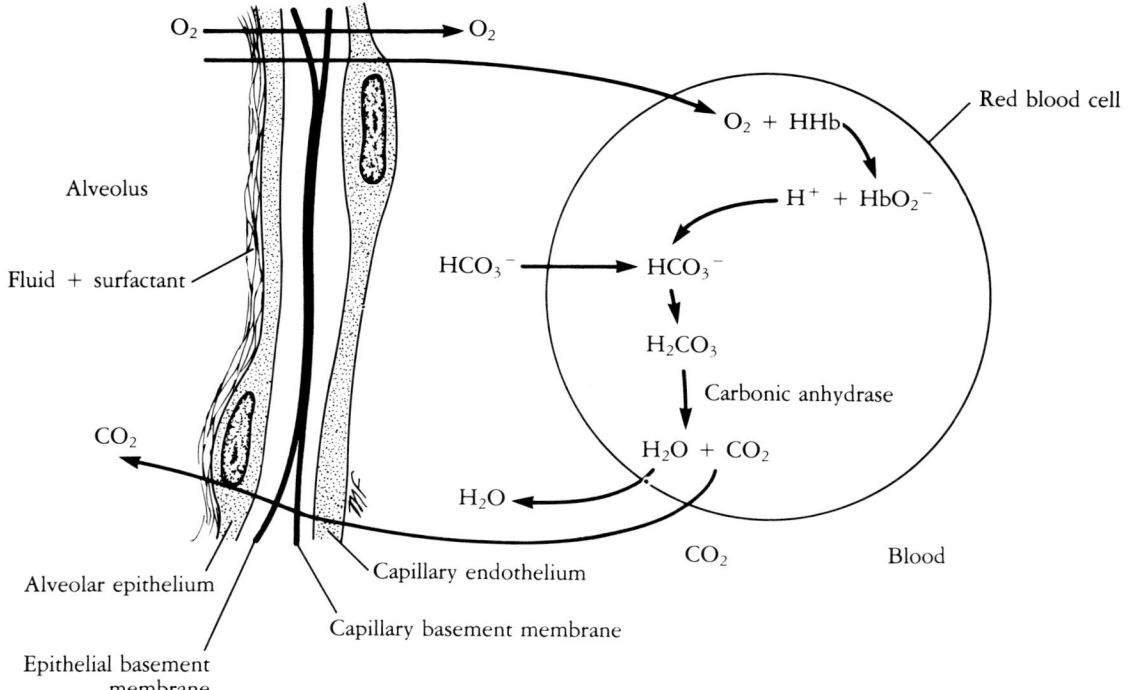
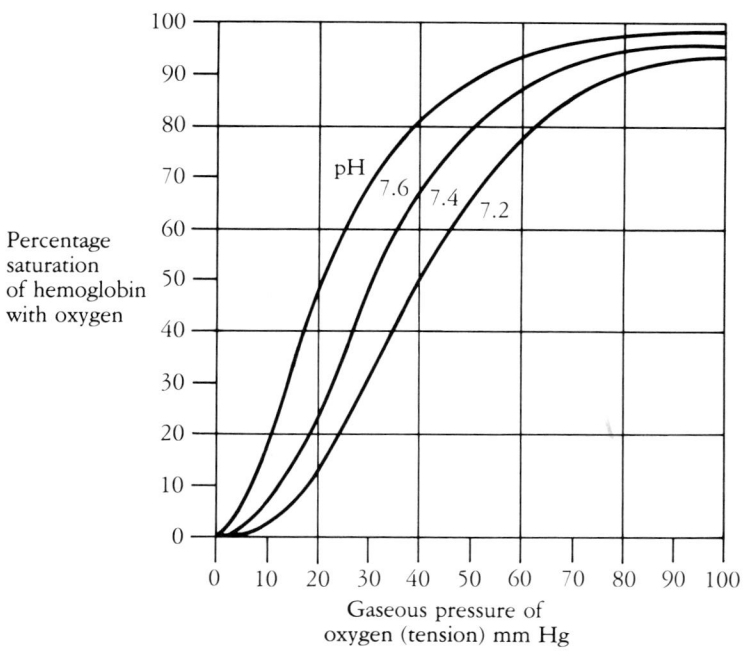

Fig. 10-33. A: Gaseous transport in the blood. B: Shift of the oxygen-hemoglobin dissociation curve in the blood to the right; such a shift can be caused by increasing the blood acidity, the carbon dioxide concentration within the blood, or the temperature of the blood.

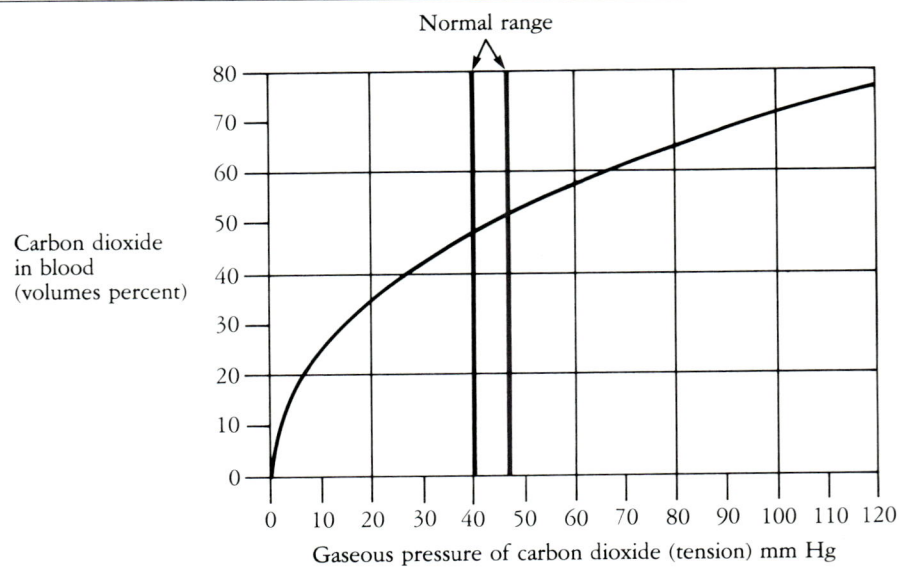

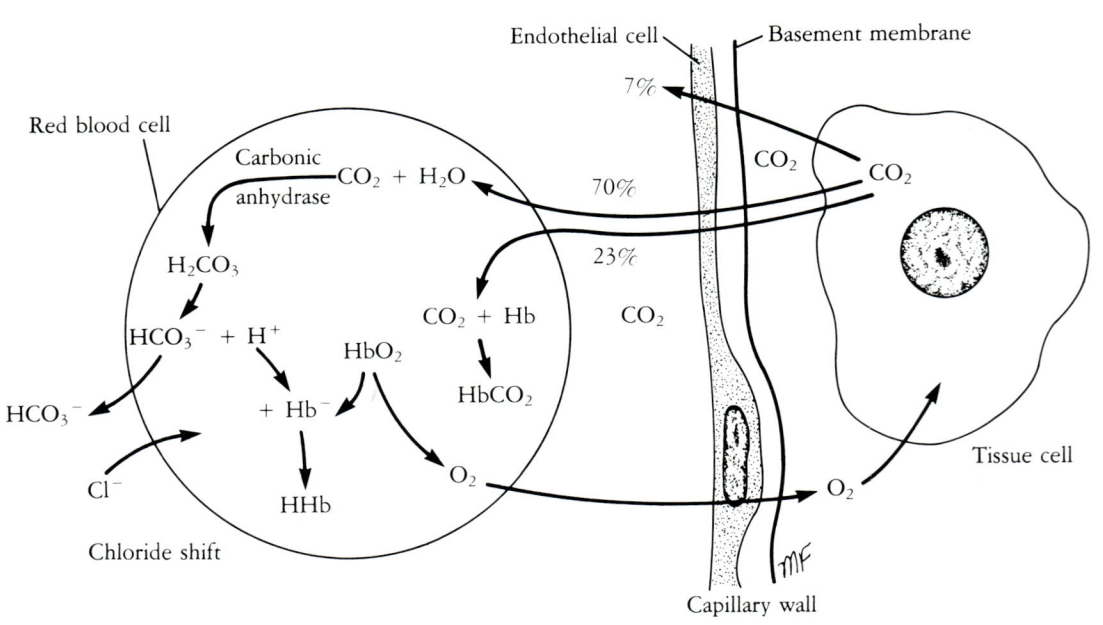

Fig. 10-34. A: *Carbon dioxide dissociation curve in the blood.* B: *Carbon dioxide transport in the blood.*

bon dioxide that combines with water to form carbonic acid in the plasma is small and that the reaction takes place very slowly, because of the absence of the enzyme carbonic anhydrase.

The carbon dioxide dissociation curve shows that the normal pressure of carbon dioxide in the venous blood leaving the body tissue is about 46 mm Hg. The pressure of carbon dioxide in the blood leaving the lungs is about 40 mm Hg. Thus, the range is small. The combination of oxygen with hemoglobin to form oxyhemoglobin tends to displace carbon dioxide from the hemoglobin and thereby aids the displacement of carbon dioxide from the blood in the lungs. This phenomenon is called the *Haldane effect.*

GASEOUS EXCHANGE WITHIN THE TISSUES (INTERNAL RESPIRATION)

When the arterial blood reaches the capillaries in the tissues, an exchange of respiratory gases (oxygen and carbon dioxide) takes place between the blood and the tissue fluid (see Fig. 10-32) because of pressure gradients of the respiratory gases.

The arterial blood entering the tissue capillaries contains oxygen at a relatively high pressure (100 mm Hg) and carbon dioxide at a relatively low pressure (40 mm Hg). The blood in the capillaries is separated from the tissue fluid by the endothelial lining and the basement membrane (see Fig. 10-32). The tissue fluid contains oxygen at a relatively low pressure (37 mm Hg) and carbon dioxide at a relatively high pressure (46 mm Hg). Because of the existing pressure gradients, gaseous equilibrium quickly is established by the diffusion of oxygen from the blood into the tissue fluid and the diffusion of carbon dioxide from the tissue fluid into the blood (see Fig. 10-32). The blood leaving the venous end of the capillary thus contains oxygen at a lower pressure (37 mm Hg) and carbon dioxide at a higher pressure (46 mm Hg) than does the blood entering the tissue capillary at the arterial end (see Fig. 10-32).

The oxygen in the tissue fluid is at a higher pressure than that within the cells. For this reason, the oxygen quickly diffuses into the cells, where it reacts with various food materials to form large quantities of carbon dioxide. This formation causes the pressure of the intracellular carbon dioxide to rise above that in the tissue fluid. Because of the pressure difference, the carbon dioxide quickly diffuses through the plasma membrane of the cell into the tissue fluid.

CONTROL OF RESPIRATION

Respiratory movements are carried out, for the most part, automatically. It is possible, however, to modify these movements by exerting voluntary control. For example, one can increase and decrease the rate of one's respiratory movements and even stop breathing for a short period of time.

The automatic control of respiratory movements is exercised by groups of nerve cells in the medulla oblongata and pons in the brain. These cells constitute the so-called *respiratory center* (Fig. 10-35). The activity of the respiratory center adjusts the rate of ventilation of the alveolar air to meet the demands of tissue metabolism so that the pressure of oxygen and carbon dioxide in the blood remains practically unchanged.

The respiratory center can be divided into three areas: (1) *medullary respiratory center,* (2) the *apneustic center,* and (3) the *pneumotaxic center.* It is believed that the nerve cells of the medullary respiratory center can be subdivided into those that control inspiratory movements—the *inspiratory center*—and those that control expiratory movements—the *expiratory center.*

The respiratory centers exert their control over the respiratory movements by discharging nerve impulses that travel to the muscles of respiration via the phrenic nerves to the diaphragm and via the intercostal nerves to the intercostal muscles. Activation of the inspiratory center causes the inspiratory muscles to contract, and the individual breathes in. Activation of the neighboring expiratory center results in the discharge of inhibitory impulses that pass to the inspiratory center and interrupt its activity. By this means, the inspiratory movements are stopped at regular intervals and the passive movements of expiration take place. In forced expiration,

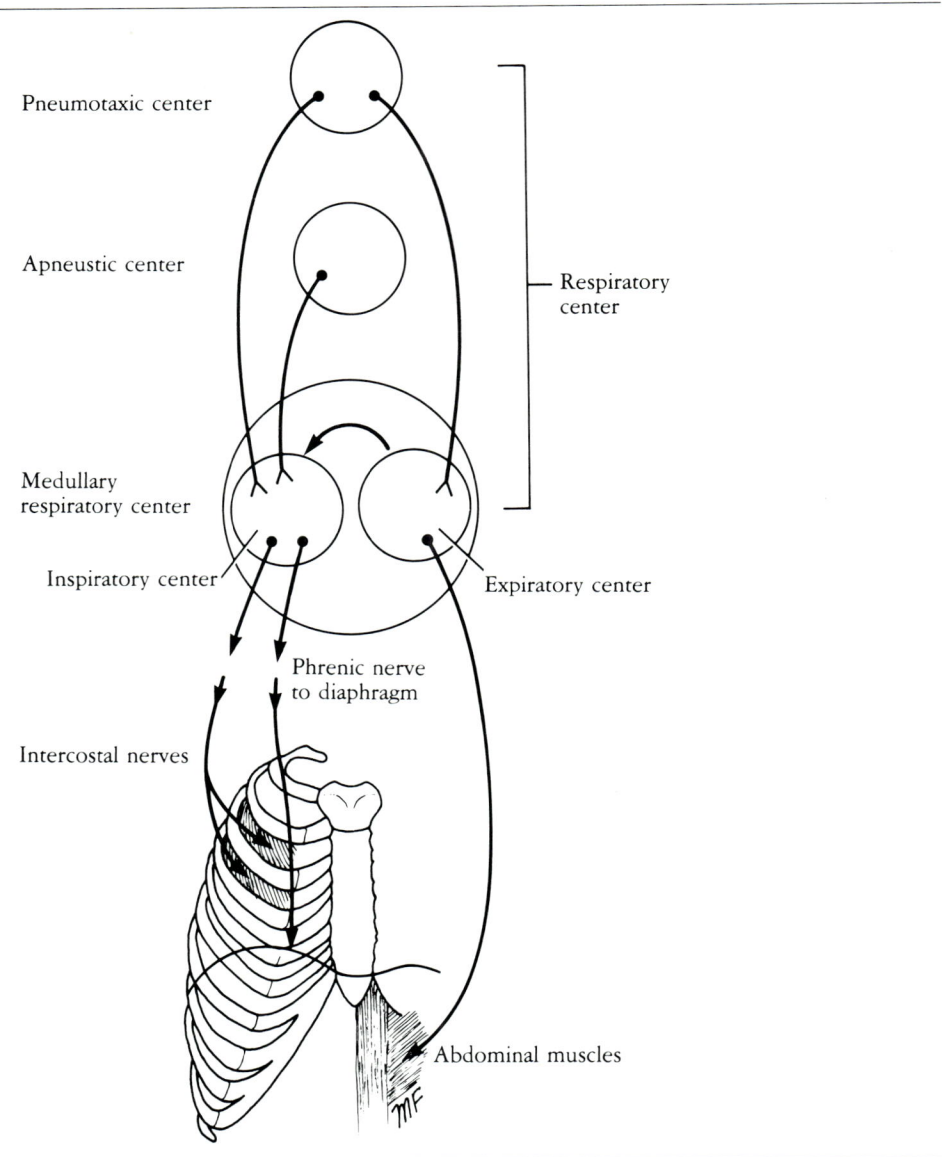

Fig. 10-35. *The working relationship among the different parts of the respiratory center in the control of respiration.*

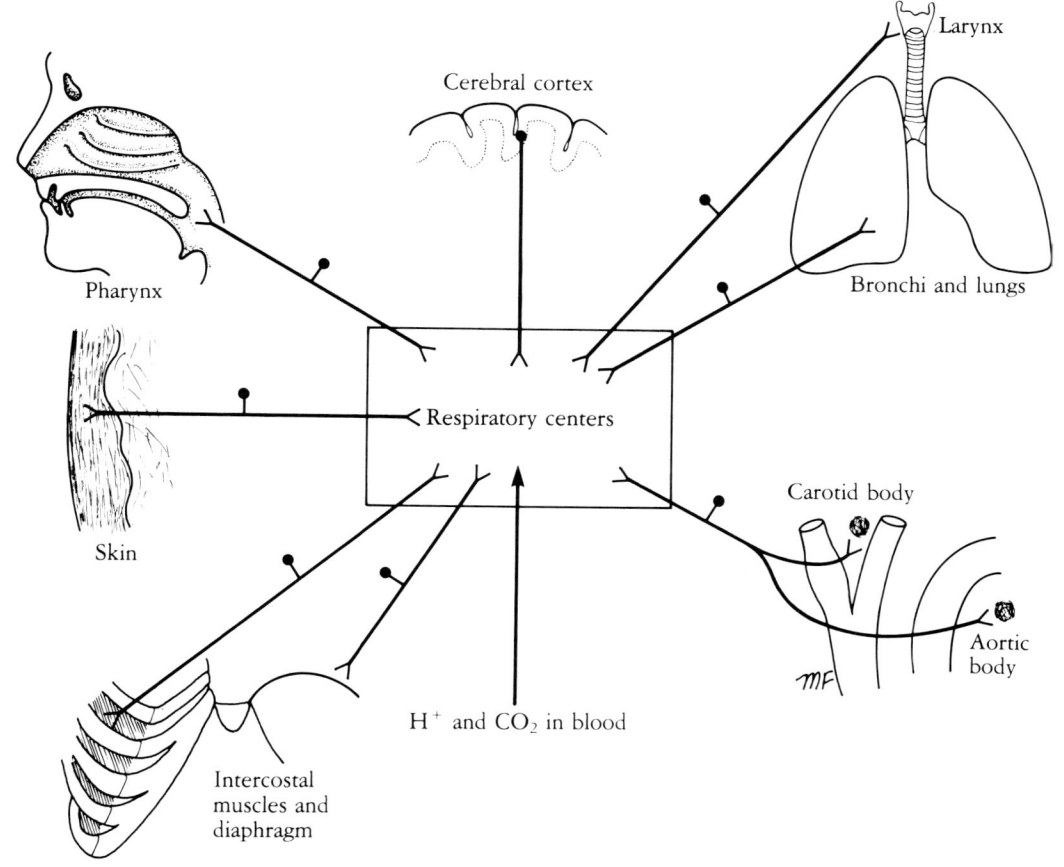

Fig. 10-36. Effects on the respiratory centers of chemical factors and nervous afferent impulses.

impulses travel from the expiratory center to the muscles involved in that activity.

The *apneustic center,* which is situated in the pons, can prolong the activity of the inspiratory center. The individual then breathes with a prolonged inspiration and a short expiration. This center is not essential for normal breathing. The *pneumotaxic center* is also situated in the pons and is believed to exert its influence on the rate of respiration by appropriately stimulating the inspiratory and expiratory centers. The pneumotaxic center is not essential for normal breathing.

Effect on the Respiratory Center of Chemical Factors and Nervous Afferent Impulses

Chemical Control of Respiration

The respiratory centers are highly sensitive to the changes in concentrations in the blood oxygen, carbon dioxide, and hydrogen ions. Oxygen exerts its control indirectly on the centers by acting on special *chemoreceptors* in the *carotid* and *aortic bodies,* which are located close to the carotid arteries in the neck and the arch of the aorta in the thorax, respectively. The chemoreceptors transmit nerve impulses that ascend to the respiratory centers of the brain via the ninth and tenth (vagus) cranial nerves. A decrease in the oxygen concentration of the blood causes stimulation of the inspiratory center (Fig. 10-36).

Carbon dioxide and hydrogen ions act directly on the respiratory center. An increase in the carbon dioxide or hydrogen ion concentration in the blood will stimulate the inspiratory center directly (see Fig. 10-36).

Nervous Control of Respiration

The respiratory centers can be influenced by general body afferent nervous impulses, by proprioceptive impulses in the respiratory muscles, and by afferent impulses originating in stretch receptors in the bronchi and bronchioles (see Fig. 10-36).

Application of hot or cold water to the skin, a pinprick, the act of swallowing, and stimulation of the nasal mucosa by an unpleasant odor are all stimuli that can alter the normal respiratory rhythm. Moreover, nervous impulses arising in the higher centers of the brain may profoundly alter respiratory movements, as, for example, in laughing and crying.

An increase in body temperature will also increase the respiratory rate.

The *Hering-Breuer inflation reflex* is a stretch reflex of great importance. When the lungs become stretched during inspiration, the stretch receptors transmit afferent inhibitory impulses to the inspiratory center via the vagus nerves (see Fig. 10-36). In this manner, further inflation of the alveoli is prevented. During expiration, the stretch receptors in the bronchial walls are no longer stimulated, and so the inspiratory center is freed from the inhibitory influence of the inflation reflex. This is the mechanism of the *Hering-Breuer deflation reflex*. Some researchers also believe that there are compression receptors in the lungs that are stimulated as the lung collapses in expiration.

COUGHING, SNEEZING, AND VOCALIZATION. These normal modifications of respiration are described on pages 372 and 373.

CLINICAL NOTES

CONDITIONS OF THE CONDUCTING PORTION OF THE RESPIRATORY SYSTEM

Nasal Cavities

Inflammation of the nasal cavities (rhinitis) is a common disorder. Acute rhinitis, or the common cold, is caused by virus infections. Allergic reactions to pollens are also common. Bacterial infections may complicate viral or allergic reactions. Initially, the mucous membrane becomes thickened and edematous and there is vasodilatation of the blood vessels. The lamina propria becomes infiltrated with neutrophils, plasma cells, lymphocytes, and eosinophils. The surface becomes excessively moist with a watery fluid that the cilia are unable to control. The nose starts to run. With a secondary bacterial infection, the nasal discharge later becomes purulent.

Paranasal Sinuses

Infection of the paranasal sinuses is a common complication of nasal infections. Rarely, the cause of maxillary sinusitis is extension from a dental abscess. Swelling of the mucous membrane at the entrances to the sinuses obstructs sinus drainage and causes severe pain.

Tumors of the nasal cavities and paranasal sinuses are very rare.

Larynx

Inflammation of the larynx (laryngitis) may occur with inflammations of the upper and lower respiratory tract. Edema of the mucous membrane covering the vocal folds may impair voice production. Swelling of the mucous membrane secondary to an allergic reaction from such causes as ingestion of an allergen or an insect bite, especially in children, may be so severe as to block the airway.

Benign and malignant tumors of the vocal folds occur. Both types of tumors usually arise from the squamous epithelium covering the vocal folds. Hoarseness of the voice is one of the first symptoms.

Trachea and Bronchi

Inhalation of *foreign bodies* into the lower respiratory tract is common, especially in children. Pins, screws, nuts, bolts, peanuts, and parts of chicken bones and toys have all found their way into the bronchi. Parts of teeth may be inhaled while a patient is under anesthesia during a difficult dental extraction. Because the right bronchus is the wider and more direct continuation of the trachea (see Fig. 10-11), foreign bodies tend to enter the right rather than the left bronchus. From there, they usually pass into the middle or lower lobe bronchi.

Bronchoscopy enables a physician to examine the interior of the trachea, its bifurcation (called the *carina*), and the main bronchi. With experience, one can examine the interior of the lobar bronchi and the beginning of the first segmental bronchi. The bronchoscope also permits collection of biopsy specimens of mucous membrane and removal of inhaled foreign bodies (even open safety pins).

The trachea and bronchi should not be regarded as rigid tubes through which air enters and leaves the lungs. With each inspiration, the bronchi elongate and dilate, and with expiration, the reverse process occurs. This is a passive mechanism caused by the inflation of the lung and its emptying of air secondary to the changing capacity of the thoracic cage. It follows that the presence of neoplasms, fibrosis, or edema fluid in neighboring lung tissue will impede this passive process seriously and thus reduce the efficiency of the respiratory function of the lungs. Bronchial asthma, a condition in which there is spasm of the bronchial smooth muscle, obstructs the airway and interferes with ventilation of the lungs. Diseases of the respiratory muscles or the joints of the thoracic wall inhibit full expansion of the lungs.

PLEURAE

As a result of disease or injury, air may enter the pleural cavity from the lungs or through the chest wall (pneumothorax). In the treatment of tuberculosis, air may purposely be injected into the pleural cavity to collapse and rest the lung. This is known as *artificial pneumothorax*. A *spontaneous pneumothorax* is a condition in which air enters the pleural cavity suddenly without its cause being immediately apparent. Investigation usually reveals that air has entered from a diseased lung.

Air in the pleural cavity associated with serous fluid is known as *hydropneumothorax;* associated with pus, as *pyopneumothorax;* and associated with blood, as *hemopneumothorax*. A collection of pus (without air) in the pleural cavity is called an *empyema*. The presence of serous fluid in the pleural cavity is referred to as *pleural effusion*.

Inflammations of the pleurae (pleuritis) are usually caused by spread of infection from the underlying lung. If the inflammatory reaction is small, the fluid exudate is resorbed. Often the fibrinous component of the exudate, which may have caused the visceral and parietal layers of pleura to adhere to each other, is invaded by capillaries and fibroblasts and converted into a permanent fibrous union, or *adhesion*. A large pleural infection may lead to an empyema.

Collections of excessive amounts of pleural fluid, which is noninflammatory in origin, may occur in cardiac failure associated with pulmonary congestion and edema.

LUNGS

Although the lungs are well protected by the bony thoracic cage, a splinter from a fractured rib may penetrate the lungs and air may escape into the pleural cavity, causing a pneumothorax and collapse of the lung. Air may also find its way into the lung connective tissue. From there, the air moves under the visceral pleura until it reaches the lung root. It then passes into the mediastinum and up into the neck, where it may distend the subcutaneous tissue, a condition known as *subcutaneous emphysema*.

Lung tissue and the visceral pleura are devoid of pain-sensitive nerve endings, so pain in the chest is always the result of conditions affecting the surrounding structures. In tuberculosis or pneumonia, for example, pain may never be experienced.

Once lung disease crosses the visceral pleura and the pleural cavity to involve the parietal pleura, pain becomes a prominent feature. Lobar pneumonia with pleurisy, for example, produces a severe, tearing pain accentuated by inspiring deeply or coughing.

A localized chronic lesion such as that of tuberculosis or a benign neoplasm may require surgical removal. If the lesion is restricted to a bronchopulmonary segment, it is possible carefully to dissect out a particular segment and remove it, leaving the surrounding lung intact *(segmental resection)*.

Defense Clearance Mechanisms in the Lungs

With each inspiration, the normal lung takes in air from the environment containing dusts, allergens, chemicals, and microorganisms. In order to protect the body from these foreign particles, the respiratory system possesses a number of clearing mechanisms. The nose, pharynx, larynx, trachea, and larger bronchi are lined for the most part with a ciliated columnar epithelium whose cilia move a thin film of mucus covering the surface toward the nasopharynx and oropharynx, where it is swallowed or expectorated. Any inspired particles eventually become stuck to the mucus like flies on flypaper.

Small foreign particles that enter the alveoli are phagocytosed by the alveolar phagocytes. The particles either are digested or are carried by the cilia up the bronchial tree to enter the oral pharynx with the mucus and then swallowed. Some phagocytes enter the lymphatic vessels and are carried to the bronchial lymph nodes. If these clearance mechanisms fail to work efficiently, pathogenic bacteria may accumulate, producing an inflammatory response with an outpouring of neutrophils.

Measurement of Volumes of Air in the Lungs

The instrument used to measure the volumes of air in the lungs is the *spirometer* (Fig. 10-37). It consists of a drum inverted over a tank of water. The drum is counterbalanced by a weight and is filled with air, and a tube connects the interior of the drum to the patient's mouth. As the patient breathes in and out, the drum rises and falls. To measure the vital capacity, the patient is asked to inspire outside air maximally and then empty his lungs as completely as possible into the spirometer. The residual volume and the total lung capacity cannot be measured by this method, because the residual air will remain in the lung even after forced expiration.

The vital capacity normally varies from one individual to another and depends on such factors as the size of the thoracic cage. Abnormal amounts of fluid in the pleural cavities, as in pleurisy or hemothorax, or excess blood in the pulmonary circulation in the lungs, as in congestive heart failure, may seriously reduce the vital capacity.

The vital capacity may be reduced gradually over a period of years in chronic emphysema. In this condition, the alveolar walls of the lungs progressively rupture, and the loss of lung tissue interferes with the elastic recoil of the lungs that normally occurs in expiration. In cases of advanced emphysema, the thoracic cage remains in a partial state of inspiration.

ARTIFICIAL RESPIRATION

If respiratory movements have stopped, as in an apparently drowned individual or as a result of electrocution or carbon monoxide poisoning, and the cardiovascular system is still functioning, it is essential that some form of artificial respiration be employed immediately. It is important to get fresh air into the lungs as soon as possible and to continue with the treatment so that the brain receives an adequate amount of oxygen and irreversible damage to the nervous tissue does not occur.

Before artificial respiration is started, it should be ascertained that the mouth and pharynx are clear of water or other foreign debris and that the tongue is pulled forward.

Mouth-to-Mouth Breathing

The first step in mouth-to-mouth breathing is to make sure that the airway is patent. To do this, the victim's head is extended by the placement of one hand beneath the head and the other on the forehead. This pulls the jaw and tongue anteriorly and opens the airway. The rescuer then takes a deep breath and breathes directly into the mouth of the patient, forcing air into the respiratory passages (see

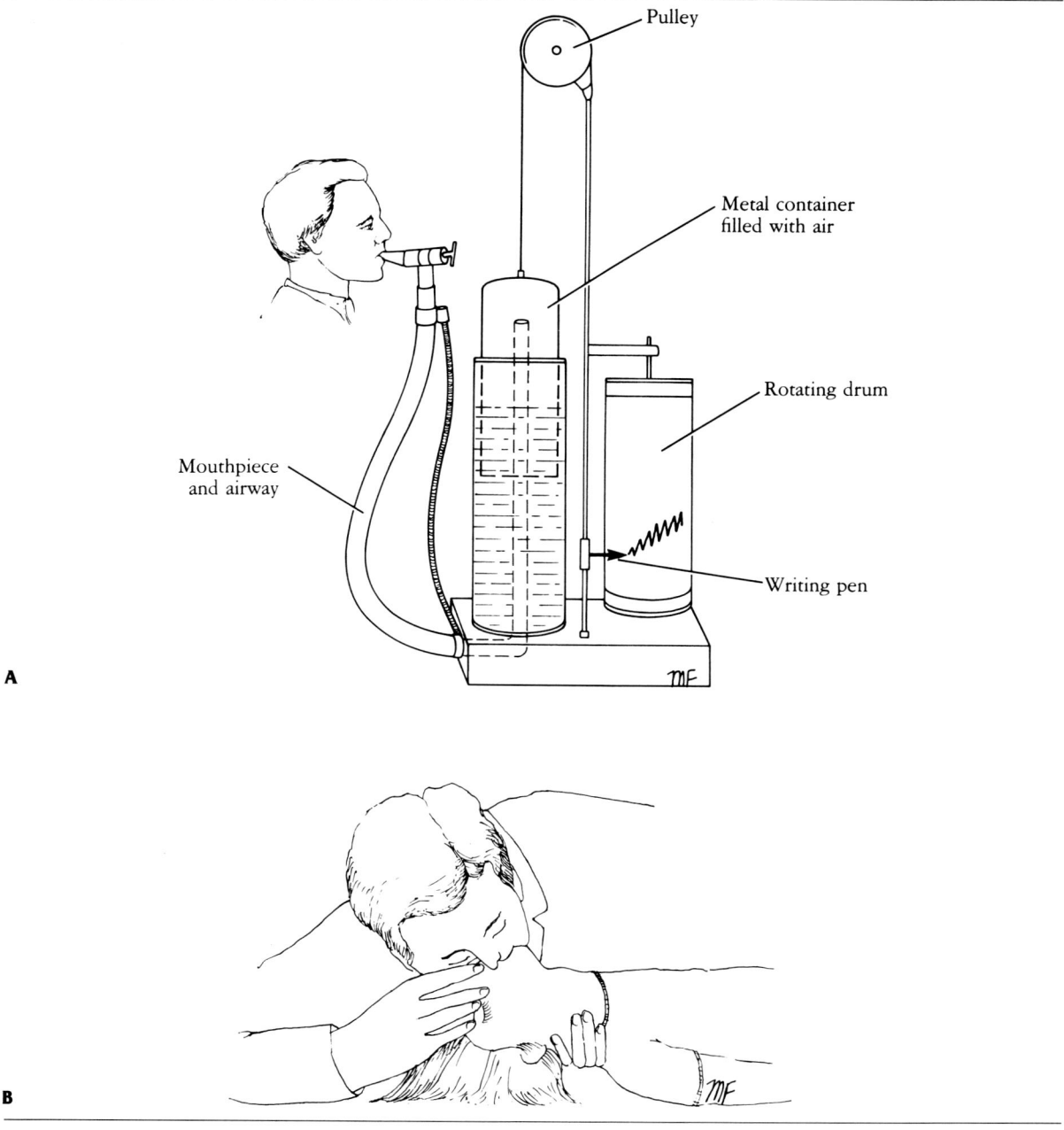

Fig. 10-37. A: General structure of a spirometer, an instrument used to measure the volumes of air in the lungs. B: Position of the rescuer and patient in mouth-to-mouth resuscitation.

Fig. 10-37). The patient's nose should be gripped between finger and thumb to prevent the escape of air. The rescuer then takes another deep breath while the patient passively expires. This process is repeated rhythmically for as long as necessary.

The normal expired air of the rescuer has sufficient oxygen to sustain life, and the carbon dioxide content assists in the stimulation of the patient's respiratory center.

Mechanical Ventilators

In medical centers, machines are available that can assist or control respiration. These are of two kinds, pressure cycled and volume cycled. These devices are indicated when the patient is unable to maintain adequate oxygen and carbon dioxide concentrations in the blood.

DISEASES THAT DECREASE RESPIRATORY EFFICIENCY

Constriction of the Bronchi as in Bronchial Asthma

One of the problems associated with bronchial asthma is spasm of the smooth muscle in the wall of the bronchioles. This spasm particularly reduces the diameter of the bronchioles during expiration. As a result, the asthmatic patient usually can inspire without difficulty but has great difficulty in expiring. Consequently, the lungs become greatly distended and the thoracic cage becomes permanently enlarged, forming the so-called *barrel chest.* In addition, the air flow through the bronchioles is impeded further by excess mucus that the patient is unable to clear because he or she is unable to produce an effective cough.

Loss of Lung Elasticity

Many diseases of the lung, such as *emphysema* and *pulmonary fibrosis,* destroy the elasticity of the lungs. Thus, the lungs are unable to recoil adequately, and expiration is incomplete. The respiratory muscles in affected patients have to assist in expiration, which is no longer a passive phenomenon.

Loss of Lung Distensibility

Diseases such as *silicosis, asbestosis, cancer,* and *pneumonia* interfere with the process of expanding the lung in inspiration. A decrease in the compliance of the lungs and the chest wall then occurs. A greater effort has to be made by the inspiratory muscles to inflate the lungs.

Pneumothorax

This condition results from the entry of air into the pleural cavity from the lungs or through the chest wall. The lung on the affected side immediately collapses because of its elastic recoil and because the pressure outside the lung is now equal to the atmospheric pressure of air within the respiratory passages. The oxygen concentration in the blood leaving the affected lung immediately falls; this explains the initial breathlessness. Assuming that the remaining lung is normal and able to compensate for the loss of respiratory efficiency, the oxygen content of the blood quickly returns to normal.

Postural Drainage

Excessive accumulation of bronchial secretions in a lobe or a segment of a lung may seriously interfere with the normal flow of air into the alveoli. Furthermore, the stagnation of such secretions often is quickly followed by infection. To aid in the normal drainage of a bronchial segment, a physiotherapist will often alter the position of the patient so that gravity will assist in the process of drainage. Sound knowledge of the bronchial tree is necessary to determine the optimum position of the patient for good postural drainage.

FACTORS THAT DEPRESS THE RESPIRATORY CENTER

Cerebral edema following severe head injuries may result in swelling of the brain tissue and compression of the neurons of the respiratory center. The neurons may become inactive and then die. Intravenous injections of hypertonic solutions often will relieve the condition by osmotically removing some of the tissue fluid from the brain.

Intracranial tumors may, by their expansion, force the medulla oblongata downward into the foramen magnum of the skull, so interfering with blood flow through the respiratory center that breathing ceases.

Anesthetics and narcotic agents at high dosages depress not only the higher centers of the brain but also the respiratory center. Sodium pentobarbital, for example, is a selective hypnotic at normal therapeutic dosage but strongly depresses the respiratory center in abnormally large doses.

FACTORS THAT STIMULATE THE RESPIRATORY CENTER

Drugs such as *Metrazol* (pentylenetetrazol), *caffeine, theophylline,* and *picrotoxin* can stimulate the respiratory center. *Coramine* (nikethamide) can stimulate the carotid and aortic body reflexes and so indirectly stimulate the inspiratory center.

BREATHING ABNORMALITIES

Cheyne-Stokes Breathing

This form is often seen in patients with advanced cerebral atherosclerosis producing cerebral ischemia. In cardiac failure, Cheyne-Stokes breathing may occur because of secondary cerebral ischemia. Massive neurological lesions, such as those caused by intracranial hemorrhage, may separate the brain stem physiologically from the cerebrum and produce this form of breathing.

Cheyne-Stokes breathing is characterized by periods of rapid and deep respiration alternating with periods of complete cessation of respiration. The underlying mechanism for this form of breathing is as follows. The rapid and deep respiration causes excessive elimination of carbon dioxide from the alveoli and blood. This decreased carbon dioxide concentration in the blood inhibits the inspiratory center, and inspiration ceases. Now the carbon dioxide concentration rises in the blood, the inspiratory center is stimulated, and the patient starts to overbreathe once again. This type of breathing occurs when the inspiratory center is excessively sensitive to changes in the carbon dioxide content of the blood and overacts, resulting in sudden and excessively great respiratory movements.

Hyperventilation and Hypoventilation

Hyperventilation can be caused by anxiety; acidosis, as in diabetes mellitus; or diseases of the central nervous system. Excessive amounts of carbon dioxide are washed out of the lungs, resulting in a lowering of the carbon dioxide pressure in the blood. The consequent alkalosis may be so severe as to cause tetany and numbness in the limbs. In patients with anxiety states, the symptoms often can be relieved by inhalation of a 5 percent carbon dioxide mixture.

Hypoventilation can be caused by any condition that reduces the volume of air entering the alveoli. Excessive amounts of carbon dioxide accumulate in the blood, and the oxygen concentration falls. Diseases of the central nervous system, neuromuscular disorders affecting the respiratory muscles, damage to the chest wall, and chronic lung diseases all can cause hypoventilation.

CARBON MONOXIDE POISONING

Hemoglobin has a much greater affinity for carbon monoxide than for oxygen.* It combines readily with carbon monoxide, forming a stable compound called *carboxyhemoglobin.* Thus, in a patient who has been exposed to carbon monoxide, the hemoglobin combines with the gas to the exclusion of oxygen, and the patient dies within a few minutes.

The treatment consists of removing the patient immediately from exposure to the carbon monoxide and commencing artificial respiration. Gradually, the carbon monoxide is liberated from the hemoglobin and the alveoli, and oxygen is taken up to form normal oxyhemoglobin. Ideally, the patient should be given an air mixture containing 40 percent oxygen and 7 percent carbon dioxide. The high oxygen concentration helps displace the carbon monoxide from the hemoglobin, and the carbon dioxide strongly stimulates the inspiratory center, which in turn increases the ventilation of the alveoli.

COMMON CLINICAL TERMS DESCRIBING ABNORMAL RESPIRATION

Dyspnea is the term used to describe difficult breathing (e.g., in asthma).

Anoxia is an absence of oxygen in the tissues (e.g., in tracheal or bronchial obstruction). *Hypoxia* is a reduced amount of oxygen in the tissues. *Anoxic anoxia* is a condition in which the blood leaves the

---

*It is interesting to note that oxygen and carbon monoxide combine at the same site on the hemoglobin molecule.

lungs without becoming normally saturated with oxygen (e.g., in high altitude flying). *Stagnant anoxia* occurs when the circulation of blood through the tissues is so slow that the oxyhemoglobin is permitted to give up a greater proportion of oxygen than normal. The venous blood leaving the tissues thus has a larger amount of reduced hemoglobin than normal (e.g., in heart failure). *Anemic anoxia* is caused by a decreased ability of the blood to carry an adequate amount of oxygen (e.g., in patients with low hemoglobin levels in the blood). *Histotoxic anoxia* occurs when the oxygen content of the blood is normal but the tissues are unable to use the oxygen (e.g., in cyanide poisoning).

Cyanosis is a blue coloration of the skin or mucous membrane caused by an excessive amount of reduced hemoglobin in the blood in the capillaries of these tissues (e.g., in heart failure).

CLINICAL PROBLEMS

For the answers to these problems, see page 799.

1. A 4-year-old boy is taken to a pediatrician because of blood-stained discharge from the right nostril of 4 days' duration. On examination, the child is found to have a piece of a plastic toy jammed in the middle meatus of his right nasal cavity. A small amount of blood-stained mucus is draining from the right nostril. Using your knowledge of microscopic anatomy, explain why foreign bodies become impacted in the nose. What is the structure of the mucous membrane in this area of the nose? Where is the mucus discharge coming from? Is the blood supply of the mucous membrane in this region scanty or profuse?

2. Following a severe cold, a patient complains of a frontal headache and a dull, aching pain on the right side of the face. What anatomical structures are likely to become secondarily infected from the nose? What is the microscopic structure of the lining of these areas?

3. A 40-year-old woman is seen by a surgeon and complains of severe pain and swelling over the left cheek. This condition, which had started 3 months previously, gradually had worsened. On examination, a large, hard swelling is found attached to the anterior surface of the left maxilla. Examination of the nose reveals a foul, purulent discharge from the left nostril that the patient states is often blood stained. A diagnosis of carcinoma of the left maxillary sinus is made. What is the structure of the mucous membrane lining the maxillary sinus (antrum)?

4. A 55-year-old man states that his wife has recently noticed an alteration in his voice. Toward the end of the day, his voice becomes husky, especially if he has been speaking a great deal. Three days previous, the huskiness had been so severe that he could speak only in a low whisper. Laryngoscopic examination reveals a papilloma of the right vocal fold. A biopsy is performed, and a subsequent diagnosis of carcinoma of the vocal fold is made. What is the normal microscopic structure of the vocal fold? Can you give a reason why the lining epithelium is different from the remainder of the larynx?

5. A 30-year-old man disturbs a hive of bees while he is painting his house. He promptly is stung on the face, neck, and arms. Knowing that he is hypersensitive to bee stings, a friend takes him to a local hospital, where he is admitted in a state of shock with extreme difficulty in breathing. Because there is edema of the larynx, it is decided to do an immediate tracheotomy. Why is edema of the larynx likely to obstruct the airway? During a tracheotomy, what structures does the knife cut through when passing through the wall of the trachea?

6. Describe the normal defense mechanisms that exist in the respiratory system. What is the likely fate of a small fragment of asbestos that has been inhaled?

7. Compare and contrast the structures of the trachea, a bronchus, a bronchiole, and a respiratory bronchiole.

8. A physician specializing in pulmonary medicine is heard to say, "As one traces the respiratory tract downward, one finds that the rigid support of its walls diminishes but the control of the size of the

lumen increases." Do you agree with that statement?

9. A 25-year-old man is found on routine chest x-ray to have a localized tuberculous lesion in the upper lobe of his right lung. It fails to respond to medication. Is it possible to remove a local area of the lung surgically? What is a bronchopulmonary segment? How does it differ from a pulmonary lobule?

10. An 18-year-old male athlete undergoing a physical examination informs his physician that at age 8 he had lobar pneumonia and pleurisy in his right lung. The physician decides to measure the vital capacity of the patient's respiratory system. Describe a simple method for taking this measurement. Define the following terms used in the description of air volumes in the lungs: (a) tidal volume, (b) inspiratory reserve volume, (c) expiratory reserve volume, (d) residual volume, (e) vital capacity.

11. Describe the structure of (a) an alveolar duct, (b) an alveolar sac, (c) an alveolus. What is the function of the different types of cells found lining the alveolar walls?

12. Describe the electron microscopic structure of the respiratory membrane. Give an account of the gaseous exchange that takes place across this membrane.

13. Blood leaving the lungs in the pulmonary veins has an oxygen saturation of about 97 percent. What is the pressure of oxygen in the blood in the pulmonary veins? What is the saturation of oxygen and the pressure of oxygen in the blood when it reaches the general tissues of the body?

14. In what form is carbon dioxide most commonly transported in the blood? What role does carbonic anhydrase play in this process? What is the chloride shift?

15. What is meant by the term *respiratory center?* Name three drugs that can stimulate and three clinical conditions that can depress the respiratory center.

16. Define the following: (a) Cheyne-Stokes breathing, (b) compliance, (c) pneumothorax, (d) surfactant.

ADDITIONAL READING

Andrews, P. M. A scanning electron microscopic study of the extrapulmonary respiratory tract. *Am. J. Anat.* 139:399, 1974.

Bradley, G. W. Control of the breathing pattern. *Int. Rev. Physiol.* 14:185, 1977.

Breeze, R. G., and Wheeldon, E. B. The cells of the pulmonary airways. *Am. Rev. Respir. Dis.* 116:705, 1977.

Cherniack, R. M. Ventilation, perfusion and gas exchange. In Frohlich, E. D. (ed.), *Pathophysiology* (2nd ed.). Philadelphia: Lippincott, 1976, p. 149.

Cohen, A. B., and Gold, W. M. Defense mechanisms of the lungs. *Annu. Rev. Physiol.* 37:325, 1975.

Davis, J. N. Control of the muscles of breathing. In Widdicombe, J. G. (ed.), *MTP International Review of Science: Physiology,* Vol. 2. Baltimore: University Park Press, 1974, p. 221.

Dermer, G. B. The pulmonary surfactant content of the inclusion bodies found within type II alveolar cells. *J. Ultrastruct. Res.* 33:306, 1970.

Fink, B. R. *The Human Larynx: A Functional Study.* New York: Raven, 1975.

Goerke, J. Lung surfactant. *Biochem. Biophys. Acta* 344:241, 1979.

Greenwood, M., and Holland, P. The mammalian respiratory tract surface: A scanning electron microscope study. *Lab. Invest.* 27:296, 1972.

Hance, A. J., and Crystal, R. G. The connective tissue of lung. *Am. Rev. Respir. Dis.* 112:657, 1975.

Jones, N. L. *Blood Gases and Acid-Base Physiology.* New York: Dekker, 1980.

Kuhn, C., III. The cells of the lung and their organelles. In Crystal, R. G. (ed.), *The Biochemical Basis of Pulmonary Function.* New York: Dekker, 1976.

Kuhn, C., III, and Finke, E. H. The topography of the pulmonary alveolus: Scanning electron microscopy using different fixations. *J. Ultrastruct. Res.* 38:161, 1972.

Macklem, P. T. Respiratory mechanics. *Annu. Rev. Physiol.* 40:157, 1978.

Mavis, R. D., Finkelstein, J. N., and Hall, B. P. Pulmonary surfactant synthesis: A highly active microsomal phosphatidate phosphohydrolase in the lung. *J. Lipid Res.* 19:467, 1978.

Michel, C. C. The transport of oxygen and carbon dioxide by the blood. In Widdicombe, J. G. (ed.), *MTP International Review of Science: Physiology*. Vol. 2. Baltimore: University Park Press, 1974, p. 67.

Mitchell, R. A. Control of respiration. In Frohlich, E. D. (ed.), *Pathophysiology* (2nd ed.). Philadelphia: Lippincott, 1976, p. 131.

Nagaishi, C. *Functional Anatomy and Histology of the Lung*. Baltimore: University Park Press, 1972.

Polyzonis, B. M., Kafandaris, P. M., Gigis, P. I., and Demetriou, T. An electron microscopic study of human olfactory mucosa. *J. Anat.* 128:77, 1979.

Ranga, V., and Kleinerman, J. Structure and function of small airways in health and disease. *Arch. Pathol. Lab. Med.* 102:609, 1978.

Takaro, T., Price, H. P., and Parra, S. C. Ultrastructural studies of apertures in the interalveolar septum of the adult human lung. *Am. Rev. Respir. Dis.* 119:425, 1979.

Thomas, E. D., et al. Direct evidence for a bone marrow origin of the alveolar macrophage in man. *Science* 192:1016, 1976.

Thurlbeck, W. M., and Abell, M. R. (eds.). *The Lung: Structure, Function, and Disease*. Baltimore: Williams & Wilkins, 1978.

Tisi, G. M. *Pulmonary Physiology in Clinical Medicine.* Baltimore: Williams & Wilkins, 1980.

Von Evler, C., and Lagercrantz, H. (eds.). *Central Nervous Control Mechanisms in Breathing*. New York: Pergamon, 1980.

Wagner, P. D. Diffusion and chemical reaction in pulmonary gas exchange. *Physiol. Rev.* 57:257, 1977.

Weibel, E. R. Morphological basis of alveolar capillary gas exchange. *Physiol. Rev.* 53:419, 1973.

Williams, M. H. (ed.). *Symposium on Disturbance of Respiratory Control*. Philadelphia: Saunders, 1980.

DIGESTIVE TRACT

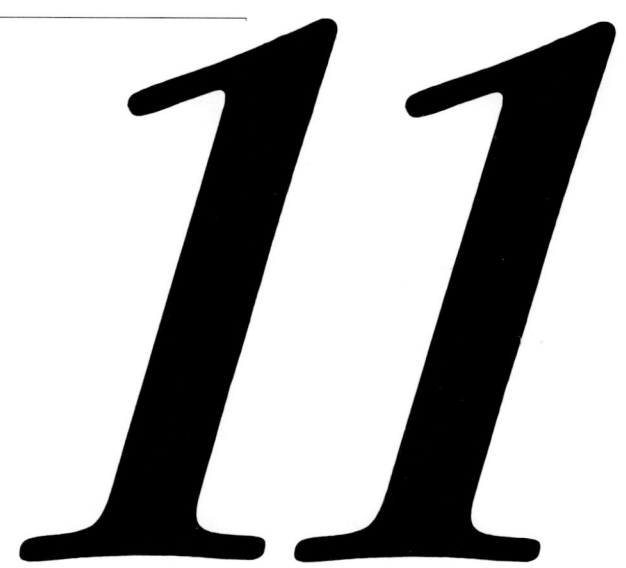

The digestive tract consists of a long, muscular tube that begins at the mouth and ends at the anus. Associated with the tube are glands that pour their secretions into the tube. The digestive process starts with the eating of food, which is followed by the mechanical and chemical breakdown of the ingested material. The products of digestion then pass readily from the intestinal lumen into the bloodstream and lymph, where they are distributed to and used by the body cells.

Digestion involves not only the decomposition of large, unabsorbable molecules into small, readily absorbable molecules, but also the mechanical processes of mastication, swallowing, and the propulsion of food along the muscular tube. In addition, the tube removes from the body the unabsorbed food residues and waste products in the form of fecal material.

The muscular tube can be divided into the mouth, pharynx, esophagus, stomach, and small and large intestines. Glandular organs involved in digestion that lie outside the alimentary tract are the salivary glands, liver, and pancreas. The liver and pancreas will be described in Chapter 12.

MOUTH

The mouth, or oral cavity, extends from the lips to the oropharyngeal isthmus. It is subdivided into the *vestibule,* which lies between the lips and cheeks externally and the gums and teeth internally, and the *mouth cavity proper,* which lies within the alveolar arches, gums, and teeth (Fig. 11-1).

Lips

Each lip is composed of a core of striated muscle, the *orbicularis oris,* embedded in fibroelastic connective tissue. The outer surface of the lips is covered with skin that contains many hair follicles, sebaceous glands, and sweat glands (Fig. 11-2; see Fig. 11-1). At the free margin of the lip is a red transitional zone between the outer skin and the mucous membrane of the mouth cavity. The redness of the lip margin is caused by the blood in the large capillary loops in the underlying connective tissue of the dermis. The epidermis of the red margin is not heavily keratinized; it is translucent, therefore, and the hemoglobin of the red cells can easily be seen. Because there are no sweat glands or sebaceous glands on the

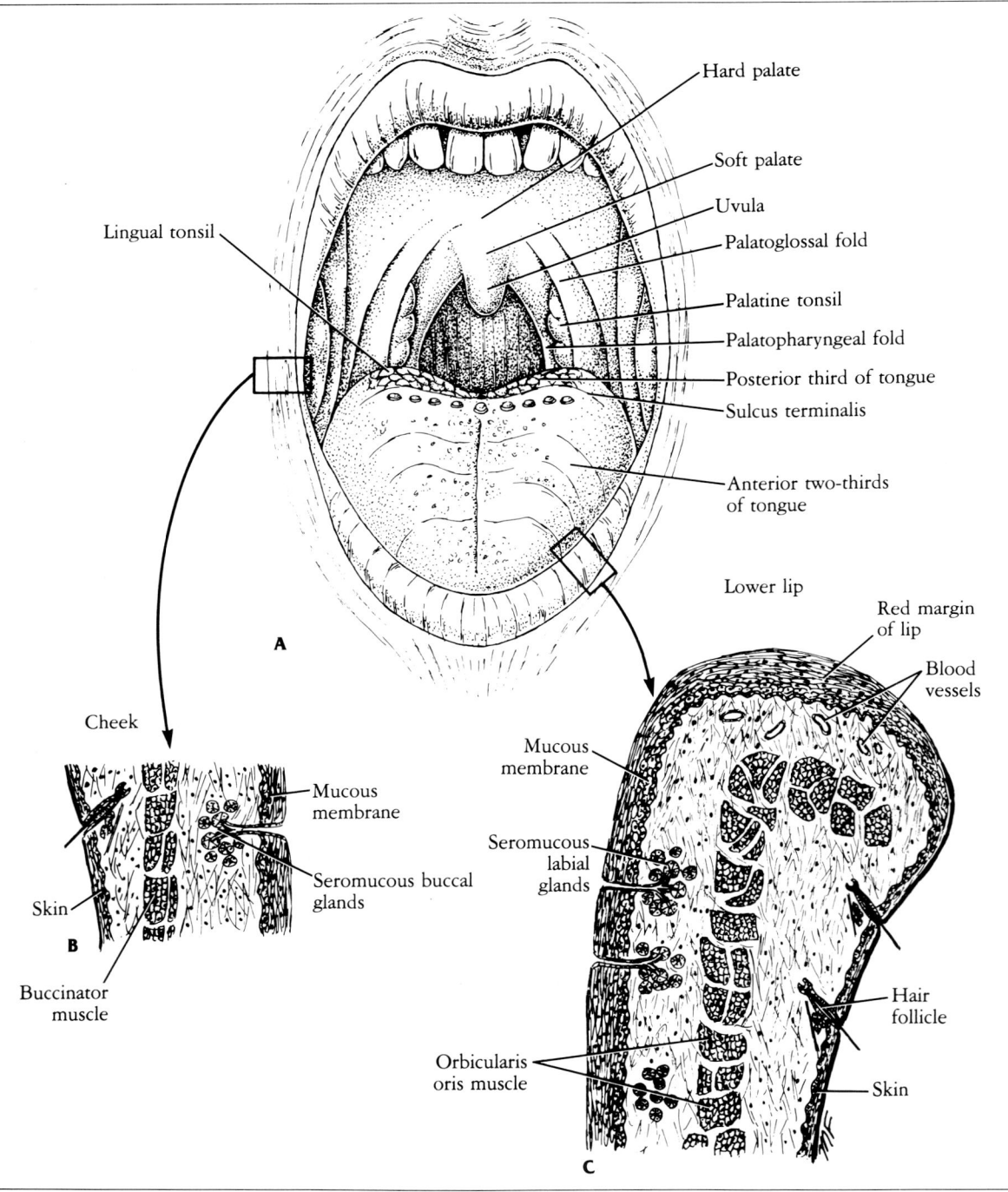

Fig. 11-1. A: Cavity of the mouth. B: Structure of the cheek. C: Structure of the lip.

lip margin, the lips must be wetted with saliva periodically by overlapping them or licking them with the tip of the tongue. Failure to do this will cause the lips to become "chapped."

The inner surface of the lip is covered with mucous membrane and consists of stratified squamous nonkeratinized epithelium lying on the connective tissue of the lamina propria. Small groups of mucous glands, the *labial glands,* are situated in the lamina propria and pour their secretions onto the surface through small ducts (Fig. 11-3; see Fig. 11-1).

The red margins of the lips are extremely sensitive to touch because of the numerous sensory nerve endings in the dermis.

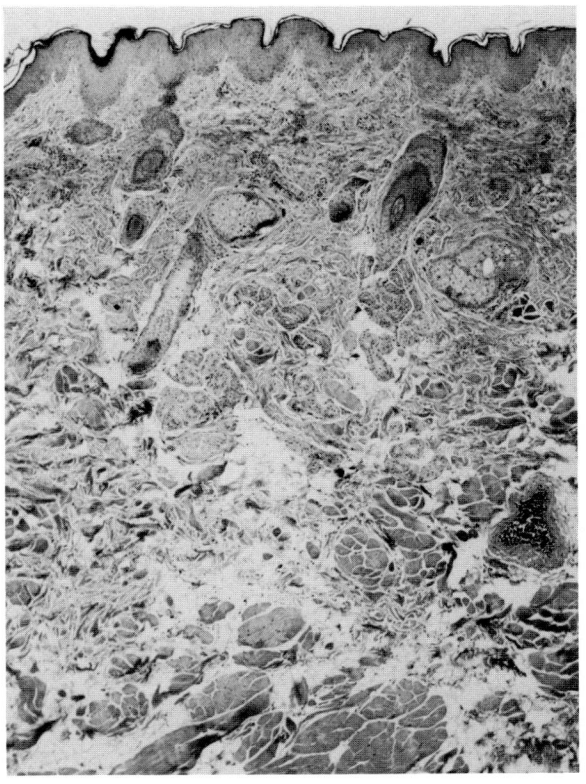

Fig. 11-2. Right: Photomicrograph of a section of the outer surface of the lip, showing skin, parts of hair follicles, and sebaceous glands. A portion of the orbicularis oris muscle is seen in the lower part of the photograph (H&E; ×40.)

Fig. 11-3. Below: Photomicrograph of a section of the inner surface of the lip, showing the thick mucous membrane covered by stratified squamous nonkeratinized epithelium. Some mucous glands in the lamina propria are just visible in the lower part of the photograph. (H&E; ×40.)

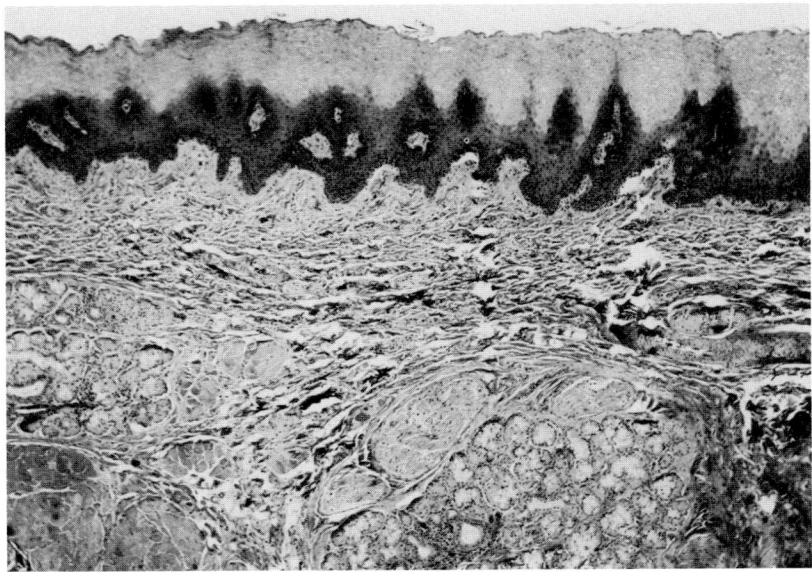

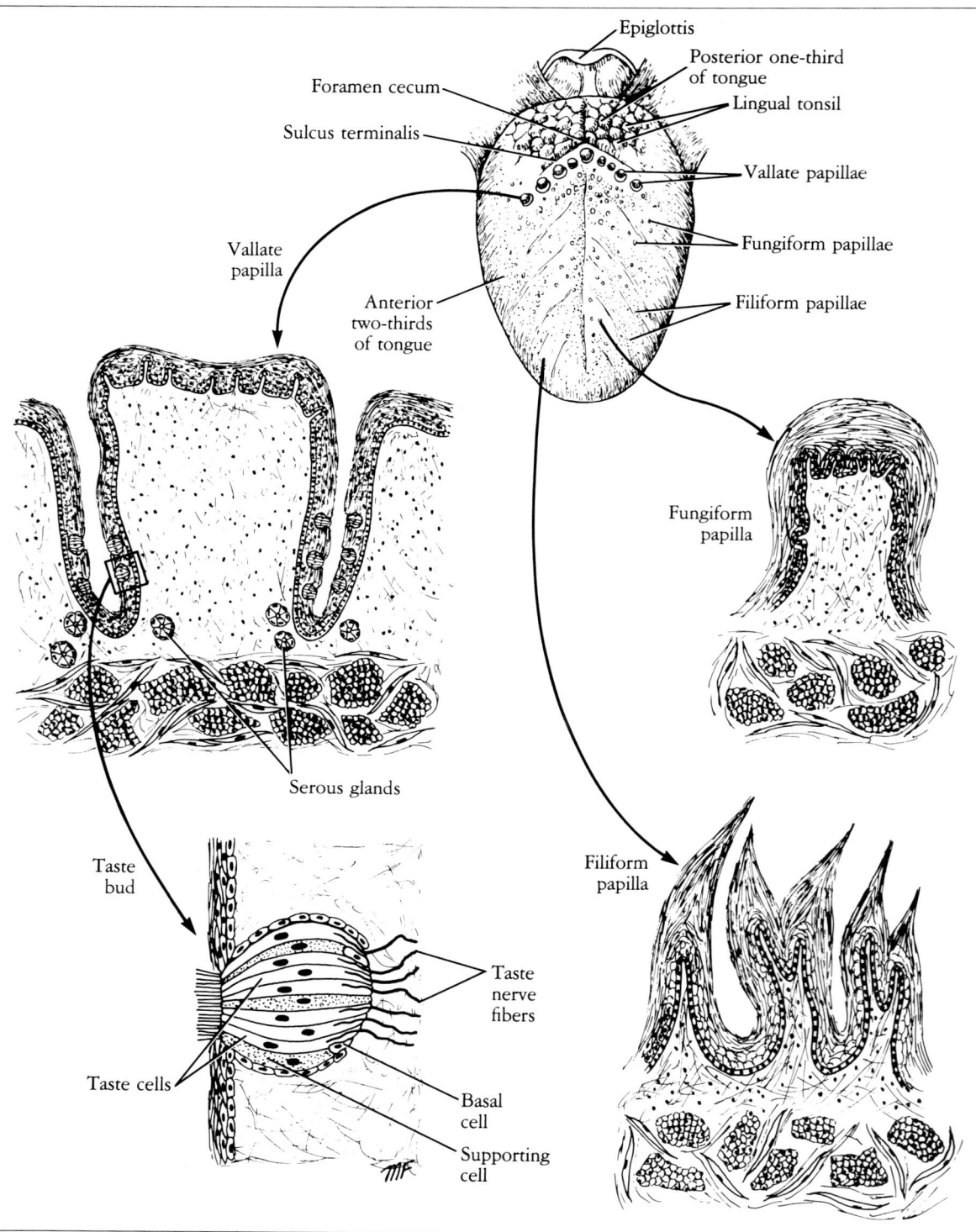

Fig. 11-4. Dorsal surface of the tongue. Shown are the location and detailed structure of the vallate papillae, fungiform papillae, and filiform papillae. The structure of a taste bud is also shown.

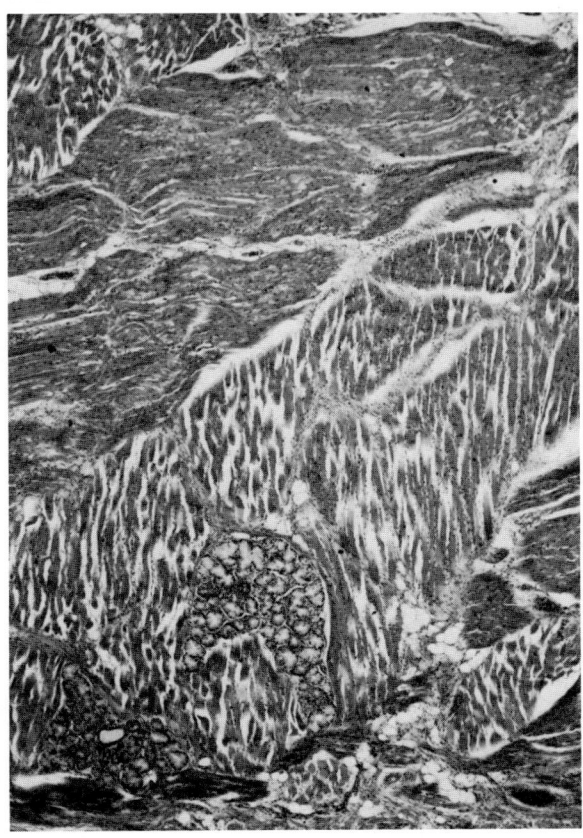

Fig. 11-5. Photomicrograph of a longitudinal section of part of the tongue. The interior of the tongue is composed of bundles of striated muscle arranged in longitudinal, transverse, and vertical directions. (H&E; ×40.)

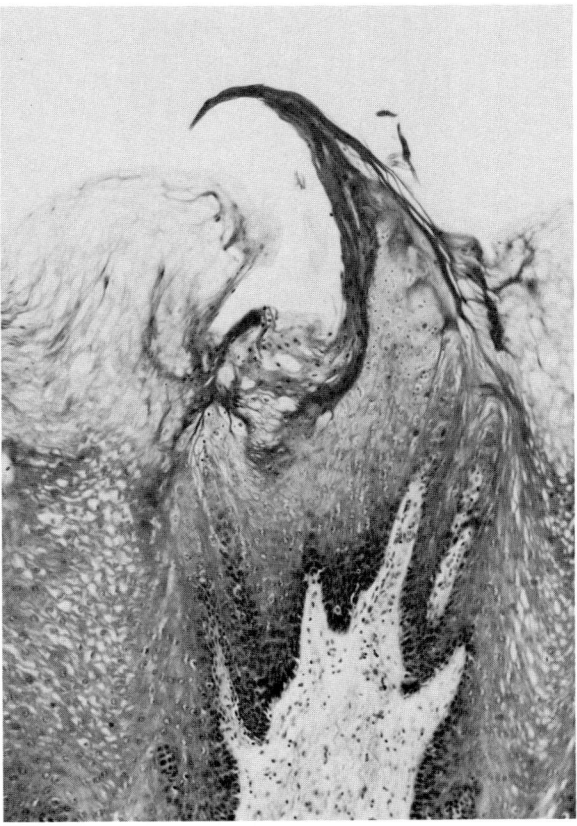

Fig. 11-6. Photomicrograph of a section of a filiform papilla in the mucous membrane of the dorsal surface of the anterior part of the tongue. Note that the papilla is covered with keratinized stratified squamous epithelium and has a core of connective tissue. (H&E; ×100.)

Cheeks

The cheeks have basically the same structure as the lips, having a core of skeletal muscle, called the *buccinator,* that is covered on the outside by skin and subcutaneous connective tissue and lined on the inside by mucous membrane (see Fig. 11-1). The mucous membrane is tethered to the bucinnator muscle by elastic fibers in the submucosa. These elastic fibers prevent redundant folds of mucous membrane from being bitten between the teeth when the jaws are closed.

Tongue

The tongue is a mass of striated muscle covered with mucous membrane (Fig. 11-4).

The muscles of the tongue are of two types, intrinsic and extrinsic. The intrinsic muscles are confined to the tongue and consist of bundles of fibers embedded in connective tissue. They are arranged in longitudinal, transverse, and vertical directions (Fig. 11-5), and they alter the shape of the tongue. The right and left halves of the tongue are separated by a septum composed of connective tissue.

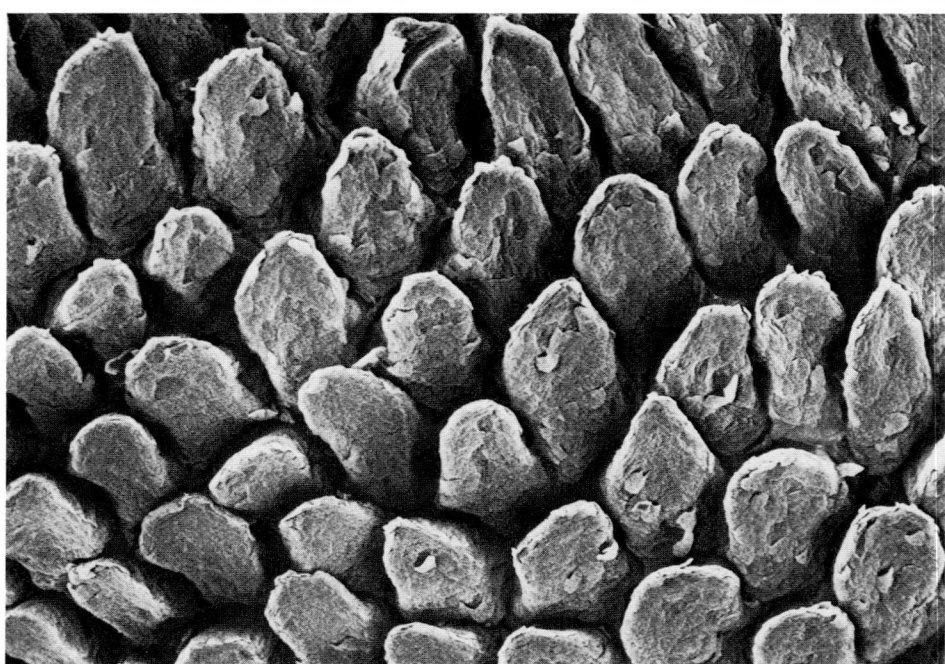

Fig. 11-7. Scanning electron micrograph of the dorsal surface of the anterior part of the tongue, showing numerous filiform papillae. (×140.) (Courtesy of Dr. M. Koering.)

The extrinsic muscles of the tongue extend from the tongue to the mandible, the styloid process of the skull, and the soft palate. The extrinsic muscles alter the position of the tongue.

The mucous membrane of the upper surface of the tongue is divided into anterior and posterior parts by a V-shaped sulcus, the *sulcus terminalis* (see Fig. 11-4). The apex of the sulcus projects backward and is marked by a small pit, the *foramen cecum*. The sulcus thus divides the tongue into the anterior two-thirds, or oral part, and the posterior third, or pharyngeal part. The foramen cecum is an embryological remnant and marks the site of the upper end of the thyroglossal duct.

The mucous membrane covering the upper surface of the anterior two-thirds of the tongue has numerous small projections, called *papillae*. The papillae are of three types: (1) filiform, (2) fungiform, and (3) vallate.

The *filiform papillae* are conical and about 2 to 3 mm long (Figs. 11-6 and 11-7; see Fig. 11-4). They are very numerous and cover the anterior two-thirds of the tongue on its upper surface. Each papilla has a connective tissue core that is covered with keratinized stratified squamous epithelium. The papillae are whitish because of the thickness of the squamous epithelium.

The *fungiform papillae* are mushroom shaped and are about the same height as the filiform papillae (Fig. 11-8; see Fig. 11-4). They are found chiefly on the sides and apex of the tongue. Each has a very vascular connective tissue core that imparts a reddish tinge to the papilla. The stratified squamous epithelium covering the surface is nonkeratinized, and occasional taste buds are present.

The *vallate papillae* are ten to twelve in number and they are situated in a row immediately in front of the sulcus terminalis (Fig. 11-9; see Fig. 11-4). Each papilla measures about 2 mm in diameter and protrudes slightly from the surface. It is surrounded by a circular furrow, in the walls of which lie taste

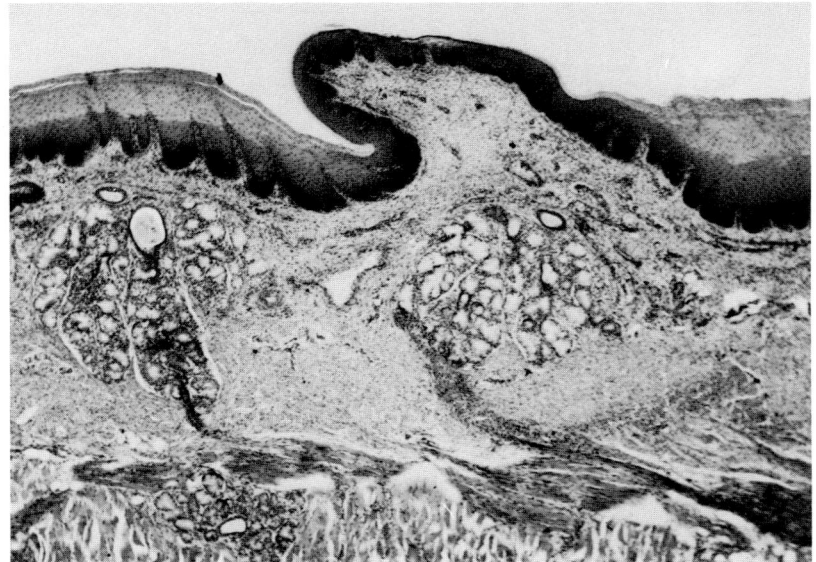

Fig. 11-8. Photomicrograph of a section of a fungiform papilla in the mucous membrane of the dorsal surface of the anterior part of the tongue. Note that the papilla is covered with nonkeratinized stratified squamous epithelium and has a core of vascular connective tissue. Some serous glands also can be seen in the lamina propria. (H&E; ×40.)

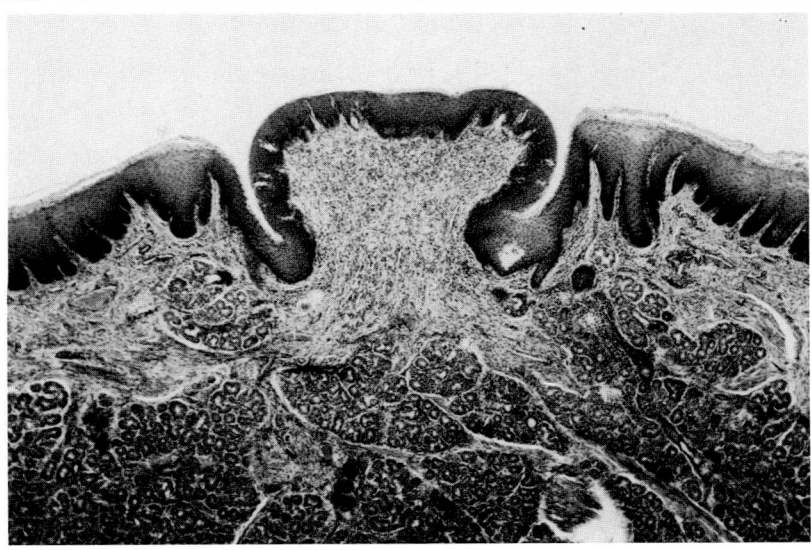

Fig. 11-9. Photomicrograph of a section of a vallate papilla in the mucous membrane of the tongue just in front of the sulcus terminalis. Note that the papilla is surrounded by a furrow, in the walls of which lie taste buds. The papilla is covered with nonkeratinized stratified squamous epithelium. Note the serous glands close to the bottom of the furrow. (H&E; ×40.)

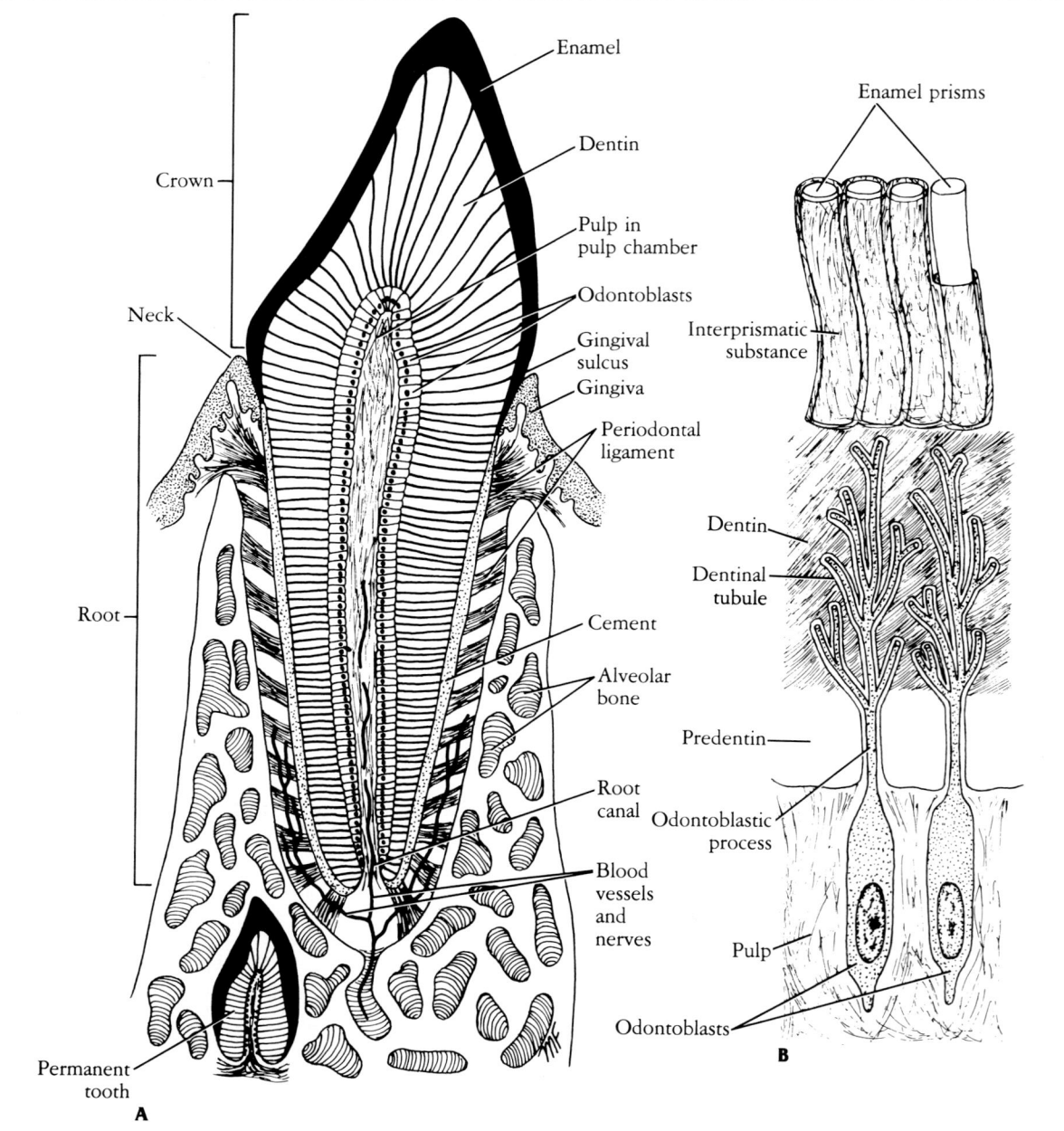

Fig. 11-10. A: Sagittal section of a deciduous incisor tooth with an unerupted permanent incisor shown below. B: Section through portions of the pulp, predentin, dentin, and enamel. Note the location of the odontoblast cell body and the odontoblastic process in the dentin.

buds. The papilla is covered by nonkeratinized stratified squamous epithelium. Serous glands open into the bottom of the furrow surrounding each papilla.

The mucous membrane covering the posterior third of the tongue is devoid of papillae but has a nodular, irregular surface because of underlying lymphatic nodules, the *lingual tonsil.*

The mucous membrane on the inferior surface of the tongue is smooth and is reflected from the tongue to the floor of the mouth. In the midline anteriorly, the undersurface of the tongue is connected to the floor of the mouth by a fold of mucous membrane, the *frenulum* of the tongue.

Taste Buds

The taste buds (see Fig. 11-4) are most numerous on the upper surface of the tongue, where they are associated with the fungiform and vallate papillae and the surface epithelium between them. Taste buds are also found scattered in the mucous membrane of the palate and pharynx. The structure of taste buds is described on page 770.

Teeth

There are two sets of teeth, appearing at different times of life. The first set, called the *deciduous teeth,* is temporary. The second set is called the *permanent teeth* (Fig. 11-10).

The *deciduous teeth* are twenty in number; four incisors, two canines, and four molars in each jaw. They begin to erupt at about the sixth month of life and have all erupted by the end of the second year. The teeth of the lower jaw usually appear before those of the upper jaw.

The *permanent teeth* are thirty-two in number, including four incisors, two canines, four premolars and six molars in each jaw. They begin to erupt at the sixth year of life. The last tooth to erupt is the third molar, however, and it does not do so until between the seventeeth and thirtieth years. Again, the teeth of the lower jaw usually appear before those of the upper jaw.

The deciduous and permanent teeth have similar microscopic structures (see Fig. 11-10). The teeth

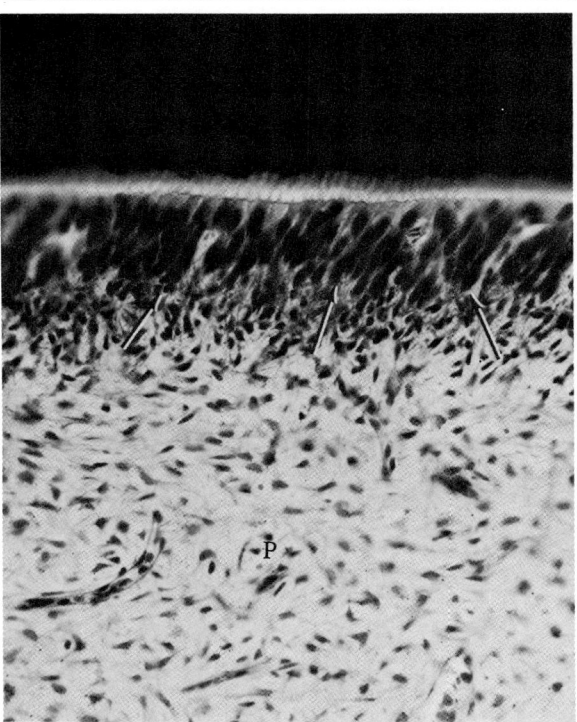

Fig. 11-11. Photomicrograph of a portion of a sagittal section of a deciduous tooth, showing the pulp (P) with odontoblasts (arrows), predentin (clear zone), and dentin (black zone). Note the dentinal tubules in the predentin. (H&E; ×200.)

are set in sockets on the alveolar processes of the mandible and the maxillae. The alveolar processes are covered by a mucoperiosteum known as the *gums* or *gingivae.* The part of the tooth that projects above the gums is the *crown*; the portion that lies within the socket is the root (see Fig. 11-10). The roots of the teeth are held securely in their sockets by bundles of collagen fibers called the *periodontal ligament.* The crown and root of a tooth join at the *neck.*

In the center of each tooth is the *pulp cavity,* which is filled with loose connective tissue containing nerves, blood, and lymph vessels. Extensions of the pulp cavity pass into the roots of the tooth and are called *root canals.* The root canals communicate with

Fig. 11-12. Photomicrograph of a section of a tooth, showing a portion of dentin with dentinal tubules. (×100.)

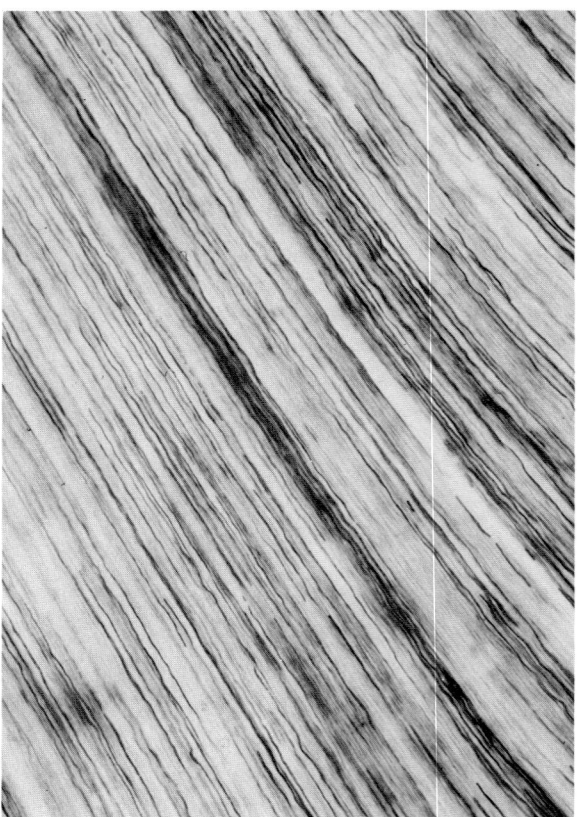

Fig. 11-13. Photomicrograph of dentin, showing dentinal tubules cut in longitudinal section. The dark wavy lines represent the odontoblastic processes within the tubules. (H&E; ×200.)

the connective tissue outside the tooth through a small foramen called the *apical foramen* (see Fig. 11-10).

The wall of the tooth is composed largely of a calcified connective tissue called *dentin* (see Fig. 11-10). The dentin is protected in the crown by a covering of tough *enamel;* in the root of the tooth, it is covered by a calcified connective tissue called *cementum*. The general structure of a tooth is shown in Figure 11-10.

Dentin

Dentin is a calcified connective tissue that is harder than compact bone. It consists of 80 percent inorganic material in the form of calcium salts (hydroxyapatite crystals) and 20 percent organic material. The dentin is formed by cells known as *odontoblasts* that line the pulp cavity (Fig. 11-11). As more and more dentin is formed during the development of the tooth, the cell bodies of the odontoblasts recede toward the center of the tooth, each leaving behind in the dentin a fine cellular process called the *odontoblastic process*. Each odontoblastic process is housed in a thin, curved *dentinal tubule* (Figs. 11-12 and 11-13), which runs from the pulp cavity to the periphery of the dentin. The walls of the dentinal tubules and the meshwork of collagen between them are

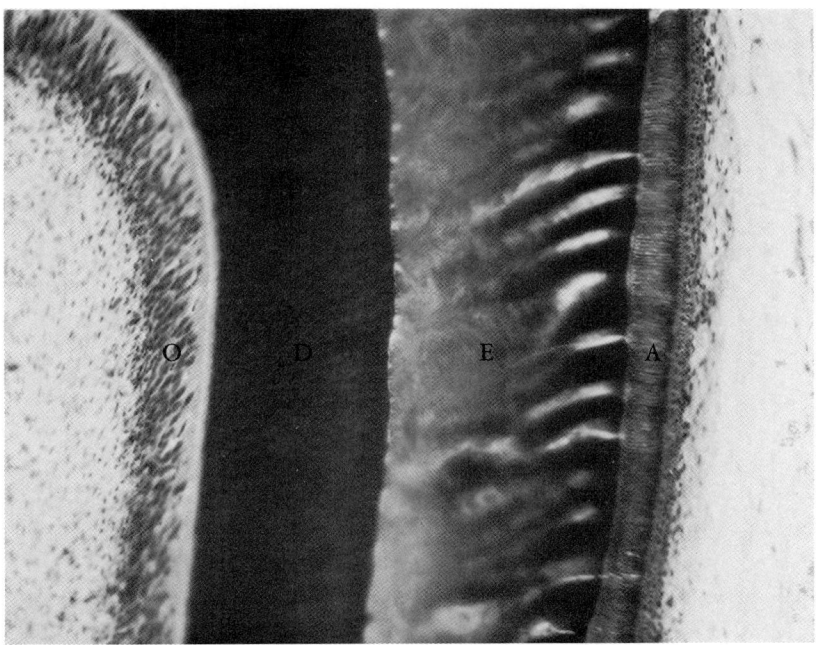

Fig. 11-14. Photomicrograph of a section of a developing tooth, showing odontoblasts (O), dentin (D), enamel (E), and ameloblasts (A). (H&E; ×100.)

embedded in calcium salts. Dentin formation continues throughout life, and the pulp cavity is progressively encroached upon with age. The newly formed dentin close to the pulp cavity that is laid down just before calcification takes place is called *predentin* (Fig. 11-14; see also Fig. 11-11).

Dentin is sensitive to touch, cold, and acid. It is believed that the odontoblastic processes transmit sensory information to the nerve endings in the pulp.

Enamel

Enamel is the hardest material found in the body, and it covers only the crown of the tooth (Fig. 11-15; see Fig. 11-10). It consists of 99.5 percent inorganic material in the form of large apatite crystals. The enamel is formed by cells called *ameloblasts*. These cells produce long, thin enamel rods, or prisms, which become calcified. Each prism is secreted at right angles to the underlying dentin and extends through the full thickness of the enamel. Surrounding each prism is a clear area of organic matrix. Once the enamel is laid down, the ameloblasts disappear.

Cementum

Cementum is similar in structure and composition to bone; it covers the root of a tooth. It is attached to the surrounding bone by the periodontal ligament (Fig. 11-16). In the region of the neck of the tooth, the cementum is acellular and consists of bundles of collagen embedded in a calcified matrix. Near the apex of the root of the tooth, the cementum is thick and cellular. The cells are called *cementocytes* and occupy lacunae in the matrix.

Pulp

The pulp fills the pulp cavity of the tooth and consists of vascular connective tissue containing star-

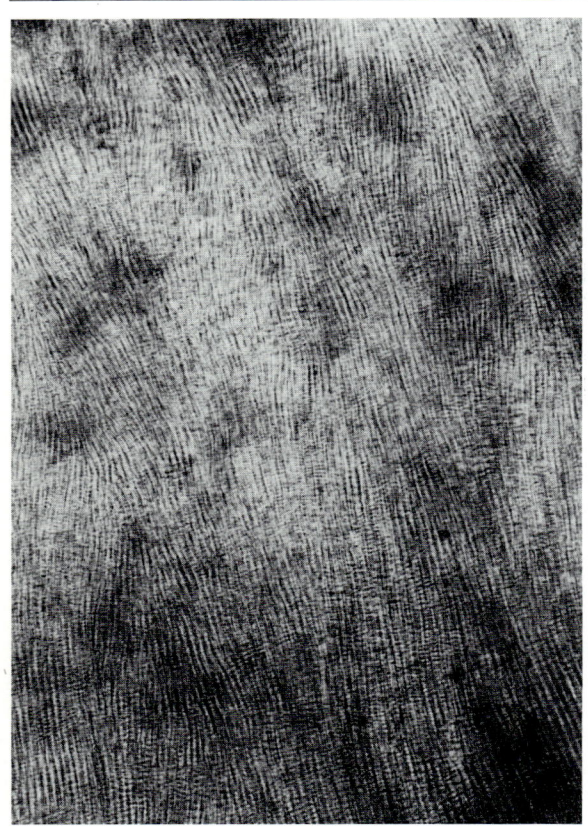

Fig. 11-15. Photomicrograph of a section of tooth enamel. The dark lines represent the organic matrix that lies between the enamel rods, or prisms. (×200.)

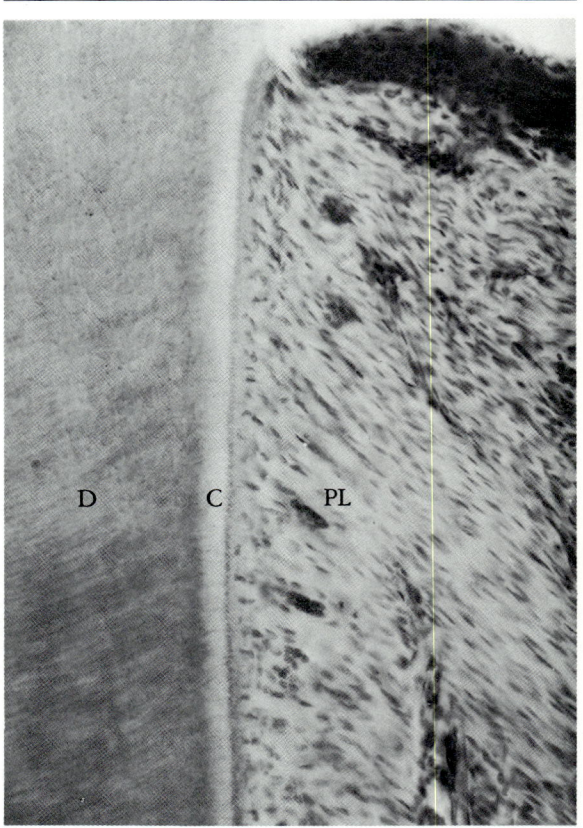

Fig. 11-16. Photomicrograph of a section of the periodontal ligament, or membrane (PL). Note on the left that the ligament is attached to the cementum (C). The dentin (D) with dentinal tubules also can be seen. A small portion of the gingiva is visible at the top. (H&E; ×200.)

shaped cells, thin collagenous fibrils, and a gelatinous ground substance (see Fig. 11-11). Lining the pulp cavity and adjacent to the dentin are the odontoblasts. The pulp contains many nerve fibers, which end in close association with the odontoblasts.

Throughout life, new dentin is deposited on the inner surface of the pulp cavity, gradually reducing its size.

Periodontal Ligament

The periodontal ligament, or membrane, surrounds the root of the tooth and suspends it within the tooth's bony socket. It consists of bundles of collagen fibers that extend from the cementum covering the root to the alveolar bone (see Fig. 11-16). When pressure is not being applied to the tooth, the collagen fibers become slack. The periodontal ligament is very sensitive to pressure and has a rich nerve supply.

Gingiva

The gingiva, or gum, is that part of the mucous membrane of the mouth that tightly surrounds the neck of the teeth like a collar. Its surface is covered with keratinized stratified squamous epithelium, and it is strongly attached to the alveolar periosteum.

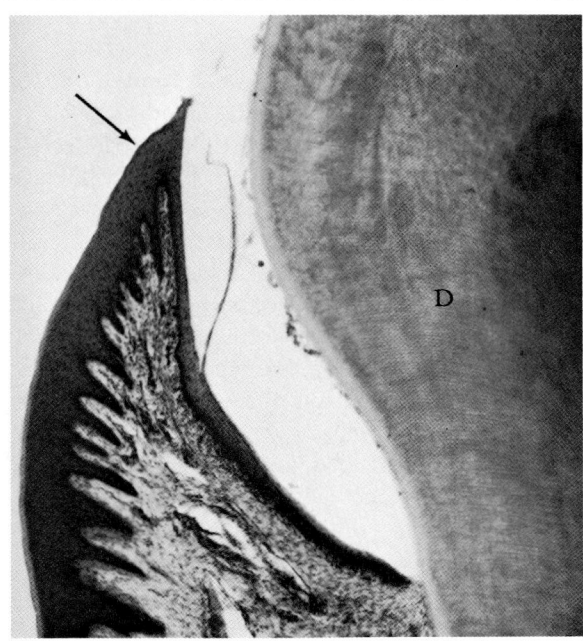

Fig. 11-17. Photomicrograph of a section through the gingival sulcus. The enamel has been dissolved, leaving a very wide sulcus. Note the gingiva (arrow) and the dentin (D). (H&E; ×40.)

Between the enamel and the superficial part of the gingiva is a shallow crevice, the *gingival sulcus,* which surrounds the tooth (Fig. 11-17; see Fig. 11-10).

Palate

The palate forms the roof of the mouth. It is divided into two parts: the hard palate, in front, and the soft palate, behind.

The *hard palate* forms a rigid surface against which the tongue can force food during mastication. It is formed by the palatine processes of the maxillae and the horizontal plates of the palatine bones. The undersurface of the hard palate is covered with mucoperiosteum and possesses a median ridge, on either side of which the mucous membrane is corrugated. The mucous membrane is covered with stratified squamous keratinized epithelium and possesses numerous mucous glands.

The *soft palate* is a mobile fold attached to the

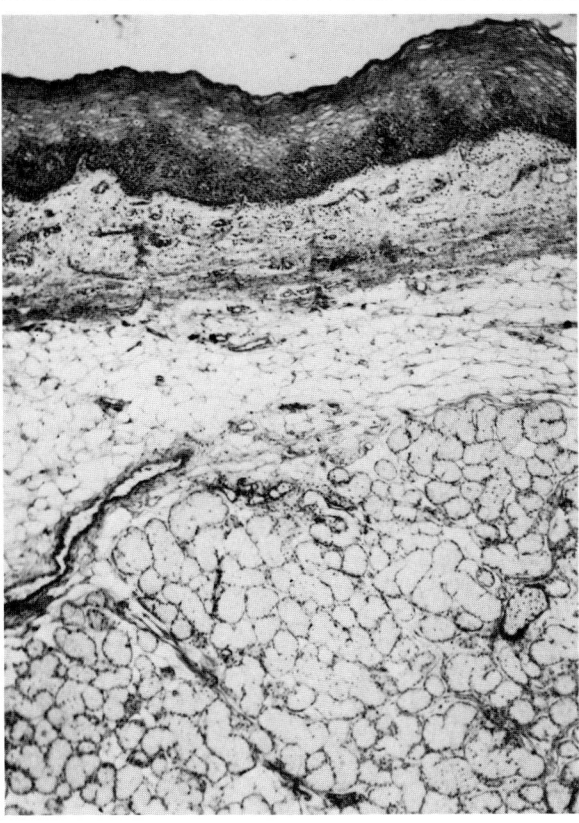

Fig. 11-18. Photomicrograph of a section through a portion of the soft palate. The oral surface (top) is covered with nonkeratinized stratified squamous epithelium. Note the numerous mucous glands in the lamina propria. (H&E; ×40.)

posterior border of the hard palate. Its free posterior border in the midline presents a conical projection called the *uvula.* The function of the soft palate is to close off the nasal part of the pharynx from the oral part during swallowing.

The soft palate is covered on its upper and lower surfaces by mucous membrane and contains an aponeurosis, voluntary muscle fibers (the musculus uvulae), lymphoid tissue (see p. 354), glands, blood vessels, and nerves. The mucous membrane lining the oral surface is covered with stratified squamous nonkeratinized epithelium (Fig. 11-18); the nasal surface is covered with pseudostratified ciliated columnar epithelium.

SALIVATION

Salivary Glands

There are numerous small salivary glands and three large pairs of salivary glands that continuously pour their secretions, the *saliva,* into the mouth cavity. The saliva moistens the lips and the mucous membrane of the mouth. The small salivary, or buccal, glands are widely scattered throughout the walls of the mouth cavity. The large salivary glands are situated outside the mouth and are called the *parotid,* the *submandibular,* and the *sublingual glands* (Fig. 11-19).

Parotid Glands

The parotid glands are the largest pair of salivary glands and are situated below the external auditory meatus and behind the mandible. The ducts of the glands pass forward and open into the vestibule of the mouth, opposite the upper second molar teeth (see Fig. 11-19).

The parotid gland is surrounded by a fibrous capsule. From the inner surface of the capsule, fibrous septa enter the gland, dividing it into lobes and lobules. One of the distinguishing features of this gland are the groups of adipose tissue cells contained in many of the septa. Delicate connective tissue containing blood vessels and nerves surrounds the ducts and acini. Myoepithelial cells are also present around the ducts and acini.

The secretory portion of the gland is composed entirely of tubulo-alveolar acini of the *serous* type (Fig. 11-20; see Fig. 11-19). The serous cells are roughly cuboidal or pyramidal in shape and surround a small tubular lumen. The nucleus of each cell is spherical and centrally located. Between the nucleus and the luminal surface of the cell, the cytoplasm contains numerous zymogen granules that stain purple with H&E. The number of secretory granules varies with the activity of the gland. Electron microscopy shows that this area of the cytoplasm also contains rough endoplasmic reticulum and a well-developed Golgi apparatus. Large amounts of rough endoplasmic reticulum are found in the cytoplasm of the basal part of the cell and are responsible for the bluish color of the cytoplasm seen with the light microscope.

The ducts of the parotid gland convey the secretions of the serous acini to the mouth cavity. The smallest ducts start within the lobules and are called *intralobular ducts* (see Fig. 11-19). Each intralobular duct is divided into an *intercalated* and a *striated duct.* The intercalated duct leads directly out of each acinus and is lined with low cuboidal epithelium. The striated duct is located distally and is lined with tall columnar cells showing vertical striations. Under the electron microscope, the vertical striations are seen to be large infoldings of the plasma membrane of the base of the cell.

The intralobular ducts join one another to form *interlobular ducts,* and they in turn join to form the final *excretory ducts.* The interlobular and excretory ducts are lined with columnar epithelium (see Fig. 11-19).

Submandibular Glands

The submandibular glands are situated below the floor of the mouth just beneath the body of the mandible (see Fig. 11-19). Their ducts extend forward and open into the mouth cavity on either side of the frenulum of the tongue just behind the lower incisor teeth.

The submandibular gland, like the parotid gland, is surrounded by a fibrous capsule and has fibrous septa that divide it into lobes and lobules. There is almost no adipose tissue within the gland.

The secretory portion of the gland is composed of tubulo-alveolar acini of the *mucous* and *serous* types (Fig. 11-21; see Fig. 11-19). The majority of the acini are serous.

The mucous cells are polyhedral in shape and surround a large lumen. The nucleus of each cell is flat and located near the base of the cell (see Fig. 11-21). Between the nucleus and the luminal surface of the cell, the cytoplasm contains large droplets of *mucigen,* which later becomes mucin. In an H&E-stained section, the mucigen is largely absent, leaving clear empty spaces. The small amount of cytoplasm in the basal region of the cell contains the rough-surfaced

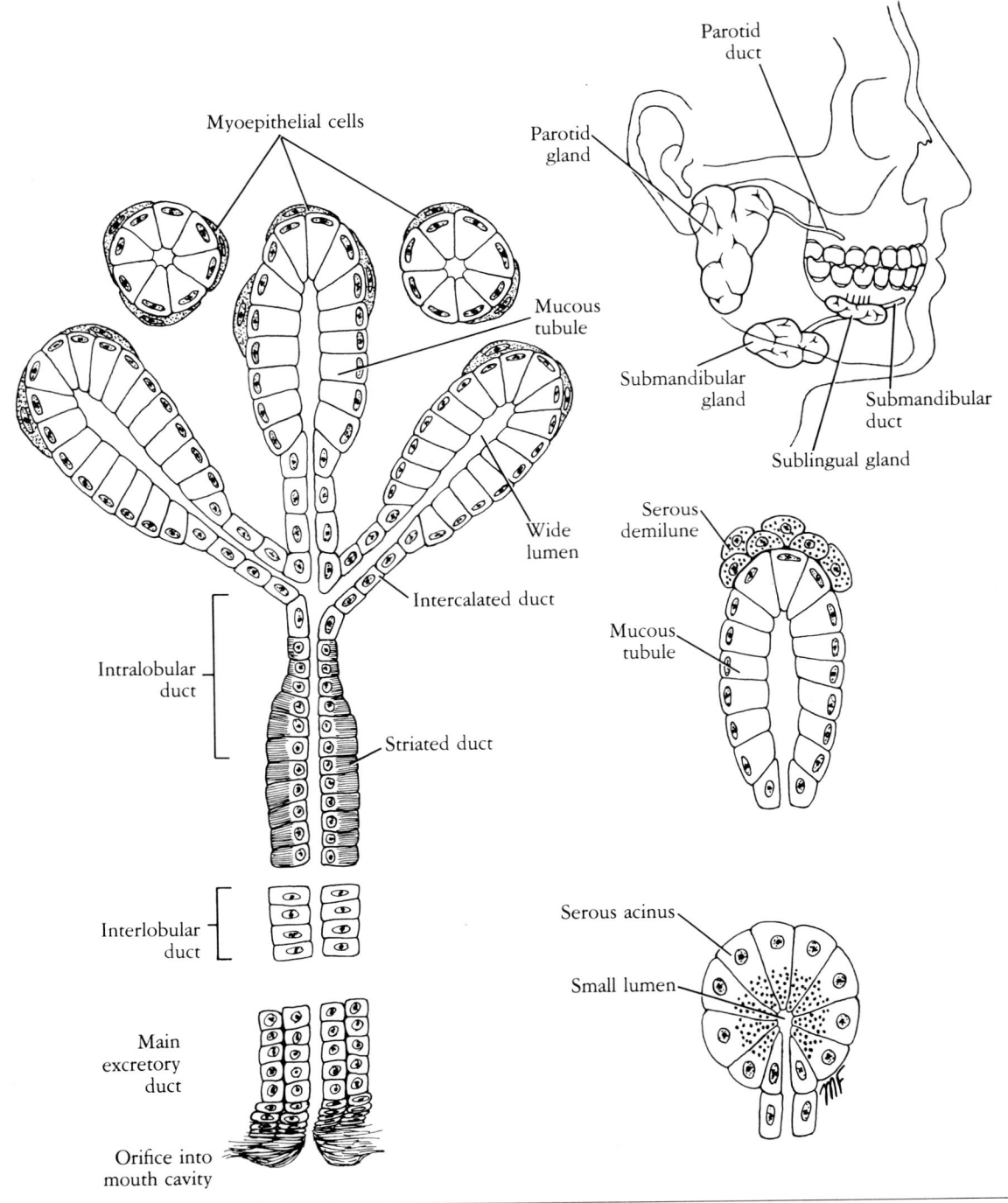

Fig. 11-19. *Location and basic structure of the parotid, submandibular, and sublingual salivary glands. Note the detailed epithelial structure of a mucous tubule, a serous acinus, a serous demilune, and the ducts.*

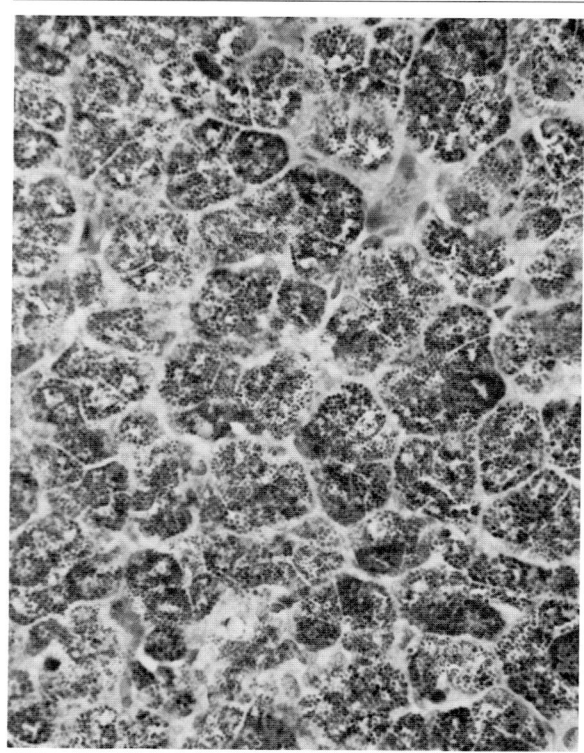

Fig. 11-20. Photomicrograph of a section of the parotid salivary gland, showing numerous serous acini whose lining cells contain zymogen granules. (H&E; ×400.)

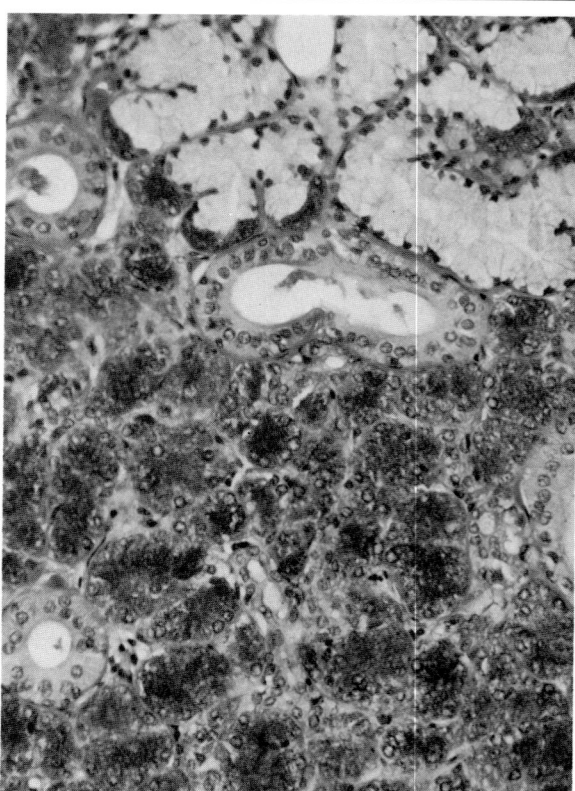

Fig. 11-21. Photomicrograph of a section of the submandibular salivary gland, showing numerous serous acini and a few mucous acini (top). The lining cells of the serous acini are filled with zymogen granules; the lining cells of the mucous acini show clear empty spaces. Note the basal position of the nuclei of the mucous cells. Several interlobular ducts also can be seen. (H&E; ×200.)

endoplasmic reticulum. The Golgi apparatus is situated between the mucigen droplets and the nucleus.

The serous cells are similar in structure to those found in the parotid gland. They are situated at the terminal end of the tubulo-alveolar acini or are arranged in small groups or crescents outside the ends of the tubules of the mucous acini (see Fig. 11-21). In the crescents, or *demilunes*, the serous cells are flattened, and their secretion passes through clefts between the mucous cells to enter the lumen of the acinus. The duct system is similar to that found in the parotid salivary gland.

Sublingual Glands

Each sublingual gland is situated below the floor of the mouth and lies anterior to the submandibular gland. The secretions enter the mouth by eight to twenty short ducts.

The sublingual gland, unlike the parotid and submandibular salivary glands, is not surrounded by a fibrous capsule; loose connective tissue septa divide the interior of the gland into lobes and lobules.

The secretory portion of the gland is composed of tubulo-alveolar acini of the mucous and serous types; the great majority of the acini are mucous (Fig. 11-22). The duct system is similar to that found in the other main salivary glands.

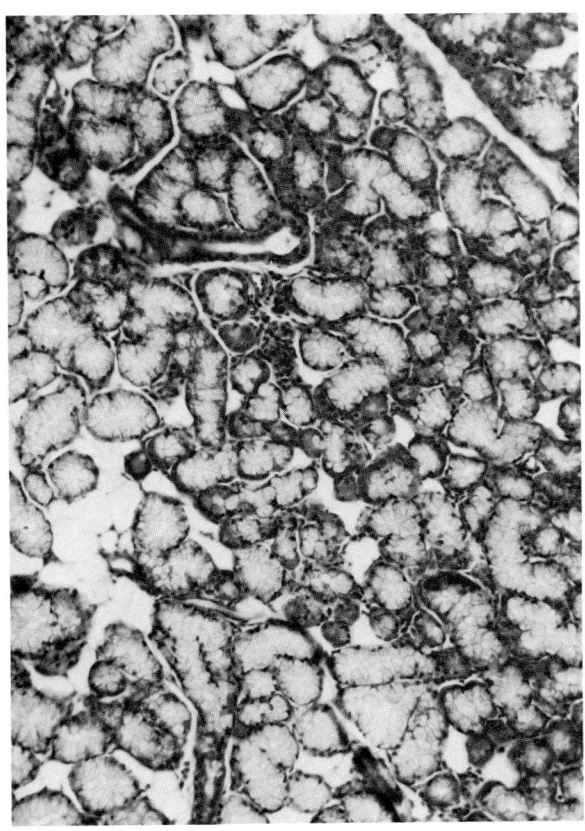

Fig. 11-22. Photomicrograph of a section of the sublingual salivary gland. Note that the great majority of the acini are mucous. (H&E; ×200.)

Saliva

The secretions of all the salivary glands are called saliva. The average adult secretes about 1,000 to 1,500 ml of saliva in 24 hours. Saliva has a pH of between 6.0 and 7.4. Saliva contains two types of secretions: (1) a serous secretion containing the enzyme *ptyalin* that digests starch and (2) a mucous secretion for lubrication and cleansing. The parotid glands are the largest salivary glands, and their secretion is entirely serous. The submandibular glands secrete a mixture of serous and mucous secretions; the sublingual and numerous buccal glands predominantly secrete mucus.

Functions

The functions of saliva are: (1) digestion, (2) lubrication of food and the mouth, (3) solvent action, (4) cleansing of the mouth, and (5) excretion.

DIGESTION. Saliva contains the enzyme *ptyalin*, which is secreted by the serous acini of the salivary glands. The enzyme hydrolyzes the polysaccharide starch into the disaccharides maltose and isomaltose. The process of starch digestion begins in the mouth and continues within the bolus after the food has been swallowed. Ptyalin is active only in an alkaline or neutral medium; its activity ceases once it is exposed to the acid of the gastric secretion.

LUBRICATION OF FOOD AND THE MOUTH. The mixing of food with saliva during mastication allows the food to be formed into a slimy mass that is swallowed easily. Lubrication of the lips, tongue, and cheeks allows them to move easily upon one another for the purposes of articulation.

SOLVENT ACTION. For substances to stimulate the taste buds and thus be tasted, they must enter into solution; saliva provides the solvent.

CLEANSING THE MOUTH. Saliva continuously bathes the teeth and the mucous membrane lining the mouth, washing off food particles, shed epithelial cells, and bacteria. Any disease process that inhibits salivary secretion results in *halitosis* (bad breath) because of the decomposing of food particles by bacteria secondary to stagnation.

EXCRETION. Organic and inorganic materials, drugs, and organisms can be excreted in the saliva. Potassium, iodine, mercury, and lead are excreted in the saliva; the lead combines with sulfur to be deposited as the characteristic blue line on the gum margins. The virus of rabies is excreted in saliva.

Control of Salivary Secretion

The salivary glands are supplied by sympathetic and parasympathetic nerves from the autonomic ner-

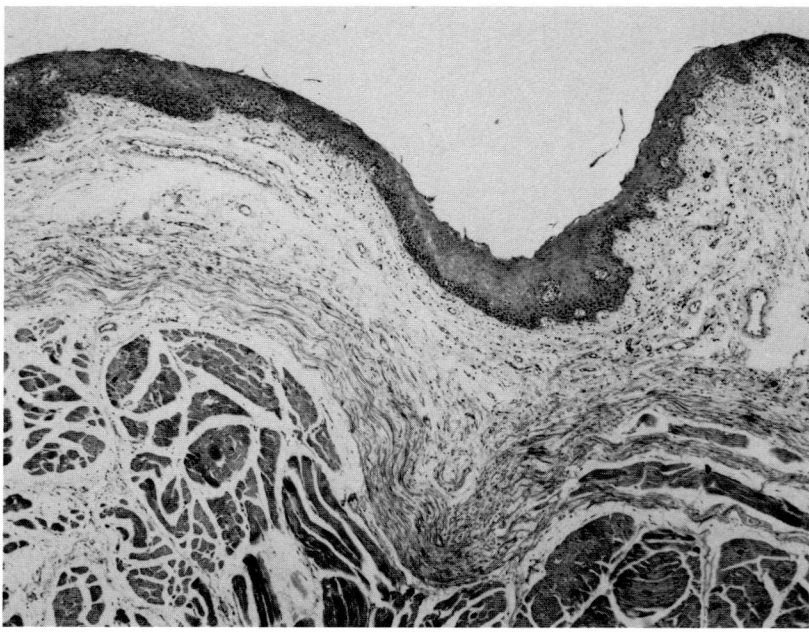

Fig. 11-23. Photomicrograph of a section of the wall of the oral part of the pharynx, showing the mucous membrane to be lined with stratified squamous nonkeratinized epithelium. A portion of the constrictor muscles can be seen in the lower part of the photograph. (H&E; ×40.)

vous system. The sympathetic nerves are derived from the superior cervical sympathetic ganglion, and the parasympathetic nerves are derived from the salivary nuclei of the facial and glossopharyngeal nerves.

Stimulation of the parasympathetic nerves produces copious secretion of saliva, whereas stimulation of the sympathetic nerves causes only a slight increase in secretion. Sympathetic stimulation also causes constriction of the blood vessels, so that sympathetic activity eventually reduces the output of saliva.

Normally, salivary secretion is a reflex phenomenon brought about by stimulation of the taste buds and sensory fibers in the mouth. Irritating foods in the stomach can stimulate excessive salivary secretion, as when an individual is nauseated. Higher centers of the nervous system can cause salivary secretion in response to the sight, smell, or thought of food or to noises associated with food preparation.

PHARYNX

The pharynx is a funnel-shaped chamber situated behind the nasal cavities, the mouth, and the larynx. For purposes of description, it can be divided into nasal, oral, and laryngeal parts (see Fig. 10-1). The pharynx conducts air from the nasal cavities to the larynx and to the middle ear via the auditory tube. It also conducts food from the mouth to the esophagus. Thus, it is an area where the respiratory and digestive systems merge and cross.

The pharynx has a musculomembranous wall that is deficient anteriorly. Here, it is replaced by the posterior nasal apertures, the oropharyngeal isthmus (opening into the mouth), and the inlet of the larynx. The wall of the pharynx has three layers, mucous, fibrous, and muscular.

The *mucous membrane* of the pharynx is continuous with that of the nasal cavities, the mouth, and the larynx (Fig. 11-23). Via the auditory tube, it is also continuous with the mucous membrane of the tympanic cavity. The upper part of the membrane is lined with ciliated columnar epithelium, the lower part with stratified squamous epithelium; where the two areas come together, there is a transitional zone. In the lamina propria, numerous mucous glands are present, especially in the nasal part.

The *fibrous layer* lies between the mucous membrane and the muscle layer. It is thicker above, where it is strongly connected to the base of the skull. Below, it becomes continuous with the submucous coat of the esophagus.

The *muscular layer* consists of the superior, middle, and inferior constrictor muscles, whose fibers run in a basically circular direction (see Fig. 11-23), and the stylopharyngeus and salpingopharyngeus muscles, whose fibers run basically longitudinally. All the muscle fibers are of the voluntary striated type.

The lymphoid tissue in the pharynx is described on page 354.

SWALLOWING

Masticated food is formed into a bolus on the dorsum of the tongue and voluntarily pushed upward and backward against the undersurface of the hard palate. This action is brought about by the contraction of the styloglossus muscles on both sides, which pull the root of the tongue upward and backward. The palatoglossus muscles now squeeze the bolus backward into the pharynx. From this point on, the process of swallowing, or deglutition, becomes an involuntary act.

The nasal part of the pharynx is shut off from the oral part by the elevation of the soft palate, the pulling forward of the posterior wall of the pharynx, and the pulling medially of the palatopharyngeal arches. These changes prevent the passage of food and drink into the nasal cavities.

The larynx and laryngeal part of the pharynx are now pulled upward by the contraction of the stylopharyngeus, salpingopharyngeus, thyrohyoid, and palatopharyngeus muscles. The main part of the larynx is thus elevated to the posterior surface of the epiglottis, and the entrance into the larynx is closed.

The bolus moves downward over the epiglottis, the closed entrance into the larynx, and reaches the lower part of the pharynx as a result of successive contractions of the superior, middle, and inferior constrictor muscles. Some of the food slides down the groove on either side of the entrance into the larynx, that is, down through the *piriform fossae*.

Finally, the lower part of the pharyngeal wall relaxes, and the bolus enters the esophagus.

DIGESTIVE TUBE FROM THE ESOPHAGUS TO THE ANUS

The esophagus, stomach, small intestine, large intestine, rectum, and anal canal have the same fundamental organizational plan (Fig. 11-24). The wall is divided into four layers, which, beginning with the luminal surface, include: (1) the *mucous membrane* or *mucosa,* which consists of the surface epithelium and an underlying layer of connective tissue, the *lamina propria*. A thin layer of smooth muscle, the *muscularis mucosae,* separates the mucous membrane from the underlying submucosa. It is arranged in two layers, an inner, circular layer and an outer, longitudinal layer.

The luminal surface of the mucous membrane is kept moist by the glandular secretions of the digestive tract. The surface cells are protective and may be secretory or absorptive. The surface of the mucous membrane may be flat where the tube serves merely to conduct the contents. In the small intestine, however, where there is a great need to increase the surface area for absorption, the mucous membrane is projected into fingerlike processes called *villi* (see Fig. 11-24). In areas where there is a need for intestinal glands, the mucous membrane is invaginated to form numerous crypts.

The surface cells of the mucous membrane are supported by the connective tissue of the lamina propria. Scattered throughout this connective tissue are collections of lymphoid tissue that serve as a defense against infection (see Fig. 11-24). The lamina propria also contains numerous blood and lymphatic capillaries that take part in the transport of

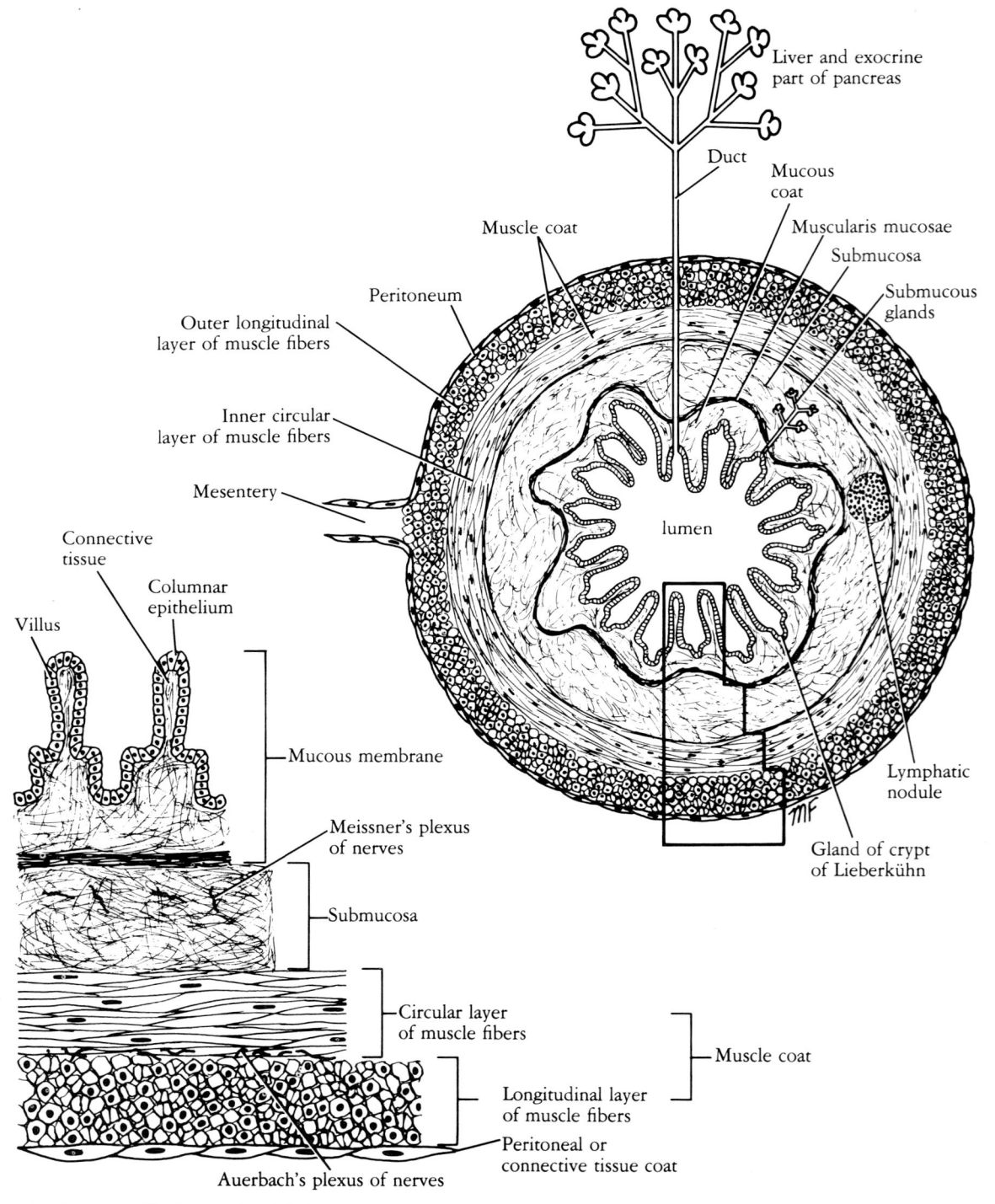

Fig. 11-24. General structure of the walls of the digestive tract. Note the four layers: (1) the mucous membrane, (2) the submucosa, (3) the muscle coat, and (4) the adventitia, or connective tissue coat.

digested food materials away from the lumen of the intestine.

The muscularis mucosae brings about local movement of the mucous membrane and may cause it to fold (see Fig. 11-24). In the small intestine, the villi are moved about by this muscular layer, and the flow of lymph in the lymphatic capillaries may be aided by the pumping action of this muscle.

(2) The *submucosa* consists of a well-developed layer of loose connective tissue containing plexuses of blood and lymphatic vessels (see Fig. 11-24). It also possesses an autonomic nerve plexus, called *Meissner's plexus,* that controls the activity of the glands and smooth muscle. The plexus consists of postganglionic sympathetic fibers and preganglionic and postganglionic parasympathetic fibers. The nerve cells are parasympathetic ganglion cells.

(3) The *muscularis coat* or *muscularis externa* consists of two layers of smooth muscle (see Fig. 11-24). In the outer layer, the muscle cells are arranged longitudinally; in the inner layer, they have a circular arrangement. This organization greatly assists the observer in determining whether the microscopic section being examined was cut in cross section or in longitudinal section. The two muscle layers are separated by a small amount of connective tissue containing an autonomic nerve plexus called the *myenteric* or *Auerbach's plexus*. This plexus controls the activity of the smooth muscle. Like Meissner's plexus, it consists of postganglionic sympathetic fibers and preganglionic and postganglionic parasympathetic fibers. The nerve cells are parasympathetic ganglion cells.

In the upper third of the esophagus, all the smooth muscle is replaced by skeletal muscle; in the middle third, there is a mixture of smooth and skeletal muscle fibers. In the stomach, there is a third layer of smooth muscle, and in the colon of the large intestine, the outer layer of longitudinal muscle fibers is grouped together to form three longitudinal bands called the *teniae coli*.

By squeezing and shortening the digestive tube, the muscular coat thoroughly mixes the food material within the lumen with the digestive enzymes. By producing a series of wavelike contractions called *peristaltic waves,* it propels the contents onward along the digestive tube.

(4) *The adventitia* is a relatively dense connective tissue layer (see Fig. 11-24) that blends with the fascia of surrounding structures. In those portions of the digestive tube that project into the peritoneal cavity, the outer surface is covered with peritoneum; in describing these areas, the term *serosa* is used in place of *adventitia*. The peritoneum consists of a single layer of flattened mesothelial cells lying on connective tissue. The peritoneum is continuous with that lining the peritoneal cavity.

Numerous blood vessels, lymphatic vessels, and nerves are present within the adventitia.

Esophagus

The esophagus is an almost straight muscular tube about 10 inches (25 cm) long that extends from the pharynx to the stomach (Fig. 11-25). Its structure contains the four layers that are characteristic of the alimentary canal: (1) mucous membrane, (2) submucosa, (3) muscular coat, and (4) adventitia (Fig. 11-26).

The *mucous membrane* is lined with stratified squamous nonkeratinized epithelium that is continuous above with that lining the pharynx (Fig. 11-27). Below, at the esophagogastric junction, there is an abrupt change as the stratified squamous epithelium gives way to simple columnar epithelium (Fig. 11-29). The stratified epithelium lining the esophagus is protective and resists the wear and tear from the passage of rough semisolid foods. The usual lamina propria and muscularis mucosae are present. *Esophageal cardiac glands* that closely resemble the cardiac glands of the stomach (see p. 436) are found at the upper and lower ends of the esophagus. They vary in number and are situated in the lamina propria; they secrete mucus.

In the empty esophagus, the mucous membrane is characteristically thrown into longitudinal folds that are eliminated during the passage of a bolus of food.

The *submucosa* contains a few tubulo-alveolar mucous glands scattered along its length (see Fig. 11-26). These are the *esophageal glands*. Their se-

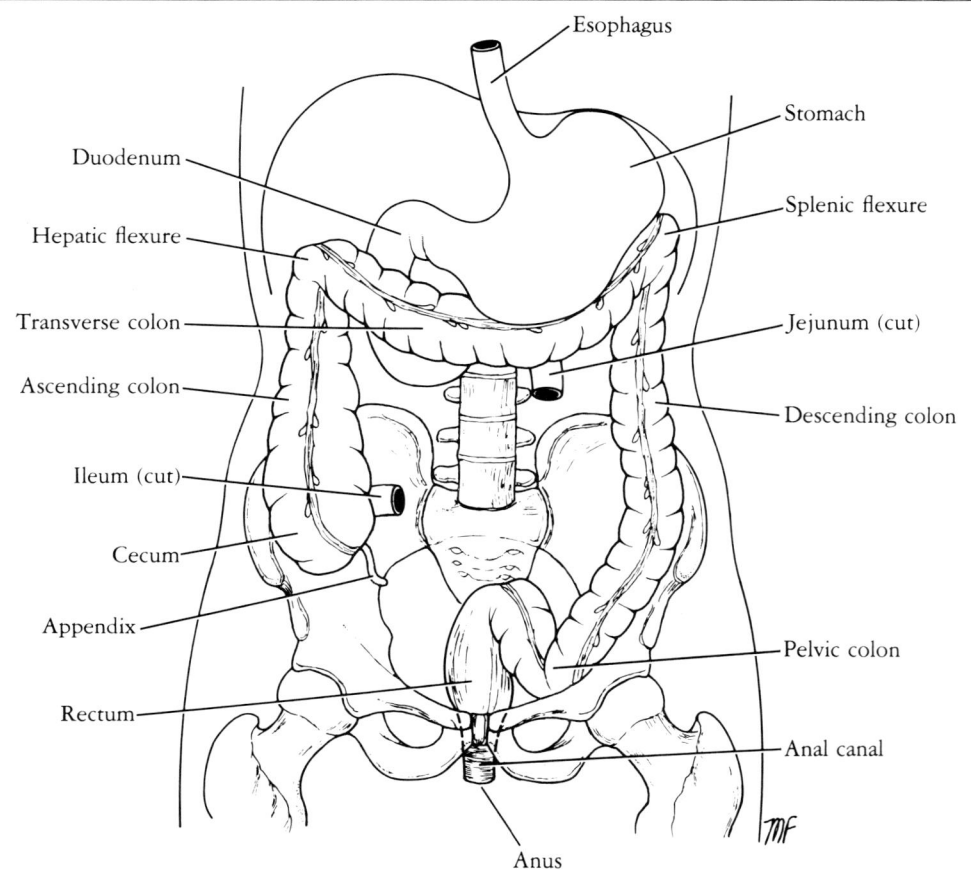

Fig. 11-25. The parts of the digestive tract from the esophagus to the anus; the greater part of the jejunum and ileum have been removed for clarity.

cretion lubricates the esophageal contents during swallowing. A Meissner's plexus of nerves is present and controls the activity of the glands and smooth muscle.

The *muscular coat* consists of the usual inner circular and outer longitudinal layers of muscle fibers (see Fig. 11-27). In the upper third of the esophagus, the muscle is skeletal (Fig. 11-28), in the lower third, it is smooth, and in the middle third, one finds a mixture of skeletal and smooth muscle. The myenteric or Auerbach's plexus of autonomic nerves lies between the circular and longitudinal muscle layers and controls the activities of the muscle. There is no thickening of the muscular coat at the cardioesophageal junction.

The *adventitia* consists of loose connective tissue that supports the esophagus (see Fig. 11-27).

Function

The esophagus conducts food from the pharynx into the stomach. Wavelike contractions of the muscular coat, called *peristalsis,* propel the food onward. Although no anatomical sphincter exists at the lower end of the esophagus, there is no doubt that the smooth muscle in this region serves physiologically as a sphincter. As the food descends through the esophagus, relaxation of the muscle at the lower end occurs ahead of the peristaltic wave, so that the food

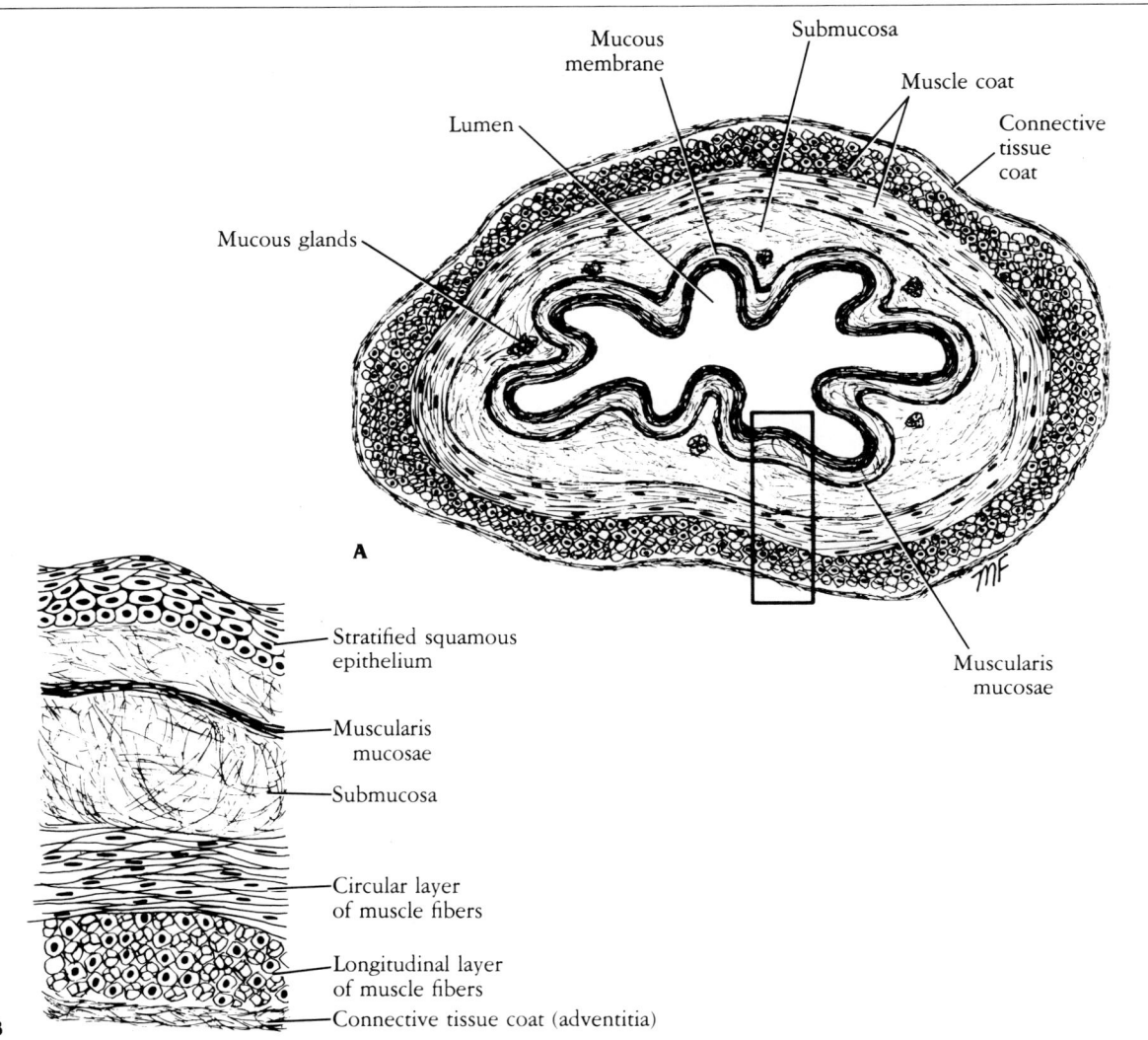

Fig. 11-26. Detailed structure of a cross section of the esophagus. A: Low-power view of the entire esophagus. B: High-power view of the structure of the wall of the esophagus.

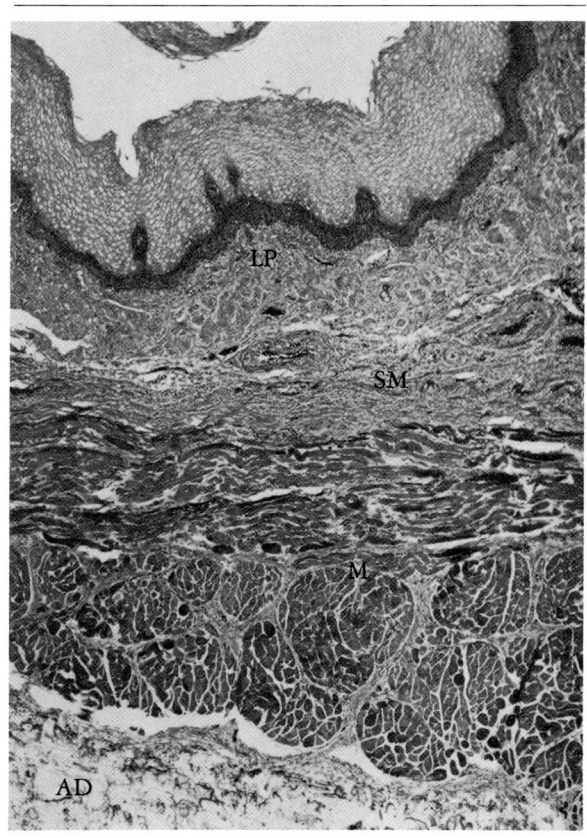

Fig. 11-27. Photomicrograph of a cross section of the lower third of the wall of the esophagus, showing mucous membrane covered with stratified squamous nonkeratinized epithelium. Also visible is the lamina propria (LP), the submucosa (SM), the muscular coat (M), and the adventitia, or connective tissue coat (AD). (H&E; ×40.)

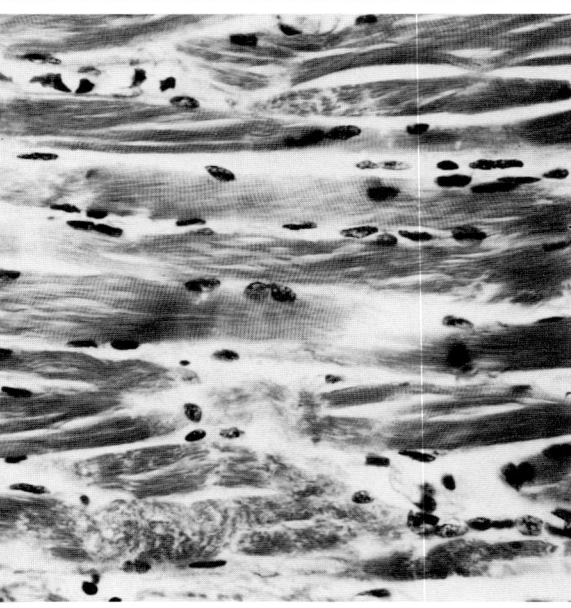

Fig. 11-28. Photomicrograph of part of the muscular coat in the upper third of the esophagus. Note the presence of striated muscle fibers in the inner circular layer of the muscle coat. (H&E; ×400.)

enters the stomach. The tonic contraction of this so-called physiological *gastroesophageal sphincter* prevents the stomach contents from regurgitating into the esophagus.

The esophageal and esophageal cardiac glands secrete mucus that lubricates the food bolus and assists its passage into the stomach.

Stomach

The stomach is a highly dilated portion of the alimentary canal and is concerned with the storage and digestion of food. For purposes of description, the stomach can be divided into several parts. The *fundus* is dome shaped and projects upward and to the left of the cardiac orifice (Fig. 11-30). It is usually full of gas. The *body* extends from the level of the cardiac orifice (esophageal opening) to the level of the *incisura angularis*, a constant notch in the lower part of the lesser curvature. The *pyloric antrum* extends from the incisura angularis to the proximal limit of the pylorus. The *pylorus* is the most tubular part of the stomach. Its thick muscular wall forms the *pyloric sphincter*. The cavity of the pylorus is called the *pyloric canal*.

The esophagus enters the stomach at the *cardiac orifice*, and the pyloric canal opens into the duodenum at the *pyloric orifice*. The *lesser curvature* forms the right border of the stomach and extends from the cardiac orifice to the pylorus (see Fig. 11-30). The *greater curvature* is much longer than the lesser curvature and extends from the left of the cardiac

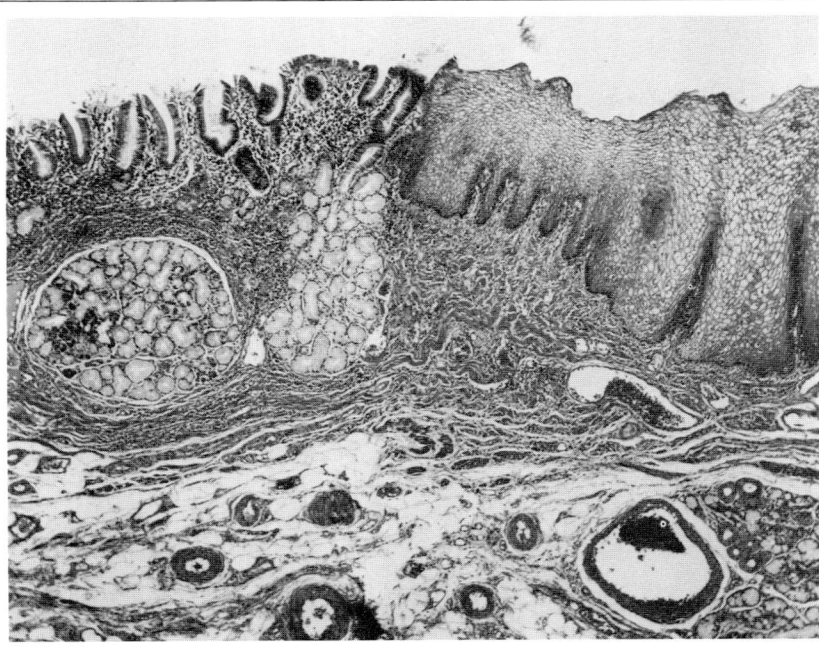

Fig. 11-29. Photomicrograph of longitudinal section of esophagogastric junction. The stomach mucous membrane and submucosa are shown at the left, and the corresponding layers of the esophagus are shown at the right. Note the abrupt change in the lining epithelium from stratified squamous in the esophagus to columnar in the stomach. Note also the compound tubular mucus-secreting cardiac gland in the mucous membrane of the stomach. (H&E; ×40.)

orifice over the dome of the fundus and then sweeps around and to the right to the inferior part of the pylorus (see Fig. 11-30).

When empty and contracted, the stomach is flattened anteroposteriorly and its lining is thrown into longitudinal folds, or *rugae*. When the stomach fills, it expands and the rugae disappear.

The stomach wall possesses the usual four layers of the alimentary canal, the (1) mucous membrane, (2) submucosa, (3) muscular coat, and (4) adventitia or serosa. The *mucous membrane* is thick and vascular and, as noted previously, in the empty stomach is thrown into longitudinal folds or *rugae*. The cores of the rugae also contain the submucosa. When the stomach fills, the rugae flatten. The surface of the mucous membrane is studded with small depressions, or pits, a few millimeters in diameter. These are known as *gastric pits,* and into the bottom of them open three to seven test-tube-shaped gastric glands (Figs. 11-31 and 11-32; see Fig. 11-30). The mucous membrane is lined with mucus-secreting simple columnar epithelial cells (Fig. 11-33). At the cardiac orifice, this epithelium abruptly changes into the stratified squamous epithelium of the esophagus (see Fig. 11-29). At the pyloric orifice, the epithelium becomes continuous with the columnar epithelium of the duodenum (see Fig. 11-38). The apical cytoplasm of the columnar epithelium usually appears empty or foamy because of the extraction of the mucous droplets and their poor staining with routine histologic dyes. The mucus stains prominently, however, with the periodic acid–Schiff procedure or mucicarmine (Fig. 11-34). The mucus secreted by these cells protects the epithelial surface from the acid contents of the stomach.

The lamina propria is composed of loose connective tissue that lies in the spaces between glands. There is a typical muscularis mucosae.

The glands of the mucous membrane are simple

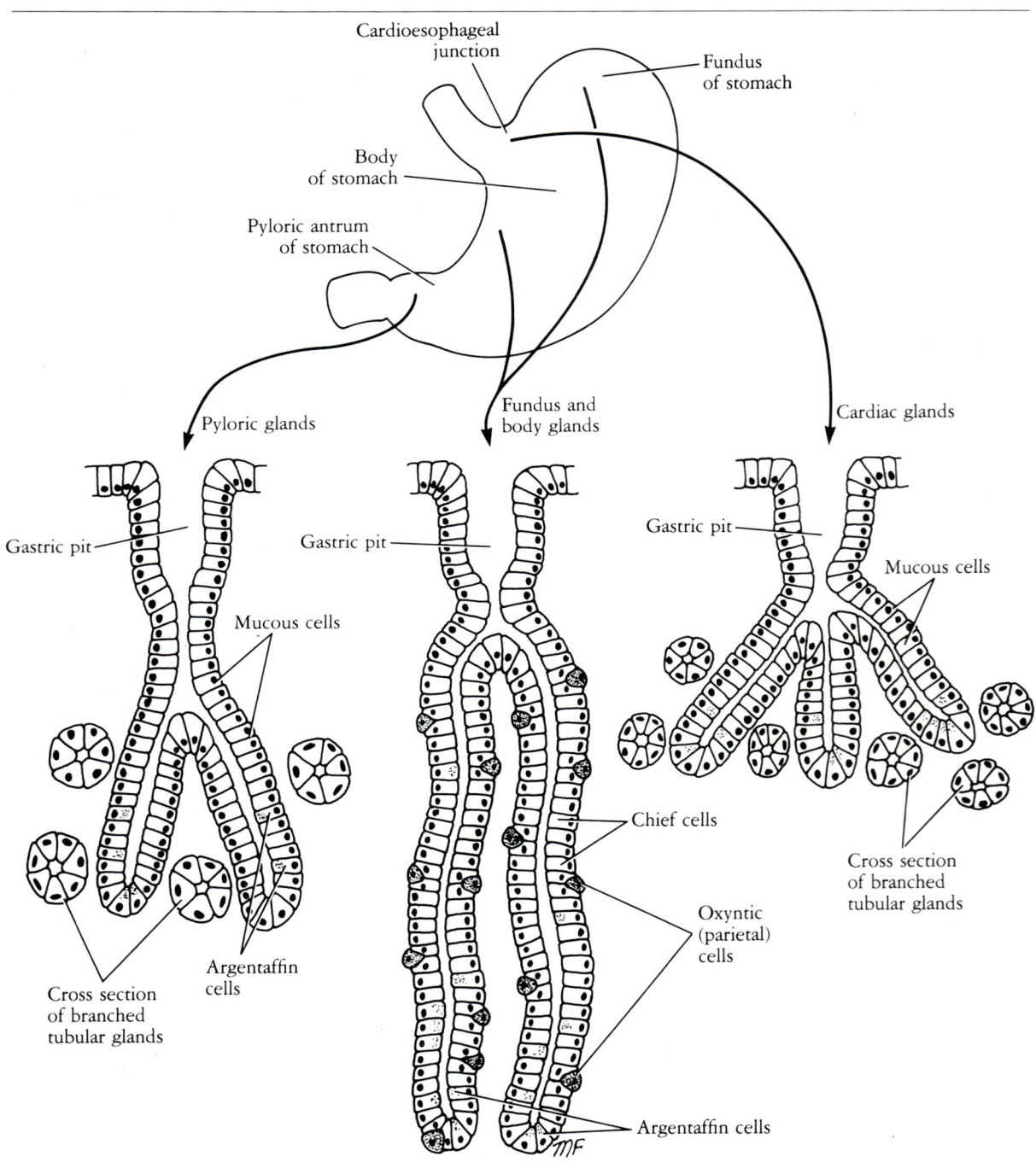

Fig. 11-30. The three types of glands found in different regions of the stomach. Note the different kinds of epithelial cells that line the glands.

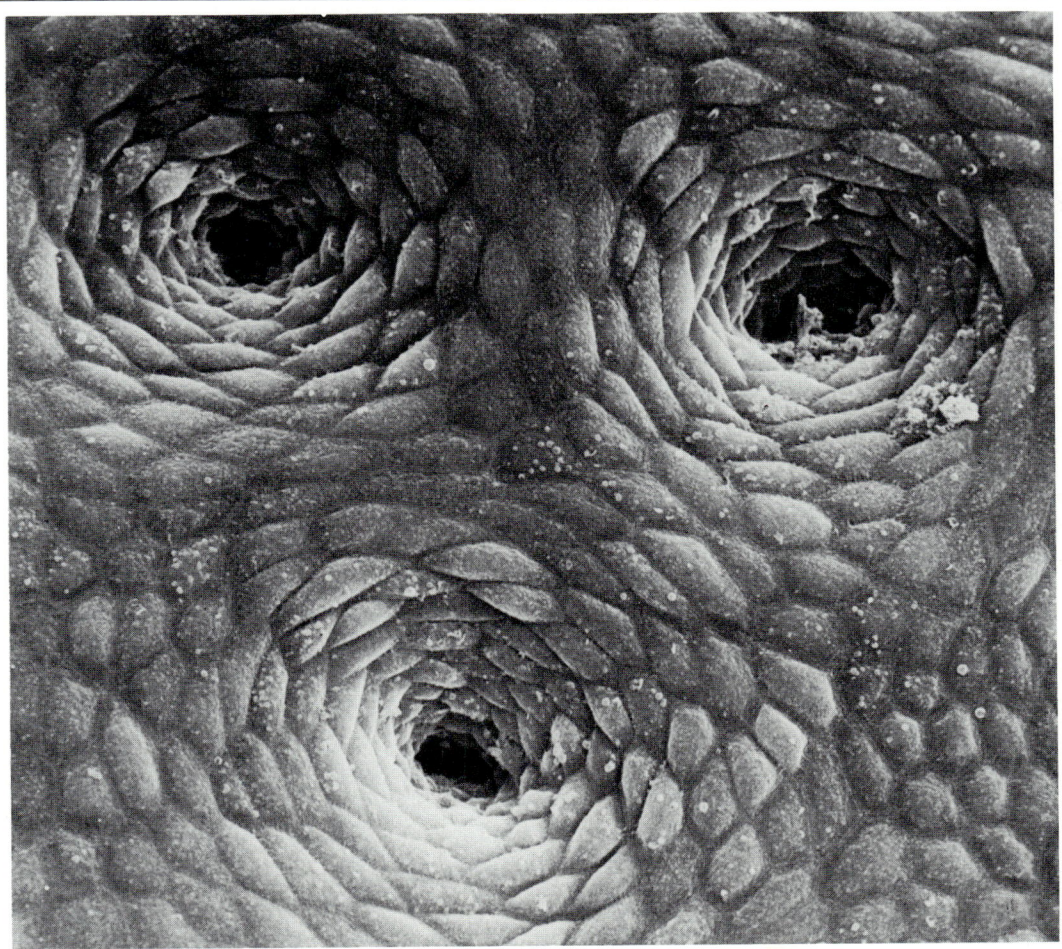

Fig. 11-31. Scanning electron micrograph of the mucous membrane of the stomach, showing the apical surfaces of the columnar cells covering the luminal surface and three gastric pits leading into the mouths of the glands. (×934.) (Courtesy of Dr. P. Andrews.)

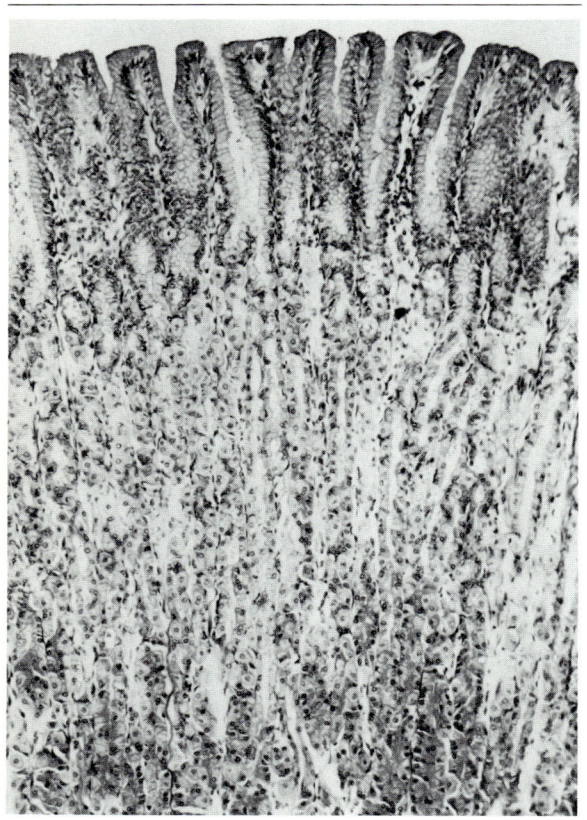

Fig. 11-32. *Photomicrograph of a longitudinal section of the mucous membrane of the fundus of the stomach, showing the gastric pits and the long tubular glands. Note that in this section, the chief or peptic cells (light cells) line most of the upper part of the glands and the parietal or oxyntic cells (dark cells) are found mainly in the lower part of the glands. (H&E; ×100.)*

tubular or branched tubular structures. There are three types of glands: (1) cardiac glands, (2) glands of the fundus and body, and (3) pyloric glands.

Cardiac Glands

The cardiac glands are found around the opening of the esophagus into the stomach. They are compound tubular glands that secrete mucous (see Fig. 11-30).

Glands of the Fundus and Body

These are simple branched tubular glands that possess four types of secretory cells: (1) chief or peptic cells, (2) parietal or oxyntic cells, (3) mucous neck cells, and (4) argentaffin cells (Fig. 11-35; see Fig. 11-33).

The *chief* or *peptic cells* (see Figs. 11-32, 11-33, and 11-35) are cuboidal or low columnar cells that line the lower half of the glands (the half located away from the stomach lumen). The cytoplasm is bluish staining and granular. Electron microscopy shows that the cells have apical microvilli; there is a supranuclear Golgi apparatus and plenty of rough endoplasmic reticulum. In the apical cytoplasm are numerous membrane-bound granules of low electron density. The granules are believed to contain *pepsinogen,* the inactive form of the enzyme *pepsin.* The basal part of the cytoplasm contains many mitochondria. The cells are also responsible for the production of the enzymes *lipase* and *amylase.*

The *parietal* or *oxyntic cells* (Fig. 11-36; see Fig. 11-33) are large, pyramid-shaped cells situated with their apical ends wedged between the chief cells. The bases of these cells tend to bulge from the lateral surface of the gland. The parietal cells are found scattered along the gland and are easily recognized because of their deeply staining eosinophilic cytoplasm.

Electron microscopy reveals a branching intracellular canaliculus that opens into the lumen of the gland through the apical plasma membrane (see Fig. 11-33). The canaliculus is lined with long microvilli that greatly increase the surface area for secretion. The cytoplasm contains numerous mitochondria, a

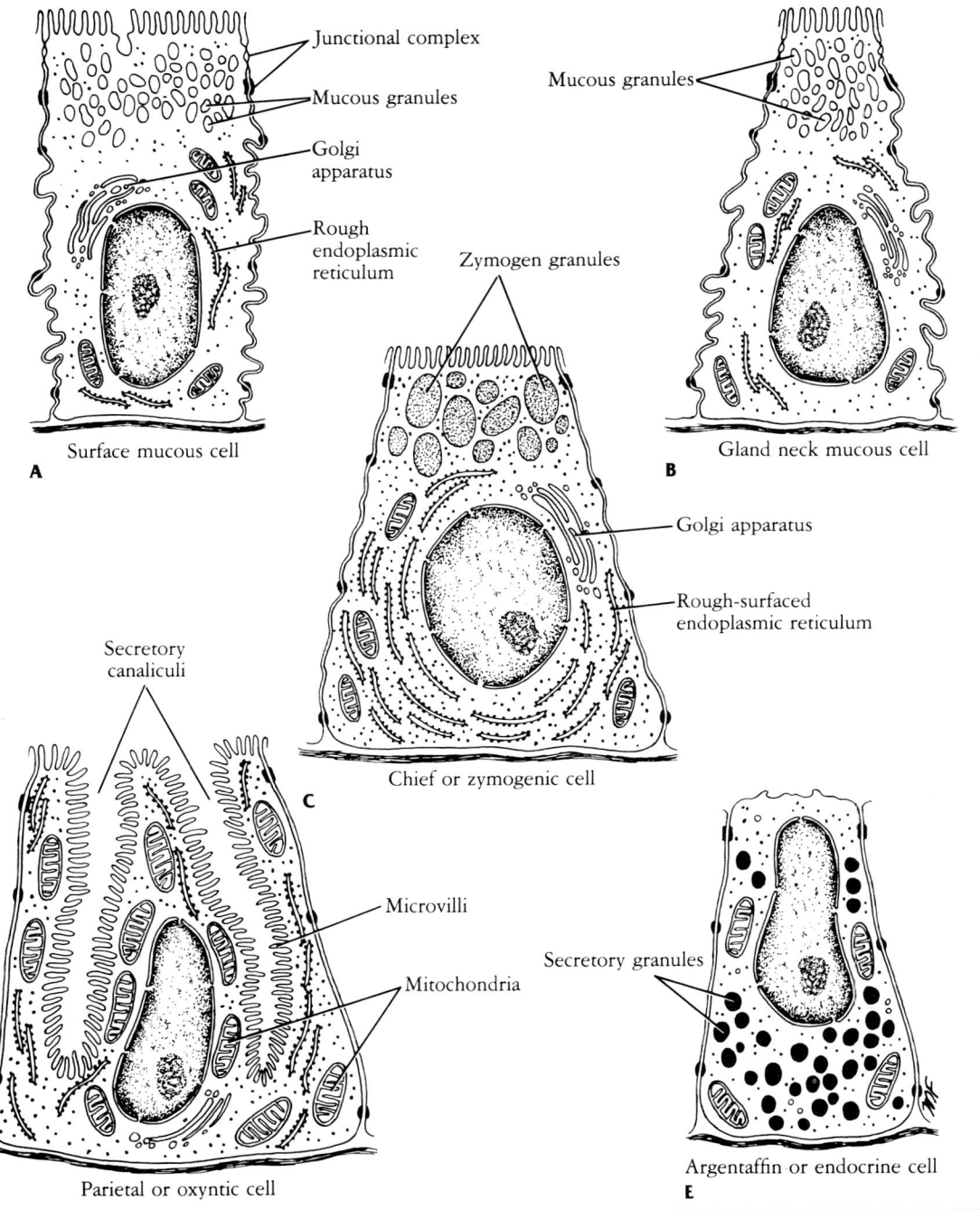

Fig. 11-33. *Main features of the different types of epithelial cells lining the stomach and its glands as seen with an electron microscope. A: Mucous surface cell. B: Gland neck mucous cell. C: Chief or zymogenic cell. D: Parietal or oxyntic cell. E: Argentaffin or endocrine cell.*

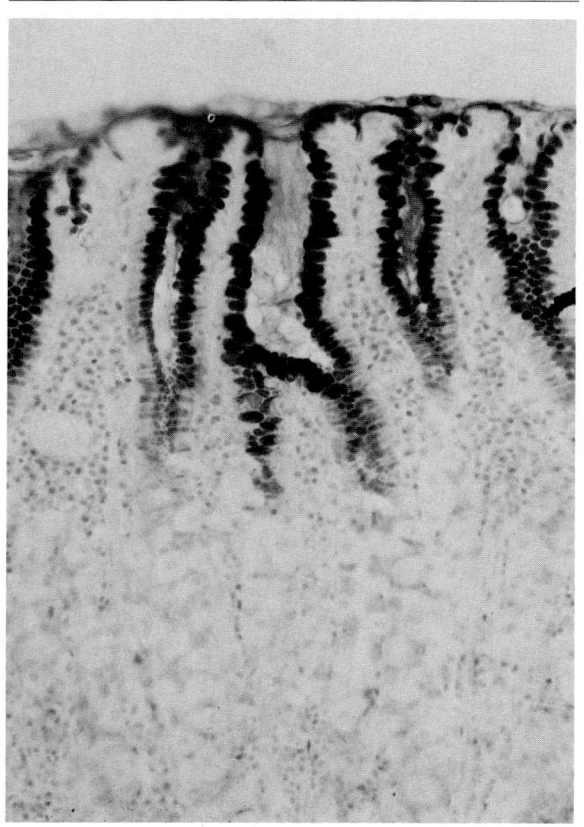

Fig. 11-34. Photomicrograph of a longitudinal section of the mucous membrane of the body of the stomach, showing the dark-staining mucus in the surface and neck cells of the glands. (Periodic acid–Schiff stain; ×100.)

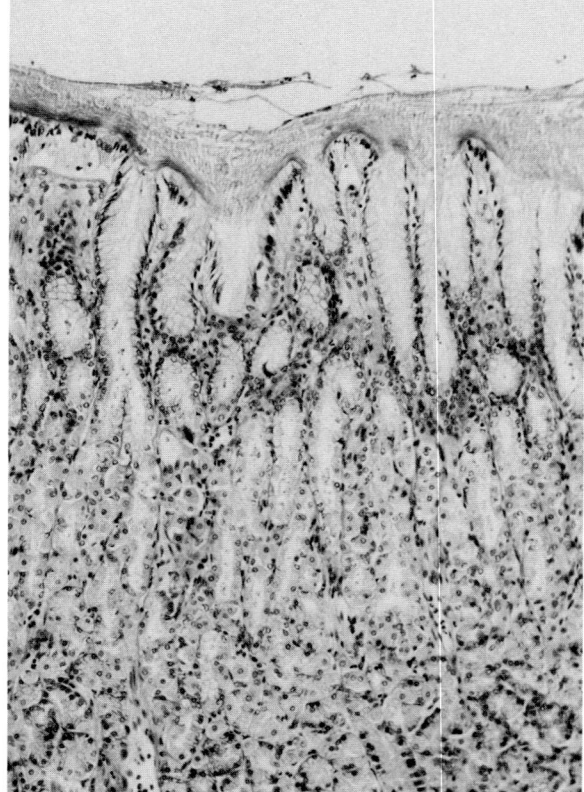

Fig. 11-35. Photomicrograph of a longitudinal section of the mucous membrane of the body of the stomach, showing the gastric pits and the tubular glands. Note the similar structures found in the fundus of the stomach (see Fig. 11-32). (H&E; ×100.)

small Golgi apparatus, little rough-surfaced endoplasmic reticulum, and no secretory granules.

The parietal cells are responsible for the production of *hydrochloric acid*. They also secrete the *intrinsic factor,* which is necessary for the normal maturation of red blood cells (see p. 185).

The *mucous neck cells* are columnar cells restricted to the neck region of the gland. They secrete mucus. It is believed that the neck cells, as a result of mitotic activity, replace the surface cells of the mucous membrane as they are worn off.

The *argentaffin cells* (see Fig. 11-33) are found scattered among the chief cells. They contain cytoplasmic granules that stain with silver or chromium salts. These cells have an endocrine function and are often referred to as *enteroendocrine cells.* One type of cell produces *serotonin,* which causes smooth muscle to contract. A second type of cell is believed to produce *enteroglucagon,* a hormone that increases blood sugar levels and is therefore antagonistic to insulin.

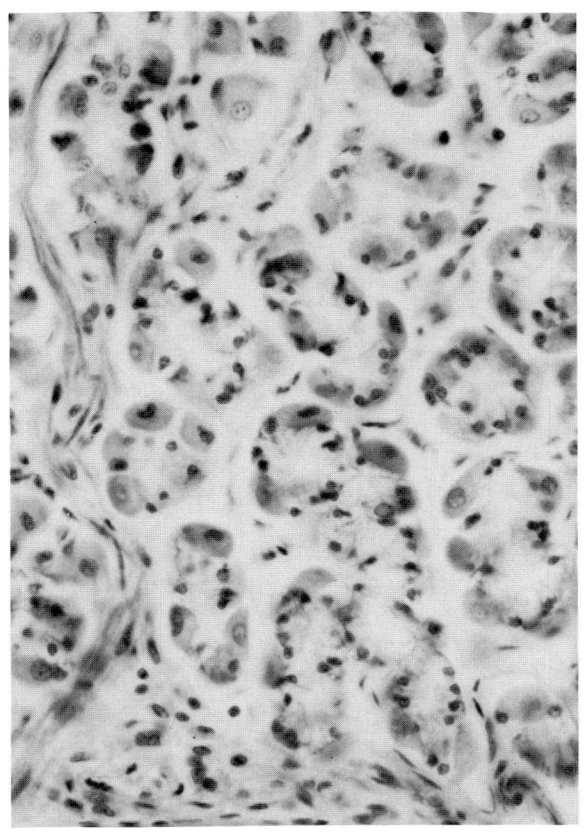

Fig. 11-36. Photomicrograph of a cross section of tubular glands found in the mucous membrane of the body of the stomach. The chief or peptic cells are the lighter-staining cells; the parietal or oxyntic cells are the darker-staining cells. (H&E; ×400.)

Pyloric Glands

These are simple branched tubular glands that are highly coiled (Fig. 11-37; see Fig. 11-30). The glands are found in the pyloric antrum and the pyloric canal (Fig. 11-38). Near the pylorus, many of the glands pass through the muscularis mucosae into the submucosa. The gastric pits in this region are longer than elsewhere and extend down into the mucosa for half its thickness. The pyloric glands are lined with columnar cells that secrete mucus and produce the hormone *gastrin*.

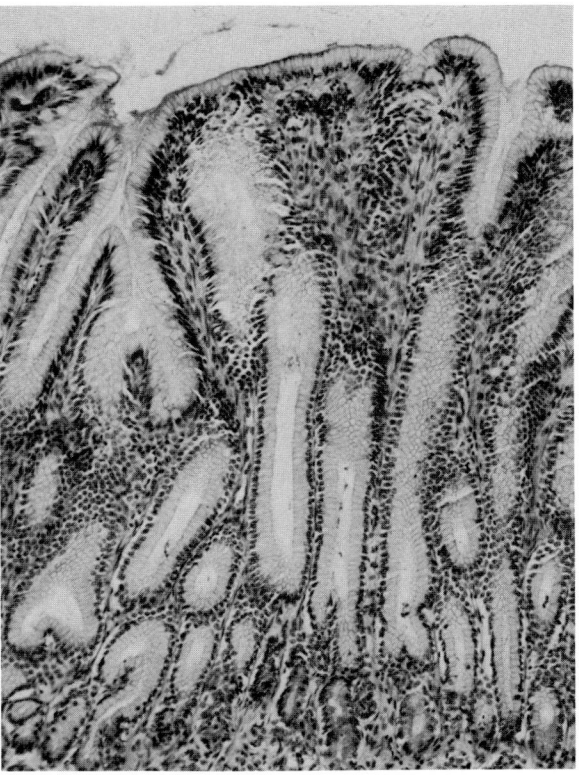

Fig. 11-37. Photomicrograph of a longitudinal section of branched tubular glands found in the mucous membrane of the pyloric antrum of the stomach. (H&E; ×100.)

The *submucosa* consists of connective tissue containing nerves, blood vessels, and lymph vessels. The blood vessels possess numerous arteriovenous shunts that are under nervous and hormonal control. When the shunts are open, blood is diverted from the mucous membrane; when this process is extensive, the mucous membrane may be predisposed to ulceration.

The *muscular coat* consists of three layers of smooth muscle: (1) longitudinal outer fibers, (2) circular middle fibers, and (3) oblique inner fibers. The longitudinal fibers are the most superficial and are concentrated along the curvatures. The middle circular fibers encircle the body of the stomach and are

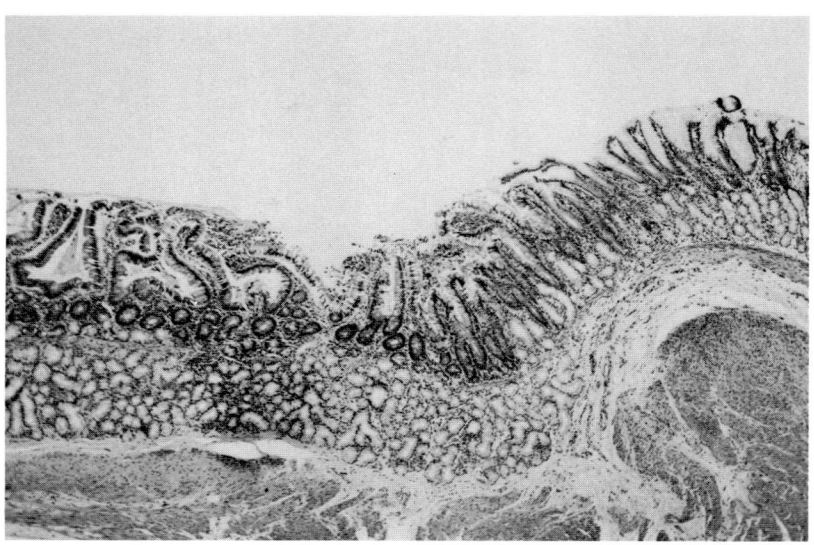

Fig. 11-38. Photomicrograph of a longitudinal section of the gastroduodenal junction. On the extreme right of the photograph is the gastric mucous membrane with the tubular glands confined to the mucous membrane. On the left is the mucous membrane of the duodenum, showing villi and Brunner's glands extending into the submucosa. (H&E; ×40.)

greatly thickened at the pylorus to form the *pyloric sphincter;* very few circular fibers are found in the region of the fundus. The oblique fibers form an incomplete layer; they loop over the fundus and pass downward along the anterior and posterior walls, running parallel with the lesser curvature.

The *serosa* is a layer of loose connective tissue covered by flattened mesothelial cells and forms the peritoneal covering of the stomach. The peritoneum completely surrounds the stomach and leaves its curvatures as double layers known as *omenta.*

Functions

The stomach has three main functions: (1) it serves as a storage or holding area for swallowed food; (2) it mixes the food with gastric secretions to form a thick fluid called *chyme;* and (3) it gradually releases the chyme into the duodenum for continued digestion and absorption from the small intestine.

MOVEMENTS OF THE STOMACH WALLS. As food passes into the stomach, the tone of the smooth muscle in the stomach wall gradually relaxes to accommodate the stomach contents. By this means, the intragastric pressure remains low until the volume of the stomach contents reaches about 1 liter; thereafter, the pressure rises.

The contents of the stomach are mixed by the peristaltic contractions of its walls, which commence at about the middle of the body and pass downward toward the pyloric sphincter. As the waves approach the pyloric region, the contractions become more powerful, and the motility in this region greatly increases as digestion proceeds.

The pyloric sphincter remains almost completely closed most of the time and prevents the flow of chyme into the duodenum. The stomach empties as the result of a wave of peristalsis that passes down through the antrum and forces the chyme through the pyloric sphincter. In this manner, the chyme is intermittently pumped into the duodenum. Excess chyme in the duodenum will inhibit the peristaltic activity in the pyloric region and stimulate the contraction of the pyloric sphincter, thus delaying the entrance of more chyme into the duodenum. Moreover, excessive amounts of acid, protein, or fat in the chyme entering the duodenum will delay further entrance of chyme into the duodenum.

GASTRIC SECRETION. The average adult secretes about 2,000 ml of gastric juice in 24 hours. The glands of the fundus and body of the stomach secrete digestive enzymes and hydrochloric acid. The most important enzyme is *pepsin,* which is produced by the chief cells in an inactive form called *pepsinogen.* Pepsinogen is converted quickly into pepsin within the lumen of the stomach by hydrochloric acid. Pepsin is a proteolytic enzyme (optimum pH, 2.0) that breaks down proteins in the stomach into polypeptides. It becomes inactive at the high pH found in the duodenum. Very small amounts of *lipase,* which acts on fat, and *amylase,* which digests starch, are also found in the gastric secretions. These enzymes are produced by the chief cells. *Hydrochloric acid* is produced by the parietal or oxyntic cells of the gastric glands; when discharged into the lumen of the stomach, it lowers the hydrogen ion concentration of the contents to a pH of about 2, permitting pepsin digestion of protein to begin. The hydrochloric acid also promotes the conversion of pepsinogen into pepsin and destroys many microorganisms that are swallowed with food.

The mucus produced by the columnar cells lining the stomach and in the cardiac and pyloric glands protects the mucous membrane from digestion by the gastric enzymes. The secretion forms a thick mucous gel layer that coats the surface of the mucous membrane. In addition, the pyloric glands produce the hormone gastrin (to be discussed).

Although a considerable amount of digestion takes place in the stomach, very little absorption occurs. Only alcohol and lipid-soluble drugs can be absorbed through the gastric mucous membrane.

Hydrochloric Acid Secretion. As stated previously, hydrochloric acid is produced by the parietal cells of the gastric glands. The plasma H^+ concentration is 0.00004 mEq/L, and the parietal cells raise the concentration in their secretion to 150 mEq/L. This secretion is highly acidic, having a pH of about 0.8.

How do these cells perform this function? The hydrogen ion is believed to be formed as follows. Carbon dioxide, either passed into the cell from the plasma or produced in the cell as a product of metabolism, combines with water in the presence of the enzyme carbonic anhydrase to form carbonic acid. Carbonic acid splits into hydrogen and bicarbonate ions. The hydrogen ion is secreted from the cell surface, and the bicarbonate ion diffuses back into the bloodstream.

The chloride ions diffuse from the blood into the parietal cells and are then secreted by the cells with the hydrogen ions. The passage of chloride ions across the cell membrane is not a passive mechanism; they are transported against an electrical gradient as well as a chemical gradient, requiring active transport. Moreover, to compensate for the movement of chloride ions, an equivalent number of bicarbonate ions moves from the parietal cells into the plasma. Thus, the blood leaving the stomach is more alkaline and the urine then becomes more alkaline, a condition known as *alkaline tide.*

It is thought that the alkaline mucus secreted by the surface cells of the mucous membrane of the stomach forms a protective layer that prevents damage to the mucous membrane by hydrochloric acid and pepsin.

Control of Gastric Secretion. Gastric secretion is controlled by nervous and hormonal mechanisms (see Fig. 11-39).

Nervous Control. The gastric glands receive nerve fibers from the vagus nerve. Stimulation of the vagi causes the glands to secrete a highly acid gastric juice rich in pepsin; there is also some increase in the secretion of mucus. Vagal stimulation increases production of the hormone gastrin.

Hormonal Control. The presence of protein foods in the stomach causes the pyloric antrum glands to secrete the hormone gastrin. Gastrin is absorbed into the blood and carried to the gastric glands, where it stimulates the parietal cells to produce hydrochloric acid; to a smaller degree, it also stimulates the chief cells to produce pepsinogen.

Phases in Gastric Secretion. There are three phases in gastric secretion: (1) cephalic, (2) gastric, and (3) intestinal.

Cephalic Phase. The sight, smell, taste, or thought

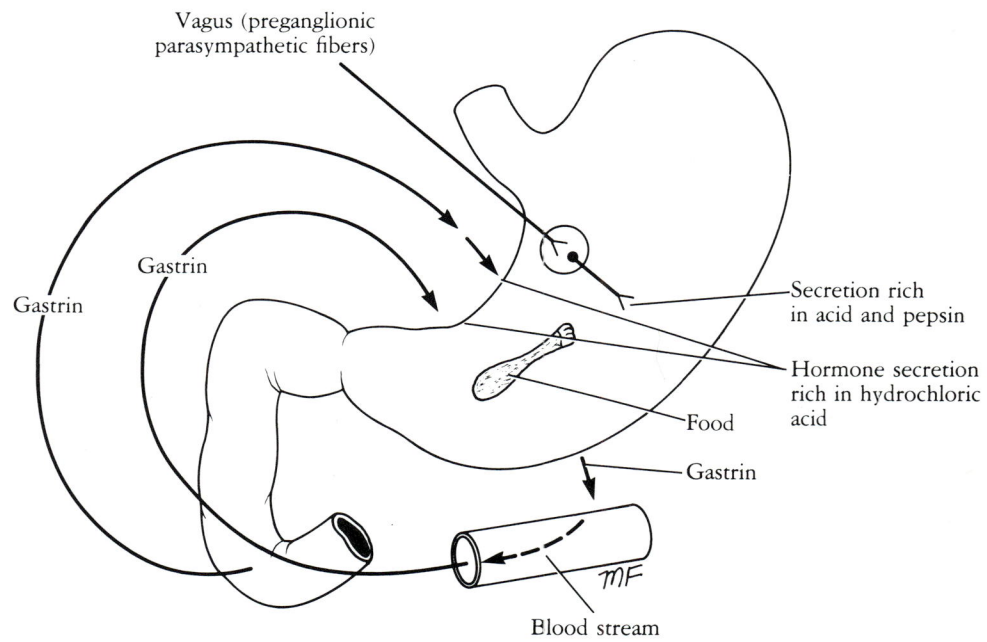

Fig. 11-39. Nervous and hormonal control of gastric secretion. Note that vagal stimulation produces a secretion rich in acid and pepsin; the hormone gastrin produces a secretion rich in acid.

of food can cause intense gastric secretion. The nervous stimuli to the cerebral cortex or the hypothalamus are relayed to the vagal nuclei. Impulses then pass to the stomach via the vagi. The cephalic phase usually initiates gastric secretion.

Gastric Phase. The presence of food in the stomach stretches the stomach wall, and nervous reflexes involving the vagus nerves or, more locally, the myenteric plexus in the stomach wall result in some stimulation of gastric secretion. The secretion during this phase, however, is caused mainly by the hormone gastrin formed in the mucosa of the stomach in response to the presence of food. The gastric phase accounts for about two-thirds of gastric secretion.

Intestinal Phase. Small amounts of gastric secretion are initiated by the presence of food in the duodenum. It is believed that gastrin is also produced in the duodenal mucosa and may be responsible for the gastric secretion.

Small Intestine

The small intestine extends from the pylorus of the stomach to the ileocecal junction. It is divided into three parts: the duodenum, about 10 inches (25 cm) long; the jejunum, about 8 feet long; and the ileum, about 12 feet long (see Fig. 11-25).

Duodenum

The duodenum is a C-shaped tube about 10 inches (25 cm) long that curves around the head of the pancreas. The first inch (2.5 cm) of the duodenum resembles the stomach in that it is covered on its anterior and posterior surfaces with peritoneum. The remainder of the duodenum is retroperitoneal, being only partially covered with peritoneum.

Jejunum and Ileum

The jejunum and ileum together measure about 20 feet (6 m) long, the upper two-fifths of this length being the jejunum. Each has distinctive features—for example, the jejunum is wider bored and thicker walled than the ileum—but there is a gradual change

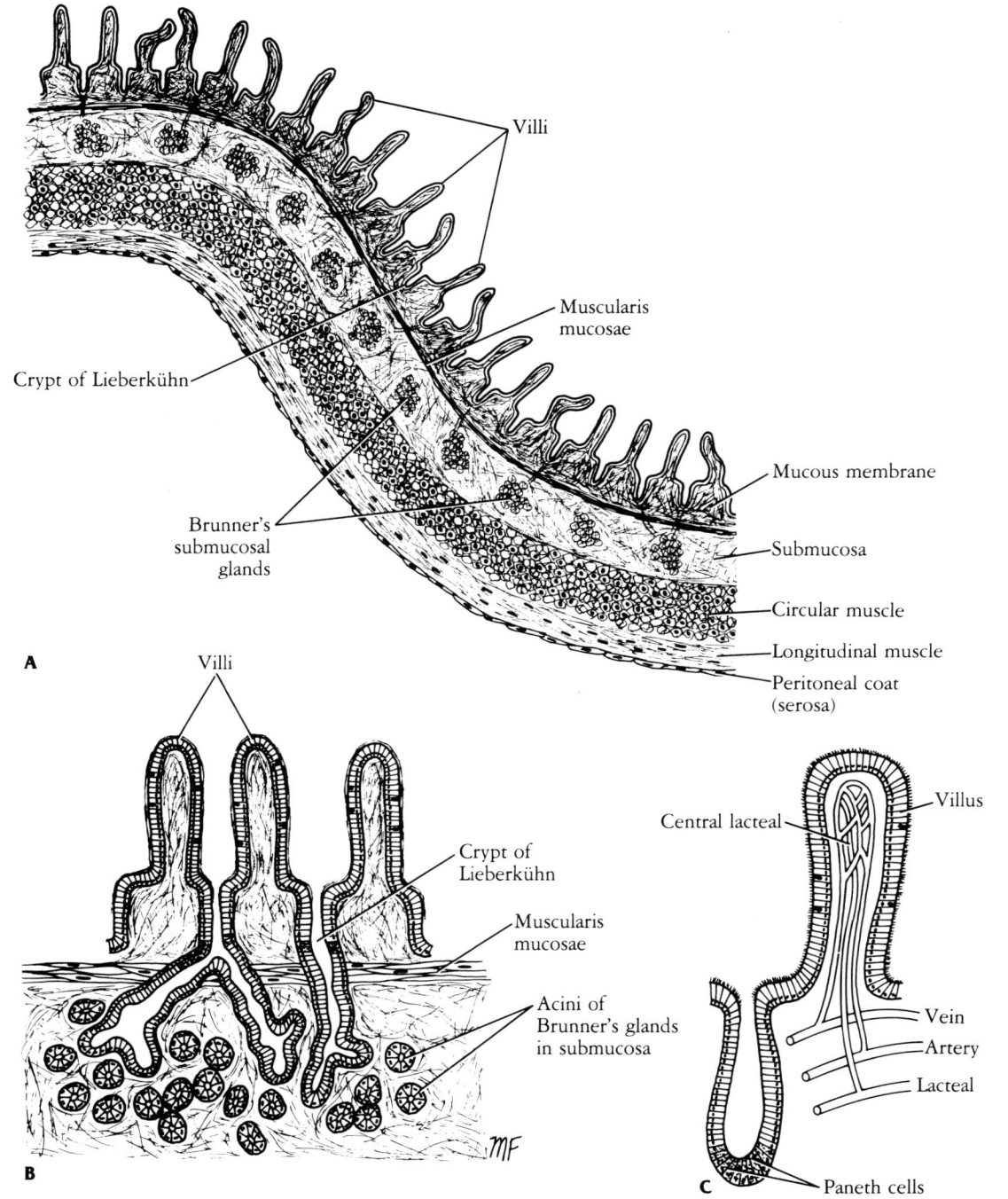

Fig. 11-40. Structure of the duodenal wall as seen on longitudinal section. A: The different layers of the wall. B: Brunner's glands opening into the crypts of Lieberkühn. C: Blood and lymphatic vessels entering and leaving a villus; note the Paneth cells in a crypt of Lieberkühn.

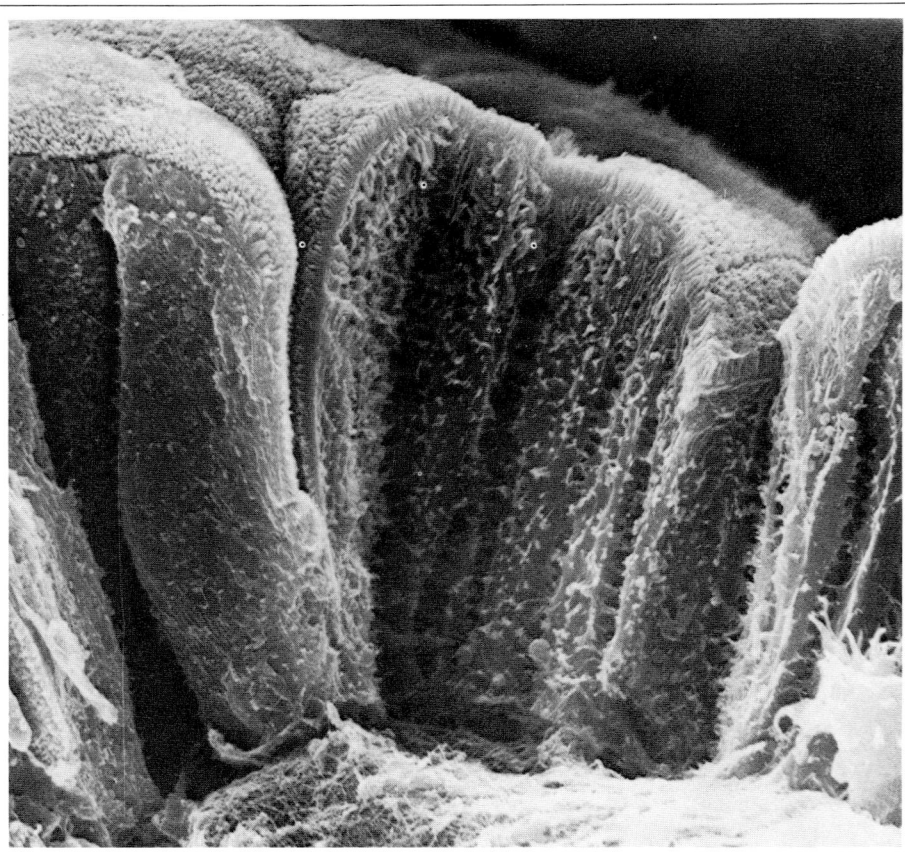

Fig. 11-41. Scanning electron micrograph of the mucous membrane of the duodenum, showing the freeze-fractured surfaces of the columnar cells covering a villus. Note the microvilli on the free surfaces of the cells. (×4,000.) (Courtesy of Dr. M. Koering.)

from one to the other. The jejunum begins at the duodenojejunal junction, and the ileum ends at the ileocecal junction.

The coils of jejunum and ileum are attached to the posterior abdominal wall by a fan-shaped fold of peritoneum known as the *mesentery of the small intestine*. The long free edge of the fold encloses the mobile intestine. The short root of the fold is continuous with the parietal peritoneum on the posterior abdominal wall. The root of the mesentery permits the entrance and exit of branches of the superior mesenteric artery and vein, lymph vessels, and nerves into the space between the two layers of peritoneum forming the mesentery.

The structure of the small intestine shows the usual four layers: (1) mucous membrane, (2) submucosa, (3) muscular coat, and (4) serosa (Fig. 11-40).

The *mucous membrane* is thrown into the numerous circular folds called the *plicae circulares*. These permanent folds extend one-half to two-thirds of the way around the lumen and serve to slow down and cause mixing of the intestinal contents. They also effectively increase the surface area. The plicae are most numerous in the distal part of the duodenum but gradually become smaller and farther apart until they disappear in the distal part of the

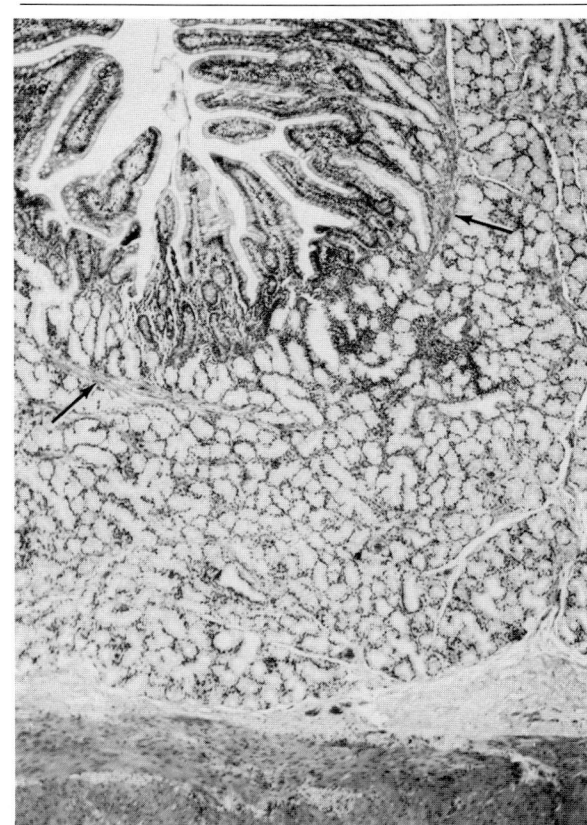

Fig. 11-42. Right: Photomicrograph of a longitudinal section of the duodenum, showing numerous villi, crypts of Lieberkühn, and Brunner's glands. Note that the Brunner's glands extend down into the submucosa and thus penetrate the muscularis mucosae (arrows). (H&E; ×40.)

Fig. 11-43. Below: Scanning electron micrograph of the luminal surface of the jejunum, showing numerous large villi covered with epithelial cells. (×75.) (Courtesy of F. G. Lightfoot.)

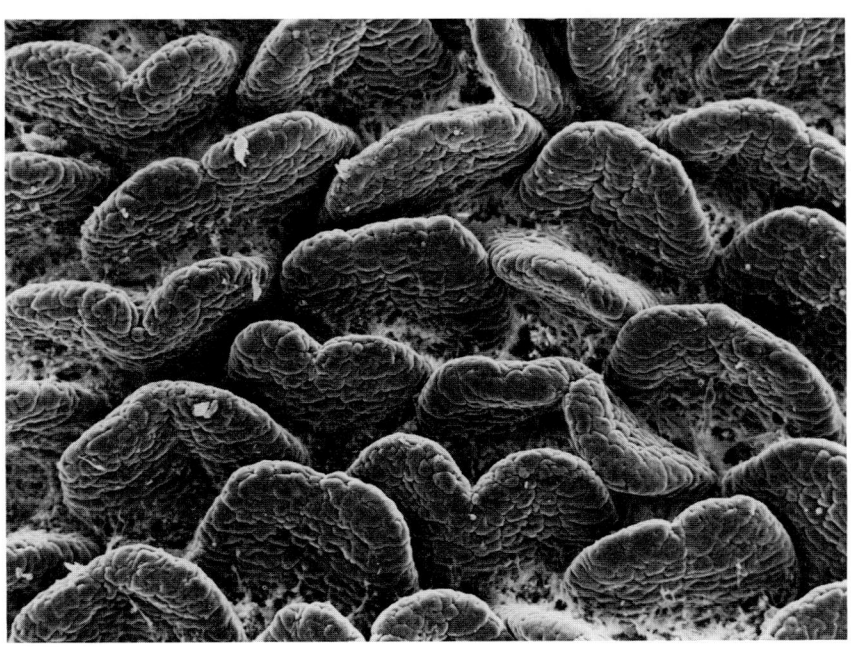

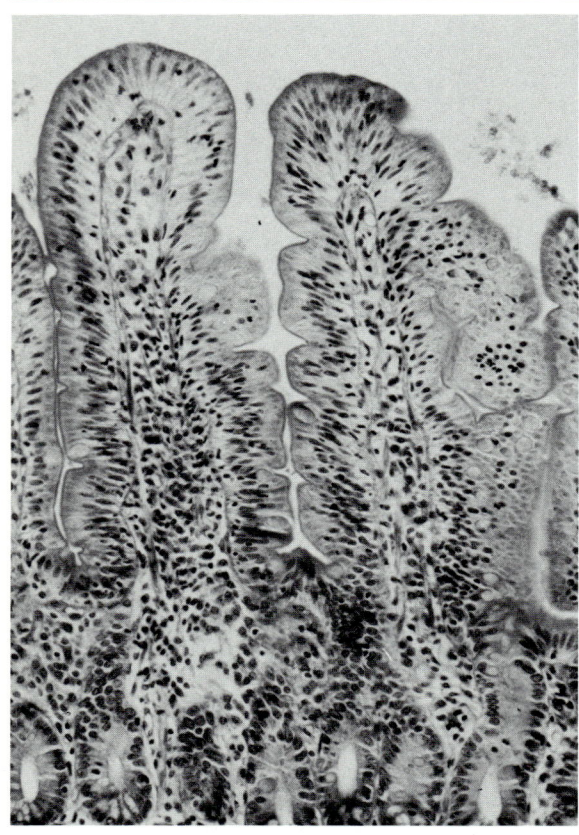

Fig. 11-44. Photomicrograph of a longitudinal section of the ileum, showing several villi and crypts of Lieberkühn. Note that the villi are covered with tall columnar cells. (H&E; ×200.)

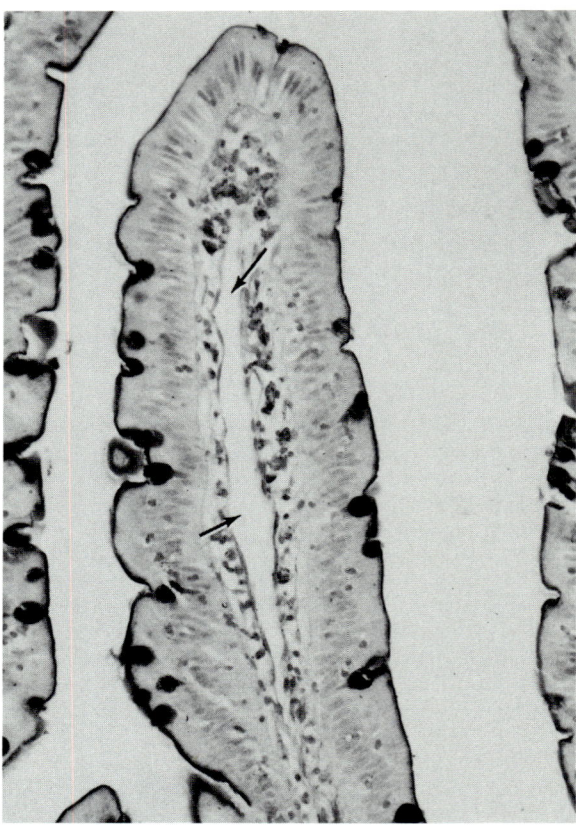

Fig. 11-45. Photomicrograph of a longitudinal section through villi of the ileum, showing dark-staining mucus in the goblet cells and covering the luminal surface of the remaining epithelial cells. Note the central lacteal (arrows). (Periodic acid–Schiff stain; ×200.)

ileum. The larger plicae have a core of submucosa.

The free surface of the mucous membrane is thrown into small, fingerlike projections called *villi* (Figs. 11-41, 11-42, and 11-43). Each villus measures about 0.5 to 1.5 mm long. In the duodenum, the villi tend to be longer and broader; they become shorter and thinner and reach a minimum size at the distal end of the ileum.

The villi are covered by simple columnar epithelium (Fig. 11-44). Each villus has a core of connective tissue containing an artery, a capillary network, and a vein as well as a central lymphatic or *lacteal* (Figs. 11-45 and 11-46). Narrow strands of smooth muscle derived from the muscularis mucosae extend into each villus and by their contraction aid the circulation of lymph through the lymphatic vessels.

The epithelium covering the villi is of three types: columnar absorptive cells, mucus-secreting goblet cells, and argentaffin cells (Fig. 11-47).

The *columnar absorptive cells* (see Fig. 11-41) possess closely packed microvilli on their free borders (Fig. 11-48) that greatly increase the surface area, furthering absorption. The outer surface of the microvilli has a well-developed cell coat formed of gly-

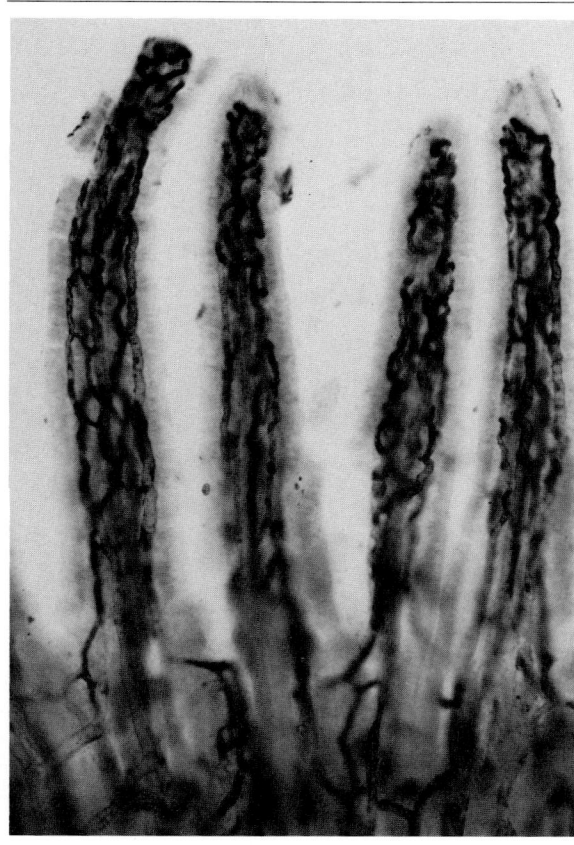

Fig. 11-46. Photomicrograph of a longitudinal section of several villi following the intravascular injection of dye material. Note that each villus contains an artery, a capillary network, and a vein as well as a central lacteal. (Eosin stain; ×100.)

coproteins that protects the cell from the action of proteolytic and mucolytic substances. It is believed that certain digestive enzymes are attached to the surface coat so that digestive processes, such as the breakdown of proteins and carbohydrates, can take place on and in the surface coat of the microvilli. Furthermore, the surface coat may have specific binding sites for certain substances, so that they are absorbed selectively. The fine cytoplasmic filaments within the microvilli not only stabilize the structures but, by shortening and lengthening, may bring about their movement.

The *goblet cells* are scattered among the absorptive cells. Their apical cytoplasm is usually filled with mucus globules (Figs. 11-49 and 11-50).

The *argentaffin cells* or endocrine cells are small and are scattered between the bases of the columnar absorptive cells. They contain dense cytoplasmic granules (Fig. 11-51; see Fig. 11-47). These cells produce the hormones *serotonin, secretin,* and *cholecystokinin,* which are thought to leave the basal ends of the cells to enter the blood capillaries of the lamina propria. The hormones *somatostatin* and *endorphin* are also believed to be produced by these endocrine cells.

Situated between the bases of the villi are the openings of the intestinal glands; these glands are known as the *crypts of Lieberkühn* (Fig. 11-52; see Fig. 11-47). The glands are tubular and extend almost to the muscularis mucosae.

The epithelium lining the upper half of the crypts is identical to that covering the villi. In the lower half of the crypts, two new types of cells are found: undifferentiated stem cells and Paneth cells.

The *undifferentiated stem cells* are continuously undergoing mitosis to replace those cells that are exfoliated from the tips of the villi. As new cells are formed, a procession of cells emerges from the mouths of the crypts and by ameboid movements ascends the sides of neighboring villi, only to be shed into the lumen from the tips of the villi (see Fig. 11-47). As the cells march up the sides of the villi, they differentiate into columnar absorptive cells, goblet cells, and argentaffin or endocrine cells. The intestinal epithelium thus constantly is being replaced by the mitotic activity of the stem cells in the bottom of the crypts.

Paneth cells are found in small groups at the bottom of the crypts (see Figs. 11-47 and 11-52). They are pyramid shaped and contain large secretory granules in the apical cytoplasm. The granules are highly visible and stain deep pink in an H&E-stained section. The function of Paneth cells is unknown, although some authorities believe they make *lysozyme,* an enzyme that dissolves bacteria.

The *lamina propria* of the mucous membrane consists of loose connective tissue that fills the intervals

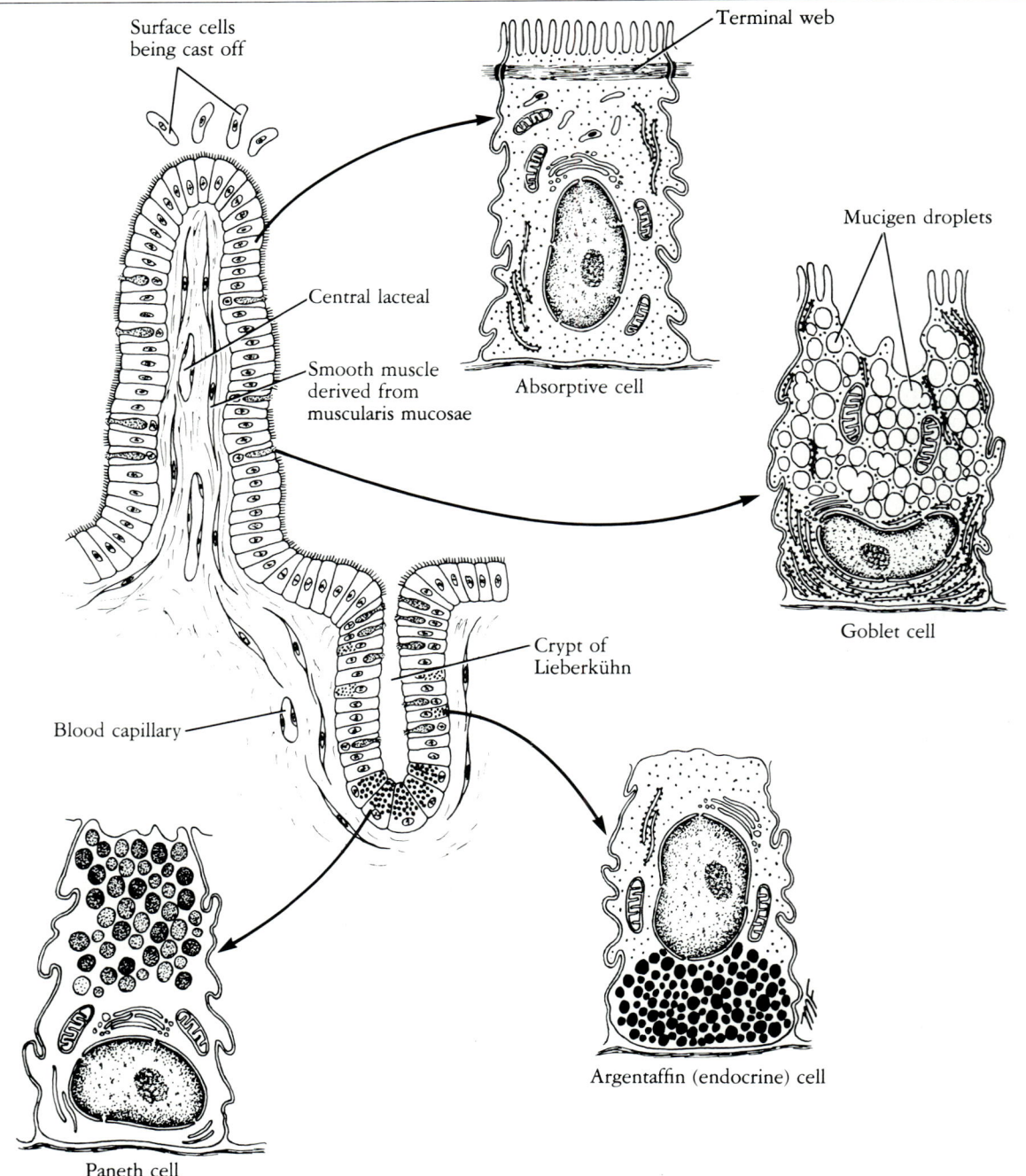

Fig. 11-47. Structure of a villus and a crypt of Lieberkühn; the electron microscopic structure of the surface epithelial cells is also shown.

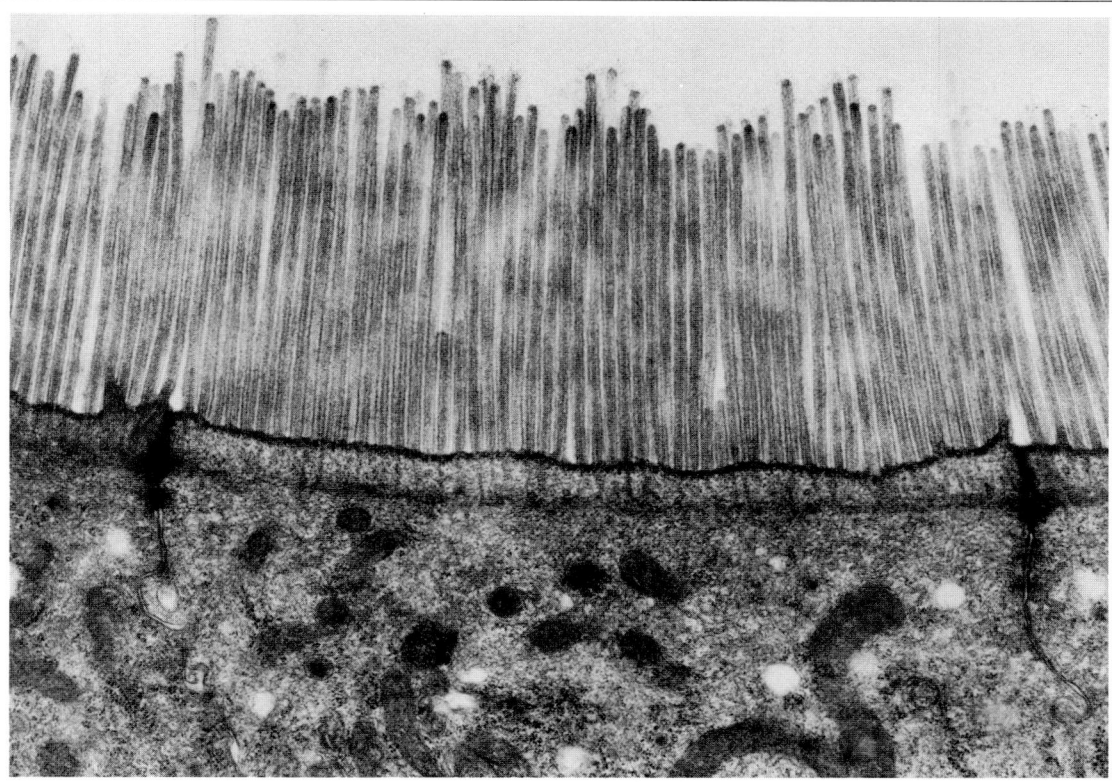

Fig. 11-48. Electron micrograph of columnar cells of the small intestine, showing apical microvilli. Note the terminal web and the junctional complexes between adjacent cells. (×16,000.) (Courtesy of Dr. L. A. Staehelin.)

between the crypts of Lieberkühn and forms the central core of the villi. Large numbers of reticular fibers and reticular cells are present, together with scattered lymphocytes, macrophages, plasma cells, and eosinophils. The eosinophils play an important protective role in preventing bacterial and viral infections from entering the tissues from the lumen of the intestine.

Nodules of lymphatic tissue are widely distributed throughout the length of the lamina propria of the small intestine and reach their greatest numbers in the ileum. The larger nodules may extend through the muscularis mucosae into the submucosa. Large confluent masses of lymphatic tissue are found in the distal part of the ileum opposite the mesenteric attachment; they are known as *Peyer's patches* (Figs. 11-53 and 11-54).

The *muscularis mucosae* is similar to that found elsewhere in the alimentary tract. As mentioned previously, strands of the smooth muscle extend up into the villi, causing their movement and aiding the circulation of lymph through the lymphatic vessels.

The *submucosa* is composed of dense connective tissue and contains the autonomic nerve plexus, *Meissner's plexus* (Fig. 11-55). In the duodenum, the submucosa contains compound tubular mucous glands, called *Brunner's glands,* that drain their alkaline secretion into the crypts of Lieberkühn. These characteristic multiple mucous acini that occupy the greater part of the submucosa in the duodenum, together with the broad mucosal villi,

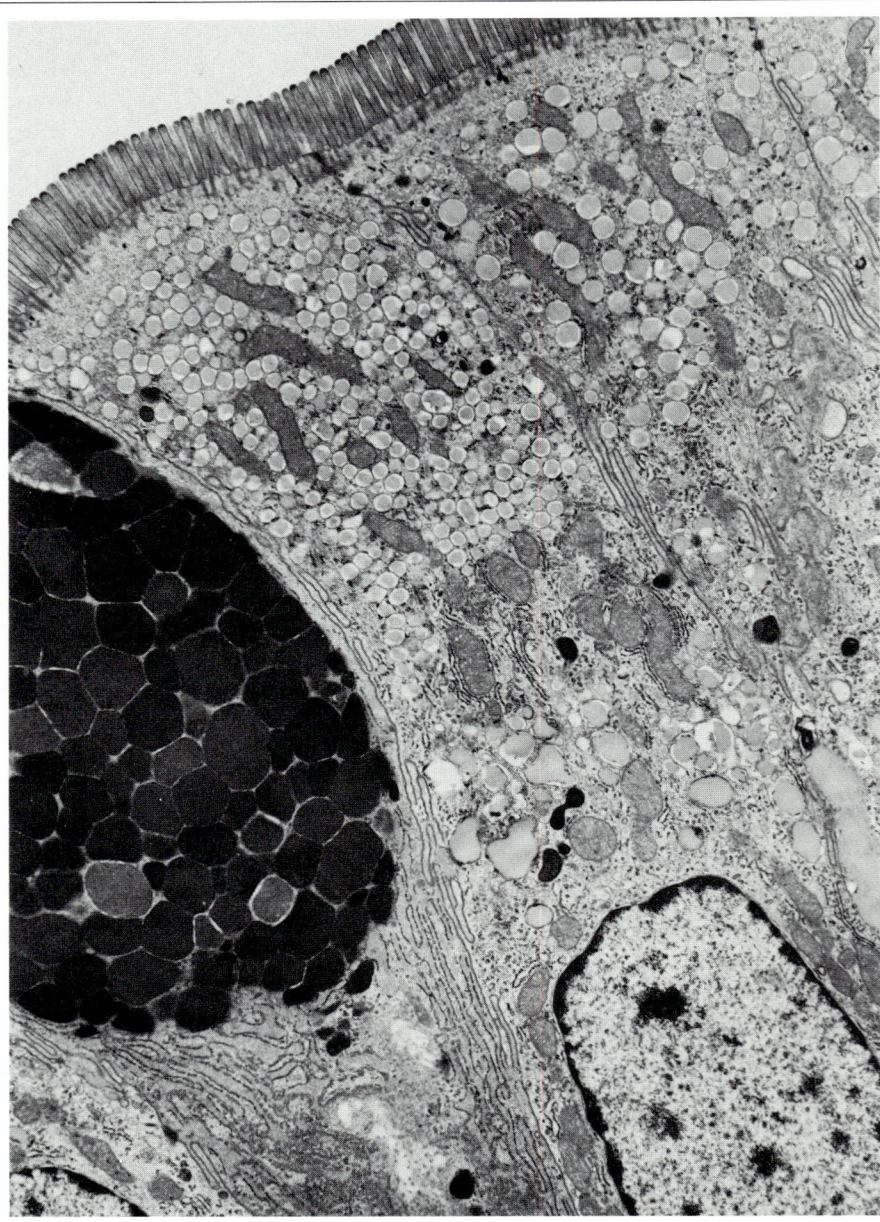

Fig. 11-49. Electron micrograph of columnar cells of the small intestine following a fatty meal. Note the large numbers of lipid droplets in vesicles of the smooth endoplasmic reticulum. An adjacent goblet cell that contains large, black-staining globules of mucin also can be seen. ($\times 5,760$.) (Courtesy of Dr. H. Friedman.)

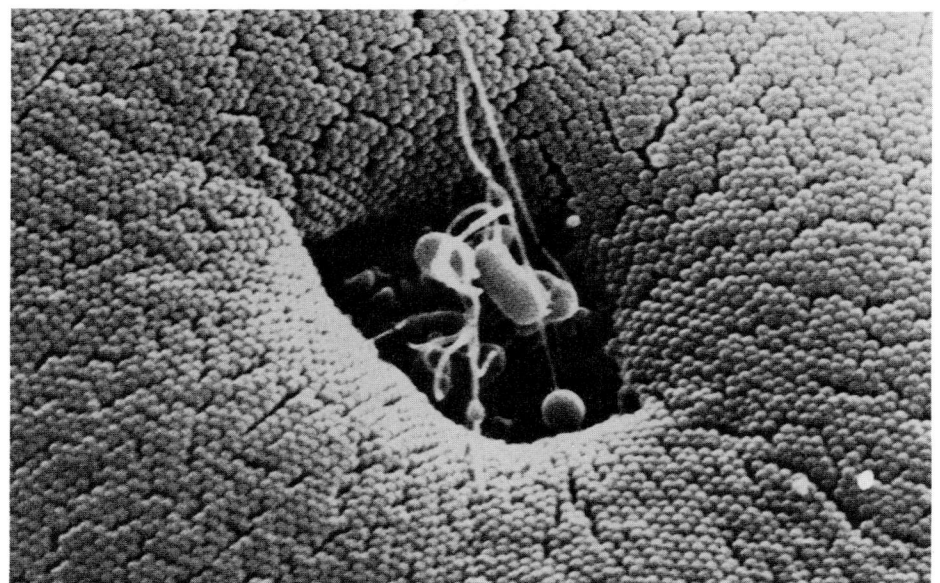

Fig. 11-50. Scanning electron micrograph of the luminal surface of the apical end of a goblet cell of the jejunum, showing several droplets of mucus about to be discharged from the cell. Note the many microvilli around the cellular opening. ($\times 12,334$.) (Courtesy of F. G. Lightfoot.)

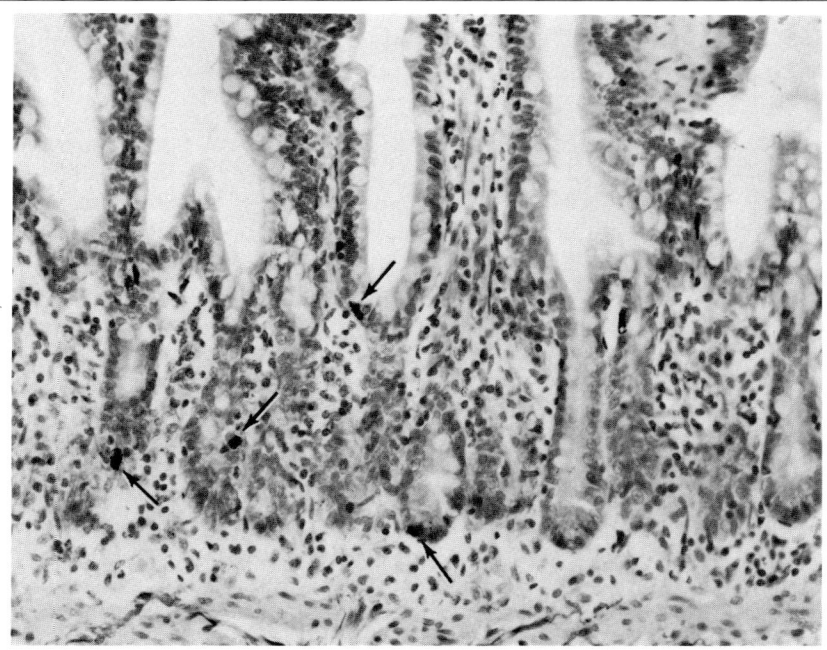

Fig. 11-51. Photomicrograph of a longitudinal section of the mucous membrane of the ileum. The heavily stained black granules are located in the cytoplasm of endocrine or argentaffin cells (arrows). (Silver stain; $\times 200$.)

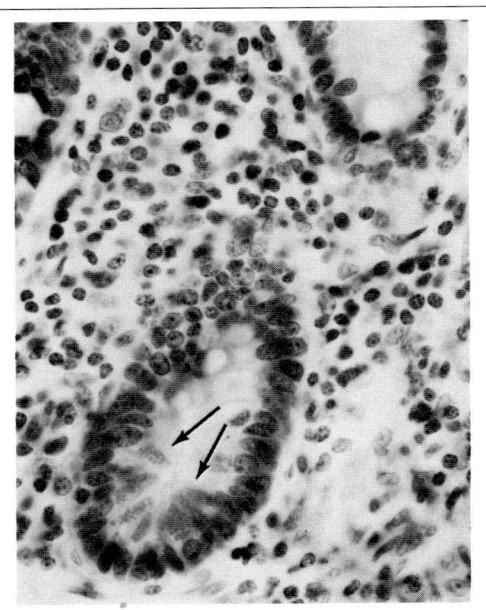

Fig. 11-52. Photomicrograph of a cross section of a crypt of Lieberkühn, showing light-staining granules in the apical cytoplasm of several Paneth cells (arrows). (H&E; ×400.)

make recognition of this area of the small intestine relatively easy (see Fig. 11-42).

The *muscular coat* consists of an inner, circular layer and an outer, longitudinal layer of smooth muscle (Fig. 11-56). Between the muscle layers is a small amount of connective tissue containing the autonomic nerve plexus, *Auerbach's plexus* (Fig. 11-57).

The *serosa* is the outermost coat of the small intestine and consists of a layer of loose connective tissue covered by flattened mesothelial cells; it forms the peritoneal covering of the small intestine. In the jejunum and ileum, the peritoneum leaves one border of the intestine as two layers to form the *mesentery of the small intestine*.

Functions

The small intestine, the part of the alimentary tract in which the greatest amount of digestion takes

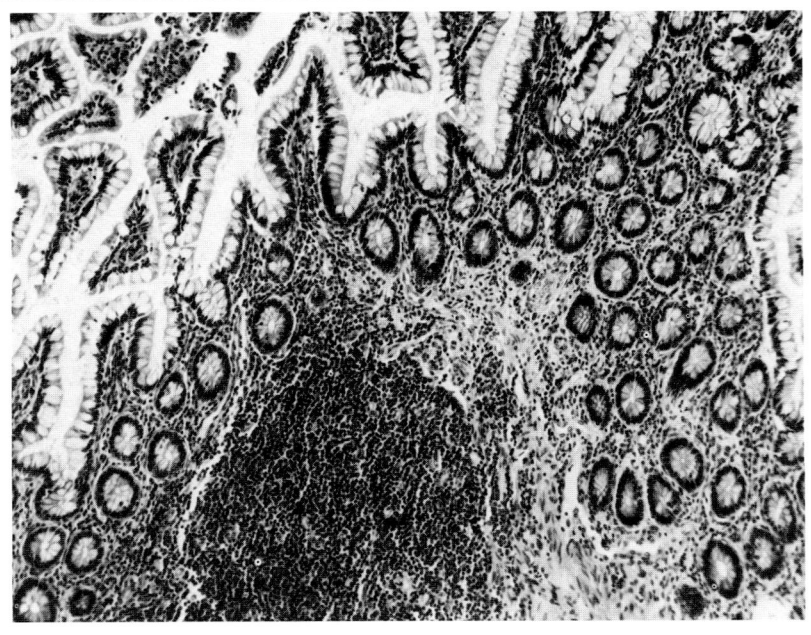

Fig. 11-53. Photomicrograph of a longitudinal section of the mucous membrane in the terminal part of the ileum. Note the large amounts of lymphoid tissue in the lamina propria (Peyer's patch). (H&E; ×100.)

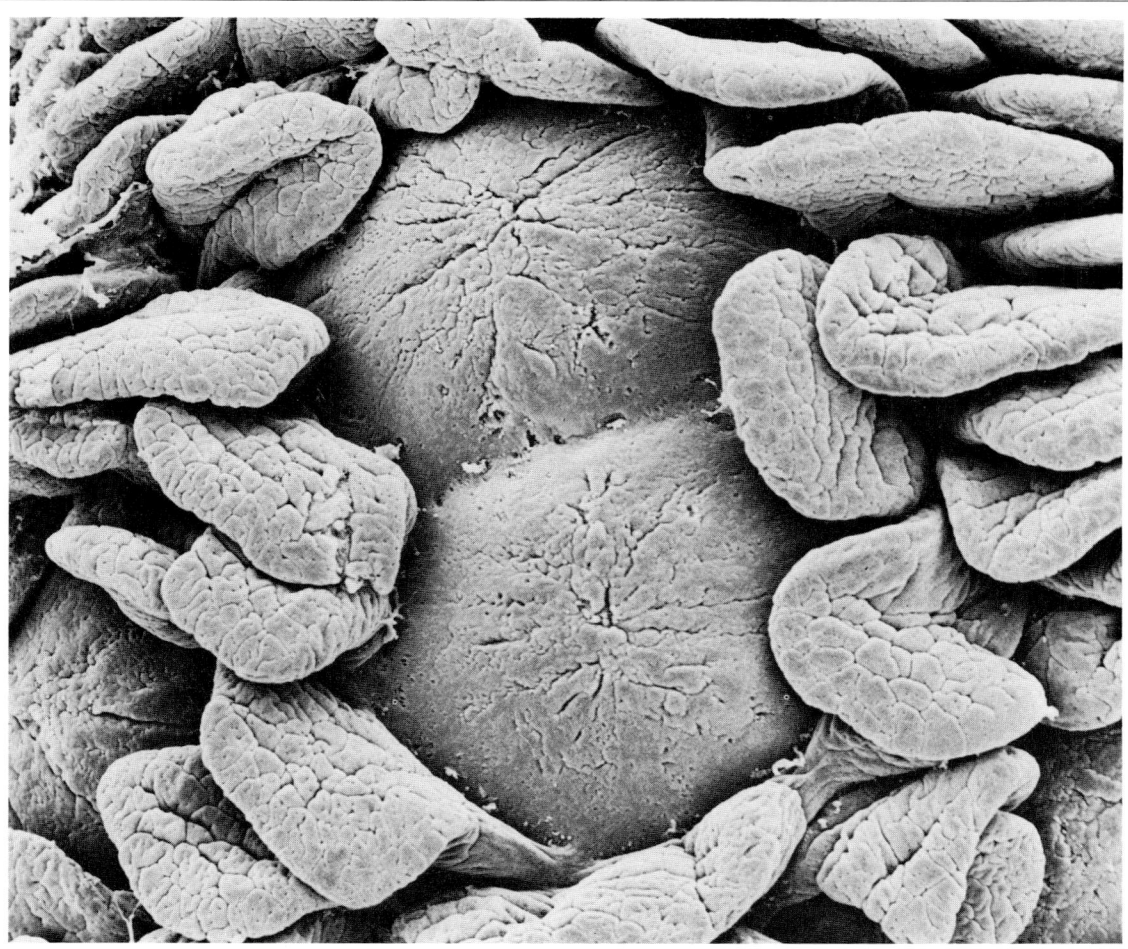

Fig. 11-54. Scanning electron micrograph of the luminal surface of the mucous membrane of the terminal part of the ileum, showing two lymph follicles of a Peyer's patch surrounded by numerous villi. (×967.) (Courtesy of F. G. Lightfoot.)

place, has four main functions: (1) it slowly conducts the digesting food from the stomach to the large intestine; (2) it thoroughly mixes the food with the secretions of the liver, pancreas, and small intestine, permitting further digestion; (3) it absorbs most of the products of digestion; and (4) it produces the hormones serotonin, secretin, cholecystokinin, and, possibly, somatostatin and endorphin.

MOVEMENTS OF THE SMALL INTESTINE. The movements of the small intestine are of two types, segmental and peristaltic.

Segmental Contractions. Segmental contractions of

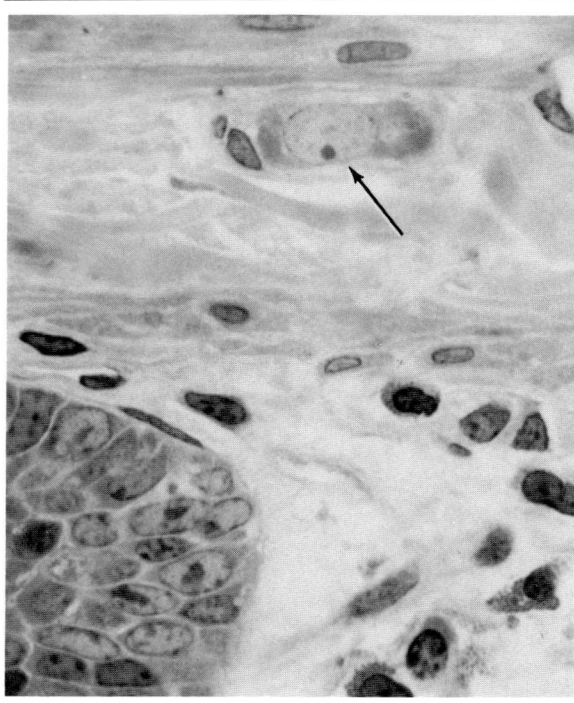

Fig. 11-55. Photomicrograph of a cross section of the submucosa of the small intestine, showing a nerve cell (arrow) of Meissner's plexus. (H&E; ×1,000.)

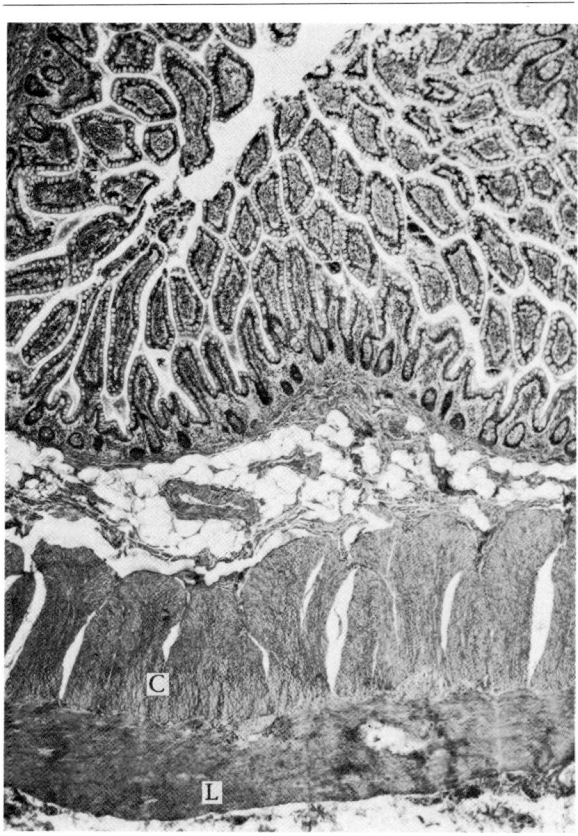

Fig. 11-56. Photomicrograph of a longitudinal section of the wall of the ileum. The villi of the mucous membrane are shown at the top. The inner, circular layer of smooth muscle (C) is visible, arranged in bundles; the outer, longitudinal layer of smooth muscle (L) can be seen below. (H&E; ×40.)

the wall of the small intestine occur once it is distended with chyme. As one set of contractions ends, a new set begins. These contractions are mainly a stationary form of movement, and there is little tendency to milk the contents along the intestinal tract. The purpose of these contractions is to mix the intestinal contents thoroughly with the secretions of the intestine, pancreas, and liver.

Peristaltic Waves. Essentially, these movements consist of a wave of contraction preceded by a wave of relaxation; they serve to propel the chyme onward through the small intestine. The wave of contraction is much faster in the proximal part of the intestine than at the distal end. It takes from 3 to 10 hours for food to travel from the stomach to the ileocecal junction.

Movements of the small intestine are stimulated by the stretching of its walls by fluid material in its lumen, bringing about a local nervous reflex involving the myenteric or Auerbach's plexus. The coordinated waves of contraction that pass down the gut are controlled by the myenteric nerve plexus. The activities of this plexus, however, can be influenced to some extent by nerve impulses from the central nervous system that reach the intestine via the vagus and splanchnic nerves. Emotional excitement or shock, for example, can stimulate an increase in intestinal movements.

A severe irritant or a cathartic can cause a sudden series of peristaltic contractions that move the food

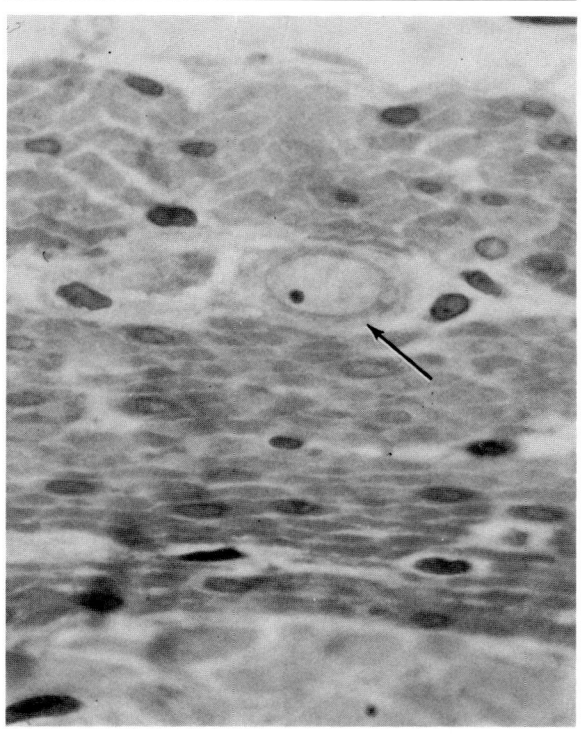

Fig. 11-57. Photomicrograph of a cross section of the muscular coat of the small intestine, showing a nerve cell (arrow) of Auerbach's plexus. (H&E; ×1,000.)

for a great distance. This special movement is referred to as a *peristaltic rush*.

SMALL INTESTINE SECRETIONS. The origins of secretions of the small intestine are threefold: (1) mucous membrane of the small intestine, (2) the pancreas, and (3) the liver.

Secretions of the Mucous Membrane of the Small Intestine. The average adult produces about 2,000 ml of secretions (succus entericus) in 24 hours; the pH of the secretions is about 7.8. Mucus is secreted by the Brunner's glands of the duodenum and the goblet cells of the mucous membrane. The mucus protects the wall of the small intestine from the acid and enzymes of the gastric juice. Enzymes secreted by the lining cells of the small intestine are enterokinase and amylase. Enterokinase is responsible for activating trypsinogen into trypsin in the pancreatic secretion (see p. 494). Amylase acts on the polysaccharide starch and breaks it down into disaccharides.

In addition, there are a number of enzymes produced in the region of the microvilli of the absorptive cells that hydrolyze food substances as they are absorbed from the intestinal lumen. These are: (1) *sucrase, maltase,* and *lactase* for hydrolyzing disaccharides into monosaccharides that can be absorbed readily; (2) *lipase* for hydrolyzing neutral fats into glycerol and fatty acids; and (3) *peptidases,* which hydrolyze polypeptides into amino acids (Figs. 11-58 to 11-61).

Control of Intestinal Secretions. The following factors control secretion: (1) direct chemical stimulation by food; (2) mechanical stretching of intestinal walls by food; (3) activation of the local myenteric nerve plexus, which is influenced by the vagus nerves; and (4) the hormone secretin.

Large Intestine

The large intestine is divided into the cecum, the vermiform appendix, the ascending colon, the transverse colon, the descending colon, the pelvic colon, the rectum, and the anal canal (see Fig. 11-25). The large intestine is a continuation of the small intestine at the ileocecal valve; it terminates on the body surface at the *anus*.

Ileocecal Valve

The ileocecal (ileocolic) valve is a rudimentary structure situated at the junction of the ileum and the colon (see Fig. 11-25). It consists of two horizontal folds of mucous membrane that project around the orifice of the ileum.

The ileal surfaces of the valve are covered with microscopic villi; the large intestine surfaces show no villi and have the histological characteristics of the large intestine.

The valve plays little or no part in the prevention of the reflux of colic contents into the ileum. The circular muscle of the lower end of the ileum (called the *ileocecal sphincter* by physiologists) serves as a sphincter and controls the flow of contents from the ileum into the colon. The smooth muscle tone is

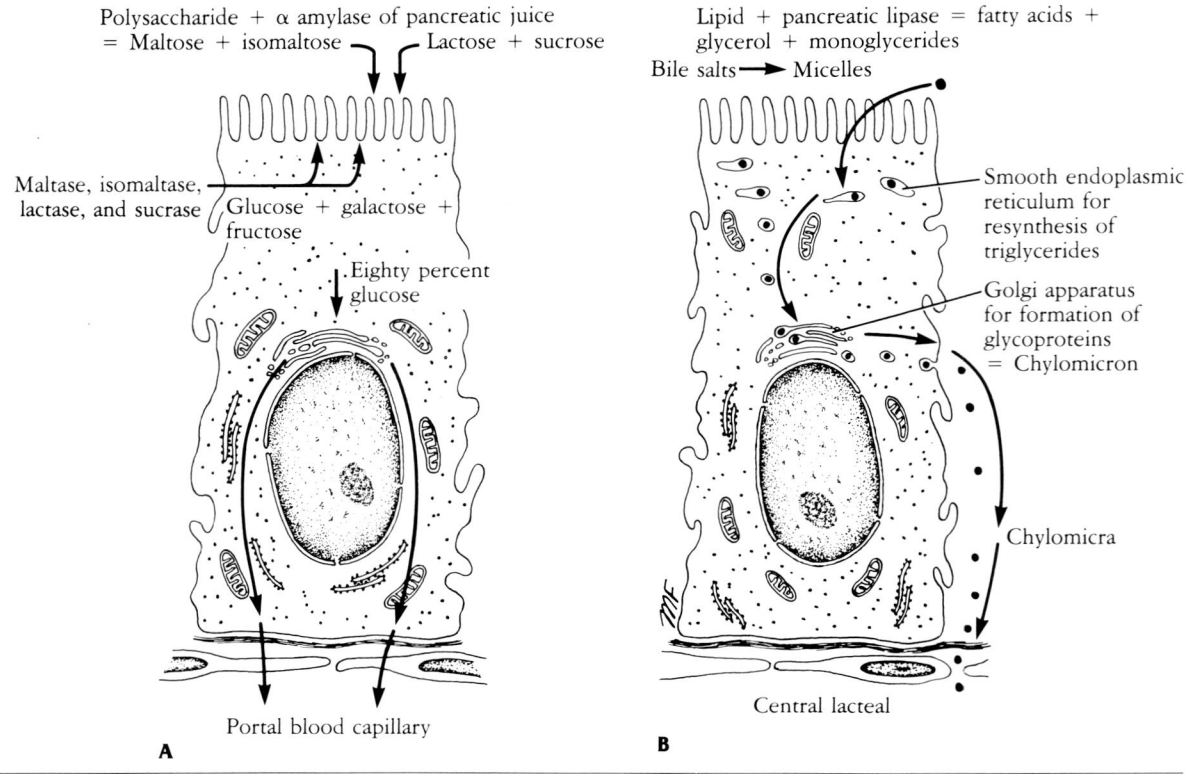

Fig. 11-58. Processes of (A) the digestion and absorption of carbohydrates and (B) the digestion and absorption of fats in the small intestine.

reflexly increased when the cecum is distended. The arrival of the hormone gastrin, produced by the stomach, will cause relaxation of the muscle tone, however.

Cecum, Colon, and Rectum

The structure of the large intestine shows the usual four layers of mucous membrane, submucosa, muscular coat, and serosa but differs from that of the small intestine in many respects (Figs. 11-62 to 11-66).

1. There are no permanent folds of mucous membrane (plicae circulares).
2. There are no villi on the surface of the mucous membrane.
3. The mucous membrane is thicker and possesses long tubular crypts of Lieberkühn that have no Paneth cells but more goblet cells. Although numerous solitary lymphatic nodules are present, there are no Peyer's patches.
4. The muscular coat differs from its counterpart in the small intestine by the arrangement of its outer, longitudinal layer into three thick bands called the *teniae coli*. In the rectum, these three longitudinal bands again become continuous around the intestinal tract. The teniae coli are shorter than the intestine and gather its wall into *sacculations*, or *haustra*. In the rectum, the longitudinal muscle is also shorter than this portion of the bowel and causes the rectal wall to bulge into the rectal lumen, forming three permanent folds

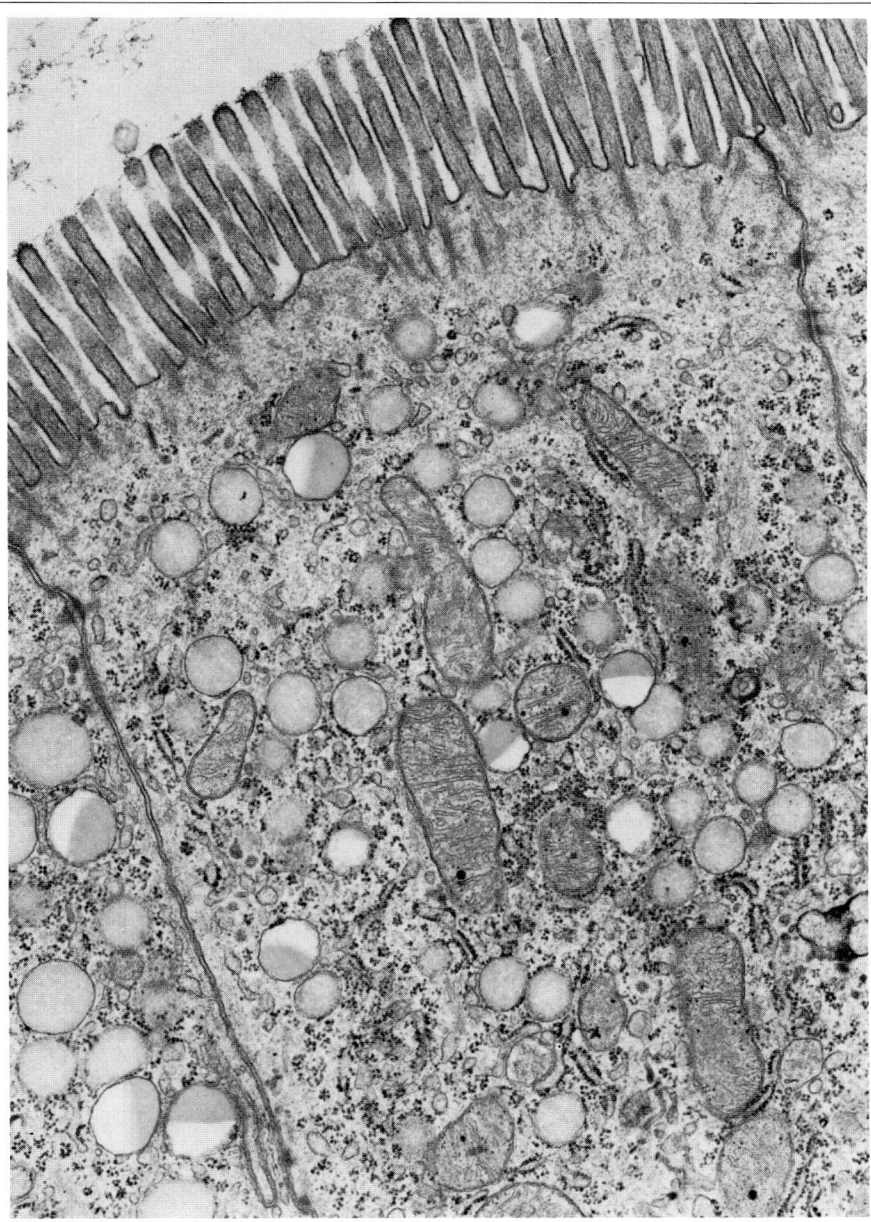

Fig. 11-59. Electron micrograph of columnar cells of the small intestine following a fatty meal. Note the large numbers of membrane-bound lipid droplets in the apical cytoplasm. ($\times 14,300$.) (Courtesy of Dr. H. Friedman.)

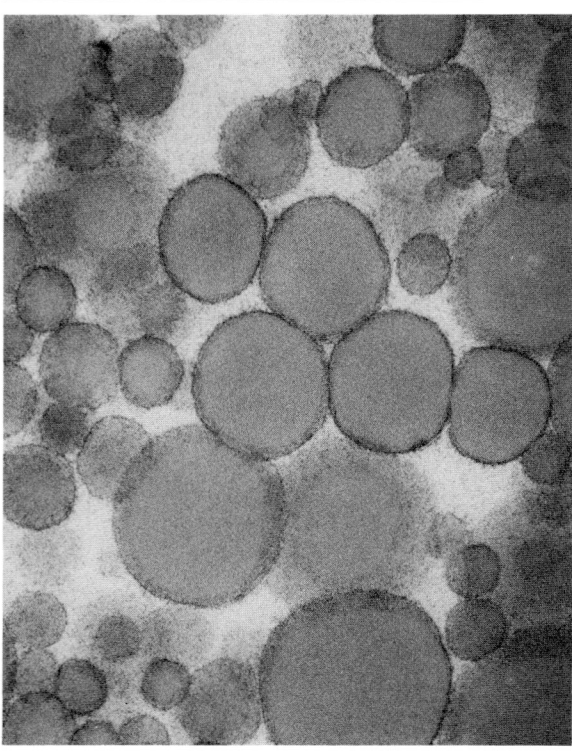

Fig. 11-60. Electron micrograph showing numerous chylomicrons in the lymph of the thoracic duct. Chylomicrons are formed in the columnar cells lining the small intestine (see Fig. 11-59) and then enter the central lacteal to be transported in the lymph to the blood via the thoracic duct. (×75,000.) (Courtesy of Dr. E. J. Blanchette-Mackie.)

called the *transverse folds of the rectum*. These folds are semicircular; two are placed on the left rectal wall and one on the right wall. They assist in supporting the feces within the rectal lumen.

5. The serosa is arranged differently in the different parts of the large intestine. It forms a complete covering of peritoneum for the cecum; it covers the anterior surface and sides of the ascending and descending colon; it covers the anterior surface and sides of the upper third of the rectum and only the anterior surface of the middle third of the rectum. The lower third of the rectum is devoid of peritoneum. In the transverse colon and pelvic colon, the peritoneum leaves the

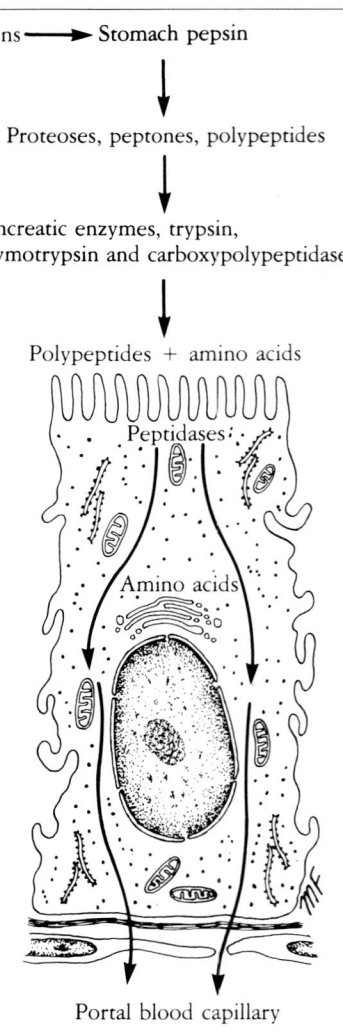

Fig. 11-61. Process of the digestion and absorption of protein.

bowel as a two-layered fold called the *transverse mesocolon* and the *pelvic mesocolon,* respectively. Large local accumulations of adipose tissue in the serosa produce characteristic fatty tags, called the *appendices epiploicae,* that protrude from the outer surface of the large intestine.

APPENDIX. The appendix is a wormlike diverticulum of the cecum and contains a large amount of lymphoid tissue. It varies in length from 3 to 5

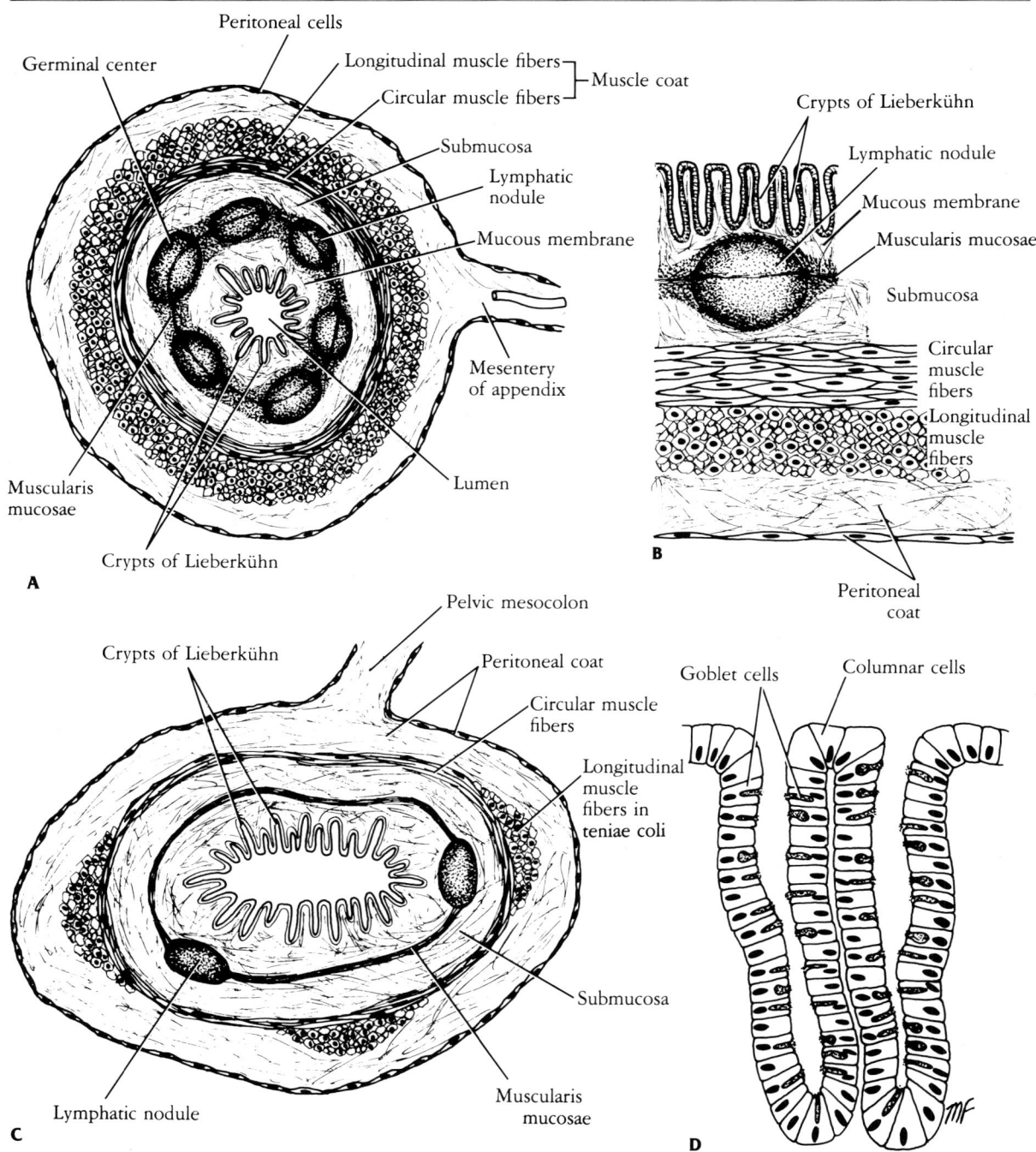

Fig. 11-62. A: General structure of the appendix as seen in cross section. B: Enlarged view of the mucous membrane and submucosa of the appendix as seen in cross section. C: General structure of the pelvic colon as seen in cross section. D: Structure of two crypts of Lieberkühn of the colon.

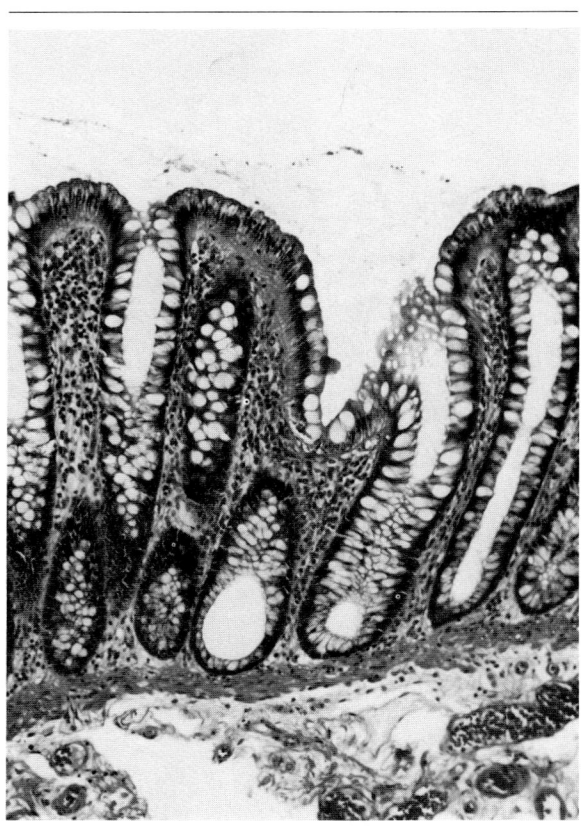

Fig. 11-63. Photomicrograph of a longitudinal section of the colon, showing the mucous membrane and part of the submucosa. Note the absence of villi and the presence of long, straight mucous glands, or crypts of Lieberkühn, and numerous mucus-secreting goblet cells. (H&E; ×100.)

inches (8 to 13 cm). The base is attached to the posteromedial surface of the cecum about 1 inch (2.5 cm) below the ileocecal junction (see Fig. 11-25). The remainder of the appendix is free.

The appendix has the usual four-layered structure of the alimentary canal. The mucous membrane is identical to that of the large intestine, possessing long tubular crypts of Lieberkühn (see Figs. 11-62, 11-63, and 11-65). The lamina propria contains very large amounts of lymphoid tissue, so that the lymph nodules may surround the lumen completely. In many areas, the lymphoid tissue extends through the muscularis mucosae into the submucosa.

The muscular coat consists of an inner, circular layer and an outer, longitudinal layer of smooth muscle. Unlike those of the cecum and colon, the longitudinal fibers form a complete coat, the teniae coli of the cecum becoming confluent at the base of the appendix.

The serosa completely surrounds the appendix. The peritoneum leaves the appendix as a two-layered fold, forming a small mesentery called the *mesoappendix*. The size of the mesoappendix varies; sometimes as much as the distal third of the appendix is devoid of mesentery. The mesoappendix is attached to the mesentery of the small intestine.

The structure of the appendix changes with age. In the elderly, the lymphoid tissue atrophies and largely is replaced by connective tissue; also, the lumen narrows.

FUNCTIONS OF THE CECUM, COLON, AND RECTUM. The main functions of the large intestine are absorption of water and storage of the undigested food residue that enters the large intestine at the ileocecal junction. By the time the contents reach the descending colon, they acquire the consistency of *feces*.

Functions of Bacteria within the Colon. Bacteria in the lumen of the colon form vitamin K, vitamin B_{12}, thiamine, riboflavin, and gas. Vitamin K is necessary for the formation of prothrombin in the liver and the production of clotting factors VII, IX, and X. Vitamin B_{12} is essential for the normal maturation of red blood cells.

Movements of the Colon. The movements of the colon are (1) segmental and (2) peristaltic.

Segmental Movements. Segmental contraction of the circularly arranged smooth muscle fibers in the large intestine and the contractions of the teniae coli serve to mix the luminal contents thoroughly and facilitate absorption of water. The bulging of the intestinal wall between the contracted segments produces saclike structures referred to as *haustrations*.

Peristaltic Movements. Periodic mass peristaltic waves, usually initiated by the presence of food in the stomach or duodenum (*gastrocolic* or *gastroduodenal reflex*), occur in the large intestine. Such waves of contraction, which progressively move the feces

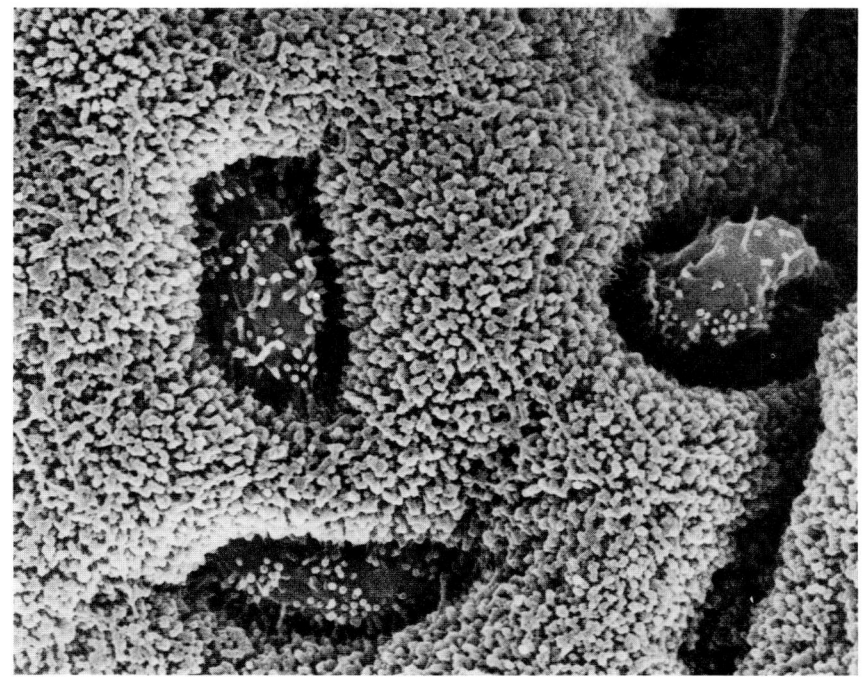

Fig. 11-64. Scanning electron micrograph of the luminal surface of the mucous membrane of the colon. Note the many microvilli covering the surface of the columnar cells, and the fewer numbers and smaller size of the microvilli over the goblet cells. (×4,750.) (Courtesy of F. G. Lightfoot.)

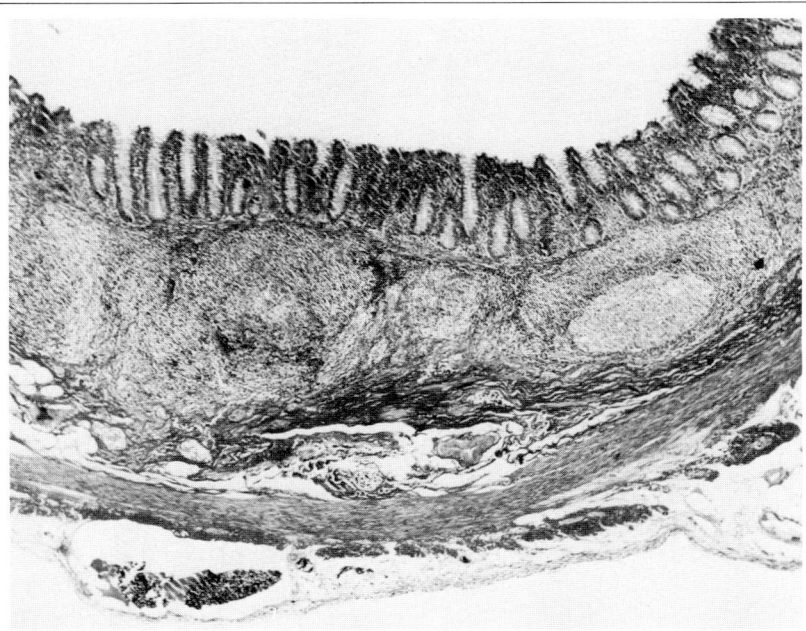

Fig. 11-65. Photomicrograph of a transverse section of the wall of the appendix. The mucous membrane contains numerous mucous glands, or crypts of Lieberkühn, and the lamina propria and submucosa are densely packed with lymphatic tissue. (H&E; ×40.)

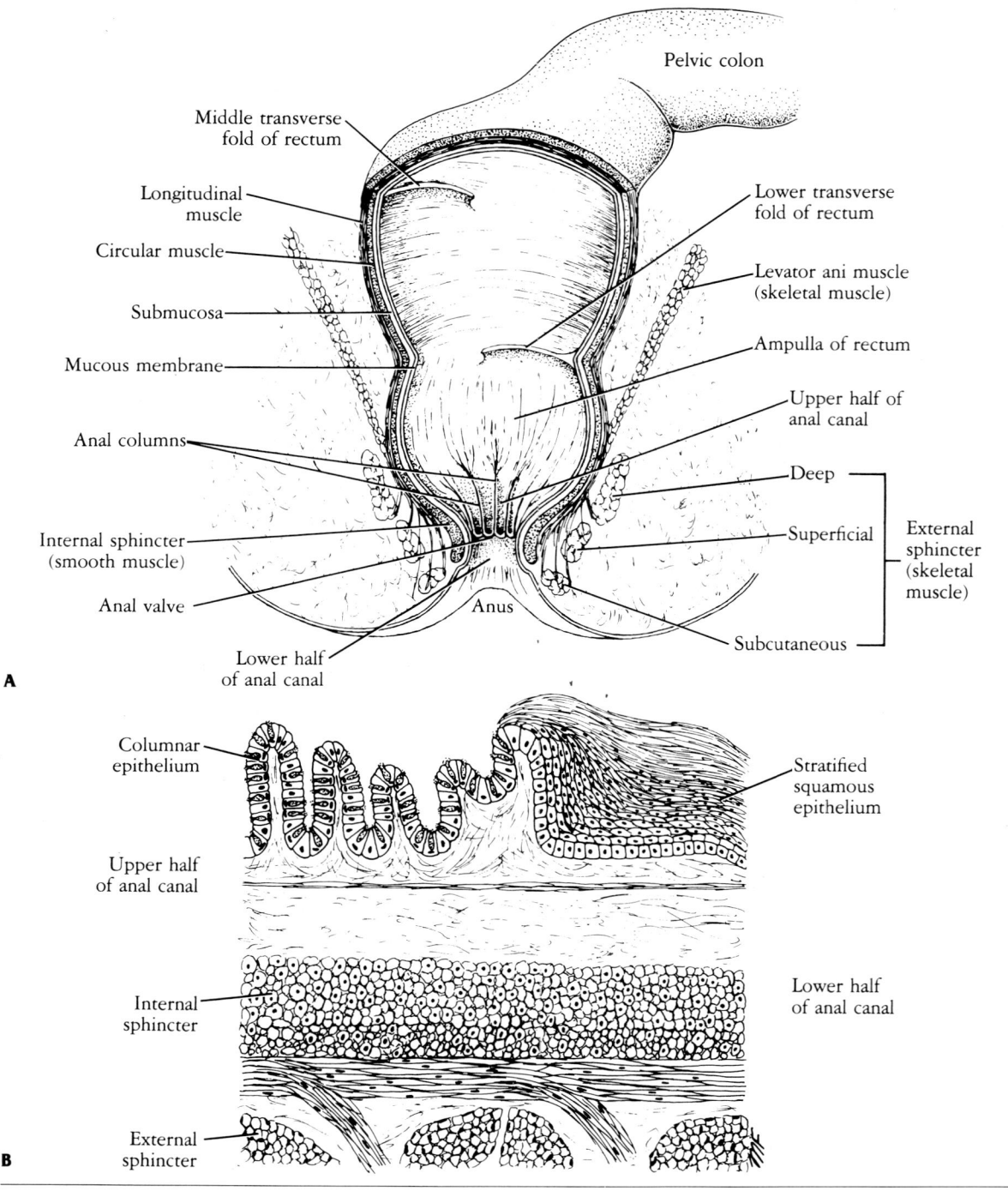

Fig. 11-66. A: *General structure of the rectum, anal canal, and sphincters of the anal canal. B: Structure of the junction of the upper and lower halves of the anal canal as seen on longitudinal section.*

onward toward the anus, result in the temporary disappearance of the haustrations. This mass peristalsis probably is controlled by the myenteric nerve plexus and the hormone gastrin. Irritation of the colon by some chemical agent or distention of the colon also can initiate this type of peristaltic movement.

Anal Canal

The anal canal is the most distal part of the alimentary canal and is continuous above with the rectum as the latter pierces the levator ani muscle. The anal canal is about 1.5 inches (4 cm) long and opens onto the surface of the *anus* (see Fig. 11-66).

The anal canal is composed of the usual four layers: mucous membrane, submucosa, muscular coat, and adventitia.

The *mucous membrane* of the upper half of the anal canal is identical in structure to that of the colon and rectum, having long tubular crypts of Lieberkühn. The surface cells are simple columnar epithelium (Fig. 11-67). The mucous membrane is thrown into vertical folds, called *anal columns,* that are joined together at their lower ends by small semilunar folds called *anal valves* (see Fig. 11-66). Each column contains a branch of the superior rectal artery and a tributary of the superior rectal vein.

In the mucous membrane of the lower half of the anal canal, the tubular crypts of Lieberkühn abruptly cease and the columnar epithelium on the surface changes to stratified squamous epithelium (see Fig. 11-67). The stratified squamous epithelium gradually merges at the anus with the perianal epidermis (Fig. 11-68). There are no anal columns.

The *submucosa* is composed of connective tissue and contains branches of the rectal blood vessels. In the region of the anal valves, several tubular glands called *anal glands* extend into the submucosa. They secrete mucus.

The *muscular coat* is composed of a circular inner and a longitudinal outer layer of smooth muscle. In the upper three-quarters of the canal, the circular coat is greatly thickened to form the *involuntary internal anal sphincter* (see Fig. 11-66). The layer of longitudinal muscle continues distally, losing many of its muscle cells and becoming fibroelastic. This layer eventually divides into slips that are attached to the dermis of the perianal skin. Some of the slips pass medially to attach to the mucous membrane.

The *voluntary external anal sphincter* is formed of skeletal muscle and surrounds the entire length of the anal canal (see Fig. 11-66). It is divided into three parts: (1) a subcutaneous part, which encircles the lower end of the anal canal; (2) a superficial part, which lies deep to the subcutaneous part; and (3) a deep part, which encircles the upper end of the anal canal. The puborectalis part of the levatores ani muscles blends with the deep part of the external sphincter (see Fig. 11-66).

Defecation. The time, place, and frequency of defecation are very much a matter of habit. Some adults defecate once a day, some several times a day, and some perfectly normal people only once in several days.

The act is preceded by a wave of peristalsis that passes down the descending and pelvic parts of the colon. The rectum becomes distended by the entrance of the feces, giving rise to the desire to defecate.

Assuming that the time and place are favorable, a coordinated reflex act occurs that results in the emptying of the descending colon, pelvic colon, rectum, and anal canal. The intra-abdominal pressure is raised by the descent of the diaphragm, the closure of the glottis, and the contraction of the muscles of the anterior abdominal walls and the levatores ani muscles. The external pressure applied to the colon and the waves of peristalsis in the wall of the colon force the feces onward. The tonic contraction of the internal and external sphincters, including the puborectalis muscles, is now voluntarily inhibited. The feces are now evacuated through the anal canal. Depending on the laxity of the submucous coat, the mucous membrane of the lower part of the canal is extruded through the anus ahead of the fecal mass. At the end of the act, the mucosa is returned to the anal canal by the tone of the longitudinal fibers of the anal walls and the contraction and upward pull of

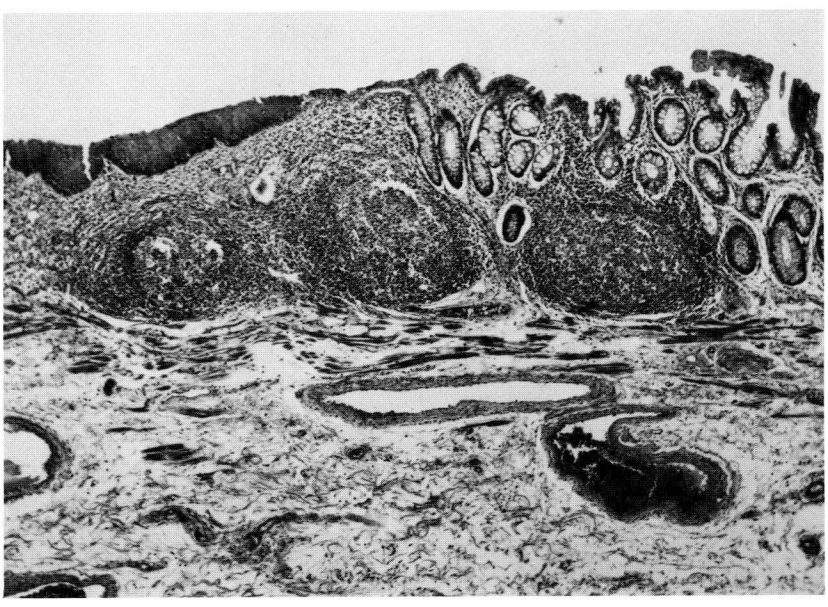

Fig. 11-67. Photomicrograph of a longitudinal section of the junction of the upper and lower halves of the anal canal, showing the mucous membrane and submucosa of the lower half on the left and that of the upper half on the right. Note that the mucous membrane of the lower half is covered with stratified squamous epithelium and has no glands, whereas the upper half is lined with columnar cells and possesses numerous mucous glands. Note also three lymphatic nodules in the lamina propria of the mucous membrane. (H&E; ×40.)

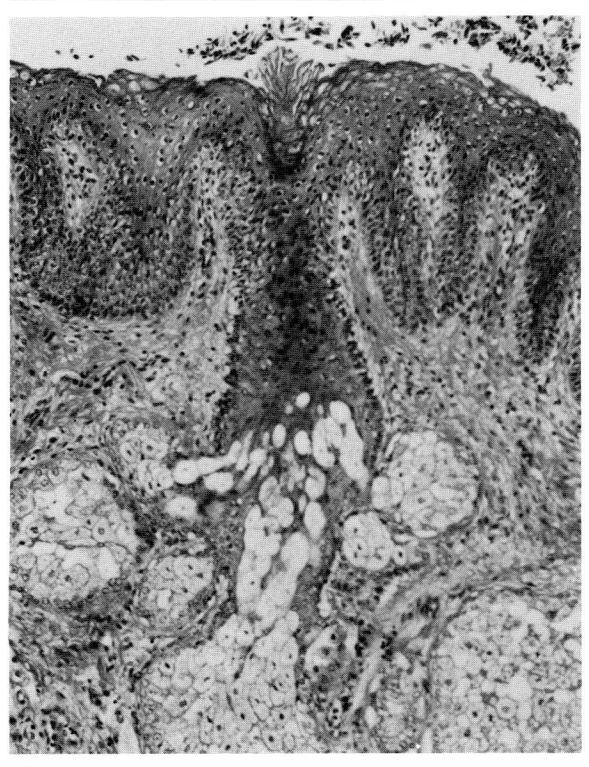

Fig. 11-68. Photomicrograph of a longitudinal section of the mucous membrane of the lower half of the anal canal near the anal margin, showing the lining of stratified squamous keratinized epithelium and part of a large hair follicle with sebaceous glands. (H&E; ×100.)

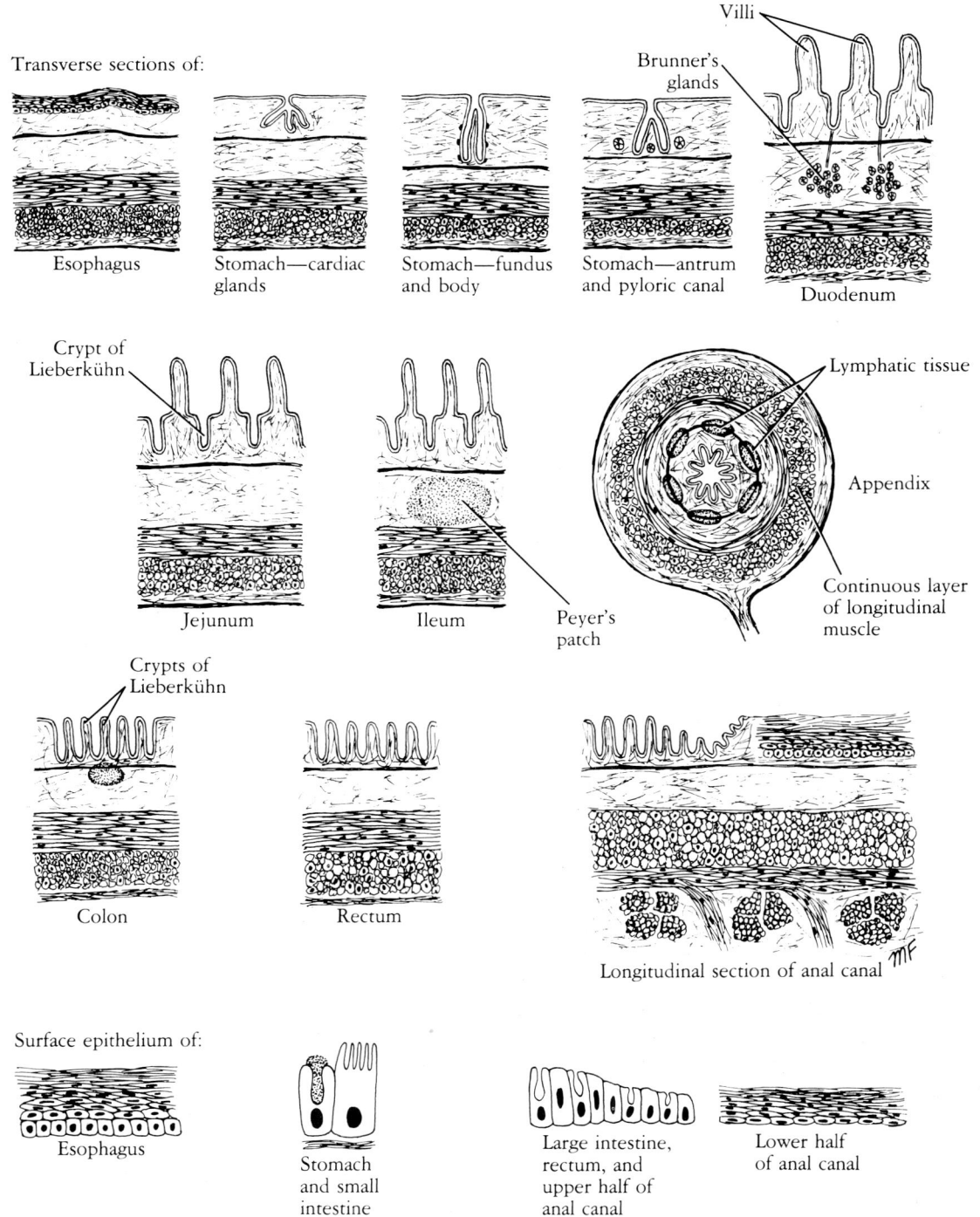

Fig. 11-69. A: *General structure of the digestive tract.* B: *Shape of the surface of epithelial cells lining the digestive tract, from the esophagus to the anal canal.*

the puborectalis muscle. The empty lumen of the anal canal is now closed by the tonic contraction of the anal sphincters.

Secretions of the Large Intestines. The crypts of Lieberkühn and the goblet cells of the mucous membrane produce large amounts of mucus that protect the mucous membrane against trauma from the hard feces and bacteria. The alkalinity of the mucus also neutralizes any residual acid within the feces and so further protects the mucous membrane. The viscous property of the mucus helps to bind the feces together.

A summary of the structure of the digestive tract is shown in Figure 11-69.

CLINICAL NOTES

MOUTH

The mouth is one of the most important areas of the body that the physician is called upon to examine. One must be able to recognize all the structures visible in the mouth and be familiar with the normal variations in the color of the mucous membrane covering the underlying structures. The oral mucous membrane can show localized disease as well as manifest disease elsewhere in the body. For example, the red margin of the lips may show cyanosis in heart disease or may have cracks at the angles of the mouth in vitamin deficiency. In digestive disorders, the tongue may be covered with a white fur (coated tongue) because of excessively long filiform papillae. The tongue also may be shiny and smooth because of the absence of these papillae in certain anemias, such as pernicious anemia.

Ulcers of the mucous membrane of the tongue are quite common, and many are overlooked by the patient. The ulcers of syphilis and malignant ulcers should not be missed. Brownish areas of pigmentation of the mouth are common in Addison's disease and are caused by the excessive stimulation of melanocytes in the mucous membrane by excessive quantities of circulating adrenocorticotropic hormone.

Teeth

Examination of the teeth should never be omitted in patients with symptoms suggestive of gastrointestinal disorders. Make sure that the patient has sufficient molars to grind up the food effectively.

Dental caries is a very common abnormality. Essentially, it is a destruction of the calcified structure of the tooth. The enamel surface of the tooth becomes eroded by a mixture of bacteria and fungi referred to as the enamel *plaque*. The organic framework of the enamel is destroyed, and the enamel is decalcified. The bacteria and fungi require the presence of carbohydrate on the tooth surface for their metabolism. Adequate amounts of saliva and its mucolytic enzymes, coupled with adequate dental hygiene, can reduce the incidence of caries.

Examine the gums carefully. Remember that healthy gums are bright pink, firm, and closely adherent to the necks of the teeth. In cases of severe abdominal pain, lead poisoning can be diagnosed by observing a black stippled line on the gums at or near the point where the teeth emerge from the gums.

SALIVARY GLANDS

Disease of the salivary glands results in the reduction of salivary flow and a dry mouth. A dry mouth can be caused by nervousness, which is normal, but it can also be caused by dehydration stemming from a number of conditions, such as vomiting and severe diarrhea. Anticholinergic, hypotensive, antidepressive drugs may inhibit the flow of saliva pharmacologically. Secretion from the submandibular gland may be obstructed by a stone in the submandibular duct.

The sublingual gland is rarely involved in disease. Benign tumors are common in the parotid and less common in the submandibular glands. The most common benign tumor arises from the epithelial and myoepithelial components, giving rise to a mixed, or pleomorphic, tumor. Malignant tumors of these glands also occur, but they are less common than benign tumors.

PHARYNX

At the junction of the mouth and the oral part of the pharynx, and the nose and the nasal part of the pharynx, there are collections of lymphoid tissues of considerable clinical importance. The palatine tonsils and the nasopharyngeal tonsils are the most important.

The *palatine tonsils* reach their maximum normal size in early childhood. After puberty, together with other lymphoid tissues in the body, they gradually atrophy. The palatine tonsils are a common site of acute infections with streptococci, producing the characteristic sore throat and pyrexia. The blood vessels of the tonsil show extreme vasodilatation and edema, causing the tonsils to appear red and enlarged. Pus tends to accumulate in the crypts of the tonsil, producing the characteristic creamy yellow dots at the orifices of the crypts. Rapid spread to the deep cervical lymph nodes is a common sequela. The giving of antibiotics is the treatment of choice; tonsillectomy is reserved for those cases with recurrent attacks of tonsillitis with complications. A peritonsillar abscess (quinsy) is caused by the spread of infection from the palatine tonsil to the loose connective tissue outside the capsule.

The *nasopharyngeal tonsil* is situated beneath the epithelium lining the roof of the nasal part of the pharynx. Like the palatine tonsil, it is largest in early childhood and starts to atrophy after puberty. Excessive hypertrophy of the lymphoid tissue, usually associated with infection, causes these tonsils to become enlarged; they are then commonly referred to as *adenoids*. Marked hypertrophy blocks the posterior nasal openings and causes the patient to snore loudly and to breathe through the open mouth. The close relationship of the infected lymphoid tissue to the auditory tube may be the cause of deafness and recurrent otitis media. Adenoidectomy is the treatment of choice in cases of hypertrophied adenoids with infection.

Abnormalities Associated with Swallowing

The swallowing reflex may be interfered with by lesions involving the ninth and tenth cranial nerve nuclei in the medulla oblongata. Such lesions will cause paralysis of the soft palate and pharynx and regurgitation of fluid through the nose. Aspiration of food into the larynx may also occur. *Myasthenia gravis,* a disease caused by an abnormality in the neuromuscular junction, may present with difficulty in swallowing as an early symptom.

ESOPHAGUS

The esophagus, as we have seen, consists of a muscular tube connecting the pharynx to the stomach. The tone of its muscle coat, together with the pressure from other mediastinal viscera, keeps its anterior and posterior walls in contact except during the passage of food or liquid.

The esophagus passes through the cavity of the thorax, where the pressure is negative compared with the atmospheric pressure, and enters the abdomen, where the pressure is positive, especially when the person coughs or strains at stool. Why, then, does gastroesophageal reflux not occur all the time? Microscopically, there is no evidence of an increased amount of stomach muscle at the lower end of the esophagus. This does not rule out the possibility of a sphincteric mechanism at the lower end of the esophagus, however. Several factors are thought to play an important role in this mechanism:

1. The angle of the entrance of the esophagus into the stomach
2. The looping fibers of the right crus of the diaphragm, which encircle the esophageal opening in the diaphragm
3. The circular smooth muscle fibers at the lower end of the esophagus, which may act independently of the remaining muscle and thus serve as a physiological sphincter

The last factor is considered by many to be the most important. It is possible that there exists a reflex arc involving the vagus nerve such that an increase in intragastric pressure is followed by an increase in tone of the muscle of the lower end of the esophagus. Hormones are also known to influence this esophageal muscle. The gastrin produced by the stomach causes the muscle to contract, whereas the secretin and cholecystokinin produced by the small intestine cause it to relax.

Achalasia of the Lower End of the Esophagus

In this disorder, there is an absence of normal peristaltic waves in the lower two-thirds of the esophagus and a spasm or failure to relax of the muscle at the lower end of the esophagus. The result is that the patient experiences progressive difficulty in swallowing (dysphagia). Eventually, the patient regurgitates food that has remained in the esophagus and has not entered the stomach. Postmortem histological examination of the esophagus has revealed a loss of ganglion cells in Auerbach's myenteric plexus. The cause of the loss of the nervous tissue is unknown.

Malignant Disease of the Esophagus

This condition is common and usually arises as a tumor of the squamous cells lining the mucous membrane. The clinical course is a progressive difficulty in swallowing solids and then liquid foods. It is associated with extreme weight loss.

STOMACH

The mucous membrane of the body of the stomach and, to a lesser extent, that of the fundus produces acid, pepsin, and the intrinsic factor. The antrum and pyloric canal mucous membrane produces weakly alkaline mucus and the hormone gastrin.

The secretion of acid and pepsin is controlled by two mechanisms, nervous and hormonal. The vagus nerves are responsible for the nervous control, and the gastrin produced by the antral mucosa is responsible for the hormonal control. It is now generally believed that the two mechanisms work closely together in each phase of gastric secretion. The nervous phase—when one is anticipating food—is mediated by the vagus nerve, which directly stimulates the gastric glands to liberate acid and pepsin and also stimulates the antral and pyloric glands to liberate gastrin. When food actually enters the stomach—the gastric phase—both the nervous and hormonal mechanisms, but especially the latter, come into play.

The role of histamine in gastric secretion is not understood, although it is known to be a powerful stimulant of acid secretion. It is possible that vagal or gastrin stimulation causes the release of histamine by the argentaffin endocrine cells, which in turn stimulates the parietal cells to produce more acid.

The so-called mucosal barrier that prevents the diffusion of acid from the lumen of the stomach into the underlying tissues and blood is of pathological importance. Clearly, this barrier is formed by the apical plasma membrane of the lining cells and the integrity of the tight junctions that unite the adjacent surfaces of these cells. The surface of the mucous membrane is also protected by the alkaline mucus secreted by the surface cells and the reflux of alkaline duodenal secretions through the pyloric sphincter.

Unfortunately, the mucosal barrier and the alkaline mucus barrier can be damaged severely by agents such as alcohol, cigarette smoke, and drugs (for example, aspirin). These substances cause death and desquamation of the surface cells and exposure of the lamina propria to the acid gastric contents.

Ulcer

Although we will not consider in detail here the various causes of gastric and duodenal ulcer, one observation is important. Without gastric acidity, chronic peptic ulcer does not occur. The medical treatment of peptic ulcer is directed toward the regulation of the diet so that the gastric secretion is not excessively stimulated; because of the consumption of small, frequent meals, the stomach lumen does not remain empty for long periods. Together with the appropriate use of antacids and drugs to inhibit gastric secretion, this treatment tends to result in healing. If medical treatment fails, surgical treatment attempts to reduce the amount of acid secretion by section of the vagus nerves and removal of the gastrin-bearing area of the mucosa, namely, the antrum.

The great majority of chronic gastric ulcers occur in the alkaline-bearing area of the antrum on the lesser curvature. A chronic ulcer gradually penetrates the mucous membrane, the submucosa, and the muscular coats and will, in time, involve the peritoneum, causing the stomach to adhere to neighboring structures. Some of the common complications include bleeding, perforation of the stomach wall, obstruction caused by excessive production of fibrous tissue in an attempt to heal the ulcer, and malignant change.

The sensation of pain in the stomach is caused by the stretching or spasmodic contraction of the smooth muscle in its walls and is referred to the epigastrium. It is believed that the pain-transmitting fibers leave the stomach in the company of sympathetic nerves. They pass through the celiac ganglia and reach the spinal cord via the greater splanchnic nerves.

Carcinoma

Carcinoma is the most common form of malignant tumor of the stomach. It arises from columnar cells of the mucous membrane or gastric cells that have undergone metaplasia so that they resemble intestinal goblet cells. Because the lymphatic vessels of the mucous membrane and submucosa of the stomach are in continuity, it is possible for cancer cells to travel to different parts of the stomach some distance from the primary site. For these reasons, malignant disease of the stomach is treated by total gastrectomy.

Achlorhydria of the stomach is very common in carcinoma of the stomach and is caused by the associated atrophy of the gastric mucous membrane.

Pernicious Anemia

This condition is caused by a failure of the parietal cells of the gastric glands to secrete adequate amounts of the intrinsic factor. The intrinsic factor (see p. 185) is necessary for the normal absorption of vitamin B_{12} from the intestine. Adequate amounts of vitamin B_{12} are required for the maturation of red blood cells.

SMALL INTESTINE

Duodenum

As the stomach empties its contents into the duodenum, the acid chyme is squirted against the anterolateral wall of the first part of the duodenum. This is thought to be an important factor in the production of a duodenal ulcer at this site. Duodenal ulcers are much more common than gastric ulcers.

Although peptic ulcers (gastric and duodenal ulcers) can have many causes, the basic cause appears to be an imbalance between the production of acid gastric secretion and the mechanisms responsible for protecting the mucous membrane from autodigestion. The large outpouring of alkaline secretions by the Brunner's glands of the mucous membrane greatly assists in the neutralization of the acid chyme, but there is no evidence that the volume of the alkaline secretions is reduced in patients with duodenal ulcer.

Like the treatment of gastric ulcer, the medical treatment here is designed to combat the acidity of the gastric juice and keep the acid diluted by having multiple small meals. Surgical treatment may be needed if the medical treatment fails or if the patient develops complications, such as perforation or bleeding.

Jejunum and Ileum

Tumors of the small intestine are rare. Infections and malabsorption syndromes are relatively common.

It was emphasized when discussing the lining cells of the mucous membrane that they are continually being cast off into the lumen as a result of simple wear and tear. The undifferentiated stem cells within the crypts of Lieberkühn continuously undergo mitosis to replace these cells; the whole process of migration and maturation of the daughter cells takes about 2 to 6 days. The inhibitory action of irradiation and chemotherapeutic drugs on mitosis in the treatment of malignant disease would interfere seriously with the replacement of these lining cells; consequently, unpleasant side effects related to the small intestine are common in these forms of treatment.

Paralytic Ileus

Paralytic ileus is a condition in which the small intestine fails to transmit peristaltic waves. It is caused by a failure of the myenteric plexus that effectively blocks the passage of intestinal contents, resulting in the accumulation of fluid and gas in the intestine. Distention of the intestine, vomiting, absence of peristaltic bowel sounds audible through a stethoscope applied to the abdominal wall, and absolute constipation with failure to pass flatus all may occur. The following are common causes of paralytic ileus:

1. *Surgical procedures.* Following abdominal operations, intestinal peristalsis may not return for 16 hours. This is normal. Should the patient have a peritoneal infection, however, paralytic ileus may occur.
2. *Reflex.* Such paralytic ileus may occur following fractures of the vertebral column or application of an abdominal plaster cast. It is presumed that in spinal cord injuries, the myenteric plexus is inhibited by afferent nervous impulses. With a plaster cast, an absence of external movement or pressure on the bowel may be the cause.
3. *Renal failure.* The accumulation of the toxic products of metabolism in renal failure is the probable cause of such paralytic ileus.
4. *Hypokalemia.* A low blood potassium level can cause paralytic ileus.

Malabsorption from the Small Intestine

In this condition, there is a malabsorption of fats, resulting in an increased excretion of fat in the feces (steatorrhea). The condition is usually associated with some diminished absorption of proteins, carbohydrates, and vitamins A, D, and K. There are many disorders that give rise to this condition, but they basically depend on three malfunctions: (1) a failure of the digestive process within the lumen of the bowel, (2) a failure of the lining cells of the small intestine to absorb the products of digestion, and (3) a failure to transport the absorbed products of digestion away from the site of absorption. Two examples will be considered briefly.

LIVER DISEASE AND BLOCKAGE OF THE BILIARY DUCTS. In liver and biliary tract disease, there may be impaired synthesis of bile salts or failure of the bile salts to reach the duodenum. Either would result in impaired digestion and absorption of fat from the small intestine and a reduced absorption of vitamins.

NONTROPICAL SPRUE AND CELIAC DISEASE. Gluten, a high-molecular-weight protein found in wheat and rye, exerts a toxic effect on the jejunal mucosa of some individuals, causing a degeneration of the villi and a reduction in the absorptive capabilities of the small intestine. As a result, such patients lose weight and suffer from steatorrhea. Other complications may arise, such as demineralization of bones because of lack of calcium absorption, macrocytic anemia caused by lack of vitamin B_{12} and folic acid absorption, and excessive bleeding time caused by vitamin K deficiency.

Typhoid Fever

This serious condition, which is caused by the ingestion of food or water contaminated with gram-negative typhoid bacilli, produces hyperplasia of the reticuloendothelial system throughout the body. There is a resultant enlargement of lymph nodes and lymph follicles in the intestine, especially the Peyer's patches of the small intestine. The hypertrophied *Peyer's patches* compress the blood supply of the mucous membrane causing ischemia and severe ulceration. Perforation of the wall of the small intestine is a complication.

Short Bowel Syndrome

Massive death of the small bowel following injury or occlusion of the superior mesenteric vessels may necessitate resection of long lengths of the small intestine. Provided that adequate amounts of vitamins B_{12}, A, B, D, E, and K are administered, about three-quarters of the small intestine can be removed without resultant nutritional defects. Calcium and iron should also be given.

Dumping Syndrome

Following removal of the stomach (gastrectomy) and esophageal jejunostomy or gastrojejunostomy, 5 to 10 percent of patients experience a collection of symptoms and signs known as the *dumping syndrome*. This syndrome is attributable to the loss of the reservoir function of the stomach and altered physiology of the small intestine. The symptoms usually start within 10 minutes of ingesting a meal and may continue for an hour. They include weakness, sweating, nausea, abdominal distention, and diarrhea.

Following gastrectomy, there is a reduction in the secretion of hydrochloric acid, pepsin, intrinsic factor, and pancreatic enzymes. There is an inadequate mixing of food with enzymes. The food passes directly into the small intestine, causing increased intestinal motility with reduced digestion and absorption of protein, fat, and carbohydrate. The presence of hypertonic chyme in the small intestine in a patient with a partial gastrectomy results in an outpouring of extracellular fluid into the intestinal lumen, causing abdominal distention. Weight loss, steatorrhea, diarrhea, iron deficiency anemia, and megaloblastic anemia (lack of vitamin B_{12} absorption) may all occur in severe cases.

The giving of small, dry meals and the possibility of joining the remains of the stomach to the proximal part of the duodenum in place of the jejunum should be considered in patients with severe symptoms and signs.

LARGE INTESTINE

Appendix

Acute appendicitis is a very common disease. Bacterial organisms invade the wall of the appendix from either the lumen or the arterial supply. Obstruction of the lumen by a hard pellet of feces (fecalith) may cause local mucosal vascular congestion and predispose to the condition. Acute inflammation spreads through the appendicular wall and may lead to suppuration, gangrene, and perforation.

Mucocele of the appendix is a condition usually caused by blockage of the lumen with a fecalith and the accumulation of mucus from the goblet cells distal to the blockage. The appendix gradually becomes distended and may measure as much as 5 cm in diameter.

Colon and Rectum

The functions of the colon and rectum are storage of food residues and feces and absorption of water. The large bowel, however, is not essential to life, so large segments may be removed surgically. As in the small intestine, the cells lining the mucous membrane constantly are sloughed off as a result of wear and tear. They are rapidly replaced by the mitotic activity of cells lying within the crypts of Lieberkühn. Unfortunately, this method of replacement leaves the lining cells extremely vulnerable to antimitotic agents used in the treatment of cancer of the abdomen, such as radiotherapy and chemotherapy.

Cancer of the colon and rectum is a very common cause of death. It arises as columnar cell adenocarcinoma and often produces mucus. In the cecum and ascending colon, large papillomatous masses tend to form that protrude into the lumen; in the descending colon and rectum, a flat elevation often forms that slowly encircles the wall and eventually ulcerates and obstructs the bowel.

Megacolon (Hirschsprung's disease) is a congenital condition in which there is a failure in the development of the ganglion cells of Meissner's and Auerbach's plexuses in the region of the lower end of the rectum. This condition produces a functional obstruction at the distal end of the rectum and a gross dilatation of the colon proximal to the obstruction. The treatment is operative excision of the aganglionic segment of the rectum.

Diverticulosis of the colon is a common clinical condition. It consists of a herniation of the lining mucosa through the circular muscle between the teniae coli at points where the circular muscle is weakest, and this is where the blood vessels pierce the muscle. It is most commonly found in the pelvic (sigmoid) colon, where the luminal diameter is narrowest and the pressure greatest.

Hemorrhoids

In the submucosa of the anal canal is a plexus of veins that principally is drained upward by the superior rectal vein. The small tributaries of the middle and inferior rectal veins communicate with each other and with the superior rectal vein through this plexus. The venous plexus therefore forms an important anastomosis between the portal venous system and the systemic venous system. *Internal hemorrhoids* (piles) are varicosities of the tributaries of the superior rectal (hemorrhoidal) vein and are covered with mucous membrane. At first, hemorrhoids are contained within the anal canal (first degree). As they enlarge, they are extruded from the canal on defecation but return at the end of the act (second degree). With further elongation, they prolapse on defecation and remain outside the anus (third degree).

External hemorrhoids are varicosities of the tributaries of the inferior rectal (hemorrhoidal) vein as they run laterally from the anal margin. They are covered by skin and commonly are associated with well-established internal hemorrhoids.

Vomiting

Vomiting is a reflex emptying of the stomach and may be caused by a number of factors, including (1) irritation of nerve endings in the stomach or duodenum, (2) excessive pain from almost any organ in the body, (3) excessive stimulation of the utricle of the inner ear, as in seasickness, (4) unpleasant odors or the observation of unpleasant scenes, or (5) administration of emetic drugs.

Nervous impulses reach the medulla oblongata of the brain via the vagus and sympathetic nerves and stimulate the *vomiting center.* A deep breath is taken, followed by closure of the glottis. The larynx is raised and its entrance thereby closed. The pyloric sphincter of the stomach closes. The act of vomiting is carried out by the sudden, simultaneous contraction of the diaphragm and the muscles of the abdominal wall. The stomach is strongly compressed from without, and the gastroesophageal sphincter is relaxed. By this means, the gastric contents are violently expelled upward through the esophagus and pharynx.

Diarrhea and Constipation

Individuals show great variation in their defecation habits. Some adults defecate once a day; others defecate once every 3 or 4 days. When the time and place are suitable, a wave of peristalsis that is set in motion reflexly passes down the colon to the rectum. Distention of the rectum caused by the entrance of the feces gives rise to the desire to defecate ("the call of the colon").

Physicians should be alert to a change in an individual's bowel habits, rather than trying to determine whether the defecation habits lie outside the wide range of the normal.

Diarrhea may be defined as the frequent passing of unformed stools and may be caused by infection or the ingestion of chemicals or drugs. Chronic diarrhea may stem from such disorders as *ulcerative colitis* and *ileitis,* and in children, *celiac disease* and *cystic fibrosis of the pancreas* should be considered. Prolonged acute diarrhea can be dangerous, especially in infants, because of the associated dehydration and loss of electrolytes.

Constipation is an excessive delay in the evacuation of the feces. The symptoms of constipation include foul breath, furred tongue, loss of appetite, nausea, loss of power of attention, and irritability. It is believed that most of these symptoms are produced by distention and irritation of the rectum. The causes of constipation are many and include malignant disease of the large bowel, fecal impaction, cerebrovascular accidents, and the action of certain drugs.

CLINICAL PROBLEMS *For the answers to these problems, see page 801.*

1. A 63-year-old farmer visits his physician because of a small ulcer he has had on the outer edge of his lower lip for the past 6 months. The ulcer is found to be shallow and has hard, everted edges. The pa-

tient says that the ulcer is painless but is worrying him because it is gradually increasing in size. Excision biopsy reveals that the ulcer is malignant. Using your knowledge of histology, describe the surface epithelium of the lip from which the carcinoma has originated. Explain why the margins of the lips are red. Why are the lips of patients sometimes blue?

2. Eskimos, who live almost entirely on fish and meat, are almost free of dental decay. In people who eat large amounts of carbohydrate and candies, dental caries is very common. What is the probable explanation for this observation? Briefly describe the structure of dental enamel and dentin. Would you expect to experience pain in disease of the dentin? When giving a general anesthetic, special care must be taken to prevent loosening of the patient's teeth. Normal teeth are held firmly in position. Describe the structure of the periodontal ligament.

3. A 24-year-old woman asks her dentist about a cyst that she has had on the inner surface of her right cheek for 4 weeks. She says that she had had a similar cyst 1 year previously that had reached a size of about half a centimeter. The previous cyst was bluish and had ruptured spontaneously while she was cleaning her teeth, discharging sticky material into her mouth. The dentist diagnoses a mucous cyst of the buccal mucous membrane. Using your knowledge of histology, describe the structure of the mucous membrane of the cheek. Are mucous glands normally present in the cheek?

4. While performing a routine physical examination of a 53-year-old woman, a physician notices that the dorsal surface of her tongue is smooth, glazed, and tender to the touch. Closer examination reveals a complete absence of papillae. What are the different types of papillae found on the dorsal surface of the tongue, and what is their structure? Do you know of any deficiency disease or diseases that may be responsible for their absence? What is the structure of a taste bud?

5. A 35-year-old woman visits her physician complaining of a left-sided submandibular swelling of 2 weeks' duration. She states that the swelling becomes worse before and during a meal and is then tender to the touch. Later, the swelling subsides, only to become more obvious at the next meal. Examination of the mouth cavity reveals a small, hard, stonelike structure just beneath the opening of the left submandibular duct into the mouth. A diagnosis of a calculus in the left submandibular duct is made, and it is concluded that the accumulation of salivary secretion and back pressure in the salivary gland is responsible for the swelling of the gland at meal times. Describe the microscopic structure of the submandibular salivary gland. Why are calculi much more common in the submandibular gland than in the parotid salivary gland?

6. An 8-year-old girl is taken to a pediatrician because she is complaining of a sore throat and has a fever of 101°F. On examination, the tonsils are red and swollen and show numerous yellow spots exuding from the tonsillar crypts. The cervical lymph nodes on both sides are enlarged and tender. A diagnosis of acute tonsillitis is made. Describe the structure of the tonsil and explain the term *tonsillar crypt*. Does the tonsil contain T or B lymphocytes?

7. A 45-year-old woman is referred to a surgeon because of her history of progressive difficulty in swallowing. The problem had started 5 years previously and gradually has worsened. She has noticed recently that she vomits about 3 hours after each meal, but on closer questioning, the physician finds it is in fact a regurgitation of the food from the previous meal mixed with froth and mucus. She has no pain but experiences some retrosternal discomfort. She has lost 30 pounds in weight over the last 3 months. Radiography following a barium swallow shows a smooth, narrowed lower segment of the esophagus and a dilatation and tortuosity of the segment of the esophagus proximal to the narrowing. A diagnosis of achalasia of the cardia is made. Describe the arrangement of muscle in the wall of the esophagus. Is there a cardioesophageal sphincter? In this patient, the regurgitated food is mixed with mucus. Where did the mucus come from?

8. We know that gastric ulcer is a common clinical

condition. We also know that the enzymes present in gastric juice can digest the stomach wall. Describe the mechanisms that normally exist to protect the gastric mucous membrane from autodigestion.

9. Compare the glands found in the mucous membrane in different parts of the stomach. Name the different types of cells found in these glands, and state their function.

10. Describe the various mechanisms that exist for the control of gastric secretion.

11. The duodenum is a common site for peptic ulcer. Name the histological structures present in the duodenum that are responsible for neutralizing the acid chyme leaving the stomach.

12. Describe the process of digestion that takes place in the small intestine. Explain how carbohydrates, fats, and proteins are absorbed from the lumen of the intestine. Describe in detail the microscopic structure of the absorptive cells of the mucous membrane.

13. Most physiologists believe that the jejunum, rather than the ileum, is the main site for the absorption of the products of digestion. Do you agree? What histological structures are present in the jejunum that aid the process of absorption? A 23-year-old woman is involved in a serious automobile accident that necessitates the removal of one-third of her small intestine. Can such a patient be expected to live a normal life following such a radical procedure?

14. A 42-year-old man attends his physician for treatment of fatty diarrhea. The patient has noticed the passage of excessively large, pale, foul-smelling stools. He also complains of weight loss, lassitude, and a sore tongue. A diagnosis of idiopathic steatorrhea is made. Using your knowledge of the structure and function of the small intestine, name the important vitamins that are unlikely to be absorbed in adequate amounts in this disease. Note that in steatorrhea, the causative agent in the diet is the protein gluten, which results in damage to the cells of the villi, causing defective absorption of fat, protein, and carbohydrates.

15. Define the following: (a) crypt of Lieberkühn, (b) Paneth cell, (c) Peyer's patch, (d) argentaffin cell.

16. Acute appendicitis is a very common disease. Acute inflammation usually starts in the mucous membrane and spreads through the appendicular wall. What is the structure of the appendicular wall? Is the longitudinal muscle coat continuous or split into three bands, as in the colon? Name the tissue that dominates the mucous membrane and submucosa when a cross section stained with H&E is examined. Why are gangrene and perforation of the appendix common complications in acute appendicitis?

17. What are the functions of the large intestine? Describe the mucous membrane and explain how its structure is adapted to its function.

18. A third-year medical student is asked on a ward round in the children's hospital to describe megacolon (Hirschsprung's disease). Having explained that the condition is a functional obstruction at the distal end of the rectum causing a gross dilatation of the colon proximal to the obstruction, he is then asked the cause of this disease. Using your knowledge of histology, how would you answer this question?

19. A 50-year-old woman visits her physician because of recurrent attacks of pain and discomfort in the left iliac fossa. The condition is exacerbated by constipation and relieved by defecation. In the past 3 weeks, the pain has become more severe and almost continuous. A tender mass can be felt in the left iliac fossa on deep palpation. After a barium enema and radiological study, a number of diverticula are noted in the pelvic colon. A diagnosis of diverticulitis is made. Describe the normal arrangement of the muscular coat in the wall of the colon. Note the potentially weak areas in the wall of the colon and explain the underlying mechanism responsible for diverticulosis.

20. Hemorrhoids are very common. They are a dila-

tation of veins in the wall of the anal canal. Describe the structure of the anal canal and explain the position of these important veins.

21. Malignant disease of the lining cells of the rectum and upper half of the anal canal is a relatively common clinical condition. What type of cell is involved? Is the lower half of the anal canal lined with the same type of cell?

ADDITIONAL READING

Anderson, J. H., and Taylor, A. B. Scanning and transmission electron microscopic studies of jejunal microvilli of the rat, hamster, and dog. *J. Morphol.* 141:281, 1973.

Beidler, L. M., and Smallman, R. L. Renewal of cells within taste buds. *J. Cell Biol.* 27:263, 1965.

Bevelander, G. *Atlas of Oral Histology and Embryology.* Philadelphia: Lea & Febiger, 1967.

Binder, H. J. (ed.). *Mechanisms of Intestinal Secretion.* New York: Liss, 1979.

Bloom, S. R. (ed.). *Gut Hormones.* New York: Churchill/Livingstone, 1978.

Bortoff, A. Myogenic control of intestinal motility. *Physiol. Rev.* 56:418, 1976.

Brindley, D. N. The intracellular phase of fat absorption. *Biomembranes* 4B:621, 1974.

Cheng, H., and Leblond, G. P. (with the collaboration of G. Trigelydes, A. Grignon, and W. W. Chang). Origin, differentiation and renewal of the four main epithelial cell types in the mouse small intestine. I. Columnar cell. *Am. J. Anat.* 141:461, 1974.

Cooke, W. T. Common problems of malabsorption. *Practitioner* 216:637, 1976.

Crane, R. K. Intestinal absorption of glucose. *Biomembranes* 4A:541, 1974.

Crane, R. K. (ed.). *International Review of Physiology: Gastrointestinal Physiology II.* Vol. 12. Baltimore: University Park Press, 1977.

David, H. The mechanism of desquamation of cells from the intestinal villi: An electron miscroscopic study. *Virchows Arch. {Pathol. Anat.}* 342:19, 1967.

Dragstedt, L. R. Some comments on the cause of gastric and duodenal ulcers. *Am. J. Digestive Dis.* 21:197, 1976.

Duthie, H. S. (ed.). *Gastrointestinal Motility in Health and Disease.* Baltimore: University Park Press, 1978.

Friedman, H. I., and Cardell, R. R., Jr. Alterations in the endoplasmic reticulum and Golgi complex of intestinal epithelial cells during absorption and after termination of this process. *Anat. Rec.* 188:77, 1977.

Friedman, M. H. F. (ed.). *Functions of the Stomach and Intestine.* Baltimore: University Park Press, 1975.

Fujita, T., and Kobayashi, S. Structure and function of gut endocrine cells. *Int. Rev. Cytol. {Suppl.}* 6:187, 1977.

Garrett, J. R., Harrison, J. D., and Stoward, P. J. *Histochemistry of Secretory Process.* London: Chapman Hall, 1977.

Grossman, M. I. The gastrointestinal hormones: An overview. *Proc. Int. Cong. Endocrinol.* 2:18, 1976.

Grossman, M. I. Neural and hormonal regulation of gastrointestinal function: An overview. *Annu. Rev. Physiol.* 41:27, 1979.

Grube, D., and Forssmann, W. G. Morphology and function of the enteroendocrine cells. *Horm. Metab. Res.* 11:589, 1979.

Ito, S., and Schofield, G. C. Studies on the depletion and accumulation of microvilli and changes in the tubulovesicular compartment of the mouse parietal cells in relation to gastric acid secretion. *J. Cell Biol.* 63:364, 1974.

Johnson, L. R. (ed.). *Gastrointestinal Physiology.* St. Louis: Mosby, 1977.

Leaming, D. B., and Cauna, N. A qualitative and quantitative study of the myenteric plexus of the small intestine of the cat. *J. Anat.* 95:160, 1961.

Leblond, C. P., and Messier, B. Renewal of chief cells and goblet cells in the small intestine as shown by radioautography after injection of thymidine H^3 into mice. *Anat. Rec.* 132:247, 1958.

Lipkin, M. Proliferation and differentiation of gastrointestinal cells. *Physiol. Rev.* 53:981, 1973.

Marsh, M. N. Studies of intestinal lymphoid tissue. I and II. *Gut* 16:665, 675, 1975.

Mathews, D. M. Absorption of amino acids and peptides from the intestine. *Clin. Endocrinol. Metab.* 3:3, 1974.

Mjör, I. A., and Pindberg, J. J. *Histology of the Human Tooth.* Copenhagen: Munksgaard, 1973.

Mooseker, M. S., and Tilney, L. G. Organization of an

actin filament–membrane complex: Filament polarity and membrane attachment in the microvilli of intestinal epithelial cells. *J. Cell Biol.* 67:725, 1975.

Pfeiffer, C. J., Rowden, G., and Weibel, J. *Gastrointestinal Ultrastructure.* New York: Academic, 1974.

Phillips, S. F., and Deuroede, G. J. Functions of the large intestine. In Crane, R. K. (ed.), *International Review of Physiology: Gastrointestinal Physiology III.* Vol. 19. Baltimore: University Park Press, 1979, p. 263.

Pope, C. E., II. Diseases of the esophagus. *Gastroenterology* 69:1058, 1975.

Risnes, S. The prism pattern of rat molar enamel: A scanning electron microscope study. *Am. J. Anat.* 155:245, 1979.

Schofield, G. C., Ito, S., and Bolender, R. P. Changes in membrane surface areas in mouse parietal cells in relation to high levels of acid secretion. *J. Anat.* 128:669, 1979.

Shklar, G., and McCarthy, P. L. *The Oral Manifestations of Systemic Disease.* Boston: Butterworth's, 1976.

Snell, R. S. The histochemical appearances of cholinesterase in the parasympathetic nerves supplying the submandibular and sublingual salivary glands of the rat. *J. Anat.* 92:534, 1958.

Snell, R. S. The histochemical appearances of cholinesterase in the parotid salivary gland of the rat. *Z. Zellforsch.* 49:330, 1959.

Snell, R. S., and Garrett, J. R. The effect of postganglionic sympathectomy on the structure of the submandibular and major sublingual salivary glands of the rat. *Z. Zellforsch.* 48:639, 1958.

Solcia, E., et al. Endocrine cells of the gastric mucosa. *Int. Rev. Cytol.* 42:223, 1975.

Soll, A., and Walsh, J. H. Regulation of gastric acid secretion. *Annu. Rev. Physiol.* 41:35, 1979.

Ten Cate, A. R. *Oral Histology.* Chicago: Science Research Associates, 1979.

Troughton, W. D., and Trier, J. S. Paneth cell and goblet cell renewal in mouse duodenal crypts. *J. Cell Biol.* 41:251, 1969.

Weinstock, A., and Leblond, C. P. Elaboration of the matrix glycoprotein of enamel by the secretory ameloblasts of the rat incisor as revealed by radioautography after galactose-^{3}H injection. *J. Cell Biol.* 51:26, 1971.

Wood, J. D. Neurophysiology of Auerbach's plexus and control of intestinal motility. *Physiol. Rev.* 55:307, 1975.

12

LIVER, BILE DUCTS, GALLBLADDER, AND PANCREAS

The chief glands associated with the intestinal tract are the liver and the pancreas. Although situated outside the gut, they discharge their secretions into the duodenum by way of large ducts.

LIVER, BILE DUCTS, AND GALLBLADDER

The liver is the largest organ of the body. It is reddish-brown, soft, and pliable and occupies the upper part of the abdomen beneath the diaphragm (Fig. 12-1).

Organization

The liver receives a profuse blood supply from the hepatic artery and the portal vein. The hepatic artery, which is relatively small, supplies the liver substance with oxygenated blood; the portal vein brings to the liver venous blood from the gastrointestinal tract loaded with the products of digestion. Both blood vessels enter the liver through a transverse opening called the *porta hepatis*. Blood leaves the posterior surface of the liver through two or three large hepatic veins that drain into the inferior vena cava.

Bile, which is a secretion of the liver, leaves through the porta hepatis via the right and left hepatic ducts.

The liver is surrounded by a thin connective tissue capsule called *Glisson's capsule,* from which thin septa enter the liver at the porta hepatis. The outer surface of the capsule is covered almost completely by peritoneum, but there are areas, known as *bare areas,* where the liver is directly in contact with the diaphragm and viscera on the posterior abdominal wall.

The liver is incompletely divided on its anterior surface into a large *right lobe* and a smaller *left lobe* by the attachment of the peritoneal *falciform ligament* (see Fig. 12-1). On the inferior and posterior surfaces, the attachment of the lesser omentum and the presence of the inferior vena cava, the gallbladder, and the ligamentum teres delineate two additional lobes, the *caudate lobe* and the *quadrate lobe.* The basic anatomical and functional unit of the liver is the *classic lobule* (see Fig. 12-1). When examined at low magnification with a light microscope, each lobule is seen to consist of epithelial cells arranged as branching plates that radiate like spokes in a wheel from a vein situated in the center known as

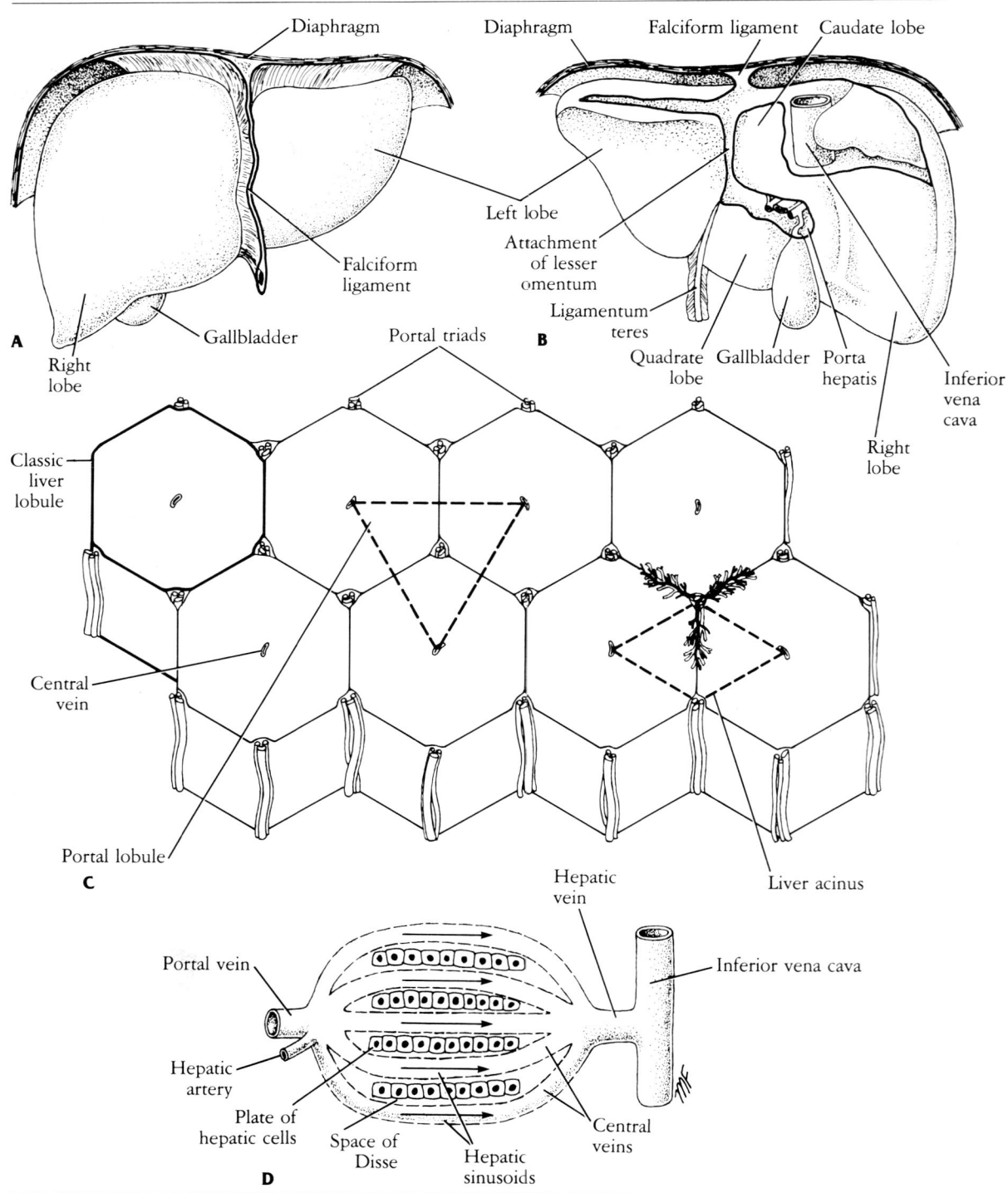

Fig. 12-1. A: Liver from the front. B: Liver from behind. C: Organization of the liver into the classic liver lobule, the portal lobule, and the liver acinus. D: Circulation of blood in the hepatic sinusoids between the plates of hepatic cells.

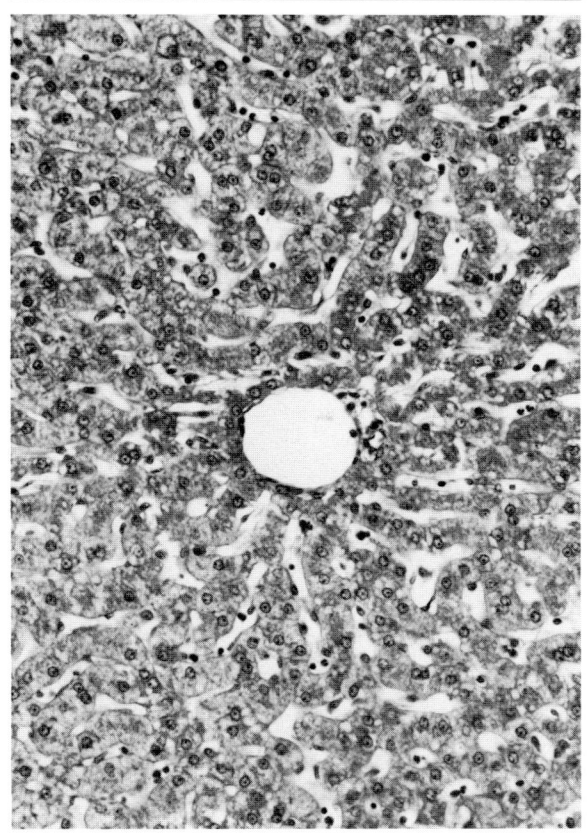

Fig. 12-2. Photomicrograph of the liver, showing the central area of a classic lobule with a central vein. (H&E; ×200.)

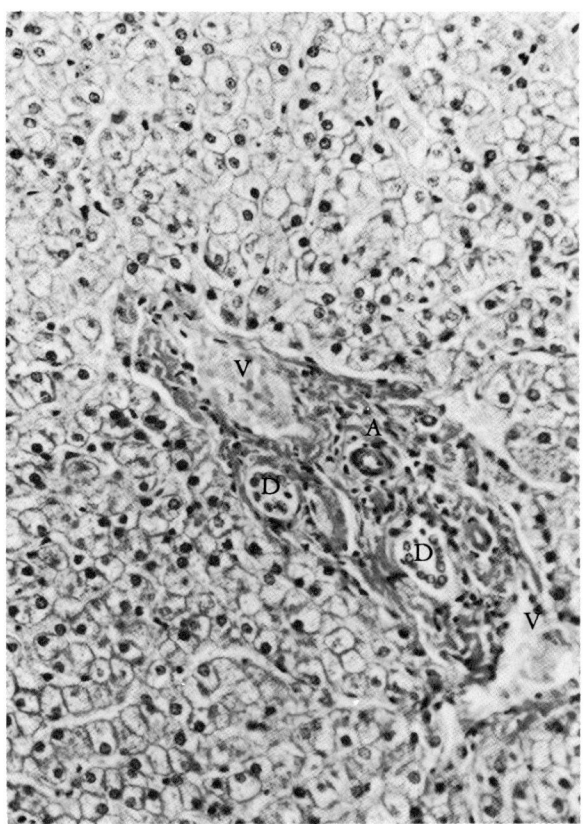

Fig. 12-3. Photomicrograph of the liver, showing the peripheral area of a classic lobule with a branch of the hepatic artery (A), a branch of the portal vein (V), and a small bile duct (D). (H&E; ×200.)

the *central vein* (Fig. 12-2). The radially arranged plates of liver cells are exposed on either side to blood sinusoids known as the *hepatic sinusoids*.

Each liver lobule is hexagonal in shape and measures about 0.5 to 2 mm in diameter; it measures several millimeters in length. At the periphery of each lobule are small branches of the hepatic artery and portal vein and a tributary of the bile duct (Fig. 12-3; see Fig. 12-1). These structures usually travel together and are known as the *portal triad*. They are supported by connective tissue and are collectively known as the *portal canal*. The presence of the portal canal at the corners of the hexagon, the central vein, and the radially arranged liver cells facilitate recognition of a liver lobule. The connective tissue of the liver lobule is confined to the portal canal. There is no connective tissue capsule separating adjacent lobules.

Blood enters the periphery of a liver lobule through the branches of the hepatic artery and portal vein in the portal canal (Fig. 12-4). The blood then flows through the sinusoids between the plates of liver cells to the central vein. The central veins from different lobules ultimately unite to form the hepatic veins, through which the blood leaves the liver. Bile secreted by the liver cells enters minute canals that run between the liver cells. Examination of a radially arranged plate of liver cells shows that

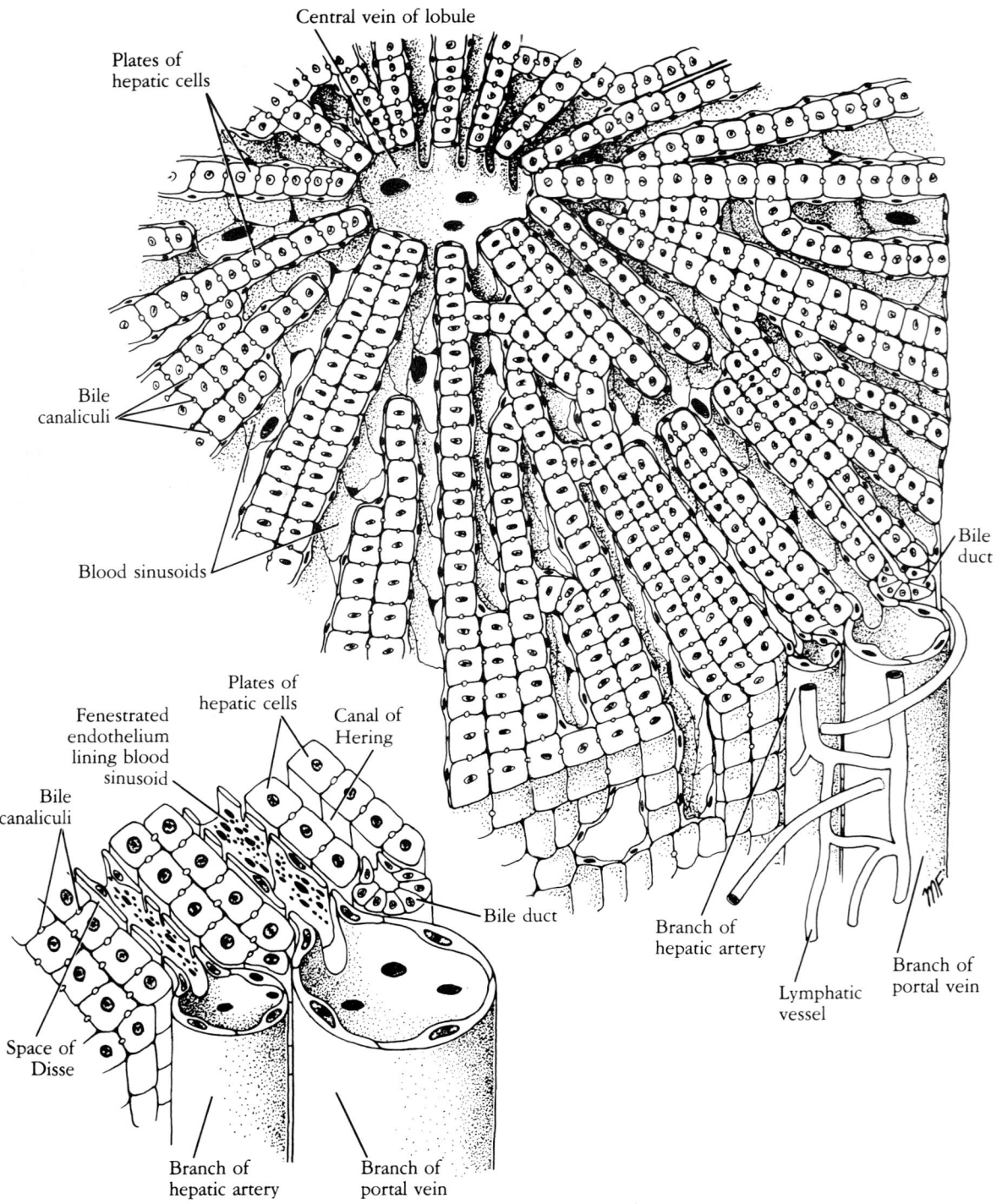

Fig. 12-4. Part of a liver lobule; an enlarged view of the portal triad is shown below. Kupffer cells have been omitted for clarity.

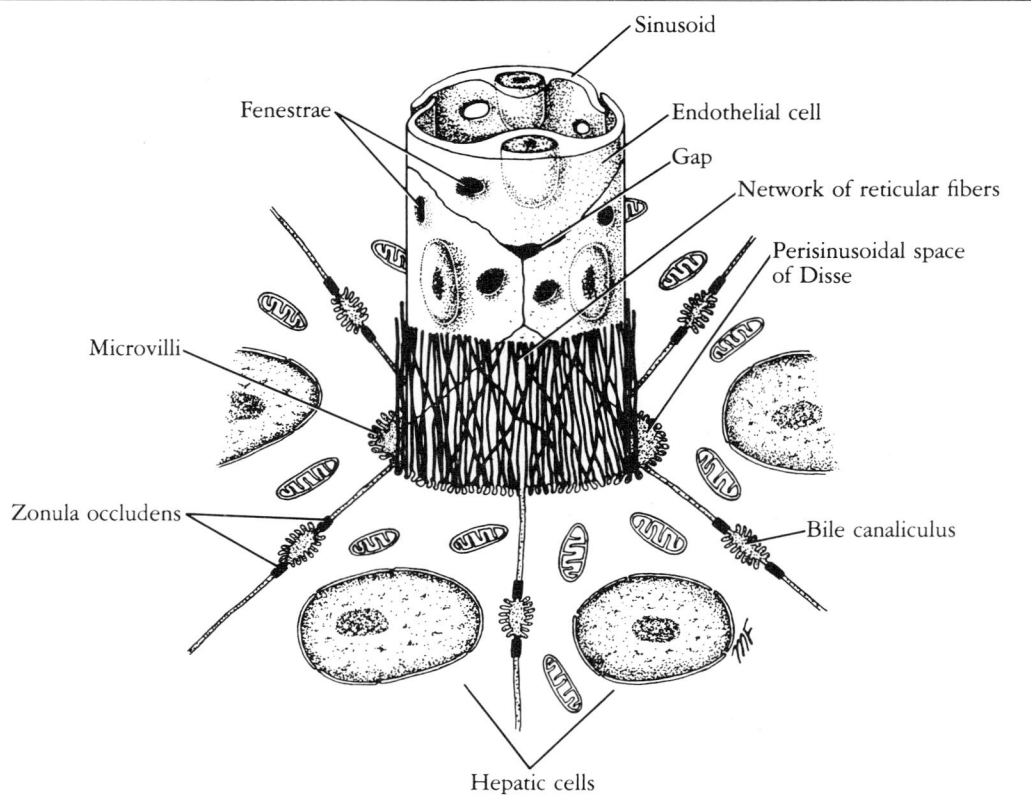

Fig. 12-5. Liver sinusoid supported by a network of reticular fibers and surrounded by hepatic cells. Note the space of Disse and the bile canaliculi. Note also the fenestrae in the endothelial cells of the sinusoids.

each plate is composed of one or two layers of liver cells, between which are the tiny canals, or *bile canaliculi* (see Fig. 12-4). The bile canaliculi are merely small intervals between adjacent cells and have no lining. Having entered a canaliculus, the bile passes to the periphery of the lobule and enters a small bile duct. In a liver lobule, the blood flows centripetally, whereas the bile flows centrifugally.

Blood Sinusoids

As noted previously, the blood sinusoids of the liver lobule run between branches of the hepatic artery and portal vein at the periphery to the central vein. They form an extensive meshwork between adjacent plates of hepatic cells (see Figs. 12-2 and 12-4). The blood sinusoids are wider than capillaries and are lined by two types of cells: (1) endothelial cells and (2) stellate cells of Kupffer.

The endothelial cells are present in greater numbers and form a discontinuous lining for the sinusoids. Large gaps occur between the endothelial cells and, together with the fenestrae through the cytoplasm of these cells and the absence of a basement membrane, allow the unformed blood elements—plasma—to percolate through the sinusoidal wall into the space between the sinusoid and the hepatic cells. This *perisinusoidal space* is known as the *space of Disse* (Figs. 12-5 and 12-6). This arrangement greatly facilitates the delivery of the products of digestion to the liver cells and the secretion of substances from the liver cells into the blood.

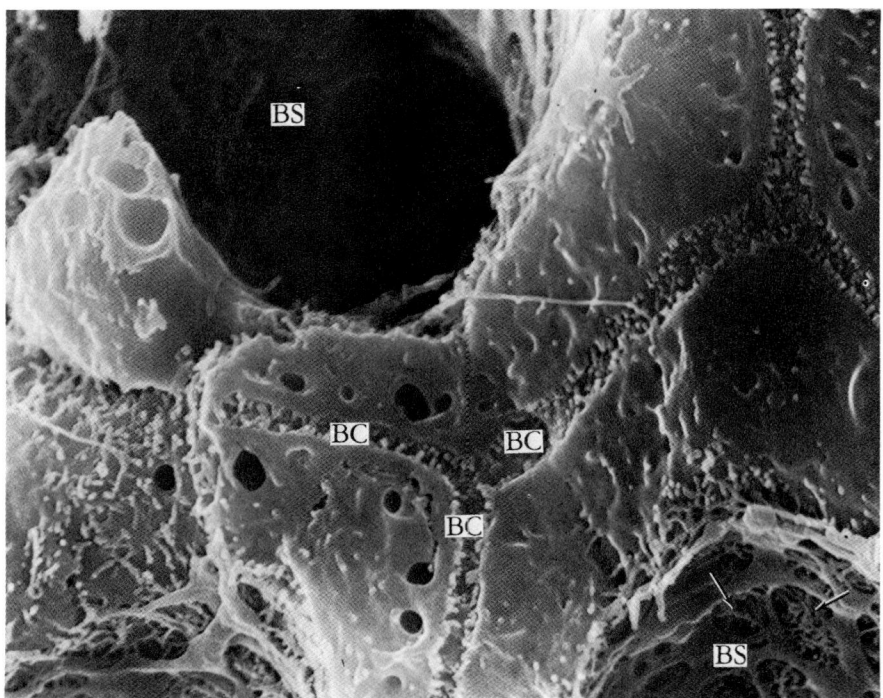

Fig. 12-6. Scanning electron micrograph of the liver, showing two blood sinusoids (BS). Note the fenestrae in the endothelial cells lining the sinusoids. Observe through the fenestrations the hepatic microvilli protruding into the space of Disse (arrows). Note also the bile canaliculi (BC) running between adjacent hepatic cells and the short hepatic microvilli protruding into the lumen of the bile canaliculi. (× 10,000.) (Courtesy of F. G. Lightfoot.)

The *Kupffer cells* are large fixed macrophages that are part of the reticuloendothelial system. They tend to bulge into the lumen of the sinusoid (Fig. 12-7) and often contain the remnants of disintegrating erythrocytes. Kupffer cells are actively phagocytic and can be easily demonstrated in animals by the intravascular injection of vital dyes such as trypan blue. Kupffer cells increase in number by mitosis.

The perisinusoidal space of Disse is filled with plasma and contains occasional reticular and collagen fibers, which support the walls of the sinusoids. The space is dominated by large numbers of microvilli that project from the free surface of the liver cells. Occasional fat-storing cells called *lipocytes* are found in the space. Their function is not known.

In the fetal liver, mesenchymal cells outside the sinusoids are involved actively in hematopoiesis. A section of fetal liver shows the sinusoids packed with red and white cells at different stages of development (see Fig. 5-27).

Liver Cells

The liver cells, or hepatocytes, as explained previously, are arranged as branching plates that radiate from a central vein within a lobule (see Figs. 12-2 and 12-4). Each liver cell surface either is in contact with a neighboring liver cell, is exposed to a perisinusoidal space, or is grooved and forms the wall of a bile canaliculus. Each cell has a large rounded nucleus with scattered chromatin and one or more nucleoli (Fig. 12-8). The majority of the cells have one nucleus, but some cells are multinucleate. The cytoplasm shows a well-developed rough-surfaced endoplasmic reticulum, and many

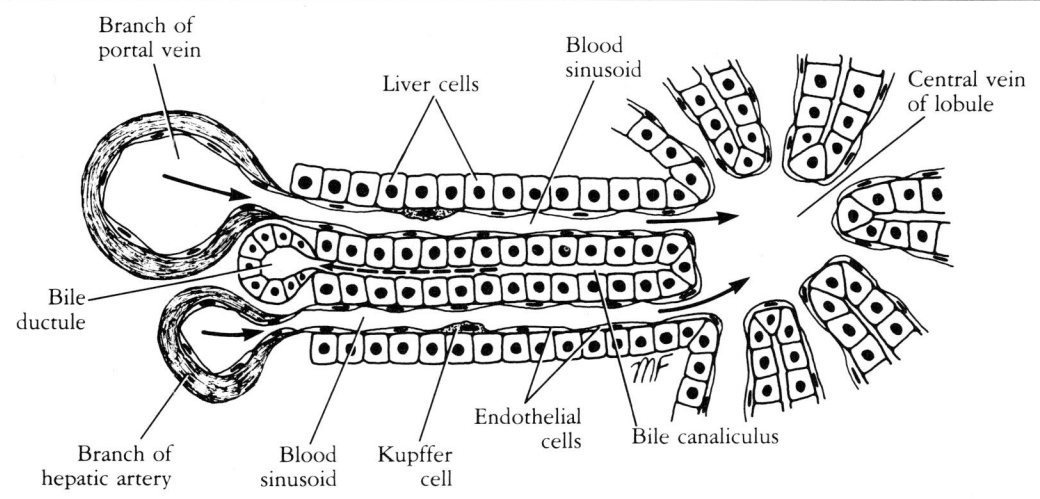

Fig. 12-7. Part of a classic liver lobule, demonstrating the direction of blood flow from branches of the portal vein and hepatic artery to the central vein (solid arrows) and the direction of bile flow in the bile canaliculus in the opposite direction (broken arrow). Note the location of the Kupffer cells in the wall of the blood sinusoid. The space of Disse is not shown.

free polyribosomes are present. There are numerous mitochondria and a moderately well formed smooth-surfaced endoplasmic reticulum. The Golgi apparatus is multiple and situated close to the bile canaliculus. Lysosomes are present, some of which contain the pigment lipofuscin. Many vacuoles containing enzymes such as peroxidase and urease also are found. Glycogen granules and lipid vacuoles are usually present in large numbers (Fig. 12-9; see Fig. 12-8).

The plasma membrane of a hepatic cell shows areas of specialization. Where a hepatic cell abuts a bile canaliculus, the plasma membrane is covered with short microvilli (see Fig. 12-8), and farther from the lumen, the plasma membranes of adjacent cells are held together by a junctional complex including zonular occludens, desmosomes, and gap junctions. Where a hepatic cell abuts a perisinusoidal space of Disse, the plasma membrane shows numerous long microvilli that are bathed by plasma that has escaped from the sinusoidal lumen.

The plasma membranes of adjacent hepatic cells show indentations and projections similar to those of a jigsaw puzzle, and this arrangement assists in holding the cells together.

Bile Canaliculi

With the light microscope, bile canaliculi are seen as very small channels that run between adjacent hepatic cells. Close examination of a liver lobule shows the canaliculus running between adjacent plates of liver cells (see Fig. 12-7). Because the plates branch and join one another, the canaliculi form a network within the liver substance and run from one lobule to another. The walls of a bile canaliculus are formed by grooves on the surfaces of adjacent liver cells; the portion of the cell membrane bounding the groove possesses short microvilli (see Figs. 12-5 and 12-8).

Near the periphery of the liver lobule, each bile canaliculus joins a ductule, or *canal of Hering*. These ductules quickly join the bile duct in the portal canal.

Connective Tissue

The liver possesses very little connective tissue, explaining its softness and pliability and its susceptibility to tearing when the abdomen is traumatized. The outer surface is covered by a thin connective tissue

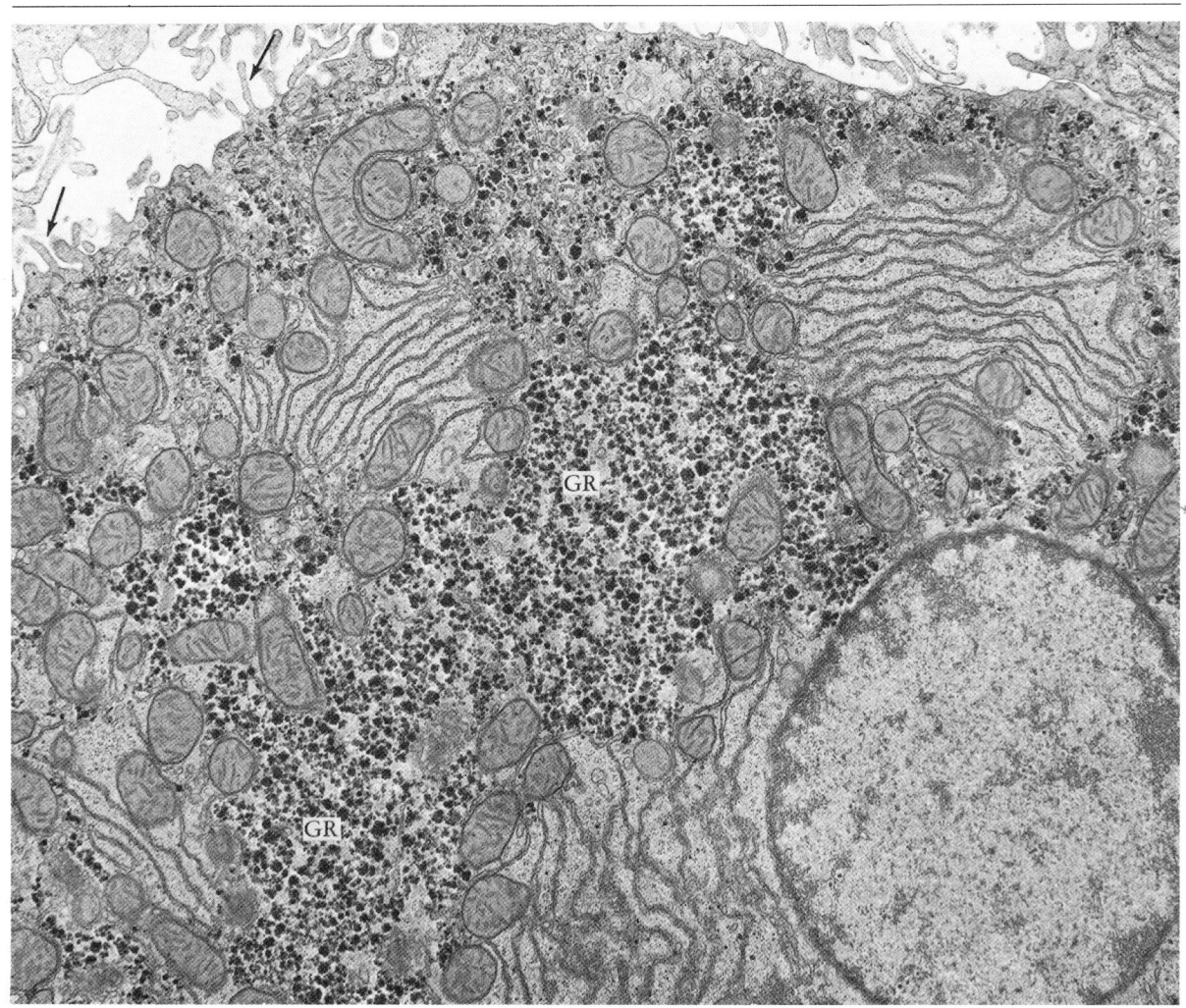

Fig. 12-8. Electron micrograph of hepatic cell (hepatocyte), showing a large, rounded nucleus with scattered chromatin, a well-developed rough-surfaced endoplasmic reticulum, many free polyribosomes, and numerous mitochondria. Note the large numbers of glycogen granules (GR). Note also the short microvilli (arrows) on the plasma membrane, which are projecting into a bile canaliculus. (Courtesy of Dr. A. L. Jones.)

capsule (Glisson's capsule), as explained previously, that extends into the liver substance at the porta hepatis. Here, it becomes continuous with the small amount of connective tissue of the portal canals, which forms a common sheath for the branches of the hepatic artery and portal vein and the bile duct. Lymphatic capillaries are also present within the portal canals. The only connective tissues within the liver lobule are the reticular (Fig. 12-10) and collagen fibers that lie outside the sinusoids. These fibers support the sinusoids and the surrounding liver cells

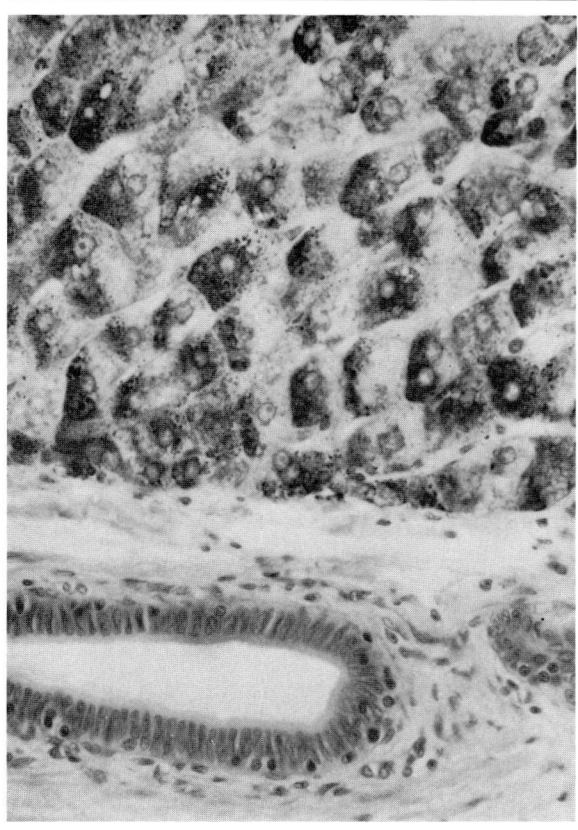

Fig. 12-9. Photomicrograph of a section of the liver and portions of a small bile duct. The liver cells have been stained to show glycogen granules, which are black in the photograph. Note the tall columnar cells lining the bile duct. (Best carmine stain; ×400.)

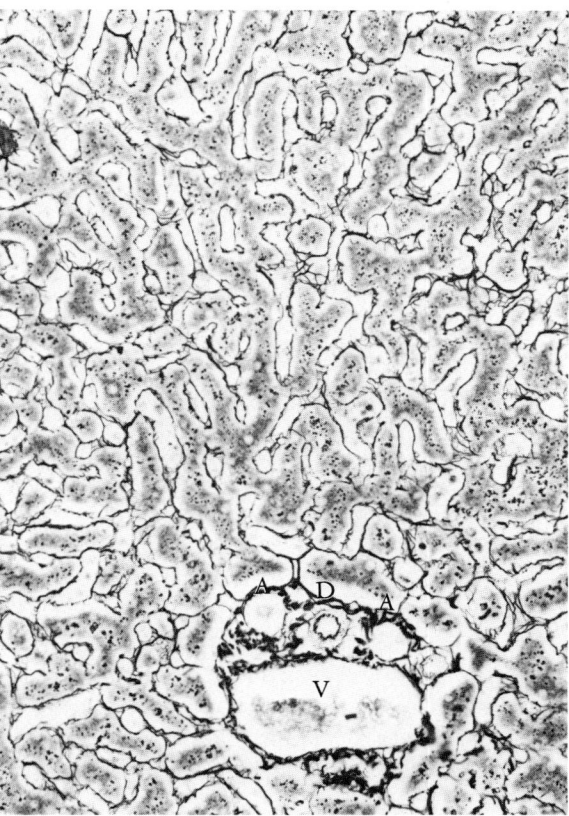

Fig. 12-10. Photomicrograph of a section of the liver, showing fine, black, wavy reticular fibers within a liver lobule. These fibers support the plates of hepatic cells and the blood sinusoids. Note the portal canal containing the portal triad: branches of the hepatic artery (A), a branch of the portal vein (V), and the bile duct (D). (Silver stain; ×200.)

and are continuous with the connective tissue in the portal canals.

Lymphatic Drainage

The liver produces a large amount of lymph (about one-third to one-half of all body lymph), which is rich in protein. The lymphatic vessels commence as capillaries within the portal canals, and these unite and leave the liver at the porta hepatis. It is now generally believed that the blood plasma, having escaped from the hepatic sinusoids through the gaps between the endothelial cells and through the fenestrae, circulates among the hepatic cells in the perisinusoidal space of Disse. Much of this plasma reaches the lymphatic capillaries in the portal canal, accounting for the large volume of lymph that leaves the liver and explaining the high protein content of the lymph.

FURTHER CONSIDERATION OF THE ORGANIZATION OF THE LIVER

Is the classic description of the liver lobule given here ideal for studying the organization of the liver in relation to disease? It must be admitted that the organization as described differs from the general arrangement of other secretory glands, where the secretion drains toward a duct lying within the center of a lobule.

Some histologists have suggested that we use the concept of a triangular *portal lobule* (see Fig. 12-1). With this arrangement, we define the peripheral limits by imaginary lines that connect three central veins. The bile duct (with its associated branches of the hepatic artery and portal vein) is then situated in the center of the lobule (see Fig. 12-1).

Pathologists, however, would prefer to relate the liver cells to their blood supply. The liver unit is then seen to occupy adjacent parts of neighboring classic hexagonal lobules and to extend between two central veins. The central veins therefore lie at the periphery of the unit rather than at its center (see Fig. 12-1). The branches of the hepatic artery and portal vein lie in the center of the unit and are at the center of functional activity. The mass of liver cells related to these vessels is referred to as a *liver acinus;* it is diamond shaped in cross section (see Fig. 12-1).

The concept of liver acini certainly helps to explain liver changes in ischemic necrosis. In this condition, the degeneration of the liver cells is seen first in those cells nearest the periphery of the acinus— that is, farthest from the branches of the portal vein and hepatic artery, where the blood is richer in oxygen.

Students of medicine nevertheless should learn the structure of a classic liver lobule, because the terminology is still widely used. They should also be aware of the concept of a portal lobule and should understand why pathologists prefer to use the liver acinus as the basic liver unit.

Functions

The liver is an extremely complex gland and has a wide variety of functions. It has, however, three basic functions: (1) production and secretion of bile, which is passed into the intestinal tract; (2) involvement in many metabolic activities; and (3) filtration of blood.

Formation of Bile

Bile is secreted by the liver cells, stored and concentrated in the gallbladder, and, later, delivered to the intestinal tract. Bile is composed of water, large amounts of bile salts, bilirubin, cholesterol, lecithin, and electrolytes. In the gallbladder, the bile is concentrated to about one-tenth its original volume as the result of absorption of water and large amounts of electrolytes.

The bile salts are important in emulsifying the fat in the intestine and in assisting in the absorption of fatty acids, monoglycerides, and lipids from the small intestine. About 94 percent of the bile salts are reabsorbed from the lower end of the ileum and return to the hepatic cells via the portal vein to be secreted promptly once again into the bile.

The bile pigment bilirubin is not formed in the liver cells but is excreted by these cells into the bile. It will be remembered that bilirubin is one of the products of hemoglobin breakdown following the phagocytosis of worn-out red blood cells by reticuloendothelial cells throughout the body (see p. 161). The bilirubin is slowly released from the phagocytes into the blood, where it combines with albumin (Fig. 12-11). The hepatic cells absorb the bilirubin-albumin complex from the blood. The bilirubin is removed from the albumin within the cells and conjugated with other substances. It is finally excreted in the bile. A small amount of the conjugated bilirubin is returned to the blood, so that this pigment always exists in the blood in both conjugated and free forms.

Metabolic Functions

CARBOHYDRATE METABOLISM. After the ingestion of the carbohydrate in a meal, excess glucose in the blood, under the influence of insulin, is stored in the liver in the form of glycogen. Under the electron microscope, it can be recognized in the hepatocytes as small dense particles arranged in clusters close to the smooth endoplasmic reticulum. When the blood glucose level starts to fall, the glycogen is broken down in the smooth-surfaced endoplasmic reticulum into glucose and returned to the blood. Should the blood glucose level fall below normal, the hepatocytes start to convert amino acids into glucose, further raising the blood glucose level. The latter process is called *gluconeogenesis.*

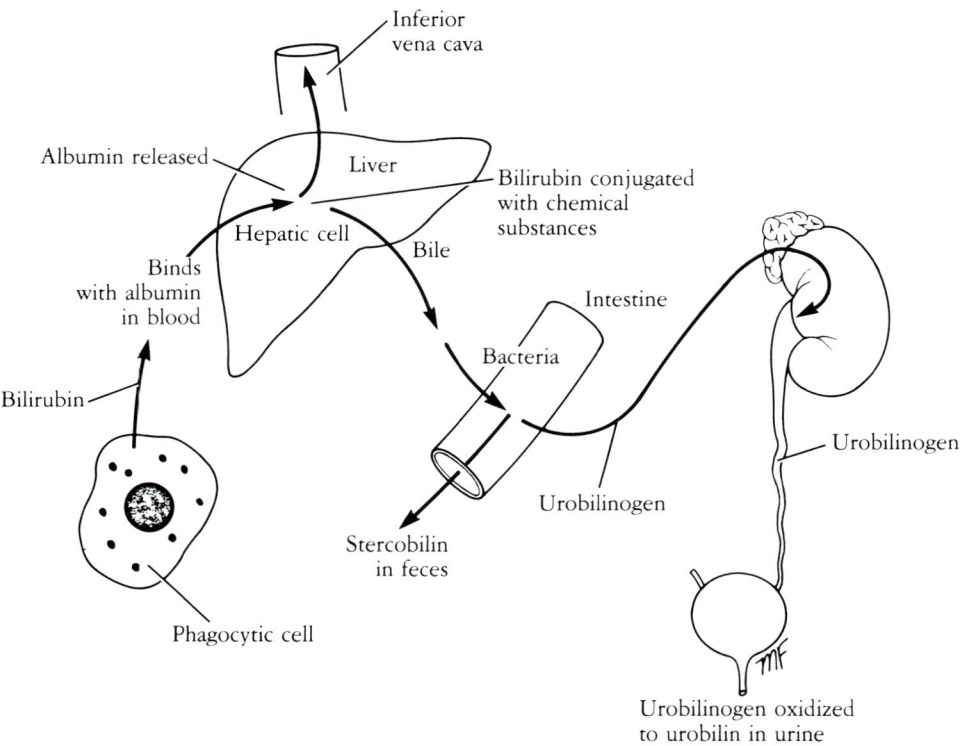

Fig. 12-11. *The formation and fate of the bile pigment bilirubin. The process is initiated when the phagocytic cells break down the hemoglobin from worn-out red blood cells and liberate bilirubin into the blood. In the liver a small amount of conjugated bilirubin is returned to the blood in the inferior vena cava, but the greater part is excreted by the hepatic cells into the bile, which passes into the intestine.*

FAT METABOLISM. *Beta Oxidation of Fatty Acids.* The presence of very large numbers of mitochondria in the hepatocytes enables the liver to play a major role in the oxidation of fatty acids, with the resultant formation of acetoacetic acid. The neutral fat is first absorbed by the hepatocytes and split into glycerol and fatty acids.

Formation of Cholesterol and Lipoproteins. Cholesterol is formed in hepatocytes largely for the purpose of conversion into bile salts. The remainder of the cholesterol is secreted into the blood with other lipoproteins and probably is used by the body in the formation of plasma membranes. The abundant smooth endoplasmic reticulum of the hepatocytes contains the enzymes necessary for the formation of cholesterol and other lipids. The rough endoplasmic reticulum forms the protein. The Golgi apparatus also participates, and the lipoproteins are transported to the cell surface in vesicles.

Synthesis of Fat from Carbohydrates and Protein. The hepatocytes are major sites of the formation of fats from carbohydrates and proteins. Once formed, the fat is carried as lipoproteins in the blood, where it is taken up and stored as depot fat in adipose tissue.

PROTEIN METABOLISM. With the exception of the gamma globulins associated with immunity and produced by the plasma cells of lymphoid tissue, all the plasma proteins are formed by the hepatocytes. Thus, the albumins, fibrinogen, and some of the globulins are formed in the rough endoplasmic reticulum of the cytoplasm. They are then transported to the cell surface via the Golgi apparatus in numerous vesicles.

The liver is also the principal organ of the body involved in deamination of amino acids and the formation of urea.

Filtration of Blood

The liver is strategically placed between the portal circulation and the inferior vena cava. It also receives blood from the hepatic artery. About 1,500 ml of blood flows through the liver each minute. As the blood permeates the hepatic sinusoids, the Kupffer cells, which are part of the reticuloendothelial system, remove by phagocytosis bacteria and other foreign particles that have gained entrance to the blood from the lumen of the intestine. Worn-out blood cells are also removed from the circulation by this method.

Bile Ducts

The smallest tributaries of the bile ducts are situated in the portal canals of the liver; they receive the bile canaliculi. The small ducts are lined with cuboidal epithelium and are surrounded by dense fibrous tissue.

The interlobular ducts join one another to form larger ducts and eventually, at the porta hepatis, form the *right* and *left hepatic ducts*. These larger ducts are lined with columnar epithelium that is surrounded by layers of connective tissue.

The extrahepatic ducts—namely, the *common hepatic duct,* formed by the union of the right and left hepatic ducts, and the *common bile duct,* formed by the union of the *cystic duct* and the *common hepatic duct*—all have similar structures and are lined with tall columnar epithelium. Near the distal end of the common bile duct, bundles of smooth muscle fibers appear in the connective tissue coat.

The common bile duct ends below by piercing the medial wall of the second part of the duodenum about halfway down its length (see Fig. 12-16). It is joined by the main pancreatic duct in 60 to 70 percent of persons, and together they open into a small ampulla in the duodenal wall called the *ampulla of*

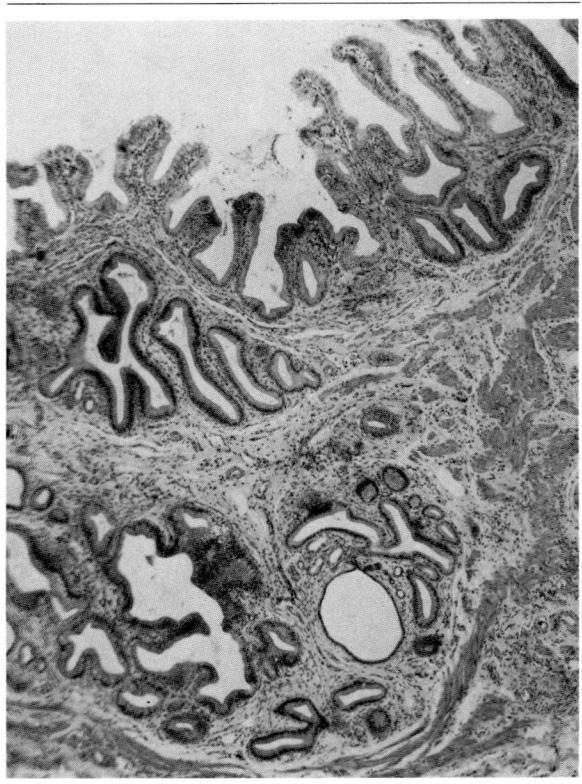

Fig. 12-12. Photomicrograph of a section of the wall of the gallbladder, showing the mucous membrane to be thrown into numerous permanent, branching folds that unite, giving the surface a honeycombed appearance. (H&E; × 40.)

Vater. The ampulla itself opens into the lumen of the duodenum by means of a small papilla, the *duodenal papilla* (see Fig. 12-16). The terminal parts of both ducts and the ampulla are surrounded by circular smooth muscle fibers known as the *sphincter of Oddi.*

The smooth muscle in the wall of the preampullary part of the common bile duct is thickened to form a separate sphincter called the *sphincter of Boyden.*

Gallbladder

The gallbladder is a pear-shaped sac lying on the visceral surface of the liver (see Fig. 12-1). For de-

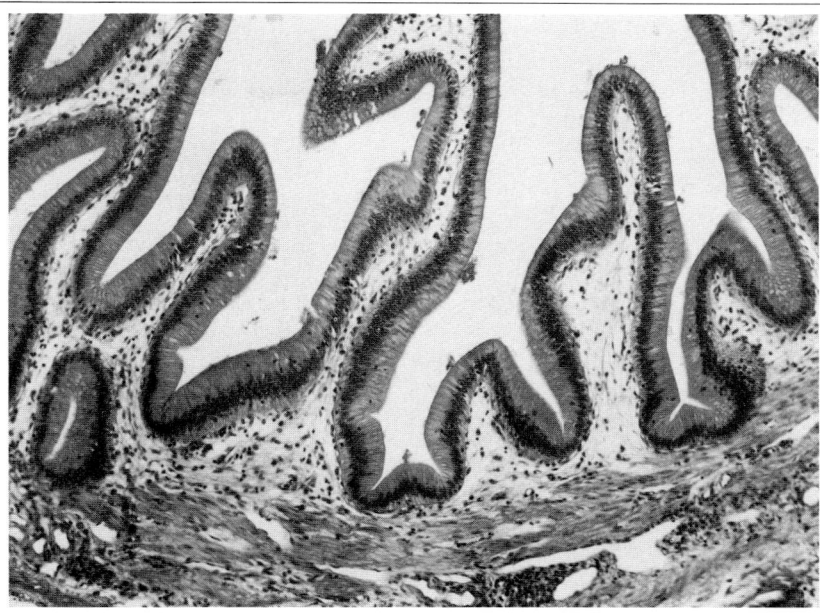

Fig. 12-13. Photomicrograph of a section of the mucous membrane of the wall of the gallbladder, showing the surface to be covered with tall columnar epithelial cells resting on a lamina propria of loose connective tissue. There is no submucosa. (H&E; ×100.)

scriptive purposes, it can be divided into the fundus, body, and neck. The *fundus* is rounded and usually projects below the inferior margin of the liver. The *body* lies in contact with the visceral surface of the liver. The *neck* becomes continuous with the cystic duct, which joins the right side of the common hepatic duct to form the common bile duct. The peritoneum completely surrounds the fundus of the gallbladder and binds the body and neck to the visceral surface of the liver.

The wall of the gallbladder is composed of three layers: (1) the mucous membrane, (2) the muscle coat, and (3) the serosa.

The *mucous membrane* is thrown into numerous permanent, branching folds that unite, giving the surface a honeycombed appearance (Fig. 12-12). The surface is covered with tall columnar epithelial cells (Figs. 12-13 and 12-14) with large numbers of microvilli on their free borders. The main function of these cells is absorption of water from the stored bile.

In the neck of the gallbladder, the mucous membrane is thrown into a number of crescentic folds forming the *spiral valve*. In this region, and only in this region, the mucous membrane has a number of tubulo-alveolar glands lined with mucus-secreting cells.

Small outpouchings of the mucous membrane extend into the muscle coat. These are known as the *Rokitansky-Aschoff sinuses*. Although some authorities believe they result from disease, others, because of their presence in otherwise normal gallbladders, believe they exist normally in small numbers. The sinuses communicate with the gallbladder lumen and are lined with columnar epithelium.

The lamina propria of the mucous membrane is composed of loose connective tissue, and there is no muscularis mucosae.

The *muscle coat* is thin and is composed of smooth muscle fibers running in many directions. The spaces between the groups of muscle fibers are filled with loose connective tissue.

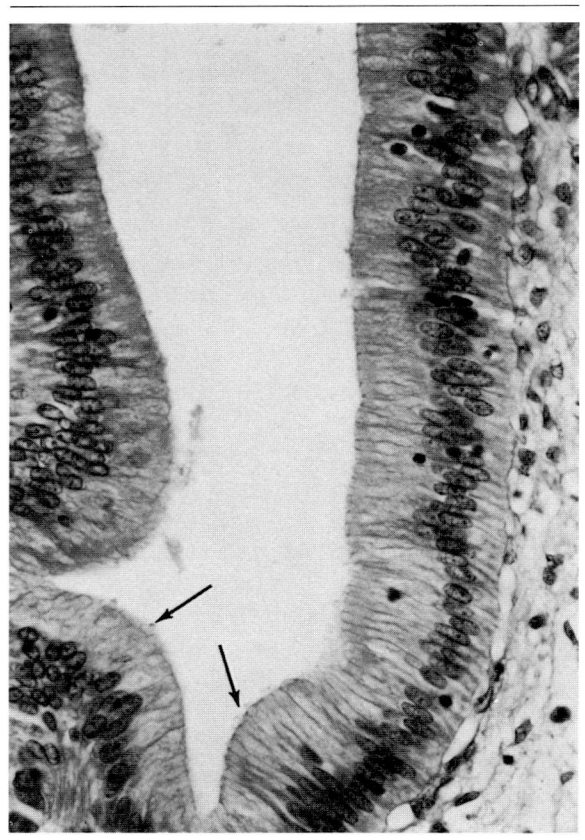

Fig. 12-14. Photomicrograph of part of the section of the mucous membrane of the gallbladder shown in Figure 12-13, showing the lining of tall columnar cells with microvilli on their free borders (arrows). (H&E; × 400.)

The *serosa* is composed of a thick layer of connective tissue that surrounds the organ. Outside the connective tissue is a layer of flattened mesothelial cells that form the peritoneum. The peritoneum completely surrounds the fundus of the gallbladder and binds the body and neck to the visceral surface of the liver.

Function

The gallbladder serves as a reservoir for bile, with a capacity of about 50 ml. Bile is continuously secreted by the liver and enters the gallbladder via the hepatic and cystic ducts. Normally, it does not enter the duodenum until the gallbladder contracts.

While the bile is stored in the gallbladder, it is concentrated, providing additional room for storage. The concentration of bile is brought about by the selective absorption of water and inorganic salts by the mucous membrane (Fig. 12-15). This process is aided by the permanent folds of the mucous membrane and the microvilli of the columnar cells, both of which increase the surface area. The final volume of bile is five to ten times smaller than that produced by the liver.

Bile is delivered to the duodenum as a result of contraction and partial emptying of the gallbladder. This mechanism is initiated by the entrance of fatty foods into the duodenum. The fat causes the release of the hormone cholecystokinin from the mucous membrane; the hormone then enters the blood, causing the gallbladder to contract. At the same time, the sphincter of Boyden and the sphincter of Oddi are relaxed, thus allowing the passage of concentrated bile into the duodenum. Hydrochloric acid in the duodenum stimulates the liver cells to increase their secretion of bile. The absorption of bile salts from the small intestine also enhances the production of bile by the liver.

PANCREAS

The pancreas is a soft, lobulated organ that lies on the posterior abdominal wall behind the peritoneum. For purposes of description, it can be divided into a *head, neck, body,* and *tail* (Fig. 12-16). The head lies within the concavity of the duodenum, and the neck, body, and tail extend to the left; the tail lies in contact with the hilus of the spleen.

Fig. 12-15. A: Possible mechanism of the extraction of water from the bile by the cells lining the gallbladder; note that sodium is pumped into the intercellular space and the water molecules follow. B: Processes within a hepatocyte during the secretion of bilirubin and the storage of carbohydrate as glycogen. C: Processes within a hepatocyte during protein and bile salt synthesis.

Bile in lumen of gallbladder
is stored and concentrated
H2O +
electrolytes
H2O +
electrolytes
Tight
junction
Columnar cell
Na+
Na+
Na+
Na+
H2O
H2O
H2O
H2O
Endothelium of
blood capillary
A
Blood
Blood
Bilirubin –
albumin complex
Urea
Albumin
Bilirubin
Deamination
Bilirubin
Synthesis
of glycogen
Amino
acids
Gluconeogenesis
Insulin
Glucose
Glucose
B
Blood
Bile canaliculus
Blood
Lipoproteins
Neutral fats
Cholesterol
Cholesterol
Fatty acids
+ glycerol
Beta-oxidation
Fats
Bile salts
Protein synthesis
Glucose
Amino acids
Albumins
Fibrinogen
Blood
Some globulins (remainder
formed by plasma cells)
C

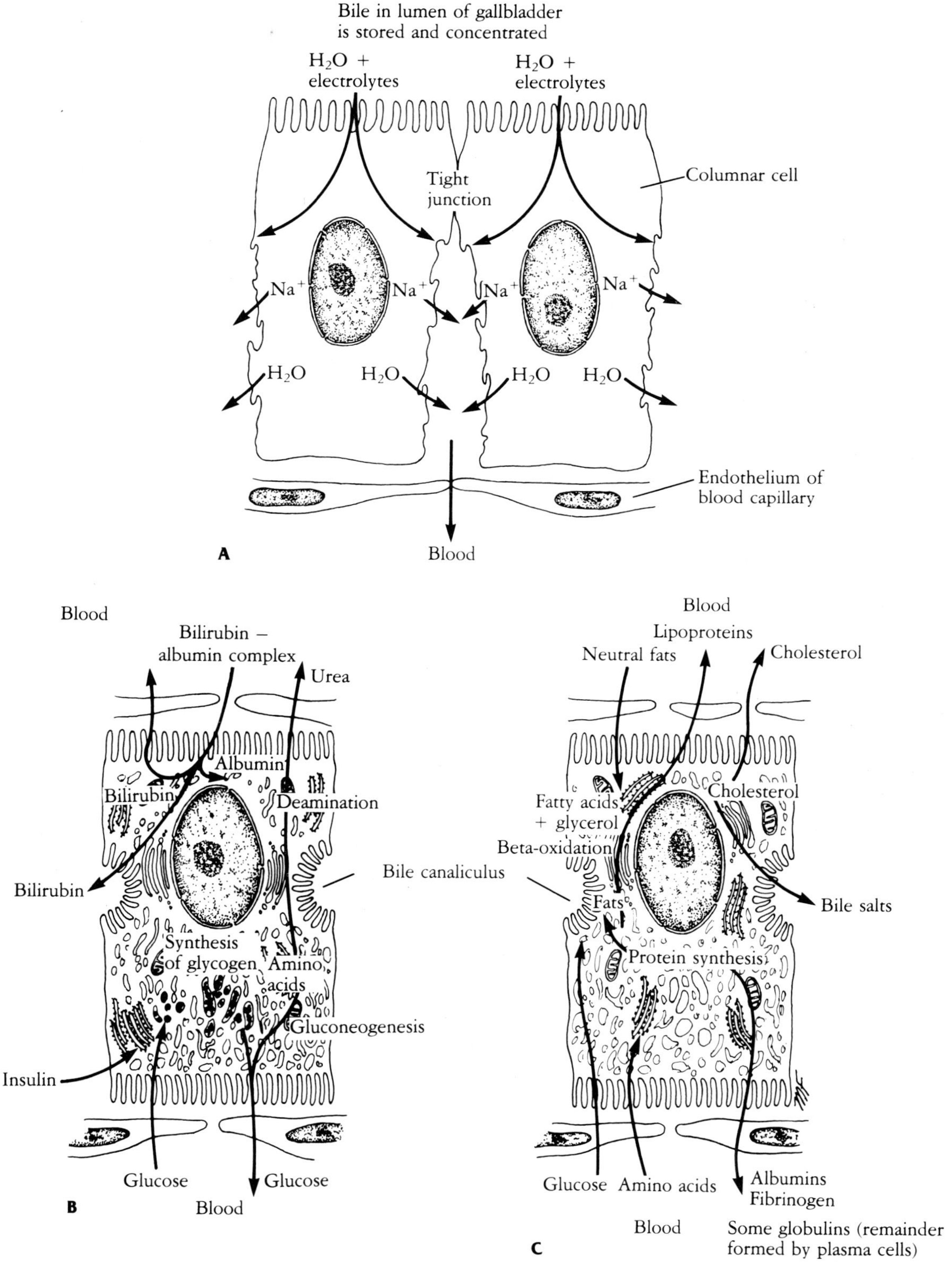

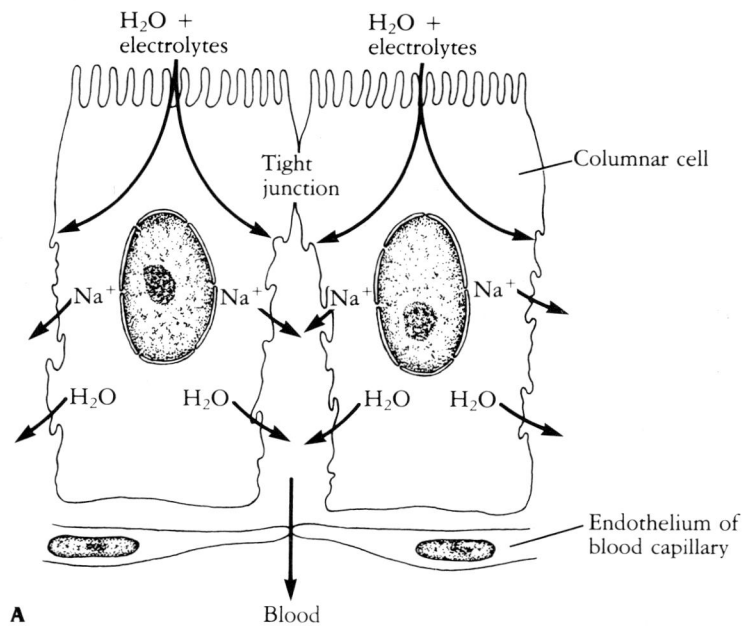

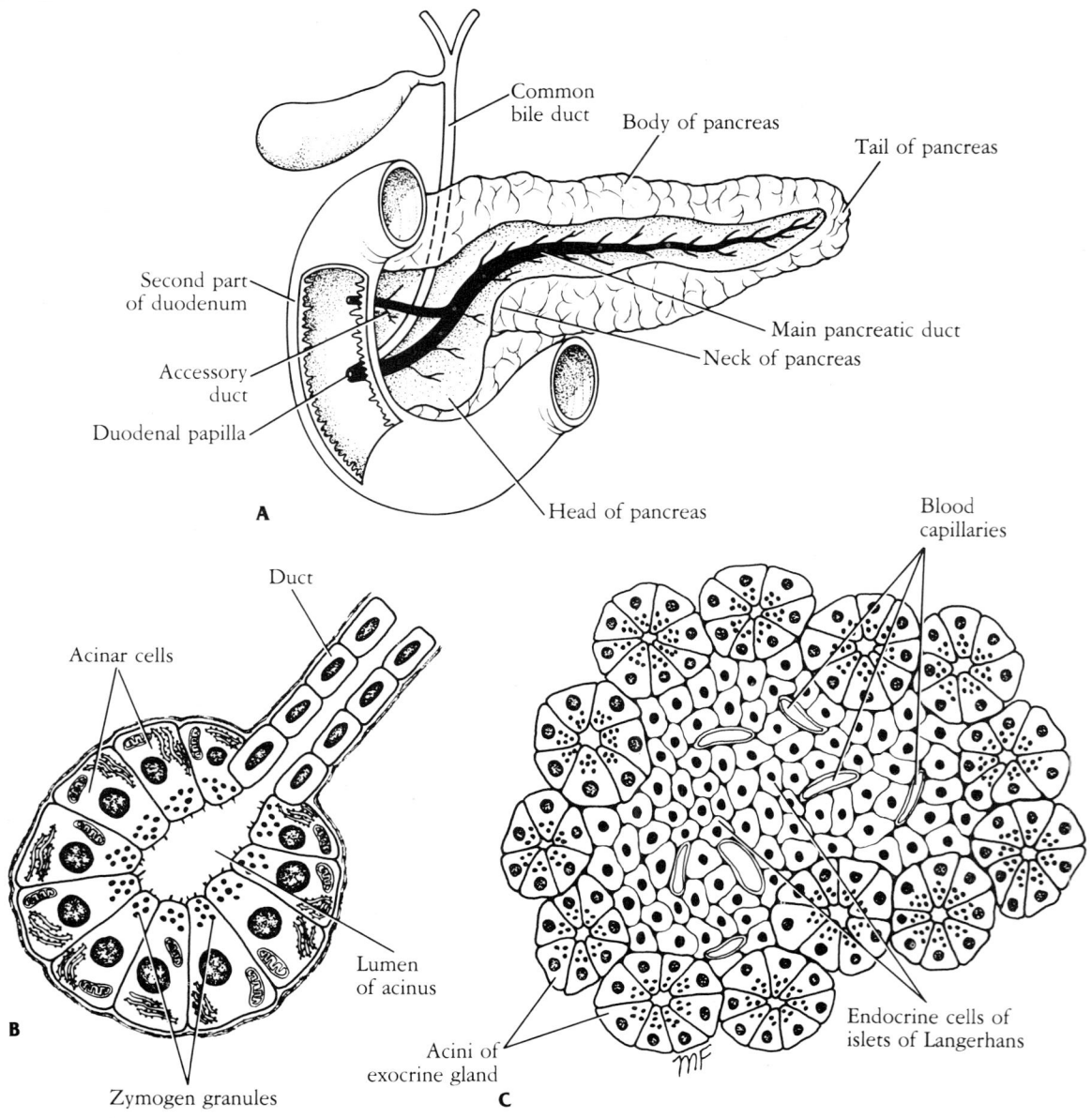

Fig. 12-16. A: The parts of the pancreas and the relationship of this organ to the duodenum and the common bile duct. Note that the pancreas has been dissected to show the pancreatic ducts; the anterior wall of the second part of the duodenum has been removed to show the opening of the accessory duct and the duodenal papilla. B: Section through the acinus of the exocrine part of the pancreas. C: Section through an islet of Langerhans, the endocrine part of the pancreas.

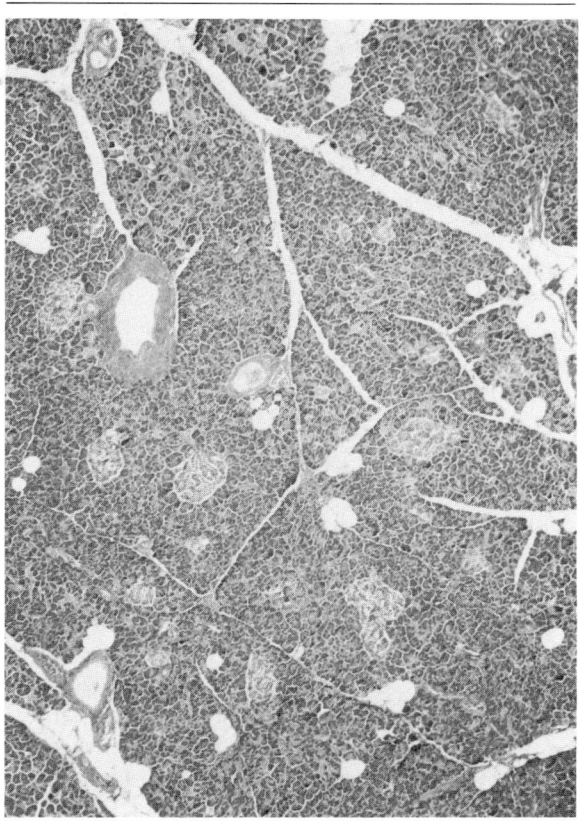

Fig. 12-17. Photomicrograph of a section of the pancreas, showing the lobules separated by connective tissue septa. The greater part of the gland is made up of dark-staining exocrine acini. Note several lightly stained islets of Langerhans. (H&E; × 10.)

The pancreas is both an exocrine and an endocrine gland. It has a thin connective tissue capsule that sends fibrous septa into the substance of the gland, dividing it into lobules. The connective tissue septa contain blood vessels, nerves, lymphatic vessels, and the ducts from the secretory acini.

The exocrine portion of the gland is a compound acinar gland. The secretory acini are lined with pyramid-shaped cells arranged around a small lumen (Fig. 12-17; see Fig. 12-16). The cells rest on a basal lamina that is supported by reticular fibers. The acinar cell possesses a spherical nucleus situated near the base of the cell. The cytoplasm between the nucleus and the apex of the cell contains zymogen granules, which stain pink with eosin, and a well-developed Golgi apparatus. The cytoplasm between the nucleus and the base of the cell is bluish when stained with hematoxylin, because of the high concentration of rough endoplasmic reticulum (see Fig. 12-16). The basal cytoplasm also has a striated appearance because of the large numbers of filamentous mitochondria. Electron microscopy of the cells reveals that the zymogen granules are membrane bound and leave the apical surface of the cell by exocytosis. A number of short microvilli project from the apical surface of the cell. Thus, the acinar cells are designed to produce large amounts of protein in the form of proteolytic enzymes.

The endocrine portions of the gland are easily recognized under the light microscope as large, pale areas among the darker-staining secretory acini (see Fig. 12-17). Each pale area consists of irregular clusters of cells known as the *islets of Langerhans*. The islets are more numerous in the tail of the pancreas than in its body, neck, or head. The cells of the islets are arranged as anastomosing cords that are profusely supplied by fenestrated capillaries. The islets are not encapsulated but are supported by reticular fibers. The islets of Langerhans have no ducts; the cells pour their secretion directly into the bloodstream.

In routine H&E-stained sections, no secretory granules can be identified in the islet cells (Fig. 12-18). When special staining techniques are used, however, four cell types can be recognized by the staining and structure of the granules. These are referred to as beta, alpha, delta, and pp (pancreatic polypeptide) cells. Specific antibody techniques have enabled researchers to localize specific hormones to individual cells.

The *beta cells,* which are centrally placed and constitute the majority of the islet cells, secrete *insulin*. The secretory granules, as seen with the electron microscope, are rectangular crystals surrounded by a loose-fitting membrane (Fig. 12-19). Insulin lowers the blood sugar level by promoting the transfer of glucose across plasma membranes, especially in muscle, liver, and fat cells.

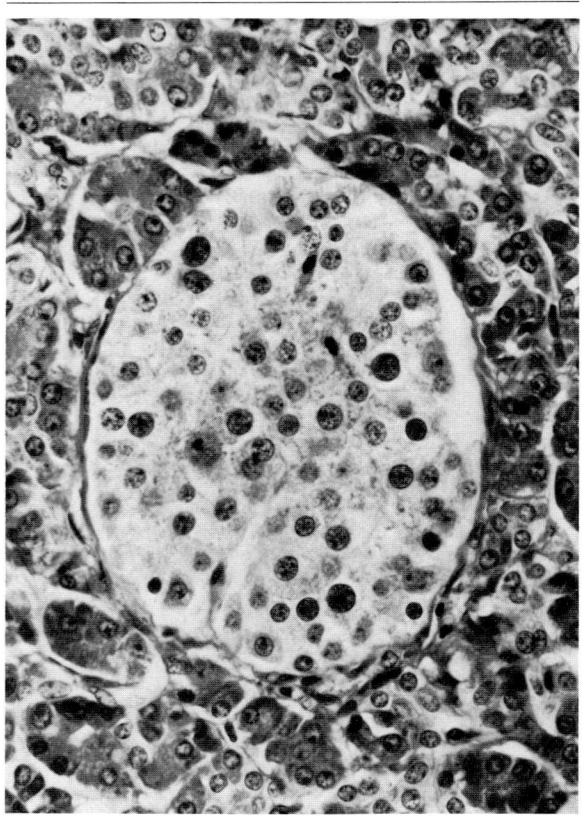

Fig. 12-18. Photomicrograph of a section of the pancreas, showing a pale-staining islet of Langerhans surrounded by numerous dark-staining exocrine acini. (H&E; ×400.)

The *alpha cells* are situated at the periphery of the islets and secrete *glucagon*. The granules have a rounded dense center surrounded by a less dense area (see Fig. 12-19). The granules are membrane bound. Glucagon raises the blood sugar level by inducing gluconeogenesis and glycolytic activity in the liver.

The *delta cells* are found among the alpha cells and secrete *somatostatin*. The delta cells have large, pale granules with closely applied membranes (see Fig. 12-19). Somatostatin inhibits the release of insulin and glucagon.

The *PP cells* are located in the islets but are also found scattered among the surrounding acini. These cells produce a polypeptide that, when injected into animals, increases peristalsis of the gut. Its function in humans is not known.

Ducts

The small lumina of the secretory acini are drained by ducts that join one another to form *intralobular ducts*. These are lined by cuboidal epithelium. The intralobular ducts join one another to form interlobular ducts. The interlobular ducts join the main and accessory ducts of the pancreas. The larger ducts are lined with tall columnar cells (Fig. 12-20), some of which are mucus-secreting goblet cells.

The main duct of the pancreas begins in the tail and runs the length of the gland, receiving numerous tributaries along the way. It pierces the posteromedial wall of the second part of the duodenum at about its middle and opens into the ampulla of Vater with the common bile duct (see Fig. 12-16) or drains separately into the duodenum.

The *accessory duct* of the pancreas drains the upper part of the head and then opens into the duodenum a short distance above the main duct (see Fig. 12-16). The accessory duct frequently communicates with the main duct and occasionally is absent. The actions of the sphincter of Oddi in relation to the flow of bile and pancreatic secretions into the duodenum are discussed on page 490.

Functions

The endocrine functions of the pancreas are fully described on page 662; their control is discussed in Chapter 16.

Exocrine Function: Pancreatic Secretion

The average adult produces about 1,200 ml of pancreatic secretion every 24 hours. The pH of the secretion is about 8.2. It contains large amounts of bicarbonate ions, which effectively neutralize the hydrochloric acid of the gastric chyme.

The enzymes present are capable of hydrolyzing proteins, fats, and carbohydrates. The proteolytic enzymes are *trypsinogen, chymotrypsinogen,* and *procarboxypolypeptidase.* Trypsinogen is inactive when it enters the duodenum but is quickly converted into

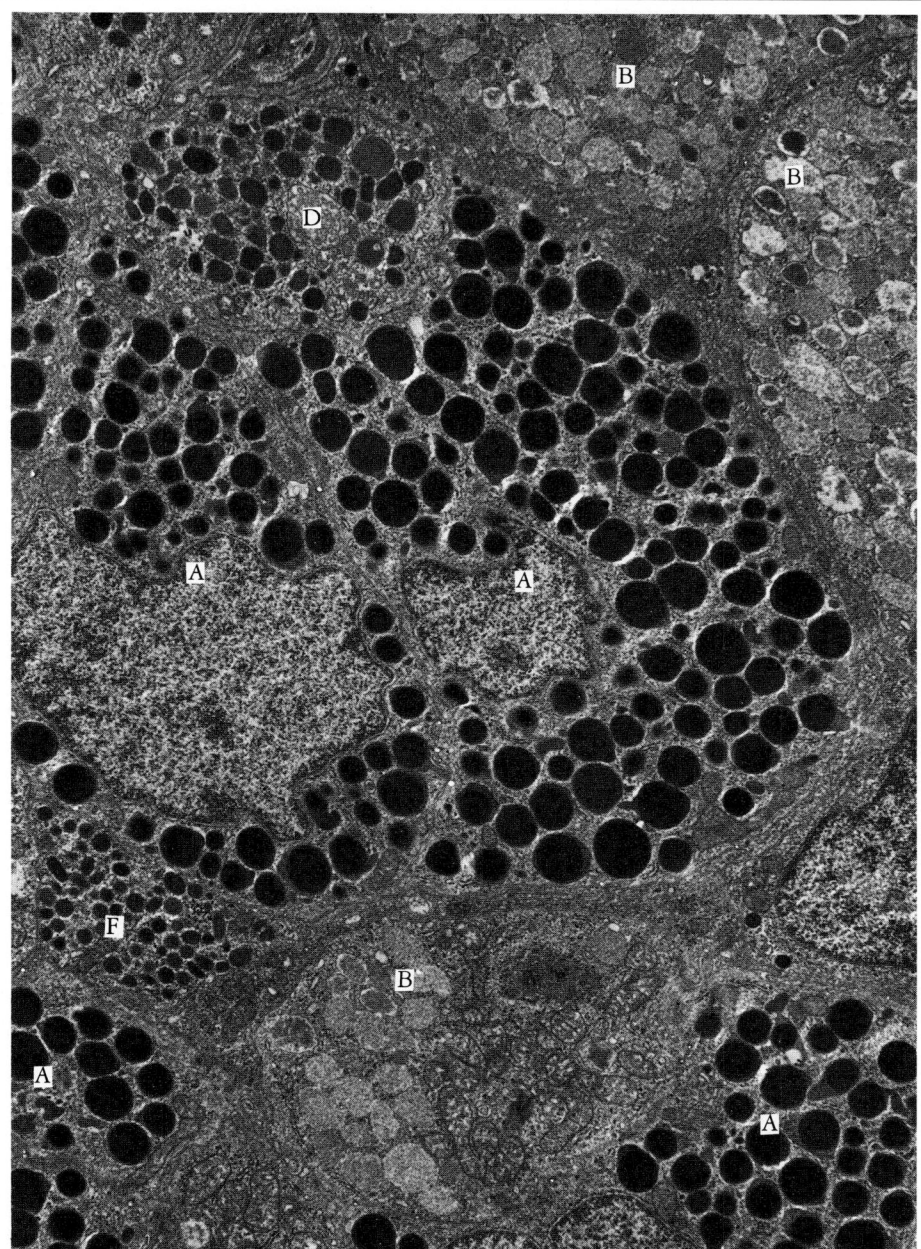

Fig. 12-19. Electron micrograph showing the four endocrine cell types present in an islet of Langerhans. In this specimen, the insulin-secreting beta cells (B) have heterogeneous granules; the glucagon-secreting alpha cells (A) have large, rounded dense granules surrounded by a less dense area; the somatostatin-secreting delta cells (D) have large, less dense granules. The pp cells, or F cells (F), which produce polypeptides, have small secretory granules. (×13,500.) (Courtesy of Dr. W. B. Rhoten.)

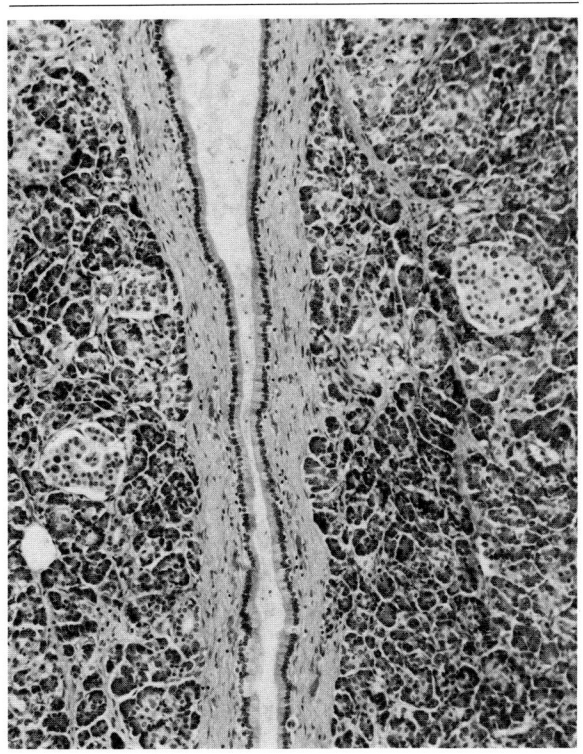

Fig. 12-20. Photomicrograph of a section of the pancreas, showing an interlobular duct, multiple dark-staining exocrine acini, and several pale-staining islets of Langerhans. Note that the duct is lined with tall columnar epithelial cells resting on connective tissue. (H&E; ×100.)

trypsin by an enzyme produced by the mucous membrane of the small intestine called *enterokinase*. The other enzymes are converted by trypsin into *chymotrypsin* and *carboxypolypeptidase*, respectively; these latter enzymes can hydrolyze proteins and polypeptides to form amino acids. *Nucleases* that split the nucleic acids are also present. The fat-splitting enzymes are *lipase* and *cholesterol esterase*. Lipase hydrolyzes neutral fat into glycerol and fatty acids, and cholesterol esterase splits cholesterol esters. The carbohydrate-splitting enzyme is amylase, which hydrolyzes all polysaccharides except cellulose to form disaccharides.

CONTROL OF PANCREATIC ACINAR SECRETION. *Nervous Control.* Stimulation of the parasympathetic nerve fibers traveling in the vagus nerves produces a pancreatic secretion rich in enzymes.

Hormonal Control. The hormone secretin is released from the mucous membrane of the upper part of the small intestine in response to the entrance of chyme into the small intestine. The hormone is quickly absorbed into the blood and stimulates the pancreatic acinar cells to produce a watery secretion rich in bicarbonate ions. The hormone cholecystokinin, also produced by the intestinal mucosa, stimulates the acinar cells to increase their secretion of enzymes.

Protective Inhibition of Trypsin Formation. To prevent the premature formation of the powerful proteolytic enzyme trypsin from its inactive precursor trypsinogen while the latter is still within the pancreas, the pancreatic cells produce a substance called *trypsin inhibitor.* This inhibition protects the pancreas from autodigestion.

SUMMARY OF DIGESTION AND ABSORPTION IN THE ALIMENTARY CANAL

Mouth

The enzyme ptyalin hydrolyzes the polysaccharide starch into maltose and isomaltose. No absorption occurs in the mouth.

Stomach

The enzyme pepsin starts to hydrolyze proteins into polypeptides in the stomach. Small quantities of lipase start to break down neutral fats into glycerol and fatty acids. Amylase continues to split starch into maltose and isomaltose. The ptyalin in the swallowed bolus continues to act on the starch for a few hours after the bolus has entered the stomach. Only water, alcohol, and some drugs can be absorbed from the stomach.

Small Intestine

Pancreatic Secretions

The enzymes trypsin, chymotrypsin, and carboxypolypeptidase can hydrolyze proteins and polypeptides to form peptides and amino acids. Nucleases split the nucleic acids. Lipase hydrolyzes neutral fat into glycerol and fatty acids. Cholesterol esterase splits cholesterol esters. Amylase splits polysaccharides to form disaccharides.

Secretions of the Small Intestine

Amylase hydrolyzes the polysaccharide starch into disaccharides; sucrase, maltase, and lactase hydrolyze the disaccharides into monosaccharides. Lipase hydrolyzes neutral fats into glycerol and fatty acids, and peptidases hydrolyze polypeptides into amino acids.

Fate of the Products of Digestion
Carbohydrates

The large polysaccharide molecules are first split by digestive enzymes into smaller disaccharide molecules. Lactose is split into galactose and glucose, sucrose is split into fructose and glucose, and maltose is split into glucose. Glucose forms the greater part of the monosaccharides found in the intestinal lumen. The monosaccharides are readily absorbed through the mucous membrane and enter the portal circulation. They are then taken to the liver or are circulated throughout the body and taken up by the tissues. Large amounts of glucose are transported to the liver and converted to glycogen for storage.

Fats

Neutral fats (the triglycerides) are hydrolyzed by the digestive enzymes into monoglycerides, free fatty acids, and glycerol. As soon as the monoglycerides and free fatty acids are formed, they are dissolved in the micelles formed by the bile salts. The bile salt micelle then transports the monoglycerides and the fatty acids across the lining epithelium of the intestine, and the micelle diffuses back into the intestinal lumen. The monoglycerides are now further digested by lipase within the epithelial cell into glycerol and fatty acids. The free fatty acids are synthesized into triglycerides, and these, together with phospholipid, cholesterol, and protein, are formed into protein-coated globules, called chylomicrons, that pass into the central lacteal of the villi. In addition, a number of short-chain fatty acids are absorbed directly from the intestinal lumen into the portal blood.

Proteins

The proteolytic enzymes of the stomach, pancreas, and intestinal epithelium break down ingested protein into amino acids. The amino acids then are rapidly absorbed from the lumen of the small intestine and transported to the liver and other tissues, where most are synthesized into body proteins. Excess amino acids are deaminated in the liver.

Feces

Feces is the name given to the semisolid contents of the descending colon. They are composed of 75 percent water and 25 percent solid material. Thirty percent of the solid materal is dead bacteria, and about 15 percent is fat. Thirty percent is undigested cellulose and sloughed epithelial cells. The remainder is a small amount of protein and some inorganic matter.

The brown color of the feces results from the presence of *stercobilin,* a derivative of bilirubin. The odor is caused by bacterial decomposition.

CLINICAL NOTES

LIVER

The liver consists of a large mass of parenchymal cells traversed by systems of blood vessels, bile ducts, and lymphatics. The liver is unique among the abdominal viscera in having a double blood supply. The portal vein supplies about two-thirds of the hepatic circulation; the hepatic artery supplies the remainder. It has been emphasized that the incoming blood flows from these vessels through the sinusoids and between the hepatocytes and leaves via the central vein. The dual blood supply is the reason infarction of the liver is extremely rare.

The blood flow through the liver in normal subjects is about 1,500 ml per minute. Impaired blood flow to the right atrium in right-sided heart failure is quickly referred back to the liver, causing a rise in intrahepatic venous pressure. Venous congestion in the liver causes edema of the parenchyma and loss of fluid from the peritoneal-covered surfaces. The fluid accumulates in the peritoneal cavity, a condition known as *ascites*. In addition, there is a very great increase in the flow of lymph away from the liver.

In cirrhosis of the liver, the hepatocytes undergo necrosis and then disorganized regeneration, and there is extensive fibrosis. In addition, portal venous blood flow through the liver is obstructed. The obstruction involves not only the portal canals but the venous sinusoids and the venous outflow. Portal hypertension develops and is followed by ascites, and opening up of the portal systemic anastomoses, and enlargement of the spleen.

The acinar organization of the liver readily explains why hepatocytes near the portal canal normally receive blood that is richer in oxygen than that received by hepatocytes lying close to the central vein. In hypoxia caused by a poor cardiac output, therefore, the hypoxic damage is greatest in those cells nearest the central vein. When the cells die, the condition is referred to as *centrilobular necrosis*. This condition should be contrasted with *midzonal necrosis*—cell death midway between the central vein and the portal canal—which occurs in yellow fever. In phosphorus poisoning, the cells closest to the afferent blood supply are affected first, and the cell death is called *peripheral necrosis*.

Liver regeneration is a remarkable phenomenon. In the normal adult, the hepatocytes rarely undergo mitosis, but destruction of the liver by disease or removal of part of the liver is quickly followed by regeneration. For example, removal of two-thirds of the liver in man is followed by complete regeneration in about 5 months. There is evidence that a hepatotrophic portal blood factor, possibly produced by the pancreas, is responsible for stimulation of liver regeneration. Destruction or removal of liver tissue allows this factor to act free of inhibition.

Liver Function Tests

A number of laboratory tests are valuable in detecting liver disease.

Serum Bilirubin Test

Bilirubin is carried to the liver in the blood in the unconjugated form. The hepatocytes conjugate it and excrete it into the bile ducts. The conjugated form can be detected in the blood by performing a red diazo test called the *direct van den Bergh reaction*. If hepatocyte disease has interfered with the uptake of unconjugated bilirubin in the blood, or if there is increased breakdown of hemoglobin, the increased amount of unconjugated bilirubin can be detected in the blood by pretreating the blood with alcohol before performing the diazo reaction. The procedure then is referred to as the *indirect van den Bergh reaction*.

An increase in the conjugated form of bilirubin occurs in bile duct obstruction when the conjugated bilirubin, having been excreted by the hepatocytes, is held back at the obstruction and is absorbed or escapes into the bloodstream (see p. 500).

Serum Alkaline Phosphatase Test

In patients with hepatocyte disease or bile duct obstruction, the serum alkaline phosphatase level is raised.

Serum Glutamic Oxalacetic Transaminase (SGOT) Test

Glutamic oxalacetic transaminase is involved in the transfer of an amino group from glutamic acid to oxalacetic acid and is found in large quantities in the liver. Liver cell injury results in the escape of this enzyme into the blood stream.

Serum Glutamic Pyruvic Transaminase (SGPT) Test

Glutamic pyruvic transaminase facilitates the transfer of an amino acid group from glutamic acid to pyruvic acid and is found in very large quantities in liver cells. This enzyme may escape into the bloodstream in liver cell injury.

Serum Plasma Protein Levels

The ability of hepatocytes to synthesize serum albumin and globin can be measured. A fall in serum albumin levels occurs in hepatocyte disease, but the test is not sensitive. Conversely, there may be a rise in beta and gamma globulins in liver disease.

Bromsulphalein (BSP) Excretion Test

Bromsulphalein is a synthetic dye that is removed from the blood by the liver. Failure of the hepatocytes to perform this function as the result of disease can be detected readily. This test is very sensitive.

Liver Biopsy

When there is doubt about a diagnosis, it may be necessary to perform a liver biopsy. A large aspirating needle is inserted into the right lobe through the eighth intercostal space on the right side under local anesthesia. Precise histological examination of the diseased hepatocytes can then be performed, provided the disease is widespread throughout the liver. Small lesions are easily missed.

Bile Ducts and Gallbladder

Pain from the gallbladder and bile ducts is caused by distention and by spasm of the smooth muscle in the wall. The pain is often very severe and colicky in nature and is referred to the epigastrium.

Radiological Investigation of the Bile Ducts

The bile passages normally are not visible on a radiograph. Their lumina may be outlined by the oral or subcutaneous administration of various iodine-containing compounds. When taken orally, the compound is absorbed from the small intestine, carried to the liver, and excreted with the bile. On reaching the gallbladder, it is concentrated with the bile. The concentrated iodine compound, mixed with the bile, is now radiopaque and will reveal the gallbladder as a pear-shaped opacity. If the patient is given a fatty meal, the gallbladder contracts, and the cystic and common bile ducts will become visible as the opaque medium passes down to the duodenum.

Gallstones

The great majority of gallstones are formed in the gallbladder; only a few originate in the bile ducts. The stones are formed of cholesterol, calcium bilirubinate, and calcium carbonate. Many stones are formed of mixtures of these substances. Between 10 and 20 percent of adults in the United States have gallstones; the incidence is higher in women. Two factors are important in the formation of stones: (1) abnormal composition of bile (excess cholesterol and insufficient bile salts and lecithin to keep it in suspension) and (2) stasis caused by biliary obstruction.

Cholecystitis, or inflammation of the gallbladder, is a common complication of gallstones. Obstruction of the biliary passages by a stone, the excessive concentration of bile, and the consequent irritation of the mucous membrane of the gallbladder cause chemical inflammation of the gallbladder wall. Later, bacterial infection of the static bile may complicate the problem.

Carcinoma of the gallbladder is a common malignancy in the elderly. Most cases are preceded by gallstones, suggesting that chronic irritation of the mucous membrane is a predisposing factor. The carcinoma is a columnar cell carcinoma.

Jaundice

Jaundice is a yellow discoloration of the body tissues caused by a raised concentration of bilirubin within them. The condition is seen most easily in the sclerae and the skin of the face and neck. The condition results from a rise in the concentration of conjugated or unconjugated bilirubin in the blood. The skin starts to look yellow when the plasma concentration of bilirubin is about 2 mg/100 ml.

As has been explained, bilirubin is formed from the breakdown of hemoglobin in the reticuloendothelial system. The unconjugated bilirubin is then transported to the liver in the blood. It follows that the excessive breakdown of hemoglobin, as in hemolytic anemia, will cause jaundice.

Once the unconjugated bilirubin reaches the liver, the hepatocytes take it up and conjugated bilirubin is formed. The conjugated bilirubin is then excreted into the biliary ducts and transported to the duodenum. In obstructive jaundice, the bile ducts may be obstructed by an impacted gallstone. If so, the conjugated bile is dammed and returns to the bloodstream (probably as a result of rupture of the bile canaliculi). The plasma concentration of conjugated bilirubin rises in this condition.

In liver disease in which the hepatocytes are unable to take up the unconjugated bilirubin from the plasma or are unable to conjugate or excrete the bilirubin into the bile canaliculi, the concentration of both forms of bilirubin in the plasma may rise, producing jaundice.

PANCREAS

The most common disease of the pancreas is diabetes mellitus. Fibrocystic disease, pancreatitis, and tumors also occur.

Diabetes mellitus is considered in some detail in the chapter on endocrine glands (see p. 680). The majority of affected patients show a loss of cytoplasmic granules within the beta cells and consequent diminished storage of insulin.

Acute pancreatitis is an enzymatic destruction of the pancreas caused by the escape of active pancreatic enzymes into the substance of the gland. This sudden event is often associated with a large intake of alcohol or a very large meal. Gallstones are present in about half of affected patients. It is thought that reflux of bile from the common bile duct into the main pancreatic duct brings about the activation of trypsinogen into trypsin, which then activates many proteases, lipase, and elastase. These enzymes then cause proteolysis, lipolysis, and destruction of pancreatic blood vessels. Alcohol may activate the whole process by causing the sphincter of Oddi to relax and permitting duodenal reflux, or by causing hypersecretion and congestion of the pancreas, producing pancreatic duct obstruction. Gallstone impaction or damage to the duodenal papillae also may allow biliary reflux into the pancreatic ducts.

The symptoms include very severe abdominal pain. The condition is a serious abdominal emergency; a number of patients die of vascular collapse and shock.

Carcinoma of the pancreas is common and arises from the duct epithelium and not from the acini or pancreatic islets. Most of the malignancies arise in the head and body of the pancreas and are adenocarcinomas. The tumors may grow silently, with no signs or symptoms, or, of they arise close to the ampulla of Vater, they may press upon the common bile duct, causing obstruction and jaundice.

CLINICAL PROBLEMS

For the answers to these problems, see page 805.

1. Describe the different classifications that exist for the basic histological unit of the liver. Which of these classifications is preferred by the pathologist?

2. A 60-year-old male bartender is diagnosed as suffering from cirrhosis of the liver. Using your knowledge of histology, explain the distribution of connective tissue in a normal liver. Explain also how necrosis and regeneration of the hepatocytes and fibrosis of the liver lobule can bring about portal hypertension and ascites in patients with cirrhosis.

3. Define the following: (a) intrahepatic bile canaliculus, (b) space of Disse, (c) Kupffer cell, (d) portal triad, (e) Glisson's capsule, (f) Rokitansky-Aschoff sinuses.

4. Trace a molecule of bilirubin from a cell in the reticuloendothelial system through the liver to the lumen of the duodenum. What is the difference between a direct and an indirect van den Bergh test, and how can this reaction be used to distinguish between jaundice caused by hemolytic anemia and that produced by biliary obstruction?

5. What is the structure and function of the gallbladder? Using your knowledge of the function of the gallbladder, how would you investigate the gallbladder radiologically? Occasionally, in surgical operations on the gallbladder, a mucocele

is found. This is a condition in which the lumen is distended with mucus. Where has the mucus come from?

6. What role do bile salts play in the process of digestion? Where are bile salts normally produced? Is there any causal connection between bile salts and gallstones? Can you think of any physiological reasons for the prevalence of gallstones in "fat, fertile females of forty"?

7. Describe mechanisms that control the delivery of bile to the duodenum. What is cholecystokinin?

8. The pancreas is said to be both an exocrine and an endocrine gland. Explain that statement. What is the light microscopic structure of the endocrine pancreas? How would you distinguish between an H&E-stained slide of the pancreas and one of the parotid salivary gland?

9. Give a detailed description of the electron microscopic structure of an islet of Langerhans. Which cell type is diseased in diabetes mellitus? Using your knowledge of the histology and physiology of the pancreatic ducts, explain a way by which trypsinogen can be activated within the pancreas and cause acute pancreatitis.

ADDITIONAL READING

Babcock, M. B., and Cardell, R. R., Jr. Hepatic glycogen patterns in fasted and fed rats. *Am. J. Anat.* 140:299, 1974.

Baltens, D., Malaisse-Lagae, F., Perrelet, A., and Orci, L. Endocrine pancreas: Three dimensional reconstruction shows two types of islets of Langerhans. *Science* 206:1323, 1979.

Berk, P. D., et al. Disorders of bilirubin metabolism. In Bondy, P. K., and Rosenberg, L. E. (eds.), *Metabolic Control and Disease* (8th ed.). Philadelphia: Saunders, 1980, p. 1009.

Blouin, A., Bolender, R. R., and Weibel, E. R. Distribution of organelles and membranes between hepatocytes and nonhepatocytes in the rat liver parenchyma: A stereological study. *J. Cell Biol.* 72:441, 1977.

Boyer, J. L. New concepts of mechanism of hepatocyte bile formation. *Physiol. Rev.* 60:303, 1980.

Brandborg, L. L. The pancreas. In Sleisenger, M. H., and Fordtran, J. S. (eds.), *Gastrointestinal Disease* (2nd ed.). Philadelphia: Saunders, 1978, p. 1388.

Braner, R. W. Liver circulation and function. *Physiol. Rev.* 43:115, 1963.

Brooks, S. E. H., and Haggis, G. H. Scanning electron microscopy of rat's liver. *Lab. Invest.* 29:60, 1973.

Bruni, C., and Porter, K. R. The fine structure of the parenchymal cells of the normal rat liver. I. General considerations. *Am. J. Pathol.* 46:691, 1965.

Burke, M. D. Progress in human pathology: Liver function. *Hum. Pathol.* 6:273, 1975.

Burkel, W. E. The fine structure of the terminal branches of the hepatic arterial system of the rat. *Anat. Rec.* 167:329, 1970.

Caro, L. G., and Palade, G. E. Protein synthesis, storage, and discharge in the pancreatic exocrine cell: An autoradiographic study. *J. Cell Biol.* 20:473, 1964.

Chapman, G. B., Chiardo, A. J., Coffey, R. J., and Weineke, K. The fine structure of the human gallbladder. *Anat. Rec.* 154:579, 1966.

Dubois, M. P. Immunoreactive somatostatin is present in discrete cells of the endocrine pancreas. *Proc. Natl. Acad. Sci. USA* 72:1340, 1975.

Erlandson, S. E., et al. Pancreatic islet cell hormones: Distribution of cell types in the islet and evidence for the presence of somatostatin and gastrin within the D cell. *J. Histochem. Cytochem.* 24:883, 1976.

Fitzgerald, P. J., and Morrison, A. B. (eds.). *The Pancreas*. Baltimore: Williams & Wilkins, 1980.

Greenway, C. V., and Stark, R. D. Hepatic vascular bed. *Physiol. Rev.* 51:23, 1971.

Howard, J. G. The origin and immunological significance of the Kupffer cells. In Van Furth, R. (ed.), *Mononuclear Phagocytes*. Oxford, Eng.: Blackwell, 1970.

Jamieson, J. D., and Palade, G. E. Intracellular transport of secretory proteins in the pancreatic exocrine cell. I. Role of the peripheral elements of the Golgi complex. *J. Cell Biol.* 34:577, 1967.

Jamieson, J. D., and Palade, G. E. Intracellular transport of secretory proteins in the pancreatic exocrine cell. II.

Transport to condensing vacuoles and zymogen granules. *J. Cell Biol.* 34:597, 1967.

Jones, A. L., and Schmucker, D. L. Current concepts of liver structure as related to function. *Gastroenterology* 73:833, 1977.

Jones, R. S., and Myers, W. C. Regulation of hepatic biliary secretion. *Annu. Rev. Physiol.* 41:67, 1979.

Kay, G. I., Wheeler, H. O., Whitlock, R. T., and Lane, N. Fluid transport in rabbit gallbladder: A combined physiological and electron microscope study. *J. Cell Biol.* 30:237, 1966.

Lacy, P. E. Islet cell functional pathology. *Pathol. Annu.* 12(1):1, 1977.

Lin, C., and Chang, J. P. Electron microscopy of albumin synthesis. *Science* 190:465, 1975.

Ma, M. H., and Biempica, L. The normal human liver cell. *Am. J. Pathol.* 62:353, 1971.

Motta, P. A. Scanning electron microscopic study of the rat sinusoids. *Cell Tissue Res.* 164:371, 1975.

Motta, P., et al. *The Liver: An Atlas of Scanning Electron Microscopy.* Tokyo: Igaku-Shoin, 1978.

Mueller, J. C., Jones, A. L., and Long, J. A. Topographical and subcellular anatomy of the guinea pig gallbladder. *Gastroenterology* 63:856, 1972.

Palade, G. Intracellular aspects of the process of protein secretions (Nobel prize lecture). *Science* 189:347, 1975.

Rappaport, A. M. The microcirculatory hepatic unit. *Microvasc. Res.* 6:212, 1973.

Rappaport, A. M. The microcirculatory acinar concept of normal and pathologic hepatic structure. *Beitr. Pathol.* 157:215, 1976.

Sarles, H. The exocrine pancreas. *Int. Rev. Physiol.* 12:173, 1977.

Sasse, D., and Schenk, A. A 3-dimensional presentation of the functional liver unit. *Acta Anat.* 93:78, 1975.

Schmid, R. Bilirubin metabolism: State of the art. *Gastroenterology* 74:1307, 1978.

Sherlock, S. *The Human Liver.* Burlington, N.C.: Carolina Biological Supply Co., 1978.

Tanikawa, K. *Ultrastructural Aspects of the Liver and Its Disorders.* New York: Igaku-Shoin, 1979.

Unger, R. H., et al. Insulin, glucagon and somatostatin secretion in the regulation of metabolism. *Annu. Rev. Physiol.* 40:307, 1978.

Wisse, E. An electron microscopic study of the fenestrated endothelial lining of rat liver sinusoids. *J. Ultrastruct. Res.* 31:125, 1970.

Wisse, E., and Knook, D. L. (eds.). *Kupffer Cells and Other Sinusoidal Cells.* Amsterdam: Elsevier North-Holland, 1977.

Wisse, E., and Knook, D. L. The investigation of sinusoidal cells: A new approach to the study of liver function. In Popper, H., and Schaffner, F. (eds.), *Progress in Liver Diseases.* Vol. 4. New York: Grune & Stratton, 1979.

URINARY SYSTEM

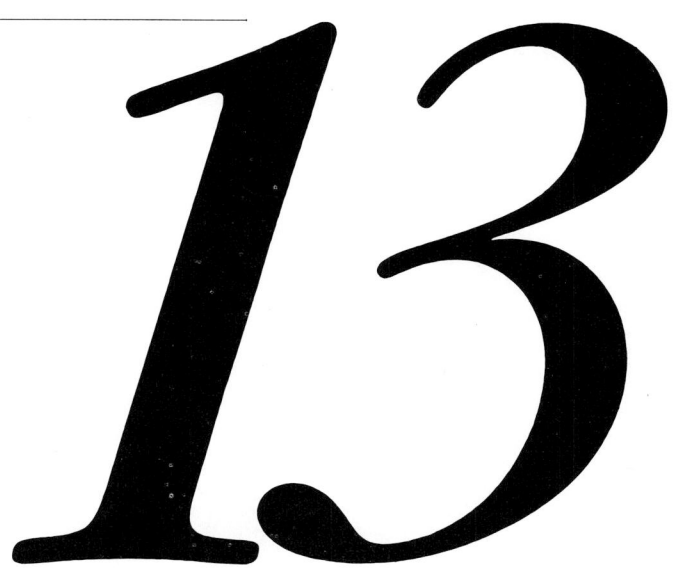

The urinary system consists of two kidneys, situated on the posterior abdominal wall; two ureters, which run down on the posterior abdominal wall and enter the pelvis; one urinary bladder, located within the pelvis; and one urethra, which traverses the perineum (Fig. 13-1). The function of the kidneys is to excrete most of the waste products of metabolism. They play a major role in controlling the water and electrolyte balance within the body and maintaining the acid-base balance of the blood. The kidneys are also endocrine glands, producing the hormones *erythropoietin,* concerned with blood formation, and *renin,* concerned with control of blood pressure.

The urethra in the male not only serves to conduct urine to the surface but is an excretory duct for the reproductive system, conveying the semen to the exterior.

KIDNEYS

The kidneys lie behind the peritoneum high on the posterior abdominal wall, largely under cover of the costal margin (see Fig. 13-1). The kidneys are surrounded by a *fibrous capsule* that is applied closely to its outer surface (Fig. 13-2). Outside the fibrous capsule is a covering of fat known as the *perinephric fat.* The *perinephric fascia* surrounds the perinephric fat and encloses the kidneys and suprarenal glands. The perinephric fascia is a condensation of areolar tissue.

On the medial border of the kidney is a vertical slit that is bounded by thick lips of renal substance and is called the *hilus* (see Fig. 13-2). Extending in from the hilus is a large cavity called the *renal sinus.* The hilus transmits the renal artery, the renal vein, the ureter, lymph vessels, and sympathetic nerve fibers.

Within the renal sinus, the upper expanded end of the ureter, called the *pelvis of the ureter,* divides into two or three *major calyces,* each of which divides into two or three *minor calyces* (see Fig. 13-2).

A coronal section through the kidneys shows it to be composed of a dark, reddish-brown outer *cortex* and a lighter-colored inner *medulla* (see Fig. 13-2). The medulla is composed of about a dozen *renal pyramids,* each with its base oriented toward the cortex and its apex, the *renal papilla,* projecting into a minor calyx. The cortex extends into the medulla between adjacent pyramids as the *renal columns* (see Fig. 13-2). Extending from the bases of the renal

13. URINARY SYSTEM

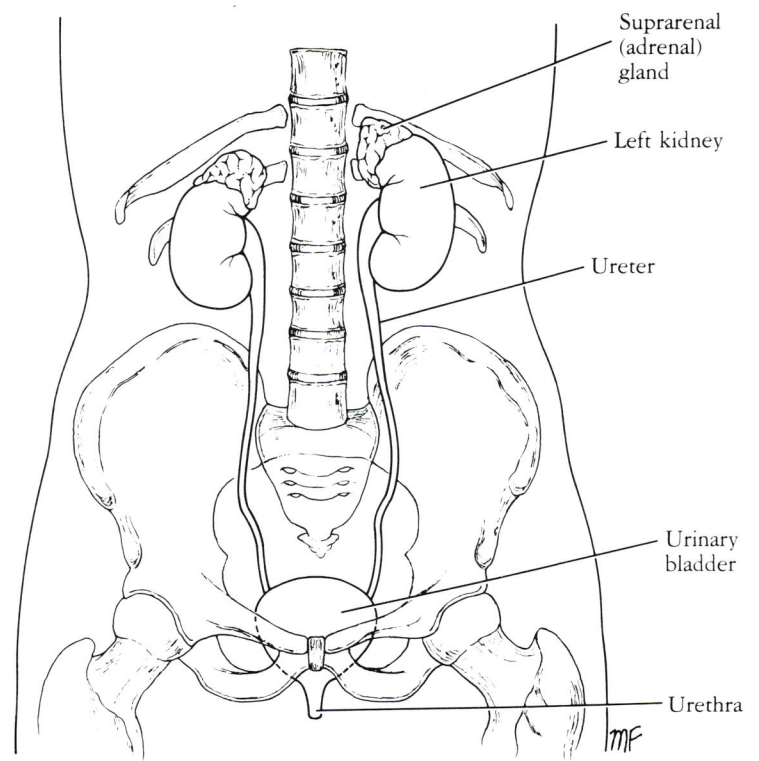

Fig. 13-1. *The parts of the urinary system.*

pyramids into the cortex are striations known as *medullary rays*.

A *renal lobe* may be defined as a renal pyramid together with the cortical tissue overlying its base and lying along its sides. It is not delineated by connective tissue. A *renal lobule* is a medullary ray and its neighboring cortical tissue. Here again, the lobules are not separated from one another by connective tissue septa.

The connective tissue of the kidney is inconspicuous and is almost absent in the cortex. It consists of fine collagen fibers and branched cells and is most obvious in the renal papillae.

Uriniferous Tubules

The kidney is composed of large numbers of microscopic units called *uriniferous tubules*. Each tubule is composed of two functional regions, the *nephron*, which produces an excretion known as urine, and the *collecting tubule*, which concentrates the urine and conveys it to the calyces (Fig. 13-3).

Nephron

There are over a million nephrons in one kidney. Each consists of four distinct parts: (1) the renal corpuscle, which contains the glomerulus, (2) the proximal convoluted tubule, (3) the loop of Henle, and (4) the distal convoluted tubule (see Fig. 13-3). The parts of the nephron form a continuous tubule that measures about 50 mm in length and runs from the cortex to the medulla and then returns to the cortex.

RENAL CORPUSCLE. The *renal corpuscle* is situated in the cortex. It is formed by the upper end of the uriniferous tubule, which is expanded into a structure called a *Bowman's capsule* (Figs. 13-4–13-7; see

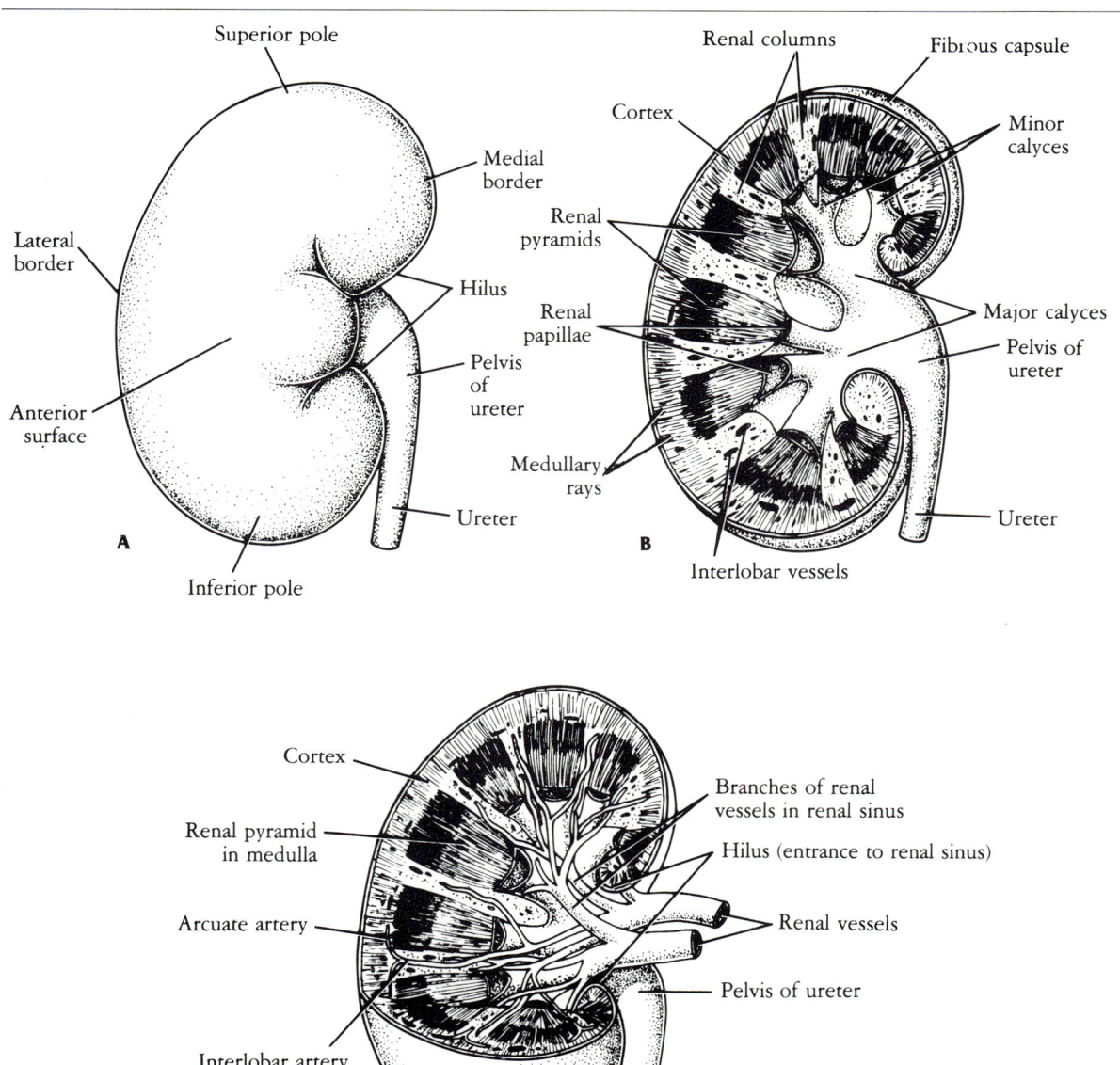

Fig. 13-2. Right kidney: (A) anterior view; (B) coronal section, showing the cortex, medulla, pyramids, renal papillae, and calyces; (C) combined coronal and transverse sections, showing renal vessels and the pelvis of the ureter.

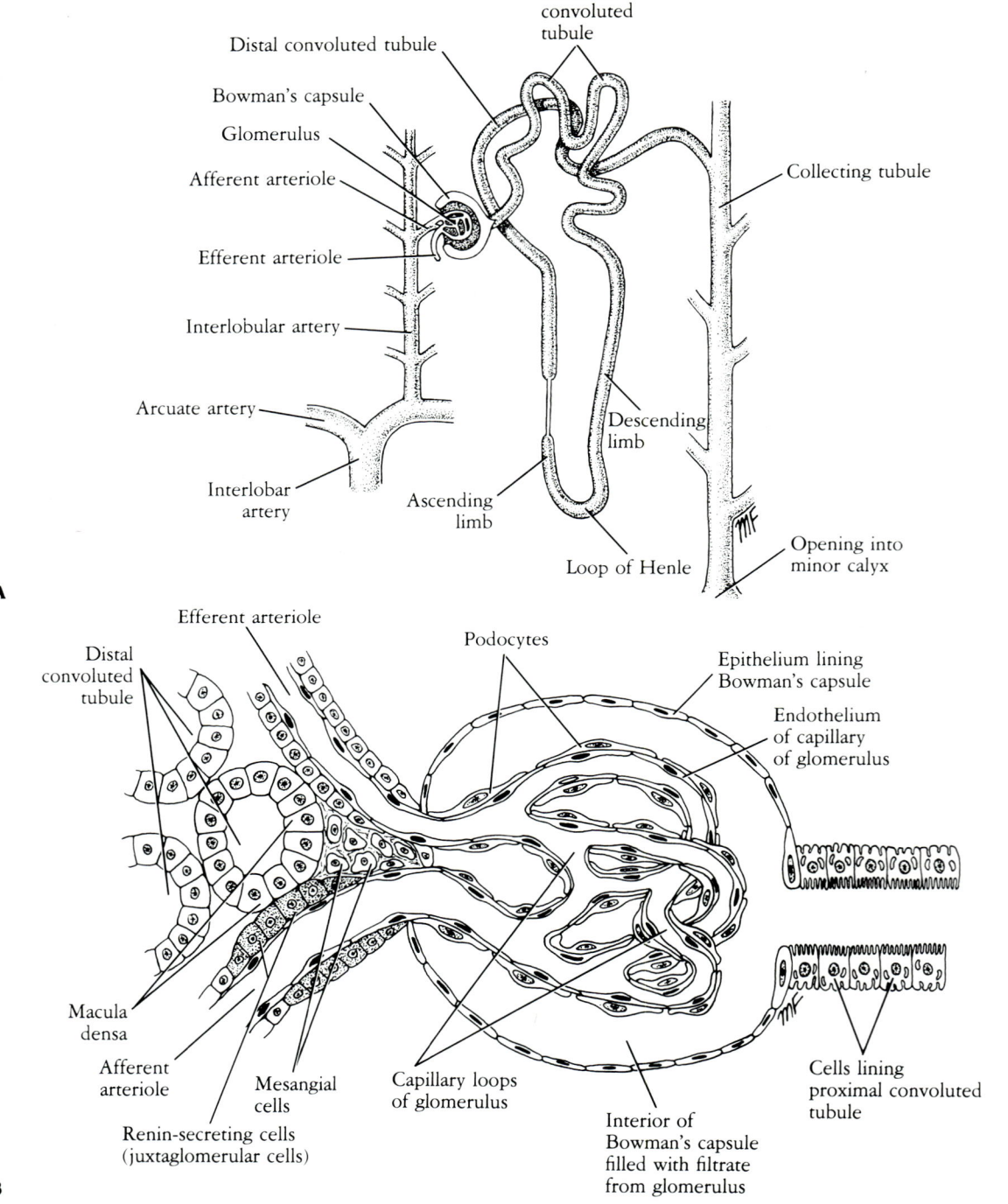

Fig. 13-3. A: The parts of a nephron and a collecting tubule. B: Detailed structure of a renal corpuscle.

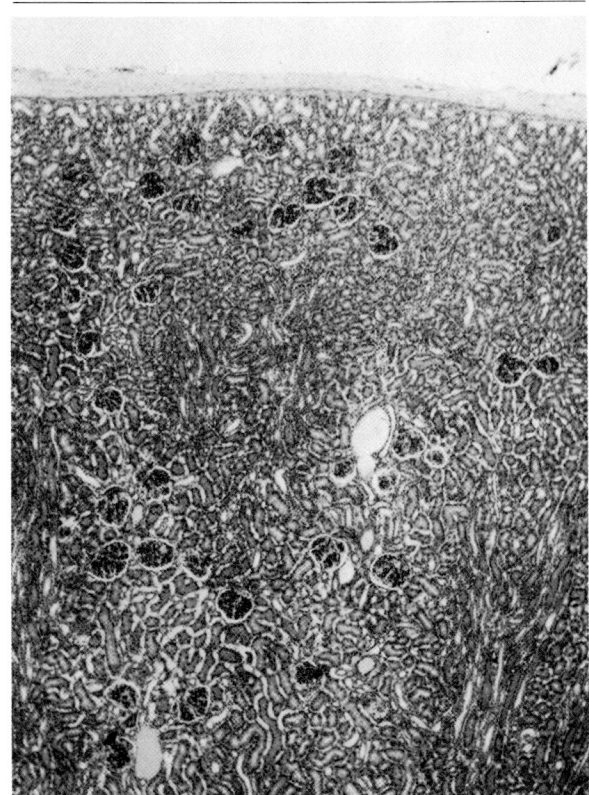

Fig. 13-4. Right: Photomicrograph of the cortex of the kidney; the fibrous capsule is seen in the upper part of the photograph. Note the numerous renal corpuscles and their associated tubules. (H&E; ×40.)

Fig. 13-5. Below: Scanning electron micrograph of the cortex of the kidney, showing numerous renal corpuscles (arrows), tubules, and blood vessels. (×50.) (Courtesy of F. G. Lightfoot.)

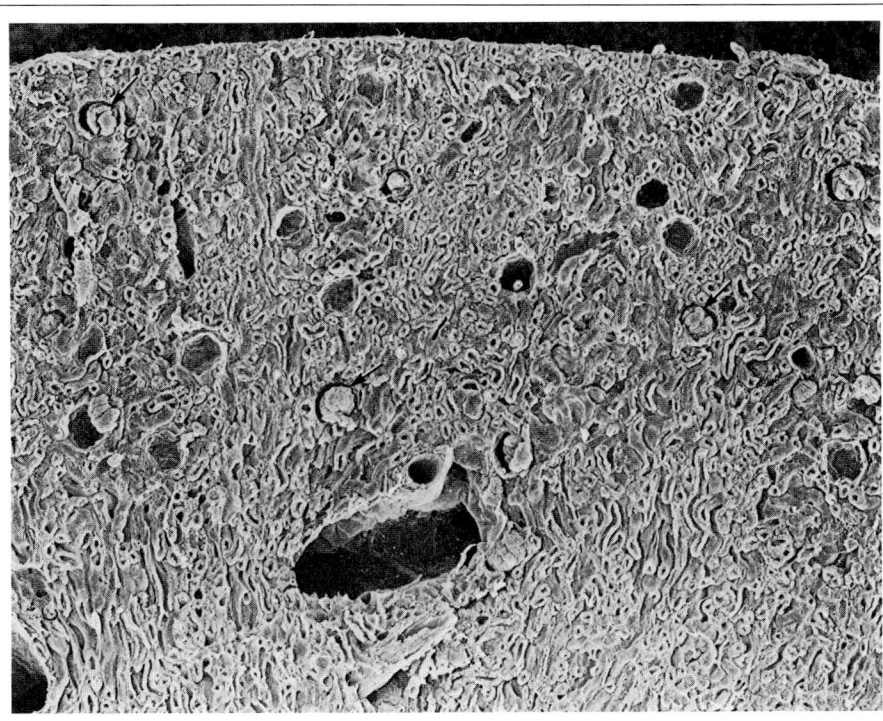

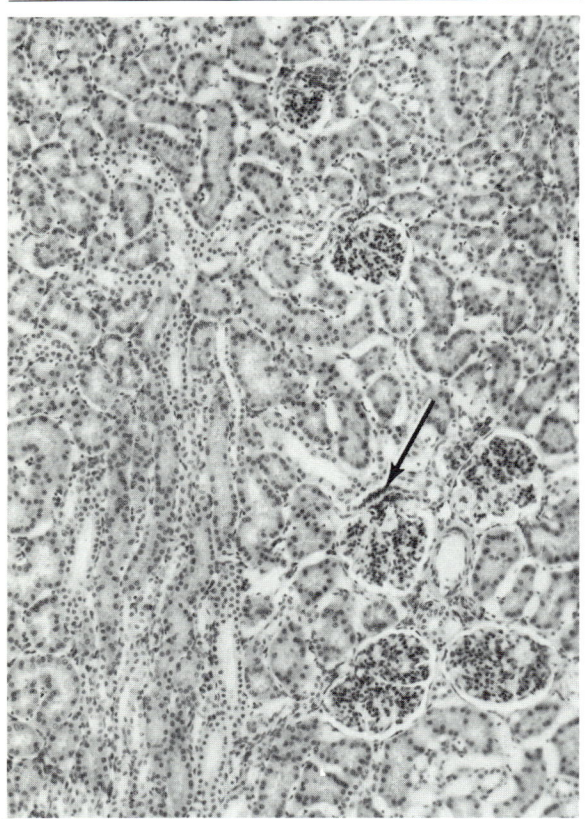

Fig. 13-6. *Photomicrograph of the cortex of the kidney, showing several glomeruli and proximal and distal convoluted tubules. Note a macula densa (arrow). (H&E; ×100.)*

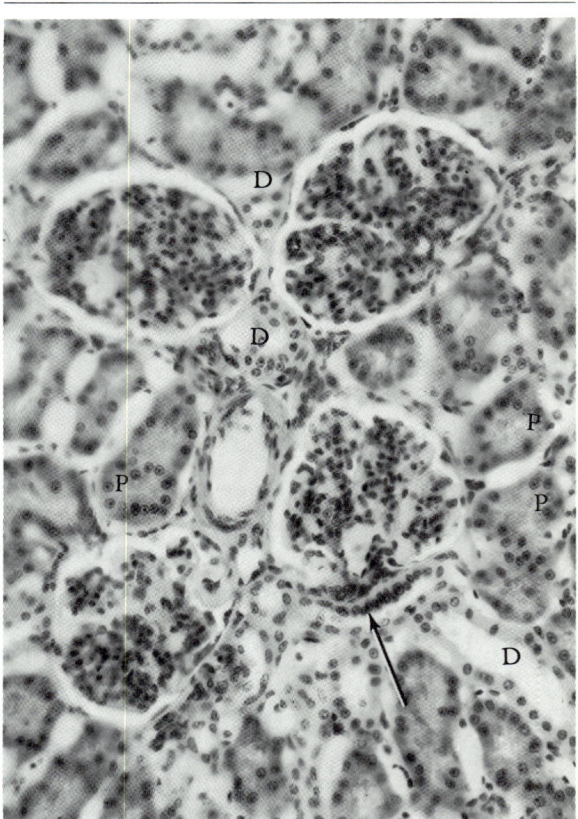

Fig. 13-7. *Photomicrograph of the cortex of the kidney, showing four renal corpuscles with their glomeruli and Bowman's capsules. Note the proximal convoluted tubules (P), the distal convoluted tubules (D), and the macula densa (arrow). (H&E; ×200.)*

Fig. 13-3). The renal corpuscle contains the glomerulus, which is a network of capillaries into which blood enters by an *afferent arteriole* and leaves through a smaller *efferent arteriole*.

The glomerulus indents the wall of the Bowman's capsule as a fist might press into the side of a balloon (Fig. 13-8). The epithelial cells that form the wall of the Bowman's capsule also serve as a covering for the glomerulus. The renal corpuscle thus consists of the Bowman's capsule and the glomerulus (see Figs. 13-4–13-7).

The outer wall of the Bowman's capsule is lined with simple squamous epithelium that abruptly changes into cuboidal epithelium at the start of the proximal convoluted tubule. Where the capsular wall is reflected onto the glomerulus, the squamous cells change into star-shaped cells with multiple processes. These cells, called *podocytes,* have large *primary processes* that tightly clasp the glomerular capillaries (Figs. 13-9 and 13-10). From the primary processes, smaller *secondary processes* arise that interdigitate with the secondary processes of other podocytes. This arrangement leaves small slitlike gaps between the processes that measure about 25 nm

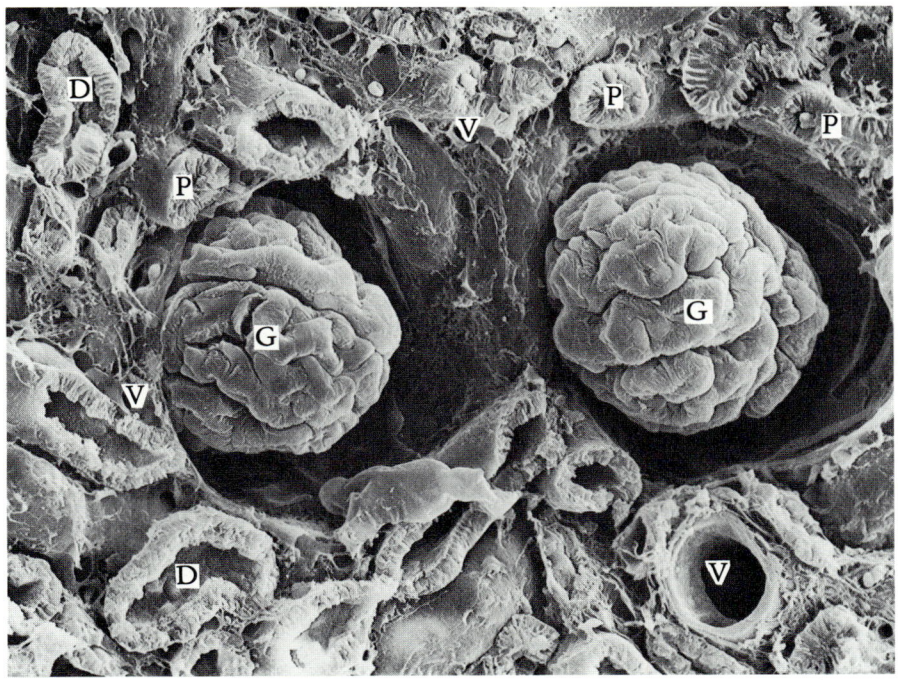

Fig. 13-8. Scanning electron micrograph of the cortex of the kidney, showing two renal corpuscles, each containing a glomerulus (G). Proximal (P) and distal (D) convoluted tubules also can be seen. Note the large and small blood vessels (V). (×400.) (Courtesy of F. G. Lightfoot.)

across and are called *slit pores* (Fig. 13-11). The secondary processes end in *feet* that are applied firmly to the basement membrane of the capillary wall of the glomerulus. Extending across the slip pores between adjacent feet is a thin *slit diaphragm* about 6 nm thick (Fig. 13-12).

The blood in the glomerular capillaries is separated from the cavity of the Bowman's capsule by: (1) the fenestrated endothelial cells lining the capillaries (Fig. 13-13), (2) a thick basement membrane (Fig. 13-14), and (3) the slit pores of the podocytes. Together these structures are known as the *filtration barrier* (see Fig. 13-11). The holes, or fenestrae, in the endothelial cells permit the passage of plasma but hold back the cells of the blood. The smaller molecules of the plasma readily pass through the basement membrane and the slit diaphragm of the podocytes to enter the cavity of the Bowman's capsule. Particles with a molecular weight greater than 160,000 are held back by the slit diaphragm. The plasma protein albumin, which has a molecular weight of 69,000, would be expected to pass through without difficulty. We know, however, that in a normal individual, it does not. The probable explanation is that the filtration mechanism is blocked by proteins with larger molecules and that the electric charge on the filter repels the albumin molecules. The fluid that finally crosses the filtration barrier and enters the capsular space is called the *glomerular filtrate*.

Lying between the glomerular capillaries are small groups of star-shaped cells that are contractile and capable of phagocytosis. These cells are called *mesangial cells* (see Fig. 13-3) and support the capillary walls by producing intercellular substance. They are also thought to remove by phagocytosis any mac-

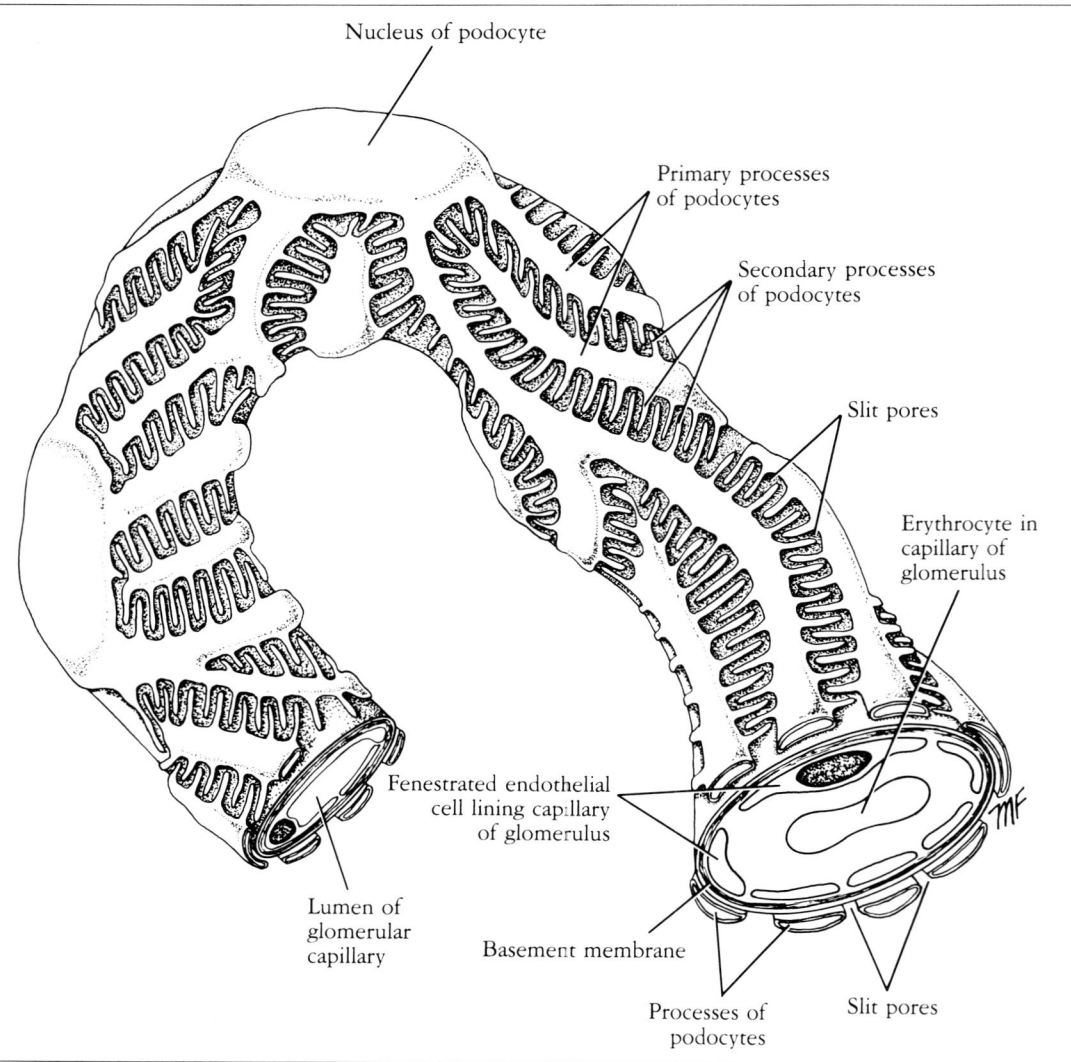

Fig. 13-9. Relationship between a podocyte and a glomerular capillary.

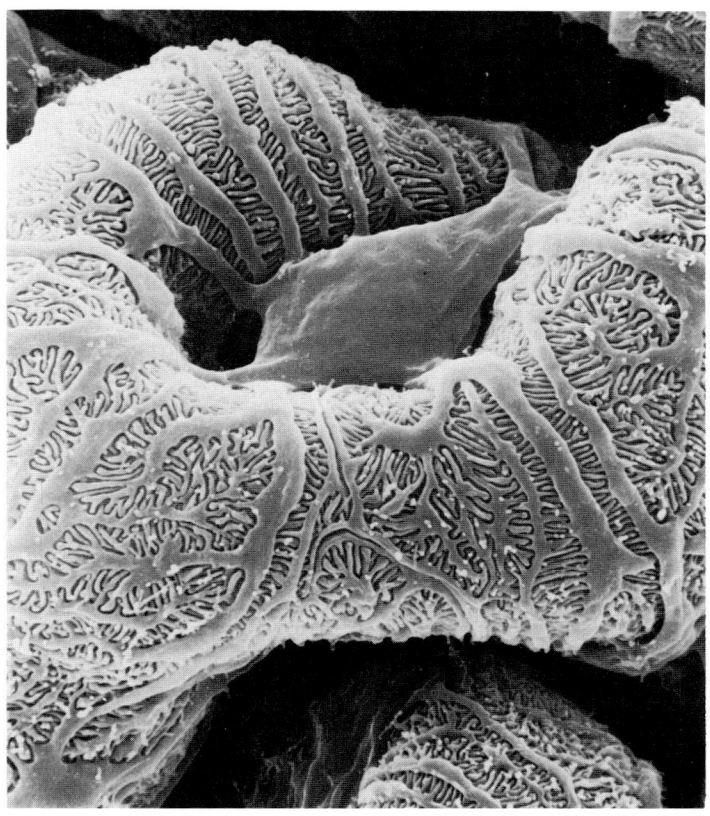

Fig. 13-10. Electron micrograph of a podocyte with large primary processes that tightly clasp a glomerular capillary. Note the smaller secondary processes that interdigitate and the slit-like gaps between them that form the slit pores. (×2,250.) (Courtesy of Dr. P. Andrews.)

romolecules that escape from the capillaries into the tissue space.

Function of the Renal Corpuscle. The rate of blood flow through both kidneys is about 1,200 ml per minute, or about 25 percent of the cardiac output. The blood enters the glomeruli under high pressure, and fluid is driven through the filter into the Bowman's capsule (see Fig. 13-3). The fenestrated capillaries of the glomeruli form the coarse filter; the basement membrane, the slit diaphragm, and the slit pores of the podocytes form the ultrafilter. The glomerular filtrate differs from the plasma in that it has almost no proteins. In 24 hours, both kidneys produce about 180 L of glomerular filtrate; about 99 percent of the filtrate is reabsorbed by the renal tubules, and only 1 percent will be excreted as urine (Fig. 13-15).

PROXIMAL CONVOLUTED TUBULE. The proximal convoluted tubule is about 14 mm long. It begins at the Bowman's capsule and follows a tortuous course in the region of the renal corpuscle (see Fig. 13-3). It ends by becoming continuous with the loop of Henle in the nearest medullary ray. In histological sections, the tubules are seen in oblique and cross sections and are the most numerous tubules in the kidney cortex. The tubule is lined with cuboidal epithelium whose free surface is covered with a

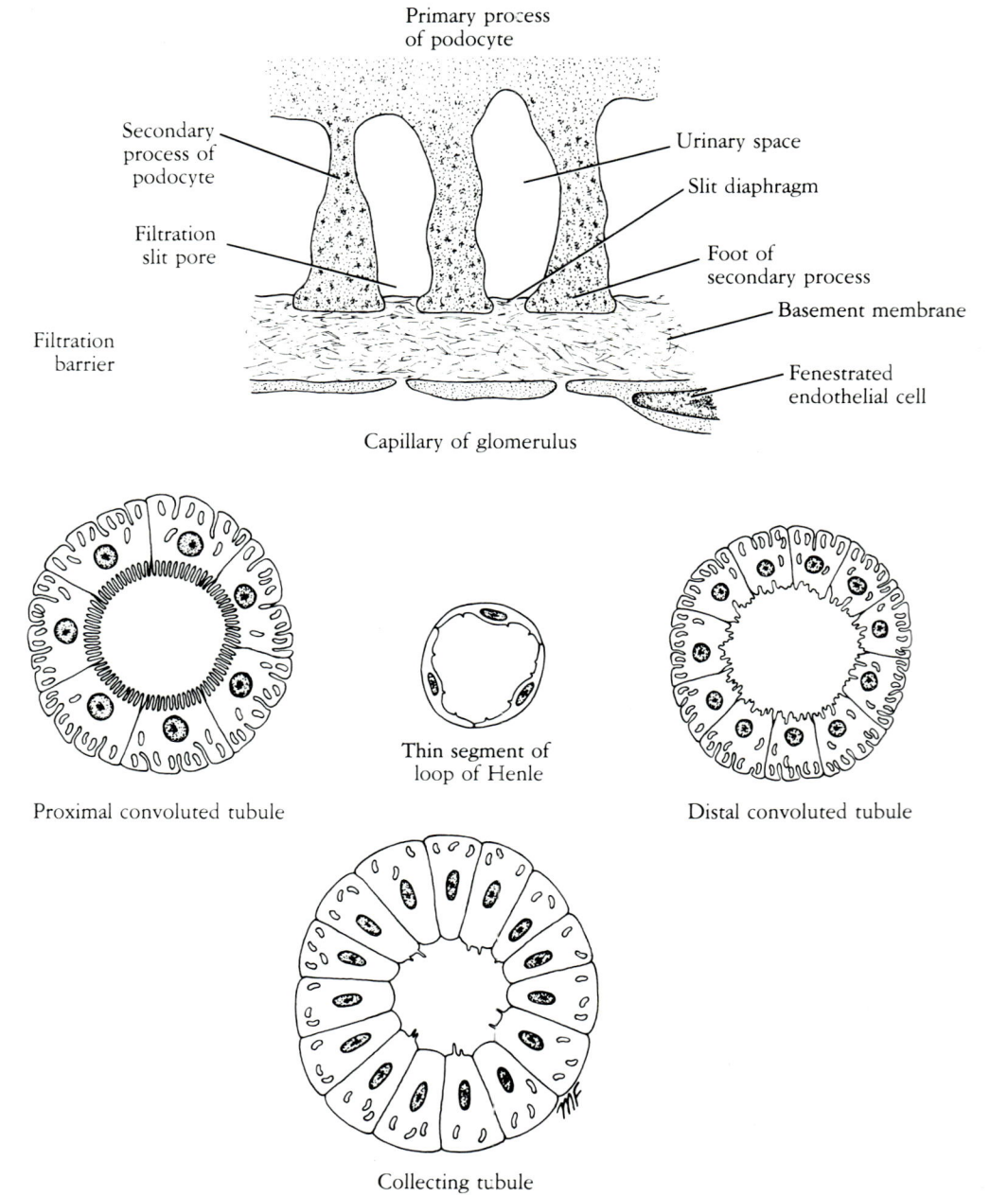

Fig. 13-11. *Structure of the filtration barrier between the urinary space in the Bowman's capsule and the lumen of the glomerular capillary; the proximal convoluted tubule; the thin segment of the loop of Henle; the distal convoluted tubule and the collecting tubule.*

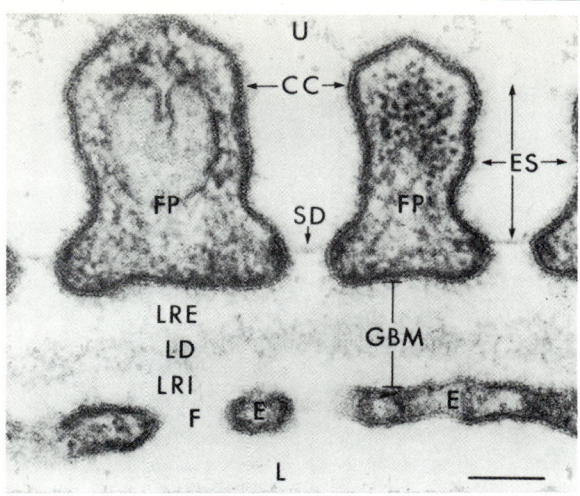

Fig. 13-12. Electron micrograph showing the foot processes (FP) of a podocyte. (U = urinary space; CC = cell coat covering the foot processes; ES = slit pores between the foot processes; SD = slit diaphragm; GBM = glomerular basement membrane; E = endothelial cell; F = fenestrae of endothelial cell.) (×82,080.) (Courtesy of Dr. M. J. Karnovsky.)

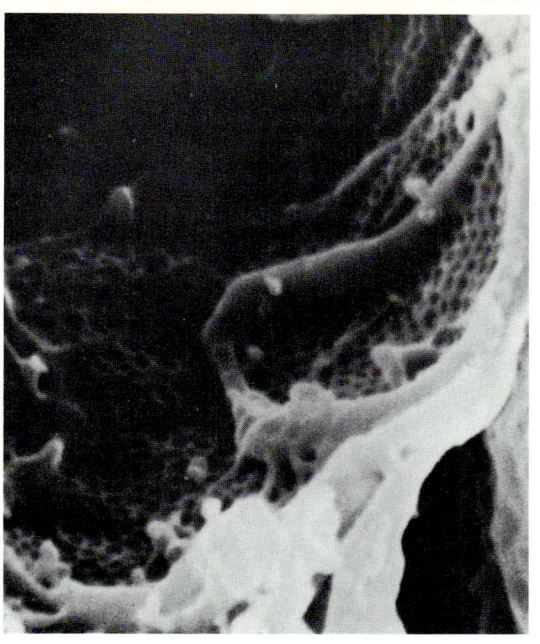

Fig. 13-13. Scanning electron micrograph of a glomerular capillary, showing the fenestrae on the luminal surface of the endothelial cells. (×20,000.) (Courtesy of F. G. Lightfoot.)

Fig. 13-14. Scanning electron micrograph of a renal corpuscle, showing the acellular connective tissue matrix of the glomerulus and Bowman's capsule; all epithelial cells have been dissolved before preparation of the specimen. (Courtesy of Dr. E. C. Carlson.)

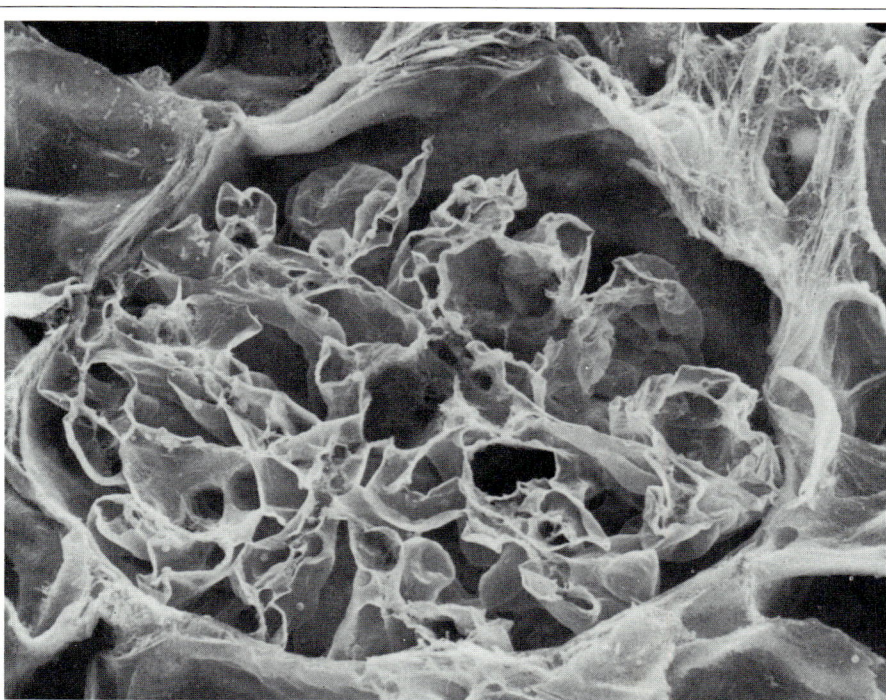

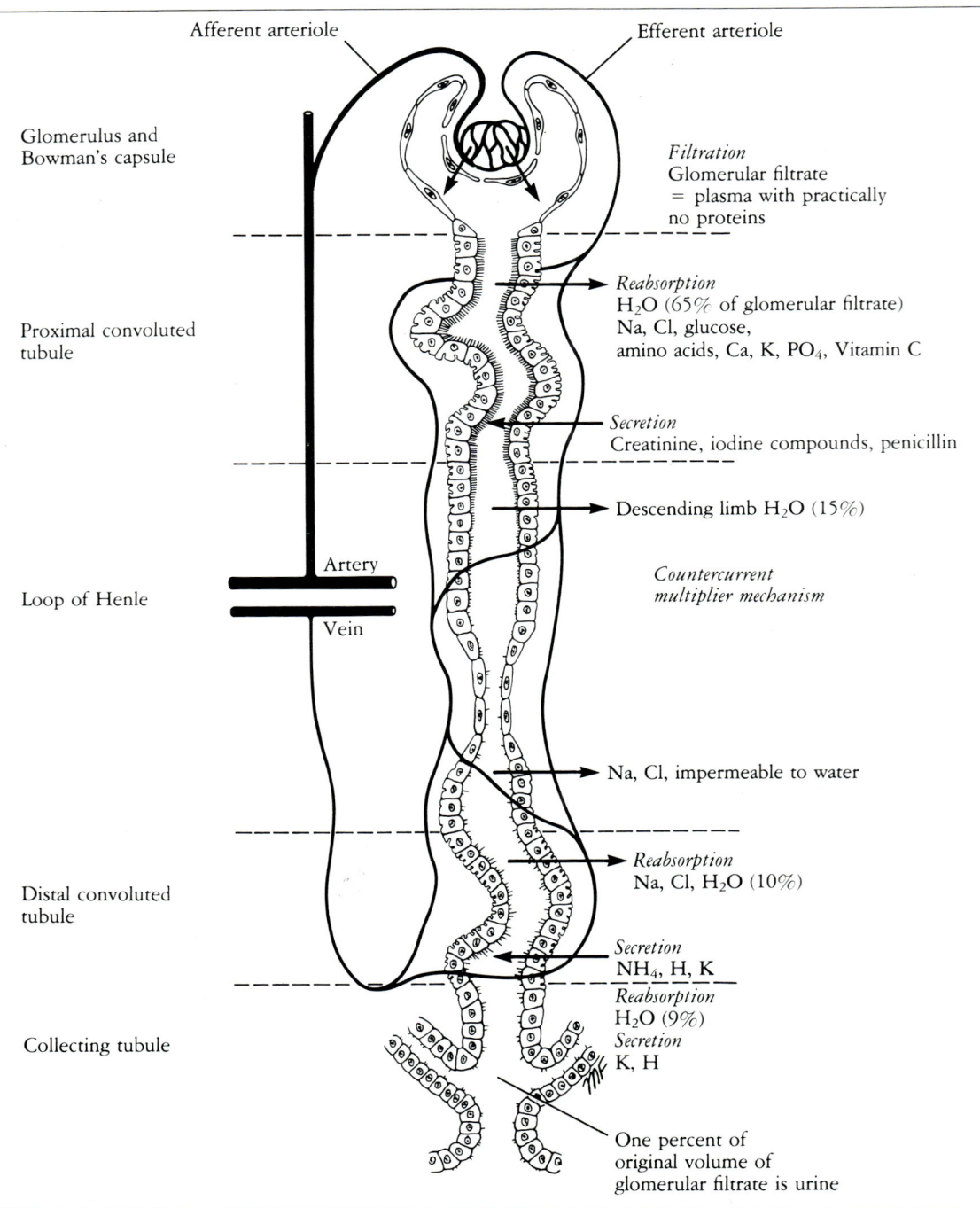

Fig. 13-15. *The basic mechanisms of filtration, reabsorption, and secretion taking place at different sites along the uriniferous tubule. Only 1 percent of the original volume of the glomerular filtrate leaves the tubule as urine.*

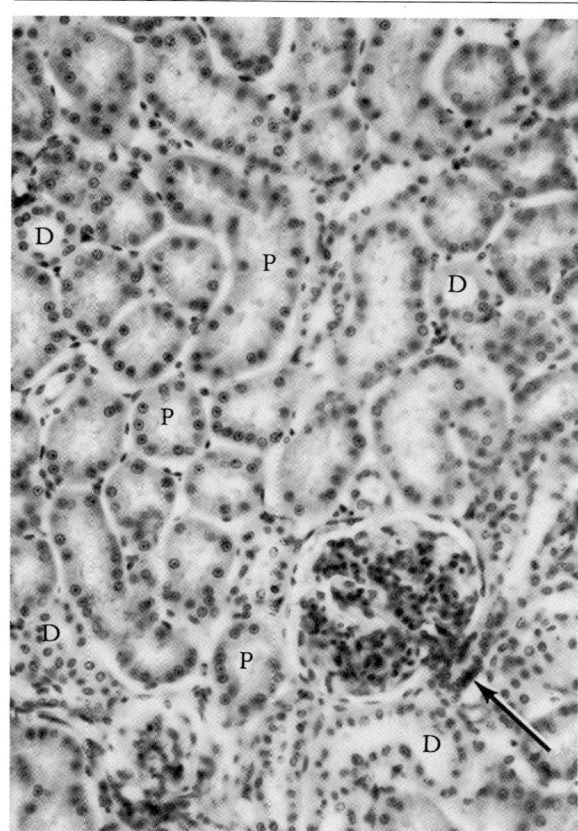

Fig. 13-16. Photomicrograph of a renal corpuscle surrounded by numerous proximal convoluted tubules (P) cut in section; several distal convoluted tubules also are shown (D). The arrow indicates the macula densa. (H&E; ×200.)

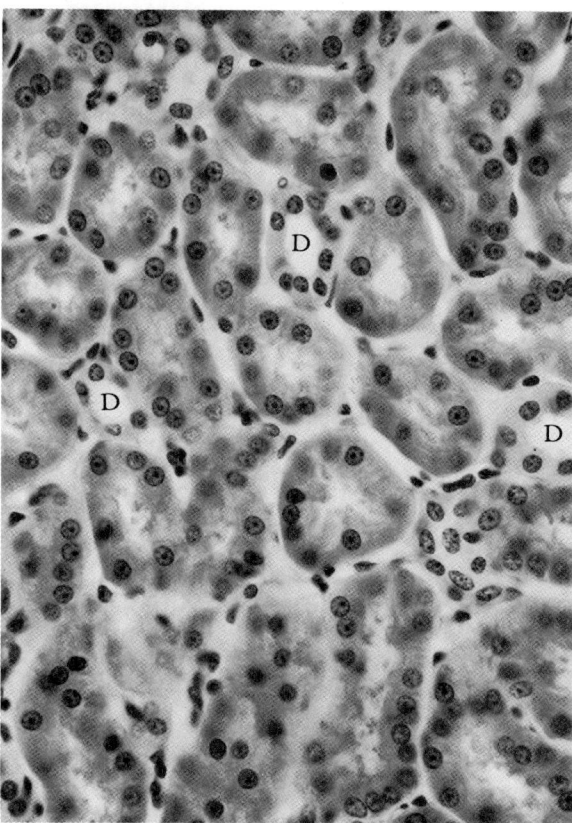

Fig. 13-17. Photomicrograph showing many proximal convoluted tubules cut in oblique and cross sections. Note that each tubule is lined with cuboidal epithelium and the cytoplasm stains strongly with eosin because of the many mitochondria (not shown). The nuclei are centrally placed, and the luminal cell surfaces have indistinct brush borders formed of microvilli. Three distal convoluted tubules are also present (D). Note that the cytoplasm of the cuboidal cells lining the distal convoluted tubules stains lighter with eosin. (H&E; ×400.)

brush border of microvilli (Fig. 13-16; see Fig. 13-11). The nucleus of each cell is centrally placed, and the cytoplasm stains intensely pink with eosin (Fig. 13-17).

Electron micrographs show a Golgi apparatus on the apical side of the nucleus and numerous rodlike mitochondria in the basal cytoplasm. The plasma membrane, especially on the base of the cell, shows much infolding and interdigitating with neighboring cells (see Fig. 13-11). The microvilli are long and densely packed at the apex of the cell, and there are small clefts between the bases of the microvilli that extend into the apical cytoplasm. Numerous vesicles

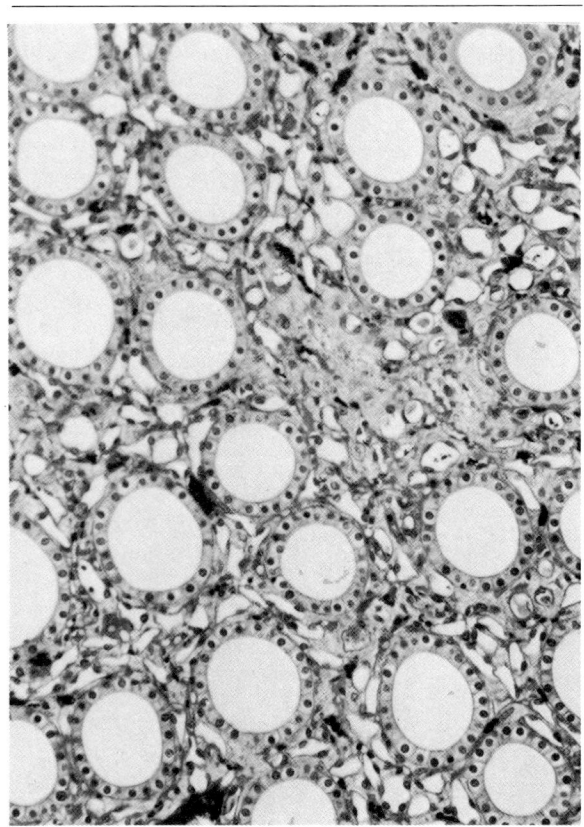

Fig. 13-18. Photomicrograph of the medulla of the kidney, showing numerous collecting tubules and thin segments of the loops of Henle in cross section. The collecting tubules are lined with cuboidal epithelial cells, and the thin segments of the loops of Henle are lined with flattened cells. (H&E; ×200.)

also are visible close to these clefts. It is thought that the clefts and vesicles are involved in the absorption of water and protein from the lumen of the tubule. Adjacent cells are attached to one another by tight junctions.

Functions of the Proximal Convoluted Tubule. The functions of the proximal convoluted tubule are reabsorption and secretion (see Fig. 13-15).

Reabsorption. About 65 percent of the glomerular filtrate is reabsorbed by the proximal convoluted tubule. The lining cells drive sodium ions out into the intercellular spaces at the sides and base of the cell by the sodium pump mechanism, reducing the sodium concentration within the cell and causing sodium ions to diffuse from the lumen of the tubule into the cell through the microvilli. The energy for the sodium pump is provided by the numerous mitochondria. Chloride ions and water are drawn osmotically out of the cell to join the sodium ions. The water and sodium chloride then diffuse into the surrounding cortical capillaries.

Active transport mechanisms bring about the reabsorption of glucose. Small protein molecules that have escaped from the blood in the glomerular filtrate are reabsorbed by pinocytosis. The protein-containing vesicles then fuse with lysosomes, and the enzymes break down the proteins into amino acids. Other substances, such as amino acids, calcium, potassium, phosphate, and vitamin C, are also reabsorbed.

Secretion. The cells of the proximal convoluted tubule secrete creatinine and certain dyes, such as the organic iodine-containing compound Diodrast (iodopyracet). They also secrete drugs such as penicillin. Although the total volume of the glomerular filtrate has been reduced by about 65 percent as it passes through the proximal convoluted tubule, it is still approximately isotonic with the blood plasma, because both water and solutes are passed from the tubular lumen into the tissue fluid.

LOOP OF HENLE. The tortuous proximal convoluted tubule straightens and becomes continuous with the loop of Henle. The loop of Henle in turn becomes continuous with the straight part of the distal convoluted tubule. Most authorities consider the loop of Henle to include the following parts of the uriniferous tubule: (1) the straight terminal part of the proximal convoluted tubule; (2) a long, thin segment; and (3) the straight commencing part of the distal convoluted tubule (see Fig. 13-3).

The loop of Henle has a descending and an ascending limb, and the two parts lie close together in a medullary ray. Those renal corpuscles situated at the periphery of the cortex just beneath the capsule have short loops that extend only into the outer part

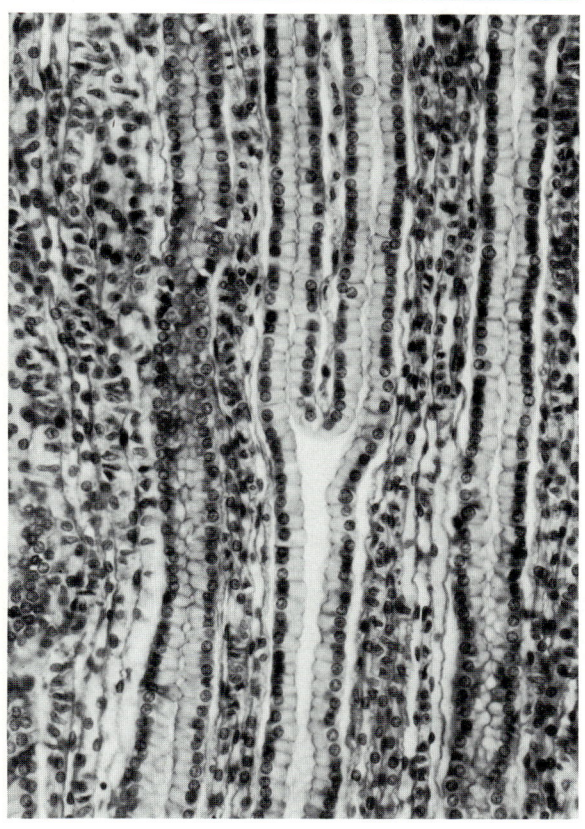

Fig. 13-19. Photomicrograph of the medulla of the kidney close to the papilla, showing two collecting tubules joining together to form a straight papillary duct. Note that the ducts are lined with tall columnar epithelial cells with dark-staining nuclei and pale cytoplasm. (H&E; ×200.)

of the medulla, whereas those corpuscles that lie close to the medulla, the *juxtamedullary glomeruli*, have long loops that extend toward the apex of the pyramids.

The thin segment of the descending and ascending limbs of the loop of Henle have a narrow lumen and squamous lining cells (Figs. 13-18 and 13-19; see Fig. 13-11). Cross sections of the tubules show a resemblance to a cross section of a capillary (see Fig. 13-18). The absence of red cells within the lumen makes identification easy, however. Electron micrographs of the lining cells show a few microvilli on their luminal surface and much folding of the plasma membranes, with interdigitation of neighboring cells.

Functions of the Loop of Henle. The loops of Henle, especially those of the juxtamedullary glomeruli, which extend deeply into the medulla, play a major role in concentrating the urine passing through the collecting tubules via the *countercurrent multiplier mechanism* (Fig. 13-20).

A countercurrent multiplier mechanism depends on the flow of fluid through a long U tube in which the two limbs of the U lie side by side and close to each other. The walls of the limbs of the U tube must be permeable so that fluid and solutes can pass between the two limbs.

In the loop of Henle, the walls of the greater part of the descending limb are lined with squamous cells that are freely permeable to sodium and water. The walls of the thicker part of the ascending limb are *impermeable to water;* chloride ions are transported actively from the tubule, and sodium ions follow. Thus, the osmotic pressure of the tissue fluid is increased greatly. Because the descending and the ascending limbs are close together, water continuously is drawn passively out of the descending limb, and the fluid within the descending limb becomes increasingly concentrated as it passes down to the hairpin turn of the loop. As the tubular fluid ascends the ascending limb, the lining cells of the thicker part remove more sodium chloride by active transport, so that the tubular fluid, which was hypertonic, becomes isotonic once again. It is at this point that the tubular fluid enters the convoluted part of the distal convoluted tubule in the renal cortex.

The whole purpose of this mechanism is to create in the tissue fluid of the medullary pyramids a continuous gradient of tonicity that starts by being isotonic at the border of the cortex with the medulla and becomes very hypertonic at the apices of the medullary pyramids. It is the hypertonicity of the medullary tissue fluid that draws the water out of the fluid within the collecting tubules, forming a concentrated urine. The countercurrent multiplier is assisted by the countercurrent exchange mechanism operating in the vasa recta of the tubular blood

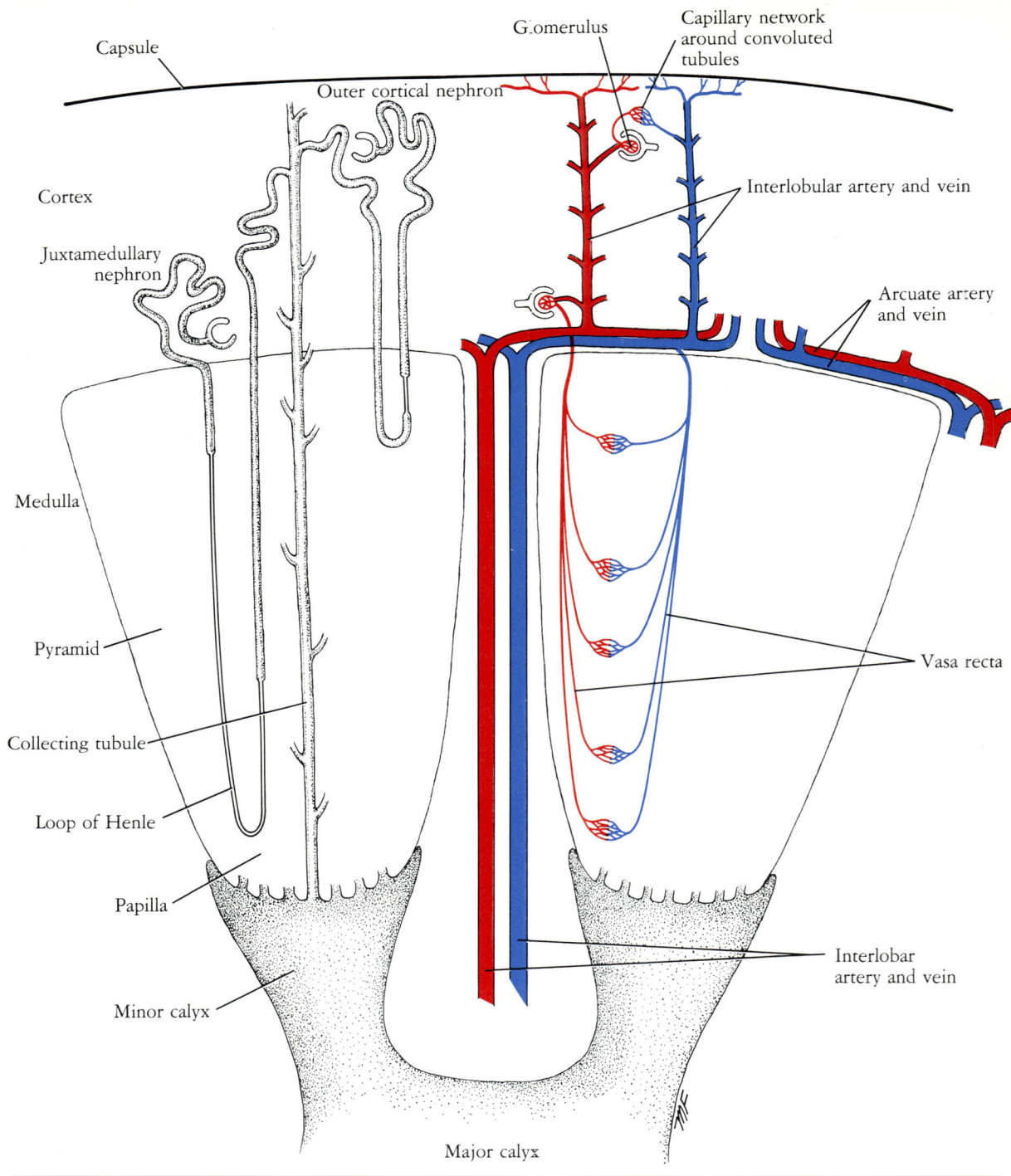

Fig. 13-20. Outer cortical and juxtamedullary nephrons with their associated blood vessels. Note the collecting tubules and ducts, and observe that they open onto the apex of the papilla into the cavity of the minor calyx.

vessels (see p. 524), which helps maintain the high osmotic pressure within the medulla.

DISTAL CONVOLUTED TUBULE. The distal convoluted tubule consists of three parts: (1) the straight segment (ascending thick segment of loop of Henle), (2) the macula densa, and (3) the convoluted portion.

The straight segment and the convoluted portion have similar structures. The lining cells are cuboidal (see Figs. 13-11 and 13-17) and possess only a few short microvilli on their free surface. The transverse diameter of the lumen is greater than that of the proximal convoluted tubule. Electron micrographs show an absence of apical clefts between the microvilli, but the plasma membranes on the sides and base of the cell show considerable infolding. Mitochondria are present in the basal cytoplasm, giving a striated appearance to this part of the cell. The cytoplasm of the cells of the distal convoluted tubule stains lighter with eosin than that of the cells of the proximal convoluted tubule, perhaps because of the smaller numbers of mitochondria in the cells of the distal tubule.

Macula Densa. The initial straight segment of the distal convoluted tubule ascends to the region of the renal corpuscle from which the tubule originated. Here, it lies close to the glomerulus between the afferent and efferent arterioles. The lining cells in this region of the tubule are packed together and are columnar. This area of the tubule is referred to as the macula densa (see Figs. 13-3 and 13-16).

Functions of the Distal Convoluted Tubule. The function of the straight segment of the distal convoluted tubule (ascending thick part of the loop of Henle) has already been considered in our discussion of the loop of Henle. It will be remembered that its walls are impermeable to water and that chloride ions are actively pumped out and sodium ions passively follow. This process effectively increases the osmotic pressure of the tissue fluid and reduces the osmotic pressure of the fluid within the tubule.

The function of the macula densa is considered with the juxtaglomerular apparatus on page 523.

The functions of the convoluted part of the distal convoluted tubule are reabsorption and secretion (see Fig. 13-15).

Reabsorption. The active transport of sodium and the passive transport of chloride out of the tubular fluid take place here. This activity is controlled by *aldosterone* secreted by the suprarenal cortex. The permeability of this part of the tubule to water is believed to be controlled by the antidiuretic hormone (ADH) secreted by the posterior lobe of the pituitary.

Secretion. Hydrogen ions and ammonium ions are secreted to assist in the process of regulating the hydrogen ion concentration of the blood. Potassium ions are also secreted.

Collecting Tubule

The collecting tubule is the most distal part of the uriniferous tubule and is not part of the nephron. Each distal convoluted tubule of a nephron becomes continuous with a collecting tubule that runs a short, arched course and enters a medullary ray. Here, a number of the short collecting tubules join a main collecting tubule as side tributaries. The main collecting tubule then passes down in the medullary ray to enter the medullary pyramid. When the collecting tubules reach the inner zone of the pyramid, groups of them join at acute angles to form *straight papillary ducts* that open on the apex of the renal papilla into a minor calyx.

The cells lining the collecting tubules are at first cuboidal (Fig. 13-21; see Fig. 13-18); later, in the straight papillary ducts, they are tall columnar (see Fig. 13-19). The cell borders are regular, with few interdigitations. The nuclei are dark staining, but the cytoplasm is pale staining because there are relatively few cytoplasmic organelles. On the apex of the renal papilla, the columnar epithelium changes to the transitional epithelium lining the minor calyx (Fig. 13-22).

FUNCTIONS OF THE COLLECTING TUBULE. The collecting tubules concentrate the urine and conduct it to the calyces and the ureter. Their primary func-

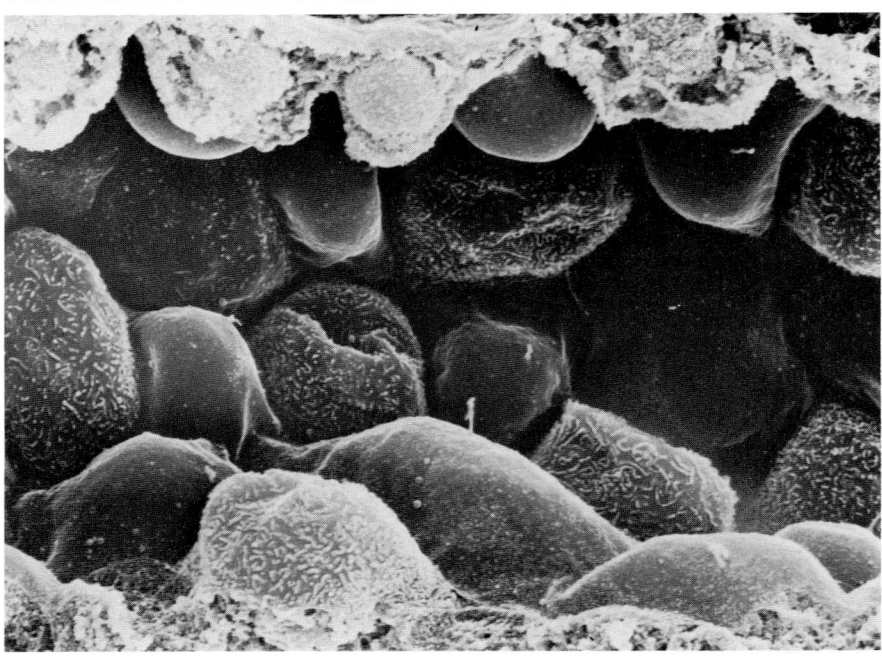

Fig. 13-21. Scanning electron micrograph of the luminal surface of a collecting tubule, showing the surfaces of the lining cuboidal cells and their microvilli. (×2,700.) (Courtesy of F. G. Lightfoot.)

tions are reabsorption and secretion (see Fig. 13-15).

Reabsorption of Water. The wall of the collecting tubule is permeable to water. The permeability is controlled, however, by ADH of the posterior lobe of the pituitary. If we remember that the countercurrent multiplier mechanism of the loop of Henle causes the tissue fluid around the collecting tubules to be hypertonic, we can understand how water diffuses from the collecting tubules into the tissue fluid under the influence of ADH, and from there is removed by the blood capillaries. The degree of concentration of the urine in the collecting tubules can never exceed the hypertonicity of the tissue fluid around the tubules. Because the permeability of the walls of the tubules is controlled by ADH, this hormone controls the degree of concentration of the urine.

The secretion of ADH is controlled by the osmotic pressure in the blood circulating through the supraoptic nuclei of the hypothalamus. Should the osmotic pressure of the blood become too high, the hormone is released by the pituitary and acts on the collecting tubules to increase reabsorption of water. Should the osmotic pressure of the circulating blood fall, the release of ADH into the blood would be diminished, and increased amounts of water would be lost from the body in the form of dilute urine.

Secretion. Potassium ions and hydrogen ions are secreted actively by the cells of the collecting tubules (see Fig. 13-15).

CONCENTRATING THE URINE. To delineate the processes involved in concentrating urine, we will follow a drop of glomerular filtrate as it leaves the Bowman's capsule to enter the proximal convoluted tubule in the renal cortex. Here, sodium and other cations are pumped out into the tissue fluid by active transport of the lining cells. The chloride ions follow the sodium passively. Water is now reabsorbed from

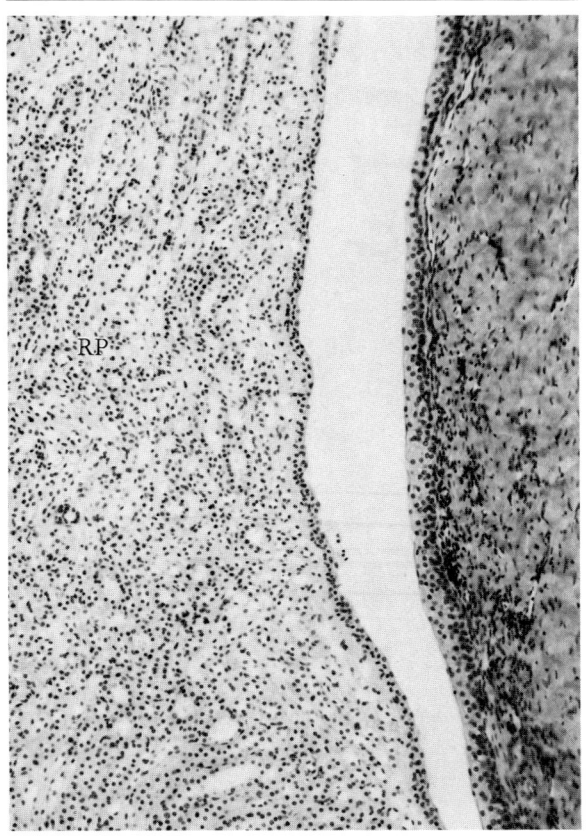

Fig. 13-22. Photomicrograph of the renal papilla (RP) near its apex as it projects into the cavity of a minor calyx; the wall of the calyx is shown on the right of the photograph. The epithelial cells covering the outer surface of the papilla and lining the calyx are of the transitional type. (H&E; ×100.)

the tubular lumen to maintain the osmotic balance; 65 percent or more of the water in the glomerular filtrate is reabsorbed by this mechanism in the proximal convoluted tubule (see Fig. 13-15). It is not controlled by ADH.

The drop of fluid now leaves the proximal convoluted tubule and enters the descending limb of the thin segment of the loop of Henle in the renal medulla. The cells lining the descending limb are highly permeable to water and to sodium chloride and other ions. The water passively diffuses from the drop of fluid by osmosis and enters the hypertonic tissue fluid in the renal medulla. About 15 percent of the water is absorbed from the descending limb by this method. Again, this mechanism is not controlled by ADH.

On entering the thickened portion of the ascending limb of the loop of Henle (i.e., the beginning of the distal convoluted tubule), the drop comes into contact with cells that are impermeable to water but actively pump out negative chloride ions. The slight positive potential that has been created within the tubular cells causes the sodium ions to diffuse into the tissue fluid. At this point, the volume of the fluid drop has not changed but the concentration of sodium chloride within it has been reduced. The fluid drop is now isotonic with the tissue fluid (see Fig. 13-15).

The fluid drop now enters the convoluted portion of the distal convoluted tubule in the renal cortex. Here, more sodium ions (and other cations) are pumped out of the fluid by the lining cells, and the chloride ions passively follow. Another 10 percent of the water passes out by diffusion (see Fig. 13-15). It is possible that the permeability of this part of the tubule is controlled by ADH. At this stage, the original fluid drop has lost about 90 percent of its water content.

The drop now passes into the collecting tubules, whose lining cells are permeable to water. It will be remembered that the collecting tubules leave the renal cortex and enter the medulla, where the tissue fluid is hypertonic. Here, a further 9 percent of the water diffuses through the lining cells and enters the tissue fluid by osmosis. The small drop of fluid remaining, which is about 1 percent of the original volume of the glomerular filtrate in the Bowman's capsule, is the urine that finally leaves the kidney.

The permeability to water of the cells lining the collecting tubules is controlled by ADH.

Composition of Urine. Urine is a watery yellow or amber solution. In an individual on a mixed diet, the urine is acid, the *average pH* being about 6.0; in a person on a vegetable diet, it is alkaline. Its *specific gravity* is about 1.002 to 1.04. The *quantity* of urine voided in 24 hours is about 1.5 L. The composition of urine is shown in Table 13-1. The urinary con-

Table 13-1. Composition of urine

Constituent	Total Excreted in 24 Hours (gm)
Inorganic Constituents	
Sodium chloride	15.0
Potassium	2.2
Sulfate (as sulfur)	2.7
Phosphate (as phosphorus)	1.2
Calcium	0.2
Magnesium	0.2
Organic Constituents	
Urea	30.0
Creatinine	1.5
Uric acid	0.7
Glucose	None

stituents are variable and are related to dietary intake. The urea content is produced mainly from the breakdown of food proteins in the body; consequently, a low protein diet will result in a low output of urea in the urine. Creatinine is derived almost entirely from the breakdown of the tissues of the body; therefore, its content in the urine is practically constant. The color of urine is caused by *urobilinogen* and *urobilin*.

Renal Blood Vessels

Each kidney is supplied by a large branch from the aorta called the *renal artery* (see Fig. 13-2). At the hilus of the kidney, the renal artery divides into branches that give rise to five *segmental arteries*. These arteries do not anastomose with one another and are therefore end arteries. They are distributed to different segments or areas of the kidney.

Lobar arteries arise from each segmental artery, one for each renal pyramid (see Fig. 13-20). Before entering the renal substance, each lobar artery gives off two or three *interlobar arteries*. The interlobar arteries run toward the cortex on each side of the renal pyramid. At the junction of the cortex and the medulla, the interlobar arteries give off the *arcuate arteries*, which arch over the bases of the medullary pyramids (see Fig. 13-20). No anastomoses take

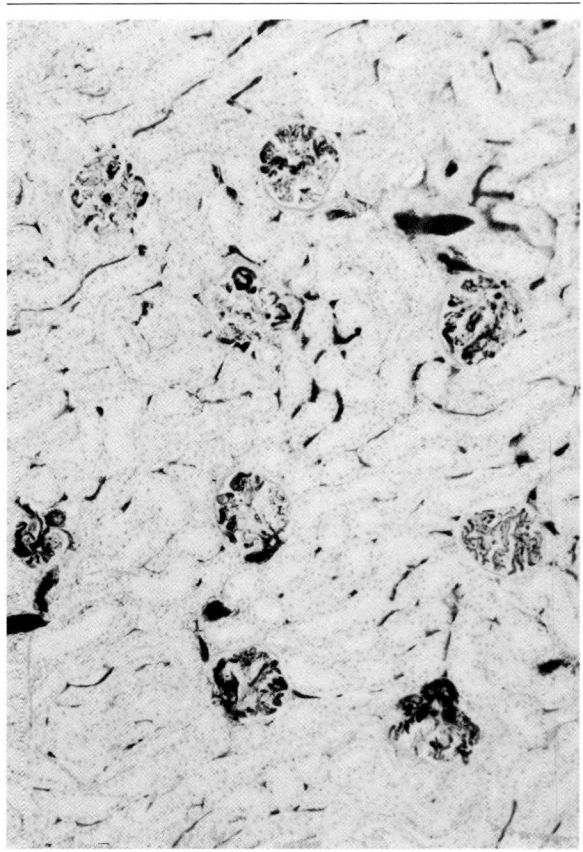

Fig. 13-23. Photomicrograph of a section of the renal cortex following an injection of a red colloidal dye into the renal artery. Note that the blood vessels and the glomerular capillaries are filled with dye, which is black in the photograph. (Hematoxylin stain; ×100.)

place between the arcuate arteries of adjacent interlobar arteries.

The arcuate arteries give off a number of *interlobular arteries* that ascend in the cortex (see Fig. 13-20). They run between adjacent renal lobules and, therefore, between adjacent medullary rays. The *afferent glomerular arterioles* arise as side branches from the interlobular arteries and quickly join the glomeruli (Fig. 13-23).

Emerging from each glomerulus is an *efferent glomerular arteriole*. The efferent arterioles arising from glomeruli in the superficial part of the cortex drain into capillary plexuses that run between and around the proximal and distal convoluted tubules. Those that emerge from more deeply placed glomeruli (the juxtamedullary glomeruli) contribute to the capillary plexuses of the cortex and then divide into a number of long, straight branches, the *descending vasa recta,* that descend into the medullary pyramids (see Fig. 13-20). These arteries give off side branches to an elongated capillary plexus that surrounds the descending and ascending limbs of the loops of Henle and the collecting tubules. The capillary plexuses in the medulla are drained by long, straight veins, the *ascending vasa recta,* that end in the arcuate or interlobular veins (see Fig. 13-20). The close relationship of the descending and ascending vasa recta, the loops of Henle, and the collecting tubules is important in that it explains the physiology of the countercurrent exchange and countercurrent multiplier mechanisms responsible for the hypertonicity of the tissue fluid in the renal medulla.

The renal veins are formed by the union of the lobar, interlobar, arcuate, and interlobular veins. These veins have a course similar to that of the arteries but, unlike them, tend to anastomose with one another.

Juxtaglomerular Apparatus

The distal convoluted tubule lies between and in close contact with the afferent and efferent arterioles of the glomerulus (Fig. 13-24). In this region, the smooth muscle cells of the tunica media of the arterioles (mainly the afferent arterioles) are large and rounded and possess cytoplasmic granules. These cells are known as *juxtaglomerular cells* and are innervated by adrenergic nerve fibers (see Fig. 13-3).

The cells lining the distal convoluted tubule in this region are columnar and are closely packed. They form the *macula densa.* The juxtaglomerular cells and the macula densa together are called the *juxtaglomerular apparatus.*

The granules in the juxtaglomerular cells contain *renin,* an enzyme that converts angiotensinogen in

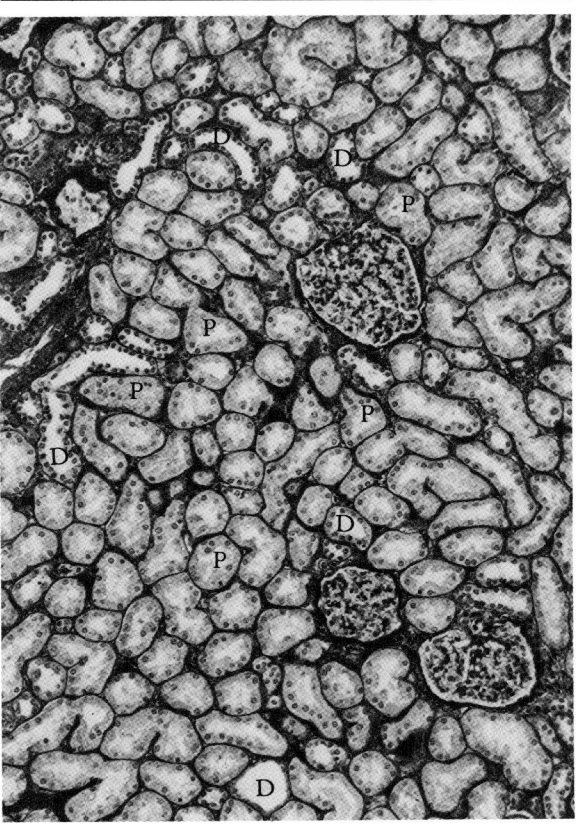

Fig. 13-24. Photomicrograph of the renal cortex, stained to show the basal laminae (black lines) of the glomeruli, Bowman's capsule, and the proximal (P) and distal (D) convoluted tubules. (Periodic acid–Schiff stain; ×100.)

the blood to angiotensin I. This substance is converted into angiotensin II, which is capable of raising the arterial blood pressure. Angiotensin II can also bring about the release of aldosterone from the adrenal cortex.

Although the precise function of the juxtaglomerular apparatus is not known, it is believed that the cells in the arterial wall are sensitive to blood pressure changes and can liberate renin from their granules, which can alter the blood pressure. It will be remembered that the filtration rate of the renal corpuscle is related to the pressure of the blood flowing through the glomerulus. It is possible that the cells of the macula densa are sensitive to the composition of the fluid passing through the distal convoluted tubule and, when appropriate, can activate the release of renin from the juxtaglomerular cells, thus changing the rate of production of the glomerular filtrate. Another possibility is that renin can initiate the release of aldosterone, which in turn causes the cells of the distal tubule to increase their removal of sodium from the fluid flowing through the tubule.

Blood Flow through the Renal Cortex and Medulla

As mentioned previously, the kidneys receive a very large blood supply, the two kidneys receiving about 25 percent of the cardiac output. The glomeruli in the cortex receive a rapid flow of blood through the afferent arterioles, but the glomerular capillary beds and the efferent arterioles offer resistance to the flow. By the time the blood reaches the vasa recta around the loops of Henle, the rate of flow has slowed considerably. Because only the efferent arterioles of the juxtamedullary glomeruli send branches down into the medulla, the medulla receives only an estimated 2 percent of the blood reaching the kidney. The blood supply to the medulla is thus small and slow compared with that to the cortex.

COUNTERCURRENT EXCHANGE MECHANISM IN THE BLOOD VESSELS SUPPLYING THE MEDULLA. As the blood vessels descend from the renal cortex into the medulla, they pass through tissue fluid that becomes increasingly hypertonic as the apex of the pyramid is approached. In fact, the tonicity of the tissue fluid at the renal papilla is about four times greater than that at the corticomedullary boundary.

Because the walls of the descending and ascending vasa recta are permeable to water and electrolytes, and the vessels are arranged as a series of long U tubes whose limbs are close together, a countercurrent exchange mechanism can operate. As the blood descends into the renal pyramid, water diffuses out and sodium chloride and other substances diffuse in. At the hairpin bend of the U, the concentration of sodium chloride in the blood is very high. As the blood ascends back to the cortex, the sodium chloride and other substances that diffuse in along the descending limb diffuse out, and water returns to the bloodstream. The result is that the blood flows through the medulla and returns to the cortex without removing the solutes of the tissue fluid in the medulla. These solutes are important in maintaining the high tonicity of the tissue fluid necessary for the countercurrent exchange multiplier mechanism to operate in the loop of Henle.

Nervous Control of the Kidney

The kidney is innervated by sympathetic and parasympathetic nerve fibers. The sympathetic fibers innervate the smooth muscle in the walls of the blood vessels. Stimulation of the sympathetic nerves causes constriction of the afferent arterioles to the glomeruli and decreases the filtration rate. A decrease in sympathetic activity causes an increase in urine output. The function of the parasympathetic fibers is not known.

Endocrine Function of the Kidney

Renin is an enzyme present in the granules of the juxtaglomerular cells. Its mode of action is described on page 523. *Erythropoietin* is a glycoprotein that stimulates the bone marrow to increase red blood cell production. It cannot be isolated from the kidneys, but the kidneys are responsible for its formation. It is thought that during hypoxia, the kidneys release an enzyme that causes the release of erythropoietin from a plasma protein.

Main Functions of the Kidney

The function of the kidneys is to clear from the blood most of the waste products of metabolism, such as urea, uric acid, urates, and creatinine. They also remove sodium, potassium, chloride, and hydrogen ions, when these are present in excess quantities, by filtering off large quantities of the plasma and then reabsorbing most of the water and all the wanted substances. In addition, unwanted substances are secreted by the kidney tubules. The final product is a small volume of fluid, called urine, con-

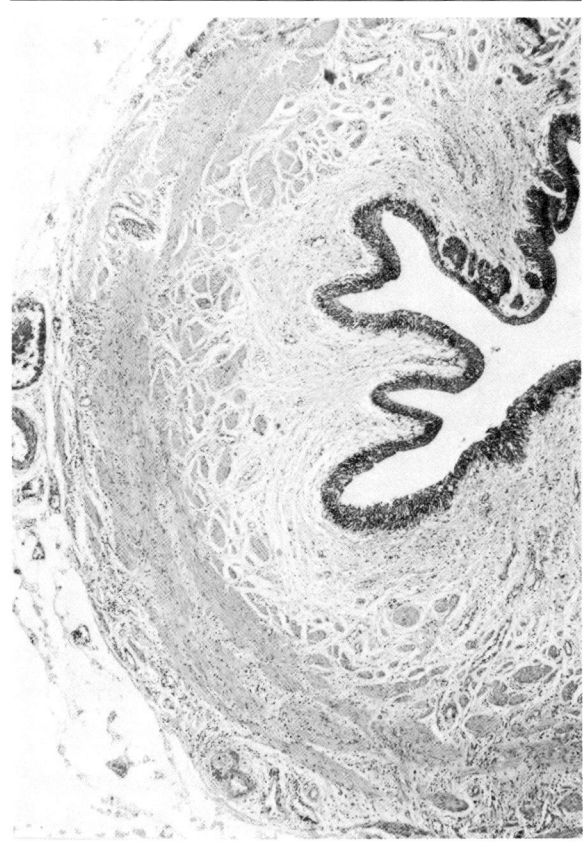

Fig. 13-25. Photomicrograph of a transverse section through the ureter, showing the mucous membrane, the muscle coat, and the fibrous coat. (H&E; ×40.)

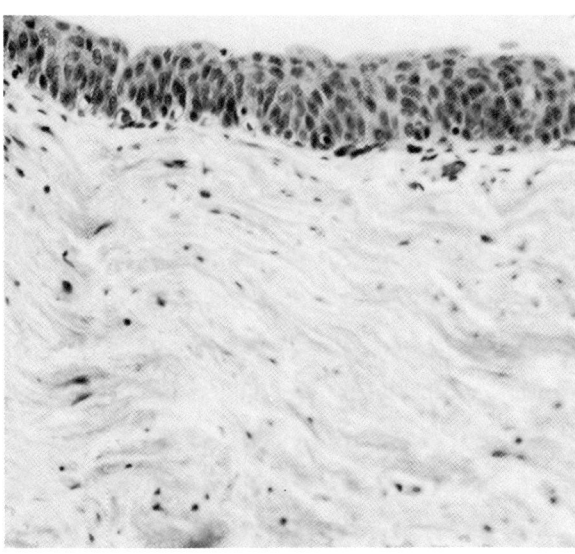

Fig. 13-26. Photomicrograph of a section of the mucous membrane of the ureter, showing the transitional epithelium lining the surface. (H&E; ×100.)

taining the unwanted substances. The kidney is also concerned with the maintenance of a normal blood pressure and erythropoiesis.

EXCRETORY PASSAGES AND MICTURITION

Calyces, Pelvis, and Ureter

The upper expanded end of the ureter, the *pelvis of the ureter,* divides within the renal sinus of the kidney into two or three *major calyces,* each of which divides into two or three *minor calyces* (see Fig. 13-2). Each minor calyx is indented by the apex of a medullary pyramid, the *renal papilla.* The calyces and pelvis of the ureter are lined with mucous membrane consisting of transitional epithelium resting on a lamina propria (see Fig. 13-22). Outside the mucous membrane is a thin muscle coat composed of outer longitudinal and inner circular smooth muscle fibers. Surrounding the muscle is a connective tissue layer that merges into the surrounding connective tissue.

Ureter

The *ureter* has three coats: a mucous membrane, a muscle coat, and a fibrous coat (Fig. 13-25).

The *mucous membrane* is thrown into a number of longitudinal folds that disappear if the ureter is distended. The mucous membrane is lined with transitional epithelium, about five cells thick, resting on a lamina propria of connective tissue (Fig. 13-26).

The *muscle coat* in the upper two-thirds of the ureter is composed of two layers of smooth muscle fibers, a longitudinal inner and a circular outer layer (note that this is the reverse of the arrangement in the intestinal tract). In the lower third of the ureter, an additional, longitudinal outer layer is present (see Fig. 13-25). Because the muscle layers are infiltrated with connective tissue, it may be difficult to recognize the individual layers on an ordinary histologic section.

The *fibrous coat* is continuous above with the fibrous tissue of the pelvis and calyces and below with the outer fibrous coat of the urinary bladder. It is composed of loose connective tissue.

FUNCTION OF THE URETERS. The ureters convey the urine from the kidneys to the urinary bladder. The urine is propelled along the ureter by peristaltic contractions of the muscle coat, aided by the filtration pressure of the glomeruli. Intermittent spurts of urine enter the bladder. Reflux of urine from the bladder cannot occur, because the ureter passes obliquely through the wall of the bladder for about three-quarters of an inch (1.9 cm) before opening into the bladder cavity. A flap of the bladder mucous membrane effectively closes the orifice as the bladder fills with urine.

Urinary Bladder

The urinary bladder is situated immediately behind the pubic bones within the pelvis (see Fig. 13-1). Its function is the storage of urine, and it has a capacity of about 500 ml. The empty bladder is pyramidal in shape, having an apex, a base, and a superior and two inferolateral surfaces; it also has a neck. When the bladder fills, it loses its pyramidal shape and becomes ovoid; the posterior surface and neck are largely unchanged in position, but the superior surface rises into the abdomen.

The bladder wall has three coats: a mucous membrane, a muscle coat, and a fibrous coat (Fig. 13-27).

The *mucous membrane* is continuous above with that of the ureters and below with that of the urethra. In the empty bladder, the mucous membrane is thrown into folds, but these disappear when the bladder is full. The area of mucous membrane covering the internal surface of the base of the bladder is referred to as the *trigone*. Here, the mucous membrane is always smooth, even when the viscus is empty, because the mucous membrane over the trigone adheres firmly to the underlying muscular coat.

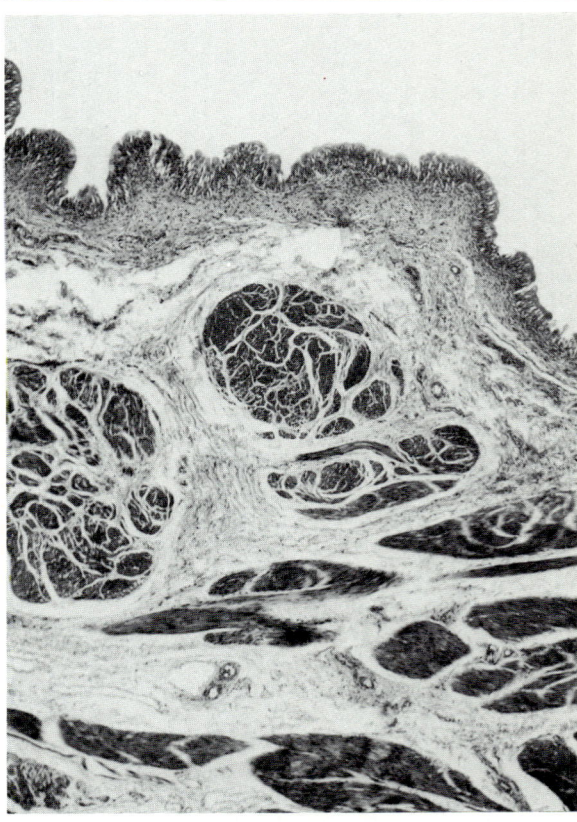

Fig. 13-27. Photomicrograph of a portion of the wall of the urinary bladder, showing the folded mucous membrane and the interlacing bundles of smooth muscle fibers forming the muscle coat. (H&E; ×40.)

The mucous membrane is lined with transitional epithelium resting on a lamina propria of connective tissue (Fig. 13-28). When the bladder wall is relaxed, the surface cells are large and rounded; as the bladder wall becomes stretched, the surface cells flatten (Fig. 13-29).

The *muscle coat,* called the *detrusor muscle,* consists of three layers of smooth muscle fibers: an outer longitudinal layer; a middle, circular layer; and an inner longitudinal layer. Because the different layers intermingle with one another, the layers are not easily recognized (see Fig. 13-27). Near the neck of the

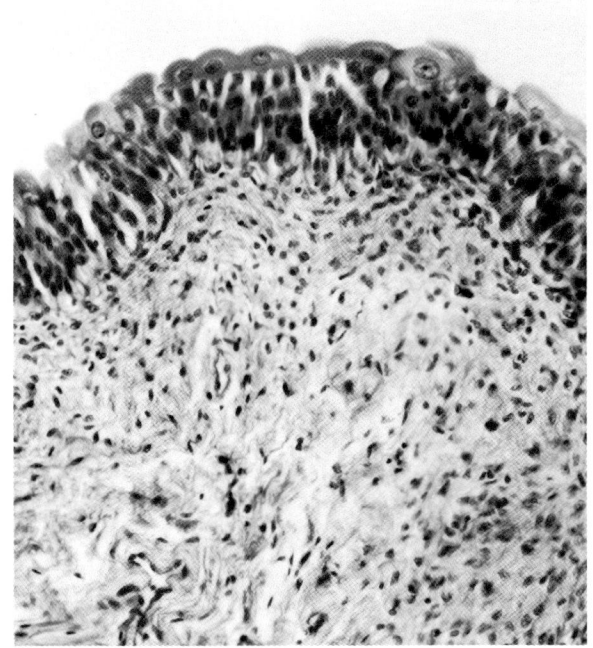

Fig. 13-28. Right: Photomicrograph of a portion of the mucous membrane lining an empty urinary bladder. Note that the mucous membrane is lined with transitional epithelium that rests on a lamina propria of connective tissue. The surface cells are large and oval. (H&E; ×200.)

Fig. 13-29. Below: Scanning electron micrograph of the luminal surface of the mucous membrane of a distended urinary bladder, showing the flattened surface epithelial cells. (×1,000.) (Courtesy of F. G. Lightfoot.)

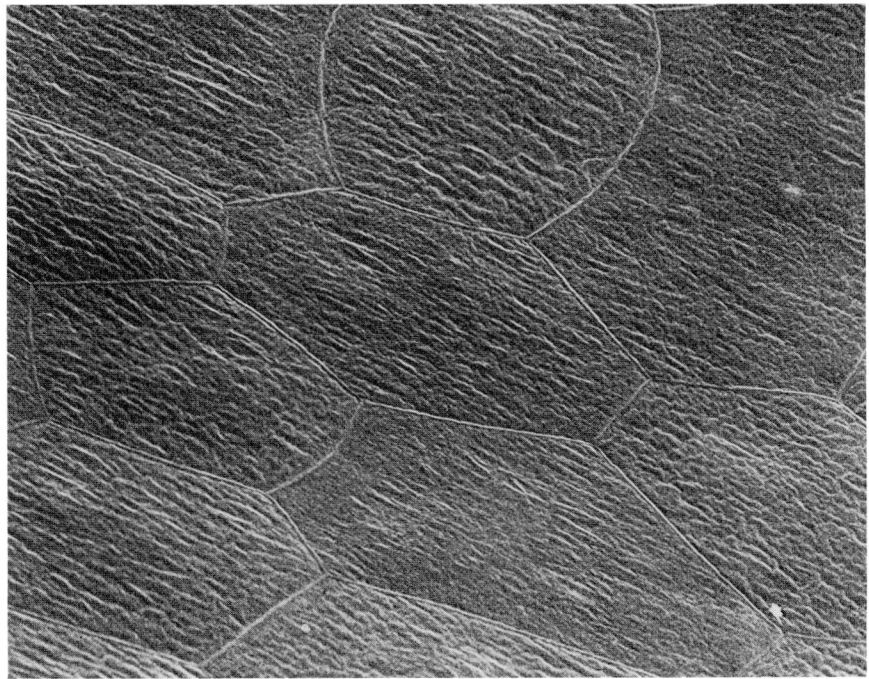

bladder, the middle layer of circular muscle fibers forms the *sphincter vesicae* around the opening into the urethra.

The *fibrous coat* is formed of loose connective tissue. On the superior wall of the bladder, it is covered by the mesothelial cells of the peritoneum.

NERVE SUPPLY OF THE BLADDER. The bladder wall is supplied by sympathetic and parasympathetic nerve fibers from the pelvic plexuses.

Urethra

Male Urethra

The male urethra is about 8 inches (20 cm) long and extends from the neck of the bladder to the external meatus on the glans penis. It is divided into three parts: (1) prostatic, (2) membranous, and (3) penile.

The *prostatic urethra* is the widest and most dilatable part of the urethra. It lies within the prostate and receives the numerous openings of the prostatic glands. The *membranous urethra* lies within the urogenital diaphragm and is surrounded by the sphincter of skeletal muscle called the *sphincter urethrae*. The membranous urethra is the least dilatable portion of the urethra. The *penile urethra* is enclosed in the bulb and the corpus spongiosum of the penis. The external meatus is the narrowest part of the entire urethra.

The mucous membrane of the urethra is lined with epithelium resting on a lamina propria of loose connective tissue. The epithelium of the prostatic urethra is transitional; in the membranous urethra, it is stratified or pseudostratified columnar. In the penile urethra, it is stratified or pseudostratified columnar, but in the glans penis, it becomes stratified squamous epithelium (Fig. 13-30).

The surface epithelium of the mucous membrane continues into the ducts of the urethral, bulbourethral, and prostatic glands. The urethral glands are numerous small mucous glands situated in the submucous connective tissue. In addition, there are a number of small diverticula, into which open branched mucous glands (glands of Littré).

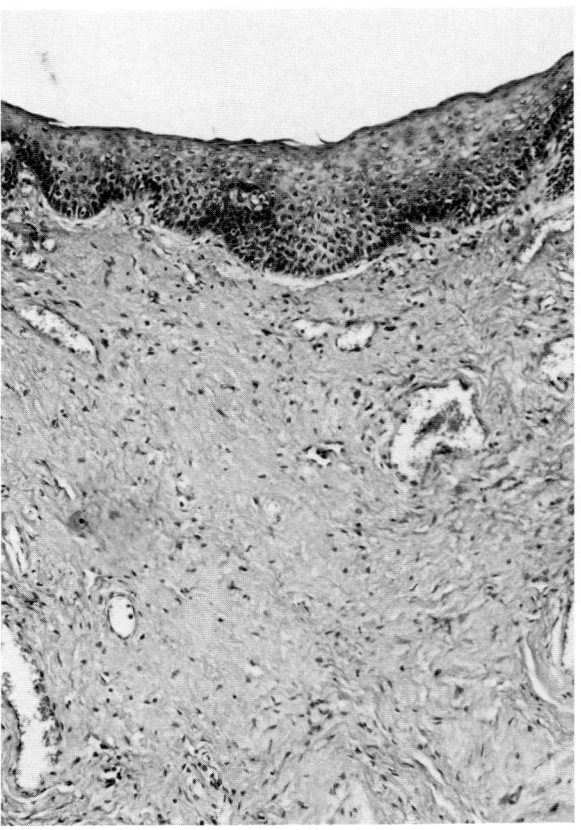

Fig. 13-30. Photomicrograph of a cross section of the male urethra in the glans penis. Note that this part of the urethra is lined with stratified squamous epithelium. (H&E; ×100.)

Female Urethra

The female urethra is about 1.5 inches (3.8 cm) long. It extends from the neck of the bladder to the vestibule, where it opens about 1 inch (2.5 cm) below the clitoris. It traverses the urogenital diaphragm, as in the male, and is surrounded here by the sphincter of skeletal muscle called the *sphincter urethrae*. The urethra lies immediately in front of the vagina.

The mucous membrane of the urethra is continuous above with that of the bladder and distally with that of the vulva. The surface epithelium is transi-

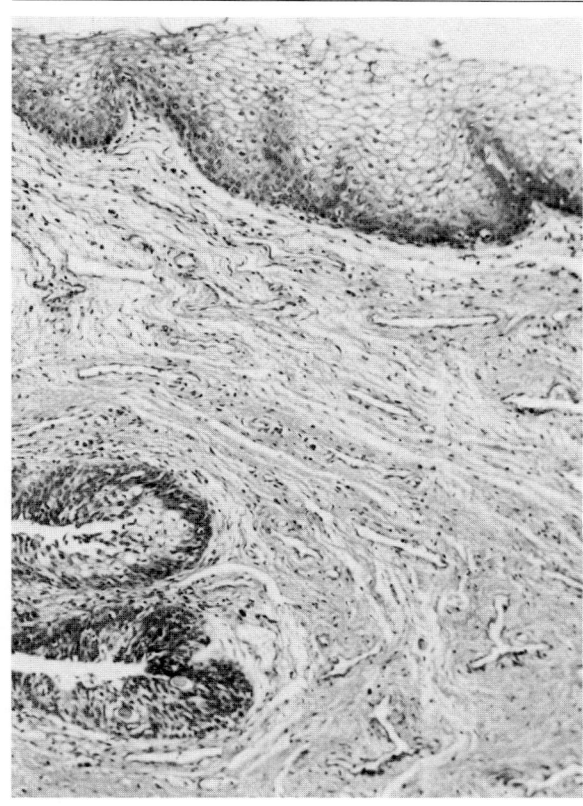

Fig. 13-31. Photomicrograph of a cross section of the lower part of the female urethra; a portion of a diverticulum of the mucous membrane is shown below. Note that this part of the urethra is lined with stratified squamous epithelium. (H&E; ×100.)

tional above, pseudostratified columnar in the middle part of its course, and stratified squamous at its lower end (Fig. 13-31). Numerous diverticula are present, many lined with mucous cells. Beneath the mucous membrane, the loose connective tissue contains a plexus of large veins. There is a muscular layer consisting of a longitudinal internal and a circular external layer of smooth muscle; the muscle is continuous above with that of the bladder wall.

Micturition

Micturition is a reflex action that, in the toilet-trained individual, is controlled by higher centers in the brain. The reflex is initiated by the stretching of the bladder muscle as the organ fills with urine. The afferent impulses pass up the pelvic splanchnic nerves and enter the second, third, and fourth sacral segments of the spinal cord. Efferent impulses leave the cord from the same segments and pass via the parasympathetic preganglionic nerve fibers through the pelvic splanchnic nerves and the pelvic plexuses to the bladder wall, where they synapse with postganglionic neurons. Nerve impulses moving along this nervous pathway cause the smooth muscle of the bladder wall (the detrusor) to contract and the sphincter vesicae to relax. Efferent impulses also pass to the urethral sphincter via the pudendal nerve (S2, S3, and S4), and the sphincter relaxes. Once urine enters the urethra, additional afferent impulses pass to the spinal cord from the urethra and reinforce the reflex action.

In young children, micturition is a simple reflex act and takes place whenever the bladder becomes distended. In the adult, this simple stretch reflex is inhibited by the activity of the cerebral cortex until the time and place are favorable for micturition. The inhibitory fibers descend with the pyramidal tracts to the second, third, and fourth sacral segments of the cord. The contraction of the sphincter urethrae, which closes the urethra, is under voluntary control, but it is not possible to relax this muscle voluntarily; this occurs reflexly.

Voluntary control of micturition is normally developed during the second or third year of life.

CLINICAL NOTES

KIDNEYS

Renal Blood Supply

The kidneys are richly supplied with blood and receive about 25 percent of the cardiac output. About 98 percent of the blood goes to the cortex, leaving only about 2 percent for the medulla. The segmental arteries are large and supply specific areas of the kidney, knowledge of which is invaluable to the urological surgeon performing a partial nephrectomy. The arteries do not anastomose with one another, so that occlusion of the lumen by an embolus will cause infarction of the area of the kidney supplied. Because the blood supply to the medulla is relatively poor and is dependent on blood that first has circulated through glomeruli in the cortex, it is not surprising that ischemic necrosis of the medulla can occur easily.

Conditions Affecting the Glomeruli

In the normal individual, approximately 125 ml of filtrate is separated from the 650 ml of plasma that flows through both kidneys in 1 minute, a filtration fraction of about 0.2. The glomerular filtrate contains all the ultrafiltrable substances in the plasma, together with a little protein. The passage of large molecules through the filtration barrier is determined largely by molecular size; it also is determined partly by molecular charge, however, and this factor is particularly important in reaction to albumin, which is normally held back because of its anionic charge.

Glomeruli can be damaged by a number of diseases. Some of these involve the glomeruli alone; others, such as hypertension, secondarily affect the glomeruli.

Acute and Chronic Glomerulonephritis

In glomerulonephritis, the glomerulus may increase in size as a result of endothelial proliferation, mesangial proliferation, or proliferation of the podocytes. This disease is often preceded by an infection somewhere in the body, commonly the throat, by β-hemolytic group A streptococci. When the antibodies react with the antigens of these organisms, a precipitate is formed that damages the glomerular filtration membrane. As a result, either the filtration is blocked or the filtration membrane's permeability is greatly increased. In some glomeruli, the membrane is actually ruptured.

Damage to glomeruli results in the escape of blood into the Bowman's capsule. The blood then appears in the urine (hematuria). Protein also escapes through the altered filtration barrier and appears in the urine (proteinuria). Severe damage will result in fewer functioning glomeruli and thus diminished urine production (oliguria). Mild hypertension occurs, because of increased cardiac output and an increase in extracellular fluid volume. The great majority of patients with acute glomerulonephritis recover. Sometimes, however, so many glomeruli have been destroyed that the signs persist. In some patients with chronic glomerulonephritis, the glomeruli are progressively destroyed and replaced by fibrous tissue, leading to renal failure.

Conditions Affecting the Tubules

Tubules

Acute tubular necrosis, a common cause of renal failure, is a destruction of the epithelial cells lining the tubules. There are two forms, ischemic and toxic.

Ischemic tubular necrosis commonly follows severe circulatory shock stemming from severe bacterial infections, severe burns, or crush injuries. As a result of the fall in blood pressure, the blood flow through the kidney and, in particular, the renal medulla is impaired severely. The result is death of the tubular epithelium, which is cast off and forms intratubular plugs, or casts.

Toxic tubular necrosis can be produced by a large number of substances, such as heavy metals (lead, gold, and arsenic), organic solvents (carbon tetrachloride, methyl alcohol), and antibacterial agents (neomycin and polymyxin). Microscopically, the tubular epithelium shows degenerative changes; if cellular death occurs, the cells are cast off into the lumen. In this form of necrosis, if the patient recovers, the epithelium recovers.

Nephrotic Syndrome

The *nephrotic syndrome* is characterized by: (1) large quantities of protein in the urine, (2) a diminished concentration of albumin in the plasma, and (3) edema. The disease is caused by damage to the glomerular filtration membrane and may be secondary to glomerulonephritis.

Essentially, the syndrome occurs when the plasma protein albumin leaks across the glomerular membrane into the Bowman's capsule. When the plasma level of albumin falls below a certain level, the colloid osmotic pressure fails to retain the fluid volume within the blood vessels and the volume of tissue fluid increases beyond the normal limit, a condition known as *edema*. As a result of these changes, the plasma volume falls. The kidney tubules attempt to restore the plasma volume by increasing the reabsorption of sodium and water. Unfortunately, much of the reabsorbed fluid passes into the tissue spaces and increases the edema.

Hypertensive Conditions
Arteriolar Nephrosclerosis

Kidney disease often leads to hypertension, but severe hypertension itself can cause renal damage and renal failure. Arteriolar nephrosclerosis is characterized by thickening and occasional necrosis of the renal arterioles, glomerular damage, and replacement fibrosis. There is a loss of glomerular and tubular function, and protein and blood appear in the urine.

Hypertension Associated with an Ischemic Kidney

In patients with chronic renal disease, the blood flow through diseased areas may be impeded by fibrous scar tissue. This lack of blood flow stimulates the production of renin, which in turn leads to the formation of angiotensin in the blood. The angiotensin increases the peripheral resistance by causing vasoconstriction of the arterioles throughout the body, and the blood pressure is raised. The vasoconstriction of the afferent arterioles in the normal glomeruli reduces the filtration of water and salt, which in turn raises the blood pressure by increasing the plasma volume.

Unilateral renal disease can cause hypertension by means of the renin-angiotensin mechanism just described. It is important to diagnose correctly this form of hypertension, because removal of the diseased kidney may cure the hypertension.

Pyelonephritis

Pyelonephritis is a severe infection of the kidney caused by the spread of infection from the ureter and pelvis of the ureter into the kidney tissue. A single infection may subside without serious functional defects, but repeated infection leads to extensive destruction of renal tissue and scarring. The renin-angiotensin mechanism often leads to hypertension, which in turn is followed by further renal damage.

Diabetes Insipidus

This disease is characterized by the production of very dilute urine, causing a constant thirst. The disease is caused by damage to the hypothalamohypophyseal tract or failure of the posterior pituitary to release ADH, causing decreased reabsorption of water from the glomerular filtrate by the distal convoluted tubules and collecting tubules. Intracerebral tumors, trauma, and surgery are possible causes of diabetes insipidus.

Renal Failure
Acute Renal Failure

Acute renal failure can be caused by a wide variety of conditions, such as toxic drugs or severe body trauma, as in crush injuries. It is characterized by a sudden decrease in the glomerular filtration rate and is accompanied by a diminution in the daily volume of urine (an oliguria of 400 ml of urine or less in 24 hours). The syndrome is associated with a rising concentration of blood urea and creatinine. The treatment in severe cases is to assume renal function by artificial means, using either peritoneal or renal dialysis.

Chronic Renal Failure

The functional reserve of renal tissue is so great that one kidney and a large portion of the second can be destroyed by disease before serious signs and symptoms of renal failure appear. If one kidney is removed, the remaining normal glomeruli and tubules increase in size (hypertrophy) to compensate. In cases of progressive renal disease, it is only when the excretory process fails to keep pace with production of waste products that the blood urea gradually rises and the patient becomes uremic.

Patients with chronic renal failure present with a wide variety of symptoms and signs, including blood disorders (such as anemia and coagulation defects), high blood pressure (hypertension), endocrine dysfunction, anorexia, nausea, and hiccups. If treatment is not instituted, the signs of increasing lethargy, coma, and death occur.

Renal Stones

Renal stones are a common clinical condition and occur more often in males than in females. Most renal stones arise in the pelvis of the ureter and either remain there or descend to lower levels within the urinary tract. A renal stone is composed of urinary salts bound together by a colloid matrix of organic material. The most common constituents are uric acid, calcium oxalate, and ammonium magnesium phosphate. These constituents occur either alone or in combination.

Many factors can be responsible for renal stone formation, but the most important are: (1) increased concentration of urinary salts and decreased production of urinary colloids; (2) diminished intake of fluids; (3) urinary infection, the common bacteria found in the nuclei of urinary calculi being staphylococci and *Escherichia coli*; (4) prolonged immobilization, resulting in decalcification of the skeleton and increased output of calcium salts, and recumbency and inactivity, favoring the stagnation of urine, with precipitation of the urinary salts; (5) urinary obstruction; (6) hyperparathyroidism, resulting in a great increase in the excretion of calcium salts; and (7) inborn errors of metabolism, such as cystinuria.

Small stones commonly pass into the ureters, where they give rise to intense colic and may cause obstruction and back-pressure effects in the kidneys. Larger stones remain in the pelvis of the ureter, where they gradually enlarge and often ulcerate the mucous membrane, producing blood in the urine (hematuria). Stones tend to obstruct the flow of urine, and the condition may be complicated by infection.

Kidney Tumors

Benign tumors are rare. Malignant tumors in the adult are adenocarcinomas that arise in the tubular epithelium. They are more common in males and are rare before the age of 50. The malignant tumor in children is Wilms's tumor, which occurs most often in the first four years. It arises from the metanephric mesoderm. Kidney tumors are diagnosed by palpating an abdominal mass or noting the onset of hematuria. Hypertension may be a presenting sign and is caused by increased renin secretion.

Benign and malignant tumors also arise from the transitional epithelium lining the calyces and pelvis of the ureter, but these form only a small percentage of kidney tumors.

Renal Pain

The afferent nerves from the kidney enter the spinal cord at segments T10 to T12. Most common diseases of the kidney, such as nephritis, are unaccompanied by pain. If pain does occur, as with renal stones, it is usually a dull ache referred to the lumbar region.

Treatment of Renal Disease

Diuretics

Diuretics are chemical substances that increase the rate of urine formation by either increasing the glomerular filtration rate or decreasing the tubular reabsorption rate. They are used to reduce the amount of fluid within the body in such conditions as edema (especially that caused by heart failure) and ascites caused by hepatic cirrhosis. The majority of diuretics used clinically act directly on the tubules of the kidney, inhibiting the reabsorption of water and sodium chloride. *Theophylline* and *caffeine*, however, increase the urinary output by dilating the afferent glomerular arterioles and thereby increasing the glomerular filtration rate.

Ethacrynic acid and *furosemide* cause rapid diuresis by inhibiting the reabsorption of salt in the ascending limb of the loop of Henle. The *thiazides* are popular diuretics and inhibit the absorption of salt and water in the distal convoluted tubules and collecting tubules.

Spironolactone antagonizes the action of aldosterone and blocks the absorption of sodium in the ascending limb of the loop of Henle, the distal convoluted tubule, and the collecting tubule. This drug also increases the reabsorption of potassium (see p. 514).

Acetazolamide is a carbonic anhydrase inhibitor and prevents the reabsorption of bicarbonate ions and water from the proximal tubules.

Dialysis

Irreversible renal failure can be treated by dialysis, which makes it possible to keep patients alive for years even after bilateral kidney function has ceased.

Dialysis is commonly used as an interim measure until a suitable live donor kidney or a cadaver kidney becomes available. In patients for whom transplantation is contraindicated for medical or immunological reasons, dialysis can be used as a permanent life-saving procedure.

HEMODIALYSIS. In this form of dialysis, the patient's arterial blood is pumped through coils of plastic tubing or allowed to flow between sheets of plastic and then returned to the patient's circulation by way of a vein. The thin plastic serves as a semipermeable membrane. It allows all constituents of the plasma, except the proteins, to diffuse freely in both directions from the plasma into the dialyzing fluid that bathes the other side of the semipermeable membrane. The composition of the dialyzing fluid is such that substances present in abnormal excess in the blood can be removed, whereas the levels of electrolytes present in normal amounts remain unchanged.

PERITONEAL DIALYSIS. In this form of dialysis, the dialyzing fluid flows into the peritoneal cavity by gravity, and it is the peritoneum that serves as a semipermeable membrane between the fluid and the blood. Because of the risk of infection, this method is used less commonly.

Evaluation of Renal Function

Examination of Urine

Serious renal disease almost invariably is accompanied by abnormalities in the urine. The use of simple and reliable methods of examination can result in the early detection of renal disease. The specimen of urine should be passed into a clean glass or plastic vessel. If a bacteriological examination is to be made, a midstream specimen should be collected after the vulva or glans penis has been cleaned with antiseptic solution.

The following simple tests should be performed: volume, color, opacity, smell, specific gravity, pH, and tests for blood, protein, and glucose. If protein is present, the centrifuged deposit should be examined microscopically. If glucose is present, the presence or absence of hydroxybutyric acid, aceto-acetic acid, and acetone should be determined (see p. 681).

Examination of Blood

Renal failure can be detected by measuring the rise in the concentrations of the nitrogenous waste products in the blood, especially creatinine and urea. These substances are the normal end-products of protein metabolism, and they are excreted in the urine by the normal kidney.

Clearance Tests

Clearance tests for urea and creatinine are used commonly to measure the glomerular filtration rate. Essentially, these tests measure the volume of blood that is cleared completely of a substance in 1 minute. It is calculated by estimating the concentration of the substance in the blood plasma and the amount excreted in the urine in a given time.

Tubular Reabsorption Tests

These tests measure the ability of the tubules to concentrate the urine. The patient is deprived of water for a given time, and the specific gravity of the urine is measured. The ability of the kidney to produce dilute urine is measured by giving the patient excess water to drink.

Tubular Secretion Tests

Phenolsulfonphthalein and organic iodine compounds that are foreign to the body are secreted actively by the renal tubules when given by injection. Their concentration in the urine can then be measured. The iodine compounds are used to obtain an *intravenous pyelogram*. They are secreted by the kidney in concentrations in the urine that produce a radiological contrast shadow.

Unilateral Renal Function Tests

Because one kidney is more than adequate to maintain normal renal function, the usual tests for renal function may be normal despite one nonfunctioning kidney. For this reason, before a nephrectomy is performed, it is essential to determine if a patient has a second kidney, and if so, whether it is functioning normally.

Intravenous pyelography enables one to compare the tubular secretory power of the two kidneys. Cystoscopy and ureteric catheterization allow the investigation of the urine of each kidney separately.

URETER

There are three sites of anatomical narrowing of the ureter where urinary calculi may be arrested: the pelvi-ureteral junction, the pelvic brim, and the entrance of the ureter into the bladder.

Ureteric Pain

The pelvis of the ureter and the ureter send their afferent nerves into the spinal cord at segments T11, T12, L1, and L2. In ureteral colic caused by a calculus or blood clot passing down the ureter, strong peristaltic waves of contraction of the smooth muscle fibers pass down the ureter in an attempt to pass the stone or clot onward. The spasm of the smooth muscle causes an agonizing, colicky pain that is referred to the skin areas supplied by the indicated segments of the spinal cord. The pain extends from the loin to the groin.

Ureter and Pregnancy

Relaxation of the smooth muscle in the wall of the ureter caused by the heightened levels of circulating blood progesterone in pregnancy frequently causes ureteral dilatation and stasis of urine in the ureters. A greater incidence of right ureteral dilatation occurs, because the enlarging uterus tends to press on the right ureter, obstructing it from the outside. A dilated obstructed ureter is very prone to secondary infection of the urine.

URINARY BLADDER

The urinary bladder is the reservoir for urine and lies halfway between the kidney and the exterior. Infection (cystitis) may reach it from the kidney or through the urethra. Moreover, small stones arising in the pelvis of the ureter may descend into the bladder, where they may be voided or grow into large vesical calculi.

Cystitis

Cystitis, or inflammation of the bladder, is a common disease and much more common in the female than in the male. Normal urine arriving in the bladder from the ureters is sterile, and, apart from a few saprophytic bacteria lodged at the distal end of the urethra, bacteria are absent from the urinary tract. The mucous membrane lining the bladder is very resistant to infection. Thus, inflammation of the bladder can occur only if the wall is weakened by such conditions as ulceration from a calculus or damage from trauma. Cystoscopy or the introduction of instruments such as infected catheters can also be responsible.

The shorter urethra in the female (with the greater likelihood of bacteria ascending from the vulva), together with the possibility of urethral trauma during sexual intercourse, explain the high incidence of infection in the female. The stagnation of urine accompanying prostatic enlargement in elderly men accounts for the increased incidence of the disease in this age group.

Bladder Tumors

The great majority of bladder tumors arise from the transitional epithelium lining the bladder. Most such tumors are malignant. Industrial carcinogenic agents have been found in the urine of many patients with malignant tumors. Not only are these agents concentrated in the kidney, but the storage function of the bladder permits them to act on the exposed transitional epithelium. Ingested dietary additives, such as nitrates and nitrites, may also be responsible. The local irritation produced by calculi or the presence of parasites such as *Schistosoma haematobium,* which is common in Egypt, may bring about histological changes (metaplasia) that progress to neoplasia.

Effects of Spinal Cord Injuries

Following injuries to the spinal cord, the nervous control of micturition is disrupted. In the innervation of the *normal bladder,* the *sympathetic outflow* is from the first and second lumbar segments of the spinal cord. The *parasympathetic outflow* is from the second, third, and fourth sacral segments of the spinal cord. *Sensory nerve fibers* enter the spinal cord at all of these segments.

Atonic bladder occurs during the phase of spinal shock immediately following the injury and may last for a few days or for several weeks. The bladder wall muscle is relaxed, the sphincter vesicae tightly contracted, and the sphincter urethrae relaxed. The bladder becomes greatly distended and finally overflows. Depending on the level of the cord injury, the patient may or may not be aware that the bladder is full.

Automatic reflex bladder occurs after the patient has recovered from spinal shock, provided that the cord lesion lies above the level of the parasympathetic outflow (S2, S3, S4). It is the type of bladder normally found in infancy. The bladder fills and empties reflexly. Stretch receptors in the bladder wall are stimulated as the bladder fills, and the afferent impulses pass to the spinal cord (segments S2, S3, and S4). Efferent impulses pass down to the bladder muscle, which contracts; the sphincter vesicae and the urethral sphincter both relax. This simple reflex occurs every 1 to 4 hours.

Autonomous bladder is the condition that occurs if the sacral segments of the spinal cord are destroyed. The bladder is without any external reflex control. The bladder wall is flaccid, and the capacity of the bladder is increased greatly. It merely fills to capacity and overflows; continuous dribbling is the result. The bladder may be emptied partially by manual compression of the lower part of the anterior abdominal wall, but infection of the urine and back-pressure effects on the ureters and kidneys are inevitable.

URETHRA

In the male, the urethra is a common site for gonococcal and nonspecific bacterial and viral infections. The mucous diverticula, the numerous small mucous glands, the bulbo-urethral glands, and the prostatic glands provide ideal sites for the organisms to lodge and proliferate. Creamy urethral discharge, burning pain on micturition, and reflex frequency of micturition are the usual clinical findings.

In the female, the short urethra, which is dilated without difficulty, facilitates the passage of catheters and cytoscopes. The fact that the urethra is embedded in the anterior wall of the vagina makes it vulnerable to traumatic injury during sexual intercourse. The shortness of the urethra is probably the main reason cystitis in the female is much more common than in the male. Any pathological organism residing in the vulva has only a short distance to travel to enter the bladder. As in the male, the numerous mucosal diverticula and their accompanying glands provide locations for gonococci and other nonspecific organisms to cause a urethritis.

CLINICAL PROBLEMS

For the answers to these problems, see page 807.

1. A 12-year-old girl is kept home from school because she complains of a severe sore throat. She is seen by a pediatrician, a throat swab is taken, and she is given a course of antibiotics. Two weeks later, her parents notice that her eyelids look puffy and swollen. Although her throat is no longer sore, she says that she feels strengthless and generally tired. She complains of a dull, aching pain on both sides in the lower part of the back. Four days later, she observes that her urine is smoky-brown in color. Using your knowledge of renal anatomy and physiology, explain what could be causing this condition. Why

does the patient have edema of her eyelids? Is there any connection between your diagnosis and the history of sore throat? Why is the urine smoky-brown in color?

2. Using your knowledge of histology, describe the following structures and their function: (a) glomerulus, (b) medullary ray, (c) renal papilla, (d) nephron, (e) podocyte, (f) mesangial cell.

3. A 49-year-old man is admitted to the coronary care unit with a diagnosis of coronary thrombosis (myocardial infarction). After 4 hours, the cardiac output deteriorated and the patient experienced heart failure and died. A large infarct was identified postmortem in the right kidney. What is the possible connection between myocardial infarction and renal infarction? Why is the blood supply to the kidney vulnerable when we know that it receives such a large proportion of the cardiac output? A renal infarct is usually triangular in shape and is white with a darker peripheral zone. Why is the infarct triangular in shape?

4. Define the following histological terms: (a) slit pore and slit diaphragm, (b) filtration barrier, (c) juxtaglomerular apparatus, (d) macula densa.

5. What are the countercurrent multiplier and the countercurrent exchanger? Where in the kidney do these mechanisms function, and what is their significance?

6. The kidney has been classified as an endocrine gland. What hormonal substances are produced by the kidney, and what is their action?

7. A 43-year-old man with chronic glomerulonephritis is asked to provide a sample of urine for analysis. What is the normal specific gravity of urine? Which protein escapes from the blood into the urine in this disease? In severe cases of this disease, does the blood level of urea or creatinine change; if so, why? Is the blood pressure of this patient likely to be normal? Why should kidney disease sometimes cause hypertension?

8. Compare and contrast the structure of the proximal and distal convoluted tubules of the kidney. Give a brief account of the functions of these two segments of the uriniferous tubule.

9. A 48-year-old woman is operated on for a cerebral tumor. Five weeks after the operation, she tells her physician that she is excessively thirsty. For the past 2 weeks, she has been drinking, on the average, 20 L a day. She also says that she is having to micturate very frequently. In fact, she is afraid to leave her house, because the desire to micturate is so frequent. The nurse examines a sample of urine and finds the specific gravity to be 1.001. What could be causing this condition? Is there any connection between the patient's symptoms and signs and her recent operation?

10. Patients with severe vascular collapse or circulatory insufficiency undergo certain physiological changes involving their kidneys: (a) decreased glomerular filtration rate; (b) increased production of renin; (c) increased proximal tubular absorption of sodium, water, and urea; and (d) increased release of ADH from the posterior pituitary. Explain each of these renal physiological changes. What are the effects on the patient's renal output and vascular system?

11. Following a partial gastrectomy, a patient is having his duodenal contents removed by means of continuous suction through a nasal tube. What are the approximate volumes of salivary, gastric, and duodenal secretions in a normal individual per day? In order to keep the water balance in this patient stable, about how much fluid would you expect him to be given intravenously over a 24-hour period, assuming there are no other medical problems?

12. A patient with advanced renal failure is waiting for a suitable kidney donor for a transplant. His blood urea nitrogen level is high, and he is developing some of the signs of uremia. What methods are available to keep this patient alive until a suitable donor can be found?

13. A 53-year-old woman is seen in the outpatient clinic and found to be suffering from cirrhosis of the

liver. Her doctor, finding that she has ascites (excess fluid in the peritoneal cavity), prescribes a diuretic. How will a diuretic reduce this excess body fluid? Name three different types of diuretics, and explain their modes of action. Why is the salt content of food restricted in these cases?

14. A medical student doing a rotation through the radiology department is asked by a radiologist to explain the procedures involved in performing an intravenous pyelogram. How would this test be used to determine the efficiency of renal function in a patient with suspected renal disease?

15. A 50-year-old man awakens one morning with severe abdominal pain. The pain is agonizing and comes in waves. It extends from his left loin to his groin. After about an hour, the pain becomes so intense that he feels nauseated, and vomits. The pain recurs every 3 or 4 minutes and extends down to his glans penis. In the emergency room, an anteroposterior radiograph of the abdomen reveals a calculus in the left ureter. (a) What causes the pain when a ureteral calculus is present? (b) Why is the pain felt in such an extensive area? (c) Where along the ureter is a calculus likely to be arrested?

16. An experienced rock-climber attempting a particularly difficult climb slips and falls 200 feet down a ravine. Although roped to his companion, he strikes a projecting ledge as he falls. After a difficult rescue operation, he is flown to a nearby hospital. Radiographic and neurological examination reveals a severe fracture dislocation of the lower thoracic region of the vertebral column and extensive local damage to the spinal cord. Assuming that the patient has a complete transection of the spinal cord, (a) will he ever again be able to tell if his urinary bladder was full? (b) will he have an automatic bladder or an autonomous bladder?

17. A 60-year-old man is examined by a urologist because he has passed blood in his urine on three occasions. Examination of a urine sample reveals the presence of blood. The patient emphasizes that he feels perfectly fit and has experienced no pain. A cystoscopic examination reveals five papillomas growing from the trigone and lateral walls of the bladder. Describe the structure of the bladder wall. Which cells give origin to the papillomas?

18. Women frequently suffer from cystitis. Can you explain why this is so, using your knowledge of the histology and anatomy of the urethra?

19. A 25-year-old sailor is treated for gonorrhea with a short course of antibiotics. Three weeks later, while on board ship, he reports to sick bay complaining of discharge from the urethra, frequency of micturition, and burning pain on micturition. Can you explain why the symptoms and signs of gonorrhea tend to recur if the disease has been treated inadequately? What is peculiar about the histological structure of the male urethra that encourages infections of the mucous membrane to become chronic?

20. Describe the different types of epithelium that line the male and female urethra. What type of muscle forms the sphincter urethrae?

ADDITIONAL READING

Andrews, P. M. Scanning electron microscopy of the kidney glomerular epithelium after treatment with polycations in situ and in vitro. *Am. J. Anat.* 153:291, 1978.

Andrews, P. M., and Porter, K. R. A scanning electron microscopic study of the nephron. *Am. J. Anat.* 140:81, 1974.

Arakawa, M., and Tokunaga, J. Further scanning electron microscopic studies of the human glomerulus. *Lab. Invest.* 31:436, 1974.

Aukland, K. Renal blood flow. *Int. Rev. Physiol.* 11:23, 1976.

Barajas, L. The ultrastructure of the juxtaglomerular apparatus as disclosed by 3-dimensional reconstruction from serial sections. *J. Ultrastruct. Res.* 33:116, 1970.

Barger, A. C., and Herd, J. A. The renal circulation. *N. Engl. J. Med.* 284:482, 1971.

Boyarsky, S. *Ureteral Dynamics.* Baltimore: Williams & Wilkins, 1972.

Boyarsky, S., et al. *Care of the Patient with Neurogenic Bladder.* Boston: Little, Brown, 1979.

Brenner, B. M., and Rector, F. C. (eds.). *The Kidney.* Vol. 1. Philadelphia: Saunders, 1976.

Brenner, B. M., et al. Transport of molecules across renal glomerular capillaries. *Physiol. Rev.* 56:502, 1976.

Burg, M. B. The nephron in transport of sodium, amino acids, and glucose. *Hosp. Pract.* 13:99, 1978.

Deetjen, P., et al. *Physiology of the Kidney and of Water Balance.* New York: Springer-Verlag, 1975.

Dirks, J. H., and Wong, N. L. M. Acute functional adaptation to nephron loss: Micro puncture studies. *Yale J. Biol. Med.* 51(3):255, 1978.

Drukker, W., et al. (eds.). *Replacement of Renal Function by Dialysis.* Boston: Nijhoff, 1979.

Fujita, T., Tokunaga, J., and Edanaga, M. Scanning electron microscopy of the glomerular filtration membrane in the rat kidney. *Cell Tissue Res.* 166:299, 1976.

Ganong, W. F. Formation and excretion of urine. In *Review of Medical Physiology* (10th ed.). Los Altos, Calif.: Lange, 1979, p. 549.

Giebisch, G., and Stanton, B. Potassium transport in the nephron. *Annu. Rev. Physiol.* 41:241, 1979.

Heptinstall, R. H. *Pathology of the Kidney* (2nd ed.). Boston: Little, Brown, 1975.

Hicks, R. M. The mammalian urinary bladder: An accommodating organ. *Biol. Rev.* 50:215, 1975.

Karnovsky, M. J., and Ryan, G. B. Substructure of the glomerular slit diaphragm in freeze-fractured normal rat kidney. *J. Cell Biol.* 65:233, 1975.

Katz, A. I., and Lindheimer, M. D. Actions of hormones on the kidney. *Annu. Rev. Physiol.* 39:97, 1977.

Knox, F. G. (ed.). *Textbook of Renal Pathophysiology.* Hagerstown, Md.: Harper & Row, 1978.

Kriz, W., and Lever, A. F. Renal countercurrent mechanisms: Structure and function. *Am. Heart J.* 78:101, 1969.

Latta, H. The glomerular capillary wall. *J. Ultrastruct. Res.* 32:526, 1970.

Latta, H., Maunsbach, A. B., and Osvaldo, L. The fine structure of renal tubules in cortex and medulla. In Dalton, A. J., and Haguenau, F. (eds.), *Ultrastructure of the Kidney.* New York: Academic, 1967.

Maul, C. G. Structure and formation of pores in fenestrated capillaries. *J. Ultrastruct. Res.* 36:768, 1971.

Michielsen, P., and Creemers, J. The structure and function of the glomerular mesangium. In Dalton, A. J., and Haguenau, F. (ed.), *Ultrastructure of the Kidney.* New York: Academic, 1967.

Miyoshi, M., Fujita, T., and Tokunaga, J. The differentiation of renal podocytes: A combined scanning and transmission electron microscope study in rats. *Arch. Histol. Jpn.* 33:161, 1971.

Morel, F., and deRouffignac, C. Kidney. *Annu. Rev. Physiol.* 35:17, 1973.

Osvaldo, L., and Latta, H. The thin limb of the loop of Henle. *J. Ultrastruct. Res.* 15:144, 1966.

Rodewald, R., and Karnovsky, M. J. Porous substructure of the glomerular slit diaphragm in the rat and mouse. *J. Cell Biol.* 60:423, 1974.

Stephenson, J. L. Countercurrent transport in the kidney. *Annu. Rev. Biophys. Bioeng.* 7:315, 1978.

Vander, A. J. *Renal Physiology.* New York: McGraw-Hill, 1980.

MALE REPRODUCTIVE SYSTEM

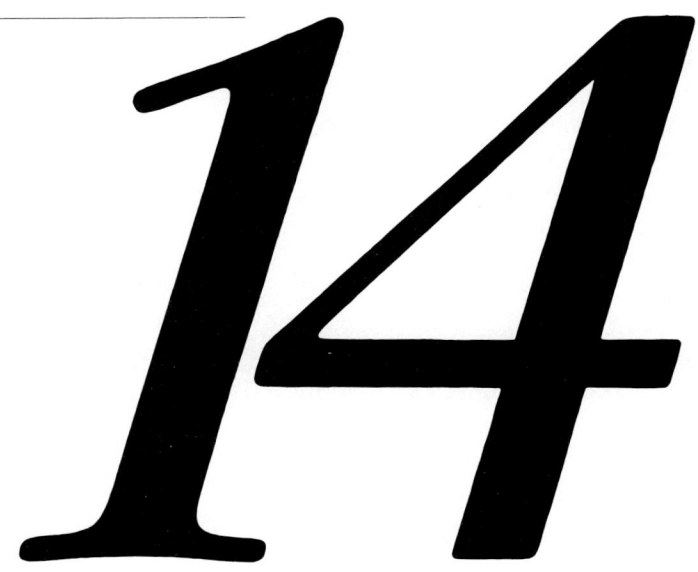

The male reproductive system consists of a pair of testes, their excretory ducts, the accessory glands, and the penis (Fig. 14-1). The excretory ducts on each side are the epididymis, the vas deferens, and the ejaculatory duct. The accessory glands are a pair of seminal vesicles, a pair of bulbo-urethral glands, and the prostate gland.

TESTES

The testes are paired organs that produce the male germ cells, the *spermatozoa,* and the male sex hormones, the *androgens.* The testes are situated in the scrotum. In early fetal life, the testes are situated in the abdominal cavity, near the kidneys. As the fetus matures, the testes descend and, just before birth, pass through the inguinal canal to enter the scrotum. The descent of the testes from the abdominal cavity into the scrotum is important, because the development of spermatozoa (spermatogenesis) will take place normally only if the testes are at a temperature lower than that of the abdominal cavity.

Each testis has a thick fibrous capsule, the *tunica albuginea* (Fig. 14-2), which thickens posteriorly to form the *mediastinum testis.* Extending from the inner surface of the capsule to the mediastinum is a series of fibrous septa that divide the interior of the organ into about two hundred and fifty lobules. Lying within each lobule are one to three coiled *seminiferous tubules* (Figs. 14-3 and 14-4; see Fig. 14-2). Each tubule is in the form of a loop, each end of which is continuous with a *straight tubule.* The straight tubules open into a network of channels within the mediastinum testis called the *rete testis* (see Figs. 14-2 and 14-5). Within each lobule, between the seminiferous tubules, are delicate connective tissue and groups of rounded or polyhedral *interstitial cells* that produce the male sex hormones.

The rete testis is drained by *efferent ductules* into a long, much-coiled duct, the *epididymis* (see Fig. 14-2), that is situated on the posterior surface of the testis.

Seminiferous Tubule

The wall of the seminiferous tubule (Figs. 14-6–14-8) has a basement membrane lined with two types of cells: (1) numerous germinal cells, the *spermatogonia,* and (2) supporting cells, the Sertoli cells.

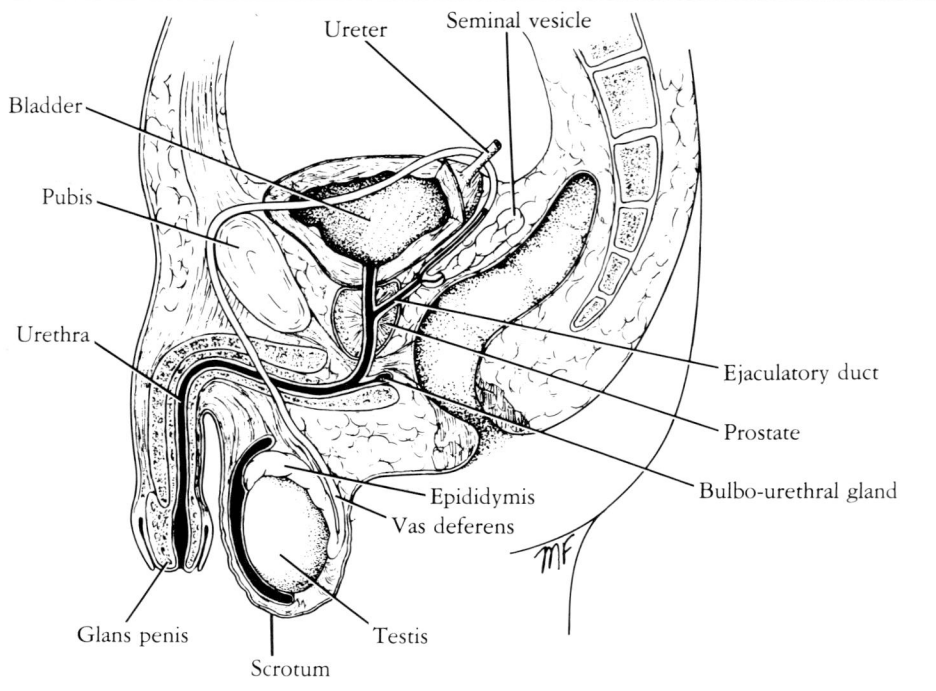

Fig. 14-1. *Male reproductive system in sagittal section.*

Spermatogenesis

The term *spermatogenesis* is applied to the sequence of events by which spermatogonia are transformed into spermatozoa (Fig. 14-9; see Fig. 14-8). The spermatogonia are stem cells situated along the basement membrane of the seminiferous tubule. They are large, rounded cells, and three types can be recognized, according to their nuclear appearance: type A dark (dark-staining nucleus), type A pale (pale-staining nucleus), and type B (spherical nucleus with clumps of chromatin along the nuclear membrane). Type A dark spermatogonia divide to maintain the numbers of spermatogonia and also to form some type A pale spermatogonia. Type A pale spermatogonia divide and differentiate into type B spermatogonia. After this division, type B spermatogonia divide by mitosis into *primary spermatocytes.* The latter cells migrate toward the middle zone of the seminiferous epithelium and then undergo meiotic division (the first meiotic division) into smaller *secondary spermatocytes,* each containing half the number of chromosomes of the primary cell (Fig. 14-10). The secondary spermatocytes soon divide (the second meiotic division) to form the smallest cells, the *spermatids,* which become embedded in the cytoplasm of the sides of the Sertoli cells. The spermatids now undergo a series of morphological changes leading to the formation of *spermatozoa.*

A spermatid (Fig. 14-11) has a centrally placed spherical nucleus, a well-defined Golgi apparatus, numerous mitochondria, and two centrioles. Several small granules appear within the Golgi apparatus, and these coalesce into a single large granule called the *acrosomal granule* (see Fig. 14-11). The acrosomal granule, with its surrounding membrane, then adheres to the outer surface of the nuclear envelope. The acrosomal membrane spreads over the anterior pole of the nucleus, finally covering its anterior half. The acrosomal granule then gradually spreads within the acrosomal membrane to form a thin layer over the anterior half of the nucleus known as the

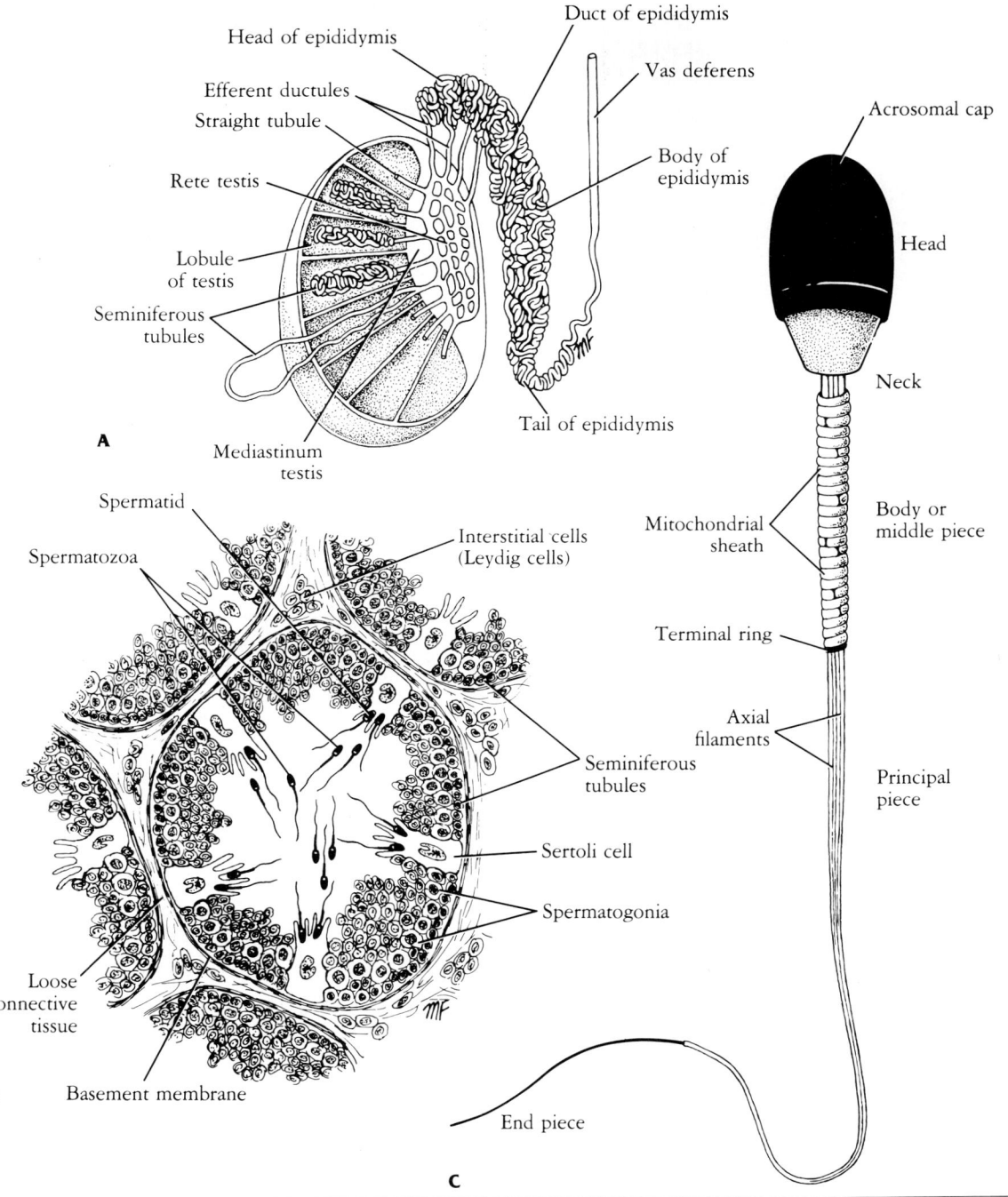

Fig. 14-2. A: General structure of the testis and the epididymis. B: Microscopic structure of a seminiferous tubule, showing interstitial cells (Leydig cells). C. Structure of a mature spermatozoon.

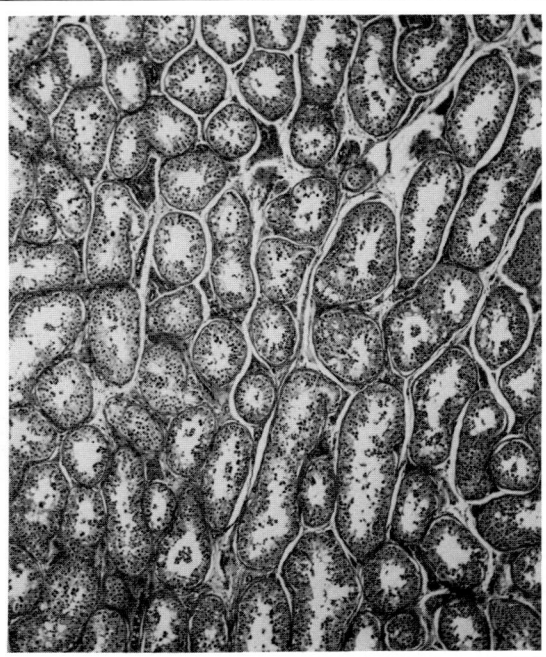

Fig. 14-3. Photomicrograph of a section of the testis, showing numerous seminiferous tubules cut in cross section. The tubules are supported by loose connective tissue. (H&E; ×40.)

acrosomal cap (see Fig. 14-11). The acrosomal cap is rich in carbohydrate and contains hydrolytic enzymes.

Meanwhile, the nucleus of the spermatid elongates and flattens (see Fig. 14-11). The centrioles migrate to the end of the nucleus opposite the acrosomal cap, and a flagellum grows out from one of them. A tube of cytoplasmic filaments, called the *caudal tube,* then appears. This is attached to the nuclear membrane and surrounds the flagellum. At the same time, the mitochondria migrate toward the flagellum and become arranged around it in the form of a sheath or collar. At the distal end of the mitochondrial collar, a ringlike structure, called the *terminal ring,* appears (see Fig. 14-11). The collar and terminal ring lie within the middle piece, or body, of the spermatozoon. The cytoplasm now forms a thin covering for the nucleus, middle piece, and tail piece. The remainder of the cytoplasm is

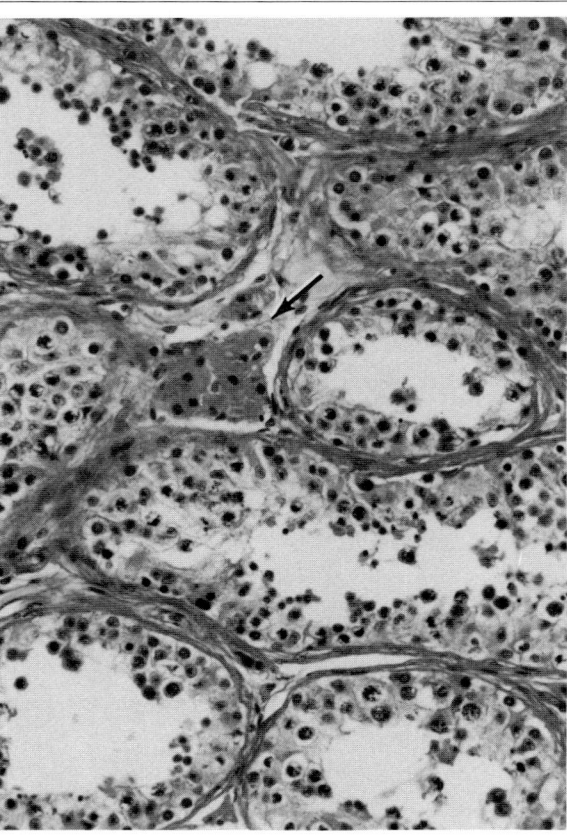

Fig. 14-4. Photomicrograph of cross sections of several seminiferous tubules. Note that each tubule is lined with several layers of cells. Only an occasional spermatozoon can be seen. Note also the Leydig cells (arrow) in the interstitial connective tissue. (H&E; ×200.)

cast off as a *residual body* from the developing spermatozoon and is phagocytosed by the Sertoli cells. The fully formed spermatozoon now leaves the Sertoli cell and lies free within the lumen of the seminiferous tubule (see Fig. 14-10). The total duration of spermatogenesis is about 64 days.

Spermatogenesis begins at about 14 years of age (Fig. 14-12) as the result of stimulation by the gonadotropic hormones of the anterior lobe of the pituitary, but it does not start at that time unless the testes are in the scrotum. Spermatogenesis is a con-

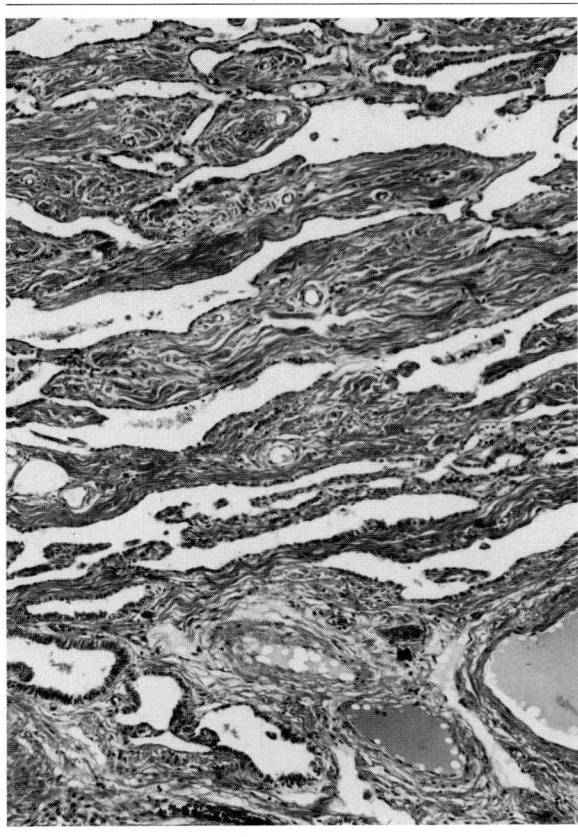

Fig. 14-5. Photomicrograph of a section of the mediastinum testis, showing the network of channels called the rete testis. The channels, or small tubes, are lined with squamous or low cubical epithelium. (H&E; ×100.)

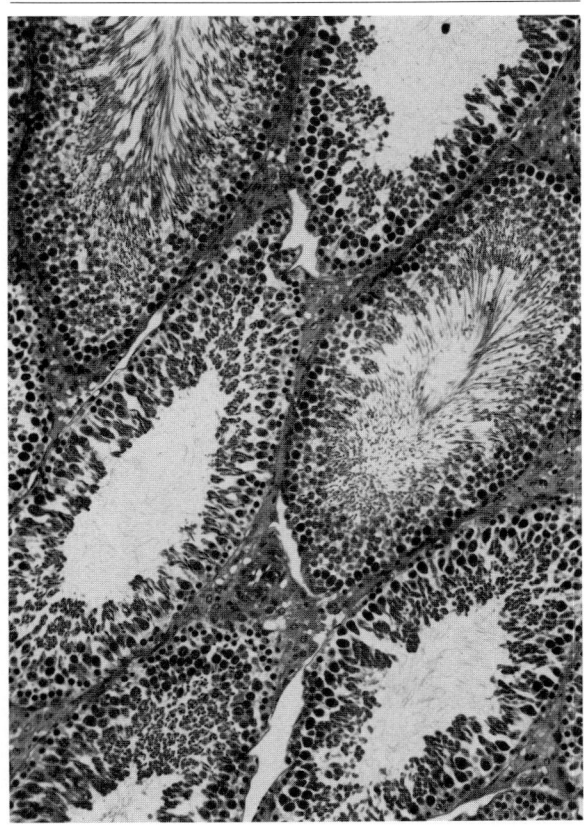

Fig. 14-6. Photomicrograph of a plastic section of several seminiferous tubules. Note the multiple spermatozoa within their lumina. (H&E; ×100.)

tinuous process, but the stages of spermatogenesis are not identical along the length of a seminiferous tubule. Spermatogenesis continues into advanced old age, but after middle age, increasing numbers of atrophic tubules are found.

CHROMOSOMAL CHANGES DURING SPERMATOGENESIS. In the human somatic cell, there are 46 chromosomes, consisting of 22 pairs of *autosomes* and one pair of *sex chromosomes* (XY). The different pairs of autosomes vary in size, but the two members of any given pair are identical. The sex chromosomes in the female (XX) are also identical, but in the male, there is one X and one much shorter Y chromosome. The spermatogonia possess 46 chromosomes (see Fig. 14-10). When these cells divide mitotically and form primary spermatocytes, each chromosome splits longitudinally, so that each new cell receives the same number of chromosomes contained in the mother cell. When the primary spermatocytes divide meiotically, the secondary spermatocytes are haploid—that is, they receive only half the number of chromosomes, 23. Thus, 22 + X chromosomes go to one secondary spermatocyte

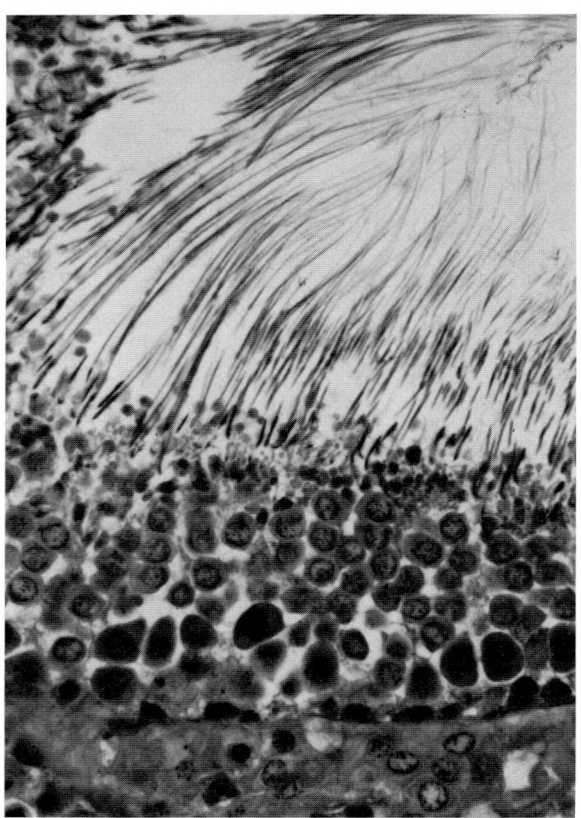

Fig. 14-7. Photomicrograph of a high-power view of the wall of a seminiferous tubule shown in Figure 14-6, showing the different layers of cells that form the germinal epithelium. Note the different types of spermatogonia, i.e., those with dark- and those with light-staining nuclei. Note also the many spermatozoa whose heads are still embedded in the Sertoli cells. (H&E; ×400.)

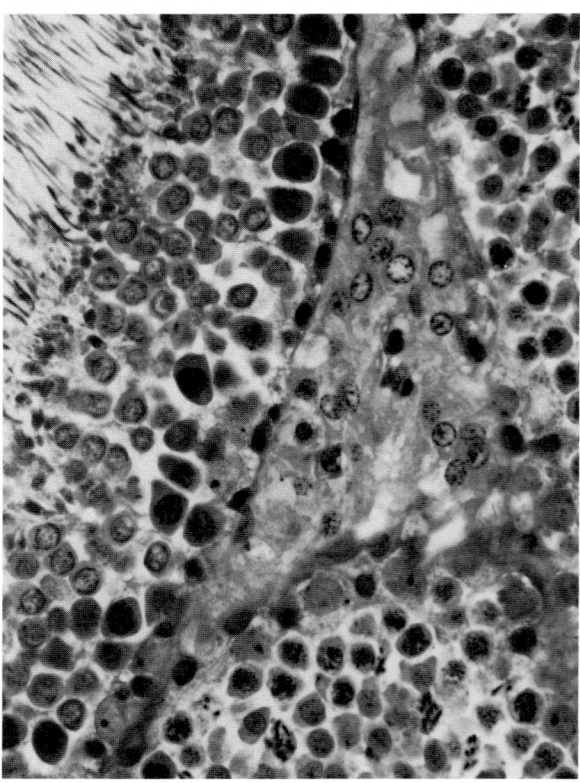

Fig. 14-8. Photomicrograph of a high-power view of the interstitial cells (Leydig cells) present in Figure 14-6. Note that these cells are large and are embedded in loose connective tissue between the seminiferous tubules. (H&E; ×400.)

and 22 + Y chromosomes pass to the other (see Fig. 14-10).

The second meiotic division, of the secondary spermatocytes to form spermatids, is such that two spermatids are produced with 22 + X chromosomes and two with 22 + Y chromosomes. By this means, one spermatogonium, with 44 autosomes and one pair of XY chromosomes, eventually gives rise to eight spermatozoa. Four of the spermatozoa have 22 autosomes and one X sex chromosome, and four have 22 autosomes and one Y sex chromosome (see Fig. 14-10).

If a spermatozoon with 22 + Y chromosomes penetrates an ovum and fertilization occurs, a male child will result. If the spermatozoon has 22 + X chromosomes, a female child will result. The described chromosomal changes are depicted in Figure 14-10.

MATURE SPERMATOZOON. The mature spermatozoon is smaller than the ovum and is about 60 μm long. It consists of a *head, neck, body,* and *tail* (Fig. 14-13; see Fig. 14-2). The head is formed largely by the condensed nucleus and is covered by the cell

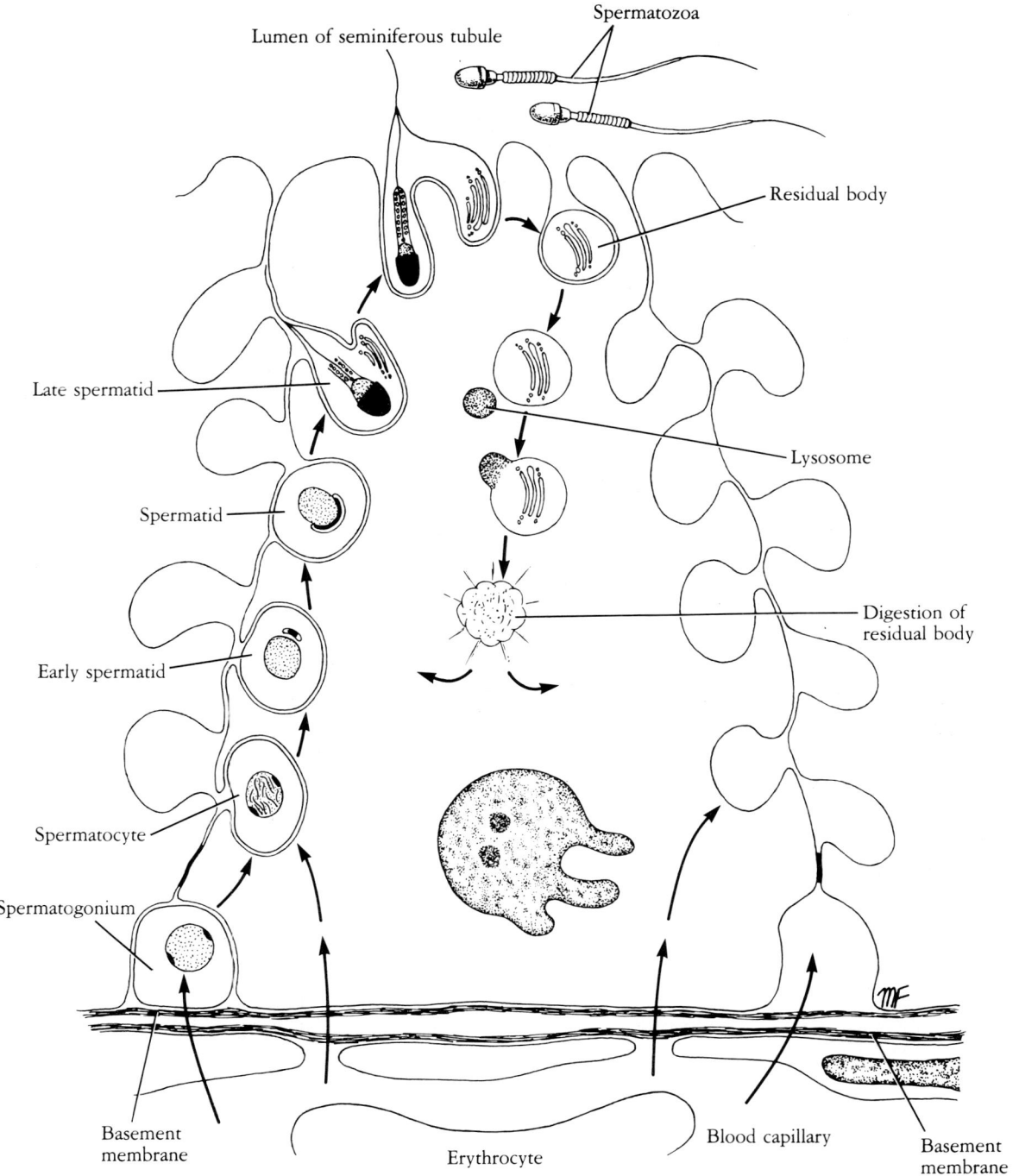

Fig. 14-9. Sertoli cell and the part it plays in spermatogenesis. Note the tight junctions situated near the base of the cell that separate the spermatogonia from the more superficial spermatocytes and spermatids. The arrows passing upward from the capillary indicate the pathways taken by nutrients and hormones.

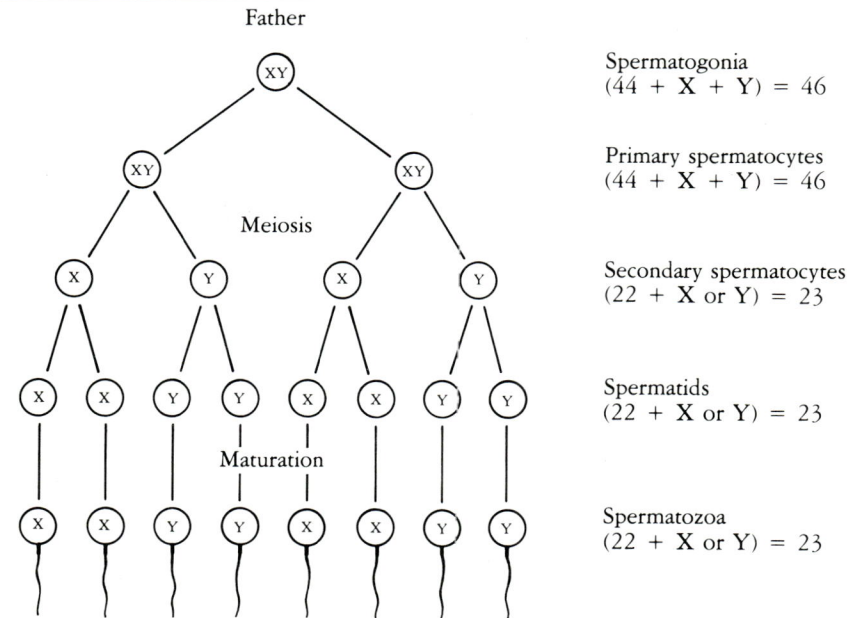

Fig. 14-10. Chromosomal changes during spermatogenesis.

membrane. Covering the anterior two-thirds of the nucleus is the acrosomal cap, which contains several enzymes, including hyaluronidase and proteases, that are involved in the penetration of the ovum. Behind the head, the spermatozoon is constricted slightly to form the neck, which contains the two centrioles. The axial filament arises from the distal centriole and in the body consists of a pair of central fibrils surrounded by two concentric rings of nine fibrils. Outside the concentric rings, a further ring of coarse fibrils is present. Mitochondria are arranged spirally around the axial filament within the middle piece, or body. The spiral collar of mitochondria ends distally at a terminal ring.

The tail forms the greater part of the spermatozoon and is the motile part of the cell. It contains the pair of central fibrils surrounded by the two concentric rings of nine fibrils. The outer coarse fibrils are present only at the proximal end of the tail. The fibrils of the tail are enclosed in a sheath of transversely oriented fibrils. Near the end of the tail, the sheath is absent. The spermatozoon has a thin layer of cytoplasm and a cell membrane. Thus, the head of the spermatozoon contains the structures responsible for the transmission of genetic information (haploid number of chromosomes) and the remainder of the spermatozoon is concerned with locomotion.

The mature spermatozoon can live for several weeks in the ducts of the male reproductive system but can live only 2 to 3 days in the ducts of the female reproductive tract.

MATURATION OF SPERMATOZOA. Once a spermatozoon has been formed and lies free in the lumen of the seminiferous tubule, it shows very little motility and at this stage is incapable of fertilizing an ovum. The spermatozoon is moved successively through the straight tubules, rete testis, and efferent ductules to the epididymis by the contraction of smooth muscle in the walls of these tubes. While lying within the epididymis, the spermatozoon undergoes further maturation, resulting in increased motility and fertilizing power.

At the time of ejaculation, the spermatozoa become very active, and it is believed that the alkaline

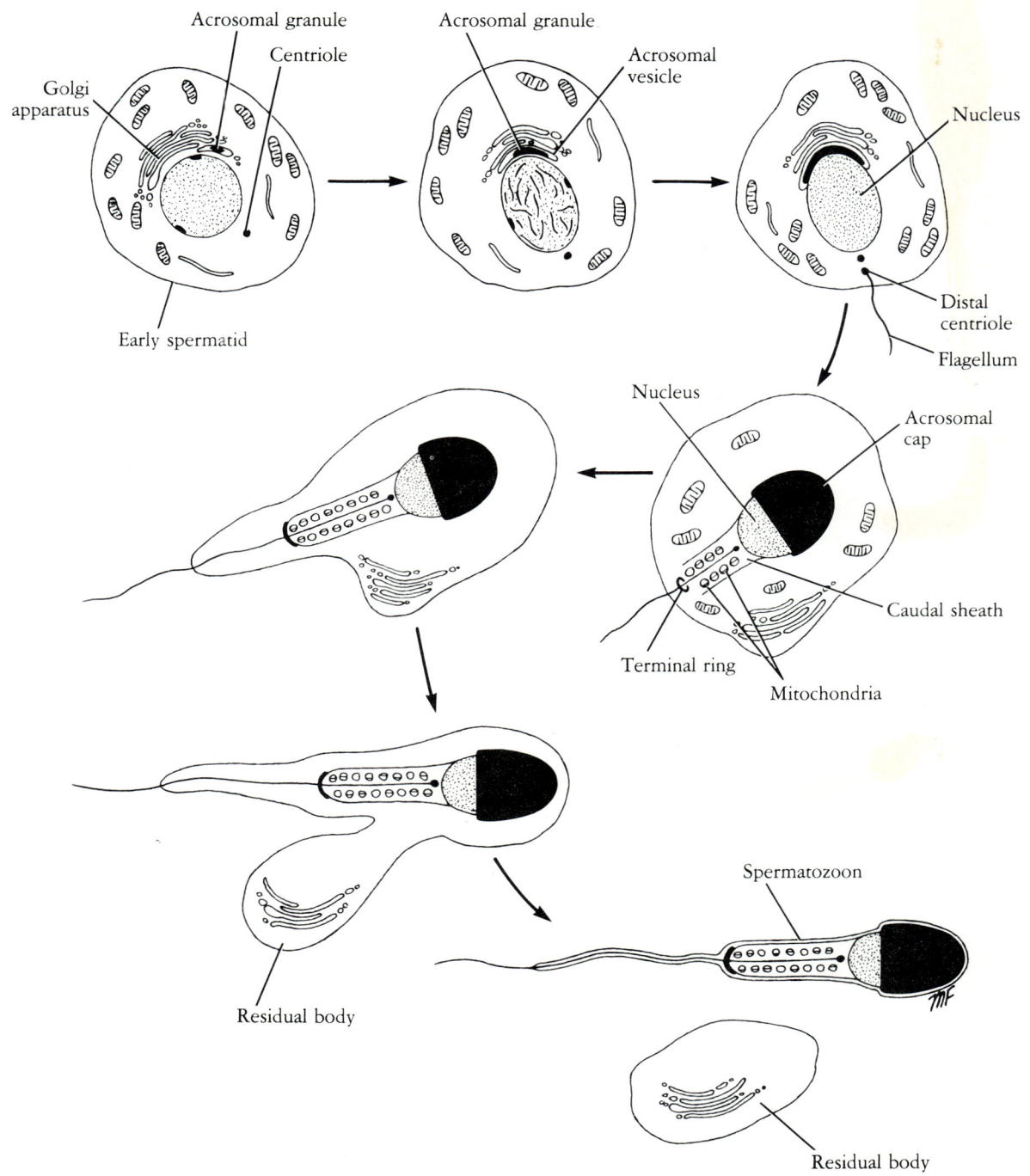

Fig. 14-11. Changes in a spermatid during the formation of a spermatozoon.

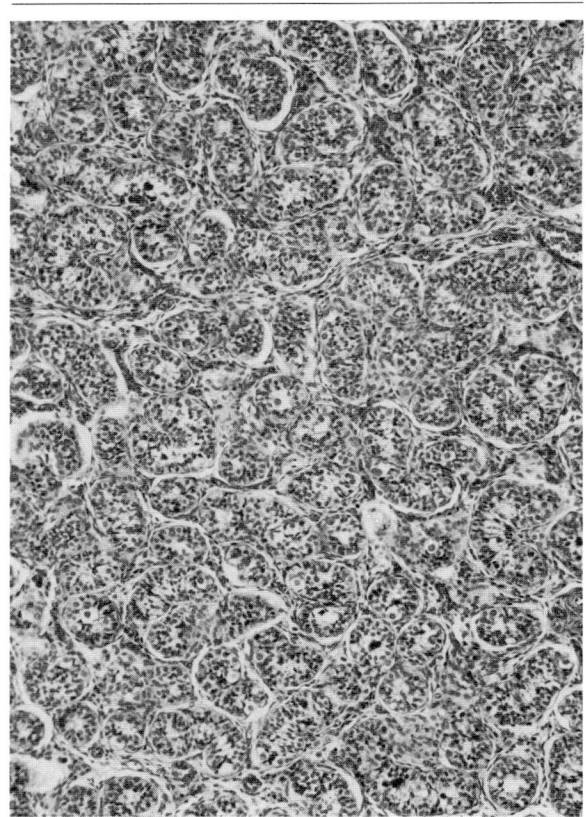

Fig. 14-12. Photomicrograph of a section of a young boy's testis. The seminiferous tubules are small, and in many the lumen is absent. (H&E; ×100.)

secretions of the seminal vesicles and prostate influence this process. (It should be remembered that the vaginal fluid is acid and tends to inhibit sperm motility.) The final process of maturation, called *capacitation*, occurs once the spermatozoa have entered the female genital tract. The spermatozoa are propelled forward by the undulating movements of their tails, and at the same time, they are rotated on their long axis. Their speed varies with the environmental conditions, but is about 2 to 3 mm a minute.

Testicular Temperature and Fertility

Normal spermatogenesis can occur only if the testes are at a temperature lower than that of the abdomen. When they are located in the scrotum, they are at a temperature about 3°C lower than the abdominal temperature. The control of testicular temperature in the scrotum is not fully understood, but the surface area of the scrotal skin can be changed reflexly by the contraction of the dartos and cremaster muscles. It is now recognized that the testicular veins in the spermatic cord that form the pampiniform plexus—together with the branches of the testicular arteries, which lie close to the veins—probably assist in stabilizing the temperature of the testes by a countercurrent heat exchange mechanism. By this means, the hot blood arriving in the artery from the abdomen loses heat to the blood ascending to the abdomen within the veins.

Supporting Cells of Sertoli

The Sertoli cells are situated on the basement membrane of the seminiferous tubule (see Fig. 14-9). They are relatively few in number and occur at intervals between the spermatogonia (Fig. 14-14). Each cell is somewhat columnar in shape and extends from the basement membrane to the lumen of the tubule. Along the sides of each cell, a stream of proliferating and differentiating germ cells moves slowly toward the lumen (see Fig. 14-9). A very close relationship exists between the Sertoli cells and the germ cells; in fact, the germ cells occupy deep recesses in the lateral and, later, the apical surfaces of the supporting cells.

The Sertoli cell possesses an ovoid or indented nucleus. The cytoplasm contains numerous organelles, including mitochondria, rough and smooth endoplasmic reticulum, Golgi complex, granules, microfilaments and microtubules (see Fig. 14-14). The filaments and tubules probably play a part in bringing about the changes in the Sertoli cell that permit the germ cells to ascend the sides of the cell in their deep recesses, to be released finally as spermatozoa.

Adjacent Sertoli cells are held together by gap junctions and multiple tight junctions (see Fig. 14-9). The tight junctions are situated near the base of the cell and separate the intervening spermatogonia from the more superficial spermatocytes and spermatids. This arrangement is important, because

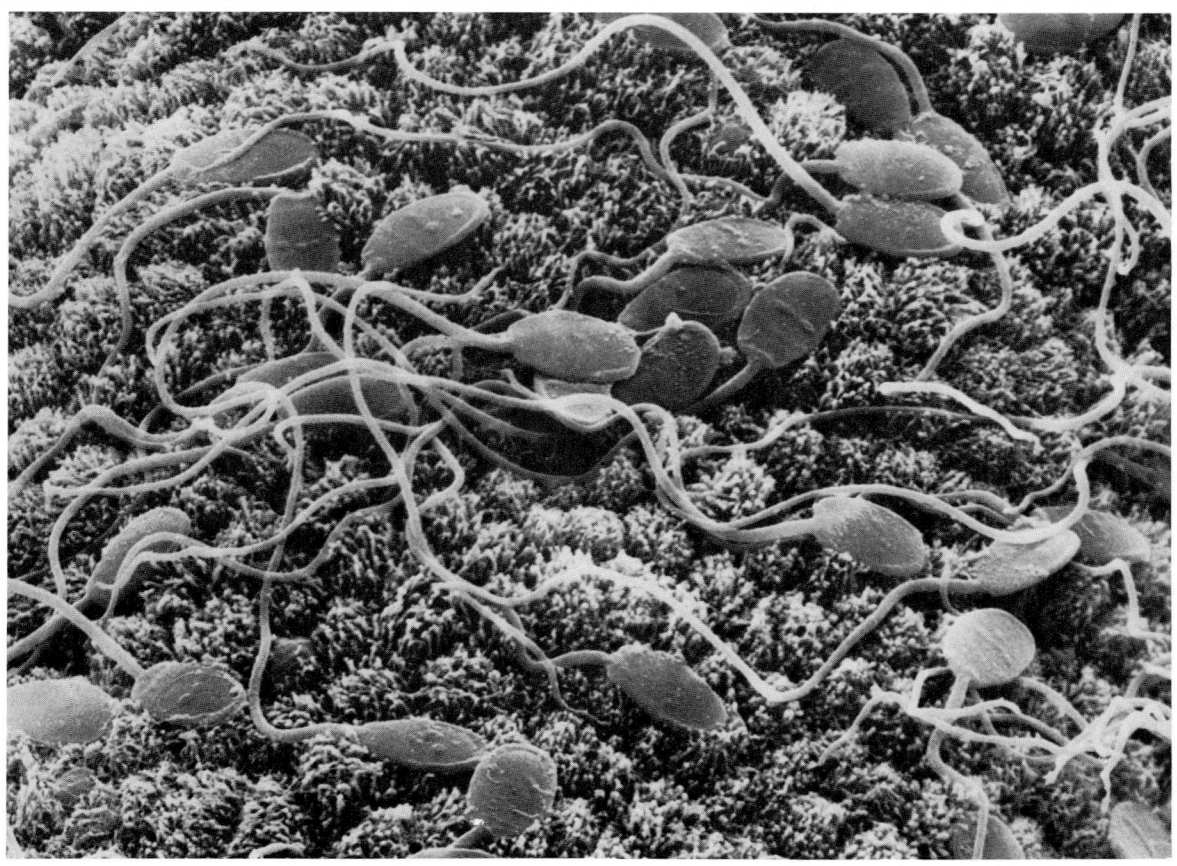

Fig. 14-13. Scanning electron micrograph showing numerous spermatozoa in the uterine cavity. (×1,000.) (Courtesy of Dr. D. M. Phillips.)

spermatogonia must be located so that hormones from the blood can have access to them (Fig. 14-15). The follicle-stimulating hormone (FSH) produced by the anterior lobe of the pituitary, for example, must reach these cells to stimulate their activity.

The spermatocytes, the spermatids, and the spermatozoa that have resulted from the division of the spermatogonia lie near the lumen of the tubule and are separated from the tissue fluid by the tight junctions between adjacent Sertoli cells. These tight junctions have been referred to as the *blood-testis barrier,* because they protect the spermatogenic cells from noxious substances that may be present within the blood. The antigens of the differentiated sperm cells are prevented from gaining access to the general body circulation, however. If they were not, it might be possible for the individual to develop an autoimmune response to his own spermatozoa.

With the presence of the blood-testis barrier, how is it possible for the spermatocytes, spermatids, and spermatozoa to receive nourishment from the bloodstream? They do so as a result of their close association with the sides of the Sertoli cells. Their presence in the recesses of the Sertoli cells allows nutrients to pass through the plasma membrane and cytoplasm of the Sertoli cells to enter the germ cells.

When spermatogonia divide by mitosis to give rise to the primary spermatocytes, the blood-testis barrier, or tight junction between adjacent Sertoli

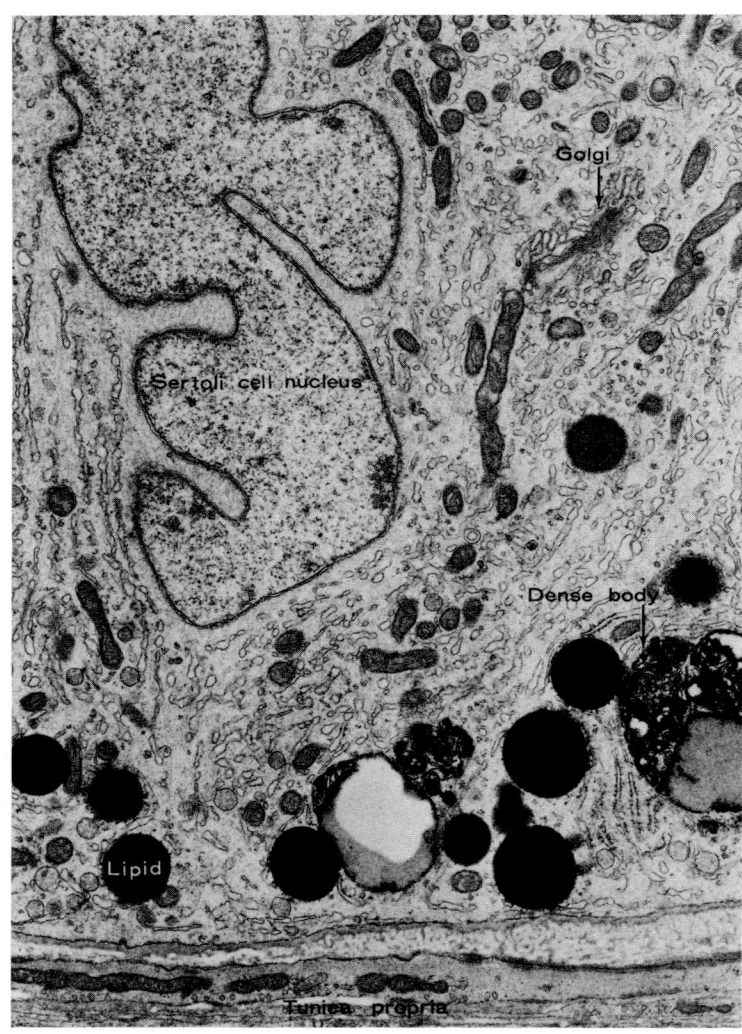

Fig. 14-14. Electron micrograph of a portion of a Sertoli cell. Note the irregularly shaped nucleus, the abundant smooth endoplasmic reticulum, the Golgi complex, many mitochondria, the lipid droplets, and the dense bodies. (×2,300.) (Courtesy of Dr. M. Dym.)

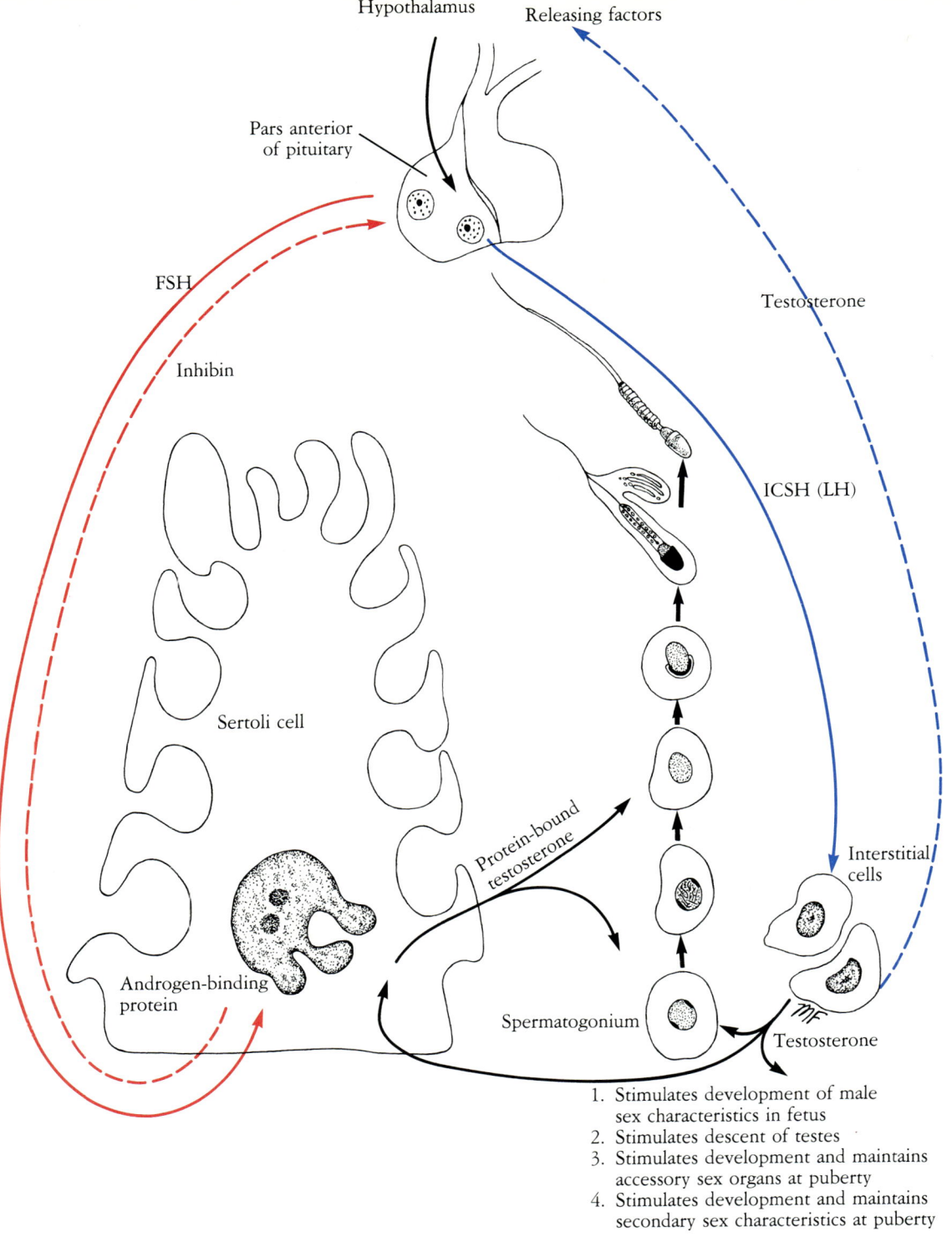

Fig. 14-15. Hormonal pathways that influence spermatogenesis and testosterone production by the interstitial cells (Leydig cells).

cells, disappears, only to reappear between the spermatocyte and the spermatogonia. This process can be likened to a barge traveling along a canal with a series of locks. The lock gates open ahead of the barge but close behind it to hold back the water.

The functions of the Sertoli cells include: (1) the support, protection, and release of the spermatogenic cells; (2) the nourishment of the spermatocytes, spermatids, and spermatozoa; (3) the phagocytosis of the residual bodies derived from the spermatids; (4) the secretion of fluid into the lumen of the seminiferous tubule for the transport of spermatozoa; and (5) the formation of small quantities of estrogens.

Effect of the Follicular Stimulating Hormone on the Sertoli Cells

The follicular stimulating hormone (FSH) acts on the Sertoli cells to form a protein that binds to androgen (see Fig. 14-15). By this process, the Sertoli cells are able to concentrate the androgens, which in turn stimulate spermatogenesis. The Sertoli cells are believed to release a hormone called *inhibin*, which passes into the bloodstream and inhibits the production of FSH. If this is true, the Sertoli cells, by means of this feedback mechanism, play a very active part in controlling the rate of spermatogenesis.

Interstitial Cells

The interstitial cells, or Leydig cells, are situated in groups embedded in loose connective tissue between the seminiferous tubules (see Figs. 14-2 and 14-8). The cells are large and polyhedral, with an eccentric nucleus and poorly staining cytoplasm. They secrete the androgens *testosterone, dihydrotestosterone,* and *androstenedione;* the most important and abundant of these is testosterone. The interstitial cells are stimulated to produce these androgens by the interstitial cell–stimulating hormone (ICSH) of the anterior lobe of the pituitary, which is identical to the luteinizing hormone (LH) in the female (see Fig. 14-15). The FSH of the anterior lobe of the pituitary is also thought to have some effect.

The interstitial cells are present in large numbers in the fetus, but they atrophy to some extent after birth. They reappear in large numbers at puberty. In the fetus, the chorionic gonadotropin from the placenta stimulates the interstitial cells of the testes to produce testosterone, which is important in the development of the male genitalia and the suppression of female genitalia formation. It also brings about the descent of the testes.

The testosterone produced by the interstitial cells is responsible for the growth, development, and maintenance of the accessory male sex organs, including the prostate, seminal vesicles, bulbourethral glands, and penis. It is also responsible for the secondary sexual changes that occur at puberty, including the growth of facial, axillary, and pubic hair, the enlargement of the larynx, and musculoskeletal growth.

For a discussion of additional functions of testosterone, see page 665.

Straight Tubules and Rete Testis

The seminiferous tubules, which are coiled, become less convoluted as they approach the mediastinum testis. They unite to form several straight tubules. These are lined with Sertoli cells and contain no spermatogonia.

The straight tubules, on entering the mediastinum testis, unite to form a network of anastomosing tubes called the *rete testis*. The tubes are lined with squamous or low cubical epithelium (see Fig. 14-5).

Efferent Ductules

At the superior end of the mediastinum testis, the tubules of the rete testis are drained by about a dozen ductules called the *efferent ductules.* These pierce the tunica albuginea and join the epididymis. The efferent ductules are lined with ciliated columnar epithelium. Beneath the basement membrane is a layer of circularly arranged smooth muscle fibers embedded in loose connective tissue.

EXCRETORY DUCTS

Epididymis

As the efferent ductules approach the epididymis, they become enlarged and convoluted and are held together by loose connective tissue to form masses

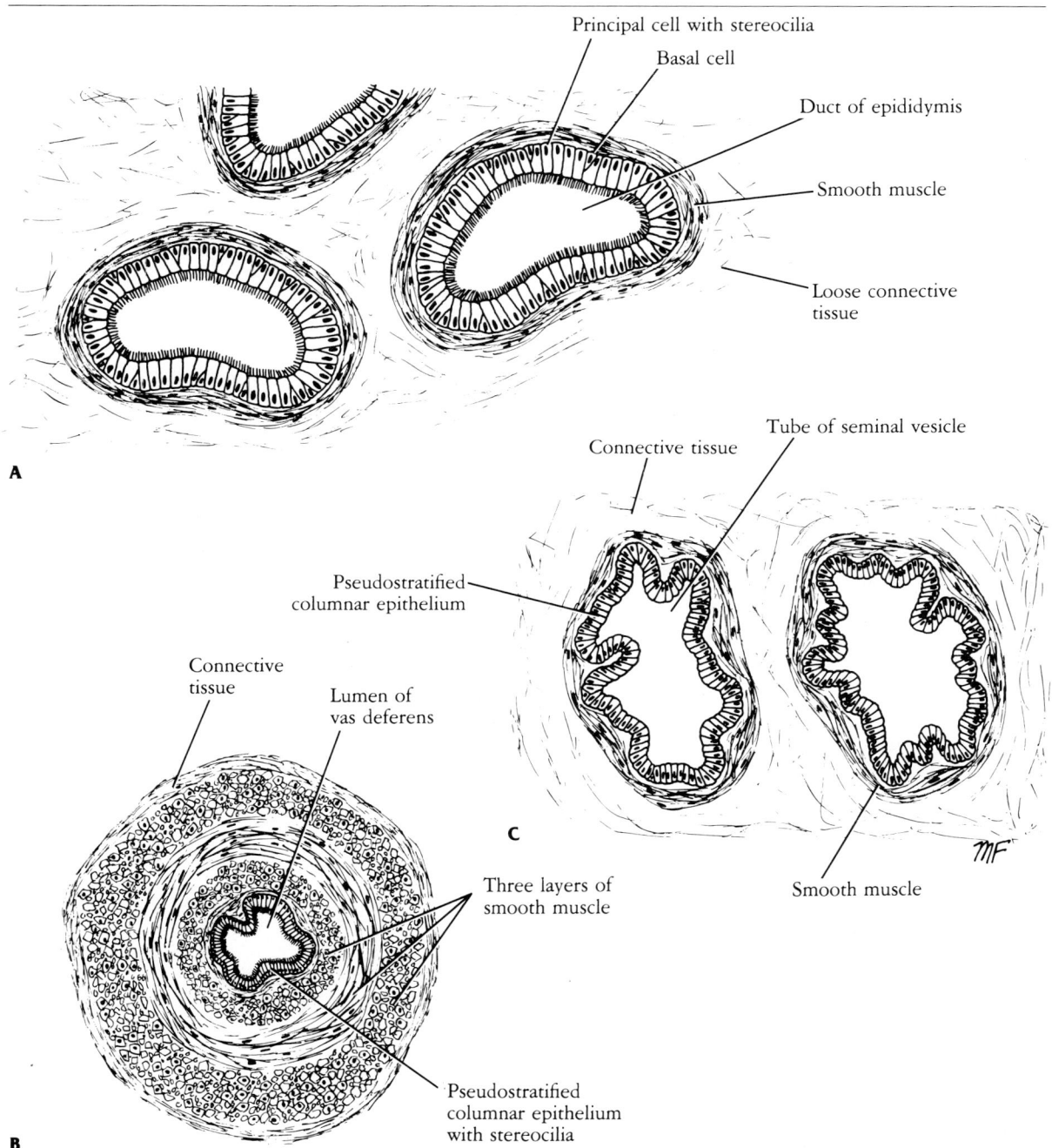

Fig. 14-16. Microscopic structure of (A) the duct of the epididymis, (B) the vas deferens, (C) the tube of the seminal vesicle.

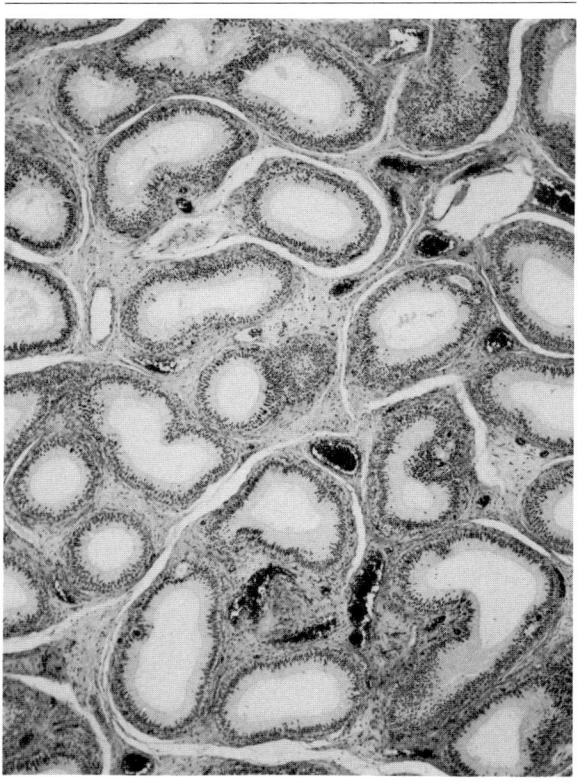

Fig. 14-17. Photomicrograph of a section of the epididymis. Note that the much-coiled duct of the epididymis has been sectioned many times. The coils of the duct are held together by delicate connective tissue. (H&E; ×40.)

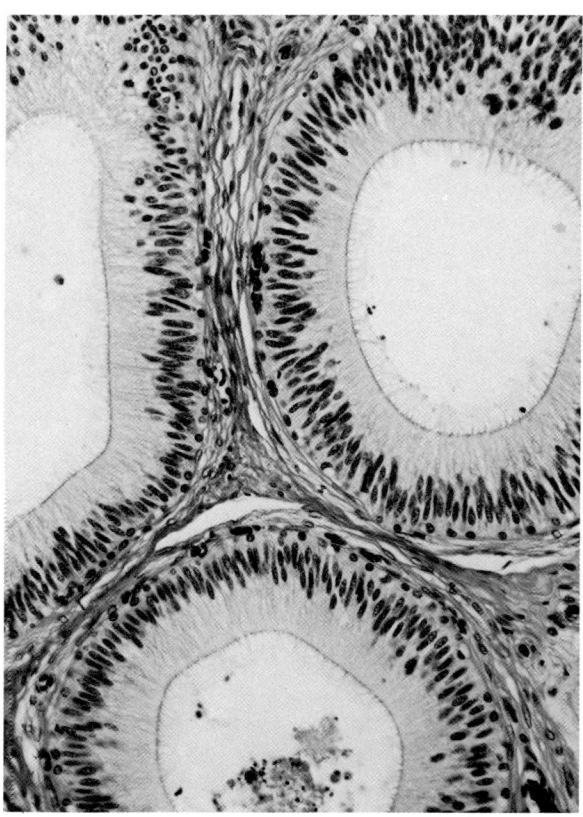

Fig. 14-18. Photomicrograph of a high-power view of a section of the coiled duct of the epididymis. The duct is lined with pseudostratified columnar epithelium. Note that the principal cells possess very long microvilli that project into the lumen. (H&E; ×200.)

known as the *lobules of the epididymis*. These ductules now join to form a single tube called the *duct of the epididymis* (see Fig. 14-2).

The duct of the epididymis is about 6 m (20 feet) long and is coiled to form the *body* and the *tail of the epididymis*. The coils of the duct are held together by delicate connective tissue. Emerging from the tail of the epididymis is the thick-walled, tubular vas deferens (see Fig. 14-2).

The duct of the epididymis is lined with pseudostratified columnar epithelium composed of two types of cells, the principal cells and the basal cells (Figs. 14-16–14-18). The *principal cells* possess extremely long microvilli that project from the free margin of the cells. These villi are so long that they are often called *stereocilia*. The basal cells are small and rest on the basement membrane; they do not extend to the luminal surface of the lining. The epithelium is surrounded by a layer of smooth muscle (see Figs. 14-16 and 14-18) that becomes thicker toward the tail of the epididymis. Most of the smooth muscle fibers in the head of the epididymis are arranged circularly, but toward the tail, three multidirectional layers can be recognized.

Function of the Epididymis

One of the main functions of the epididymis is the absorption of fluid. This process is greatly assisted

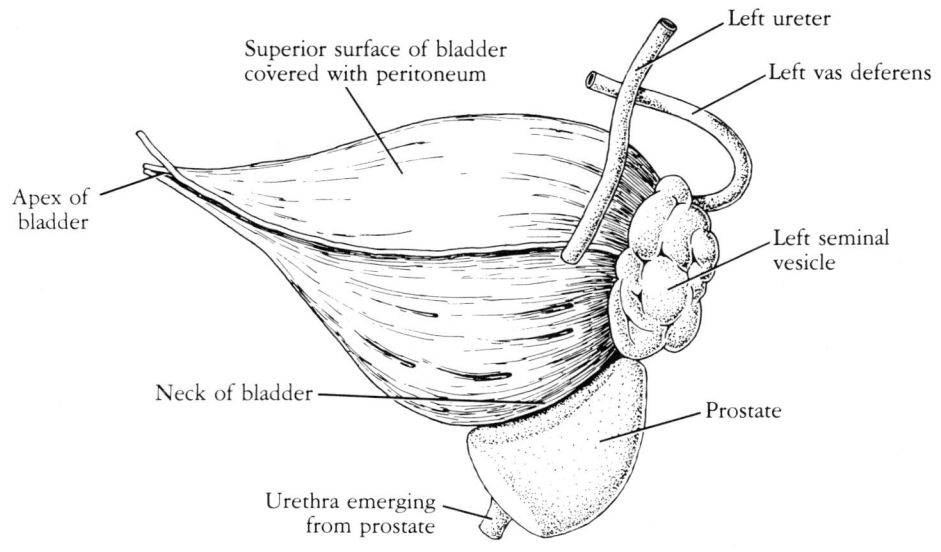
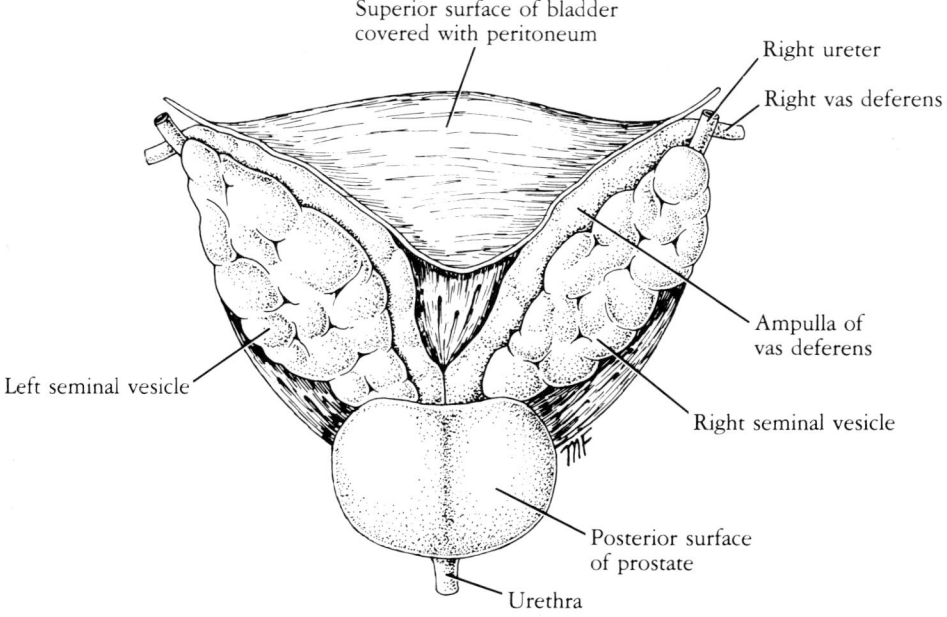

Fig. 14-19. General arrangement of the bladder, ureter, vas deferens, seminal vesicle, and prostate: (A) lateral view; (B) posterior view.

by the long microvilli of the principal cells. The long length of the duct of the epididymis provides storage space for the spermatozoa and allows them to mature. It will be remembered that testicular spermatozoa have little motility, whereas sperm removed from the tail of the epididymis are fully motile. Another function of the epididymis may be the addition of substances to the seminal fluid to nourish the maturing sperm. It is also possible that some of the cells are phagocytic, because fragments of spermatozoa have been seen within the cytoplasm of the lining cells.

Vas Deferens

The vas deferens, or ductus deferens, is a continuation of the duct of the epididymis (see Fig. 14-2). It emerges from the lower end, or tail, of the epididymis and ascends along the posterior border of the testis. It then passes up within the spermatic cord through the inguinal canal into the abdomen (see Fig. 14-1) and then descends into the pelvis to reach the posterior surface of the bladder (Fig. 14-19). Here it expands to form the *ampulla* and then joins the duct of the seminal vesicle to form the *ejaculatory duct*. The vas deferens has a mucous membrane, a very thick muscular coat, and a fibrous coat (Fig. 14-20; see Fig. 14-16).

The *mucous membrane* is arranged in longitudinal folds (see Fig. 14-20) and is lined with columnar epithelium. Toward the distal end, the epithelium is pseudostratified and the columnar cells bear stereocilia (Fig. 14-21). The lamina propria is formed of connective tissue and is fairly prominent.

The *muscular coat* is very thick and consists of three distinct layers of smooth muscle (see Fig. 14-20). The inner and outer layers are arranged longitudinally; between them is a well-defined circular layer (see Fig. 14-21).

The *fibrous coat* is thick and supports the blood vessels and nerves. The vas deferens can be palpated easily between the finger and thumb through the skin of the scrotum. Its cordlike, firm consistency is caused entirely by the thick muscular coat.

The function of the vas deferens is to convey the

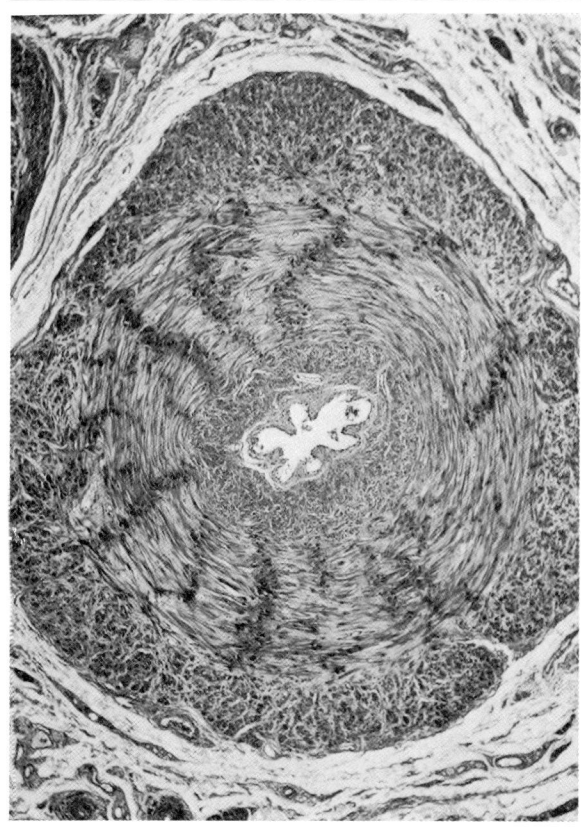

Fig. 14-20. Photomicrograph of a cross section of the vas deferens, showing the very thick muscular wall and the small lumen. (H&E; ×40.)

spermatozoa by peristalsis from the epididymis to the ejaculatory duct during ejaculation.

Ejaculatory Ducts

There are two ejaculatory ducts. Each is formed by the union of the vas deferens and the duct of the seminal vesicle (see Fig. 14-1). The ejaculatory ducts pierce the base of the prostate and run anteroinferiorly, opening into the prostatic urethra just within the orifice of the prostatic utricle (Fig. 14-22). The ducts are lined with simple or pseudostratified columnar epithelium, which is surrounded

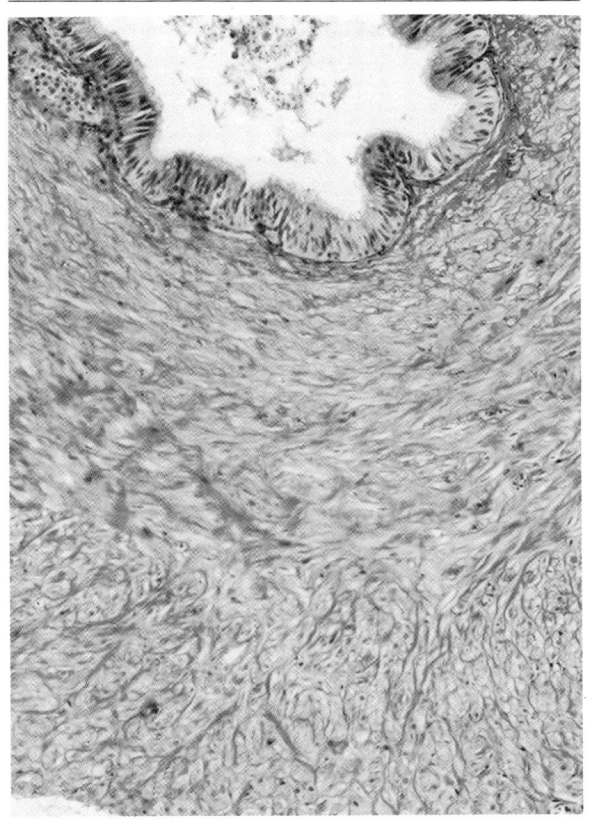

Fig. 14-21. Photomicrograph of a high-power view of a section of the distal part of the vas deferens shown in Figure 14-20. The mucous membrane is arranged in longitudinal folds and is lined with pseudostratified columnar cells that bear stereocilia. The smooth muscular coat is very thick and consists of an inner and an outer layer of longitudinally arranged fibers and a middle circular layer. (H&E; ×100.)

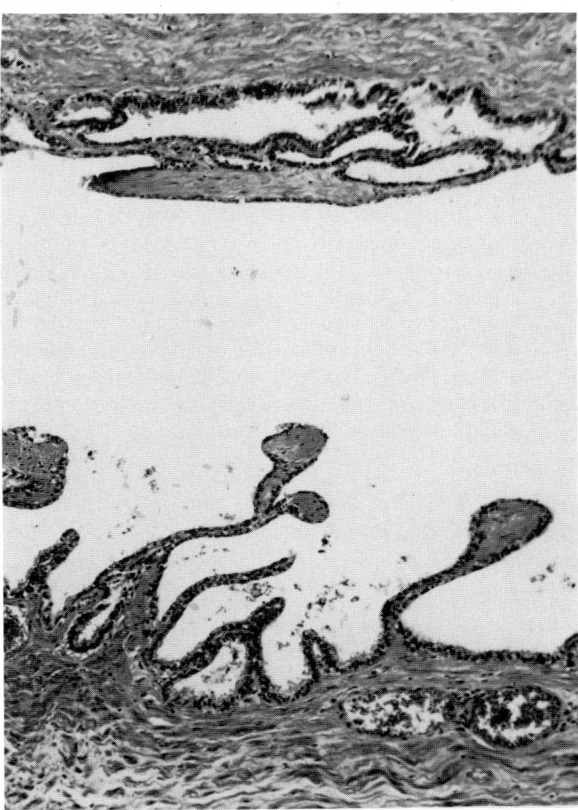

Fig. 14-22. Photomicrograph of part of the tube of the seminal vesicle, showing the mucous membrane that is formed into complex folds. (H&E; ×100.)

by connective tissue. There is no muscle in the wall of the ejaculatory ducts, the propulsive power for the seminal fluid being provided by the smooth muscle in the walls of the vas deferentia, seminal vesicles, and prostate.

The function of the ejaculatory ducts is to convey the spermatozoa and the secretions of the seminal vesicles to the prostatic urethra.

ACCESSORY GLANDS

Seminal Vesicles

The seminal vesicles are paired organs situated within the pelvis between the base of the bladder and the rectum (see Figs. 14-1 and 14-19). Each seminal vesicle consists of a much-coiled tube embedded in connective tissue (see Fig. 14-16). The seminal vesicles have a mucous coat, a muscular coat, and a fibrous coat.

The *mucous membrane* is thrown into many complex folds (Figs. 14-22 and 14-23) and is lined with pseudostratified columnar epithelium that secretes a yellowish viscous liquid. The *muscular coat* is com-

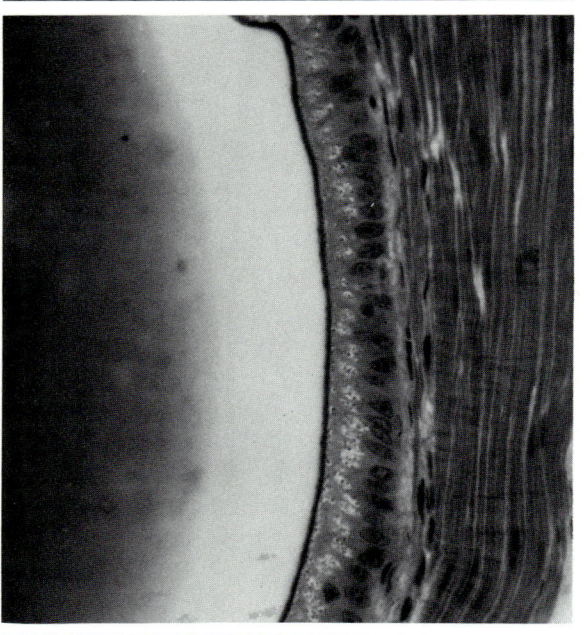

Fig. 14-23. Photomicrograph of a plastic section of the wall of the tube of the seminal vesicle. The mucous membrane is lined with columnar epithelium. Note the circularly arranged smooth muscle fibers outside the mucous membrane. (H&E; ×400.)

posed of smooth muscle fibers arranged in inner circular and outer longitudinal layers. The *fibrous coat* is composed of loose connective tissue.

The function of the seminal vesicles is controlled by testosterone; castration results in atrophy of the vesicles. The secretions of the mucous membrane contribute to the seminal fluid; they contain fructose and other important substances, such as ascorbic acid, inositol, and amino acids, that are essential for nourishment of the spermatozoa. Prostaglandins are also secreted, and it is possible that they assist fertilization by making the mucus of the cervix of the uterus more receptive to spermatozoa. The walls of the seminal vesicles contract during ejaculation and expel their contents into the ejaculatory ducts, thus washing the spermatozoa out of the urethra.

Prostate

The prostate is a single large gland that surrounds the prostatic urethra and lies within the pelvis below the neck of the bladder (see Fig. 14-19). It possesses a thin capsule composed of connective tissue and smooth muscle. The interior of the organ is made up of a large number of glands, whose ducts open into the prostatic urethra (see Fig. 14-24). The glands are embedded in a mixture of smooth muscle and connective tissue.

The interior of the prostate is divided incompletely into a number of lobes by the passage of the two ejaculatory ducts (see Fig. 14-24). These lobes are: (1) The small middle, or median, lobe, which is the wedge of gland situated between the urethra and the ejaculatory ducts. Its upper surface is related to the trigone of the bladder; it is rich in glands. (2) The posterior lobe is situated behind the urethra and below the ejaculatory ducts and also contains glandular tissue. (3) The right and left lobes lie on either side of the urethra and are separated from each other by a shallow, vertical groove on the posterior surface of the prostate. The lateral lobes contain many glands. (4) The anterior lobe lies in front of the urethra and is almost devoid of glandular tissue (see Fig. 14-24).

The glands of the prostate are tubulo-alveolar (Fig. 14-25), and the majority open by ducts into the prostatic sinuses on either side of the urethral crest (see Fig. 14-24). The glands situated in the periphery of the prostate are large and branched, and the ducts curve posteriorly to open into the sinuses. The inner zone of the prostate contains smaller submucosal glands that also open into the sinuses. A number of even smaller mucosal glands surround the prostatic urethra and open into its lumen. The epithelium lining the glands is columnar (Fig. 14-26), and the cytoplasm contains numerous secretory granules; they are strongly positive for acid phosphatase. The epithelium rests on loose connective tissue. In older men, concretions, which may be partially calcified, may be found in the lumen of a secretory gland (Fig. 14-27). They are probably formed of precipitated secretory material.

The smooth muscle in the stroma is concentrated in two areas. Just beneath the capsule is a well-defined layer that surrounds the gland. Another

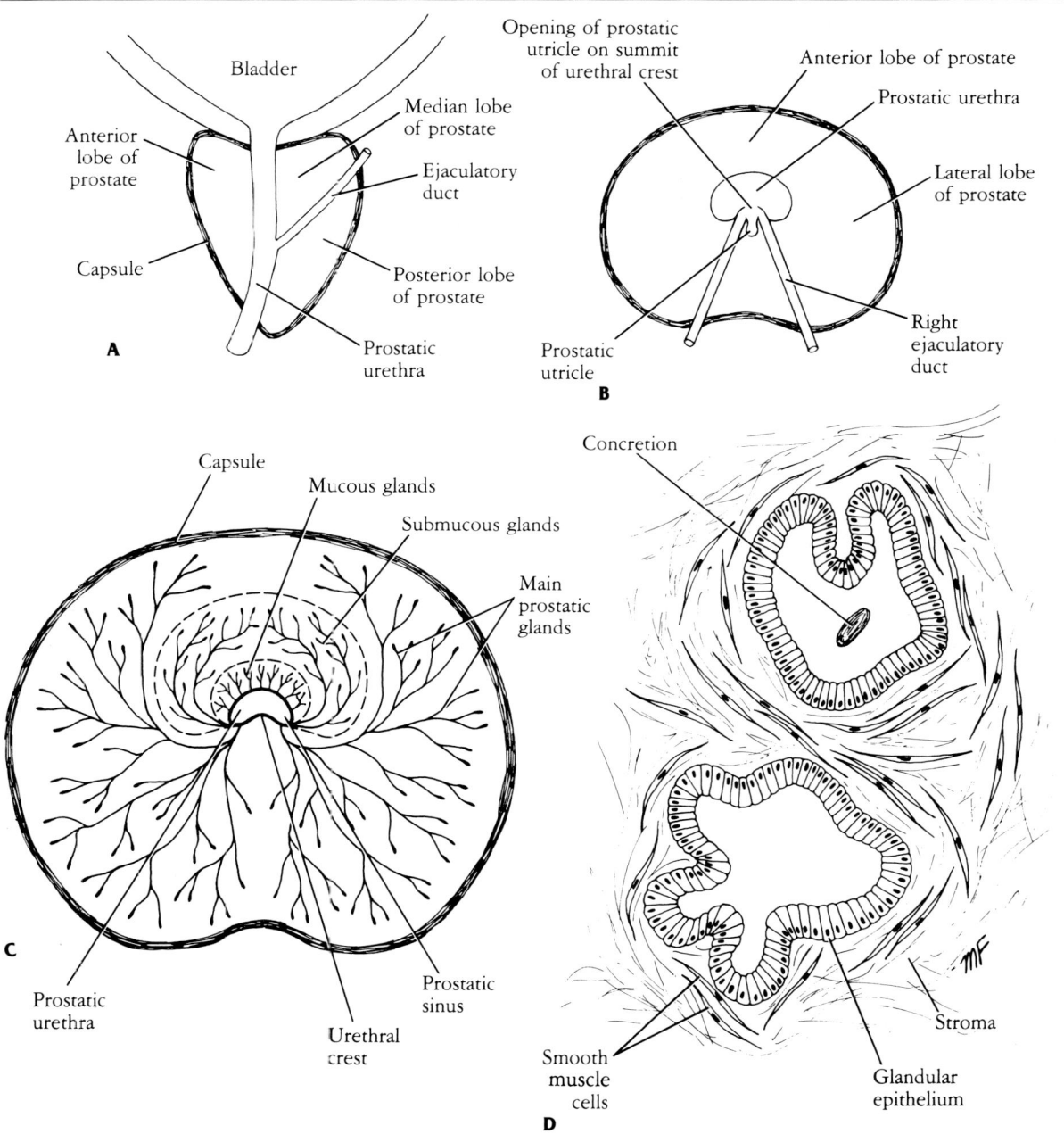

Fig. 14-24. A: Sagittal section of the prostate. B: Horizontal section of the prostate. C: Opening of the prostatic glands into the urethra as seen in horizontal section. D: Structure of the prostatic glands, which are embedded in a mixture of smooth muscle and connective tissue.

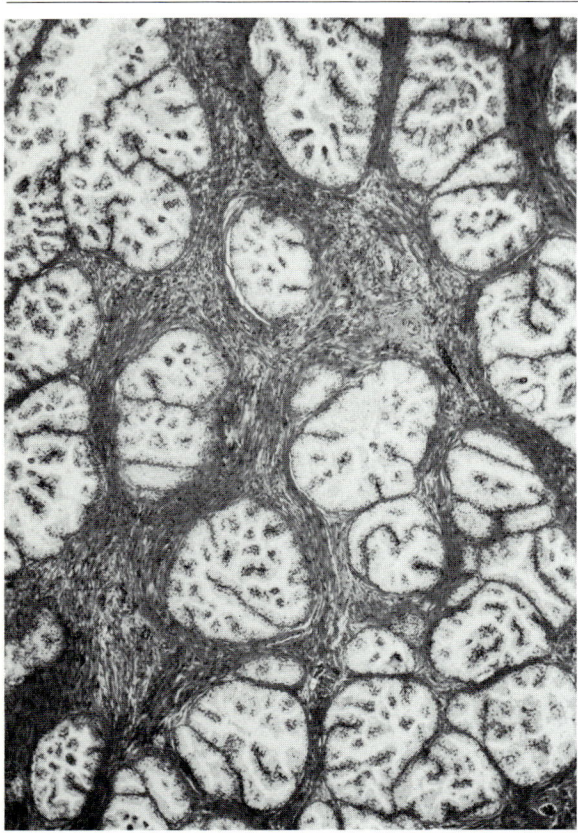

Fig. 14-25. *Photomicrograph of a portion of the prostate. Note the large number of glands embedded in a mixture of smooth muscle and connective tissue. (H&E; ×40.)*

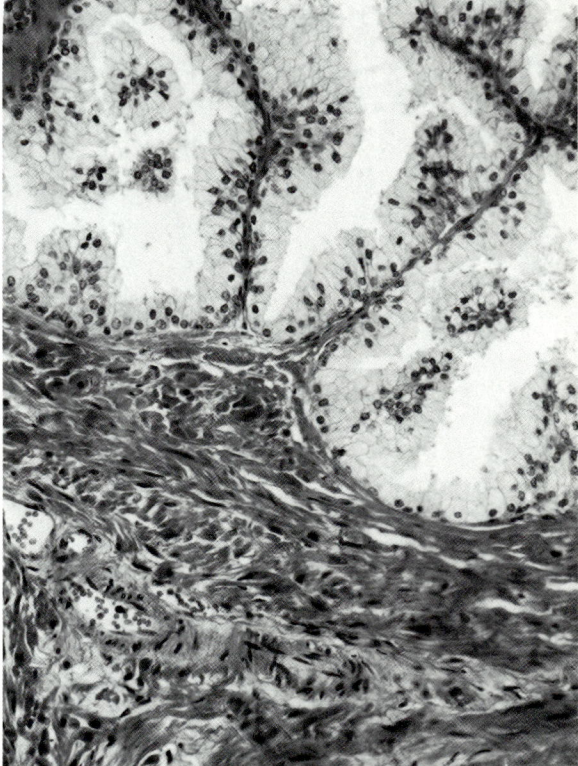

Fig. 14-26. *Photomicrograph of a high-power view of part of the prostate section seen in Figure 14-25, showing the tubuloalveolar glands lined with columnar epithelial cells. The epithelium rests on connective tissue. (H&E; ×100.)*

layer surrounds the urethra and is continuous with the smooth muscle of the bladder above and that surrounding the membranous urethra below.

The function of the prostate is controlled by testosterone, and castration produces atrophy of the gland. The secretion is a thin, milky fluid containing citric acid and acid phosphatase. It is added to the seminal fluid at the time of ejaculation. The smooth muscle in the capsule and stroma contract, and the secretion from the many glands is squeezed into the prostatic urethra. The prostatic secretion is alkaline and helps to neutralize the acidity in the vagina.

Bulbo-urethral Glands

The bulbo-urethral glands, or Cowper's glands, are two small glands located in the deep perineal pouch (see Fig. 14-1). These glands are tubulo-alveolar, and their columnar cells secrete mucus. The ducts of the glands open into the penile part of the urethra. The secretion is poured into the urethra as the result of erotic stimulation.

The *function of the bulbo-urethral glands* is controlled by testosterone, and castration produces atrophy of the glands. The secretion of the glands is added to the seminal fluid. The precise function of the secretion is unknown.

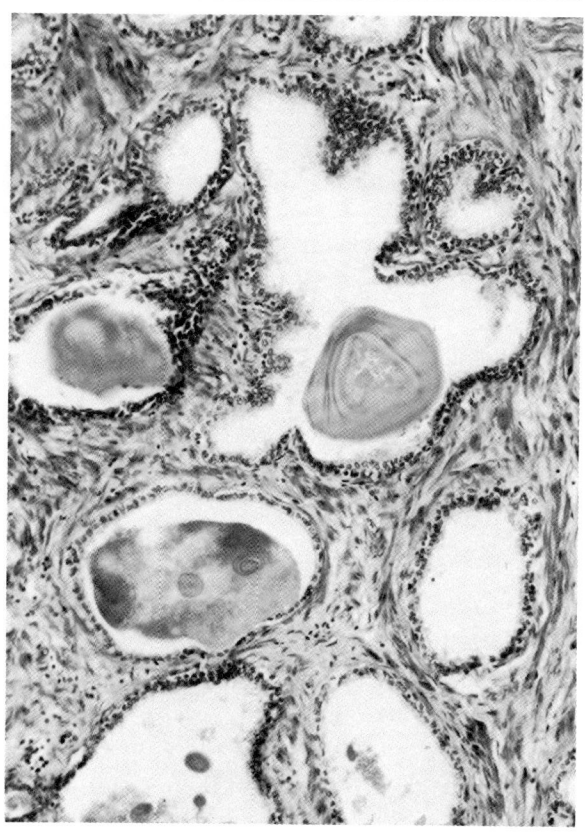

Fig. 14-27. Photomicrograph of a portion of the prostate removed from an old man. Note several concretions in the lumina of the glands. (H&E; ×100.)

PENIS

The penis has a fixed *root* and a *body*, which hangs free (Fig. 14-28; see Fig. 14-1).

The root of the penis is made up of three masses of erectile tissue: the *bulb* of the penis and the *right* and *left crura* of the penis (see Fig. 14-28). The bulb is situated at the midline. It is traversed by the urethra and is covered on its outer surface by sheets of skeletal muscle, the *bulbo-spongiosus muscles*. Each crus is attached to the side of the pubic arch and is covered on its outer surface by a sheet of skeletal muscle, the *ischiocavernosus muscle*. The bulb and crura continue forward into the body of the penis.

The body of the penis essentially is composed of three cylinders of erectile tissue enclosed in a tubular sheath of fascia. The erectile tissue consists of two dorsally placed *corpora cavernosa* and a single *corpus spongiosum* applied to their ventral surface (see Fig. 14-28). At its distal extremity, the corpus spongiosum expands to form the *glans penis,* which covers the distal ends of the corpora cavernosa. The *prepuce* is a hoodlike fold of skin that covers the glans (see Fig. 14-28).

Each cylinder of erectile tissue is composed of a tough wall of dense fibrous tissue. The walls of the adjacent corpora cavernosa fuse at the midline to form a median septum. In the glans penis, the dermis of the covering skin forms the fibrous wall. Inside the erectile tissue is a spongework of connective tissue and smooth muscle (Fig. 14-29). The vascular spaces in the sponge are lined with endothelium and are filled with blood from branches of the internal pudendal artery; the spaces are drained by veins that enter the internal pudendal vein. The cylinders of erectile tissue are enclosed in fascia and surrounded by thin skin. The skin on the distal part of the body is devoid of hair.

Erection

Erection in the male is built up gradually as a consequence of various sexual stimuli. Pleasurable sights, sounds, smells, and other psychic stimuli, fortified later by direct tactile stimuli from the general body skin and genital skin, result in a bombardment of the central nervous system by afferent stimuli. Efferent nervous impulses pass down the spinal cord to the parasympathetic outflow in the second, third, and fourth sacral segments. The parasympathetic preganglionic fibers enter the pelvic plexuses and synapse on the postganglionic neurons. The postganglionic fibers join the internal pudendal arteries and are distributed along their branches, which enter the erectile tissue at the root of the penis. Vasodilatation of the arteries now occurs, greatly increasing blood flow through the blood spaces of the erectile tissue. The corpora cavernosa and corpus spongiosum become engorged with blood and expand, compressing their draining veins against the

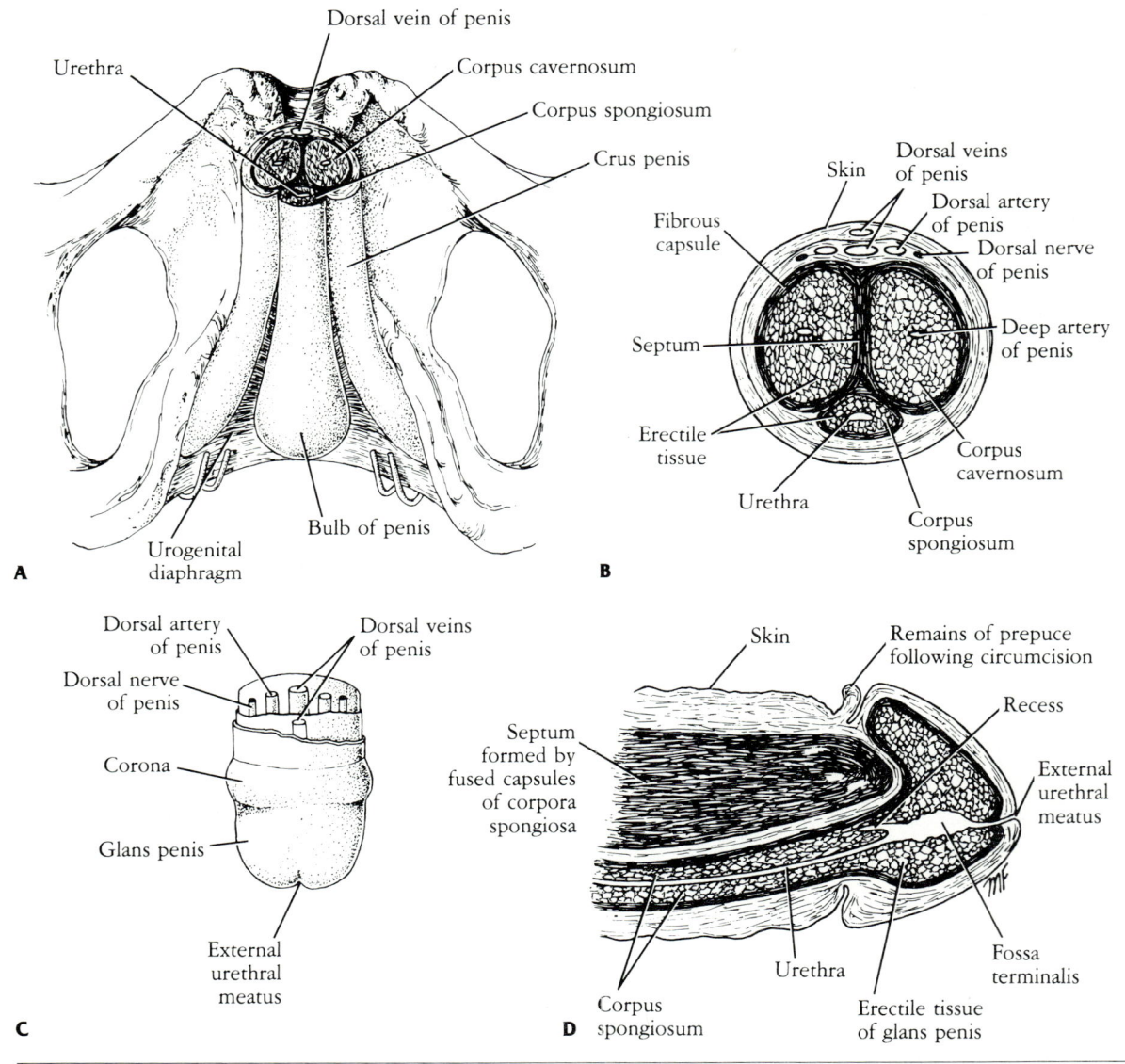

Fig. 14-28. A: General arrangement of the erectile tissue in the root of the penis. B: Cross section of the body of the penis. C: Opening of the external urethral meatus on the glans penis. D: Longitudinal section of the glans and body of the penis, showing the urethra within the corpus spongiosum.

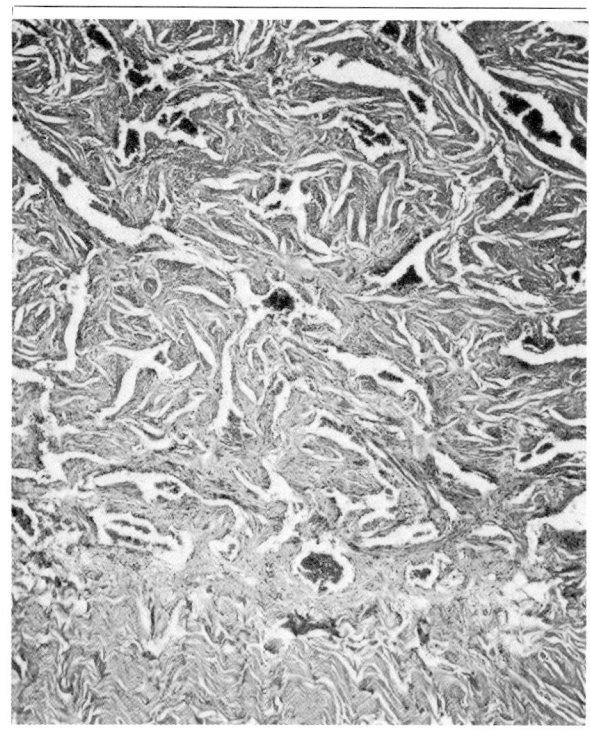

Fig. 14-29. Photomicrograph of a section of the erectile tissue of the corpus cavernosum, showing a spongework of connective tissue and smooth muscle. The vascular spaces of the sponge are lined with endothelium. (H&E; ×40.)

surrounding fascia. By this means, the outflow of blood from the erectile tissue is retarded, and the internal pressure thus is accentuated further and maintained. The penis thus increases in length and diameter and assumes the erect position.

Once the climax of sexual excitement is reached and ejaculation takes place, or the excitement passes or is inhibited, the arteries supplying the erectile tissue undergo vasoconstriction. The penis then returns to its flaccid state.

STORAGE AND TRANSPORT OF SPERMATOZOA

At the conclusion of spermatogenesis, the spermatozoa become detached from the Sertoli cells and lie free in the fluid in the seminiferous tubules. At this stage of their development, they are nonmotile and are transported passively in groups into the efferent ductules of the testis and the duct of the epididymis by the contraction of smooth muscle in the walls of these passages and by the action of the ciliated epithelium. The spermatozoa accumulate in the epididymis and are nourished with the secretion of the lining epithelium. About 20 days are required for the spermatozoa to traverse the 6-meter length of the tortuous duct of the epididymis. During this period, they become motile and attain their full physiological state, which they retain only for a limited time. If ejaculation does not occur, the sperm degenerate and die.

The introduction of spermatozoa into the vagina involves erection of the penis and ejaculation of the seminal fluid.

Ejaculation

During the increasing sexual excitement that occurs during sex play, the external urinary meatus of the glans penis becomes moist because of the secretions of the bulbo-urethral glands.

Friction on the glans penis, reinforced by other afferent nervous impulses, results in a discharge that travels along the sympathetic nerve fibers to the smooth muscle of the duct of the epididymis and the vas deferens on each side, the seminal vesicles, and the prostate. The smooth muscle contracts, and the spermatozoa, together with the secretions of the seminal vesicles and prostate, are discharged into the prostatic urethra. The fluid now joins the secretions of the bulbo-urethral glands and is ejected from the penile urethra by the rhythmic contractions of the bulbospongiosus muscles, which compress the urethra. Meanwhile, the sphincter of the bladder contracts and prevents a reflux of spermatozoa into the bladder. The spermatozoa and the secretions of the several accessory glands constitute the *seminal fluid,* or *semen.*

At the climax of male sexual excitement, a mass discharge of nervous impulses takes place in the central nervous system. Impulses pass down the spinal cord to the sympathetic outflow (T1 to L2). The nervous impulses that pass to the genital organs are thought to leave the cord at the first and second lumbar segments in the preganglionic sympathetic fibers. Many of these fibers synapse with postganglionic neurons in the first and second lumbar ganglia. Other fibers may synapse in ganglia in the lower lumbar or pelvic parts of the sympathetic trunks. The postganglionic fibers are then distributed to the vas deferens, the seminal vesicles, and the prostate via the hypogastric and pelvic plexuses.

Semen

The average volume of the ejaculate is about 3.5 ml. The spermatozoa are suspended in the secretions of the accessory glands, termed the *seminal plasma*. The average concentration of spermatozoa is about 100 million per milliliter; of these, about 20 percent are morphologically abnormal and almost 25 percent are nonmotile. The secretion of the seminal vesicles contributes substantially to the volume of the semen. It is rich in fructose, which is a source of energy for the highly motile spermatozoa. The alkaline secretions of the other accessory glands help neutralize the acid contents of the male urethra and the vagina. Following ejaculation, the spermatozoa become actively motile; their tails undulate and propel them forward and at the same time rotate them on their long axis.

It has been estimated that 10 to 20 percent of marriages are sterile, and in about one-third to one-half of these, the male is the sterile partner. For this reason, microscopic and biochemical examination of the semen is important in childless marriages.

CLINICAL NOTES

Testes

The testes develop high up on the posterior abdominal wall, and in late fetal life they descend behind the peritoneum, dragging their blood supply, nerve supply, and lymphatic drainage after them. During the seventh fetal month, the testes pass through the inguinal canal to their final position in the scrotum. If neither testis descends into the scrotum, the person will be sterile. The higher temperature in the abdominal cavity and in the inguinal canal will cause irreversible destructive changes in the seminiferous tubules of the testes. The organs will become smaller, and the interior gradually will be replaced by fibrous tissue. The normal stimulus for the descent of the testis through the inguinal canal into the scrotum is testosterone, which is secreted by the fetal testes.

Cryptorchidism

Cryptorchidism (undescended testes) may be unilateral or bilateral. Two forms of imperfect descent are recognized, incomplete descent and maldescent.

Incomplete descent, in which the testis, although traveling down its normal path, fails to reach the floor of the scrotum. The testis may be found within the abdomen, within the inguinal canal, at the superficial inguinal ring, or high up in the scrotum.

Maldescent, in which the testis travels down an abnormal path and fails to reach the scrotum. The testis may be found in the superficial fascia of the anterior abdominal wall above the inguinal ligament, in front of the pubis, in the perineum, or in the thigh.

Because of the sensitivity of spermatogenesis to temperature, it is necessary to bring the testis down into the scrotum. If the testis is brought down into the scrotum surgically before puberty, it will develop and function normally. A maldescended testis, although often developing normally, is very susceptible to traumatic injury and for this reason should be placed in the scrotum. Many authorities believe that there is a greater incidence of tumor formation in testes that have not descended into the scrotum.

Male Infertility

As we have discussed, normal spermatogenesis may be prevented by excessive temperatures. Orchitis, or inflammation of the testis, is a common complication of mumps; when bilateral, it may cause sterility. The orchitis in this case usually develops about 1 week after the swelling of the parotid salivary glands. The inflammatory reaction is accompanied by severe edema, which raises the pressure inside the tough fibrous tunica albuginea and causes intense pain. Pressure atrophy of the seminiferous tubules occurs.

Should the number of spermatozoa fall below 20 million per milliliter, or one-fifth the normal concentration, a man is likely to be infertile.

Abnormal-looking spermatozoa frequently are found in the semen. Spermatozoa may have abnormally small or large heads. They may have tapering or narrow heads, two or more tails, or one tail and two heads. Spermatozoa with a normal appearance may lack normal motility. Normal spermatozoa move rapidly and in a straight line; abnormal forms are sluggish and tend to move in a circle or an irregular pattern. The percentage of spermatozoa that can be abnormal without loss of fertility is difficult to estimate but is believed to be as high as 10 percent.

Tumors of the Testes

The great majority of tumors of the testes arise from spermatogonia; these tumors are almost always malignant. The *seminomas* are the most common form; they remain localized for a long time before metastasizing to the para-aortic lymph nodes. Fortunately, such tumors are radiosensitive, and if they are diagnosed early, the prognosis is good. *Embryonal carcinomas* are another form of malignant tumor; they give rise to cell types derived from ectoderm, mesenchyme, and endoderm. These tumors are more malignant than seminomas, and they are not very sensitive to radiation. *Choriocarcinomas* are rare and are formed of cytotrophoblast and syncytiotrophoblast cells. They are highly malignant, and the prognosis is very poor.

Benign tumors of the interstitial cells are rare; they may elaborate androgens.

EPIDIDYMIS

Infection of the epididymis is common after puberty and can be caused by gonococcal or nonspecific infection, usually following retrograde spread of infection from the urethra, prostate, and seminal vesicles. Chronic infection, in the form of tuberculosis, does occur and is usually spread via the bloodstream from tuberculosis of the lungs.

VAS DEFERENS

The vas deferens conveys spermatozoa from the epididymis to the ejaculatory duct on each side of the body. Any inflammatory lesion of this structure or mechanical obstruction (such as a vasectomy) on both sides may produce infertility. Joining the normal, patent part of the vas to the epididymis or to a more distal segment of the vas (vasovasostomy) may correct the obstruction. Unfortunately, the vas deferens also serves as a duct for the retrograde spread of infection from the prostatic urethra to the epididymis and testis. For this reason, bilateral vasectomy routinely is performed by urologists prior to prostatic surgery.

Bilateral vasectomy is a simple surgical method of making a male sterile. Both vasa are ligated and divided through a small incision under local anesthesia. The patient is pronounced sterile when a masturbation specimen of semen is found to contain no spermatozoa. The procedure of vasovasostomy, mentioned earlier, is a microsurgical procedure that can make the male fertile again. The procedure is difficult, however, and is not always successful.

PROSTATE

Inflammation of the prostate is a common condition. The infecting organisms reach the prostate by ascending through the urethra. If many of the numerous glands become infected, the result is often persistence of the infection, a condition known as *chronic prostatitis*. E. coli is the most common infecting organism. Chronic prostatitis frequently leads to recurrent urinary infections, with spread to the epididymis.

Benign enlargement of the prostate is common in men over 50 years of age. The cause of the enlargement is unknown but may be an imbalance in the hormonal control of the gland involving both androgens and estrogens. It will be remembered that androgens are produced by the interstitial cells of the testis and that estrogens can also be produced by

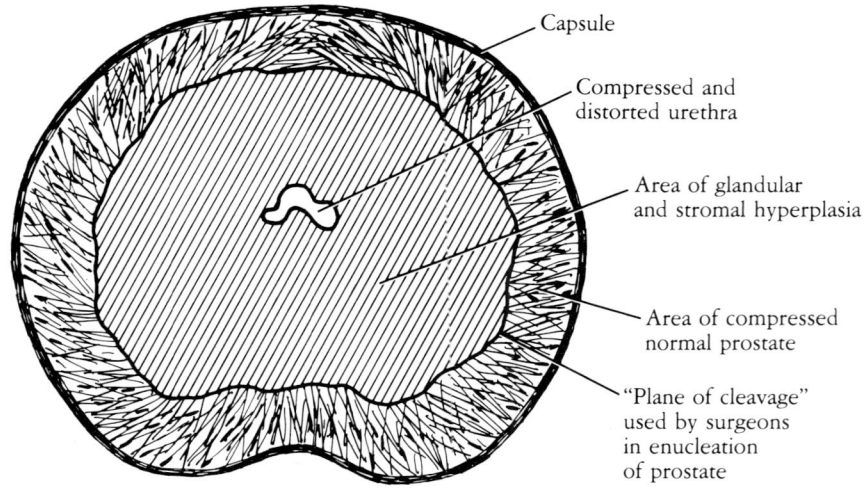
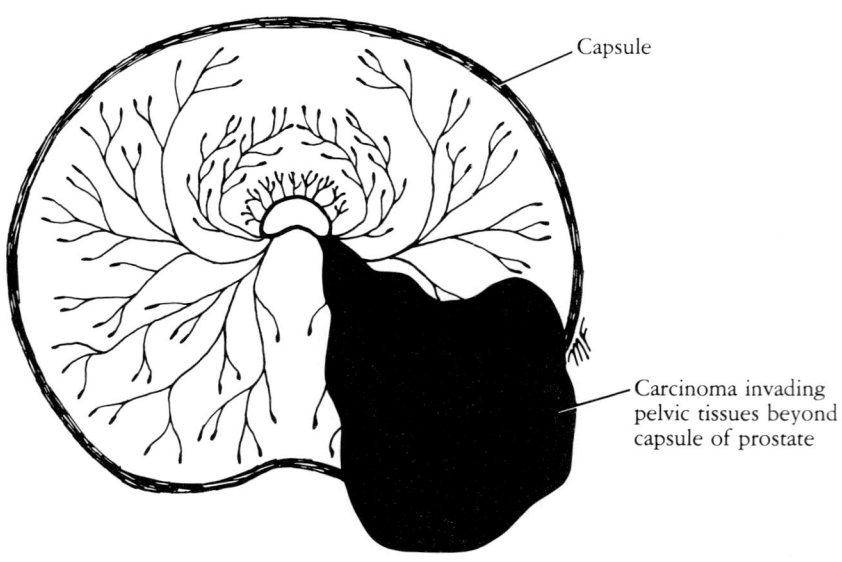

Fig. 14-30. Cross sections of two prostates, showing a benign enlargement and a carcinoma.

these cells, the Sertoli cells, and the suprarenal cortex. The enlargement results from the appearance of nodules arising in the inner zone of the prostate. The nodules are composed of a mixture of fibromuscular hypertrophy and hyperplasia and glandular hypertrophy and hyperplasia. Many of the glands become cystically dilated. As the nodules in the inner zone of the gland enlarge, they compress the surrounding outer glandular tissue, creating a kind of false capsule. This process provides the surgeon with a line of cleavage that permits enucleation of the inner zone of the prostate, with the outer zone being left behind (a suprapubic prostatectomy) (Fig. 14-30).

Fortunately, only a few men with benign enlargement of the prostate possess clinical symptoms. The median lobe may enlarge upward and encroach within the sphincter vesicae, located at the neck of the bladder. The resultant leakage of urine into the prostatic urethra causes an intense reflex desire to micturate. Enlargement of the median and lateral lobes of the gland produces elongation and lateral compression and distortion of the urethra, so that the patient experiences difficulty in passing urine, and the stream is weak. Back-pressure effects on the ureters and both kidneys are a common complication. Enlargement of the median lobe results in the formation of a pouch of stagnant urine behind the urethral orifice within the bladder. The stagnant urine frequently becomes infected, and bladder inflammation (cystitis) adds to the patient's symptoms.

Carcinoma of the prostate is very common in men over 50 years of age and usually arises in the peripheral areas of the gland (see Fig. 14-30). The lesion is an adenocarcinoma. The normal prostate produces small amounts of acid phosphatase, which escapes into the bloodstream. New radioimmunoassay techniques have been developed that can detect a rise in enzyme production in cases of prostatic cancer. As many as 30 percent of men over the age of 50 have a small carcinoma of the prostate that is producing no clinical signs or symptoms.

For many years, it has been recognized that carcinoma of the prostate is androgen-dependent. Although it is not possible to cure prostatic cancer with hormonal treatment, the administration of estrogens, bilateral orchidectomy, or both can increase the survival rate greatly.

PENIS

Phimosis. The prepuce normally provides a covering for the glans and can be retracted easily, exposing the glans. Should the orifice of the prepuce be too small, retraction is impossible, a condition known as *phimosis.* Phimosis can be a congenital defect or can result from infection and inflammation of the prepuce with secondary fibrosis and constriction. In severe cases of phimosis, secretions from the undersurface of the prepuce become trapped beneath it, leading to infection and further scarring. In severe instances, obstruction of the urethra may result.

Infections of the penis are common and include the various venereal diseases.

Tumors of the penis are rare. Squamous cell carcinoma of the glans is the usual form, and protection against this malignant tumor can be obtained by circumcision in infancy. It is thought that circumcision, by preventing the accumulation of secretions (smegma) beneath the prepuce, removes the possibility of chronic irritation and infections, which are thought to be responsible for the malignant change in the squamous epithelium.

Impotence. Erection of the penis is a vascular phenomenon and depends on the dilatation of the arteries supplying the erectile tissue and the simultaneous constriction of the veins draining the tissue. A normal man should be able to experience an erection (be potent) until he is at least 90 years old. Impotence can be caused by a circulatory failure, such as obstruction of the common or internal iliac arteries, or by interference with the innervation of the arteries following a spinal cord injury. Adrenergic blocking agents, such as the phenothiazines, can cause impotence. Many individuals with impotence have psychological problems.

EJACULATORY PROBLEMS

A patient may have problems with erection (impotence), may have an abnormal seminal fluid with insufficient numbers of healthy spermatozoa (infertility), or may be unable to ejaculate normally. An individual who has had a bilateral vasectomy can ejaculate without difficulty; the emission consists of the secretions of the seminal vesicles, prostate, and bulbo-urethral and urethral glands. The sexual act is completed satisfactorily, but the person is sterile.

Retrograde ejaculation can occur in a patient with a malfunctioning bladder sphincter. It may be caused by diabetic neuropathy or spinal cord injuries in which the nerve supply to the bladder sphincter is altered. Any surgical damage to the bladder neck can also cause this problem. On ejaculation, the seminal fluid enters the bladder rather than the penile urethra.

Premature ejaculation can cause extreme frustration to the man and his sexual partner. Consultation with a sex counselor may be required to overcome this functional disorder.

CLINICAL PROBLEMS

For the answers to these problems, see page 810.

1. An 80-year-old man visits his physician and asks his advice about marrying a 25-year-old woman. He says they are devoted to each other and want to raise a family. He is concerned that his advanced age may interfere with his ability to have intercourse and to produce viable spermatozoa. Using your knowledge of histology and physiology, what advice would you give this patient?

2. A 16-year-old boy is diagnosed as having mumps. He has swelling in the right parotid region and notes some discomfort on opening and closing his mouth. One week later, he develops severe pain in the left testicle. On examination, the left testicle is slightly swollen, tense, and acutely tender. He has a pyrexia of 100°F. A diagnosis is made of left-sided orchitis secondary to the mumps infection. Using your knowledge of histology and physiology, do you think that sterility will follow this infection?

3. Describe in detail the process of spermatogenesis. Indicate at what stage the number of chromosomes is reduced to the haploid number. What are the advantages to the human race of having a meiotic division of the gametes prior to fertilization?

4. A 10-year-old boy is playing ball with a friend during school recess. While making a tackle, the boy receives a severe blow to his scrotum from his friend's knee. The boy collapses on the ground in extreme pain and has difficulty in getting his breath. The teacher helps him to his feet. He then complains of pain in the scrotum and says he feels sick. Why are the testes so sensitive to trauma, and why are the effects so widespread? Using your knowledge of histology, describe the general structure of the testes.

5. Describe the microscopic structure of a Sertoli cell. Explain the functions of these cells.

6. What special tests could you perform on a man whom you believe may be responsible for a sterile marriage?

7. An 18-year-old man is medically examined prior to entering the army. On physical examination, he is found to have bilaterally undescended testes (cryptorchidism). Based on your knowledge of anatomy and physiology, what advice would you give this patient?

8. Describe the structure and function of the epididymis. Clinically, it is a common site of infection. From where in the male reproductive tract do the organisms spread?

9. A medical student who enjoys the company of the opposite sex decides to have a vasectomy. He asks his physician if there will be any unpleasant aftereffects of the operation. He also wants to know if it will be possible for him to have another operation later to restore the continuity of the vas deferens and allow him to reproduce. What would you tell the student? Describe the structure and function of the vas deferens.

10. A 63-year-old man has a history of prostatic disease. His latest symptoms include difficulty in starting to micturate, a poor urinary stream, and dif-

ficulty in stopping the flow of urine. Which lobe or lobes of the prostate are likely to interfere with the sphincter vesicae? Describe the histological structure of the prostate gland. What is the function of the prostatic secretion, and what controls the activity of this gland? What is benign enlargement of the prostate, and what mechanism is thought to be responsible for it? When performing a suprapubic prostatectomy for benign enlargement of the gland, the urological surgeon feels for a line of cleavage in the prostate that will permit enucleation of the prostate. What is this so-called line of cleavage?

11. A 68-year-old man with a history of prostatic disease is found on radiography of his skeleton to have extensive carcinomatous metastases in his pelvis and lumbar vertebrae. His serum acid phosphatase level is abnormally high, and a rectal examination reveals a hard nodule on the posterior surface of the prostate. A carcinoma of the prostate arises from which cells in the gland? Which part of the prostate commonly is first involved in this disease? What part can hormonal therapy play in the treatment of this common and fatal disease?

12. Describe the structure of the penis as seen in cross section on a microscopic slide. Describe the mechanisms involved in erection of the penis. What is the difference between impotence and infertility? Give an account of the mechanisms involved in ejaculation.

ADDITIONAL READING

Arimura, A. Hypothalamic gonadotropin-releasing hormone and reproduction. *Int. Rev. Physiol.* 13:1, 1977.

Bardin, C. W. Pituitary-testicular axis. In Yen, S. S. C., and Jaffe, R. B. (eds.), *Reproductive Endocrinology*. Philadelphia: Saunders, 1978, p. 110.

Camatini, M., Franchi, E., and deCurtis, I. Sertoli junctions in human testes: A freeze fracture lanthanum tracer study. *J. Submicrosc. Cytol.* 11:511, 1979.

Christensen, A. K. Fine structure of testicular interstitial cells in humans. In Rosemberg, E., and Paulsen, C. A. (eds.), *Advances in Experimental Medicine and Biology: The Human Testis.* New York: Plenum, 1970, p. 75.

Clark, R. V. Three dimensional organization of testicular interstitial tissue and lymphatic space in the rat. *Anat. Rec.* 184:203, 1976.

Clermont, Y. Renewal of spermatogonia in man. *Am. J. Anat.* 118:509, 1966.

Dym, M. The fine structure of monkey Sertoli cells in the transitional zone at the junction of the seminiferous tubules with the tubuli recti. *Am. J. Anat.* 140:1, 1974.

Dym, M. The mammalian rete testes: A morphological examination. *Anat. Rec.* 186:493, 1976.

Dym, M., and Cavicchia, J. C. Functional morphology of the testis. *Biol. Reprod.* 18:1, 1978.

Dym, M., and Fawcett, D. W. The blood-testis barrier in the rat and physiologic compartment of the seminiferous epithelium. *Biol. Reprod.* 3:308, 1970.

Fawcett, D. W. The mammalian spermatozoon. *Dev. Biol.* 44:394, 1975.

Fawcett, D. W., Neaves, W. B., and Flores, M. N. Comparative observations on intertubular lymphatics and the organization of the interstitial tissue of the mammalian testis. *Biol. Reprod.* 9:500, 1973.

Fink, G. Feedback actions of target hormones on hypothalamus and pituitary, with special reference to gonadal steroids. *Ann. Rev. Physiol.* 41:571, 1979.

Franks, L. M. Benign nodular hyperplasia of the prostate: A review. *Ann. R. Coll. Surg. (Eng.)* 14:92, 1954.

Franks, L. M. Etiology, epidemiology, and pathology of prostatic cancer. *Cancer* 32:1092, 1973.

Hafez, E. S. E., and Spring-Mills, E. (eds.). *Accessory Glands of the Male Reproductive Tract.* Ann Arbor, Mich.: Ann Arbor Science, 1979.

Johnson, A. D., and Gomes, W. R. (eds.). *The Testis.* Vols. 1–4. New York: Academic, 1970–1977.

Mann, T. Secretory function of the prostate, seminal vesicle and other male accessory organs of reproduction. *J. Reprod. Fertil.* 37:179, 1974.

Mostofi, F. K. Testicular tumors: Epidemiologic, etiologic and pathologic features. *Cancer* 32:1186, 1973.

Nagano, T., and Suzuki, F. Freeze fracture observations on the intercellular junctions of Sertoli cells and of Leydig cells in the human testis. *Cell Tissue Res.* 166:37, 1976.

Odell, W. D. The physiology of puberty: Disorders of the pubertal process. In DeGroot, L. J., et al. (eds.), *Endocrinology*. Vol. 3. New York: Grune & Stratton, 1979, p. 1363.

Riva, A. Fine structure of human seminal vesicle epithelium. *J. Anat.* 102:71, 1967.

Ross, M. H. The Sertoli cell specialization during spermiogenesis and at spermeation. *Anat. Rec.* 186:79, 1976.

Smith, K. D. Testicular function in the aging male. In DeGroot, L. J., et al. (eds.), *Endocrinology*. Vol. 3. New York: Grune & Stratton, 1979, p. 1577.

Steinberger, E. Hormonal control of mammalian spermatogenesis. *Physiol. Rev.* 51:1, 1971.

Wong, P. Y. D., and Yeung, C. H. Hormonal regulation of fluid reabsorption in isolated rat cauda epididymis. *Endocrinology* 101:1391, 1977.

FEMALE REPRODUCTIVE SYSTEM

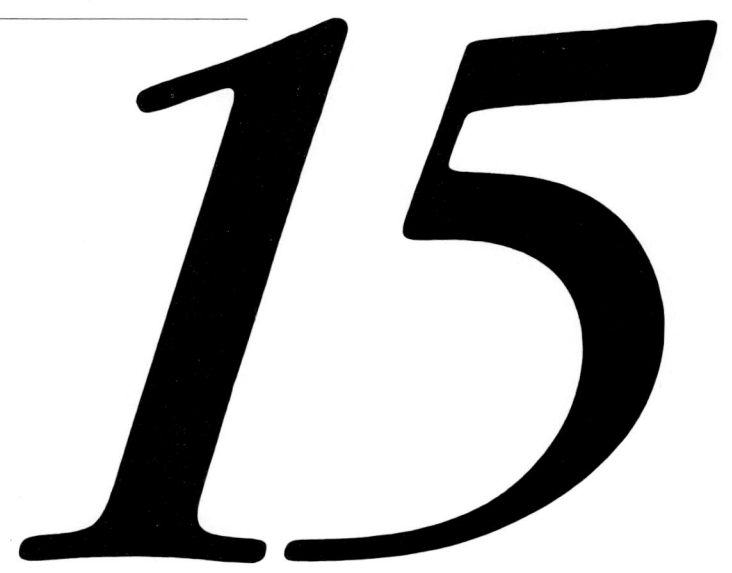

The female reproductive system consists of a pair of ovaries, a pair of uterine tubes, a uterus, a vagina, and the external genital organs. The structure of the mammary glands also will be described, because they undergo changes that are related to the reproductive system.

OVARIES

The ovaries are the organs responsible for the production of the female germ cells, the *ova*, and the female sex hormones, *estrogens* and *progesterone*, in the sexually mature female. Each ovary is an almond-shaped organ measuring 1.5 × .75 inches (4 × 2 cm) and is attached to the back of the broad ligament by the *mesovarium* (Figs. 15-1 and 15-2). Usually the ovary lies with its long axis vertical, but it shares in any movement of the broad ligament and uterus. The ovary is suspended from the lateral wall of the pelvis by that part of the broad ligament that extends between the mesovarium and the lateral pelvic wall; this structure is known as the *suspensory ligament* of the ovary and contains the ovarian vessels and nerves. The *round ligament* of the ovary lies within the broad ligament and connects the medial margin of the ovary to the lateral wall of the uterus.

The ovaries are surrounded by a thin fibrous capsule, the *tunica albuginea* (Fig. 15-3). This capsule is covered externally by a single layer of cuboid cells called the germinal epithelium (Fig. 15-4; see Fig. 15-3). The term *germinal epithelium* is a misnomer, because the layer does not give rise to ova. The germinal epithelium is a modified area of peritoneum and is continuous with the squamous mesothelial cells of the general peritoneum at the hilus of the ovary, where the mesovarium is attached. The ovary has an outer cortex and an inner medulla, but the division between the two is ill defined. The compact connective tissue stroma of the cortex is composed of a network of reticular fibers and spindle-shaped cells (see Fig. 15-4). The stromal cells may be responsible for the secretion of estrogens. The connective tissue stroma of the medulla is very vascular and contains elastic fibers and smooth muscle fibers. Embedded in the stroma of the cortex are the *ovarian follicles,* in different stages of development and degeneration (Fig. 15-5; see Fig. 15-3).

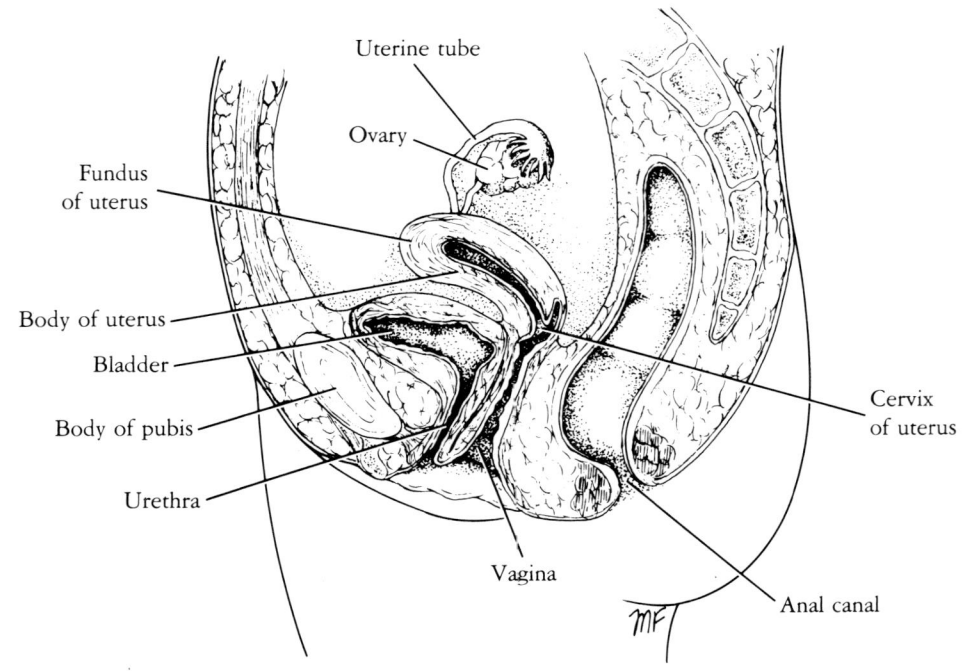

Fig. 15-1. Female reproductive system as seen in sagittal section.

Ovarian Follicles

An ovarian follicle consists of an ovum surrounded by a layer of epithelial cells.

During early fetal development, primordial germ cells migrate from the yolk sac into the developing ovaries, which are first situated in the abdominal cavity, near the kidneys. These germ cells then differentiate into *oogonia*. By the third prenatal month, the oogonia start to undergo a number of mitotic divisions within the cortex of the ovary that result in the formation of the *primary oocytes*. The oocytes now enter the prophase of their first meiotic division, and by the time of birth, they are in a late stage of prophase in their meiotic division. Each primary oocyte becomes surrounded by a single layer of flattened cells, forming a *primordial follicle* (see Fig. 15-3). The surrounding cells are termed *granulosa cells*. Many oogonia and primary oocytes degenerate during the fifth and sixth months of fetal life; most of the surviving primordial follicles occupy the periphery of the cortex. The nucleus of the oocyte is large, pale, and centrally placed. Little chromatin is seen, but the nucleolus is prominent. The cytoplasm is pale, and yolk granules are dispersed evenly throughout it. At birth there may be over 700,000 follicles present in the two ovaries. The number diminishes with age; about 40,000 survive to puberty.

During the third month of fetal development, the ovaries descend to the pelvic brim. Later, they take up their final position on the posterior surfaces of the broad ligament, where they are suspended by the mesovarium.

The Ovaries before Puberty

The ovaries gradually enlarge after birth. It is believed that the stromal cells produce a small amount of estrogen, which inhibits the hypothalamic neurosecretory cells from secreting the follicle-stimulating hormone (FSH) releasing factor.

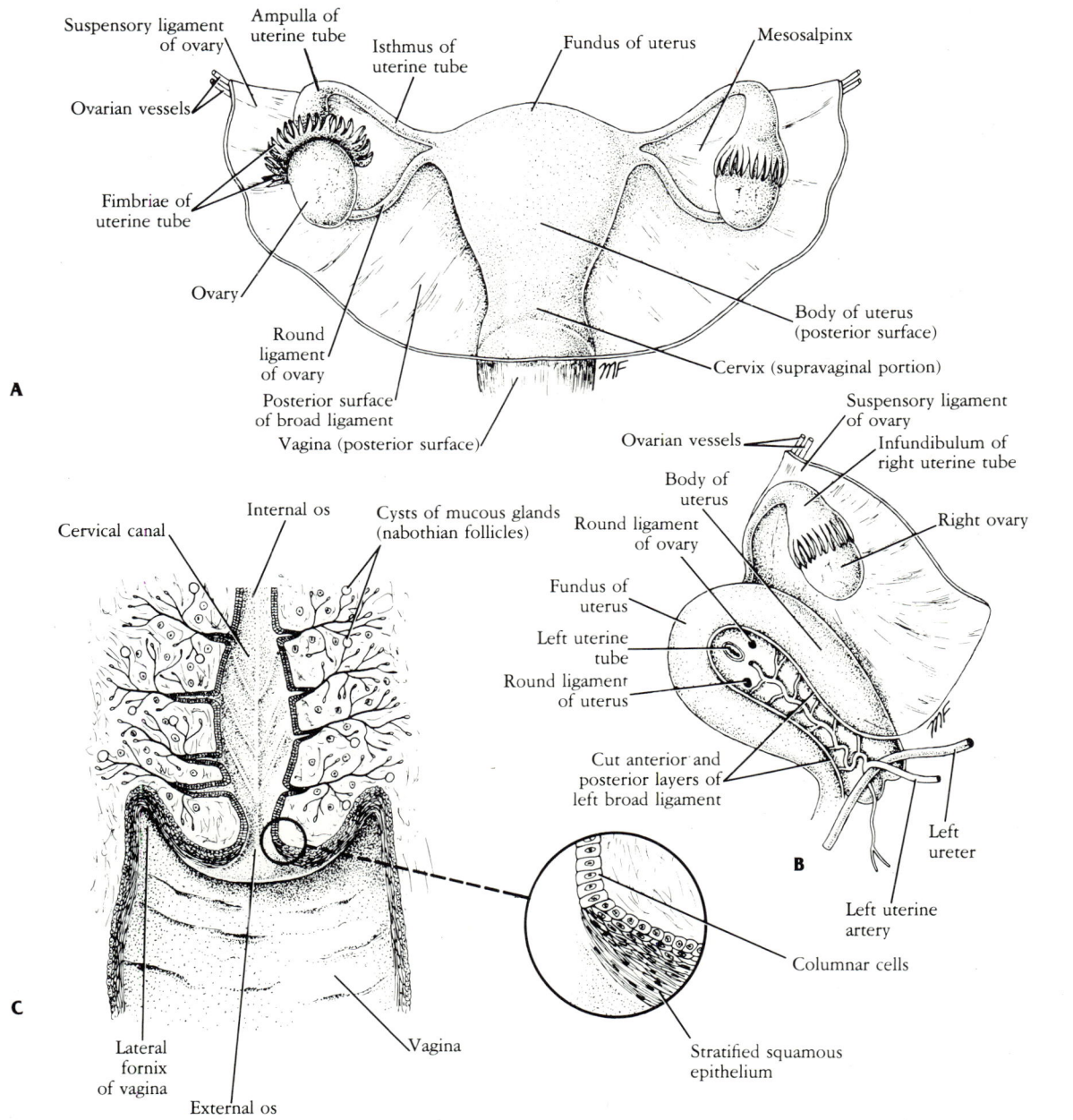

Fig. 15-2. A: Posterior surface of the uterus and the broad ligaments; note the position of the ovaries and the different parts of the uterine tubes. B: Lateral view of uterus. C: Coronal section of the cervix, showing the cervical canal and associated mucous glands; note the important changes that take place in the lining epithelial cells at the external os.

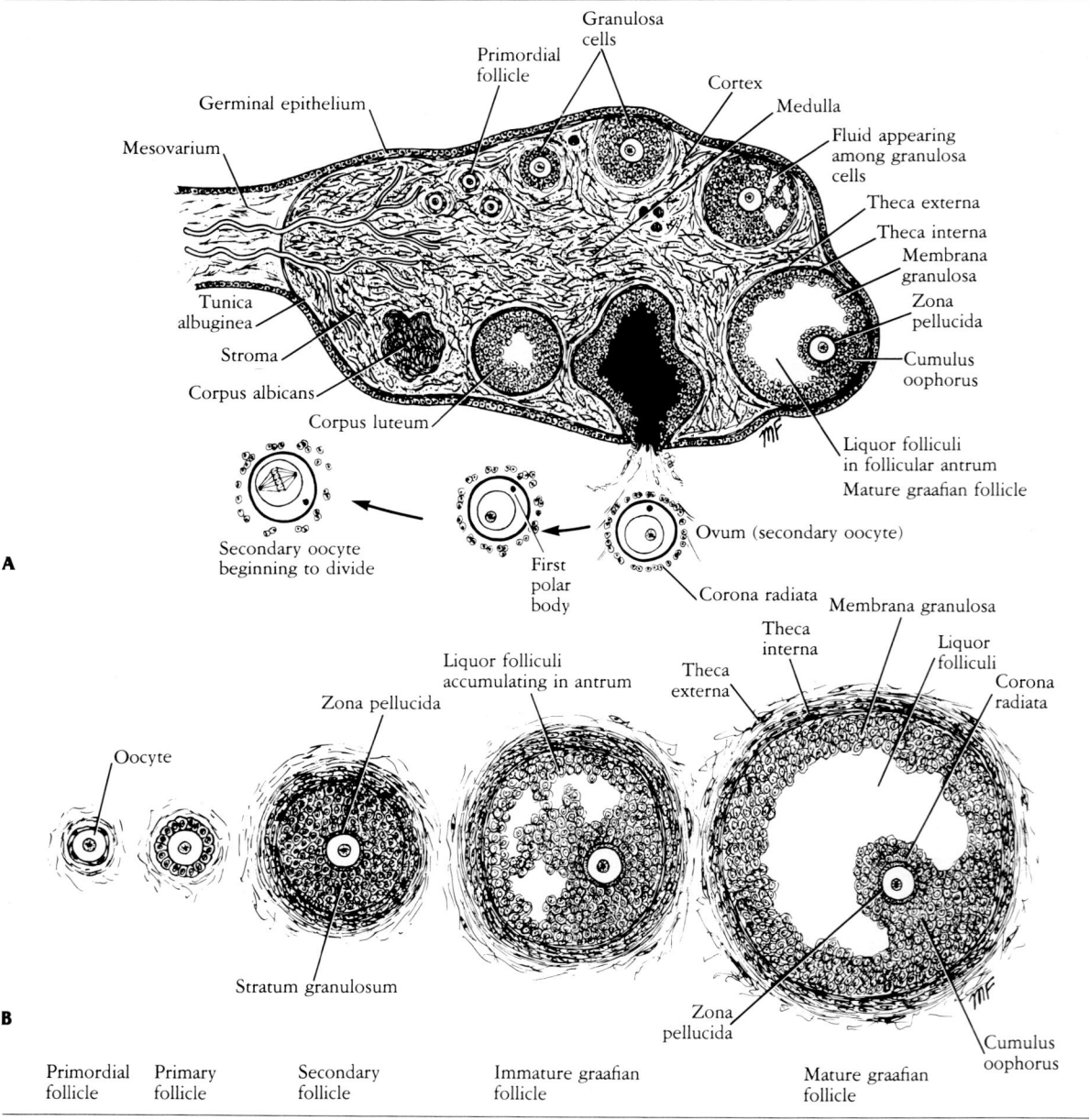

Fig. 15-3. A: Section of the ovary; note the different stages in the maturation of an ovarian follicle. B: Maturation of an ovarian follicle, starting with a primordial follicle and ending with a mature graafian follicle.

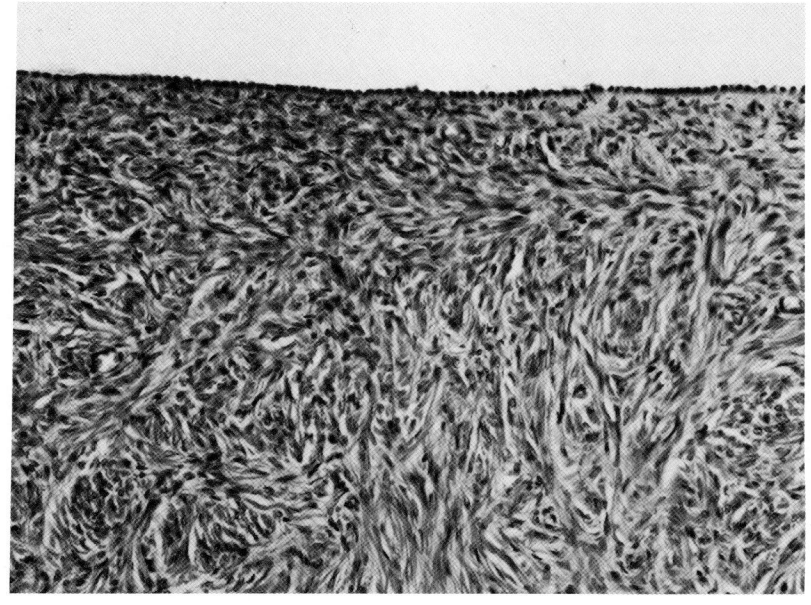

Fig. 15-4. Photomicrograph of a section of the cortex of the ovary, showing at the top the covering formed by a single layer of cuboidal cells called the germinal epithelium. Note the compact stroma of the cortex. (H&E; ×200.)

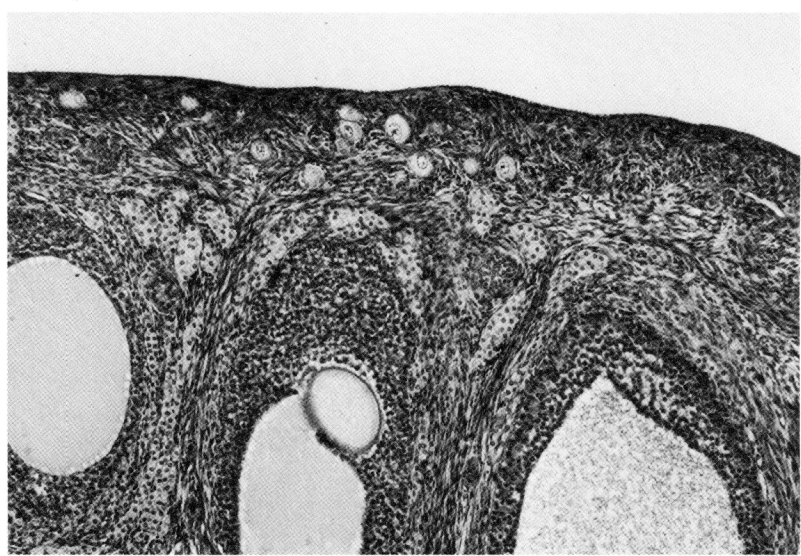

Fig. 15-5. Photomicrograph of a section of a portion of the ovarian cortex, showing several small primordial follicles and parts of three immature follicles. (H&E; ×100.)

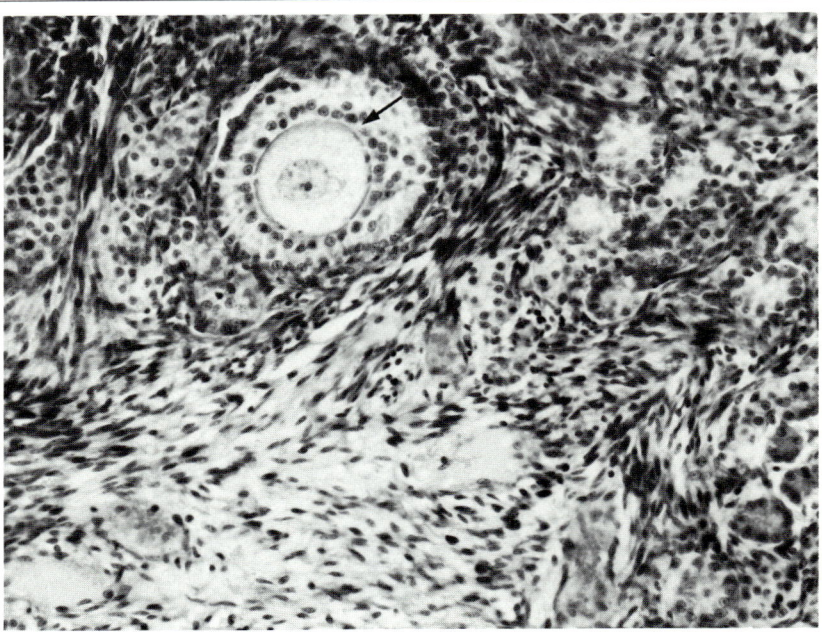

Fig. 15-6. *Photomicrograph of a section of a portion of the ovarian cortex, showing a growing follicle with an ovum. Note the large nucleus and prominent nucleolus, the zona pellucida (arrow), and the stratum granulosum. (H&E; ×100.)*

The Ovaries at Puberty: Onset of the Ovarian Cycle

At puberty the hypothalamic neurosecretory cells become less sensitive to estrogen and start secreting the *FSH releasing factor*. This substance stimulates the cells of the anterior lobe of the pituitary to produce FSH. The FSH now stimulates the ovarian follicles, and the ovarian cycles begin. During each cycle, many follicles in both ovaries start to enlarge. Gradually, one follicle gains ascendancy and reaches maturity; the remainder degenerate and become *atretic follicles*. As a result, only one ovum normally is released during each ovarian cycle. It has been estimated that only 300 to 400 follicles come to full maturity and liberate ova from the ovaries during the reproductive life of a woman.

After puberty, the primordial follicles enlarge in response to the FSH of the anterior lobe of the pituitary. The granulosa cells become cuboidal and begin to divide, so that the oocyte becomes surrounded by a number of layers of granulosa cells (Fig. 15-6; see Fig. 15-3). These cells now secrete around the oocyte a hyaline material composed of glycoproteins. This material forms the *zona pellucida*. As the oocyte increases in size, irregular spaces filled with clear fluid, the *liquor folliculi*, appear among the granulosa cells. These spaces later coalesce to form a single cavity, the *follicular antrum* (Fig. 15-7; see Fig. 15-3). The granulosa cells that line the cavity make up the *membrana granulosa*. The oocyte, still surrounded by granulosa cells now called the *cumulus oophorus*, projects into the antrum from one side. At this stage of development, the follicle is known as a *graafian follicle* (Fig. 15-8; see Fig. 15-3). While the follicle has been growing, the surrounding stroma has been differentiating into an inner, vascular layer of secretory cells, the *theca interna*, and an outer, connective tissue layer, the *theca externa*. After 10 to 14 days of growth, the follicle

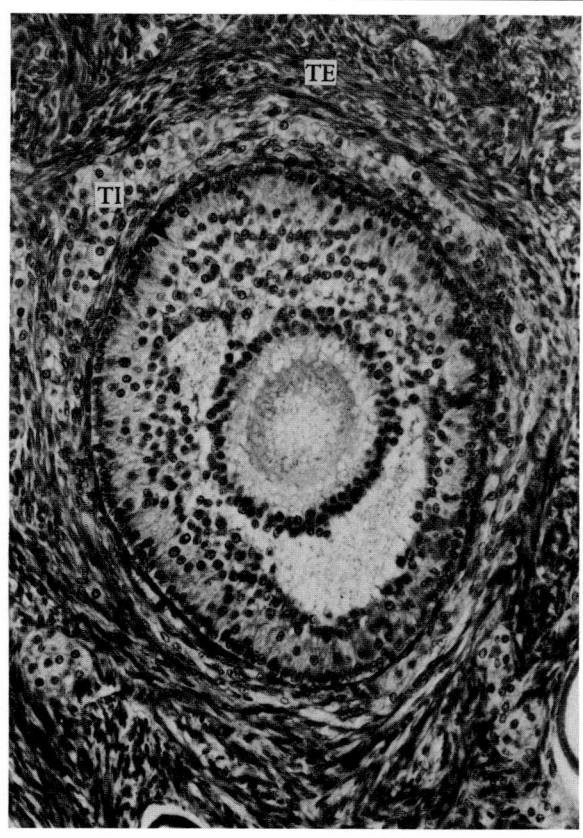

Fig. 15-7. Photomicrograph of a maturing graafian follicle, showing the liquor folliculi accumulating in the antrum. Note the theca interna (TI) and theca externa (TE) in the surrounding ovarian stroma. (H&E; ×200.)

measures about 10 mm in diameter and bulges slightly from the free surface of the ovary.

As the ovarian follicles mature under the influence of the FSH of the anterior lobe of the pituitary, the ovary begins to elaborate large amounts of estrogens. It is believed that the theca interna cells secrete most of the estrogens.

Ovulation

Ovulation in a normal woman who has a 28-day sexual cycle occurs 14 days after the onset of menstruation.

The meiotic division of the primary oocyte that began during the third month of fetal development is finally completed a few hours before ovulation, and the *secondary oocyte* and the *first polar body* are formed. The first polar body, which receives only a little cytoplasm, lies between the zona pellucida and the cell membrane of the secondary oocyte (see Fig. 15-3). As a result of the continued accumulation of liquor folliculi, the tense graafian follicle now ruptures, and ovulation occurs: the secondary oocyte, the zona pellucida, and the cumulus oophorus, now known as the *corona radiata,* escape into the peritoneal cavity. Immediately after ovulation, the secondary oocyte undergoes the second meiotic division, forming the *mature ovum* and the *second polar body;* this division is not completed unless and until fertilization occurs, however. When the second polar body is formed, the first and second polar bodies undergo rapid breakdown and disappear. The mature ovum has a diameter of about 120 μm.

Following ovulation, the walls of the follicle collapse and the cells of the membrana granulosa are thrown into folds. Blood from the ruptured capillaries of the theca interna fills the remains of the antrum, and clots. The cells of the membrana granulosa and the theca interna are stimulated by the *luteinizing hormone* (LH) of the pituitary. They enlarge, and their cytoplasm accumulates lipid. Later, a yellow pigment appears in the cytoplasm. These modified cells are known as *luteal cells,* and together they form the *corpus luteum* (Figs. 15-9 and 15-10; see Fig. 15-3). The luteinized theca interna cells continue to produce estrogens, and the luteinized granulosa cells start to produce large amounts of progesterone and estrogen. As a result of continued hormonal stimulation from the pituitary, the corpus luteum enlarges for about 10 days after ovulation, reaching a diameter of about 2 cm. At that time, it is visible on the surface of the ovary as a yellowish projection surrounded by an area of hyperemia. If fertilization does not occur, the LH of the pituitary decreases and the corpus luteum begins to involute. The secretion of progesterone diminishes, and the corpus luteum is finally converted

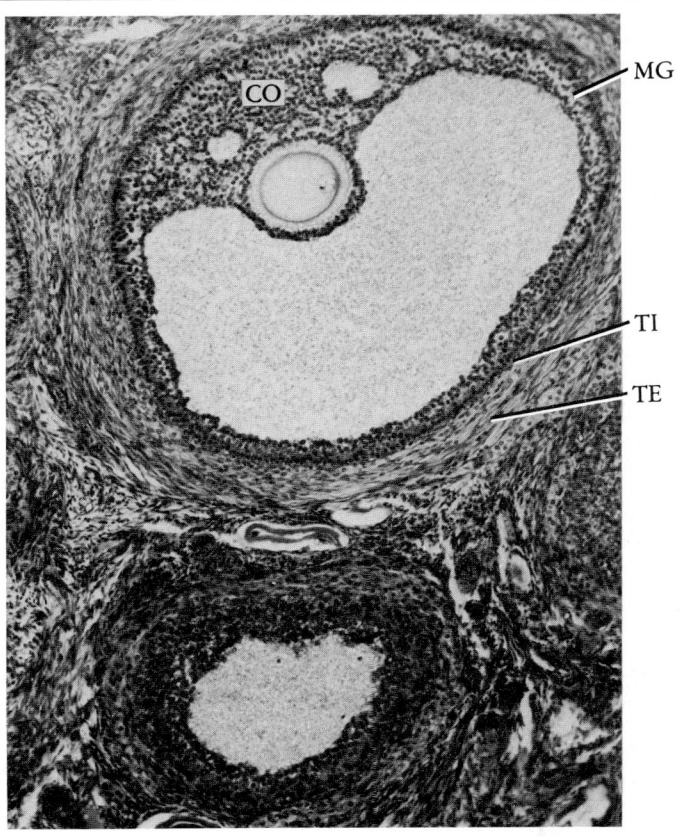

Fig. 15-8. Photomicrograph of a mature graafian follicle, showing the ovum, the cumulus oophorus (CO), and the membrane granulosa (MG). Note also the theca interna (TI) and the theca externa (TE). (H&E; ×100.)

into a fibrous scar, the *corpus albicans* (Fig. 15-11; see Fig. 15-3).

Hormonal Control of Ovulation

At the beginning of each ovarian cycle, the increased production of FSH by the anterior lobe of the pituitary causes many follicles in both ovaries to enlarge (Fig. 15-12). As stated earlier, one follicle then starts to enlarge more quickly than the others, while the remainder degenerate and become atretic. The reason for this ascendency of one follicle over the remainder is unknown, as is the cause of the atresia. Just before ovulation, the anterior lobe of the pituitary secretes increasing amounts of LH, a process necessary for the final maturation of the follicle prior to ovulation. The actual rupture of the follicle is brought about by the continued accumulation of liquor folliculi and the degeneration of the overlying theca externa.

Chromosomal Changes during Oogenesis

The human somatic cell contains 46 chromosomes, consisting of 22 pairs of autosomes and one pair of sex chromosomes (XY or XX). The different pairs of autosomes vary in size, but the two members of any given pair of autosomes are identical. The sex chromosomes in the female (XX) are identical. The

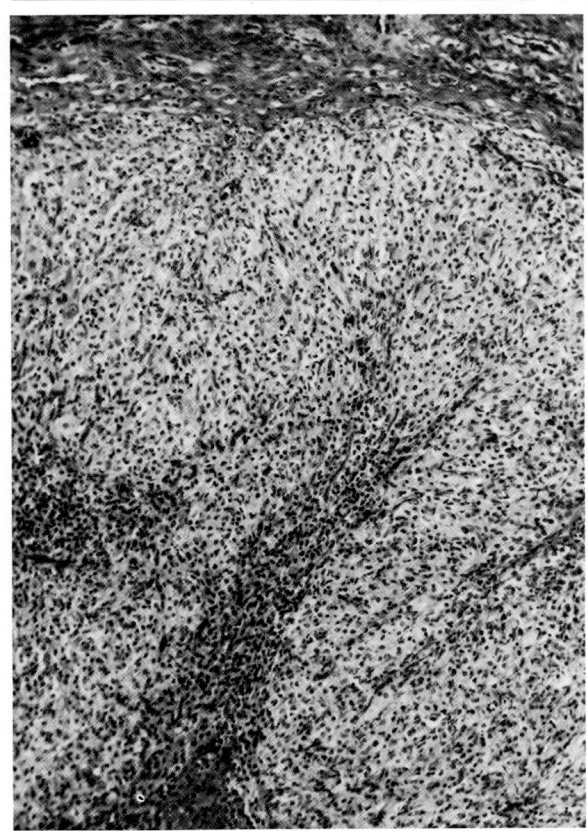

Fig. 15-9. Photomicrograph of a portion of the corpus luteum. Note the large, pale-staining luteal cells. (H&E; ×100.)

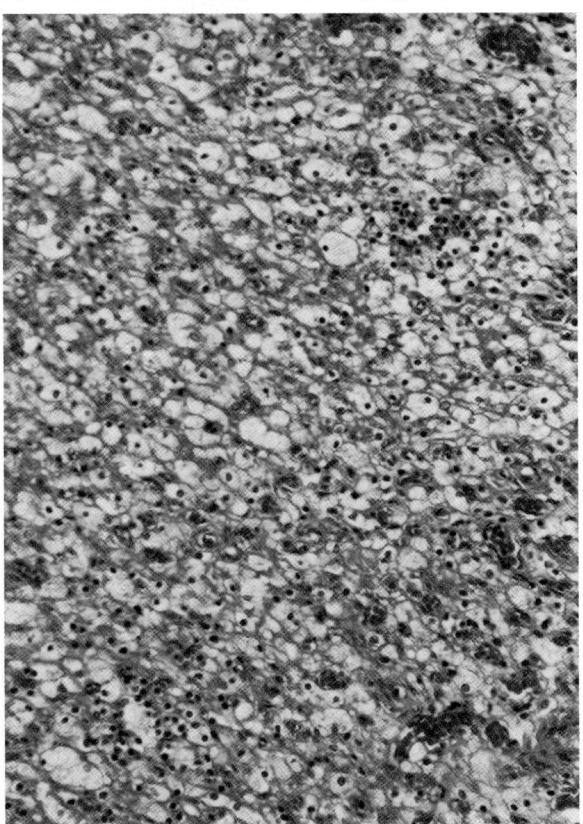

Fig. 15-10. Photomicrograph of a high-power view of the section of corpus luteum shown in Figure 15-9. Note again the very large, pale-staining cells, whose cytoplasm contains many lipid droplets and yellow pigment. The lipid was dissolved out of the section during the preparation of the slide. (H&E; ×200.)

oogonium possesses 46 chromosomes (Fig. 15-13). When such a cell divides mitotically to form primary oocytes, each chromosome splits longitudinally, so that each daughter cell receives the same number of chromosomes as possessed by the mother cell. When each primary oocyte divides meiotically (first meiotic division), the resulting secondary oocyte is haploid: it receives only half the number of chromosomes, i.e., 23. The other 22 + X chromosomes go to the first polar body, the very much smaller of the two daughter cells, which receives very little cytoplasm from the mother cell.

The second meiotic division, that of the secondary oocyte, forms one ovum with 22 + X chromosomes and a second polar body (resulting from unequal distribution of cytoplasm from the mother cell) with 22 + X chromosomes. At the same time, the first polar body may divide to form two additional secondary polar bodies. By this means, one oogonium with 44 autosomes and one pair of XX chromosomes eventually gives rise to two ova, each with 22 autosomes and one X sex chromosome.

If fertilization should occur and a spermatozoon

has been shown to be under the control of LH as well. When the corpus luteum finally degenerates after 12 days (assuming fertilization has not occurred), the secretions of progesterone and estrogens cease, the negative feedback on the pituitary comes to an end, the FSH and, later, the LH secretions from the pituitary begin again, and a new ovarian cycle commences. The sudden drop in the level of progesterone and estrogens in the blood at the end of the ovarian cycle results in the degeneration of the endometrium lining the uterus, a process known as *menstruation.*

Functions of the Ovarian Estrogens and Progesterone

The estrogens produced by the ovary are mainly β-estradiol and estrone. They are responsible for the development and maintenance of the uterine tubes, uterus, vagina, external genitalia, and breasts. They also produce and maintain the secondary sexual characteristics of the female.

Progesterone produced by the corpus luteum of the ovary, together with the estrogens, develops the secretory phase of the endometrium of the uterus. It also stimulates the secretion of mucus in the lining cells of the uterine tubes and promotes the development of the alveolar cells of the breasts (see Fig. 15-12).

The further functions of these important hormones are discussed in Chapter 16.

UTERINE TUBES

There are two uterine tubes; each is about 4 inches (10 cm) long and lies in the upper border of the broad ligament (see Fig. 15-2). Each connects the peritoneal cavity in the region of the ovary with the cavity of the uterus. The uterine tube may be divided into four parts: the infundibulum, the ampulla, the isthmus, and the intramural part.

The *infundibulum* is the funnel-shaped lateral extremity; it projects beyond the broad ligament and overlies the ovary. The free edge of the funnel is broken up into a number of fingerlike processes, known as *fimbriae,* which are draped over the ovary (see Fig. 15-2). The *ampulla* is the widest part of the

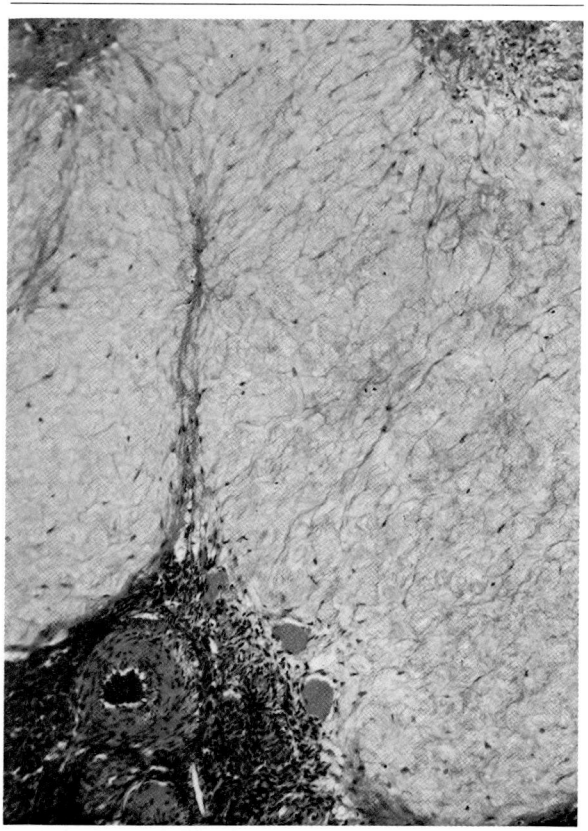

Fig. 15-11. Photomicrograph of a section of the corpus albicans. Note the replacement of the corpus luteum cells with dense fibrous tissue. (H&E; ×100.)

with 22 + Y chromosomes enters an ovum with 22 + X chromosomes, a male child will result. If a spermatozoon with 22 + X chromosomes enters an ovum, a female child will result. The chromosomal changes we have discussed are shown in Figure 15-13.

Termination of the Ovarian Cycle

We have shown how the ovarian follicle matures and how ovulation occurs as the result of stimulation first by FSH and then by FSH and LH from the anterior lobe of the pituitary (see Fig. 15-12). The development and maintenance of the corpus luteum

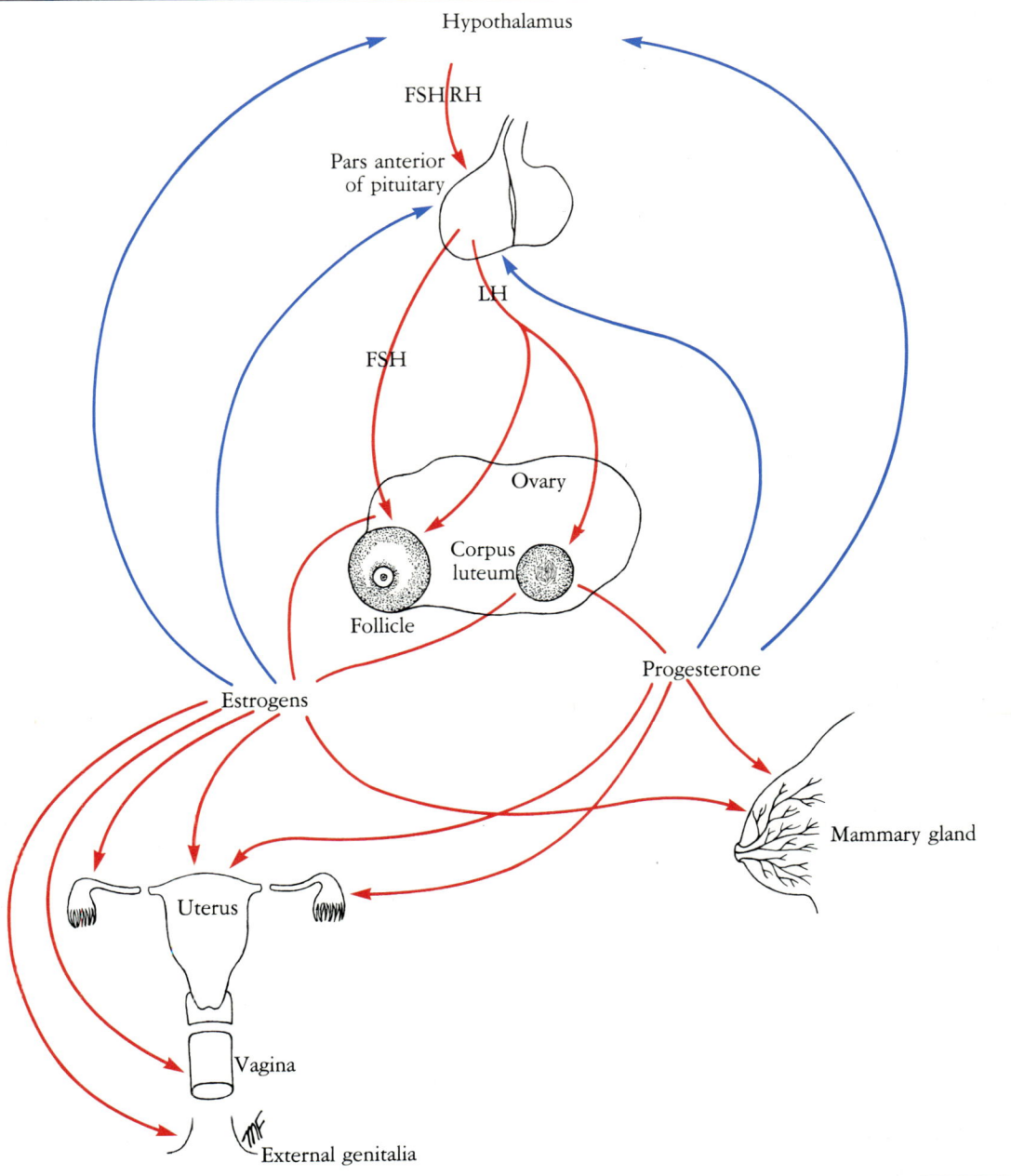

Fig. 15-12. Hormonal control of the female reproductive system, including the mammary glands. Note the important feedback mechanism involving the hypothalamus.

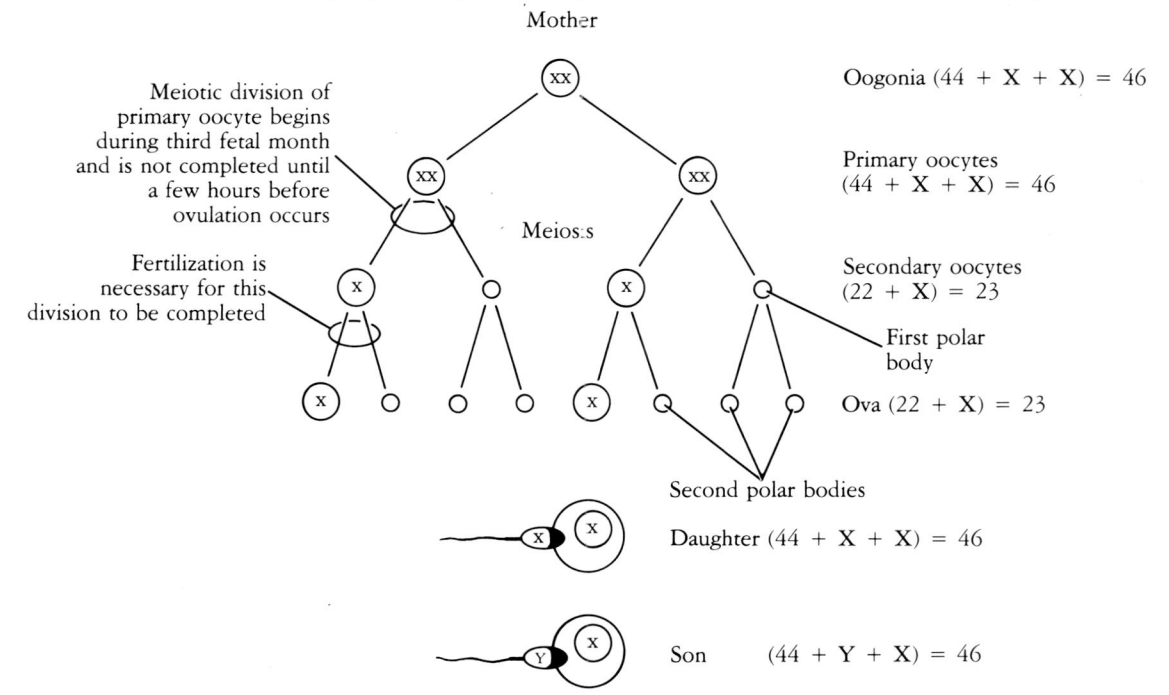

Fig. 15-13. *Chromosomal changes during oogenesis, ultimately resulting in the formation of a zygote. Note that the X or Y chromosome in the fertilizing spermatozoon determines the sex of the future child.*

tube; it is in this portion that fertilization of the ovum takes place (see Fig. 15-2). The *isthmus* is the narrowest part of the tube and lies just lateral to the uterus (see Fig. 15-2). The *intramural part* is the segment that pierces the uterine wall.

The wall of the uterine tube is made up of three layers: (1) a mucous membrane, (2) a muscular coat, and (3) a connective tissue coat. The *mucous membrane* forms numerous delicate longitudinal folds (Figs. 15-14 and 15-15). It is covered with epithelial cells that rest on a lamina propria of connective tissue (Fig. 15-16). There are three types of epithelial cells: ciliated columnar cells, nonciliated columnar secretory mucous cells (Fig. 15-17), and intercalated cells, which may be precursor or resting secretory cells. The secretory cells increase their activity and store their secretion during the follicular phase of the ovarian cycle as a result of the stimulating action of estrogens. The cells discharge their secretion during the luteal phase of the cycle in response to progesterone. The *muscle coat* consists of circular inner and longitudinal outer layers of smooth muscle fibers (see Figs. 15-14 and 15-15). The *connective tissue coat* is formed of areolar tissue covered in part by squamous mesothelial cells of the pelvic peritoneum (see Figs. 15-14 and 15-15).

Function of the Uterine Tube

The uterine tube receives the ovum from the ovary and provides a site where fertilization can occur. The secretions of the lining cells nourish the fertilized ovum, and the action of the cilia and the peristalsis of the walls of the tube transport the fertilized ovum to the cavity of the uterus. The tube also provides a conduit along which the spermatozoa

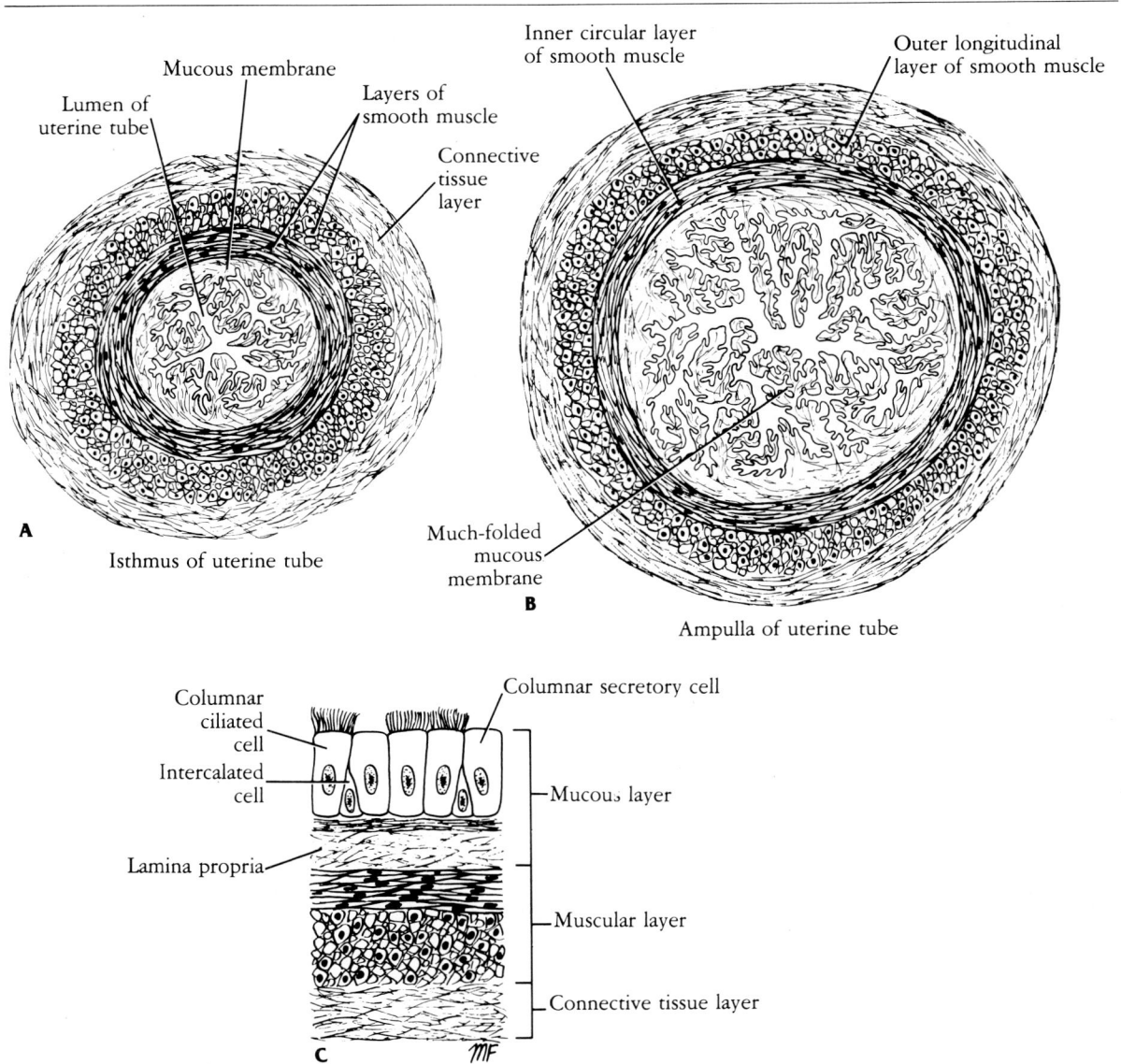

Fig. 15-14. General structure of the uterine tube in cross section at (A) the isthmus and (B) the ampulla. C: The three types of epithelial cells lining the mucous membrane.

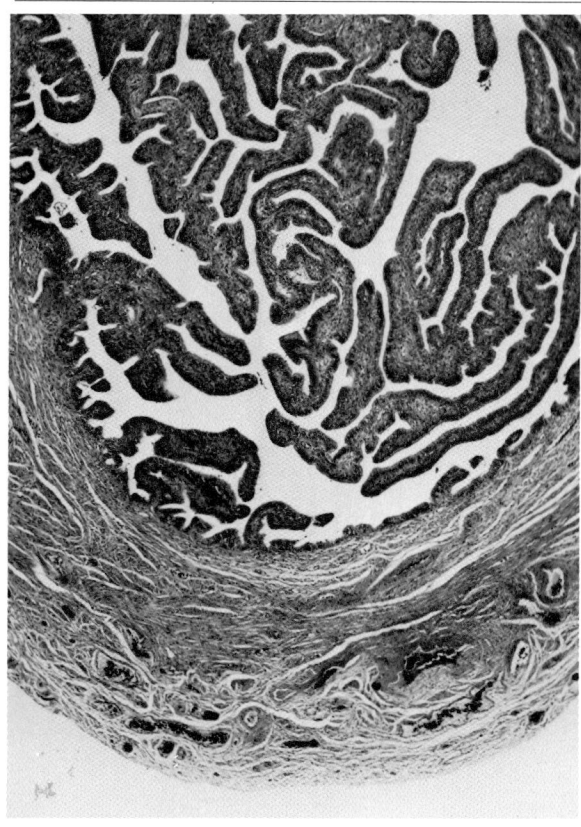

Fig. 15-15. Photomicrograph of a cross section of the ampulla of the uterine tube, showing the extensive folding of the mucous membrane. (H&E; ×40.)

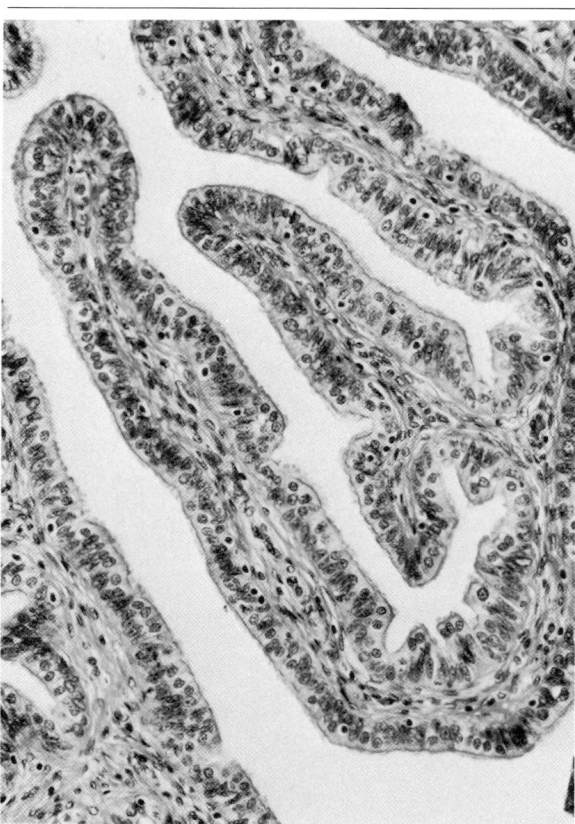

Fig. 15-16. Photomicrograph of a cross section of the mucous membrane of the ampulla of the uterine tube. The extensive folding of the mucous membrane is visible, as is the lining of ciliated columnar epithelium, which rests on a lamina propria of connective tissue. It is not possible at this magnification to identify the secretory cells or the intercalated cells. (H&E; ×200.)

travel to reach the ovum, and the secretions also, nourish the spermatozoa.

UTERUS

The uterus is located in the pelvis between the bladder and the rectum (see Fig. 15-1). It is a hollow, pear-shaped organ with thick muscular walls and serves as a site for the reception, retention, and nutrition of the fertilized ovum. In the young woman who has not had a child, it measures 3 inches (8 cm) long, 2 inches (5 cm) wide, and 1 inch (2.5 cm) thick. For purposes of description, it can be divided into the fundus, body, and cervix (see Fig. 15-2).

The *fundus* is the part of the uterus above the entrance of the uterine tubes. The *body* is the part below the entrance of the uterine tubes. It narrows below, where it becomes continuous with the *cervix*. The cervix pierces the anterior wall of the vagina and is divided into the *supravaginal* and *vaginal parts*.

The *cavity* of the uterine body is triangular in coronal section, but it is merely a cleft in the sagittal plane (see Fig. 15-1). The cavity of the cervix, the

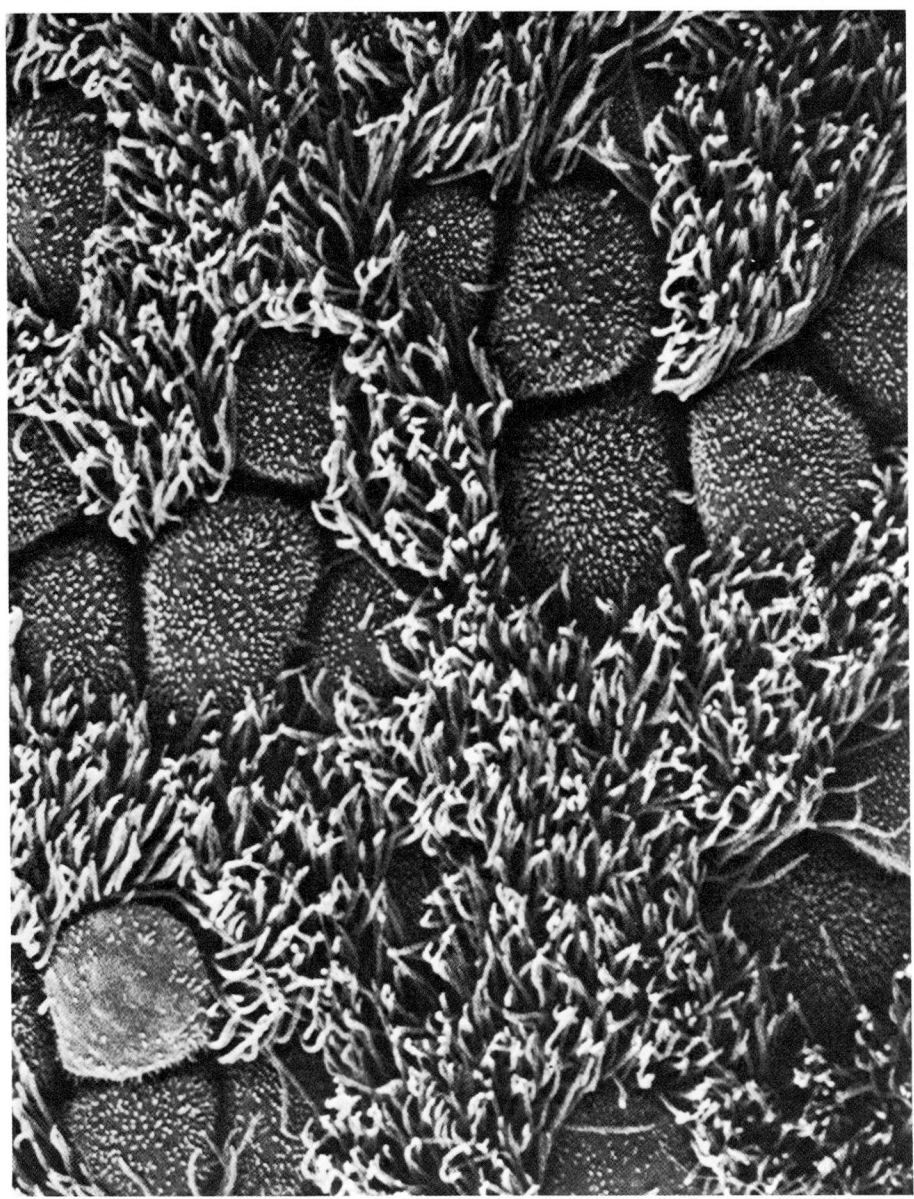

Fig. 15-17. Scanning electron micrograph of the luminal surface of the mucous membrane of the uterine tube, showing the numerous villi of the columnar ciliated epithelial cells and several secretory cells bearing short microvilli. ($\times 6,817$.) (Courtesy of Dr. M. Koering.)

cervical canal, is spindle shaped and communicates with the cavity of the body through the *internal os* and with that of the vagina through the *external os.*

Uterine Wall

The wall of the uterus has three coats: (1) the serosa, (2) the muscular coat, or myometrium, and (3) the mucous membrane, or endometrium.

Serosal Coat

The serosal coat, or peritoneum, consists of a layer of squamous mesothelial cells resting on areolar tissue. It covers the uterus and is reflected onto the bladder anteriorly. Posteriorly it continues onto the vagina and from there is reflected onto the rectum. Laterally the peritoneum extends to the lateral wall of the pelvis, forming the broad ligament.

Muscular Coat

The muscular coat, or myometrium, is very thick and is composed of smooth muscle fibers and connective tissue (Fig. 15-18). The muscle fibers interlace in many directions. There is a higher proportion of connective tissue in the cervix than elsewhere.

Mucous Membrane (Endometrium)

The mucous membrane, or endometrium, is continuous above with the mucous membrane of the uterine tubes and below with the mucous membrane of the vagina. The endometrium is applied directly to the muscle, there being no submucosa.

The endometrium in the body of the uterus and the upper third of the cervix, from puberty until the menopause, undergoes extensive changes in structure during the menstrual cycle in response to the ovarian hormones. Basically, the endometrium is lined with a simple columnar epithelium resting on a lamina propria of connective tissue (Fig. 15-19). There are numerous simple tubular glands whose mouths open into the cavity of the uterus. The glands extend almost to the myometrium and are lined with columnar mucus-secreting cells. The endometrium can be divided into a thick, superficial part that undergoes functional and structural

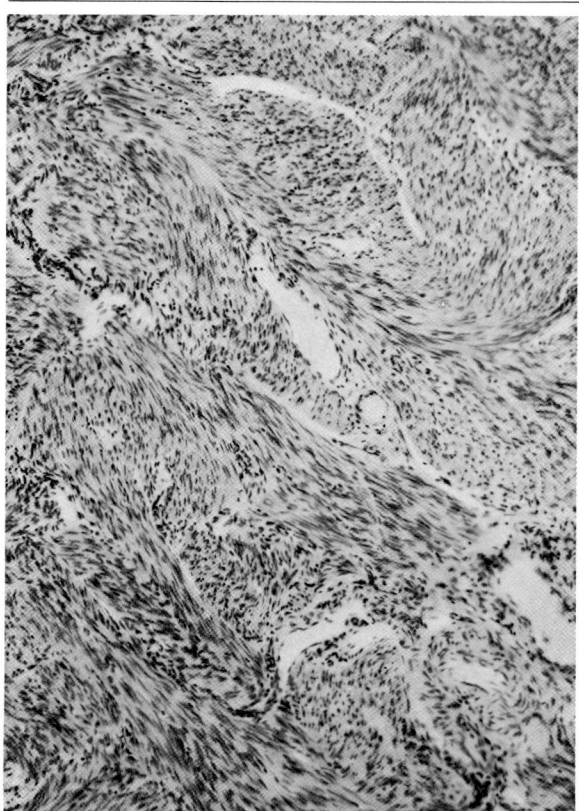

Fig. 15-18. Photomicrograph of a section through the myometrium of the body of the uterus, showing many bundles of smooth muscle fibers interlacing in many directions. (H&E; ×100.)

changes during the menstrual cycle and a thin, basal part that changes little during the menstrual cycle and is responsible for re-forming the superficial layer after the menstrual flow has ceased.

In the cervix of the uterus, the endometrium is lined with ciliated columnar epithelium. In the lower part, the cilia are absent, and at the external os, the columnar cells give way to stratified squamous epithelium (Fig. 15-20; see Fig. 15-2). The outer surface of the vaginal part of the cervix is covered by stratified squamous epithelium. The glands of the endometrium of the cervix are large

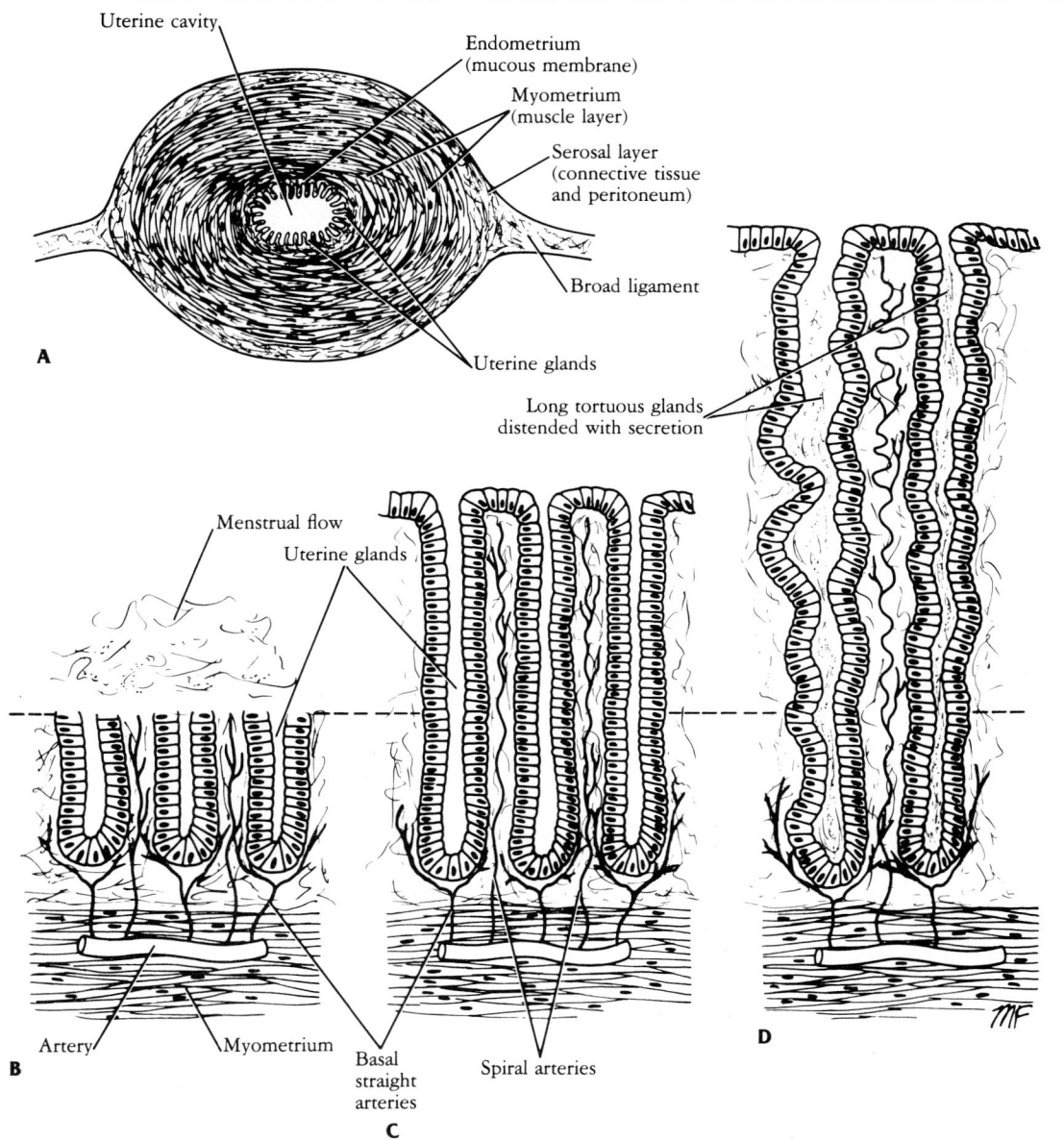

Fig. 15-19. A: *General structure of the body of the uterus as seen in cross section.* B: *Structure of the endometrium during menstruation.* C: *Structure of the endometrium during the proliferative phase of the menstrual cycle.* D: *Structure of the endometrium during the secretory phase of the cycle. In B, C, and D, note the basal straight arteries and the spiral arteries.*

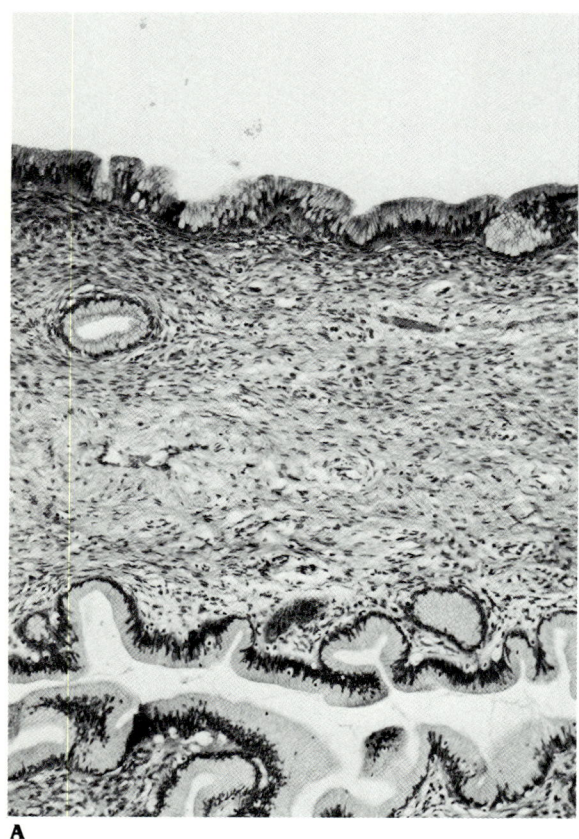 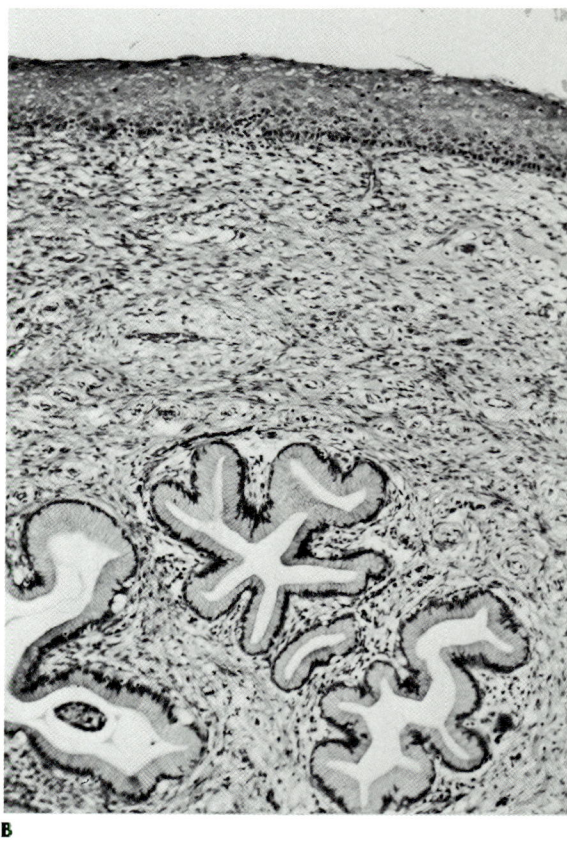

Fig. 15-20. Photomicrograph of two longitudinal sections of the cervix. A: The lining of columnar epithelial cells and the large mucus-secreting glands of the lower part of the cervical canal. B: The outer surface of the vaginal part of the cervix at the external os; note that the lining columnar cells are replaced here by stratified squamous epithelium. (H&E; ×100.)

and secrete a thick, alkaline mucus. It is normal for many of the gland orifices to be blocked, leading to retention of the secretion and cystlike spaces filled with secretion. The lining of the lower two-thirds of the cervix does not undergo extensive structural changes during the menstrual cycle.

CYCLICAL CHANGES IN THE STRUCTURE OF THE ENDOMETRIUM. Each month between puberty and the menopause, the endometrium lining the body and the upper part of the cervix of the uterus undergoes cyclical changes in structure that are known as the *menstrual cycle*. The duration of the menstrual cycle varies from one woman to another, and perfectly normal women may regularly have cycles of 26 to 32 days. In this account, we will use as an example a cycle of 28 days.

A menstrual (endometrial) cycle may be divided into three phases: menstrual, proliferative, and secretory.

Menstruation. Menstruation is the shedding of the superficial zone of the endometrium into the uterine cavity, leaving only the basal zone (see Fig. 15-19). The *menstrual flow* thus consists of blood, partially disintegrated epithelium and stroma, and secretions of the endometrial glands. Menstruation is produced by the sudden reduction in both estrogens and progesterone at the end of the ovarian cycle. The endometrium suddenly is deprived of the supporting action of these hormones, and the spiral arteries that supply the superficial zone of the endometrium constrict. After a variable time, the constricted arteries open up, the walls of the damaged vessels in the superficial part of the endometrium rupture, and blood pours into the stroma, disrupting the tissue. The process leads to hemorrhage into the uterine cavity and the shedding of all but the deepest part of the endometrium. Menstruation normally lasts about 4 to 6 days.

Proliferative Phase. At the end of menstruation, only the deep, or basal, parts of the endometrium remain. These are supplied by their own arteries, the *basal arteries,* which do not undergo constriction. The epithelial cells that form the blind ends of the glands in the basal endometrium now multiply and repair the denuded surface of the endometrium. This process is controlled by the secretions of estrogens by the ovaries. On about the sixth day of the menstrual cycle, when the damage resulting from the menstrual period has been repaired, proliferative changes begin. The endometrium initially is thin and consists of columnar epithelium that dips down into a loose stroma to form simple tubular glands (Fig. 15-21; see 15-19). From the sixth to the fourteenth day, the endometrium thickens. This thickening is caused by increasing numbers of stromal cells, elongation of the tubular glands, and growth of blood vessels; all these proliferative changes are controlled by the ovarian estrogens. At the time of ovulation, which in a 28-day cycle occurs on day 14 + or − 1 day, the endometrium is 2 to 3 mm thick.

Secretory Phase. Once ovulation has occurred, the corpus luteum is formed and starts to secrete progesterone and estrogens. The theca interna continues to secrete estrogen. The combined action of these two hormones produces the secretory changes in the endometrium. The endometrium thickens further, and the glands become long and tortuous and distended with secretion that is rich in glycogen,

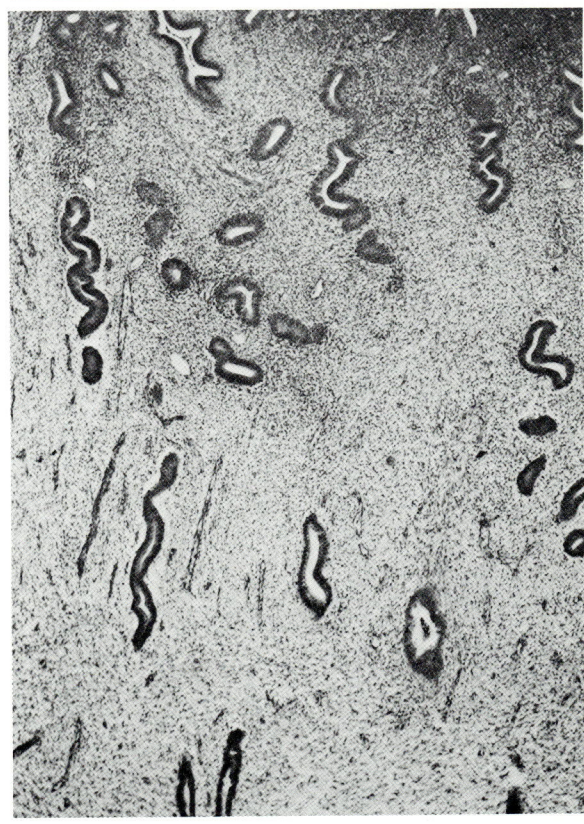

Fig. 15-21. Photomicrograph of a vertical section of the endometrium during the proliferative phase of the menstrual cycle. Note the simple tubular glands embedded in a loose stroma. (H&E; ×40.)

mucopolysaccharides, and lipid (Figs. 15-22 and 15-23; see Fig. 15-19). The stromal cells proliferate, enlarge, and become closely packed. The arteries are highly coiled and congested and are known as the spiral arteries. At the end of this phase of the cycle, the endometrium is 5 to 8 mm thick. During the last days of this phase, increasing numbers of lymphocytes are found in the stroma between the glands.

Thus, the various changes that take place in the endometrium during the second half of the menstrual cycle may be regarded as preparing the uterine lin-

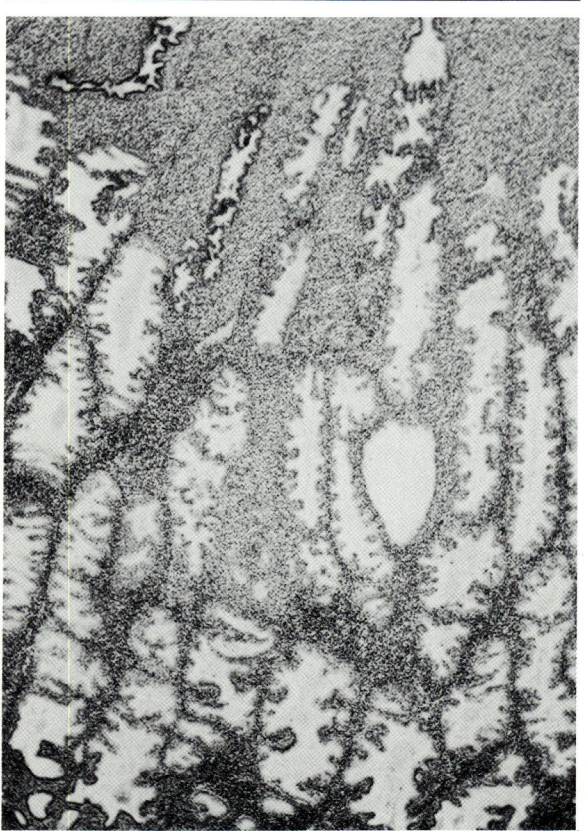

Fig. 15-22. Photomicrograph of a vertical section of the endometrium during the secretory phase of the menstrual cycle. Note the long, tortuous tubular glands distended with secretion. Compare with Figure 15-21. (H&E; ×40.)

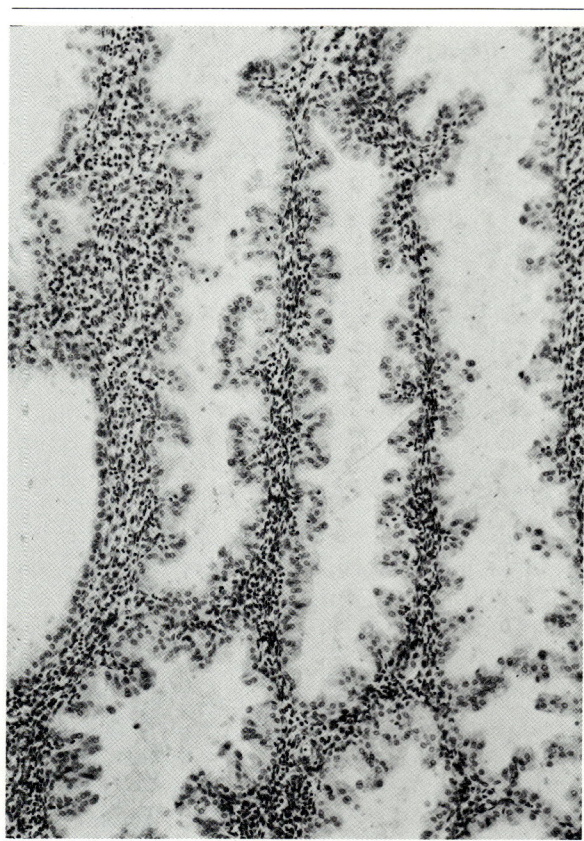

Fig. 15-23. Photomicrograph of a high-power view of the tubular glands of the endometrium during the secretory phase of the menstrual cycle. The glands are very tortuous and distended with secretion and are lined with columnar cells. The stromal cells are densely packed between the glands. (H&E; ×100.)

ing for the nourishment and reception of the fertilized ovum (blastocyst). On entering the uterine cavity, the fertilized ovum lies free within the secretion produced by the highly developed endometrial glands. This secretion is called uterine milk, and it provides an excellent medium for the rapidly dividing cells in the blastocyst.

Should fertilization not occur, the corpus luteum degenerates and the endometrium is once again deprived of the supporting action of estrogen and progesterone. Menstruation then begins again.

Uterus in the Child

The uterus remains small until puberty, when it enlarges greatly in response to the estrogens secreted by the ovaries. The endometrium in the child is lined throughout with ciliated columnar epithelium.

Uterus after the Menopause

After the menopause, the uterus atrophies and becomes smaller and less vascular and the lining of the endometrium becomes a low columnar or cuboidal epithelium. These changes occur because the ovaries no longer produce estrogens and progesterone. As we have stated, primordial follicles disappear completely at the menopause.

Uterus in Pregnancy

During pregnancy, the uterus becomes greatly enlarged and rises out of the pelvis, so that by the tenth month it has reached the xiphoid process. The increase in size is largely due to hypertrophy of the smooth muscle fibers, although some hyperplasia does take place. The enormous growth in size of the uterus is controlled by the increasing production of estrogens and progesterone, first by the corpus luteum and later by the placenta.

Implantation of the Blastocyst

The endometrium of the uterus reaches its maximum thickness (5 to 8 mm) and development during the secretory phase of the menstrual cycle (see Fig. 15-23). Three distinct layers can be recognized: a superficial *compact layer,* an intermediate *spongy layer,* and a thin *basal layer.*

The blastocyst enters the uterine cavity between the fourth and ninth days after ovulation, and, with the disappearance of the zona pellucida, the outer surface of the trophoblast comes into direct contact with the endometrium and adheres to it. The adherence and attachment of the blastocyst to the endometrium are referred to as *implantation* (Fig. 15-24). Normal implantation takes place in the endometrium of the body of the uterus, most frequently on the upper part of the posterior wall near the midline. Usually the blastocyst becomes attached between the openings of the endometrial glands, but occasionally it lodges within the mouth of one of the glands. In the region of contact between the blastocyst and the endometrium, the trophoblast cells of the blastocyst start to proliferate, so that the wall of the blastocyst becomes thickened. In this area, the trophoblast cells become differentiated into an inner *cytotrophoblast* (see Fig. 15-24), composed of a single layer of individual cells, and a thick outer layer, the *syncytiotrophoblast,* in which the cell boundaries are lost. The part of the trophoblast wall of the blastocyst that projects into the uterine cavity remains thin. The trophoblast enzymatically and physically causes the uterine epithelium in the area of attachment to start to degenerate and break down. It is believed that the trophoblast can absorb the products of cellular breakdown that are used to nourish the developing embryo. By the eleventh or twelfth day, the blastocyst sinks beneath the surface epithelium and becomes completely embedded in the stroma of the compact zone of the endometrium (see Fig. 15-24). The defect in the endometrial surface is closed by blood clot and later by proliferation of the surrounding surface epithelium.

Decidua

FORMATION. When the process of implantation is complete (day 12), the blastocyst lies in the superficial part of the compact layer of the endometrium. The stroma cells lying close to the trophoblast enlarge, become polyhedral, and are filled with glycogen and lipid material. The capillaries of the endometrium become congested and dilated and form intercommunicating sinusoids. As trophoblastic erosion of the endometrium continues, the walls of the maternal blood sinusoids are broken down (see Fig. 15-24). Meanwhile, many of the trophoblastic lacunae become confluent with one another and with the maternal blood sinusoids. In the earliest stage, the blood in the lacunae and the spaces in the endometrial stroma shows no circulation. Later, when the walls of the maternal arterioles and venules have become eroded by the trophoblast, a definite circulation of blood is established. Thus, the endometrium found in the secretory phase of the menstrual cycle undergoes further changes at the site of implantation. The changed endometrium is known as the *decidua,* and the enlarged stroma cells are called *decidual cells.*

The decidual cells first are confined to the immediate area of implantation, but they soon appear throughout the lining of the uterus. At this stage, the entire lining of the uterus is referred to as the decidua, and three different regions can be recognized: (1) the *decidua basalis,* a region lying between

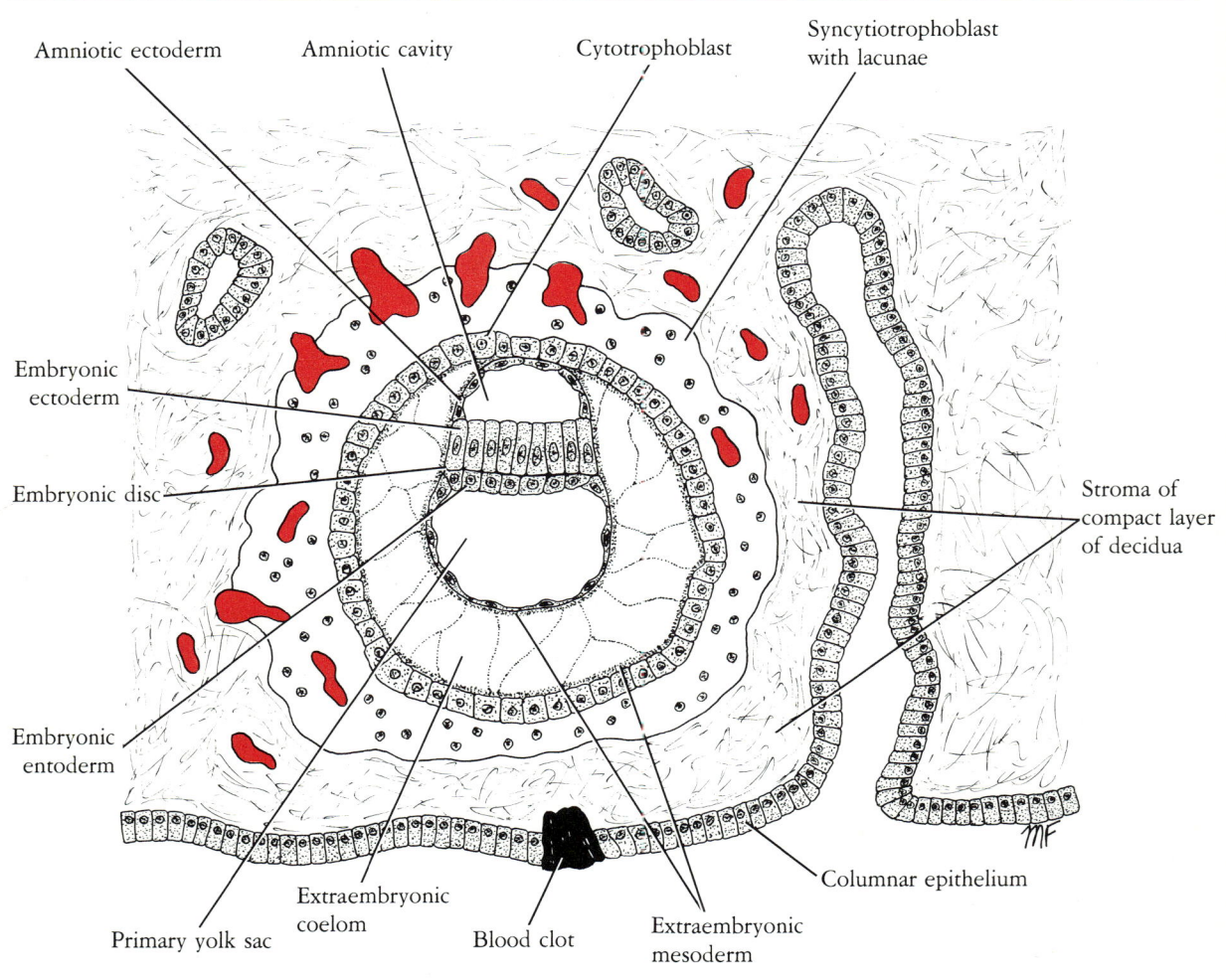

Fig. 15-24. Cross section of an 11-day-old blastocyst, showing the formation of two germ layers, the embryonic ectoderm and the embryonic entoderm. The amniotic cavity, the primary yolk sac, and the extra-embryonic coelom are also visible. The trophoblast has differentiated into the syncytiotrophoblast with lacunae and the cytotrophoblast.

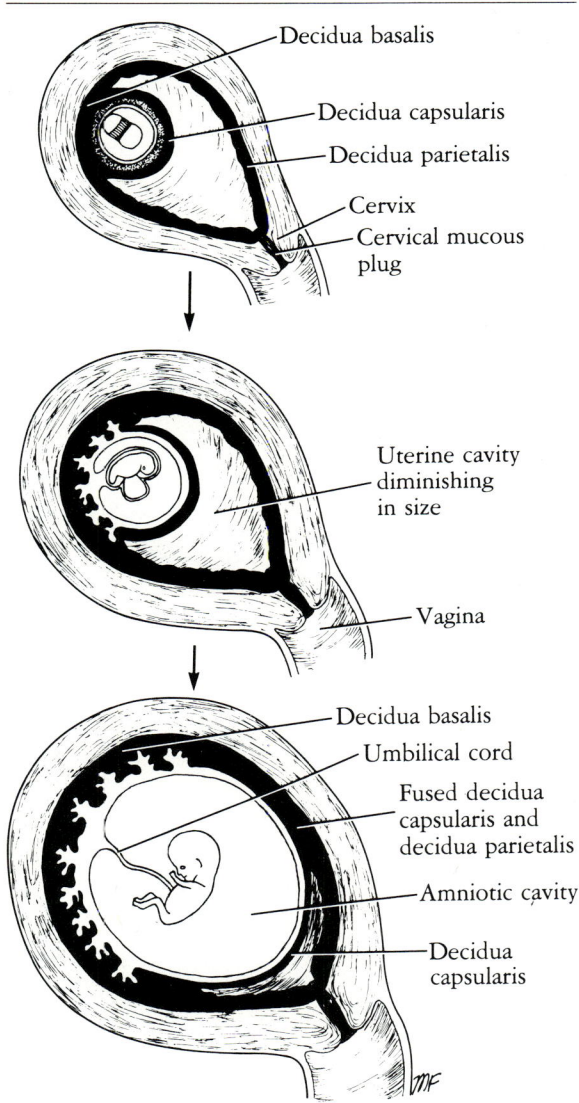

Fig. 15-25. *Developing conceptus expanding into the uterine cavity. The three different regions of the decidua can be recognized. By the fourth month, the uterine cavity is obliterated by the fusion of the decidua capsularis with the decidua parietalis.*

the blastocyst and the muscular wall of the uterus; (2) the *decidua capsularis*, a region that covers the blastocyst and separates it from the cavity of the uterus; and (3) the *decidua parietalis*, which is the remainder of the lining of the uterus (Fig. 15-25).

HORMONAL CONTROL OF THE DECIDUA. Once the ovum is fertilized, the corpus luteum continues to enlarge until the fourth month of pregnancy. During this time, it actively produces progesterone and estrogens, and the secretory activity of the endometrium, now referred to as the decidua, increases (Fig. 15-26). The corpus luteum at first is controlled by the luteinizing hormone (LH) secreted by the pituitary. Later, as the blastocyst becomes implanted in the decidua, the syncytial trophoblast starts to secrete the *chorionic gonadotropic hormone*. This hormone causes the corpus luteum to secrete large quantities of estrogens and progesterone that are responsible for maintaining the decidua.

At the end of the fourth month, the corpus luteum starts to degenerate, and, although it is still present at the end of pregnancy, estrogens and progesterone production is taken over by the placenta. This mechanism maintains the thick decidua throughout pregnancy.

Placenta

ESTABLISHMENT. During the process of implantation, lacunae appear in the syncytiotrophoblast that later become confluent. As a result of erosion of the decidual blood vessels, maternal blood enters the lacunae. Between day 9 and day 20, the trophoblast and the lining of extra-embryonic mesoderm, together known as the *chorion*, undergo intense growth and differentiation. Cords of cytotrophoblast cells migrate into the irregular processes of the syncytial layer (Fig. 15-27). At this stage, the processes are known as *primary villi*. Each villus now has an inner core of cytotrophoblast and an outer covering of syncytiotrophoblast. These villi lie between the large blood-filled spaces formed by the confluence of the trophoblastic lacunae and the excavated areas of the decidua. The blood-filled spaces

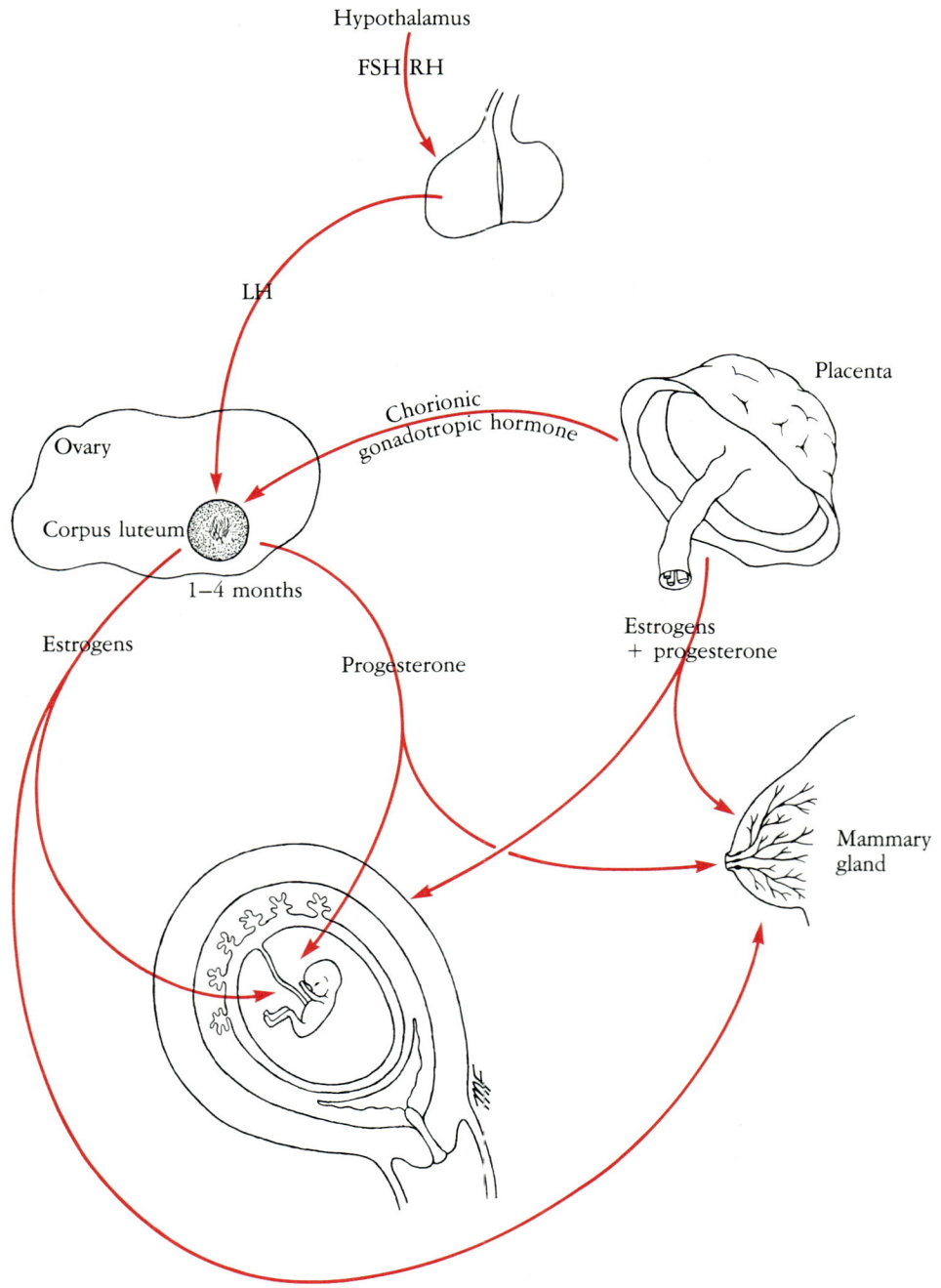

Fig. 15-26. Hormonal control of the pregnant uterus and mammary glands. Note the important part played by the hormones produced by the placenta.

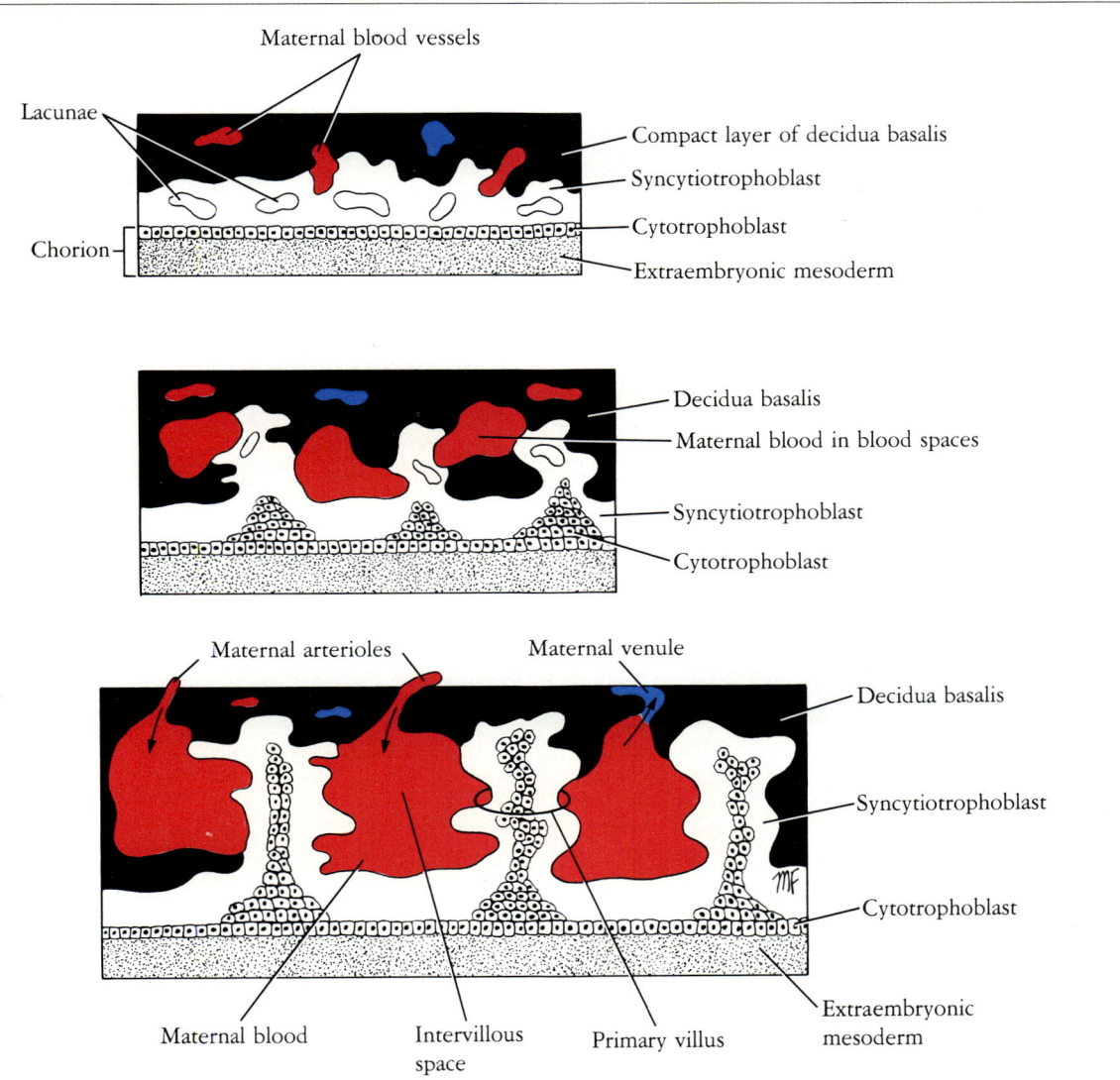

Fig. 15-27. Development of the primary chorionic villi.

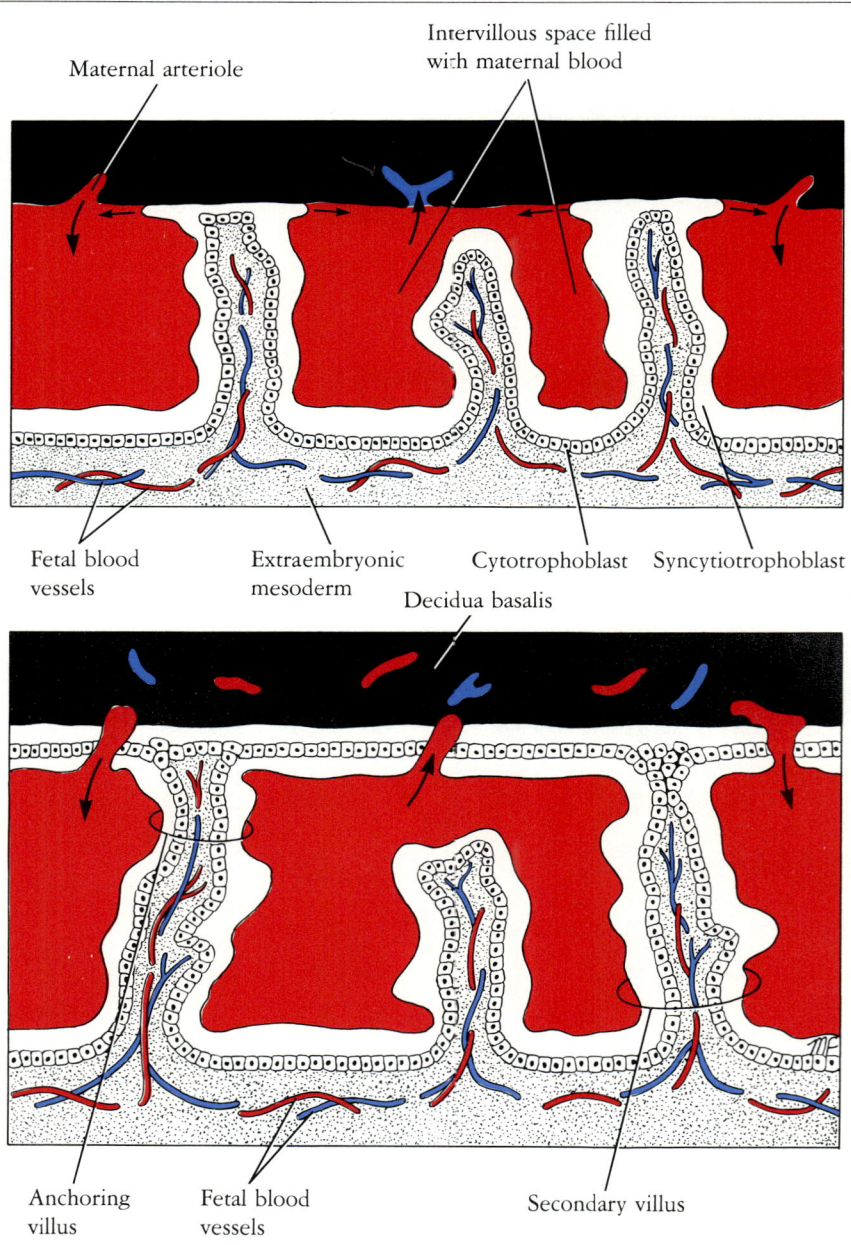

Fig. 15-28. Development of the secondary chorionic villi.

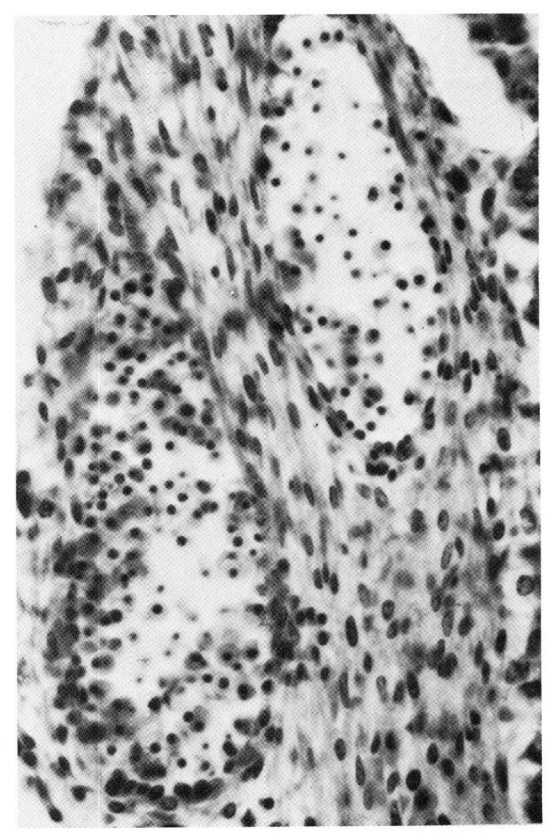

Fig. 15-29. Photomicrograph of a section of the chorion, showing the fetal blood vessels containing nucleated erythrocytes and leukocytes. (H&E; ×400.)

are known as *intervillous spaces.* The extra-embryonic mesoderm of the chorion now invades the cytotrophoblastic core of each primary villus, which becomes known as a *secondary villus* (Fig. 15-28). At this stage, the cytotrophoblast cells and the syncytiotrophblast proliferate until they contact the stroma of the decidua. With further proliferation, they come to line all the intervillous spaces. Some of the villi project freely into the spaces and are not attached to the decidua.

Later, the mesenchymal cells that form the core of each secondary villus differentiate, and small blood capillaries appear. These soon connect with the blood vessels in the chorion (Fig. 15-29) and the newly formed blood vessels in the body stalk and in the embryo. The blood vessels in the body stalk will become the *umbilical vessels* (Fig. 15-30).

As the embryo continues to grow and enlarge, the decidua capsularis stretches and the villi in the corresponding part of the chorion gradually atrophy and disappear. This area of the chorion is then known as the *chorion laeve.* In contrast, the villi opposite the decidua basalis and in the region of the body stalk (the future site of the umbilical cord) increase in size and complexity; the chorion in this region is known as the *chorion frondosum.*

The placenta, the organ that carries out respiration, excretion, and nutrition for the embryo, is fully formed during the fourth month. It is developed by mother and child in symbiosis and consists of fetal and maternal parts.

Fetal Part of the Placenta. The villi of the chorion frondosum enlarge and become elaborately branched; they project into the intervillous spaces (Figs. 15-31 to 15-33). Some of the villi are attached directly to the decidua and have the additional function of ensuring anatomical fixation of the growing embryo to the uterine wall; for this reason, they are called *anchoring villi.*

During the fourth month, the layer of cytotrophoblast begins to regress, leaving only a syncytial covering. Thus, in the mature placenta, the fetal blood within the villi is separated from the maternal blood only by the endothelium of the capillaries and the single layer of syncytiotrophoblast. In the wall of the chorion, the blood vessels anastomose with one another and the larger vessels converge to the attachment of the umbilical cord. The edge of the fetal part of the placenta is continuous with the chorion laeve.

Maternal Part of the Placenta. During the invasion of the stratum compactum of the decidua basalis by the syncytiotrophoblast, large areas were excavated to form the irregular intervillous spaces (see Figs. 15-27 and 15-30). The lacunae of the syncytiotrophoblast form a small part of these spaces. As the intervillous spaces develop, they become lined with trophoblast, as we have described. Maternal spiral arterioles containing oxygenated blood open into

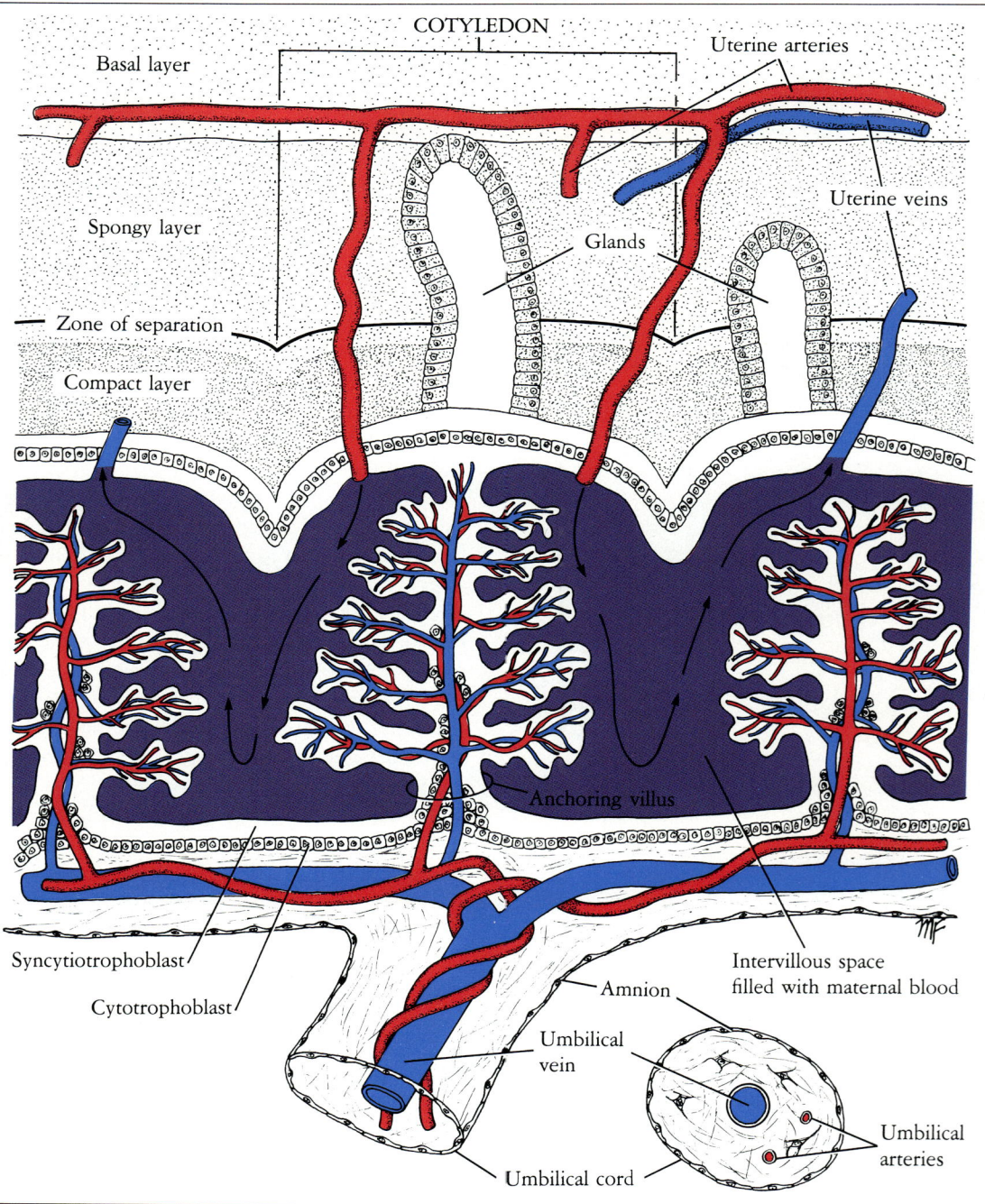

Fig. 15-30. Fetal and maternal parts of the placenta. The heavy solid line indicates the zone in the stratum spongiosum where separation occurs during the third stage of labor.

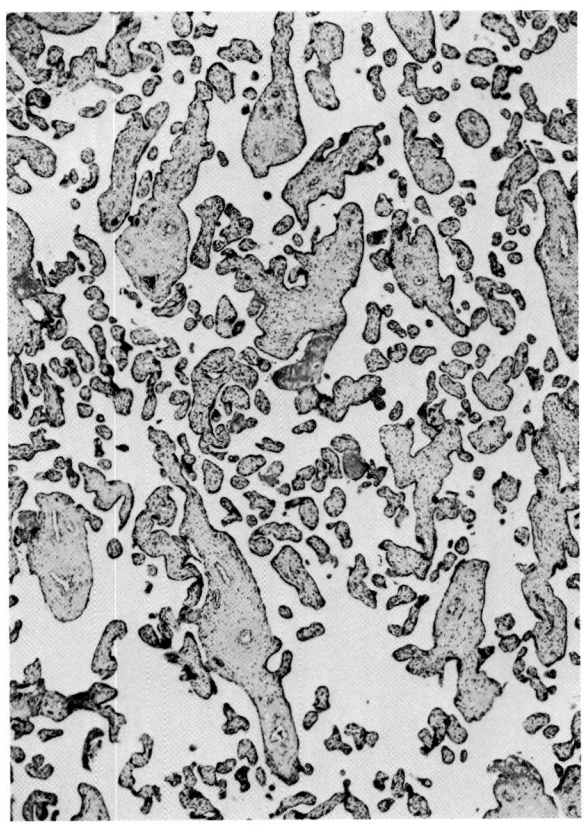

Fig. 15-31. Photomicrograph of a cross section of the fetal part of the placenta, showing the villi of the chorion projecting into the intervillous spaces. The villi contain numerous fetal blood vessels. The intervillous spaces here are empty; the maternal blood has been washed out during slide preparation. (H&E; ×40.)

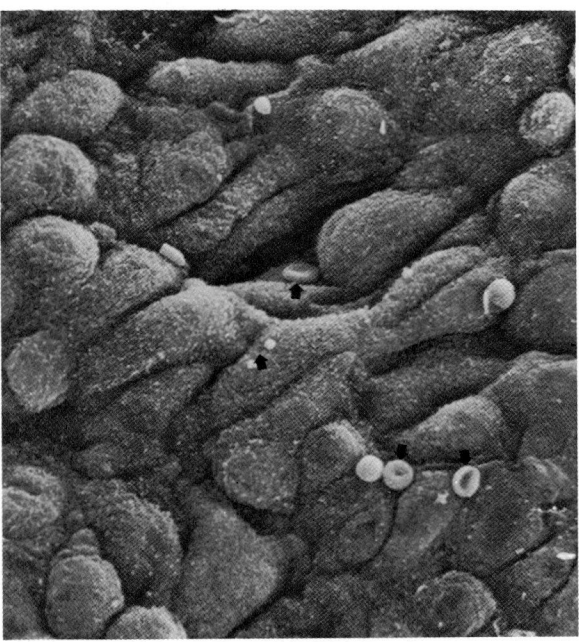

Fig. 15-32. Scanning electron micrograph of the surface of a placental villus, showing the syncytiotrophoblast covered by small microvilli. A few maternal erythrocytes (arrows) are shown in contact with the trophoblast. (×800.) (Courtesy of Drs. A. G. H. Al-Zuhair, M. E. A. Ibrahim, and S. Mughal.)

the spaces at intervals and bathe the outer surfaces of the bushy villi of the fetal part of the placenta. Venules drain the maternal blood from the spaces, aided by the mild contractions of the uterus. The *marginal sinus* is the name given to the most peripheral part of the intervillous space, i.e., the part that lies closest to the edge of the placenta. It has no particular significance.

In some areas, parts of the stratum compactum remain as solid projections, or septa, that project into the intervillous space. Such septa, called *placental septa*, mark off the territory of a major villous tree and in so doing divide the placenta into distinct lobules, or *cotyledons* (see Fig. 15-30). There may be a total of fifteen to thirty cotyledons, incompletely separated from one another by the placental septa. At the edge of the maternal part of the placenta, the decidua basalis is continuous with the decidua parietalis.

GROSS APPEARANCE OF THE PLACENTA. By the fourth month of pregnancy, the placenta is a well-developed organ. As the pregnancy continues, the placenta increases in area and thickness. The increase in placental area accompanies the steady expansion of the uterus. In fact, the placental attachment occupies one-third of the internal surface of the uterus throughout the remainder of the preg-

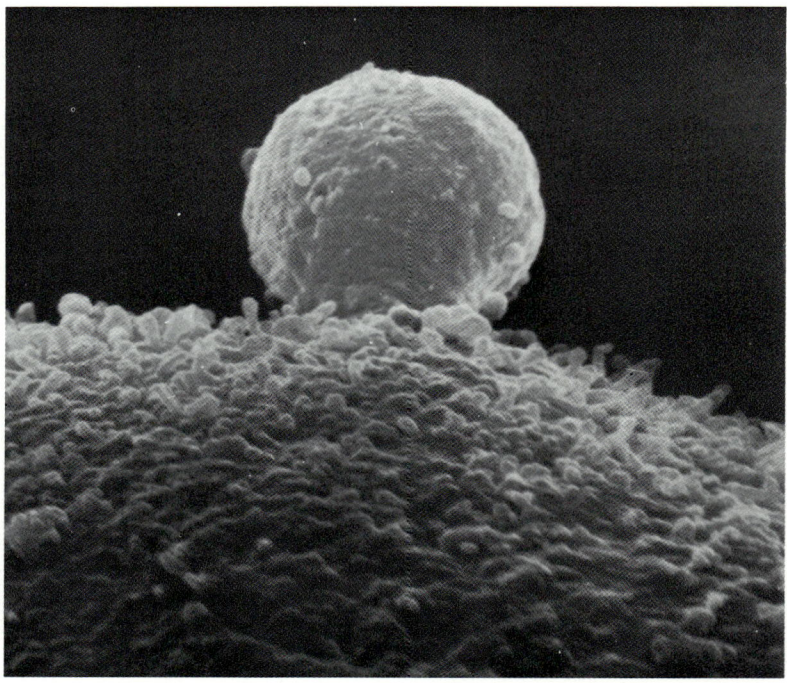

Fig. 15-33. Scanning electron micrograph of the surface of a placental villus, showing a maternal lymphocyte in contact with the trophoblast. Note the numerous small microvilli on the free surface of the syncytiotrophoblast. (×8,100.) (Courtesy of Drs. A. G. H. Al-Zuhair, M. E. A. Ibrahim, and S. Mughal.)

nancy. The increase in placental thickness is a result of elongation of the villi.

At term, the placenta has a flattened, circular shape, with a diameter of about 8 inches (20 cm) and a thickness of about 1 inch (2.5 cm), and weighs about 1 lb. (500 gm). It thins at the edges, where it is continuous with the fetal membranes (Fig. 15-34). The fetus is suspended from the placenta by the umbilical cord.

At birth, a few minutes after the delivery of the child, the placenta separates from the uterine wall and is expelled from the uterine cavity by contractions of the uterine musculature. The line of separation occurs through the spongy layer of the decidua basalis.

The outer *maternal surface* of the freshly shed placenta is dark red and oozes blood from the torn maternal vessels. It is spongy, with a rough outer surface, and margins of the cotyledons can be recognized (see Fig. 15-34).

The *fetal surface* is smooth and shiny and is raised in ridges by the umbilical vessels, which radiate from the attachment of the umbilical cord near its center. This surface is covered by amnion, which is fused with the underlying chorion.

The fetal membranes, which surround and enclose the liquor amnii, are continuous with the edge of the placenta and consist of the amnion and chorion laeve and a small amount of adherent decidua parietalis.

PLACENTAL CIRCULATION. *Maternal Circulation in the Placenta.* Maternal blood enters the intervillous spaces via the spiral arteries of the decidua basalis

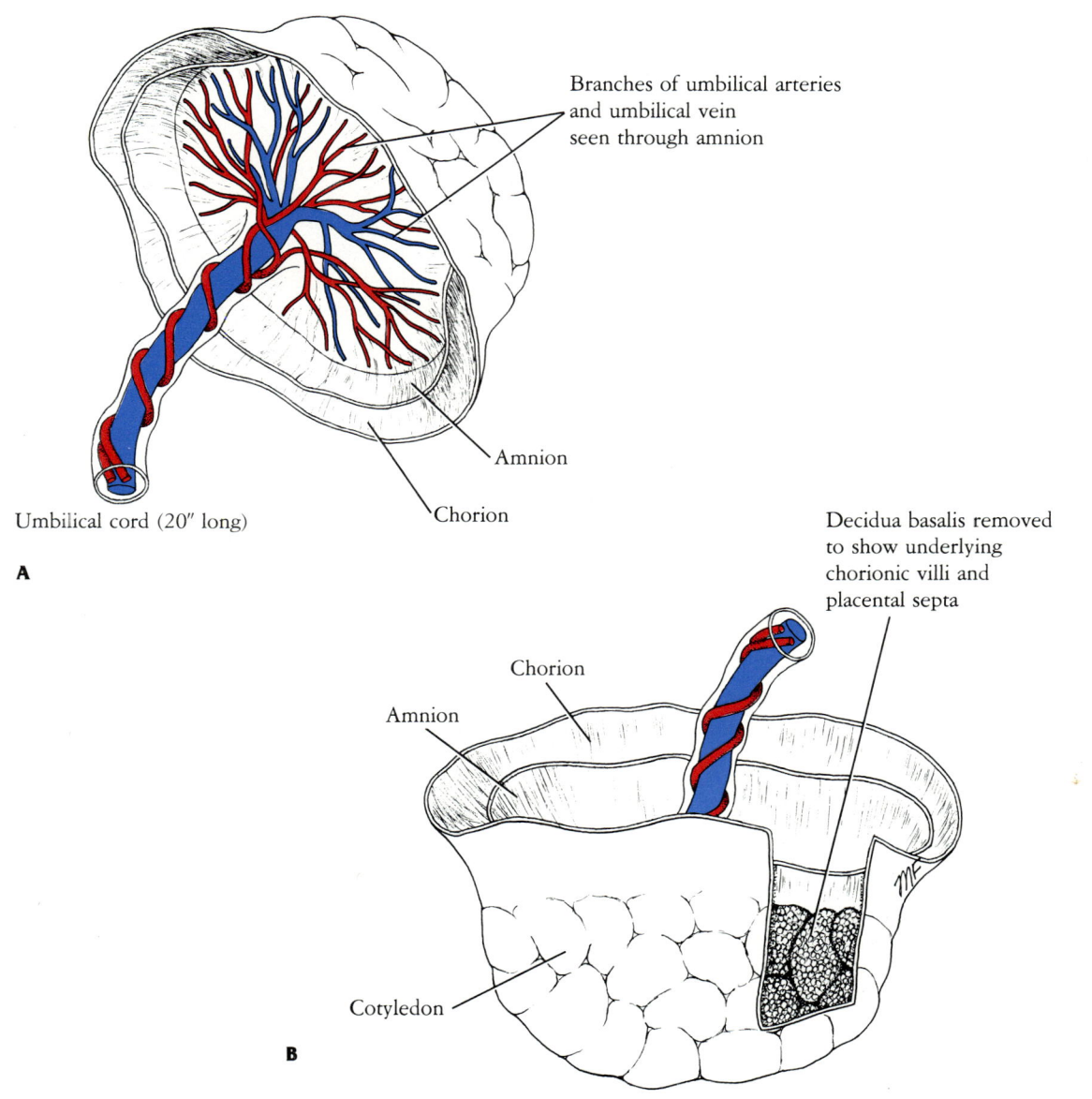

Fig. 15-34. *Mature placenta as seen from the fetal surface (A) and the maternal surface (B).*

and leaves by means of numerous thin-walled decidual veins. The total capacity of the intervillous spaces is relatively large: about 175 ml of maternal blood. In the mature placenta, the blood flow is about 500 ml per minute. The spiral arteries squirt the fresh maternal blood onto the bushy embryonic villi, and the blood is drained by the venules. The periodic uterine contractions aid this process by squeezing the intervillous spaces and forcing the blood into the venules and uterine veins.

Fetal Circulation in the Placenta. The deoxygenated fetal blood reaches the chorionic villi via the two umbilical arteries and their branches. The blood flows through the arterioles and small capillaries in the frondlike branches of the villi. Oxygenated blood now returns to the fetus via the venules and veins, which join one another and drain into the umbilical vein. Blood flows through the fetal villi at about 400 ml per minute. In the mature placenta, the fetal blood is separated from the maternal blood in the villi by the very thin syncytiotrophoblast, the mesenchymal stroma, and the endothelial lining of the capillaries. These layers constitute the *placental membrane* or *placental barrier;* the total area of this membrane is about 14 square meters.

FUNCTIONS OF THE PLACENTA. The functions of the placenta fall into several groups.

1. *Respiration.* Oxygen supplied by the mother diffuses across the placental membrane into the fetal blood. This process is aided by the greater affinity for oxygen of fetal hemoglobin compared with maternal hemoglobin. Carbon dioxide passes readily in the opposite direction. The placenta thus serves as an efficient lung for the fetus.
2. *Nutrition.* Water, inorganic salts, carbohydrates, fats, proteins, and vitamins can all pass in different forms from the maternal to the fetal blood.
3. *Excretion.* Products of fetal metabolism can cross the placenta into the maternal circulation, the placenta functioning like a kidney.
4. *Protection.* Foreign particulate matter, such as bacteria, is unable to cross the barrier unless the placenta itself becomes actively involved in the inflammatory process.
5. *Storage.* Carbohydrates, proteins, calcium, and iron are stored in the placenta. These are later released into the fetal circulation for use by the fetus.
6. *Hormonal production.* Hormones, including estrogens, progesterone, chorionic gonadotropin, and chorionic somatomammotropin are produced by the placenta.

PLACENTAL MEMBRANE. *Detailed Structure.* The placental membrane separates the fetal blood in the chorionic villi from the maternal blood in the intervillous spaces. In the early stage, it is about 0.025 mm thick and consists of the fetal capillary endothelium, the stroma of the villus, the cytotrophoblast, and the syncytiotrophoblast. After the fifth month of pregnancy, the cytotrophoblast cells disappear, the syncytiotrophoblast thins greatly, and the stroma of the villi is much reduced. In the later months of pregnancy, the membrane is only about 0.002 mm thick. Toward the end of pregnancy, fibrinoid material is deposited on the maternal surface of the chorionic villi; this tends to thicken the placental membrane.

It has been shown by the use of tracer substances that the permeability of the placental membrane alters with histological changes. It reaches its maximum during the thirty-sixth week and rapidly declines during the last few weeks of pregnancy. Electron microscopic examination of the syncytiotrophoblast shows that numerous microvilli are present on its free surface, greatly increasing the surface area and facilitating diffusion. The presence of vacuoles and pinocytotic vesicles also indicates that macromolecules and fluid are transferred across the membrane by means other than simple diffusion. Histochemical investigations of the placental membrane have revealed the presence of the enzymes cholinesterase and acid and alkaline phosphatase as well as proteolytic and glycolytic enzymes, all of which probably are involved in the transfer process.

Transfer across the Placental Membrane. Diffusion. Simple diffusion is the method used to transfer small molecules—such as gases, water, free amino acids, simple sugars, some hormones and vitamins, and inorganic substances—across the membrane.

Active Transport. The concentrations of calcium, inorganic phosphorus, and free amino nitrogen are slightly higher in fetal blood than in maternal blood, raising the possibility that some transport mechanism exists in addition to simple diffusion. The level of fructose in fetal blood is considerably higher than that in maternal blood; possibly, the placenta manufactures fructose from glucose. Vitamin C appears to be absorbed selectively across the placenta. Substances of very high molecular weight, such as protein, are known to cross the membrane, and it is now generally agreed that pinocytosis is the method of transfer. It is believed that antigens and antibodies are also transferred by this means. Maternal antibodies that have a higher molecular weight—those for such diseases as diphtheria, scarlet fever, tetanus, smallpox, and measles—are actively transferred across the barrier, conferring passive immunity to such infections on the child for a variable period after birth.

Some researchers have suggested the existence of small openings in the membrane sufficiently large to permit the passage of very large protein molecules or erythrocytes. The evidence supporting the existence of such holes, however, is unconvincing.

In Rh incompatibility, fetal erythrocyte antigens cross the membrane and result in antibody production by the mother against the Rh antigens. The maternal antibodies then cross the membrane and cause breakdown of the erythrocytes of the fetus, with consequent severe anemia, jaundice, and even fetal death.

PLACENTA AS AN ENDOCRINE GLAND. The placenta secretes estrogens, progesterone, chorionic gonadotropin, and chorionic somatomammotropin (Fig. 15-35). Extraction procedures and histochemical studies have revealed that these hormones are produced in the fetal part of the placenta in the syncytiotrophoblast.

Function of Estrogens in Pregnancy. The placental estrogens are responsible for the continuing enlargement of the uterus, the growth of the glandular ducts in the breast, and the increase in size of the maternal external genitalia. Toward the end of pregnancy, the high concentrations of circulating estrogens bring about relaxation of the sacro-iliac joints and the symphysis pubis, thus enlarging the pelvic inlet and outlet for the passage of the fetus during parturition. Estrogen also increases the contractility of the smooth muscle of the uterine wall and thus plays an important role in promoting uterine contractions when labor commences.

Function of Progesterone in Pregnancy. The placenta becomes the main producer of progesterone, assuming the role from the corpus luteum at about the fourth month of pregnancy. Progesterone is essential for the development and maintenance of the decidua throughout pregnancy. It is also responsible for the further development and growth of the glandular alveoli of the breasts. Progesterone opposes the action of estrogen on the contractility of the smooth muscle of the uterus. Toward the end of pregnancy, the amount of estrogen produced increases, whereas that of progesterone does not. The uterine muscle thus becomes more irritable and more susceptible to the influence of oxytocin from the posterior lobe of the pituitary and to other factors at the end of pregnancy.

Function of Chorionic Gonadotropin. Chorionic gonadotropin is responsible for the continued growth and maintenance of the corpus luteum at the end of the menstrual cycle once fertilization has occurred. The corpus luteum in turn produces increasing quantities of estrogens and progesterone, which further develop the secretory endometrium with the formation of the decidua. As we have mentioned, the corpus luteum starts to degenerate at about the fourth month of pregnancy, and the formation of

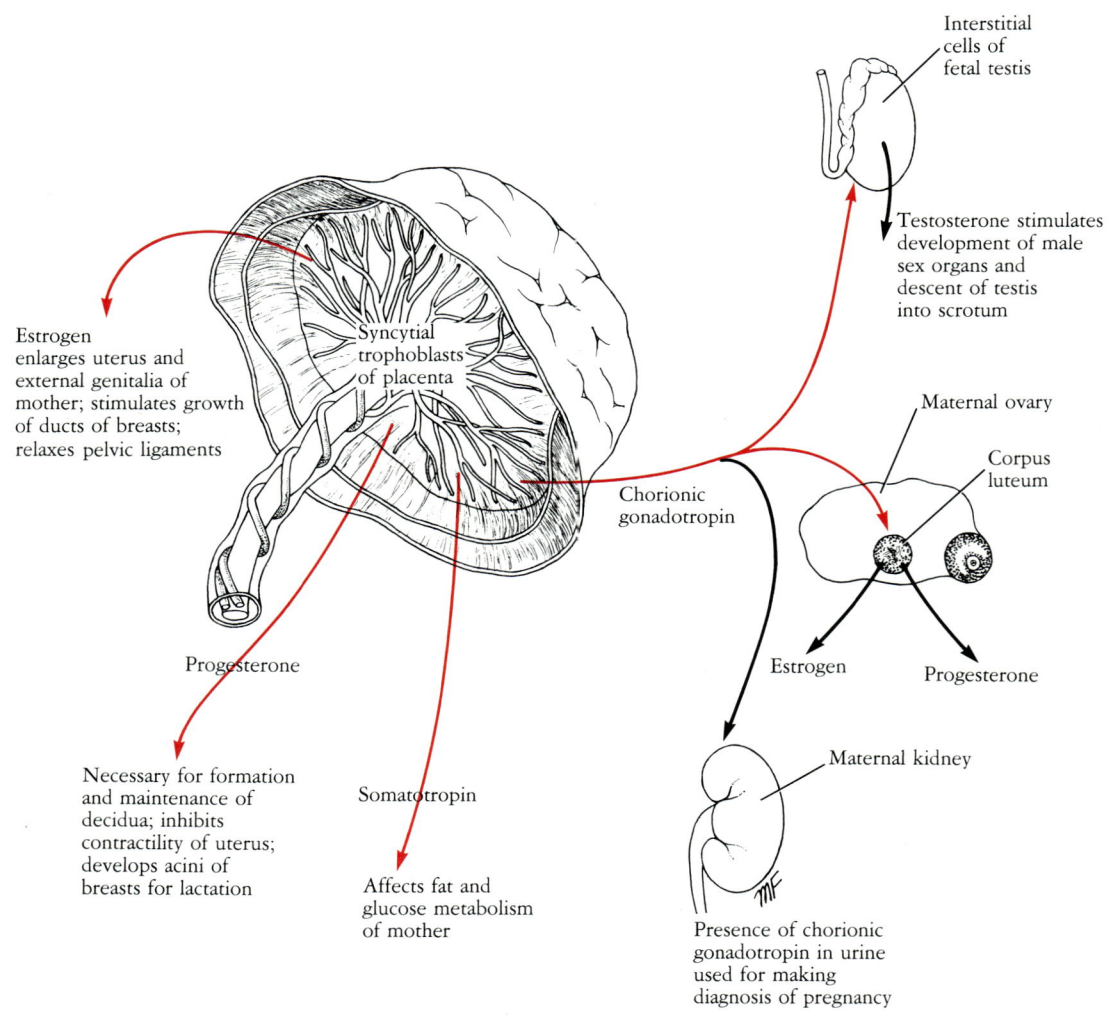

Fig. 15-35. Actions of the various hormones produced by the syncytiotrophoblast of the placenta.

large and increasing amounts of estrogens and progesterone is taken over by the placenta. The corpus luteum becomes progressively smaller but persists until parturition.

Function of Chorionic Somatomammotropin. Chorionic somatomammotropin is a recently discovered hormone that can influence the carbohydrate and fat metabolism of the mother and makes more glucose and fatty acids available for the fetus.

SEPARATION OF THE PLACENTA DURING THE THIRD STAGE OF LABOR. After the birth of the child, the rhythmic contractions of the uterus continue but are painless. Separation of the placenta from the uterine wall now takes place. As the uterus shrinks, there is a decrease in the surface area at the site of placental attachment. The placenta, unable to accommodate itself to the decreased area, begins to fold up and is squeezed off the uterine wall. Separation takes place at the spongy layer of the decidua basalis (see Fig. 15-30), and some bleeding occurs.

In a similar manner, the fetal membranes (the amnion and the chorion) and the remains of the decidua parietalis are squeezed from the remainder of the uterine wall. As the placenta is finally expelled from the uterus by the uterine contractions, the membranes attached to it are dragged along and peeled from the inner surface of the uterus. The expelled placenta and fetal membranes are often referred to as the *afterbirth*. The uterine muscle now becomes firmly contracted, and little bleeding occurs.

Role of the Uterus in Labor

Labor, or parturition, is the series of processes by which the baby, the fetal membranes, and the placenta are expelled from the genital tract of the mother. Normally this process takes place at the end of the tenth lunar month, at which time the pregnancy is said to be at *term*.

ONSET OF LABOR. The cause of the onset of labor is not definitely known. Throughout most of pregnancy, the uterus undergoes contractions that are painless, arrhythmic, and weak. Why they should suddenly become painful, rhythmic, and forceful at the onset of labor is still a matter for conjecture.

The uterine muscle in the region of the placenta remains largely inactive up to the time of birth to allow the placental circulation to function satisfactorily. In animals, the local injection of progesterone into the uterine muscle decreases its spontaneous activity. In the human subject, production of progesterone from the placenta increases after the fourth month of pregnancy, and it is probable that progesterone exerts a local inhibitory action on the uterine muscle cells near the placenta. Accompanying this local action of progesterone, the uterine muscle away from the placental site gradually hypertrophies, probably in response to a rise in estrogen influence. In the rabbit, for example, estrogen can cause hypertrophy of the uterine muscle in preparation for parturition. By the end of pregnancy, the contractility of the uterus has been fully developed in response to estrogen, and it is particularly sensitive to the actions of oxytocin at this time. In women, the onset of labor does not appear to be caused by a great change in the blood levels of either estrogen or progesterone. In some laboratory animals, the onset of parturition can be delayed by injecting large doses of progesterone. It is possible that the onset of labor in women can be attributed to the sudden withdrawal of an amount of progesterone or one of its metabolites too small to be detected by present biochemical techniques. Once the presenting part (usually the fetal head) starts to stretch the cervix, it is thought that a nervous reflex mechanism is initiated that increases the force of the contractions of the uterine body.

Uterine muscular activity is largely independent of the extrinsic innervation. In animals, normal parturition may take place following sympathectomy or section of the spinal cord. In women in labor, spinal anesthesia does not interfere with the normal uterine contractions. Severe emotional disturbances, however, may cause premature parturition.

During labor, the contractions of the uterus are assisted greatly by the contractions of the muscles of the anterior abdominal wall. The woman inhales deeply and closes the glottis of the larynx, thus preventing air from escaping from the lungs. The diaphragm is now fixed, permitting the abdominal muscles to exert their maximum force on the uterus. The abdominal muscles can be made to contract voluntarily by the mother, but as the baby descends through the birth canal, nervous impulses pass involuntarily and reflexly from the uterus and vagina to the abdominal muscles via the spinal cord.

The pain of the uterine contractions experienced in early labor almost certainly is caused by the anoxia of the uterine muscle resulting from the stronger and more prolonged contractions, which reduce the blood flow through the muscle. The pain impulses reach the spinal cord through the pelvic plexuses. During the second stage of labor, as the baby descends through the perineum, the pain is caused by stretching of the perineal structures. The pain impulses reach the spinal cord through the pudendal nerve. Blockage of the pudendal nerve and spinal or caudal anesthesia are procedures used in obstetrics to anesthetize the pain fibers.

Uterus after Parturition

The uterus after parturition rapidly shrinks in size but never completely regains its pregravid state. The smooth muscle of the uterine wall undergoes autolysis, and the end-products are removed by the phagocytic activity of histiocytes and by the bloodstream.

For about 3 weeks after birth, a discharge occurs from the genital tract of the mother. This is known as the *lochia,* and at first it is bright red and consists of blood and decidual remains; later it becomes brown, then yellow, and finally it stops. The denuded walls of the uterine cavity become lined with endometrium within 2 to 3 weeks after delivery as a result of the proliferation of the columnar cells of the glands and stroma of the decidual remains. The placental site requires a longer time for repair: about 6 to 8 weeks. The repair process is under the control of estrogens secreted by the ovary.

VAGINA

The vagina is the female organ for copulation; it serves as the excretory duct for the uterus and forms part of the birth canal. The vagina (see Fig. 15-1) extends upward and backward from the vulva to the uterus and is about 3 inches (8 cm) long. The vaginal orifice possesses a thin mucosal fold called the *hymen,* which is perforated at its center. The vagina has anterior and posterior walls, which are normally in apposition. The upper half of the vagina lies within the pelvis between the bladder anteriorly and the rectum posteriorly; the lower half lies within the perineum between the urethra anteriorly and the anal canal posteriorly.

The wall of the vagina has three coats: (1) a mucous membrane, (2) a muscular coat, and (3) a connective tissue coat. The mucous membrane has two longitudinal folds, one on the anterior and one on the posterior wall, and from these folds numerous transverse folds extend laterally on each side. The mucous membrane is lined with stratified squamous nonkeratinized epithelium (Fig. 15-36). Between puberty and the menopause, the epithelium is thick and the cells contain large amounts of glycogen in

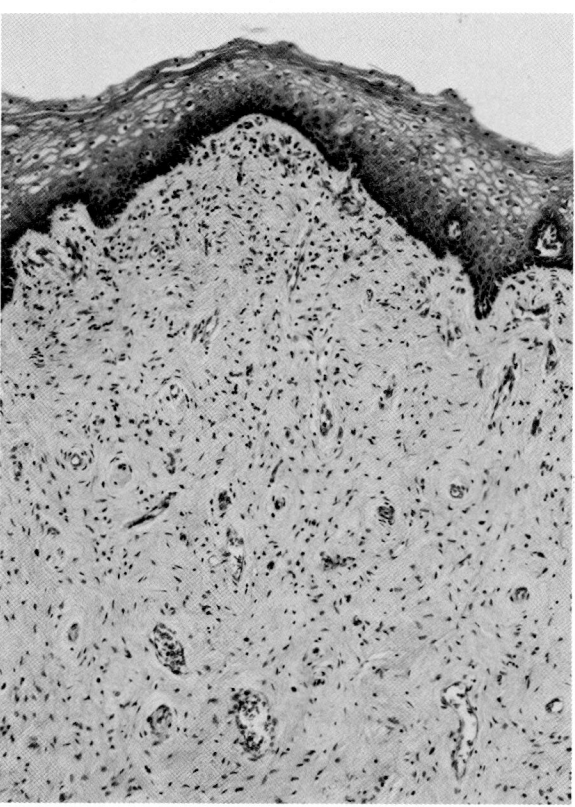

Fig. 15-36. Photomicrograph of a section of the vaginal wall, showing the stratified squamous nonkeratinized epithelium lining the mucous membrane. Note there are no glands in the mucous membrane of the vagina. (H&E; ×100.)

their cytoplasm (Fig. 15-37), giving the cytoplasm a vacuolated appearance on an H&E-stained section. As the surface cells are desquamated, the glycogen is liberated and fermented by *Döderlein's bacilli,* which convert it into lactic acid. The low pH of the vaginal lumen inhibits the growth of pathogenic bacteria. The epithelial lining and the glycogen content of the cells are controlled by the ovarian estrogens. There are no glands in the mucous membrane of the vagina. Mucous present in the vagina has been secreted by the glands of the cervix.

The muscle coat is composed of longitudinal outer and circularly arranged inner smooth muscle

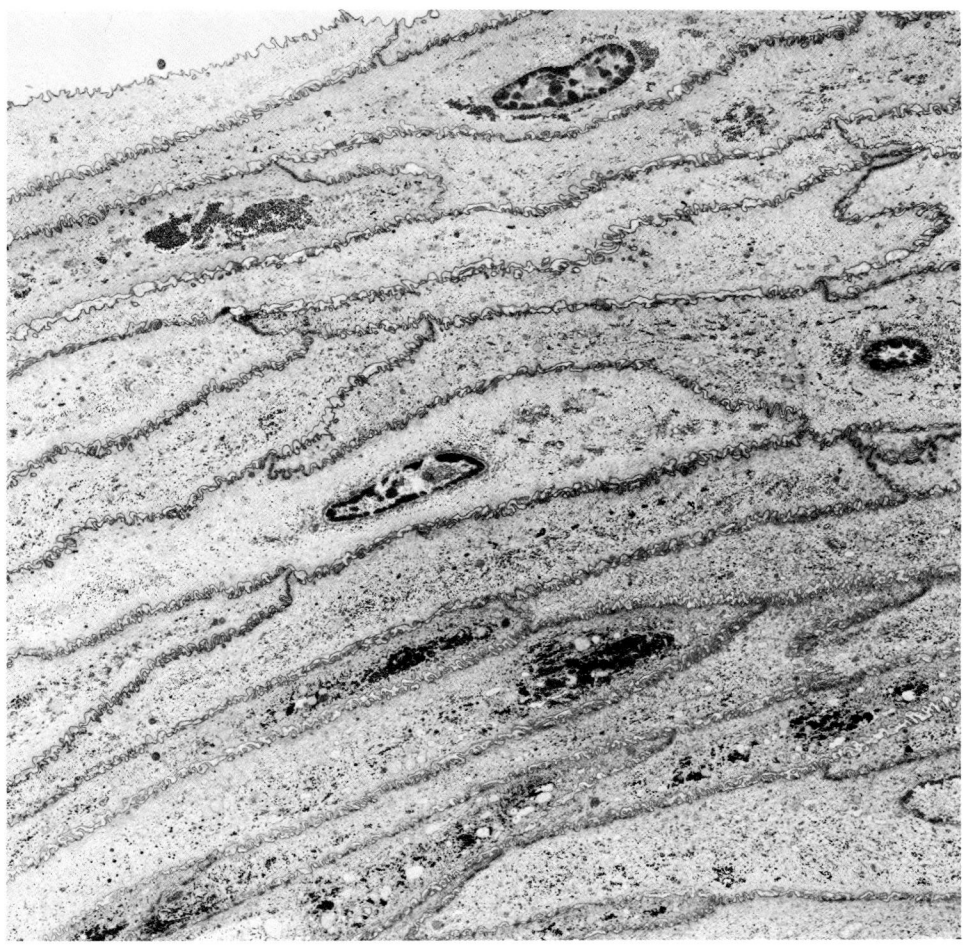

Fig. 15-37. Electron micrograph of the superficial layers of the lining epithelium of the vagina, showing the large amounts of glycogen (black dots) in the cytoplasm of the squamous cells. (×2,860.) (Courtesy of Dr. B. F. King.)

fibers. The lower end of the vagina is surrounded by a layer of striated muscle called the *bulbospongiosus muscle*. The connective tissue coat is composed of a layer of areolar tissue containing a large plexus of blood vessels.

EXTERNAL GENITALIA

The *vulva* is the name applied to the female external genitalia; the vulva includes the labia majora, the labia minora, the clitoris, and the greater vestibular glands.

Labia

The *labia majora* are prominent folds of skin extending back from the mons pubis to unite posteriorly in the midline (Fig. 15-38). They are equivalent to the scrotum in the male. The inner surface of the labia is smooth and devoid of hair; it possesses numerous hair follicles and sebaceous and sweat glands, however. Within the labia is a large amount of adipose tissue and some smooth muscle fibers, which are equivalent to the dartos muscle in the male.

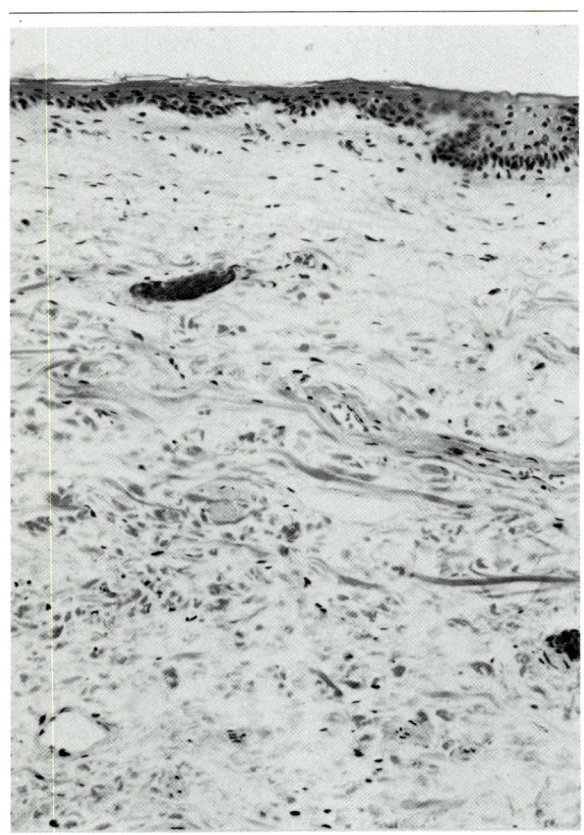

Fig. 15-38. Photomicrograph of a section of the medial surface of the labium majus, showing the covering of stratified squamous epithelium. (H&E; ×130.)

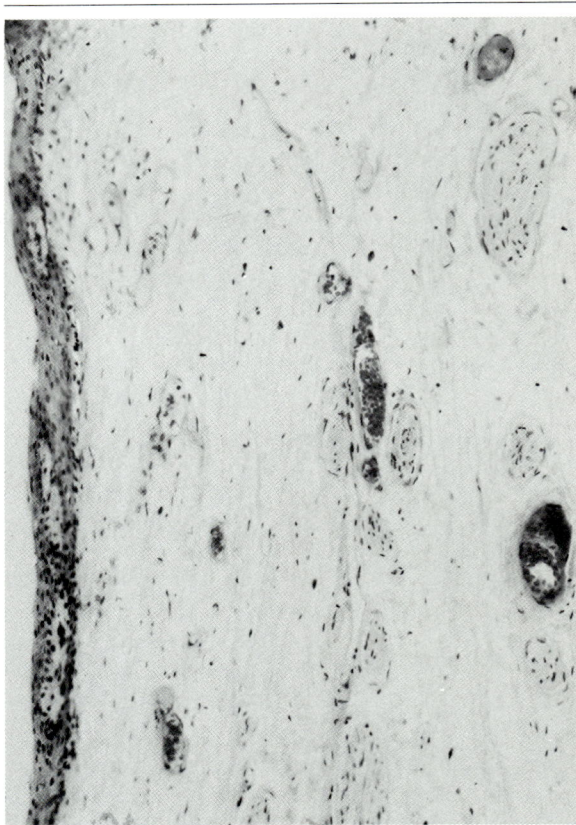

Fig. 15-39. Photomicrograph of a section of the medial surface of the labium minus. The surface can be seen to be covered by stratified squamous epithelium that rests on a very vascular connective tissue. (H&E; ×130.)

The *labia minora* are two smaller folds of soft, hairless skin that lie between the labia majora (Fig. 15-39). Their posterior ends are united to form a sharp fold, the *fourchette;* anteriorly, they split to enclose the clitoris, forming an anterior *prepuce* and a posterior *frenulum.* Numerous sebaceous glands are found on both surfaces of the fold. The core of each fold is composed of loose connective tissue that contains numerous blood vessels.

Clitoris

The clitoris, which corresponds to the penis in the male, is situated at the apex of the vestibule ante-riorly. The clitoris has a fixed *root* and a small *body,* which hangs free.

The root of the clitoris consists of the bulb of the vestibule and the crura of the clitoris. The bulb of the vestibule corresponds to the bulb of the penis, but because of the presence of the vagina, it is divided into two halves. It is composed of erectile tissue surrounded by a dense layer of fibrous tissue. It is attached to the undersurface of the urogenital diaphragm and is covered by a thin layer of striated muscle, the *bulbospongiosus muscle.* Anteriorly, the two halves of the bulb of the vestibule unite in the

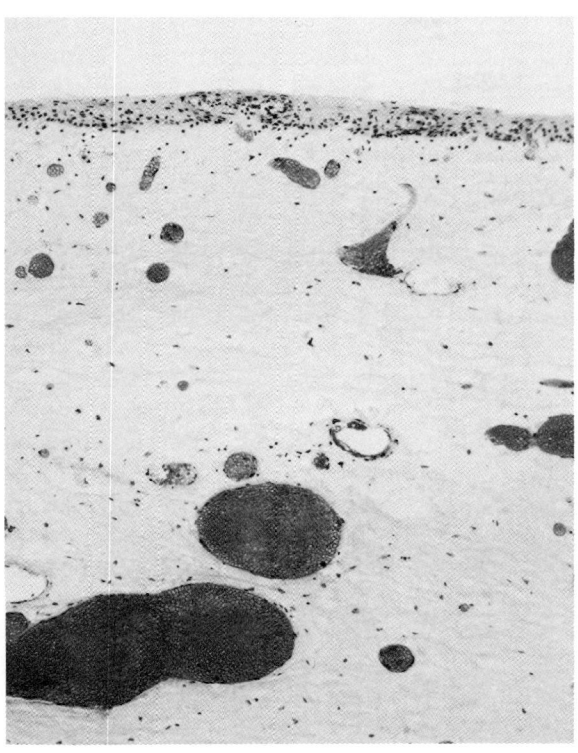

Fig. 15-40. Photomicrograph of a section of the glans clitoris. Note that the surface is covered by stratified squamous epithelium and the interior possesses erectile tissue, which is filled with blood. (H&E; ×100.)

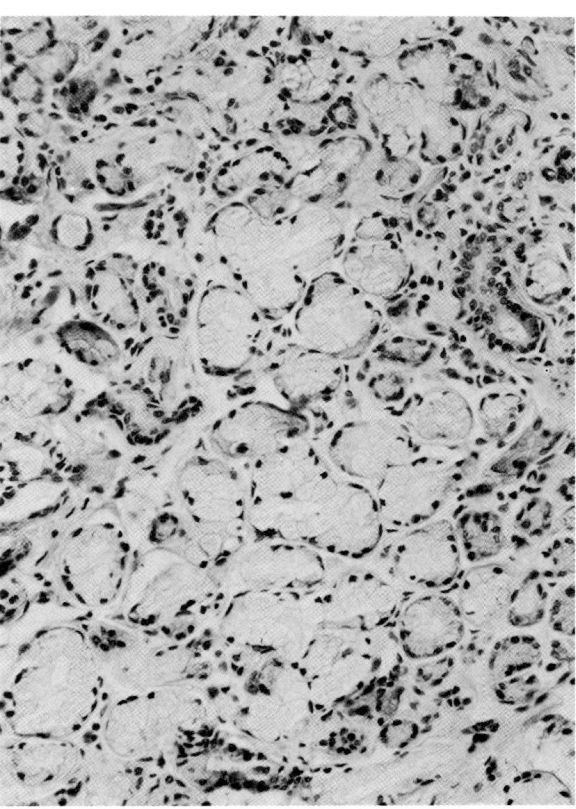

Fig. 15-41. Photomicrograph of a section of a greater vestibular gland, showing numerous tubulo-alveolar mucus-secreting units. (H&E; ×200.)

body of the clitoris to form the *glans clitoris* (Fig. 15-40).

The *crura of the clitoris* correspond to the crura of the penis. They are composed of erectile tissue surrounded by a dense layer of fibrous tissue. They continue forward into the body of the clitoris, forming the two *corpora cavernosa*. The crura are covered by a thin layer of skeletal muscle called the *ischiocavernosus* muscles.

The clitoris is surrounded by thin skin that contains numerous sensory nerve endings.

Erection of the Clitoris

Sexual excitement produces engorgement of the erectile tissue within the clitoris in exactly the same manner as it does in the penis of the male.

Greater Vestibular Glands

The greater vestibular glands are a pair of tubulo-alveolar mucus-secreting glands that lie under cover of the posterior parts of the bulb of the vestibule and the labia majora (Fig. 15-41). Each drains its secretion into the vestibule by a small duct that opens into the groove between the hymen and the posterior part of the labium minus. These glands serve to secrete a lubricating mucus during sexual intercourse.

External Genitalia of the Female Newborn

During fetal life, maternal and placental hormones enter the fetal circulation and activate the tissues of the mammary gland (see p. 618) and the reproductive system. The external genitalia show congestion and moisture, and the vaginal epithelium is hypertrophied. As the hormonal levels in the blood decrease, there may be uterine bleeding, vaginal desquamation, and a mucoid vaginal discharge. By the end of the second week after birth, the congestion of the genitalia disappears and the vaginal discharge ceases.

Orgasm in the Female

As in the male, vision, hearing, smell, touch, and other psychic stimuli gradually build up the intensity of sexual excitement. During this process, the vaginal walls become moist as a result of transudation of fluid through the congested mucous membrane. In addition, the greater vestibular glands at the vaginal orifice secrete a lubricating mucus.

The upper part of the vagina, which resides in the pelvic cavity, is supplied by the pelvic plexuses and is sensitive to stretch only. The region of the vaginal orifice, the labia minora, and the clitoris are extremely sensitive to touch.

Appropriate sexual stimulation of these sensitive areas, reinforced by afferent nervous impulses from the breasts and other regions, results in a climax of pleasurable sensory impulses reaching the central nervous system. Impulses then pass down the spinal cord to the sympathetic outflow (T1–L2).

The nervous impulses that pass to the genital organs are thought to leave the cord at the first and second lumbar segments in preganglionic sympathetic fibers. Many of these fibers synapse with postganglionic neurons in the first and second lumbar ganglia; other fibers may synapse in ganglia in the lower lumbar or pelvic parts of the sympathetic trunks. The postganglionic fibers are then distributed to the smooth muscle of the vaginal wall, which rhythmically contracts. In addition, nervous impulses travel in the pudendal nerve (S2, S3, and S4) to reach the bulbospongiosus and ischiocavernosus muscles, which also undergo rhythmic contraction.

MAMMARY GLANDS

The mammary glands are specialized accessory glands of the skin that are capable of secreting milk. They are present in both sexes. In the male and the immature female, they are similar in structure. The *nipples* are small, and each is surrounded by a colored area of skin called the *areola.* The breast tissue consists of little more than a system of ducts embedded in connective tissue; the ducts do not extend beyond the margin of the areola.

At puberty, the mammary glands in the female gradually enlarge and assume their hemispherical shape under the influence of the ovarian hormones (Fig. 15-42). The ducts elongate, but the increased size of the glands is caused by the deposition of adipose tissue. The base of the breast extends from the second to the sixth rib and from the lateral margin of the sternum to the midaxillary line. The greater part of the gland lies in the superficial fascia. A small part, called the *axillary tail,* extends upward and laterally, pierces the deep fascia at the lower border of the pectoralis major muscle, and enters the axilla. The mammary glands are separated from the deep fascia covering the underlying muscle by an area of loose areolar tissue known as the *retromammary space.*

Adult Female Resting Mammary Gland
Structure

In young women, the breasts tend to protrude forward from a circular base; in older women, they tend to be pendulous. Each gland consists of fifteen to twenty *lobes,* which radiate out from the nipple. There is no capsule. Each lobe is separated from its neighbors by connective tissue septa containing adipose tissue; the septa in the upper part of the gland are well developed, extend from the skin to the deep fascia, and serve as *suspensory ligaments.* The main lactiferous duct from each lobe opens separately on the summit of the nipple and possesses a dilated ampulla or lactiferous sinus just prior to its termination (see Fig. 15-42).

Each lobe is composed of several lobules held

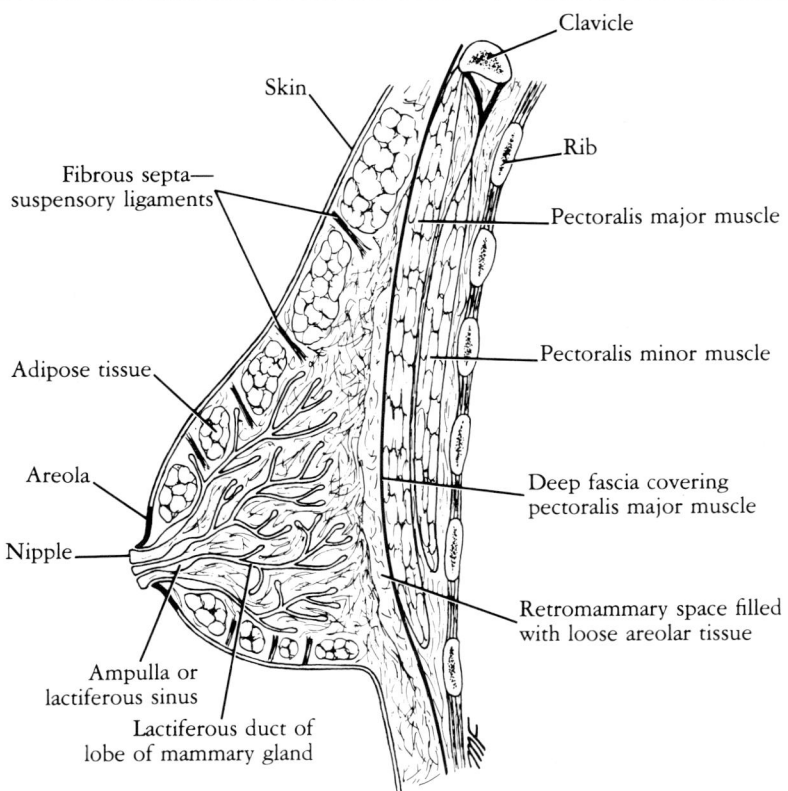

Fig. 15-42. Vertical section of the mammary gland, showing the general structure in a mature woman.

together by areolar and adipose tissue. Intralobular ducts join one another to form the main lactiferous duct (Fig. 15-43). The smaller ducts are lined with columnar epithelial cells, outside of which is a layer of myoepithelial cells resting on a basal lamina. The larger ducts are lined with two layers of epithelial cells. There are no secretory alveoli in the resting mammary gland (Fig. 15-44). The cells that close off the blind end of each intralobular duct enlarge during the second half of each menstrual cycle (Fig. 15-45), however, and some secretion may appear in the lumen. It is these cells that can develop into alveoli if appropriately activated by hormones. The greater part of the resting mammary gland is composed of adipose tissue. The increase in size of the mammary gland and the feeling of tenseness within the gland that may occur prior to the onset of menstruation is caused by the vasodilatation of the blood vessels within the glands and the accompanying edema of the connective tissue. It is during this phase of the cycle that large numbers of lymphocytes appear in the connective tissue surrounding the ducts. The nipple is a conical projection from the anterior surface of the gland and is traversed by fifteen to twenty lactiferous ducts, which open by small orifices on its tip. The skin of the nipple is pink or brown. There are numerous circular and longitudinal smooth muscle fibers in the connective tissue of the nipple, which cause the nipple to become erect when it is mechanically stimulated. The areola is an

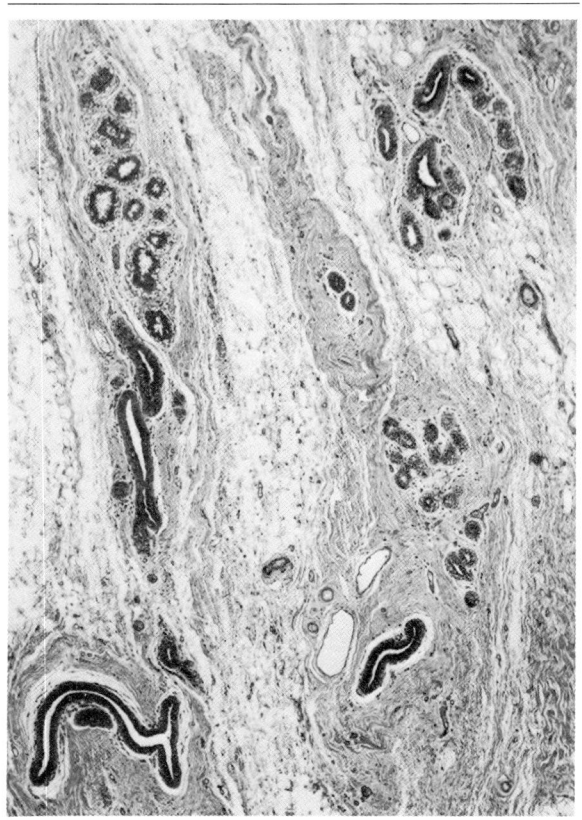

Fig. 15-43. Photomicrograph of a section of the mammary gland beneath the areola in the mature female, showing numerous large ducts supported by connective tissue. (H&E; ×52.)

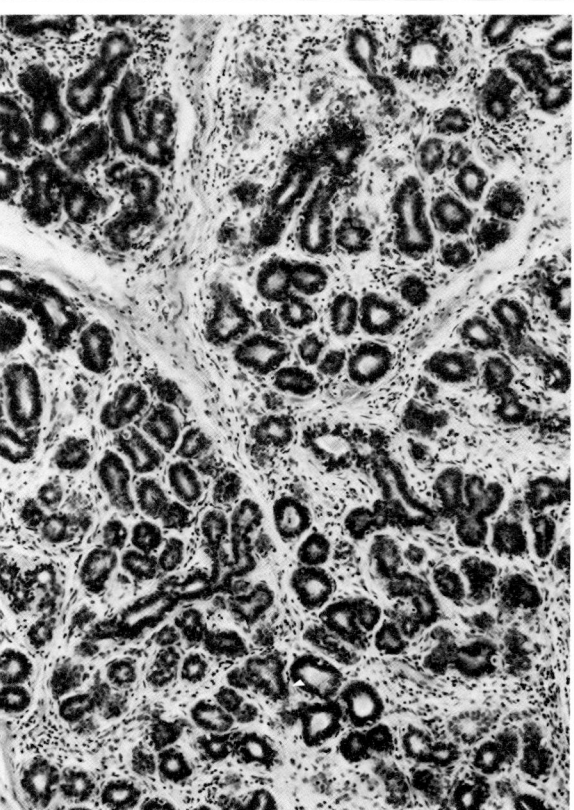

Fig. 15-44. Photomicrograph of a section of a resting mammary gland, showing numerous ducts supported by connective tissue. There are no secretory alveoli in the resting mammary gland. (H&E; ×100.)

area of pigmented skin that surrounds the base of the nipple. There are numerous sebaceous and sweat glands in the areola. The sebaceous glands, sometimes called *areolar glands,* are responsible for the tiny tubercles on the areola. Large tubercles are produced by larger modified sweat glands and are called *Montgomery's glands.*

Control of Structure of Adult Female Resting Mammary Gland

Under the influence of ovarian estrogens at puberty, the ducts of the gland elongate and some branching takes place (Figs. 15-45 and 15-46). The estrogens also increase the volume and vascularity of the connective tissue, and large amounts of adipose tissue are formed, causing the breasts to enlarge and to assume their adult shape. The nipples also enlarge. Progesterone has little or no effect on the gland, although it may cause some epithelial enlargement in the cells at the end of the duct system in the second half of the menstrual cycle. Thus, the adult resting gland undergoes cyclical stimulation by the ovarian hormones between puberty and the menopause.

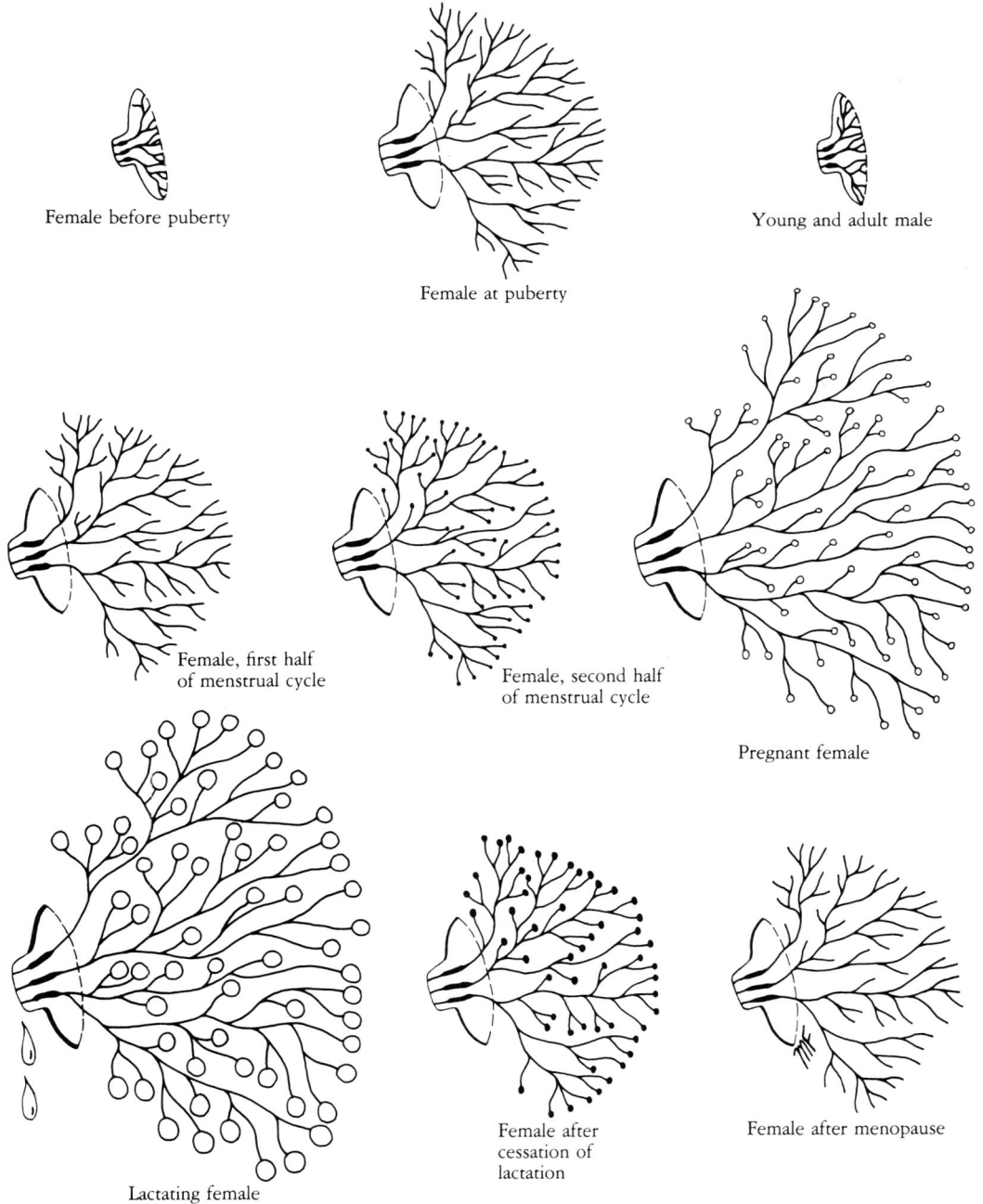

Fig. 15-45. Extent of development of the ducts and secretory alveoli in the mammary gland in both sexes at different stages of activity.

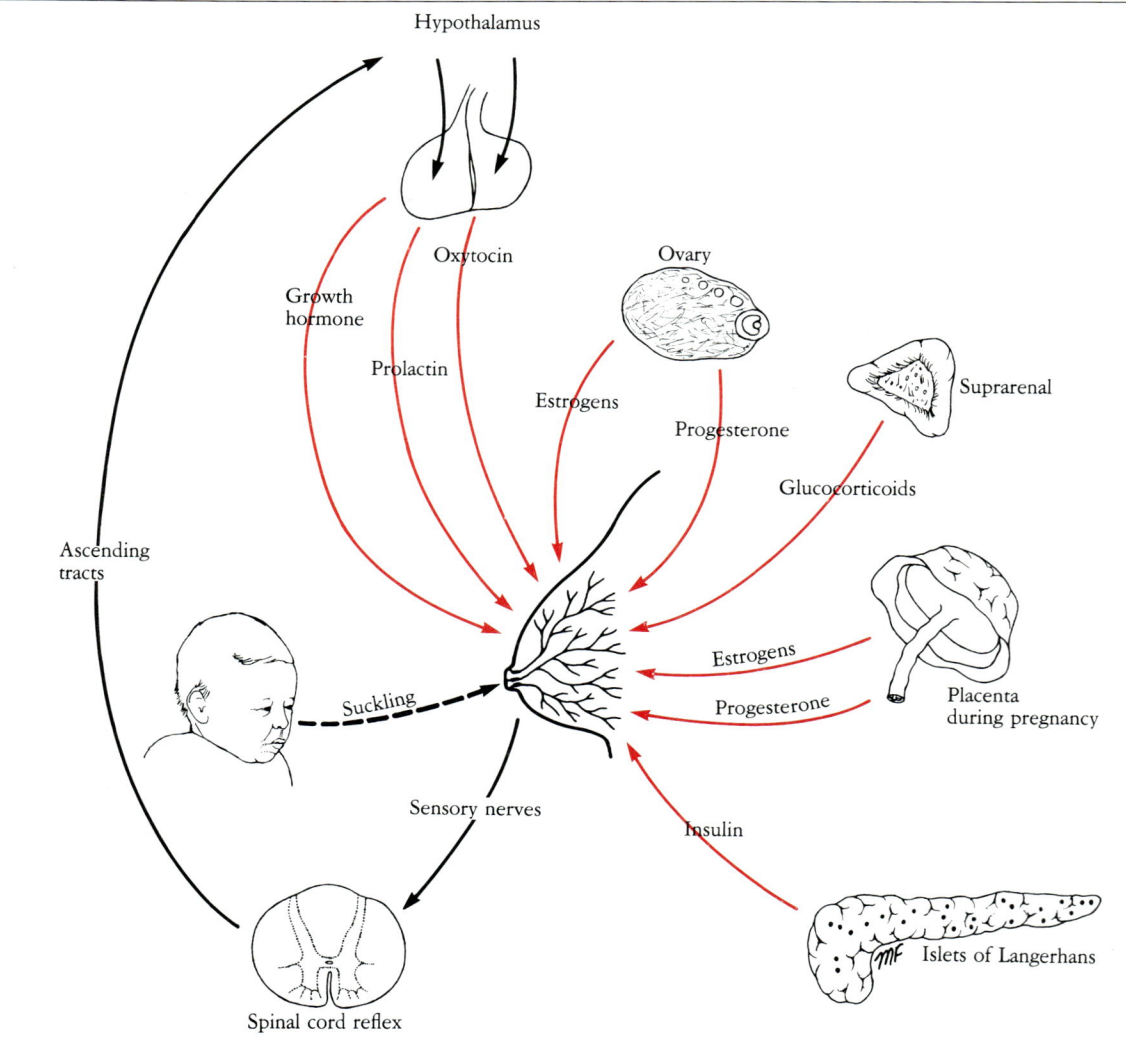

Fig. 15-46. Hormonal control of the mammary gland.

Mammary Gland during Pregnancy

Structure

During the early months of pregnancy, there is a rapid increase in length and branching in the duct system (see Fig. 15-45). In addition, secretory alveoli develop at the ends of the smaller ducts and the connective tissue becomes filled with expanding and budding alveoli. The alveoli are lined with columnar epithelial cells and are surrounded by a discontinuous layer of myoepithelial cells. The vascularity of the connective tissue also increases to provide adequate nourishment for the developing gland. The nipple enlarges, and the areola becomes darker and more extensive as a result of increased deposits of melanin pigment in the epidermis. The areolar glands enlarge and become more active.

During the second half of pregnancy, the growth process slows. The breasts, however, continue to enlarge, largely because of the distention of the al-

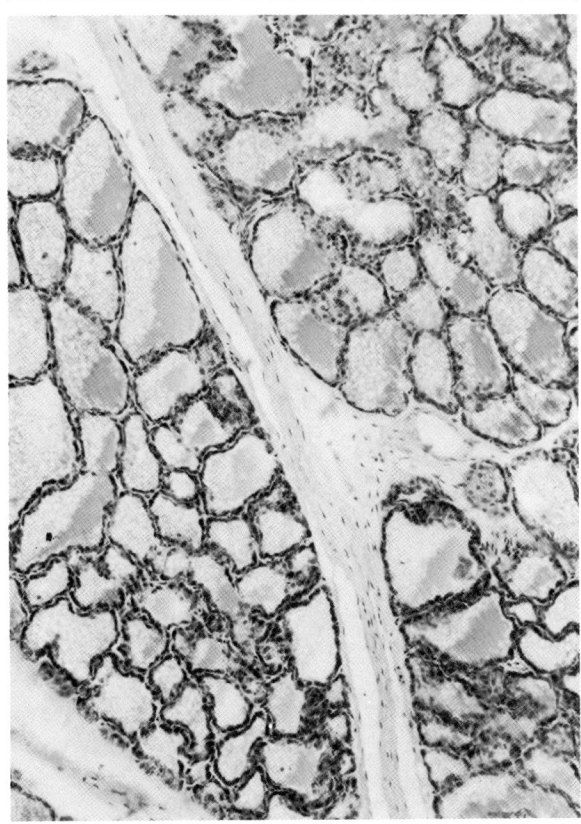

Fig. 15-47. Photomicrograph of a section of a lactating mammary gland, showing the alveoli to be distended with milk. (H&E; ×100.)

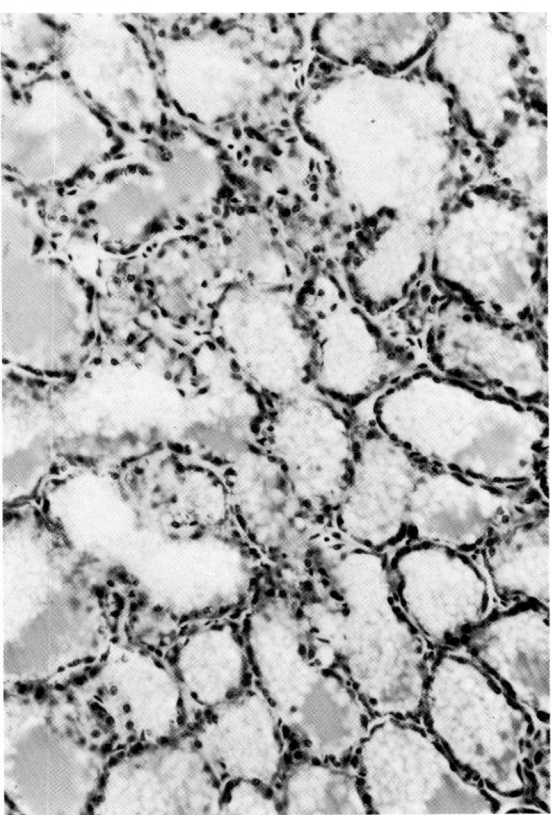

Fig. 15-48. Photomicrograph of a high-power view of the section of lactating mammary gland shown in Figure 15-47, showing the distended alveoli to be lined with flattened cuboidal epithelium. The connective tissue between the alveoli is compressed and is not easily visible. (H&E; ×200.)

veoli with fluid secretion called *colostrum*. This secretion is not milk but is rich in proteins and lactose. It contains practically no fat. Occasional cells called *colostrum corpuscles* are found in the alveolar lumina, and their cytoplasm contains numerous fat globules. These corpuscles are thought to be cells that have been shed from the walls of the alveoli or phagocytes that have entered the lumina of the alveoli.

Control of the Mammary Gland during Pregnancy

The large amounts of estrogen secreted by the placenta are responsible for the considerable growth of the duct system and the increased vascularity of the connective tissue (see Fig. 15-46). Progesterone also produced by the placenta is responsible for the extensive development of the alveoli. There is evidence as well that the growth hormone and prolactin produced by the pituitary, the adrenal glucocorticoids, and insulin take part in preparing the breasts for lactation.

Lactating Mammary Gland

Structure

The structure of the lactating gland varies in different areas. In an area that is moderately active, the alveoli are filled with milk and the walls are lined with tall columnar epithelium (Figs. 15-47 to 15-49).

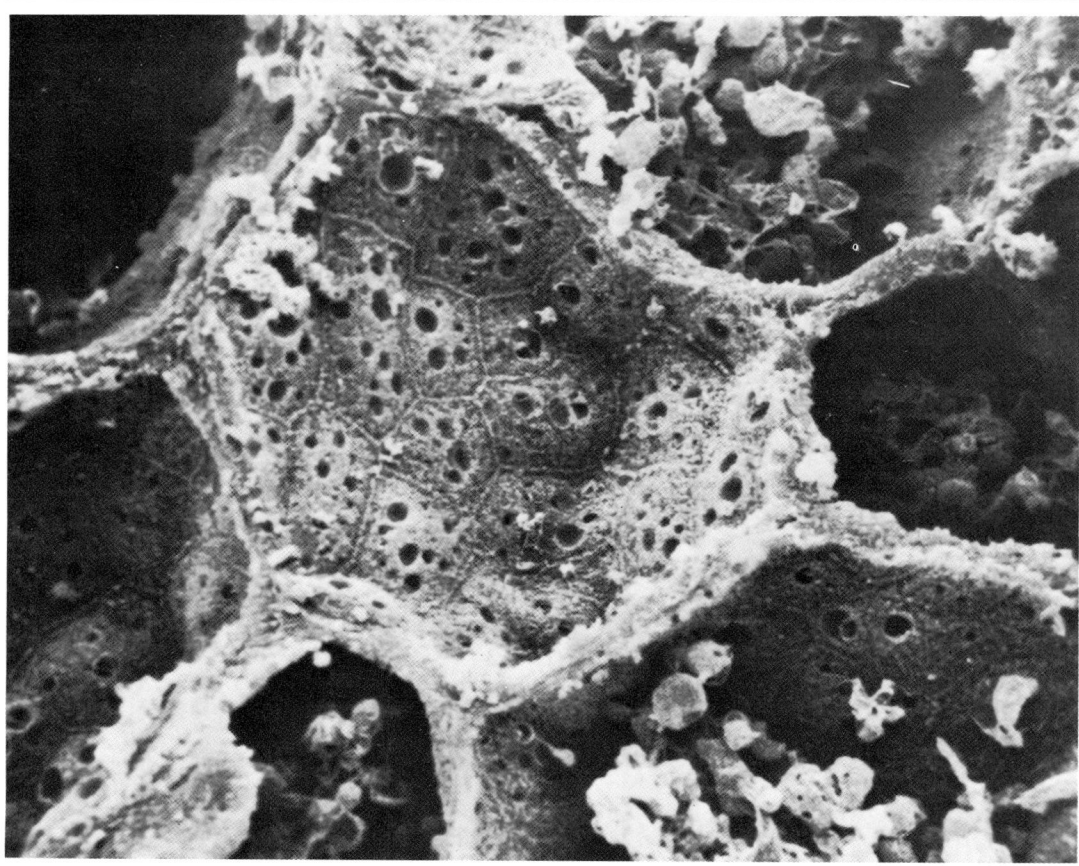

Fig. 15-49. Scanning electron micrograph of several alveoli of a lactating mammary gland. The cut alveolar walls can be recognized by their straight borders with dense microvilli. The craters in the cells lining the alveoli were left by secretory droplets in the process of leaving the cells; these droplets were removed by specimen preparation. Numerous fat droplet membrane ghosts are visible in adjacent alveoli. (×550.) (Courtesy of Dr. M. Nemanic.)

Where there is a great deal of activity, the alveoli are distended with milk and the walls are thin and lined with cuboidal epithelium; the nucleus is situated toward the base of the cell; the basal region of the cytoplasm is filled with rough endoplasmic reticulum, and the Golgi apparatus is situated on the luminal side of the nucleus.

The protein fraction of the secretion is produced by the rough endoplasmic reticulum and passed by transfer vesicles to the Golgi apparatus. The lactose of the milk is formed in the Golgi apparatus, and it, together with the protein, is passed to the luminal surface of the cell, where it is discharged by exocytosis. The fat in the milk is formed in the cytoplasm; the fat vacuoles accumulate in the apical region of the cell, where they fuse to form large milk vacuoles (see Fig. 15-49). The milk vacuoles finally protrude from the apex of the cell, which eventually ruptures and discharges the fat, surrounded by a layer of cell membrane and a little cytoplasm. The fat secretion is therefore an example of apocrine secretion. Numerous mitochondria, lysosomes, and free ribosomes are also present in the cytoplasm.

On histological section, the lobules are shown to

be very much enlarged (see Fig. 15-47), and an occasional intralobular duct is visible. The connective tissue between the lobules is compressed and thinned.

The first secretion discharged from the breasts after birth is *colostrum*. It contains protein and lactose but no fat.

Control of the Lactating Mammary Gland

We have already discussed how during pregnancy, the mammary gland undergoes great development of the ducts and alveoli in response to estrogens and progesterone secreted by the placenta, the growth hormone and prolactin secreted by the pituitary, and the adrenal glucocorticoids (see Fig. 15-46). Insulin also plays a role in the process.

Prolactin from the mother's pituitary is responsible for stimulating the alveolar cells to secrete milk. The concentration of this hormone in the mother's blood rises toward the end of pregnancy, but its action is inhibited by the high levels of estrogens and progesterone produced by the placenta.

During the third stage of labor, the placenta is expelled from the uterus and there is a sudden drop in the blood concentration of estrogens and progesterone. The action of prolactin now is uninhibited, and the alveoli start to produce large quantities of milk. The milk passes out of the alveoli into the ducts and lactiferous sinuses in response to the squeezing action of the myoepithelial cells that surround the alveoli. The myoepithelial cells are stimulated to contract by oxytocin, which is secreted into the blood from the posterior lobe of the mother's pituitary. The contraction of the myoepithelial cells occurs as a reflex act that follows the stimulation of the nipple by the suckling child. The afferent nervous impulses reach the hypothalamus via the cutaneous nerves, the ascending tracts in the spinal cord leading to the hypothalamus.

The continued production of milk by the mammary glands depends on the suckling activity of the baby. Each time the baby feeds, not only is oxytocin liberated reflexly, but large quantities of prolactin are also released from the anterior lobe of the pituitary. The prolactin results in the secretion and accumulation of milk in the alveoli between feedings. Normally, a woman who enjoys nursing her child will be able to do so for 6 months or longer. But in an unhappy mother, or one with psychological problems, the reflex hormonal mechanism breaks down and the production of oxytocin is inhibited. In a mother who decides not to breast-feed her child, the absence of suckling quickly results in a stoppage of oxytocin and prolactin production, and the alveoli lose their secretory activity.

Regression of the Lactating Mammary Gland

Once the baby has been weaned, the mammary glands return to their inactive state. The remaining milk is absorbed; the alveoli shrink, and most of them disappear. The interlobular connective tissue thickens. The breasts and the nipples shrink and return nearly to their original size. The pigmentation of the areola fades, but the area never lightens to its original color.

Suppression of the Ovarian and Menstrual Cycles during Lactation

Most lactating women do not menstruate while they are nursing. The explanation is probably that suckling, via nervous pathways already discussed, inhibits the production of the LH releasing factor and the FSH releasing factor by the hypothalamus; therefore, LH and FSH formation in the anterior lobe of the pituitary is suppressed. As a result, the ovarian cycle is never restarted and the endometrium never undergoes changes. Once the mother ceases to nurse her baby, the ovarian cycle quickly resumes.

Structure of the Mammary Gland after the Menopause

Following the menopause, the mammary gland atrophies (see Fig. 15-45). Most of the alveoli disappear, leaving behind the ducts. The glandular structure thus resembles the structure seen before puberty. The connective tissue becomes less cellular, and the collagen fibers decrease in number. The adipose tissue may increase or decrease in amount. The mammary gland tends to shrink in size and becomes more pendulous. The atrophy after the menopause is caused by an absence of ovarian estrogens and progesterone.

Structure of the Mammary Gland in the Newborn

While the fetus is in the uterus, the maternal and placental hormones cross the placental barrier and cause proliferation of the duct epithelium and the surrounding connective tissue. This proliferation may cause swelling of the mammary glands in both sexes during the first week of life, and in some cases a milky fluid, called *witch's milk,* may be expressed from the nipples. The condition is resolved spontaneously as the maternal hormone levels in the child fall.

CLINICAL NOTES

STAGES OF DEVELOPMENT

Puberty

Puberty in the female may be defined as the series of bodily and behavioral changes that take place in response to the interactions among the hypothalamus, pituitary, and gonads. Normally, puberty begins with the appearance of pubic hair and budding of the breasts at about age 10 or 11. At the same age, the external genitalia and the uterus rapidly enlarge. The axillary hair makes its appearance and cyclic menstruation begins by about age 13 or 14.

Menarche

Menarche is the onset of cyclic menstrual bleeding. It is a dramatic event, occurring at an average age of 13 years. Menarche before age 9 or after age 17 is considered abnormal.

Most girls are anovulatory for the first 12 to 18 months after menarche; the uterine bleeding during this phase results from estrogen stimulation and withdrawal. The uterus is incompletely matured at this time. A girl at this stage is thus usually infertile.

Adolescence

Adolescence is evidenced by a spurt in body height, development of secondary sexual characteristics, and gradual attainment of psychosexual maturity. The child undergoes emotional changes such as bursts of great energy, inconsistency, and unpredictability.

Menopause

Menopause is the time when the menstrual periods cease. It may occur abruptly, but more commonly the menstrual bleeding gradually becomes scanty and the periods become irregular and more widely spaced. Menopause occurs on the average between the ages of 49 and 50; the normal range is from the mid-forties through the mid-fifties. It signifies the decline in ovarian function.

OVARIES

Comprehension of ovarian structure and functioning is central to the understanding and treatment of many gynecological problems. Although it is not possible to provide in this text a comprehensive discussion of the many diseases that affect the ovaries, a few of the more important will be discussed briefly.

Malformations of the Ovaries

Ovarian Dysgenesis

Complete failure of both ovaries to develop is a characteristic of *Turner's syndrome.* The classic features of this syndrome are webbed neck, short and stocky build, increased carrying angle of the elbows, lack of secondary sex characteristics, and amenorrhea (absence of menstrual periods).

Accessory Ovarian Tissue

Accessory ovarian tissue is sometimes found along the migratory course of the gonad.

Imperfect Ovarian Descent

The ovary may fail to descend into the pelvis or, very rarely, may be drawn downward with the round ligament of the uterus into the inguinal canal or even into the labium majus.

Malformation of Ova

The formation of abnormal ova is believed to be an extremely rare condition. More than one oocyte may be found in a developing follicle, but the excess ova usually degenerate before ovulation takes place.

Primary Ovarian Failure

In individuals with primary ovarian failure, menstrual bleeding has never occurred (primary amenorrhea). The condition is associated with sexual infantilism. Ovarian dysgenesis, as in Turner's syndrome, is a good example. In diagnosis, it is very important to exclude other organ malfunctions first, such as a lesion of the hypothalamus, pituitary, adrenal, or thyroid.

Secondary Ovarian Failure

Individuals with secondary ovarian failure have secondary amenorrhea or scanty periods (oligomenorrhea). Assuming that the woman is not pregnant, disease of the hypothalamus, pituitary, and thyroid should be excluded in diagnosis. Drugs such as the phenothiazines and oral contraceptives may be responsible. In the adolescent, one of the most common causes of such failure is an emotional upset, such as leaving home for college. In such a case, the problem spontaneously resolves and a normal, regular menstrual cycle returns.

Clinical Observation of Ovarian Function and Ovulation

Recording Basal Body Temperature

In a patient who has no infections and whose menstrual cycle is regular, it is quite simple to establish the time of ovulation by measuring the body temperature each morning, either orally or rectally. At the time of ovulation, there is a sudden drop in body temperature, followed by a rise of 0.5 to 1°F that remains for 9 to 10 days. The temperature method can also be used to detect poor corpus luteum function, which is indicated by a short or irregular rise in temperature during the second, postovulatory half of the cycle.

Endometrial Biopsy

An endometrial biopsy specimen is taken easily by using a curette, which is introduced into the uterine cavity through the cervix without an anesthetic. The most satisfactory time to obtain a biopsy specimen is midway through the secretory phase of the cycle, when the combined actions of the estrogens and progesterone on the endometrium may be studied.

Cervical Mucus

Estrogens normally cause the cervical mucus to increase in amount and to become clear, acellular, and translucent. It can be seen flowing from the external os of the cervix at midcycle. A sample of mucus taken at this time can be examined on a histological slide and the presence or absence of cells noted. A lack of estrogen or the presence of progesterone inhibits the production of cervical mucus.

Vaginal Smear

In a patient who is free of vaginal infections, it is possible to detect a series of vaginal cellular changes that are related to the ovarian cycle. The Papanicolaou staining technique is used, and vaginal smears taken at different phases of the cycle can be studied.

Immediately after menstruation, the smear shows many histiocytes and neutrophil leukocytes, and few squamous cells. At midcycle, numerous large squamous cells with acidophilic cytoplasm and pyknotic nuclei are seen, and histiocytes and neutrophils are absent. During the late secretory phase of the cycle, the squamous cells are smaller, the cytoplasm is less acidophilic, and the nuclei are less pyknotic; neutrophils reappear in large numbers. Once menstruation commences, the smear is contaminated with red blood cells and endometrial cells.

Hormone Assay

Hormone assay of blood plasma is possible using modern techniques. The plasma levels of FSH, LH, the estrogens, and progesterone at different stages during the ovarian cycle can now be evaluated.

Cysts of the Ovary

Follicular cysts are very common and may reach 1.5 cm in diameter. They are unruptured graafian follicles and are filled with a clear fluid. *Luteal cysts* can be larger than follicular cysts but are much less common. The corpus luteum is replaced by clear fluid.

In *polycystic ovaries,* multiple cysts are present in both ovaries. The cysts are thought to occur in response to excess ovarian stimulation by FSH and LH. Excess androgens are produced by the theca cells, leading to virilism and secondary amenorrhea.

Tumors of the Ovary

Tumors of the ovary are common, and most are benign. The great majority of tumors arise from the peritoneal epithelium covering the ovary; the remainder arise from the germ cells and from the stroma. Benign tumors can be removed surgically. Malignant tumors extend onto the surface of the ovary and then spread rapidly throughout the peritoneal cavity, producing excessive peritoneal fluid (malignant ascites).

A rare form of tumor that occurs most commonly after the menopause is the granulosa–theca cell tumor. This tumor is of interest because it may secrete large quantities of estrogens that may lead to hyperplasia of the endometrium and cystic disease of the breast. Another rare hormone-producing tumor is the Sertoli-Leydig cell tumor, which secretes androgens that cause defeminization. It is thought that the neoplasm arises from embryonic male sex cells.

The ovary is a common site for metastatic tumors that have arisen from other pelvic or abdominal organs.

UTERINE TUBES

The uterine tube is a direct route of communication from the vulva through the vagina and uterine cavity to the peritoneal cavity. It is the route along which gonorrhea spreads to involve the pelvic peritoneum. Inflammation of the uterine tube (salpingitis) is caused most commonly by the gonococcus. Unfortunately, the inflammation causes irreparable damage to the lining epithelium, and the subsequent scarring leads to narrowing of the tube and to sterility.

Implantation of a fertilized ovum may occur outside the uterine cavity in the wall of the uterine tube. This is a variety of *ectopic pregnancy*. Because there is no decidua formation in the tube, the eroding action of the trophoblast quickly destroys the wall of the tube. Tubal abortion or rupture of the tube, with the effusion of a large quantity of blood into the peritoneal cavity, is the common result.

UTERUS

Hypoplasia

Hypoplasia of the uterus is usually caused by an ovarian or pituitary hypofunction. The inadequate growth of the uterus in this condition is caused by a lack of secretion of estrogens by the ovaries.

Infection

Although the uterine cavity communicates directly with the vulva through the vagina, it is remarkably resistant to infections. Should parts of the conceptus be retained within the uterine cavity following an abortion, however, an ideal medium for infection exists. Curettage of the remains followed by the administration of antibiotics systemically quickly results in recovery.

Endometriosis

In this condition, pieces of endometrium grow outside the uterine cavity; they may be found in the tubes or anywhere within the pelvic peritoneal cavity. The cause of this disease is not known, but the following possibilities exist: (1) fragments of endometrium have been regurgitated along the uterine tubes during menstruation and have become implanted on the pelvic peritoneum; (2) the peritoneum has undergone metaplasia; and (3) endometrial cells have spread locally via the lymphatic vessels or veins.

With each ovarian cycle, the ectopic endometrium is built up by the estrogens and progesterone and then caused to be shed, with accompanying hemorrhage. The intrapelvic bleeding causes extreme pain (dysmenorrhea), and the blood causes adhesions. Eventually the pelvic viscera, including the uterine tubes and ovaries, become embedded in a mass of fibrous tissue, leading to sterility.

Dysfunctional Uterine Bleeding

The normal buildup of the endometrium is carefully controlled by the plasma levels of estrogens and progesterone, and the concentrations of these hormones must rise and fall regularly with each menstrual cycle. A failure of this hormonal control can lead to excessive buildup of the endometrium, atrophy of the endometrium, or premature shedding of the endometrium. Moreover, the cyclical changes may become very irregular and may be accompanied by bleeding between the menstrual periods.

In anovulatory menstrual cycles, which are common at the menarche and just before the menopause, the graafian follicle fails to liberate the ovum and the corpus luteum does not form. Under these circumstances, the endometrium proliferates excessively under the influence of the estrogens alone; finally, when menstruation occurs, the hyperplastic endometrium is cast off, usually accompanied by excessive bleeding. Other endocrine disorders, such as pituitary, thyroid, and adrenal disease, may lead to ovarian dysfunction.

Low production of progesterone by the corpus luteum may lead to inadequate development of the endometrium during the secretory phase. Infertility and excessive menstrual bleeding may be the presenting symptoms and signs in these cases.

Failure of the corpus luteum to degenerate may lead to a prolonged secretory phase of the cycle; when menstruation finally occurs, it is accompanied by excessive bleeding.

The Endometrium and Oral Contraceptives

The use of oral contraceptives may produce a number of endometrial changes, some of which may be confused with the development of the decidua of pregnancy. The estrogenic and progestational agents may stimulate the glands or the stroma excessively, but when the contraceptives are stopped, the endometrium reverts to normal.

Tumors of the Uterus

The two most common uterine tumors are the leiomyomas (fibroids) and the adenocarcinomas.

The *leiomyomas* are very common benign tumors arising in the smooth muscle of the myometrium. They are thought to be caused by excessive stimulation of the smooth muscle by estrogens. They may grow rapidly during pregnancy and may complicate labor. Such tumors frequently are responsible for excessive blood loss during the menstrual period.

Adenocarcinoma of the endometrium is a common form of cancer in older women. The cause is thought to be excessive stimulation of the endometrium by estrogens, which are produced outside the ovary. The tumor arises from the columnar cells of the endometrium. The common symptom is irregular vaginal bleeding associated with excessive mucus production.

Cervix of the Uterus

Inflammations

The cervical canal is about 1 inch (2.5 cm) long; opening into it are numerous long, branching glands. The canal opens at the external os into the vagina, which normally contains many different kinds of bacteria. The trauma of childbirth, the passing of instruments through the cervix in gynecological procedures, and intercourse are some of the factors predisposing to the entrance of pathogenic organisms into the cervix and the development of an acute or chronic cervicitis. Excessive mucoid discharge from the vagina (leukorrhea) is a common sign. Epithelial thickening, inflammation and edema of the lamina propria, and blockage of the ducts of the mucous glands are common findings. Chronic cervicitis with leukorrhea is a cause of sterility, if it is left untreated, epithelial metaplasia may occur, which may progress to cervical carcinoma.

Carcinoma of the Cervix

Cancer of the cervix is very common in women. It is extremely rare, however, in women who have never had sexual intercourse and in women who have not had children. Early coitus and multiple sexual partners increase the likelihood of this disease, as does herpes virus infection. Chronic cervicitis is believed to be an important predisposing factor.

The great majority of carcinomas of the cervix arise from the squamous epithelium near the squamocolumnar junction at the external os. The remainder are adenocarcinomas that arise from the columnar epithelial cells of the lining of the cervical canal or from the glands. It is now generally accepted that carcinoma of the cervix is preceded by a dysplasia and an anaplasia of the epithelium which is a precursor of carcinoma in situ; this later becomes an invasive carcinoma.

Unfortunately, cervical carcinoma almost invariably is without signs or symptoms in its early stages. Schiller's test and the Papanicolaou test are invaluable in making an early diagnosis. Schiller's test consists of painting the external os with an iodine solution. The glycogen normally present in the cytoplasm of the squamous epithelial cells takes up the stain, turning the mucous membrane mahogony brown. If the stain is not taken up in certain areas, this indicates that the squamous cells in these areas are abnormal; a local biopsy specimen should be obtained to make a histological diagnosis. The Papanicolaou smear test involves the simple aspiration of fluid that pools in the posterior fornix of the vagina. This fluid is smeared quickly on a glass slide. Some clinicians take a sample directly from the external os of the cervix and smear it on a slide. The smear is fixed, stained, and examined by a cytologist. It is possible to detect severe anaplasia or dysplasia, carcinoma in situ, or invasive carcinoma by this method.

VAGINA

The vaginal mucous membrane possesses no glands, but its surface is kept moist by mucus draining from the cervix and by transudation of fluid through the epithelium. The epithelium, which is controlled by ovarian estrogens, is normally nonkeratinized but contains glycogen in its cytoplasm. Desquamated cells liberate the glycogen, which is broken down by the Döderlein's bacilli into lactic acid, lowering the hydrogen concentration and inhibiting the growth of pathogenic organisms. For this reason, the vagina remains relatively free from infection during the reproductive period of life. The thin epithelial lining and the absence of glycogen in the squamous cells before puberty and after the menopause make the vaginal wall prone to infection at these times. Such infections are treated with antibiotics, and the simultaneous administration of estrogens quickly thickens the vaginal epithelium. The infection then rapidly disappears.

The vaginal epithelial lining thickens in pregnancy because of the outpouring of placental estrogens. It is thicker in sexually active women as an effect of repeated intercourse. Should the vaginal wall become dry because of exposure, as in a severe vaginal prolapse, the surface cells undergo keratinization.

The vaginal smear and the changes that take place at different stages in the ovarian cycle have been described on page 619. The importance of the vaginal smear ("Pap test") in the early detection of carcinoma of the cervix has been stressed.

EXTERNAL GENITAL ORGANS

The presence of numerous glands and ducts opening onto the surface makes the region of the vulva prone to infection. The ducts of the greater vestibular glands, the vagina (with its indirect communication with the peritoneal cavity), the urethra, and the para-urethral glands all can become infected. Provided that the pH of the vagina is kept low, the vagina is capable of resisting infection to a remarkable degree.

Infection of the greater vestibular glands (Bartholin's glands) is common in gonorrheal infections. If the duct of a gland becomes blocked by infection, the secretion is dammed back and the gland becomes cystic. A *Bartholin cyst* may reach several centimeters in diameter and is a common condition.

REPRODUCTIVE CONSIDERATIONS AND ABNORMALITIES

Sterility in the Female

About 10 to 20 percent of marriages are sterile, and in one-half to two-thirds of these, the female is the responsible partner. For fertilization to occur, many different cellular processes must take place normally and the reproductive organs, including the external genitalia, must be functioning correctly. In the female, the ovaries must be capable of producing normal ova. Irregular and infrequent ovulation caused by hormonal problems may be responsible for infertility. The uterine tubes may be narrowed or blocked because of fibrosis resulting from inflammations such as gonorrhea. The uterine cavity may be distorted or narrowed by a tumor, which may interfere with normal implantation. Chronic cervicitis may alter the chemical composition of the cervical secretions to such an extent that the spermatozoa cannot survive.

Contraceptive Drugs

The use of a progesterone-containing pill as an ovulation-inhibiting agent has become an accepted method of controlling conception. The progestogens completely suppress ovulation by inhibiting the output of pituitary LH, which is necessary for the final stages of ovulation. It is probable that progesterone suppresses the release of the LH releasing factor by the hypothalamus. The combination of both progesterone and estrogen in a single pill that is taken orally each day for 21 days, or the sequential administration of estrogen for 15 days followed by progesterone for 6 days, allows the endometrium to be built up. The periodic interruption of the drug therapy for 7 days results in vasoconstriction of the endometrial blood vessels; an interval of withdrawal bleeding occurs, which may be likened to the normal menstrual flow. The interruption of the hormone therapy thus prevents excessive buildup of the endometrium and excessive stimulation of the mammary glands. On the fifth day after the onset of the withdrawal bleeding, the patient begins another 21-day pill regimen.

Abnormal Sites of Implantation

Normal implantation takes place in the endometrium of the body of the uterus, most frequently on the upper part of the posterior wall near the midline. Occasionally, implantation occurs at sites that are considered abnormal. In order of decreasing frequency, they are: (1) the region of the internal os of the cervix, (2) the ampulla of the uterine tube, (3) the isthmus of the uterine tube, (4) the angle of the uterine cavity near the entrance of the uterine tube, (5) the infundibulum of the uterine tube, (6) the ovary, (7) the intramural part of the uterine tube, and (8) the peritoneal cavity.

Implantation of the blastocyst outside the uterine cavity is referred to as an *ectopic pregnancy*. The blastocyst buries itself in the extra-uterine structure as a result of the destructive action of the trophoblast. If implantation takes place within the uterine tube, early abortion occurs, with or without rupture of the tube, and is accompanied by considerable hemorrhage. Such abortion usually takes place between the sixth and tenth weeks of pregnancy.

Placenta

Abnormalities of Size and Shape

The normal placenta is flat and circular, with a diameter of about 8 inches (20 cm) and a thickness of about 1 inch (2.5 cm). Occasionally, abnormalities occur: the placenta may be excessively thin and large, may have several incomplete lobes, or may contain a hole, in which there is an absence of placental structure. The umbilical cord may be attached at the placental margin or attached to the fetal membranes some distance from the edge of the placenta. A knowledge of these possible abnormalities is important in obstetrics, because it is essential that all parts of the placenta and the fetal membranes be expelled from the uterus during the third stage of labor. Retained fragments increase the likelihood of uterine infection and also may interfere with the contraction of the uterine wall and thus with the prevention of postpartum hemorrhage.

Abnormalities of Weight and Position

The placenta normally weighs about 1 lb. (500 gm). Very small placentas are found in women suffering from chronic hypertension. Excessively large placentas occur with *fetal hydrops*, a condition of the fetus in which severe hemolytic disease results from serological incompatibility of mother and baby (e.g., presence of Rh antigens).

Normally the placenta is situated in the upper half of the uterus. Should implantation occur in the lower half of the body of the uterus, the condition is called *placenta praevia* and is of great clinical importance. Severe painless hemorrhage occurring from the twenty-eighth week onward is the clinical sign of placenta praevia and is caused by expansion of the lower half of the uterine wall at this time and by its tearing away from the placenta.

Placental Infarction

Infarction is found to some degree in more than half of placentas at birth. Palpable, solid areas can be identified close to the decidual surface. Initially, coagulation of maternal blood occurs around a group of villi, and the vessels within the villi become engorged. At this stage, the infarct is red. Later, the villi undergo necrosis and fibrosis, and the infarct becomes white. Massive infarction of the placenta can lead to the death of the fetus. In most cases the cause of the infarction is unknown, but occasionally it may be trauma applied to the mother's abdomen that produces shearing forces on the placental-uterine junction, interfering locally with the maternal circulation.

Drugs and the Placental Membrane

Most drugs have a low molecular weight and thus cross the placental membrane by simple diffusion. Antibiotics such as sulfonamides and penicillin pass across in small amounts, as do alcohol and nicotine. Morphine, barbiturates, and general anesthetics given to the mother do cross into the fetal circulation and depress the respiratory center of the fetus. Particular attention must be paid to this fact at the time of delivery, because the child may have difficulty in breathing immediately after birth. Certain drugs taken by the mother are definitely harmful to the fetus. Thalidomide, for example, a popular tranquilizing drug given to women during the early months of pregnancy some years ago, crosses the placental membrane and causes numerous defects in fetal growth.

MAMMARY GLANDS

Male Mammary Glands

The male breast is rudimentary and is not subject to the monthly rise and fall in hormone levels found in the female. The possibility of cancer of the breast, however, should never be forgotten during physical examinations of the male. About 1 to 2 percent of breast cancers occur in males. Cancer of the male breast has a worse prognosis than that in the female, probably because the small amount of breast tissue in the male results in an early, rapid spread to the regional lymph nodes. As we have mentioned, histologically the breast tissue in the male is limited to the subareolar area.

Female Mammary Glands

Disease of the breast, especially carcinoma, is extremely common in women. The breast is also the site of different types of benign tumors and may be subject to acute inflammation and abscess formation. For these reasons, the physician should be familiar with the structure of the breast and the ways in which this structure changes throughout life. The hormonal control of this gland and the histological responses to the different hormones also should be understood.

What the physician feels on palpation of the breast is determined by the microscopical structure of this organ. Because the greater part of the gland lies in the superficial fascia, it can be moved freely in all directions. Because only about 15 percent of the adult resting gland is made up of glandular components and the remaining 85 percent is formed of connective tissue, much of which is adipose tissue, it is not surprising to find that the gland is soft. Nevertheless, on careful palpation with the open hand, the breast is found to have a firm overall lobulated consistency, produced by the fifteen to twenty glandular units that radiate from the nipple.

Normally, the skin feels completely mobile over the breast substance. But if the fibrous septa that separate the lobules become involved in a scirrhous carcinoma or in a disease, such as a breast abscess, that results in the production of contracting fibrous tissue, the septa will be pulled upon, causing dimpling of the skin.

The attachment and opening of the lactiferous ducts onto the summit of the nipple explain the presence of a retracted nipple in carcinoma of the breast. The underlying neoplasm pulls on the lactiferous ducts as it invades the surrounding breast tissue.

Supernumerary nipples occasionally occur along a line extending from the axilla to the groin; they may or may not be associated with breast tissue. This minor congenital anomaly may result in a mistaken diagnosis of warts or moles.

Congenital inverted nipple is a common anomaly and is caused by a failure of the nipple to develop completely. The inversion usually corrects itself during pregnancy or by repeated traction of the nipples. Unless it is corrected, breast-feeding of an infant is difficult or impossible. A long-standing congenital inverted nipple must not be confused with the recently occurring retracted nipple caused by an underlying carcinoma mentioned previously.

Infections

An acute infection of the mammary gland may occur during lactation. Pathogenic bacteria gain entrance to the breast tissue through a crack in the nipple. Because of the fibrous septa, the infection at first remains localized to one compartment or lobe. Should an abscess occur, it should be drained through a radial incision to avoid spread of the infection into neighboring compartments; a radial incision also will minimize the damage to the radially arranged ducts.

Fibrocystic Disease

Fibrocystic disease is the most common disorder of the female breast. It is rare before puberty and unlikely to develop after the menopause. It may involve both breasts but usually does not do so equally. The patient complains of pain, tenderness, or a lump in the breast. The disease varies in intensity but usually ceases after the menopause. Four main microscopic changes occur: (1) connective tissue hyperplasia around the ducts and in the fibrous stroma, (2) single or multiple cyst formation within the ducts, (3) glandular hyperplasia involving the proliferation of the small ducts and gland buds, and (4) hyperplasia of the duct epithelium.

The cause of fibrocystic disease is believed to be an imbalance between estrogens and progesterone in their cyclic control of the mammary gland; an excess of estrogens is thought to be the main factor. Clinically, many authorities believe that patients with fibrocystic disease have a higher incidence of carcinoma. One of the great problems of fibrocystic disease is that clinically even the most experienced surgeon sometimes cannot on palpation distinguish the lesion from a carcinoma. Repeated physical examination of the patient and yearly mammograms constitute the method of management. If there is doubt as to diagnosis, an open biopsy of the lesion followed by histological examination is essential.

Tumors of the Mammary Glands

Benign tumors of the breast are quite common. *Duct papillomas* arise from the columnar epithelium lining the larger ducts. *Fibroadenomas* are smooth, lobulated tumors resulting from hyperplasia of the connective tissue and glandular tissue.

Carcinoma of the breast is the most common form of cancer in the female. Although the cause of this condition remains a mystery, there is considerable evidence that genetic factors, infection by viruses, and hormonal imbalance probably play important roles. The repeated, cyclical hyperplasia and subsequent atrophy of the glandular tissue that occur in response to the ovarian hormones, estrogens, and progesterone throughout the reproductive life of the female appear to make this organ very susceptible to malignant change. Multiple pregnancies, late menarche, and early menopause reduce the time during which the breasts are exposed to these hormones; in such instances, the incidence of carcinoma is lower. Of the hormones that act on the breast tissue, the estrogens are known to stimulate strongly the growth of duct epithelium, and it is an excess of this hormone that is most likely to be involved in the development of carcinoma.

Most carcinomas of the breast arise in the upper outer quadrant of the gland. The great majority arise from the columnar cells lining the ducts; the remainder arise from the epithelium lining the acini. At first, the neoplastic cells remain within or near the ducts. Later, the cells become invasive and spread through the breast tissue; they then metastasize to the regional lymph nodes or beyond. The hardness of some of the tumors is caused by an increase in the fibrous connective tissue.

CLINICAL PROBLEMS

For the answers to these problems, see page 813.

1. A mother asks her physician to explain what is meant by the terms *puberty, menarche, adolescence,* and *menopause.* She also asks if her daughter can become pregnant once she has started to menstruate. What would you tell this mother?

2. A medical student is fascinated by the elaborate mechanisms involved in the maturation of the spermatozoon in the testis. He understands that the testis must descend into the scrotum before normal spermatogenesis can take place because the temperature within the abdomen or the inguinal canal is too high. He also understands that the maturing spermatids are protected by the blood-testis barrier from toxic agents that may be circulating in the blood. He asks his professor of histology if a similar blood-ovarian barrier exists in the female. He also states that he does not understand why it is not necessary for the ovary to descend into the labium majus. Can you answer these questions?

3. Describe in detail the process of ovulation. What factors control this cyclical process? Using your knowledge of histology and physiology, describe briefly some clinical tests that you could perform to determine whether a patient is ovulating normally.

4. A 20-year-old woman visits her physician for a premarital examination and to discuss conception control. Can you explain the action of contraceptive drugs?

5. A 33-year-old woman attends a gynecologist, complaining of irregular menstrual bleeding. What hormonal problems related to the ovary could be responsible for dysfunctional bleeding in this woman?

6. A medical student is asked on a ward round what therapeutic methods exist for the treatment of anovulation associated with secondary amenorrhea. He also is asked if there are any complications associated with the treatment. How would you answer these questions?

7. A 23-year-old woman admitted to the emergency room complains of severe spasmodic pain in the right iliac fossa. Just prior to admission, the pain had suddenly intensified, and the patient had collapsed. On physical examination, the patient is observed to have the signs and symptoms of internal hemorrhage. There is extreme tenderness in the right iliac fossa and some rigidity of the abdominal muscles. When questioned about her menstrual history, she discloses that she has missed her last period. The attending physician makes a diagnosis of a ruptured ectopic pregnancy. Explain where implantation normally occurs. What is the normal histological structure of the uterine tube? What changes take

place in the uterine tube if implantation occurs in the tube?

8. Give a detailed description of the structure of the endometrium (a) before puberty, (b) after puberty, and (c) after the menopause. Describe the hormonal changes that are responsible for these structural changes.

9. Following the diagnostic procedure of dilatation and curettage of a uterus for dysfunctional uterine bleeding, the histopathologist informs the gynecologist that the uterine scrapings have the appearance of the decidua. What is the decidua? Which hormones are responsible for the development and maintenance of the decidua?

10. Describe the structure and functions of the placenta. How may the efficiency of this organ be impaired?

11. The placenta is an endocrine organ. Name the hormones that are produced by the placenta and their main functions.

12. Describe the structure of the placental barrier. Name three harmful organisms and three harmful drugs that can pass from the mother through the placenta to the fetus.

13. A 26-year-old woman is admitted to the emergency room with severe vaginal bleeding. She is 33 weeks pregnant and has had repeated slight bleeding for the past 2 weeks, but this has stopped spontaneously. She has no pain associated with the bleeding. Abdominal examination reveals that the fetal head is high, and it is not possible to make the head descend into the pelvis. Examination of the genital organs shows no cause for the bleeding. A diagnosis of placenta praevia is made. What is placenta praevia? What is the cause of the bleeding? Why is the bleeding painless?

14. Describe the structure of the cervix of the uterus. Carcinoma of the cervix of the uterus is very common. From which cell type does the carcinoma usually arise?

15. Infection of the vagina is a comparatively rare condition. Why? Describe the structure of the vaginal wall and explain why, during reproductive life, the pH of the vaginal fluid is acid. What is the hormonal control of the cells lining the vaginal wall? Does the structure of the vaginal wall change in pregnancy?

16. What is a "Pap smear"? Briefly describe the main cellular changes found in a vaginal smear at different phases of the ovarian cycle. Name a particular disease that may be diagnosed early with a Pap smear.

17. The greater vestibular glands frequently are infected in cases of gonorrhea. Describe the structure of these glands and explain how they may become cystic.

18. One of the common venereal diseases is herpes simplex. This virus infection causes the repeated occurrence of blisters on the labia minora and cervix. Describe the epithelium covering the outer and inner surfaces of the labia minora. Describe also the epithelial covering of the cervix in the region of the external os.

19. Give a detailed account of the structure of the female mammary gland (a) before puberty, (b) in the adult resting state, (c) during pregnancy, (d) during lactation, and (e) after the menopause. Which hormones are responsible for these structural changes?

20. Fibrocystic disease of the female breast is a very common condition. It is believed to be caused by an imbalance in hormonal control of the gland. Can you explain this hypothesis?

21. Carcinoma of the breast is the most common form of cancer in the female. Where does this malignant condition arise? Can you explain why cancer of the breast frequently causes dimpling of the skin and retraction of the nipple?

22. Describe the structure of the male mammary gland. What is "witch's milk"?

23. A 27-year-old nursing mother is examined in

the doctor's office and found to have a large abscess in the upper outer quadrant of the right breast. The physician decides to incise the abscess and give the patient a course of antibiotics. Knowing the histological structure of the breast, explain why the physician made a radial rather than a circumferential incision in order to drain the pus from the abscess.

24. A surgeon takes a group of students on a ward round and, after examining three women with clinically detectable lumps in the breast, asks the students to explain why a woman who has had multiple pregnancies, a late menarche, or an early menopause has less likelihood of developing breast carcinoma than other women. How would you answer this question?

ADDITIONAL READING

Adams, E. C., and Hertig, A. T. Studies on the human corpus luteum. *J. Cell Biol.* 41:696, 1969.

Anderson, E., and Albertini, D. Gap junctions between the oocyte and companion follicle cells in the mammalian ovary. *J. Cell Biol.* 71:680, 1976.

Arimura, A. Hypothalamic gonadotropin-releasing hormone and reproduction. *Int. Rev. Physiol.* 13:1, 1977.

Banarjee, M. R. Responses of mammary cells to hormones. *Int. Rev. Cytol.* 47:1, 1976.

Bjersing, L., and Cajander, S. Ovulation and the role of surface epithelium. *Experientia* 31:605, 1975.

Blandau, R. J. (ed.). *The Biology of the Blastocyst.* Chicago: University of Chicago Press, 1971.

Blaustein, A. *Pathology of the Female Genital Tract.* New York: Springer-Verlag, 1977.

Boyd, J. D., and Hamilton, W. J. Electron microscopic observations on the cytotrophoblast contribution to the syncytium in the human placenta. *J. Anat.* 100:535, 1966.

Crisp, T. M., Dessouky, A. D., and Denys, F. R. The fine structure of the human corpus luteum of early pregnancy and during the progestational phase of the menstrual cycle. *Am. J. Anat.* 127:37, 1970.

Dirksen, E. R., and Satir, P. Ciliary activity in the mouse oviduct as studied by transmission and scanning electron microscopy. *Tissue Cell* 4:389, 1972.

Ferenczy, A. Anatomy and histology of the cervix; benign lesions of the cervix; cervical intraepithelial neoplasia; carcinoma and other malignant tumors of the cervix. In Blaustein, A. (ed.), *Pathology of the Female Genital Tract.* New York: Springer-Verlag, 1977, p. 102.

Greep, R. O. (ed.). *Handbook of Physiology.* Sec. 7: *Endocrinology.* Vol. II: *Female Reproductive System.* Washington, D.C.: American Physiological Society, 1975.

Greep, R. O. The female reproductive system. In Greep, R. O., Koblinsky, M. A., and Jaffe, F. S. (eds.). *Reproduction and Human Welfare: A Challenge to Research.* Cambridge, Mass.: MIT Press, 1976, p. 81.

Gregoire, A. T., Kandil, O., and Ledger, W. J. The glycogen content of human vaginal epithelial tissue. *Fertil. Steril.* 22:64, 1971.

Guraya, S. S. Recent advances in the morphology, histochemistry and biochemistry of the developing mammalian ovary. *Int. Rev. Cytol.* 51:49, 1977.

Guyton, A. C. *Textbook of Medical Physiology* (6th ed.). Philadelphia: Saunders, 1981.

Haagensen, C. D. *Diseases of the Breast.* Philadelphia: Saunders, 1971.

Hafez, E. S. E. (ed.). *Scanning Electron Microscopic Atlas of Mammalian Reproduction.* New York: Springer-Verlag, 1975.

Jones, R. E. (ed.). *The Vertebrate Ovary.* New York: Plenum, 1978.

Koering, M. J. Luteolysis in normal and prostaglandin F2 treated pseudopregnant rabbits. *J. Reprod. Fertil.* 40:259, 1974.

Koering, M. J. Structural morphological changes of the regressive corpus luteum in the rabbit. *Biol. Reprod.* 18:719, 1978.

Koering, M. J. Preantral follicle development during the menstrual cycle in the Macaca mulatta ovary. *Am. J. Anat.* 166:429, 1983.

Koering, M. J., Goodman, A. L., Williams, R. F., and Hodgen, G. D. Granulosa cell pyknosis in the dominant follicle of monkeys. *Fertil. Steril.* 37:837, 1982.

Koering, M. J., and Sholl, S. A. Changes in ovarian interstitial tissue and progestin levels in the rabbit during the periovulatory period. *Biol. Reprod.* 19:936, 1978.

MacMahon, B., et al. Etiology of human breast cancer. *J. Natl. Cancer Inst.* 50:21, 1973.

McCann, S. M. Luteinizing-hormone-releasing-hormone. *N. Engl. J. Med.* 296:797, 1977.

McNatty, K. P., et al. The production of progesterone, androgens, and estrogens by granulosa cells, thecal tissue, and stromal tissue from human ovaries in vitro. *J. Clin. Endocrinol. Metab.* 49:687, 1979.

Motta, P., and Van Blerkom, J. A scanning electron microscope study of the luteo-follicular complex. I. Follicle and oocyte. *J. Submicrosc. Cytol.* 6:297, 1974.

Nemanic, M. K., and Pitelka, D. R. A scanning electron microscope study of the lactating mammary gland. *J. Cell Biol.* 48:410, 1971.

Rock, J., and Hertig, A. T. The human conceptus during the first two weeks of gestation. *Am. J. Obstet. Gynecol.* 55:6, 1948.

Schlafke, S., and Enders, A. C. Cellular basis of interaction between trophoblast and uterus at implantation. *Biol. Reprod.* 12:41, 1975.

Segal, S. J. The physiology of human reproduction. *Sci. Am.* 231:52, 1974.

Villee, D. B. Development of endocrine function in the human placenta and fetus. *N. Engl. J. Med.* 281:473, 1969.

Vorherr, H. *The Breast: Morphology, Physiology and Lactation.* New York: Academic Press, 1974.

Wooding, F. B. P. The mechanism of secretion of the milk fat globule. *J. Cell Sci.* 9:805, 1971.

Yen, S. Neuroendocrine regulation of the menstrual cycle. *Hosp. Pract.* 14:83, 1979.

ENDOCRINE SYSTEM

16

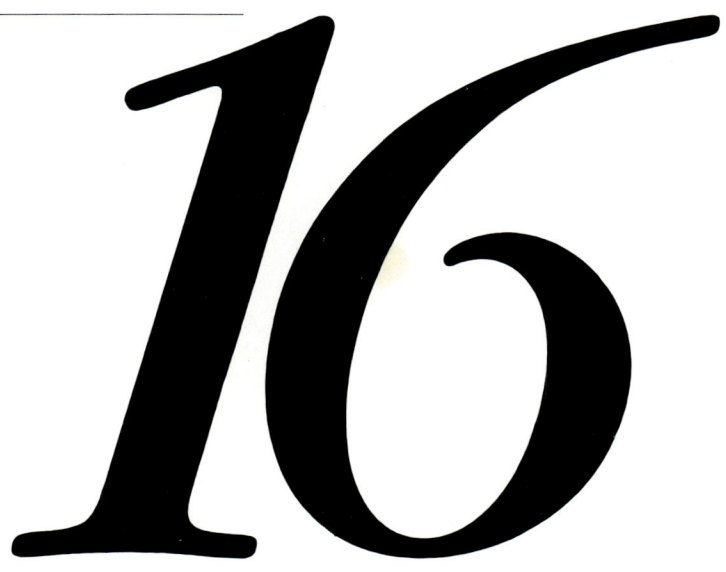

The autonomic nervous system and the endocrine system work closely together to regulate the metabolic activities of the different organs and tissues of the body so as to maintain homeostasis. The autonomic nervous system uses nervous impulses and releases neurotransmitter substances at nerve endings in order to obtain a rapid and localized response. The endocrine system exerts a slower and more diffuse response by synthesizing and releasing into the bloodstream chemical substances called *hormones*. The specific structure acted on by a hormone is referred to as its *target organ*. The activities of the autonomic nervous system and the endocrine system are integrated and coordinated by the hypothalamus.

The endocrine system is made up of several glands (Fig. 16-1): the pituitary (hypophysis), thyroid, parathyroids, suprarenals (adrenals), gonads, islets of Langerhans of the pancreas, and, when present, the placenta. In addition, there are groups of cells that form a minor part of the system and are not considered in this chapter: the gastroenteroendocrine cells, thymic cells, kidney cells, and certain cells of the lung that store and secrete amines.

The endocrine glands must be distinguished from the exocrine glands. Exocrine glands, such as the salivary, mammary, and sweat glands, pour their secretions onto a surface of the body by means of ducts. The endocrine glands have no ducts and consist of masses of cells richly supplied by blood vessels, which pour their secretion directly into the bloodstream.

HORMONES
Structure
Hormones are of three chemical types: (1) small proteins, or polypeptides, for example, the hormones of the anterior lobe of the pituitary and of the islets of Langerhans; (2) steroids, for example, the adrenocortical hormones, testosterone, and the estrogens and progesterone; and (3) amines, for example, the thyroid and suprarenal medullary hormones.

Negative Feedback Mechanism in the Control of Endocrine Glands
Once a hormone has exerted its controlling function, information is transferred back either directly

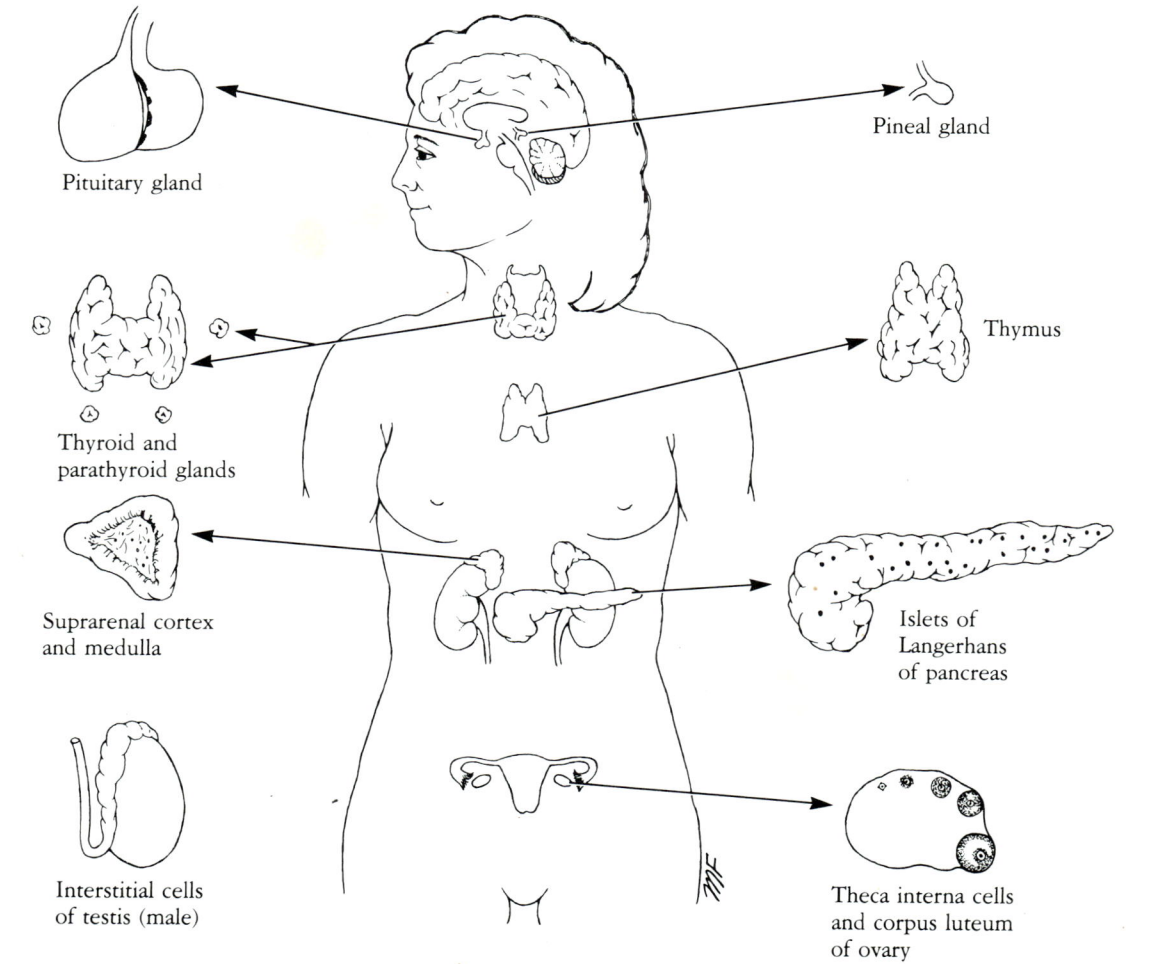

Fig. 16-1. Location of the glands of the endocrine system.

or indirectly to the endocrine gland to inhibit further secretion. Should the gland secrete insufficient hormone, the feedback mechanism decreases and the endocrine gland begins to secrete sufficient quantities of the hormone again. By this feedback mechanism, the productivity of the endocrine glands is controlled so that homeostasis is maintained.

Action of Hormones

Hormones exert their control on specific tissues at very low plasma concentrations. Many circulating hormones are bound to plasma proteins, making them biologically inactive and permitting large quantities of hormone to circulate and to be available if required quickly. Hormones are disposed of by the body by being inactivated by the target tissue or destroyed by the liver or kidneys.

Hormones exert their control at the cellular level in a variety of ways:

1. By changing membrane permeability. Insulin, for example, increases the membrane permeability

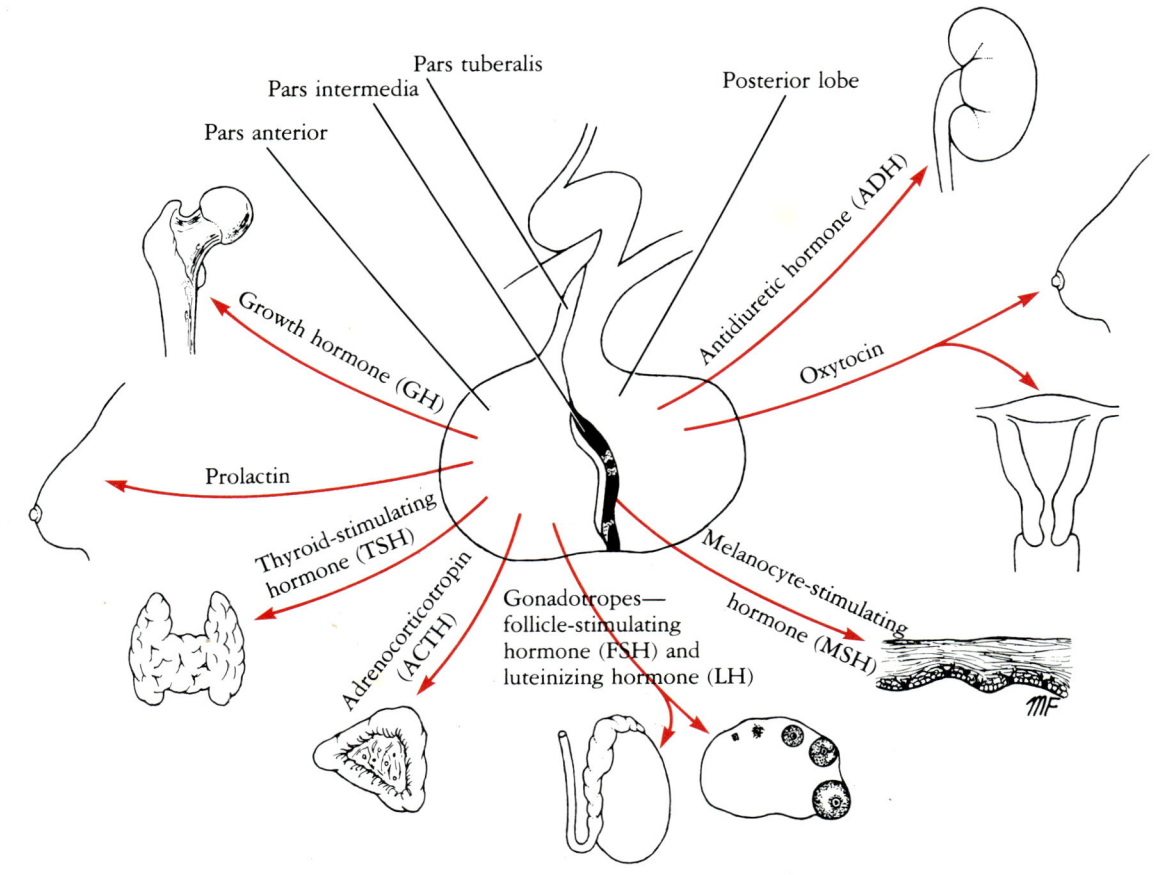

Fig. 16-2. Importance of the pituitary gland in controlling other endocrine glands and tissues in the body. The hormones secreted by the different parts of the pituitary gland in exerting this control are indicated.

of muscle cells for glucose transport. How this is accomplished is not known.

2. By the formation of cyclic 3′,5′-adenosine monophosphate (cyclic AMP) within the cell. Cyclic AMP is formed in small amounts when the hormone becomes attached to the receptors on the cell membrane. The enzyme *adenyl cyclase,* located in the membrane, becomes activated, causing increased amounts of cyclic AMP to be formed from adenosine triphosphate (ATP). The cyclic AMP serves as a *secondary hormone,* or messenger, within the cell and brings about changes in activity of certain intracellular enzymes. For example, epinephrine stimulates the liver cells to break down glycogen into glucose by this method.

3. By acting on the genes and changing the deoxyribonucleic acid (DNA)-controlled synthesis of ribonucleic acid (RNA). The steroid hormones, for example, act by causing the synthesis of proteins within the cells.

4. By changing the permeability of cell membranes to ions. Acetylcholine, which may be regarded as a local hormone, excites a muscle cell to contract by this method.

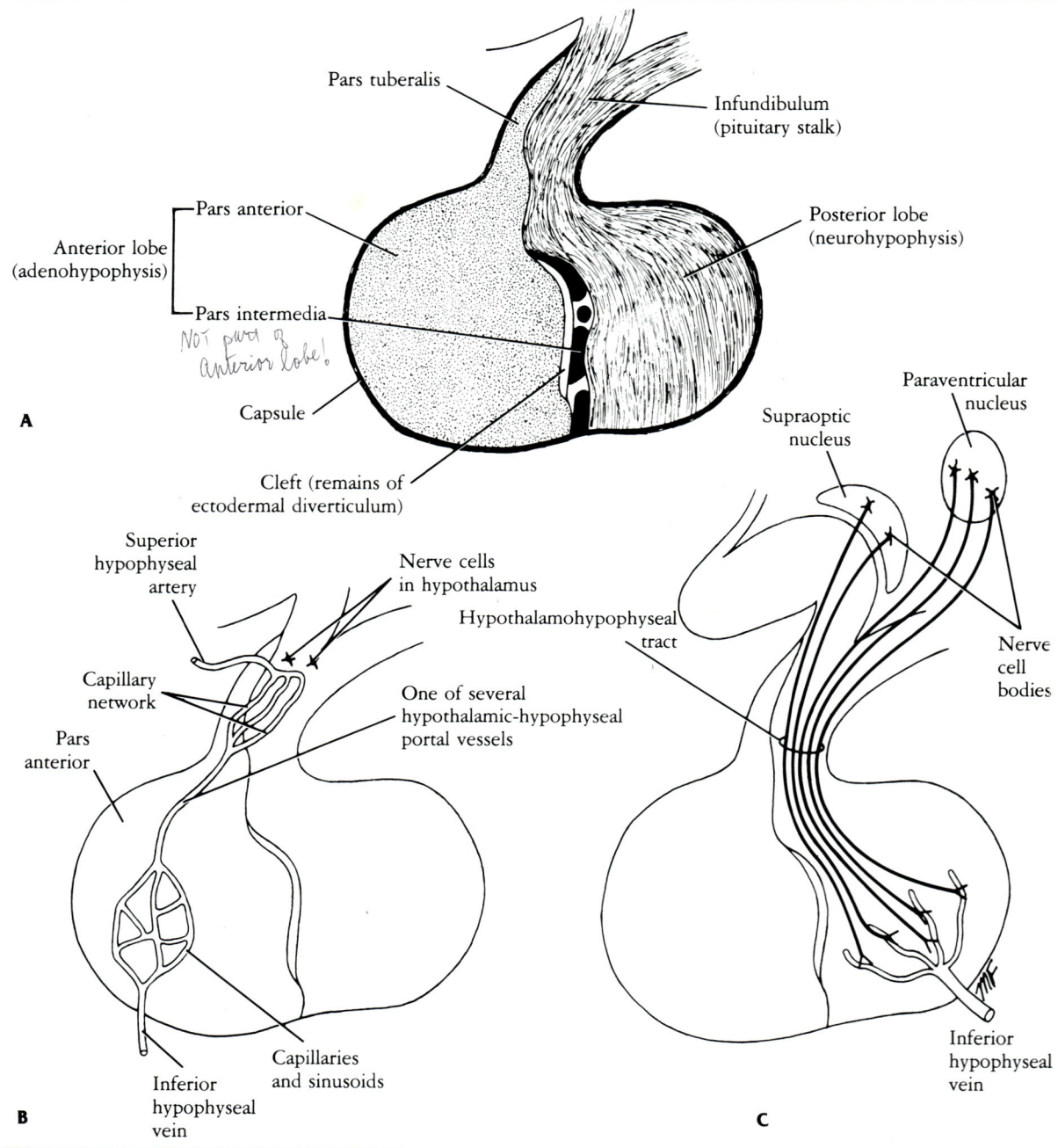

Fig. 16-3. (A) Division of the pituitary gland into the pars anterior, pars intermedia (anterior lobe), and pars nervosa (posterior lobe); (B) hypothalamohypophyseal portal vessels; (C) hypothalamohypophyseal tract.

PITUITARY GLAND

The pituitary gland, or hypophysis cerebri, is a small oval structure attached to the undersurface of the brain by the *infundibulum*. It is well protected by virtue of its location in the sella turcica of the sphenoid bone of the skull. Because the hormones produced by the gland influence the activities of many other endocrine glands (Fig. 16-2), the pituitary is often referred to as the master endocrine gland. For this reason it is of very great importance and vital to life.

The pituitary gland is divided into an *anterior lobe*, or *adenohypophysis*, and a *posterior lobe*, or *neurohypophysis* (Fig. 16-3). The anterior lobe is subdivided into the *pars anterior* (sometimes called the pars distalis) and the *pars intermedia*, which may be separated by a cleft that is a remnant of an embryonic pouch. A projection from the pars anterior, the *pars tuberalis*, extends up along the anterior and lateral surfaces of the pituitary stalk.

Control of the Pituitary Gland by the Hypothalamus

The pituitary gland is controlled by the hypothalamus, which is that part of the floor of the third ventricle from which the pituitary is suspended (Fig. 16-4). The control is exercised through two connections: (1) the *hypothalamohypophyseal portal vessels*, which join the hypothalamus to the anterior lobe, and (2) the *hypothalamohypophyseal tract*, which joins the hypothalamus to the posterior lobe (see Fig. 16-3).

The anterior lobe is controlled by *releasing* and *inhibitory hormones*, which are produced by neurons in the hypothalamus and are passed to the anterior lobe in the blood through the hypophyseal portal vessels. These hormones exert their control over the glandular cells of the anterior lobe (see Fig. 16-4). The posterior lobe contains the distal ends of the nerve fibers that form the hypothalamohypophyseal tract. The two hormones secreted by the posterior lobe actually are produced in the nerve cell bodies in the hypothalamus and descend in the nerve fibers in the tract to be released into the bloodstream in the posterior lobe (see Fig. 16-3).

The activities of the hypothalamus are themselves modified by information received along numerous afferent pathways from different parts of the central nervous system and by the plasma levels of circulating electrolytes and hormones (see Fig. 16-4). Thus, the hypothalamus, which also controls the autonomic nervous system, is the chief brain center by which normal homeostasis is maintained.

Anterior Lobe
Pars Anterior

The pars anterior consists of irregular branching cords of cells supported by reticular fibers (Figs. 16-5 and 16-6). Between the cords are sinusoids, into which open the hypothalamohypophyseal portal vessels. The sinusoids drain into the inferior hypophyseal veins. The pars anterior is covered externally by a tough fibrous capsule. There are three main cell types, which may be distinguished by the affinity of their cytoplasmic granules for different stains: *acidophils, basophils,* and *chromophobes* (Figs. 16-7 and 16-8).

The *acidophils* possess large cytoplasmic granules that stain well with eosin (see Fig. 16-8). There are two types of acidophils: *somatotropes*, which produce growth hormone, and *mammotropes*, which produce *prolactin* (see Fig. 16-4). The mammotropes are present in large numbers during pregnancy and lactation.

The *basophils* (see Fig. 16-7) possess cytoplasmic granules that stain well with methylene blue. There are three types of basophils: *thyrotropes*, which produce thyroid-stimulating hormone; *corticotropes*, which produce adrenocorticotropin; and *gonadotropes*, which produce follicle-stimulating hormone and luteinizing hormone (see Fig. 16-4).

The *chromophobes* are cells whose cytoplasm does not stain with the usual dyes (see Fig. 16-8). They tend to occur in groups in the centers of the cords and are thought to be inactive acidophil and basophil cells. When they become active, granules reappear in their cytoplasm that stain well with either acid or basic dyes.

The recognition of the cellular sites of origin of specific hormones was made possible by first study-

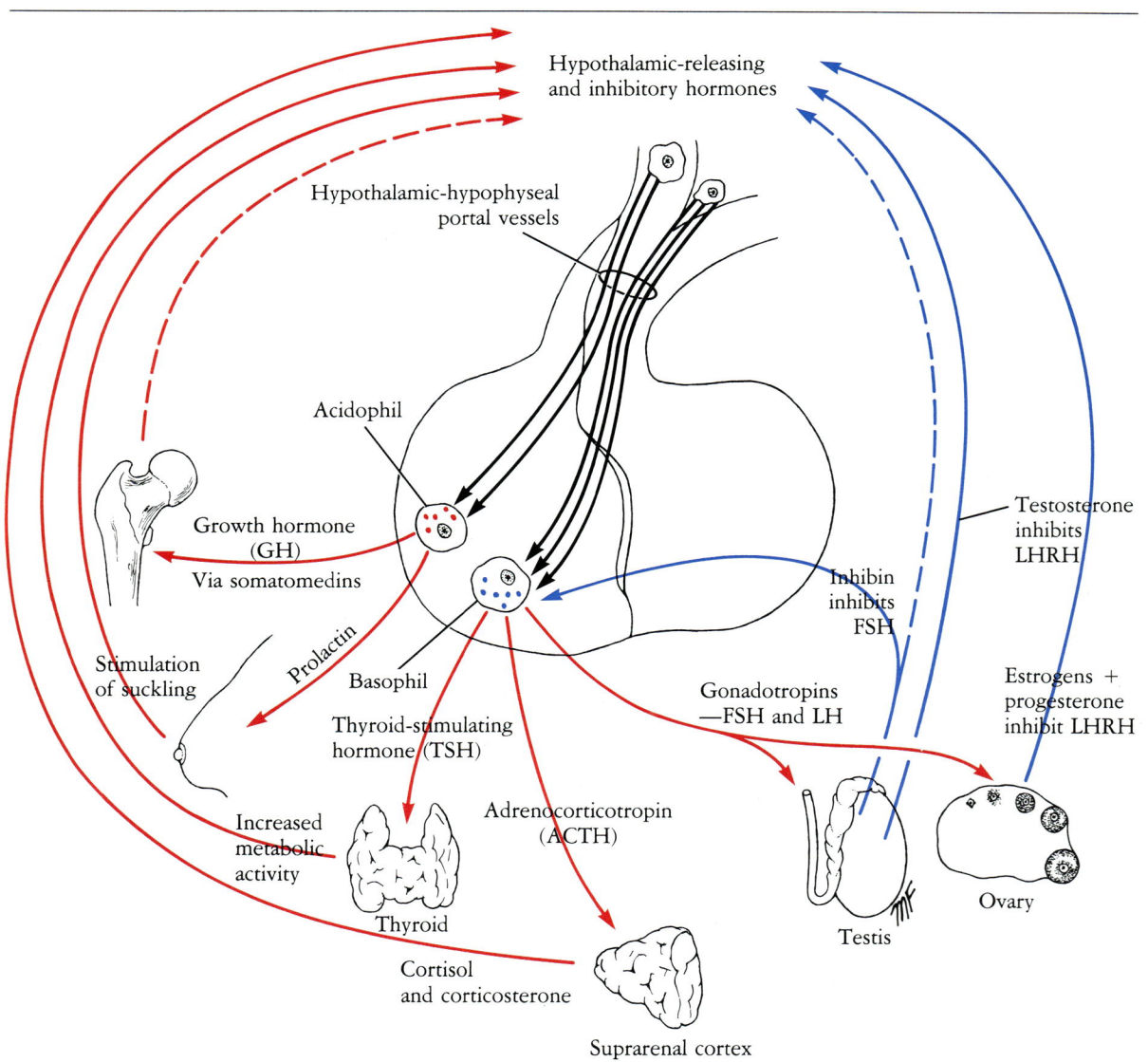

Fig. 16-4. Control of the secretions of the pars anterior of the pituitary gland by the hypothalamus. Note that the activities of the hypothalamus are modified by information received from other parts of the nervous system and by the plasma levels of circulating hormones.

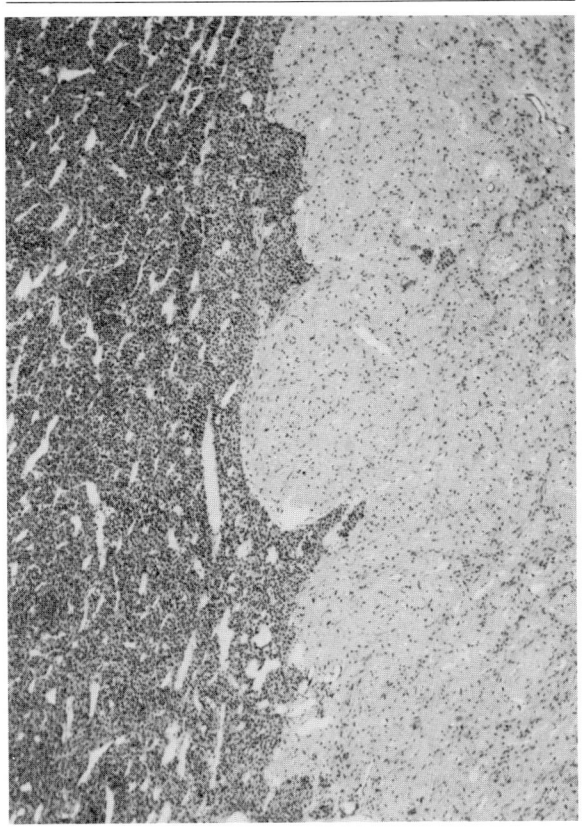

Fig. 16-5. Photomicrograph of a sagittal section of the pituitary gland, showing the dark-staining pars anterior on the left and the light-staining pars nervosa (posterior lobe, neurohypophysis) on the right. (H&E; ×40.)

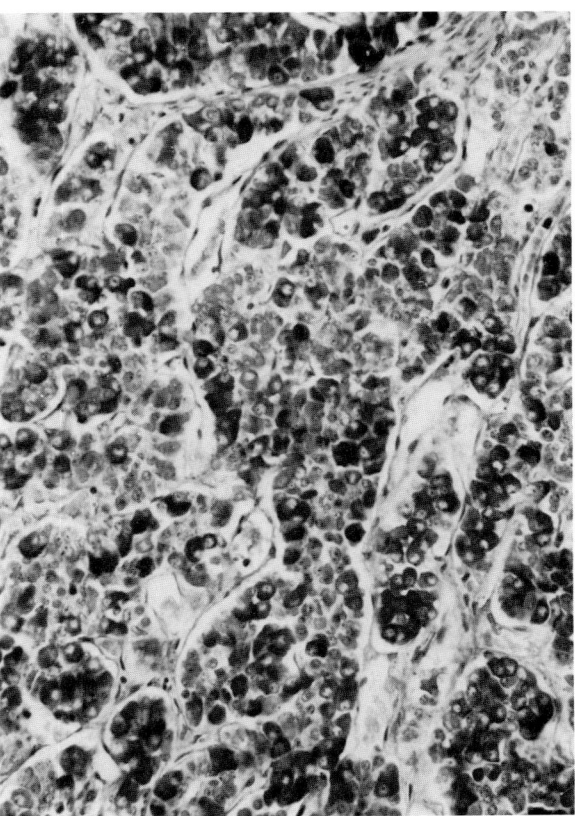

Fig. 16-6. Photomicrograph of the pars anterior of the anterior lobe of the pituitary gland, showing irregular branching cords of cells supported by delicate connective tissue. Note the blood sinusoids between the cords. Note also the unequal staining of the different cell types. The very densely stained cells are acidophils, and the moderately stained cells are basophils. (Mallory trichrome stain; ×200.)

ing the affinities of different cells for acid and basic dyes. This information was then applied to studies of pituitaries from patients who had had known hormonal defects. Later, electron microscopy provided further evidence to distinguish different types of cells. More recently, immunofluorescence techniques have enabled researchers to identify the cells of origin of most of the hormones.

CONTROL OF SECRETION AND FUNCTIONS OF THE PARS ANTERIOR HORMONES. *Growth Hormone.* The ventromedial nucleus of the hypothalamus secretes into the capillaries of the hypothalamohypophyseal portal system a *growth hormone–releasing hormone* (*GHRH*), which is carried by the blood to the somatotrope cells of the pars anterior (see Fig. 16-4). This process stimulates the release of stored growth hormone (GH), which enters the general circulation and stimulates body growth by increasing the size and number of cells. This action is not carried out directly by GH but by intermediate hormones formed in the liver called *somatomedins*. It is believed that the increased growth rate brought about by GH

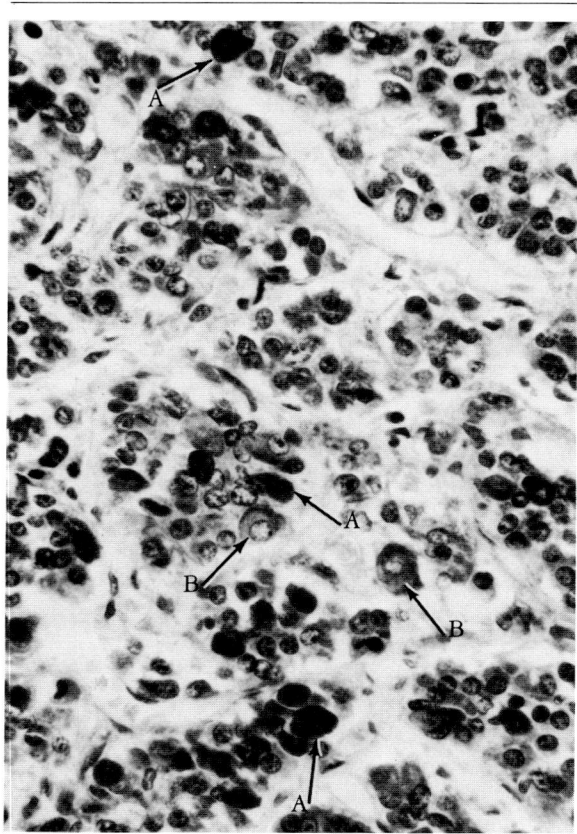

Fig. 16-7. Photomicrograph of high-power view of the pars anterior of the pituitary gland shown in Figure 16-6. The densely stained acidophil cells (A) and the less-stained basophil cells (B) can be seen clearly. (Mallory trichrome stain; ×400.)

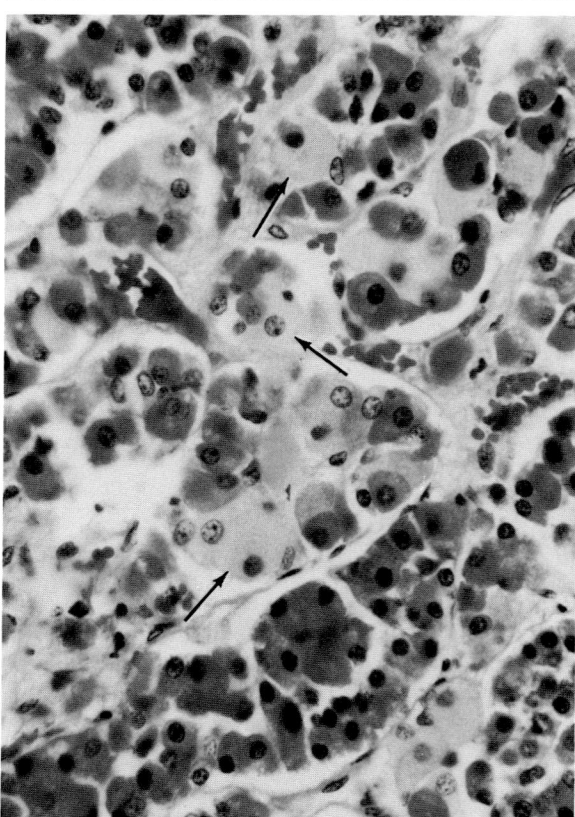

Fig. 16-8. Photomicrograph of the pars anterior of the pituitary gland, showing numerous deeply stained acidophil cells. The few poorly stained cells are chromophobe cells (arrows). (H&E; ×400.)

is accomplished mainly by increasing the synthesis of proteins.

Another region of the hypothalamus secretes into the hypothalamohypophyseal portal system a *growth hormone–inhibitory hormone* (GHIH), *somatostatin*. It is not known precisely how the secretion of GH from the pituitary is controlled. There is probably a negative feedback mechanism involving either the growth hormone–releasing hormone or the growth hormone–inhibitory hormone.

Growth hormone, by means of its intermediaries, the somatomedins, strongly stimulates the proliferation of cartilage cells in the epiphyses of growing bones. A normal person stops growing as the result of either a decrease in the amount of GH produced or a decrease in the sensitivity of the cartilage cells to the circulating somatomedins.

Prolactin. A *prolactin-inhibitory hormone* (PIH) is continuously secreted in large amounts by the hypothalamus and transported by the hypothalamohypophyseal portal system to the mammatrope cells of the pars anterior (see Fig. 16-4). Another hormone produced by the hypothalamus and passed to the pituitary is the prolactin-releasing hormone (PRH).

PRH acts only at certain times—when the baby suckles, for example.

Because the prolactin-inhibitory hormone is the dominant hormone, *prolactin* secretion by the mammatrope cells is kept at a low level. In a mother who has just delivered her child, however, suckling stimulates sensitive nerve endings in the nipple that transmit impulses to the hypothalamus, resulting in the inhibition of PIH and the release of PRH. The mammotrope cells become very active, and the increased prolactin secretion initiates and maintains lactation from the breast (see Fig. 16-4). During pregnancy, the high circulating levels of estrogens and progesterone from the placenta inhibit the secretion of prolactin. Immediately following delivery of the child and the placenta, the estrogens and progesterone levels in the blood fall and the inhibitory effect is lost. The function of prolactin in the male is unknown.

Thyroid-Stimulating Hormone. A hypothalamic hormone, the *thyrotropin-releasing hormone* (TRH), is secreted into the hypothalamohypophyseal portal system and carried by the blood to the thyrotrope cells of the pars anterior (see Fig. 16-4). Here, it stimulates the release of the *thyroid-stimulating hormone* (thyrotropin, TSH), which enters the general circulation and stimulates the thyroid gland to release the thyroid hormones (TH). The thyroid hormones increase the metabolic rate. As the metabolism of the body increases, the body temperature rises. The increase in body heat is detected by cells in the hypothalamus, which then reduce the production of TRH, TSH, and TH. Should the body temperature fall, more TRH is secreted, producing increased release of TSH, which in turn stimulates the thyroid gland to release more TH (see Fig. 16-4). Emotion can also stimulate the hypothalamus to increase the output of TRH.

Adrenocorticotropin. A *corticotropin-releasing hormone* (CRH) is produced by the hypothalamus and is transported by the hypothalamohypophyseal portal system to the corticotrope cells of the pars anterior (see Fig. 16-4). These cells are then stimulated to release adrenocorticotropin (ACTH) into the bloodstream. ACTH enters the general circulation and stimulates the cells of the adrenal cortex to synthesize and release cortisol and small amounts of corticosterone. A raised concentration of cortisol in the blood will inhibit the production of CRH and further release of ACTH. The main stimulus for increased cortisol and corticosterone production by the adrenal cortex is the exposure of the body to stress. Afferent nervous impulses from different parts of the body are conducted to the hypothalamus, immediately causing an increase in the production and secretion of CRH. By this mechanism, stress leads to the presence of large amounts of cortisol and corticosterone in the blood (see Fig. 16-4).

Gonadotropin. At puberty in both sexes, the hypothalamus starts to secrete the gonadotropin-releasing hormone (GRH), which travels to the pituitary via the hypothalamohypophyseal portal system (see Fig. 16-4). This releasing hormone stimulates the gonadotrope cells of the pars anterior to release the follicle-stimulating hormone (FSH) and the luteinizing hormone (LH).

The *follicle-stimulating hormone* enters the general circulation and induces the production of spermatozoa in the seminiferous tubules of the testes and the follicular and hormonal development of the ovaries (see Fig. 16-4). A controlling feedback mechanism exists. In the male, it is believed that the *Sertoli* cells produce a hormone called *inhibin,* which inhibits the production of FSH; it may also inhibit the production of GRH in the hypothalamus. In the female, the ovarian hormones regulate the production of GRH in the hypothalamus and, possibly, FSH production by the gonadotrope cells of the pars anterior.

The *luteinizing hormone* enters the general circulation from the gonadotrope cells of the pars anterior and, in the male, stimulates the interstitial cells of the testes to release *testosterone* (see Fig. 16-4). In the male, the luteinizing hormone is sometimes referred to as the *interstitial cell–stimulating hormone* (ICSH). The testosterone level in the blood regulates the amount of GRH produced by the hypothalamus (see Fig. 16-4).

In the female, LH assists FSH in bringing about

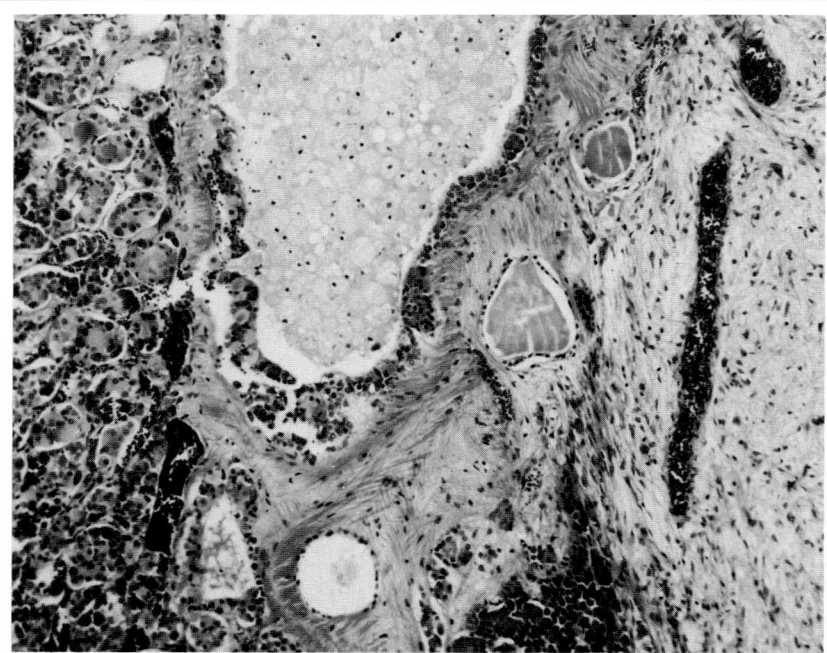

Fig. 16-9. *Photomicrograph of the pars intermedia of the pituitary gland, interposed between the pars anterior on the left and the pars posterior (posterior lobe) on the right. Note that some of the cells are arranged as follicles that contain colloid material. (H&E; ×100.)*

ovulation. It also stimulates the granulosa cells and the theca interna cells to become the corpus luteum following ovulation. The LH now stimulates the corpus luteum to secrete progesterone and estrogens. The progesterone and estrogen levels in the blood exert negative feedback on the hypothalamus and regulate the production of GRH. They also may directly affect the output of LH from the gonadotrope cells of the pars anterior (see Fig. 16-4).

Pars Intermedia

In humans, the pars intermedia is rudimentary and consists of a few irregular cords of cells with basophilic granular cytoplasm (Figs. 16-9 and 16-10). Some of the cells are arranged as follicles that contain colloid material. A few of the cells extend for a short distance into the pars nervosa. It is not certain whether the cells of the pars intermedia are the source of the melanocyte-stimulating hormone (MSH) produced by the pituitary or whether this hormone is produced by the basophil cells of the pars anterior.

FUNCTION OF THE MELANOCYTE-STIMULATING HORMONE. This hormone is a polypeptide that exists in two forms, a highly potent form, *alpha MSH*, and a less potent form, *beta MSH*. In lower animals, MSH is produced by the cells of the pars intermedia, but in humans, there is some doubt as to its origin, as we have just discussed.

The hormone stimulates the melanocytes of the epidermis of the skin to produce more melanin. As a result, the melanin granules become dispersed throughout the cytoplasm of the melanocytes and the cells darken (Fig. 16-11). Much of the melanin leaves the melanocytes to enter adjacent epidermal cells. The final result is that the skin of the individual becomes darker.

The melanocyte-stimulating hormones, together with the increased concentrations of estrogens and

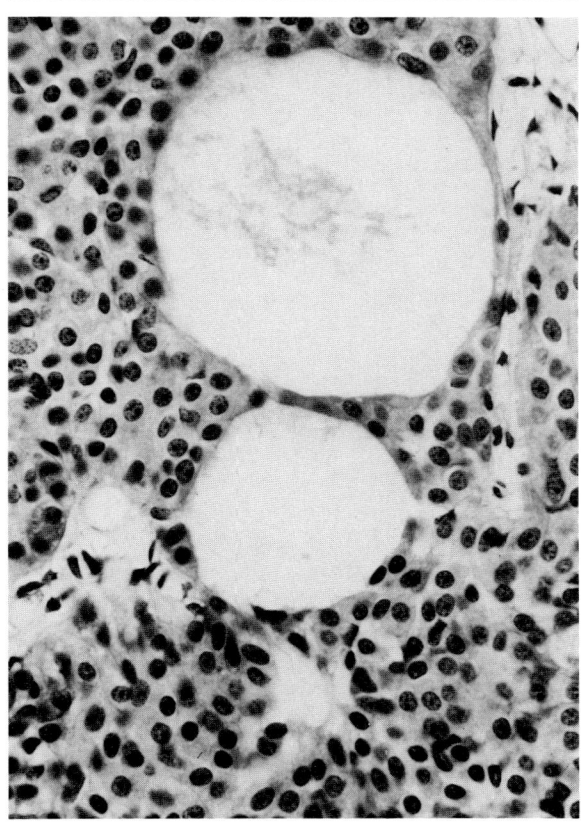

Fig. 16-10. Photomicrograph of the pars intermedia of the pituitary gland, showing irregular cords of cells. Note that some of the cells are arranged around two follicles. (H&E; ×400.)

progesterone circulating in the blood during pregnancy, are responsible for the characteristic darkening of the skin of the face, nipples, and genitalia that occurs in the pregnant woman.

Pars Tuberalis

The pars tuberalis extends superiorly like an incomplete collar along the anterior and lateral surfaces of the pituitary stalk. The cells are cuboidal and are arranged in cords between the numerous longitudinally arranged blood vessels of the hypothalamohypophyseal portal system. The cell cytoplasm contains fine granules, colloid droplets, and glycogen. The function of the pars tuberalis is unknown.

Posterior Lobe

The posterior lobe of the pituitary consists essentially of bundles of fine nonmyelinated nerve fibers that form the hypothalamohypophyseal tract, associated with glialike supporting cells called *pituicytes* (Figs. 16-12 and 16-13). The pituicytes have no known secretory function.

The nerve cell bodies of the hypothalamohypophyseal tract are situated in the supraoptic nucleus and the paraventricular nucleus of the hypothalamus. The axons of these cells descend through the stalk of the pituitary and end blindly close to blood capillaries. The nerve cells synthesize two hormones, the *antidiuretic hormone* (ADH, vasopressin) and *oxytocin*. The antidiuretic hormone is produced mainly in the paraventricular nucleus. The two hormones are transported in combination with a carrier protein called *neurophysin* down the axons to the nerve endings, where they first accumulate and are then released by exocytosis into the bloodstream (see Fig. 16-11). The hormones are released from the nerve endings when the nerve impulses from the hypothalamus reach the endings.

Hormonal Functions

ANTIDIURETIC HORMONE. This hormone conserves body water by increasing the reabsorption of water in the collecting tubules of the kidneys, as described fully on page 520. It is believed that the nerve cells of the supraoptic nucleus function as osmoreceptors. Thus, when the osmotic pressure of the body fluids rises after water deprivation, the cells are stimulated and ADH is released; a lowering of the osmotic pressure of the body fluids has the reverse effect.

This hormone is also known as vasopressin because it can cause the contraction of smooth muscle in arterial walls and thereby raise the blood pressure. It may serve an important function in restoring the blood pressure to normal after a severe hemorrhage.

OXYTOCIN. Oxytocin stimulates the smooth muscle of the uterus to contract during orgasm (see Fig. 16-11). It thus may facilitate fertilization of the ovum

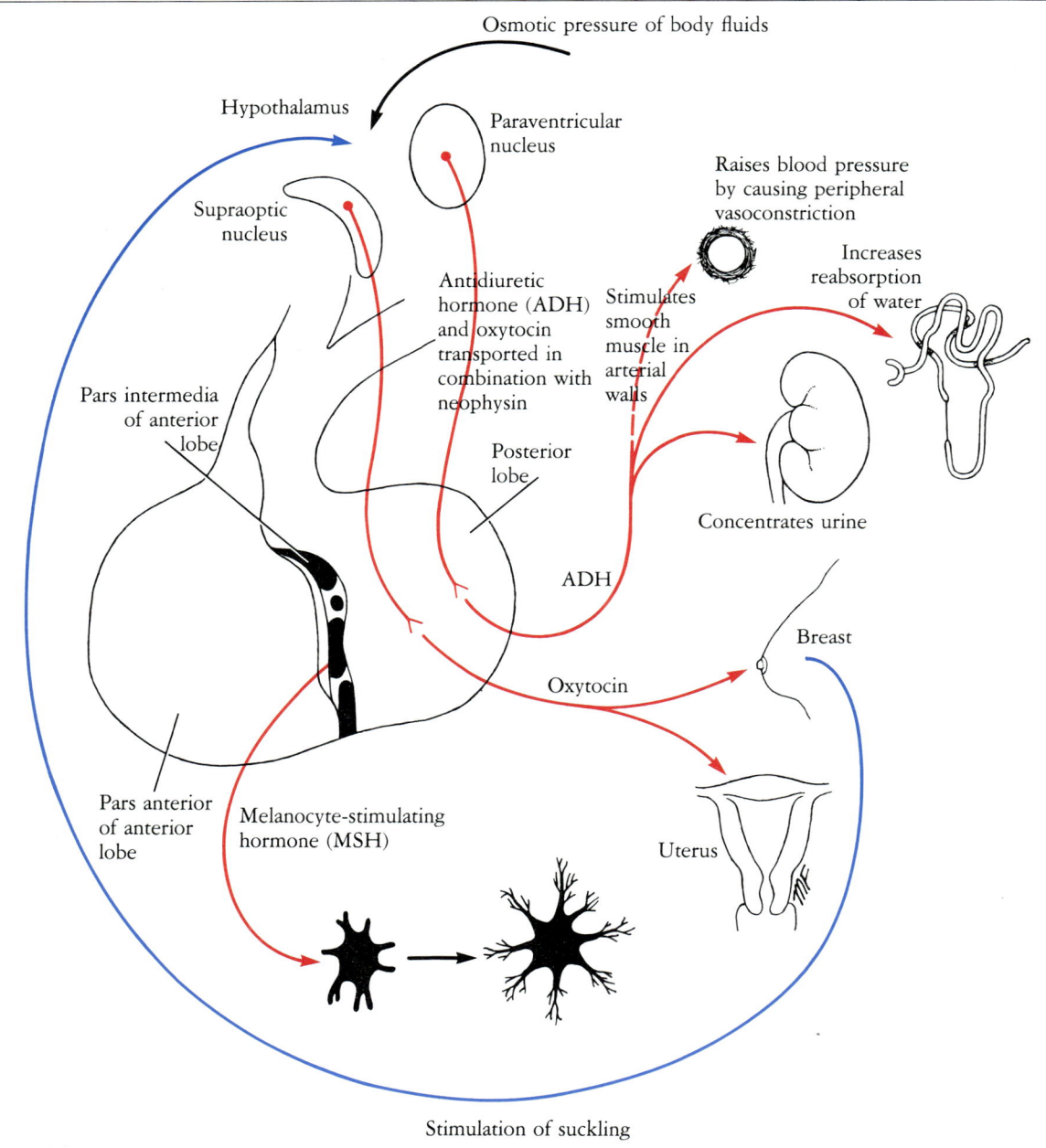

Fig. 16-11. Hormonal activities of the pars intermedia of the anterior lobe and the pars posterior (posterior lobe) of the pituitary gland. Note that the nerve cells of the supraoptic and paraventricular nuclei of the hypothalamus synthesize antidiuretic hormone and oxytocin, which are then transported to the posterior lobe in the hypothalamohypophyseal tract.

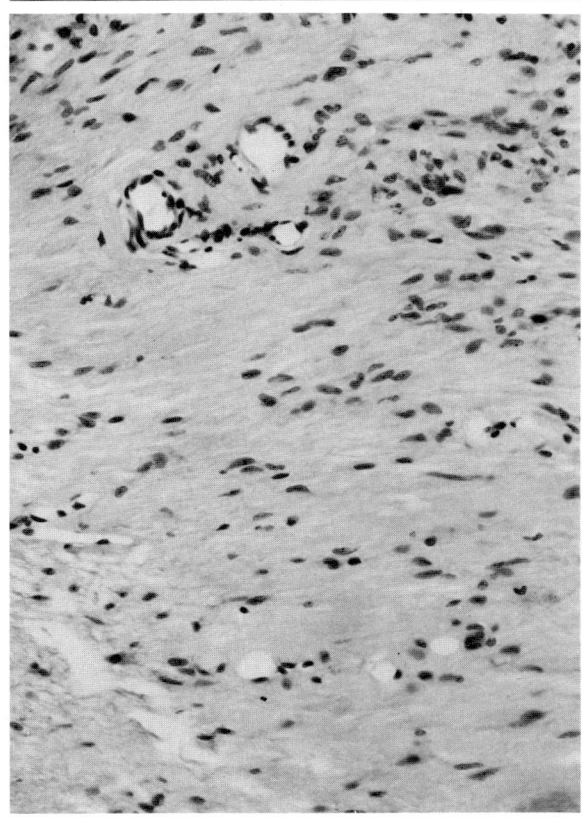

Fig. 16-12. Photomicrograph of the posterior lobe of the pituitary gland, showing bundles of nerve fibers that form the hypothalamohypophyseal tract. Some of the nuclei visible are those of glialike supporting cells, the pituicytes. (H&E; ×200.)

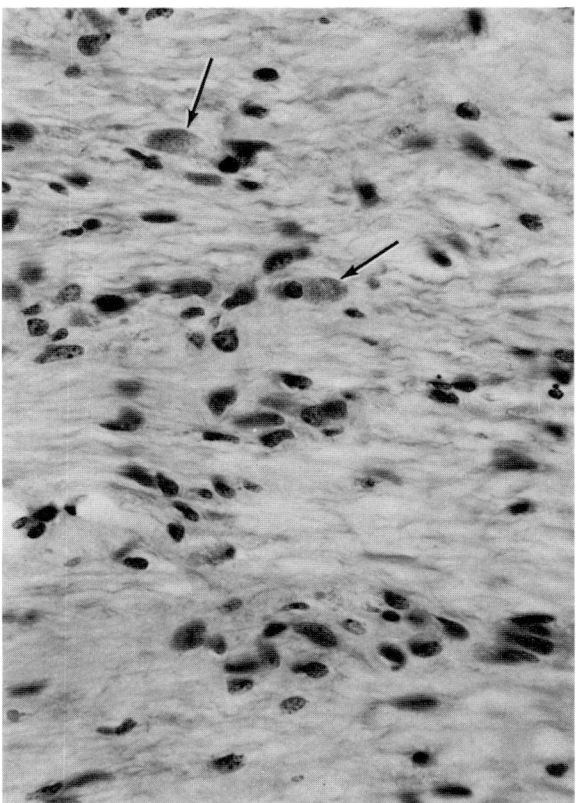

Fig. 16-13. Photomicrograph of high-power view of the posterior lobe of the pituitary gland shown in Figure 16-12, showing bundles of nerve fibers forming the hypothalamohypophyseal tract. Note the accumulation of secretion (arrows) within the nerve fibers, often referred to as Herring bodies. (H&E; ×400.)

by propelling the semen through the uterine cavity into the uterine tubes.

Oxytocin is also a powerful stimulant of the pregnant uterus and probably plays an important role in labor, especially during the second and third stages. Once the placenta and the fetal membranes have been delivered from the uterus, the uterine muscle contracts firmly, and little bleeding occurs. Here again, oxytocin is probably a strong stimulant.

Oxytocin causes contraction of the myoepithelial cells that surround the alveoli of the mammary glands (see Fig. 16-11). The suckling of the child at the breast causes nervous impulses to ascend to the brain, where they stimulate the paraventricular nucleus and cause the release of oxytocin. By this mechanism, oxytocin causes the milk to be expressed from the alveoli and made available for the baby. This same mechanism causes the smooth muscle of the uterus to contract, so that placing the newborn child to the mother's breast can reduce uterine bleeding following the delivery of the placenta and eliminate the need for drugs.

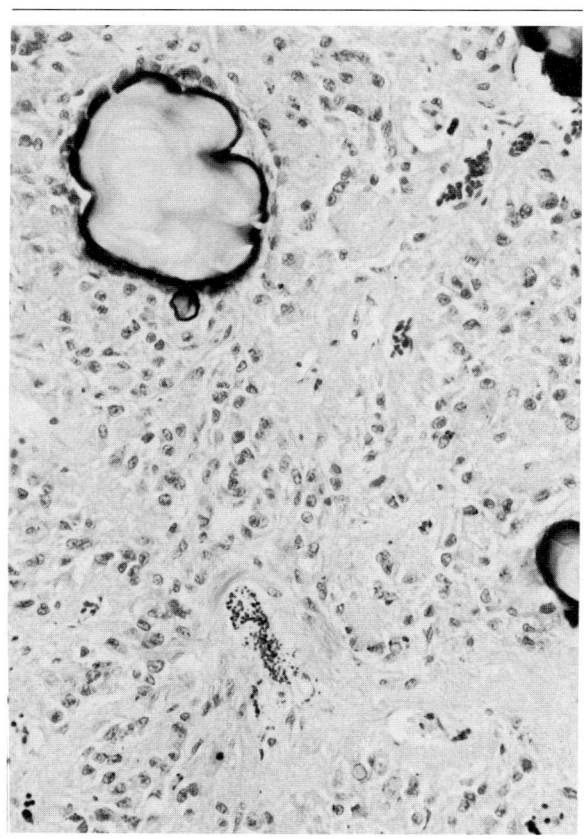

Fig. 16-14. Photomicrograph of a section of the pineal gland, showing groups of cells called pinealocytes. Note the concretions of calcified material called brain sand. (H&E; ×200.)

PINEAL GLAND

The pineal gland is a small, cone-shaped body that projects posteriorly from the posterior end of the roof of the third ventricle of the brain. It is covered on its outer surface by pia mater, which forms the capsule. Extending into the interior of the gland from the capsule are a number of fibrous trabeculae that incompletely divide it into lobules. The trabeculae carry the blood vessels and nerves into the substance of the gland. The gland is composed of groups of cells called *pinealocytes* supported by glial cells (Fig. 16-14). The pinealocytes are large cells possessing extensive processes that are intertwined with the processes of the glial cells. The pinealocyte processes end as swellings close to blood capillaries or near the ependymal cells lining the pineal recess. Stored in the terminal swellings are vesicles containing monoamines and polypeptide hormones. The gland has a rich blood supply and is innervated by postganglionic sympathetic nerve fibers. Concretions of calcified material called *brain sand* progressively accumulate within the pineal gland with age (see Fig. 16-14).

Although the function of the pineal gland is not fully understood, the gland has been shown to contain *melatonin, serotonin,* and *norepinephrine.* The enzyme necessary for the conversion of serotonin into melatonin, *serotonin*-N-*acetyltransferase,* is also present. The release of norepinephrine from the postganglionic sympathetic fibers stimulates the pinealocytes to increase their output of melatonin. The concentration of melatonin in the blood conforms to a circadian rhythm, being highest during darkness and lowest during the day.

Although melatonin has been shown to cause the aggregation of melanin granules in frog skin pigment cells, it apparently has no effect on mammalian melanocytes. Clinical observations of patients with pineal tumors have revealed that the pineal gland may have an antigonadotropic function brought about by the suppression of the secretion of the gonadotropic hormone of the pars anterior of the pituitary.

THYROID GLAND

The thyroid gland is situated in the neck and is closely related to the larynx and the trachea. It consists of right and left lobes connected by a narrow isthmus. The gland is surrounded by an outer false capsule, derived from the pretracheal layer of deep cervical fascia, that anchors the gland to the trachea and larynx. The gland also is surrounded by an inner true capsule, consisting of connective tissue, that sends septa into the gland.

The thyroid gland is composed of structural units of varying size called *follicles.* Each follicle is spherical and is lined with a single layer of cuboidal cells, the *follicular cells* (Figs. 16-15 and 16-16). The cavity

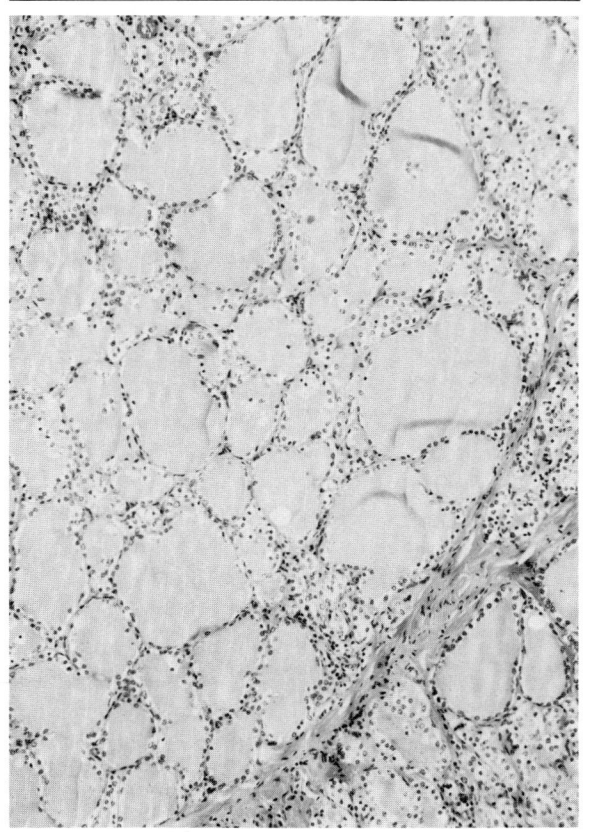

Fig. 16-15. Photomicrograph of a section of the thyroid gland, showing follicles of varying size. The cavity of each follicle is filled with homogeneous material called colloid. Connective tissue septa also can be seen. (H&E; ×100.)

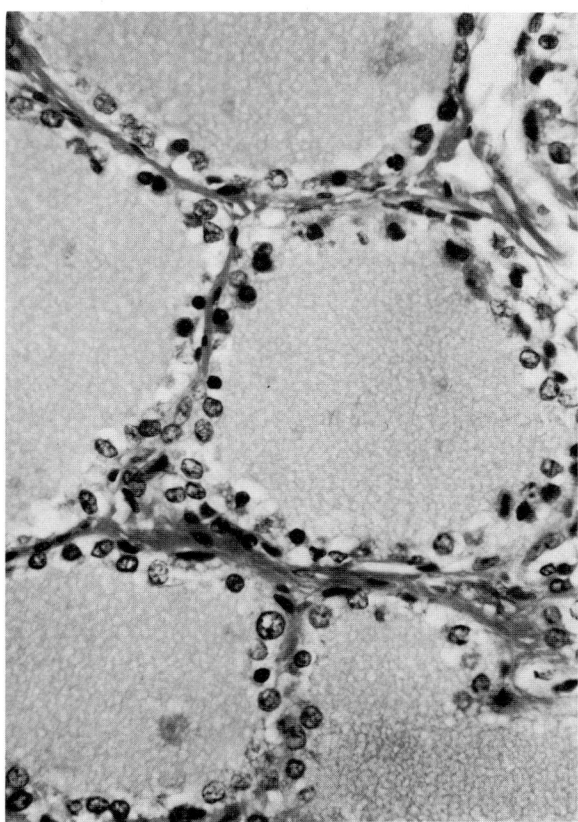

Fig. 16-16. Photomicrograph of a section of the thyroid gland, showing several follicles lined with cuboidal epithelium. The follicles are surrounded by a small amount of very vascular connective tissue. The cavity of each follicle is filled with colloid. (H&E; ×400.)

of the follicle is filled with a homogeneous material called *colloid*. The follicles are surrounded by a small amount of connective tissue that is richly supplied with blood vessels.

The follicular cells change their shape with different levels of activity. When not stimulated by thyrotropin, the cells are low cuboidal or even squamous and there is a great accumulation of colloid in the cavity of the follicle. When the cells are stimulated excessively by thyrotropin, they become columnar and may even multiply. Under these conditions, the colloid is scant and there is evidence of increased stromal vascularity. When examined with the electron microscope, the apices of the cells display microvilli that lengthen with increased activity of the cells. There are a well-developed rough endoplasmic reticulum and Golgi apparatus, which are necessary for the production and secretion of protein material.

In addition to the main epithelial cells that line the follicles, there is a smaller group of cells that are situated singly or in small groups in the spaces between the follicles. These cells are larger than the follicular cells and lie within the follicular basement membrane. They are known as the *parafollicular cells*. The parafollicular cells are oval, and their cytoplasm contains numerous membrane-bound secretory granules.

Follicular Cells
Function
The follicular cells secrete into the cavity of the follicle (1) glycoprotein molecules called thyroglobulin that contain the amino acid tyrosine (referred to as the tyrosyl radical), (2) iodine molecules, and (3) enzymes.

The glycoprotein is formed as follows: The amino acids are absorbed from the bloodstream and formed into polypeptides in the rough endoplasmic reticulum (Fig. 16-17). The carbohydrate mannose is added to the molecule within the rough endoplasmic reticulum. When the molecule arrives at the Golgi apparatus, galactose is added and the thyroglobulin molecule is completed. The thyroglobulin molecules are now packaged into vesicles that are discharged from the luminal surface of the cells by exocytosis.

The iodine secretion occurs as follows: Iodide is absorbed from the blood and is oxidized to iodine by the enzyme peroxidase within the follicular cells. The iodine molecules are then concentrated within the cells and finally passed out into the cavity of the follicle.

Once the thyroglobulin and the iodine reach the follicular cavity, formation of the two hormones *thyroxine* and *triiodothyronine* commences (see Fig. 16-17). The tyrosyl group of the secreted thyroglobulin first is combined with iodine to form *monoiodotyrosyl* and then is converted to *diiodotyrosyl*. Two molecules of diiodotyrosyl are then combined to form one molecule of thyroxine (T_4), which remains as part of the thyroglobulin molecule. In another reaction, one molecule of monoiodotyrosyl combines with one molecule of diiodotyrosyl to form *triiodothyronine* (T_3). The hormones thyroxine and triiodothyronine are now stored in the thyroglobulin colloid in the cavity of the follicle and may remain there for as long as 3 months (see Fig. 16-17).

In response to the thyroid-stimulating hormone produced by the pars anterior of the pituitary, the hormones thyroxine and triiodothyronine are liberated from the follicular colloid and enter the bloodstream via the following mechanism: The apical microvilli elongate, extend into the colloid, and fuse around small quantities of the material. By this means, portions of the thyroglobulin are absorbed into the cells by endocytosis. The thyroglobulin vesicles then fuse with lysosomes, and the lysosomal proteases split the inactive thyroglobulin molecule into the active hormones thyroxin and triiodothyronine (see Fig. 16-17). These hormones are then released into the bloodstream on the basal side of the cell. The monoiodotyrosine and the diiodotyrosine are not released but are split by a dehalogenase enzyme, and the iodine released is reused in the formation of more hormone. Thyroxine is released in much larger quantities than triiodothyronine, but the latter hormone is more potent.

Control of Secretion
The activity of the follicular cells is controlled mainly by the TSH of the pars anterior of the pituitary (see Fig. 16-17). In addition, postganglionic sympathetic nerve endings on the follicular cells and the blood vessels of the gland probably have some controlling influence. Experiments have shown that norepinephrine causes an increase in the formation of cyclic AMP, which is followed by an increase in the release of thyroid hormones.

Effect of the Thyroid Hormones on the Tissues
Once the hormones enter the blood, the greater part combines with plasma proteins to form such substances as thyroxine-binding globulin. Over a period of days, the hormones gradually are released from the protein and enter the tissues.

The thyroid hormones increase the metabolic activity of most cells of the body, increasing oxygen consumption and heat production. At puberty and during menstruation and pregnancy, the activity of the thyroid gland is increased. In patients with hypothyroidism (see p. 677), the basal metabolism (the energy output of the individual at complete rest 12 to 18 hours after a meal) is reduced to 30 to 40 percent below normal, whereas it may be increased

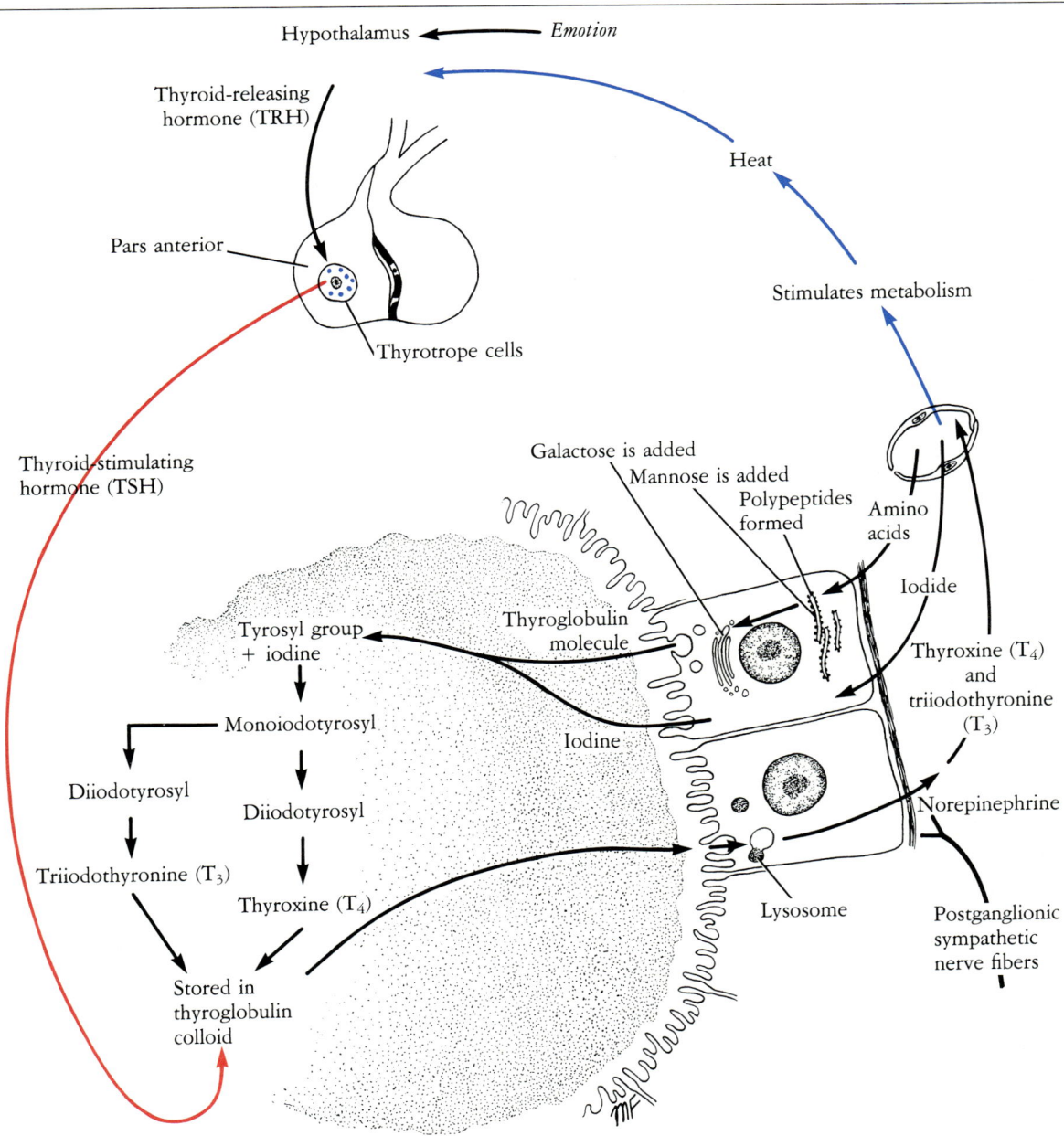

Fig. 16-17. Formation and control of follicular cell secretion in the thyroid gland. Note the feedback mechanism to the hypothalamus.

to 50 to 100 percent above normal in hyperthyroidism (see p. 676).

The thyroid hormones have many important actions, including actions on the following structures and processes:

The central nervous system. The hormones are essential for the normal activity of the nervous system.

Growth and tissue differentiation. The thyroid hormones are necessary for the growth and differentiation of most tissues of the body; they stimulate synthesis of proteins throughout the body tissues.

Protein metabolism. The thyroid hormones promote protein synthesis by increasing the rate at which the ribosomes form proteins. They also activate the DNA transcription process in the cell nuclei, which causes the formation of new proteins within cells.

Carbohydrate metabolism. The thyroid hormones stimulate the absorption of glucose from the intestine and increase the utilization of glucose by the tissues. They also stimulate the breakdown of glycogen into glucose in the liver, heart, and skeletal muscle.

Lipid metabolism. The thyroid hormones increase the mobilization of lipids from the adipose tissue and stimulate the oxidation of free fatty acids by the cells. The hormones reduce the plasma cholesterol levels by stimulating the liver to destroy cholesterol and by increasing the excretion in the bile.

Gonads. The thyroid hormones are necessary for normal gonad development. In patients with hypothyroidism, the secondary sexual characters do not develop, amenorrhea may occur, and fertility is reduced.

Function of the Parafollicular Cells

The parafollicular cells produce the hormone *thyrocalcitonin,* which lowers the level of blood calcium. The hormone acts by inhibiting the breakdown of bone by the osteoclasts, thereby reducing the return of calcium to the blood (Fig. 16-18). Thyrocalcitonin thus has an effect on blood calcium levels opposite that of the parathyroid hormone.

The parafollicular cells are not under the control of the pituitary gland but are stimulated by hypercalcemia and suppressed by hypocalcemia.

PARATHYROID GLANDS

The parathyroid glands are four small, yellowish-brown, ovoid structures that are related to the posterior border of the thyroid gland in the neck. They are intimately related to the thyroid gland, lying within its fascial capsule. The two *superior parathyroid glands* are the more constant in position and lie at the level of the middle of the posterior border of the thyroid gland. The two *inferior parathyroid glands* usually lie close to the inferior poles of the thyroid gland. They may lie within the fascial sheath, embedded in the thyroid substance, or outside the fascial sheath. Sometimes they are located somewhat caudal to the thyroid gland and may even reside in the thorax.

Each parathyroid gland is surrounded by a loose connective tissue capsule. Delicate septa pass into the gland from the capsule, carrying the blood vessels. The gland consists of branching columns of cells between which lie sinusoidal capillaries (Figs. 16-19 and 16-20). Two main types of cells are present, the *chief* or *principal cells* and the *oxyphil cells.* Until puberty, only the chief cells are present. At puberty, the oxyphil cells appear, but they remain in the minority.

The chief cells are small. They have a centrally placed nucleus with slightly acidophilic cytoplasm; that is, the cytoplasm stains pink with eosin (see Fig. 16-20). Some chief cell cytoplasm looks light colored because of the presence of large amounts of glycogen; in other chief cells, the cytoplasm is darker, and very little glycogen is present. Under the electron microscope, the cells are seen to have a well-developed Golgi apparatus, mitochondria, and numerous secretory granules.

The oxyphil cells are found scattered among the chief cells. They are slightly larger than the chief

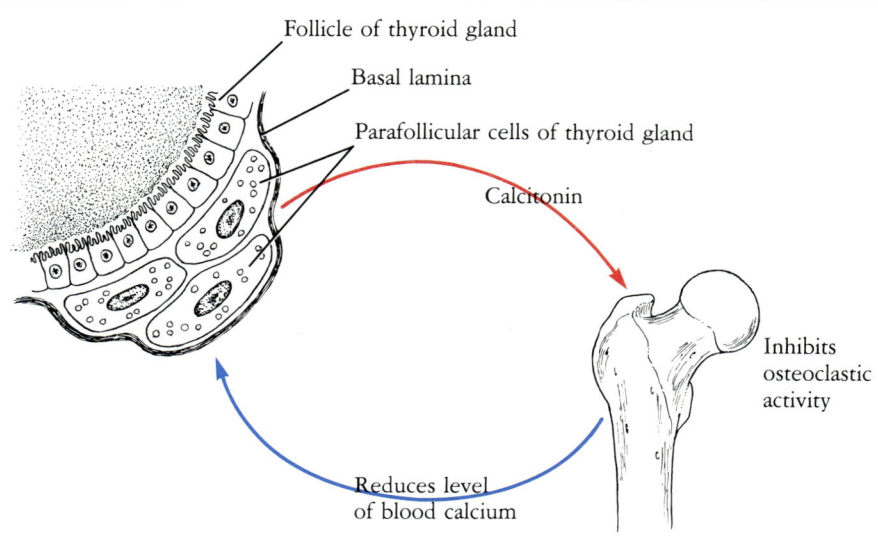
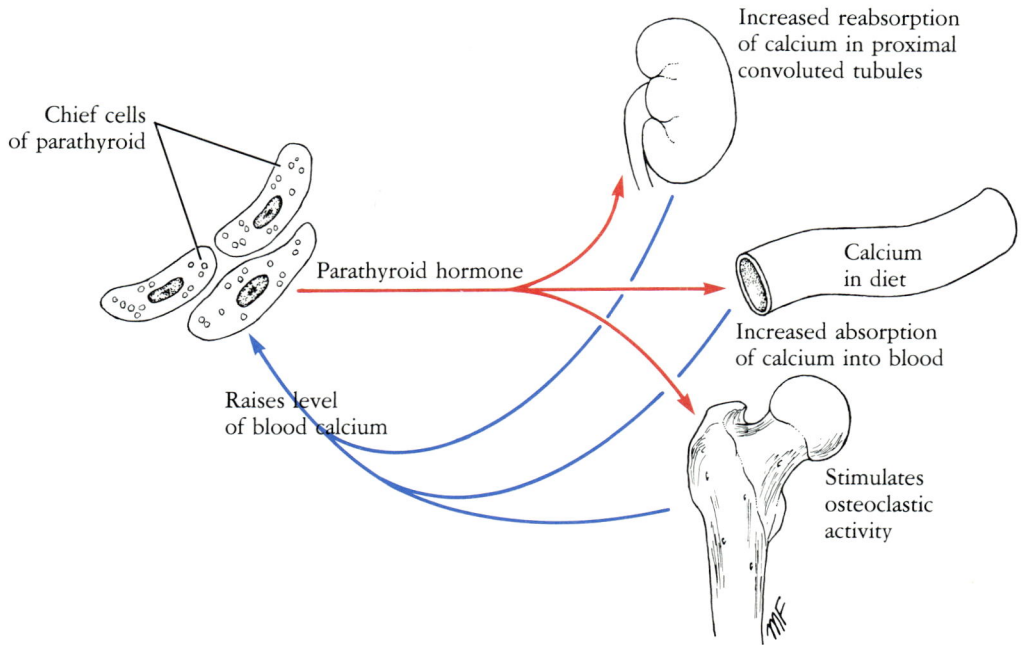

Fig. 16-18. Actions of thyrocalcitonin (A) and the parathyroid hormone (B) on calcium metabolism.

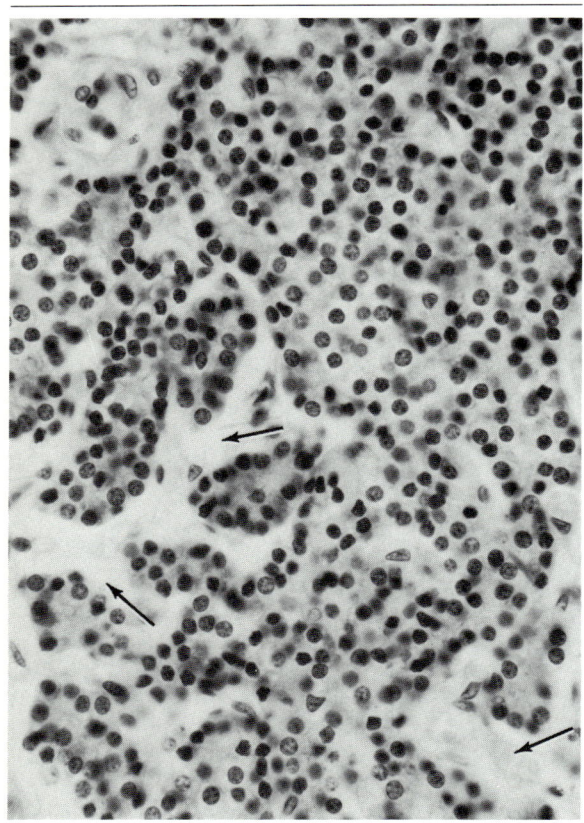

Fig. 16-19. *Photomicrograph of a section of the parathyroid gland, showing columns of cells between which lie sinusoidal capillaries (arrows). (H&E; ×100.)*

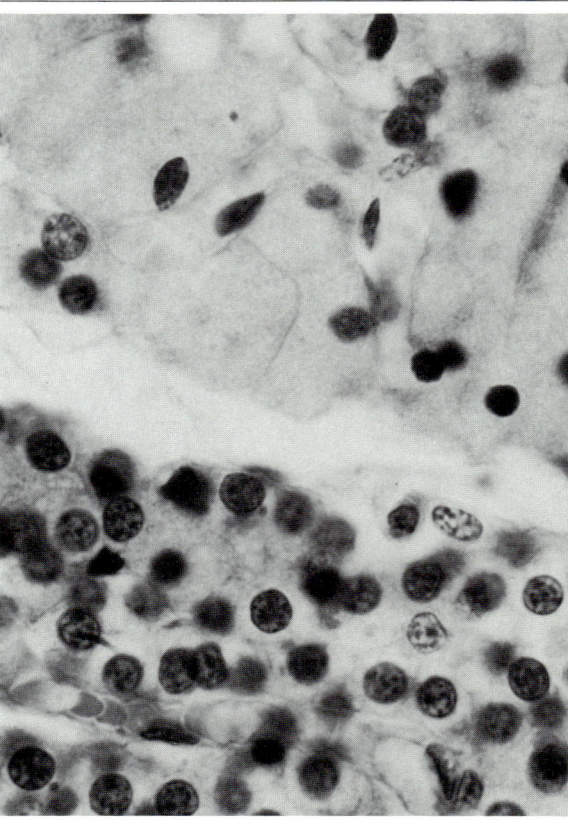

Fig. 16-20. *Photomicrograph of a section of the parathyroid gland, showing a large group of oxyphil cells (top) and a group of smaller, darker-staining chief cells (bottom). (H&E; ×400.)*

cells, and the cytoplasm stains bright pink with eosin (see Fig. 16-20). Electron microscopic examination reveals numerous mitochondria and glycogen granules, but there are no secretory granules. Cells having a structure intermediate between chief cells and oxyphil cells are also present. They are believed to be immature oxyphil cells.

In the young, the gland is packed with epithelial cells. In the adult, adipose tissue appears in the connective tissue and separates the cells into columns. In the old, the adipose tissue diminishes.

The chief cells are responsible for producing the parathyroid hormone. The function of the oxyphil cells is not known.

Functions of the Parathyroid Hormone

The parathyroid hormone stimulates osteoclastic activity in bones, thus mobilizing the bone calcium and increasing the calcium levels in the blood (see Fig. 16-18). The phosphate absorption from the bone is overshadowed by the effect of the hormone on the kidneys, which is to diminish strongly the rate of reabsorption of phosphate in the proximal convoluted tubules; the net result is that the phosphate level in the blood falls. The parathyroid hormone also stimulates the absorption of dietary calcium from the small intestine and the reabsorption of calcium in the proximal convoluted tubules of the kidney.

The relationship between vitamin D, the parathyroid hormone, and thyrocalcitonin should be understood. Vitamin D stimulates calcium absorption from the intestine and assists in the control of calcium deposition in bone. It is thought that the parathyroid hormone acts on bone by stimulating the conversion of vitamin D to 1,25-dihydroxycholecalciferol, which causes the decalcification of bone. Thyrocalcitonin, in contrast, inhibits the breakdown of bone by the osteoclasts and thus lowers the level of blood calcium.

Secretion of the parathyroid hormone is controlled by the calcium levels in the blood. After even a very small decrease in the calcium level, the parathyroid glands increase their secretion of hormone. The parathyroid glands enlarge in the mother during pregnancy and lactation, because calcium is used by the fetus and large amounts of calcium are necessary for the formation of milk.

SUPRARENAL GLANDS

There are two suprarenal (adrenal) glands. They are yellowish and lie behind the peritoneum on the upper poles of the kidneys. The right suprarenal gland is pyramidal and caps the upper pole of the right kidney (see Fig. 16-1). The left suprarenal gland is crescent shaped and extends along the medial border of the left kidney from the upper pole to the hilus. The glands are surrounded by connective tissue containing a large amount of adipose tissue. Each gland has a thick capsule of connective tissue that sends septa into the interior of the gland.

A section across the suprarenal gland reveals an outer, yellow part called the *cortex* and a smaller, inner, dark red part called the *medulla* (Fig. 16-21).

Suprarenal Cortex

The suprarenal cortex consists of three concentric layers or zones (Figs. 16-22–16-24). Immediately beneath the capsule is the *zona glomerulosa*. This is a thin layer composed of clusters of columnar cells. The nuclei are dark staining, and the cytoplasm contains some lipid droplets. Next is the *zona fas-*

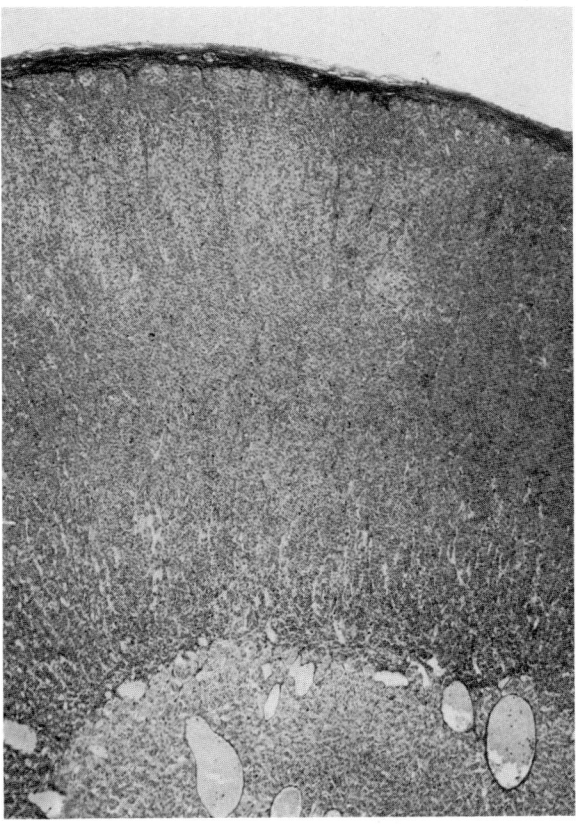

Fig. 16-21. Photomicrograph of a section of the suprarenal gland, showing the connective tissue capsule above, the dark-staining cortex and the lighter-staining medulla below. Note the sinusoidal capillaries in the cortex and the very large capillaries in the medulla. (H&E; ×40.)

ciculata, which is a thick layer composed of radially arranged columns of cells. The cells are polyhedral; the cytoplasm is basophilic and contains numerous lipid droplets (Fig. 16-25). The innermost layer is the *zona reticularis,* which consists of an anastomosing network of cells that rests on the medulla. The cells resemble those of the zona fasciculata. The cytoplasm is darkly acidophilic, and there are no lipid droplets. The cells contain large amounts of lipochrome pigment.

When examined with the electron microscope, the cells of the zona glomerulosa and zona fas-

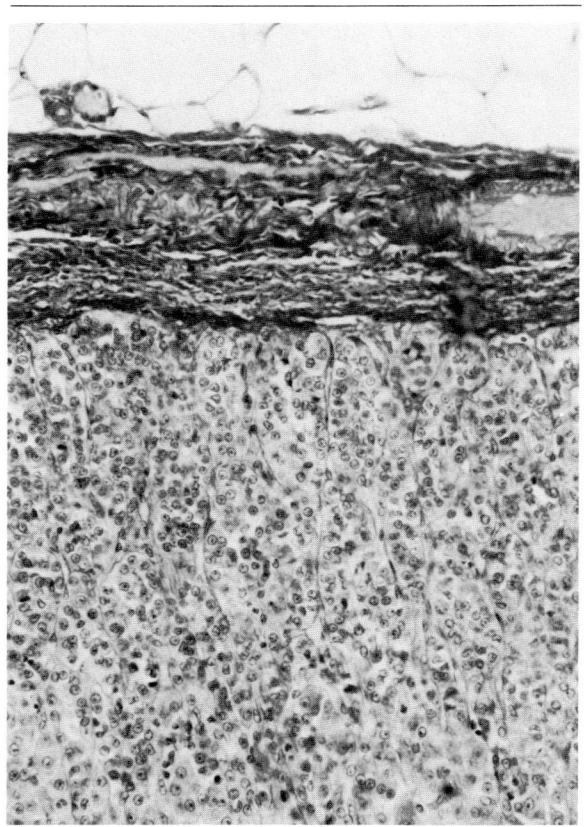

Fig. 16-22. Photomicrograph of a section of the outer portion of the cortex of the suprarenal gland, showing the zona glomerulosa and a small part of the zona fasciculata below. Note the connective tissue capsule above. (H&E; ×200.)

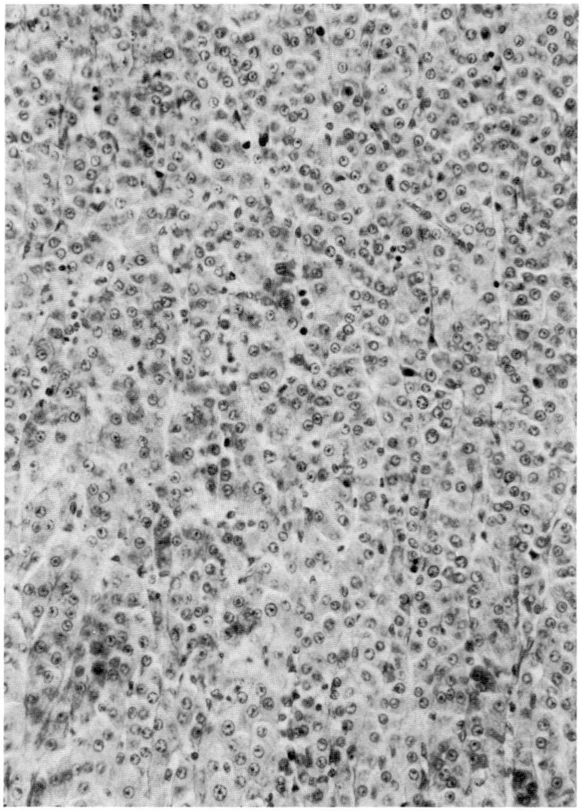

Fig. 16-23. Photomicrograph of a section of the cortex of the suprarenal gland, showing columns of cells in the zona fasciculata. The slitlike spaces situated between the columns are occupied by fenestrated blood sinusoids. (H&E; ×200.)

ciculata show large amounts of cytoplasmic agranular endoplasmic reticulum. There are also many mitochondria, whose cristae are tubular rather than flat septa. In the zona reticularis, there is a large amount of agranular endoplasmic reticulum, numerous lysosomes, and pigment bodies.

The cortical cells are supported by a delicate connective tissue containing sinusoidal blood vessels.

Function

The zona glomerulosa secretes hormones called *mineralocorticoids,* namely *aldosterone* and, in small amounts, *deoxycorticosterone,* which are concerned with the control of fluid and electrolyte balance (Fig. 16-26). The zona fasciculata and zona reticularis secrete hormones called *glucocorticoids,* namely *cortisol* and, in small amounts, *corticosterone* and *cortisone,* which are concerned with the control of the metabolism of carbohydrates, fats, and proteins. In addition, the zona fasciculata and the zona reticularis produce very small quantities of the male sex hormones, the androgens, and the female sex hormones, the estrogens and progesterone. These hormones almost certainly play a role in the prepubertal development of the sex organs; otherwise, they do not appear to have important functions.

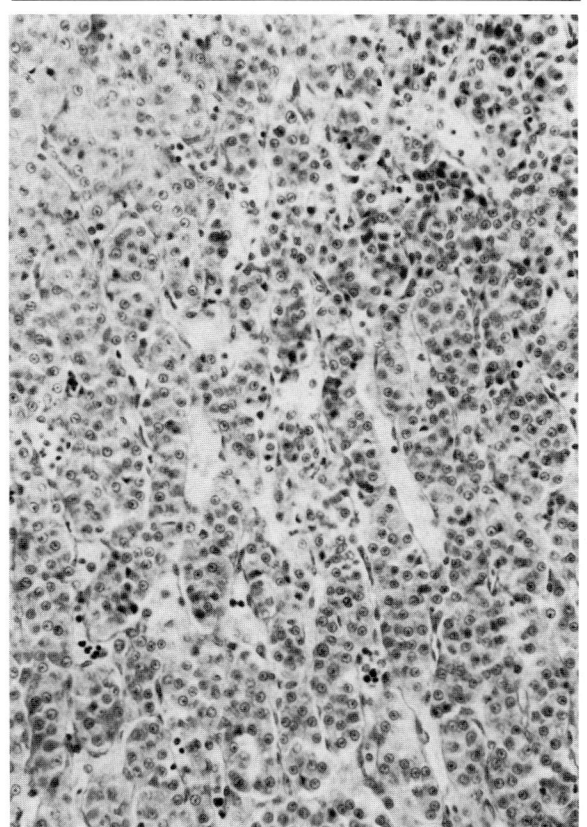

Fig. 16-24. Photomicrograph of a section of the zona reticularis of the cortex of the suprarenal gland, showing the anastomosing columns of cells separated by blood sinusoids. (H&E; ×200.)

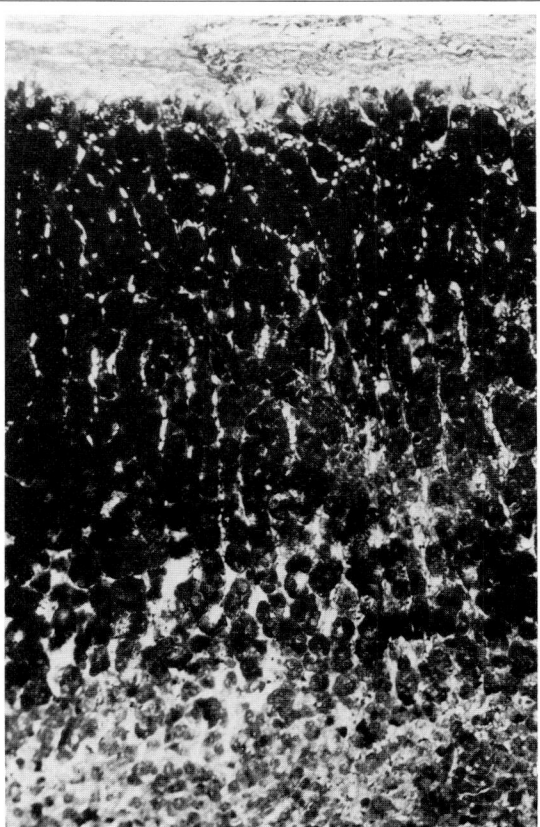

Fig. 16-25. Photomicrograph of a section of the suprarenal gland stained to show lipid material. The lipid appears black within the cytoplasm. Note that the cells of the zona glomerulosa just beneath the capsule (top) contain only a small amount of lipid, whereas the cells of the zona fasciculata are packed with lipid. In the lower part of the photograph, the cells of the zona reticularis are visible and can be seen to contain practically no lipid. (Sudan black stain; ×100.)

MINERALOCORTICOIDS. Aldosterone increases the reabsorption of sodium in the distal convoluted and collecting tubules of the kidney and increases the tubular excretion of potassium by the kidney (see Fig. 16-26). Deoxycorticosterone has almost the same actions as aldosterone. The mineralocorticoids thus assist in the control of the water and electrolyte balance of the body fluids.

Regulation of Aldosterone Secretion. The main factor controlling aldosterone secretion is the renin-angiotensin system (see p. 523). Renin is released from the juxtaglomerular cells of the kidney in response to a fall in blood pressure or a lowered sodium level in the blood. Renin then catalyzes the transformation of serum angiotensinogen into *angiotensin I*, which is changed into *angiotensin II* by an enzyme present in the plasma. The rising concentration of angiotensin II in the bloodstream stimulates the zona glomerulosa cells to increase their secretion of aldosterone (see Fig. 16-26). The resulting rise in blood pressure caused by the retention of sodium and the increase in blood volume inhibits

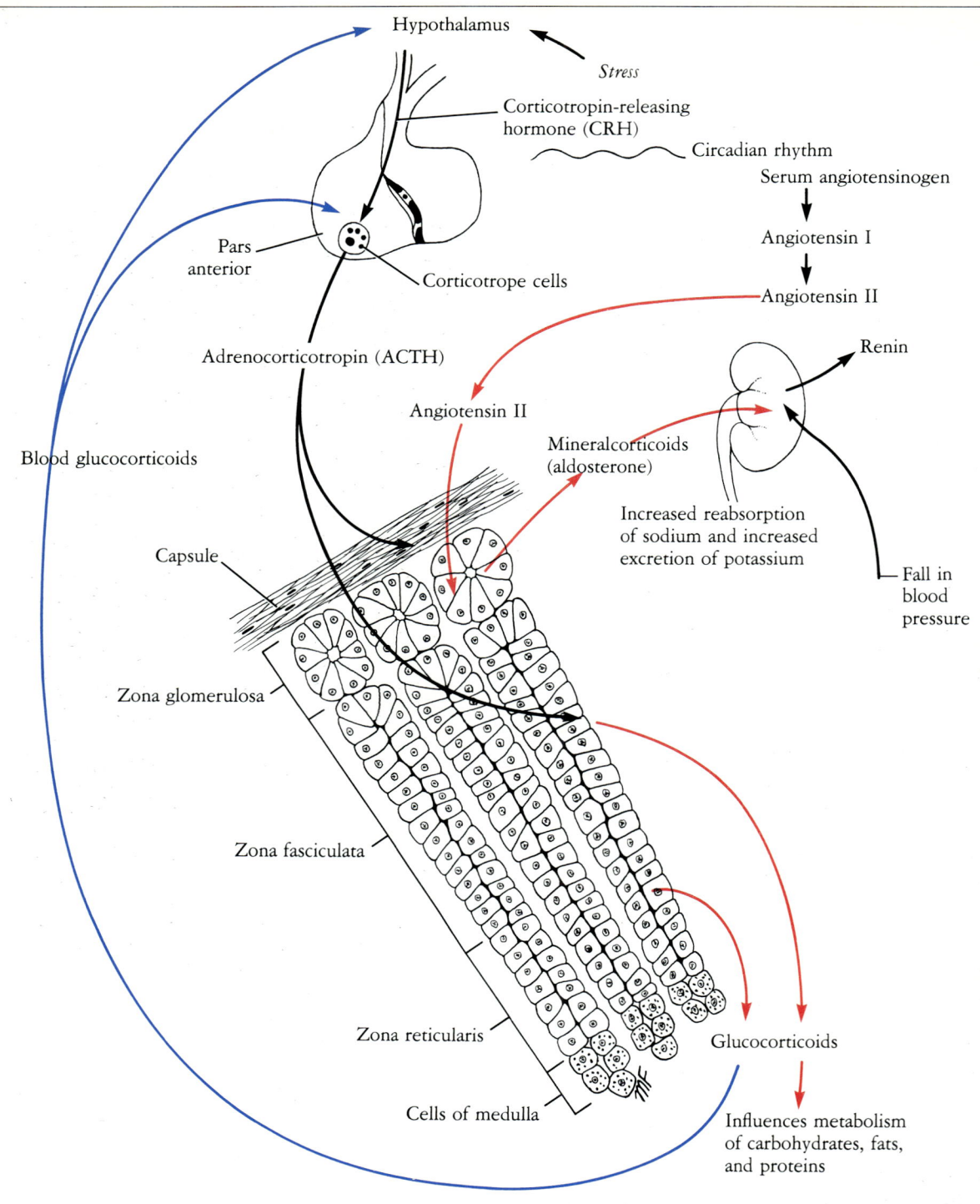

Fig. 16-26. Actions of the hormones secreted by the suprarenal cortex. The control of the suprarenal cortex by the pituitary gland and the hypothalamus is also shown, as is the renin-angiotensin control of aldosterone secretion.

the further release of renin by the juxtaglomerular cells.

A failure in the production of aldosterone quickly upsets the homeostasis of the body. The potassium ion concentration of the extracellular fluid rises, the sodium concentrations fall, and the extracellular fluid and blood volumes are reduced. Shock and death may follow rapidly.

The zona glomerulosa cells require ACTH for their normal existence. An absence of this hormone leads to atrophy of these cells and a consequent reduction in the production of aldosterone.

GLUCOCORTICOIDS. These hormones perform important actions in carbohydrate, fat, and protein metabolism (see Fig. 16-26).

In *carbohydrate metabolism,* the glucocorticoids stimulate the conversion of amino acids in the liver to glucose (gluconeogenesis). The newly formed glucose is stored in the liver as glycogen, and the excess is released into the blood. These hormones also decrease the rate at which tissue cells use glucose.

In *fat metabolism,* the glucocorticoids stimulate the breakdown of lipid in fat cells into free fatty acids. They also promote the oxidation of fatty acid in tissue cells. This mechanism enables cells to use fatty acids in the place of glucose as an energy source in times of starvation.

In *protein metabolism,* the glucocorticoids decrease the tissue protein in the body by inhibiting protein synthesis and increasing the breakdown of cellular protein.

All these actions of the glucocorticoids produce substances within the body—namely, glucose and fatty acids—that are a ready source of energy if the body is subjected to stress.

Regulation of Glucocorticoid Secretion. Secretion of the glucocorticoids is controlled by the adrenocorticotropic hormone, which is produced by the corticotrope cells of the pars anterior of the pituitary (see Fig. 16-26). Any form of bodily stress causes afferent nervous impulses to be transmitted to the hypothalamus, which results in the passage of large amounts of the corticotropin-releasing hormone to

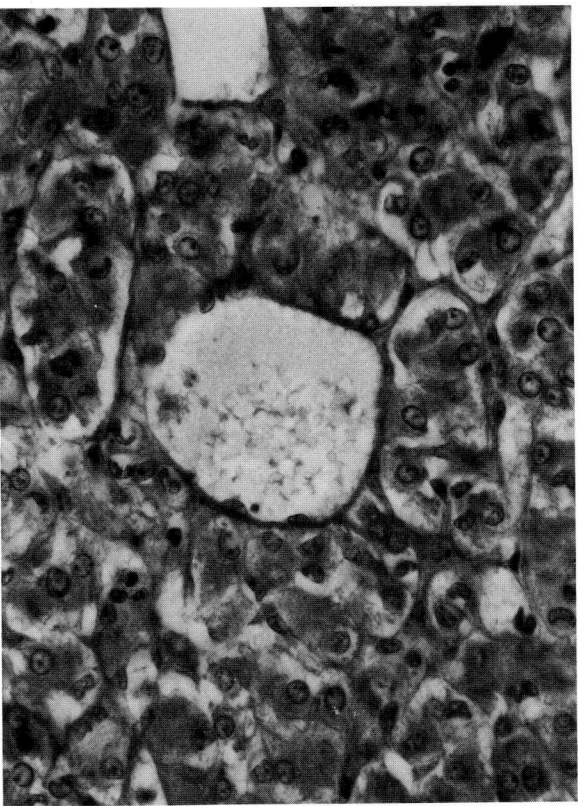

Fig. 16-27. Photomicrograph of a section of the suprarenal medulla, showing groups of cells supported by delicate connective tissue. Two blood sinusoids are visible. (H&E; ×400.)

the corticotrope cells of the pituitary. Within a very short time, the concentration of glucocorticoids in the blood rises to a high level.

The presence of large amounts of cortisol in the blood has a direct negative feedback effect on the production of CRH in the hypothalamus and the formation of ACTH in the pituitary (see Fig. 16-26). This feedback mechanism thus automatically regulates the levels of the glucocorticoids in the bloodstream.

The production of CRH by the hypothalamus takes place according to a *circadian rhythm,* the highest production occurring in the morning and the lowest in the late afternoon. In a person who sleeps

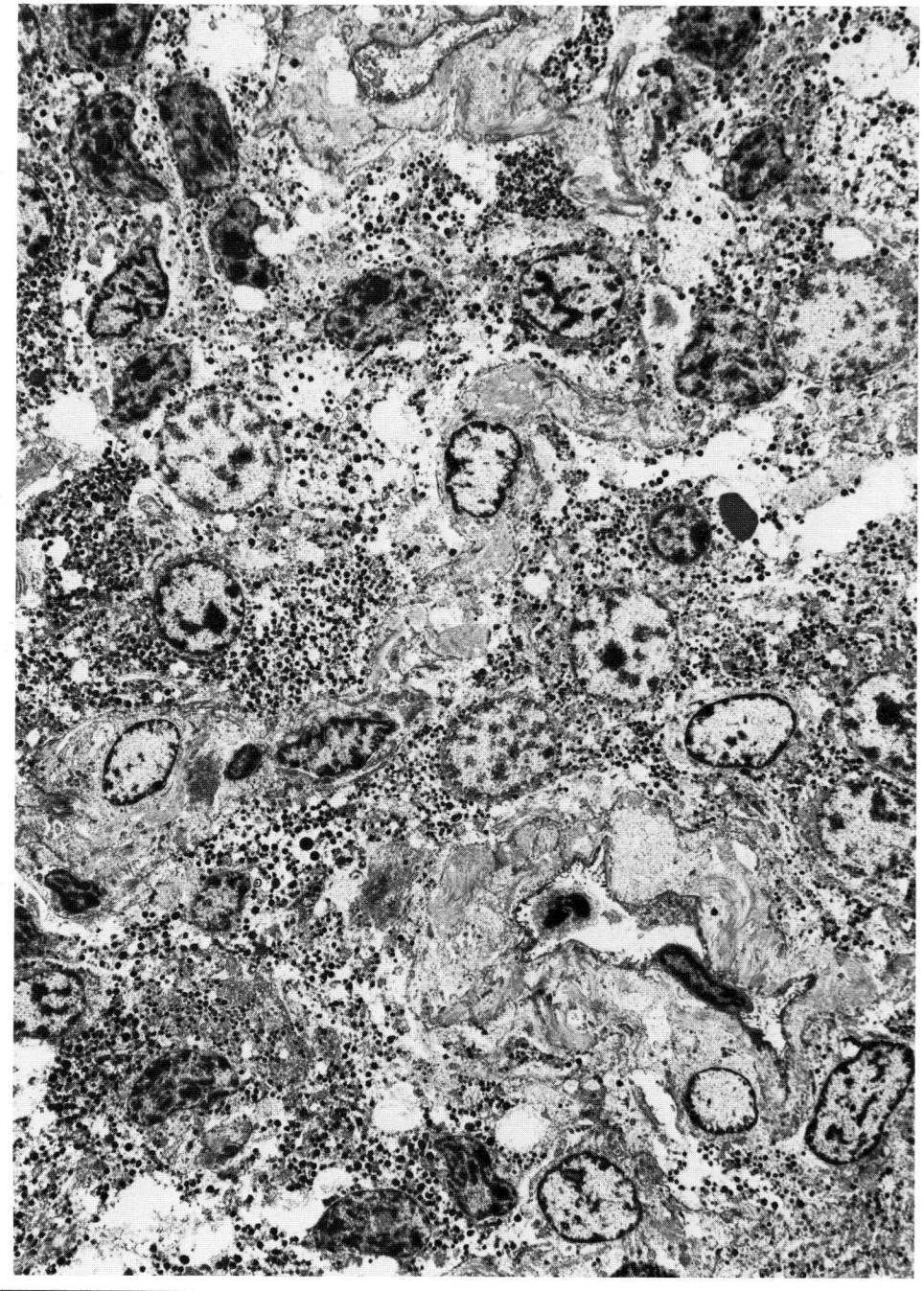

Fig. 16-28. Electron micrograph of the epithelial cells of the suprarenal medulla, showing the cytoplasm to contain numerous dense granules that store catecholamines. (×2,600.) (Courtesy of Drs. S. W. Carmichael and R. G. Ulrich.)

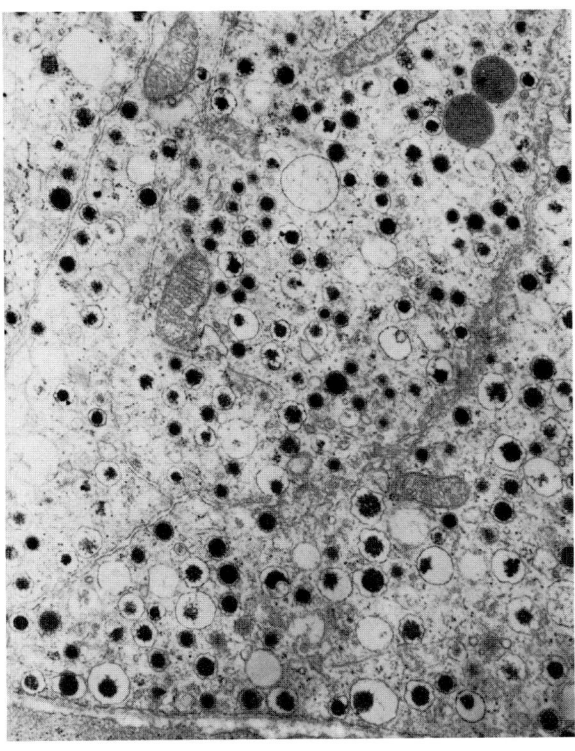

Fig. 16-29. Electron micrograph of the epithelial cells of the suprarenal medulla, showing the cytoplasm to contain numerous membrane-bound, dense granules that store catecholamines. Note that some granules are less dense than others and have a large clear zone separating them from the bounding membrane. (×12,000.) (Courtesy of Drs. S. W. Carmichael and R. G. Ulrich.)

at night and is awake during the day, the levels of the blood glucocorticoids will be highest in the morning and lowest in the late afternoon. Should a person's sleep habits change, the glucocorticoid levels in the blood will undergo corresponding changes.

Suprarenal Medulla

The suprarenal medulla is composed of groups of epithelial cells supported by a delicate connective tissue that is richly supplied by blood sinusoids (Fig. 16-27). The cells contain cytoplasmic granules that become brown when exposed to chromium salts; for this reason, they are sometimes referred to as *chromaffin cells*. The chromaffin cells synthesize and secrete norepinephrine and epinephrine. The hormones are released into the venous sinusoids in response to stimulation by the preganglionic sympathetic nerve fibers. The nerve endings are cholinergic.

Examination of the cells with an electron microscope (Figs. 16-28–16-30) shows that the cytoplasmic granules are membrane bound. There are two types of cells. The cells that produce norepinephrine have granules that possess a very dense core, whereas the cells that secrete epinephrine have granules that are homogeneous and not so dense. The hormones are released from the cells by a process of exocytosis. Some of the cells of the medulla are thought to produce serotonin in addition to epinephrine (Fig. 16-31).

In addition to the cells just described, occasional sympathetic ganglion cells are found in the suprarenal medulla.

Actions of the Catecholamines

Stimulation of the sympathetic nerve supply to the suprarenal medulla causes the release of epinephrine and norepinephrine into the blood sinusoids. About four times as much epinephrine is released as norepinephrine (Fig. 16-32). The effect on the tissues is widespread and prolonged, because the hormones circulate in the bloodstream throughout the body. This action should be compared with direct stimulation of sympathetic autonomic nerves, in which the action is localized and short lived.

The following important actions of the catecholamines should be noted:

CARDIOVASCULAR EFFECTS
1. *Blood pressure.* Both hormones raise the blood pressure by causing peripheral vasoconstriction and thereby increasing the peripheral resistance. They also cause constriction of the veins, thus increasing the venous return.
2. *Heart.* Both hormones increase the rate and force of contraction of the heart.
3. *Coronary blood flow.* Both hormones increase the

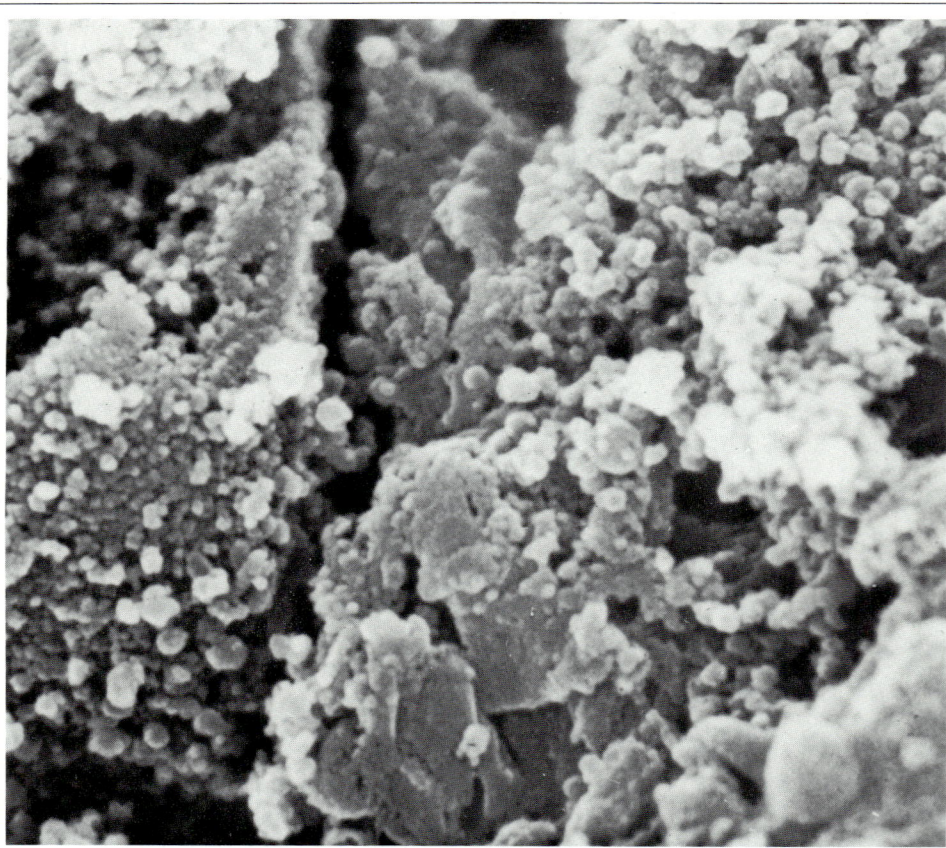

Fig. 16-30. Scanning electron micrograph of the interior of the epithelial cells of the suprarenal medulla after treatment with potassium hydroxide. Numerous catecholamine-storing vesicles of different sizes are visible. (×20,000.) (Courtesy of Drs. S. W. Carmichael and R. G. Ulrich.)

coronary blood flow by causing dilatation of the coronary arteries.

4. *Skeletal muscle blood flow.* Both hormones increase the blood flow through the muscles by causing dilatation of the arteries. The blood is thus redistributed from the skin and splanchnic areas to skeletal muscle.

RESPIRATORY SYSTEM
1. Both hormones increase the rate and depth of breathing, probably as a result of direct stimulation of the respiratory centers.
2. Both hormones relax the smooth muscle of the bronchi so that there is bronchiolar dilatation.

GASTROINTESTINAL TRACT. Both hormones cause relaxation of the general smooth muscle of the wall of the gastrointestinal tract and thereby inhibit peristalsis; they cause contraction of the smooth muscle of the pyloric and ileocolic sphincters, however.

SKELETAL MUSCLE. Both hormones increase the force of contraction of skeletal muscle.

URINARY BLADDER. Both hormones cause relaxation of the smooth muscle of the detrusor and contraction of the sphincter.

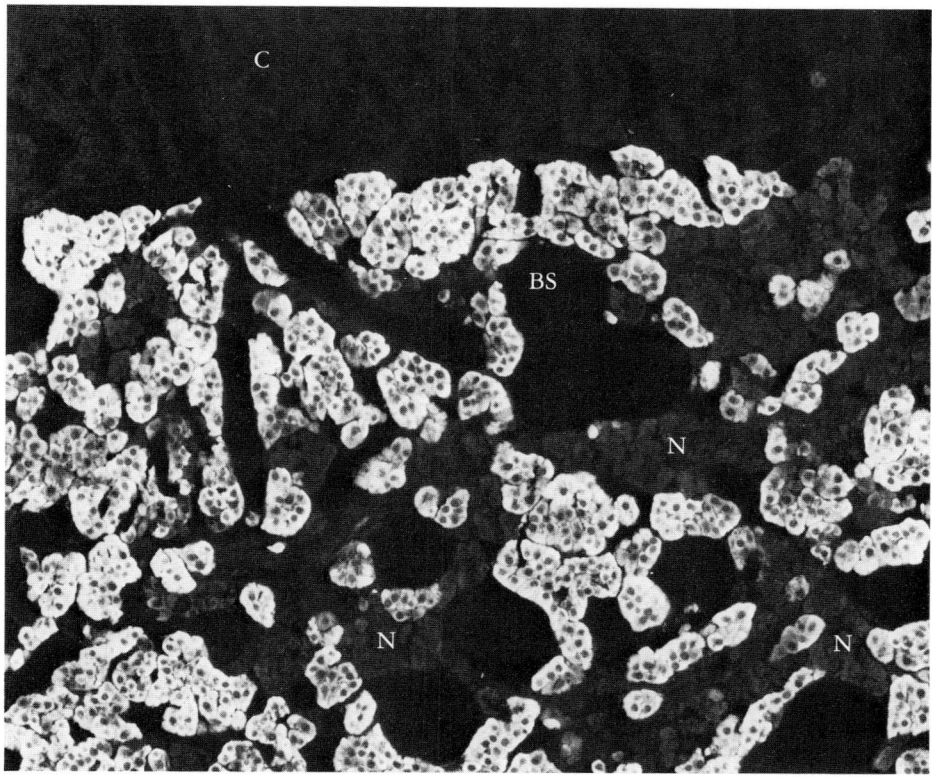

Fig. 16-31. Photomicrograph of epithelial cells of the suprarenal medulla stained by indirect immunofluorescence with an antiserum to serotonin. The serotonin immunoreactivity appears to be limited to the cytoplasm of the epinephrine-storing cells. Norepinephrine-storing cells (N) show no immunoreactivity. (BS = blood sinusoid; C = suprarenal cortex.) (Courtesy of Drs. A. Verhofstad and G. Jonsson.)

EYE. Both hormones cause dilatation of the pupil of the eye by stimulating the contraction of the smooth muscle of the dilator pupillae muscle.

METABOLISM
1. *Oxygen consumption.* Both hormones stimulate metabolism throughout the body, greatly increasing oxygen consumption.
2. *Blood sugar.* Both hormones raise the blood sugar level by stimulating the conversion of glycogen into glucose in the liver and muscle.
3. *Adipose tissue.* Both hormones stimulate the breakdown of lipids, thus releasing fatty acids into the bloodstream.

The following important differences in action between epinephrine and norepinephrine should be remembered: (1) epinephrine has a greater effect on the heart than does norepinephrine; (2) epinephrine has a much greater simulating effect on metabolism than does norepinephrine; and (3) epinephrine has only a weak action on the blood vessels of skeletal muscle compared with norepinephrine.

The effects of norepinephrine are much more prolonged than those of epinephrine, because norepinephrine is destroyed in the body more slowly.

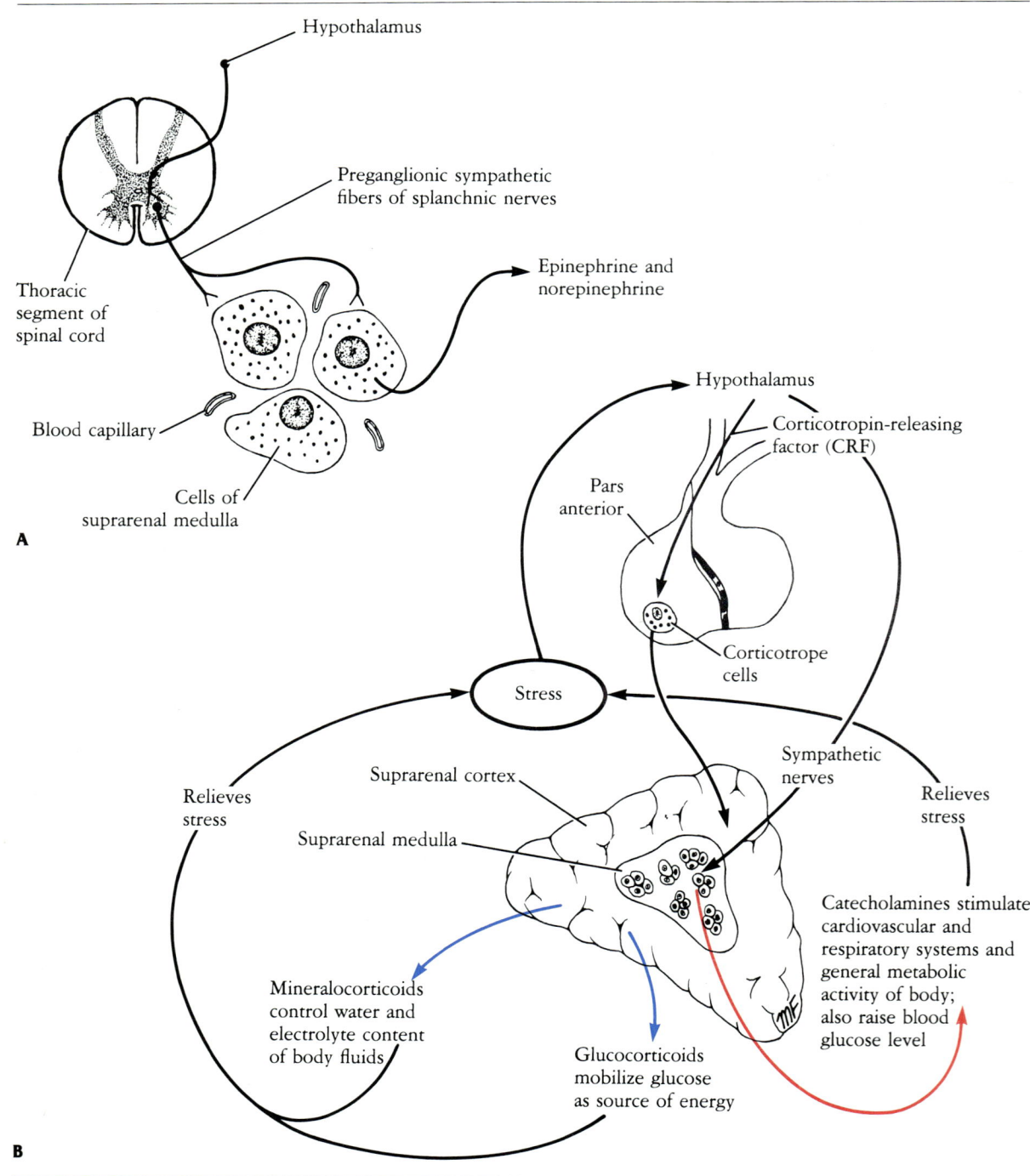

Fig. 16-32. (A) Sympathetic control of the release of catecholamines from the epithelial cells of the suprarenal medulla; (B) response of the suprarenal cortex and medulla to stress.

Regulation of Catecholamine Secretion

The suprarenal medullary cells are stimulated directly by the release of acetylcholine at the terminations of the preganglionic sympathetic fibers of the splanchnic nerves (see Fig. 16-32). The suprarenal medulla is thus mobilized at the same time as the sympathetic part of the autonomic nervous system. In fact, one can regard the cells of the suprarenal medulla as similar to the postganglionic neurons, because many of them release norepinephrine into the bloodstream, as do the postganglionic sympathetic fibers at their endings on organs.

The advantages of this duplication of effort are as follows: (1) The postganglionic sympathetic activity can be localized to a specific organ, whereas the actions of the catecholamines of the suprarenal medulla are spread throughout the body. (2) In an emergency, the effects of the sympathetic postganglionic fibers are increased and prolonged enormously by the outpouring of large amounts of the catecholamines of the suprarenal medulla into the general blood circulation. (3) The catecholamines of the suprarenal medulla can stimulate structures all over the body that are not innervated by sympathetic fibers. It is by this route that epinephrine is able to stimulate profoundly the general metabolic rate of the body.

Blood Supply of Suprarenal Gland

The blood supply to the suprarenal gland is profuse. The arteries enter the cortex from the capsule. From a capsular plexus, fenestrated sinusoids run between the columns of cortical cells. At the corticomedullary junction, the sinusoids drain into collecting veins. The small collecting veins then run between the chromaffin cells of the medulla and drain into large medullary veins. Some large arteries pass directly to the medulla along connective tissue septa and branch repeatedly to form a capillary network between the chromaffin cells. The capillaries drain into the medullary veins, which leave the suprarenal gland as the suprarenal vein. The suprarenal medulla thus receives a double blood supply, one from the cortex and a direct one from the capsular arteries.

The cortical blood supply is rich in glucocorticoids, which are necessary for the synthesis of an enzyme needed for the formation of epinephrine and norepinephrine in the medullary cells. It has been suggested that the activity of the medullary cells could be modified by altering the relative amounts of blood reaching the medulla from the two sources.

Stress and the Suprarenal Gland

When the body is stressed by fear, pain, or cold, the activities of the suprarenal gland are greatly increased to combat the effects of the stress and preserve homeostasis (see Fig. 16-32). Mineralocorticoids from the cortex assist by controlling the water and electrolyte content of the body fluids, and glucocorticoids mobilize and increase the production of glucose so that it is available as an immediate energy source. Catecholamines from the medulla stimulate the cardiovascular and respiratory systems and the general metabolic activity of the body. They also assist the glucocorticoids in raising the blood glucose level and assist the sympathetic part of the autonomic nervous system.

ISLETS OF LANGERHANS OF THE PANCREAS

The pancreas is a soft, lobulated organ that lies on the posterior abdominal wall behind the peritoneum. For purposes of description, it can be divided into a *head, neck, body,* and *tail* (see Fig. 12-16).

The head lies within the concavity of the duodenum, and the neck, body, and tail extend to the left; the tail lies in contact with the hilus of the spleen.

The pancreas is both an exocrine and an endocrine gland. The greater part of the gland produces the exocrine secretion, which passes into the duodenum (for details, see p. 490).

The endocrine portions of the gland are easily recognized under the light microscope as large pale areas among the darker-staining secretory acini (see Figs. 12-18 and 16-33). Each pale area consists of irregular clusters of cells known as the *islets of Langerhans*. The islets are more numerous in the tail of the pancreas than in its body, neck, or head. The

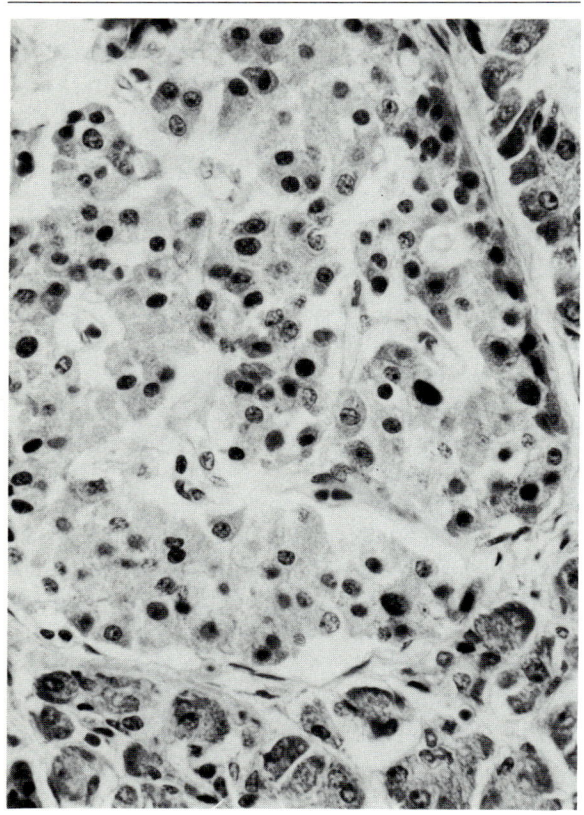

Fig. 16-33. Photomicrograph of an islet of Langerhans of the pancreas, showing irregular clusters of pale-staining cells separated by delicate connective tissue containing capillaries. No obvious granules can be identified in the islet cells. Note the dark-staining secretory acini of the exocrine part of the pancreas. (H&E; ×400.)

cells of the islets are arranged as anastomosing cords that are supplied profusely by fenestrated capillaries. The islets are not encapsulated but are supported by reticular fibers. The islets of Langerhans have no ducts; the cells pour their secretion directly into the bloodstream.

On routine H&E-stained sections, no secretory granules can be identified in the islet cells (see Fig. 16-33). When special staining techniques are used, however, four cell types can be recognized by the staining and morphological characteristics of their granules. These are referred to as beta, alpha, and delta cells and the PP cell (pancreatic polypeptide cell). Specific antibody techniques have enabled researchers to localize specific hormones to individual cells.

The *beta cells*, which are centrally placed and form the majority of the islet cells, secrete insulin. The secretory granules, as seen with the electron microscope, are rectangular crystals surrounded by a loose-fitting membrane (see Fig. 12-19). The *alpha cells* are situated at the periphery of the islets and secrete *glucagon*. The granules have a rounded, dense center surrounded by a less dense area (see Fig. 12-19). The granules are membrane bound. The *delta cells* are found among the alpha cells and secrete somatostatin. They have large pale granules with closely applied membranes (see Fig. 12-19). The PP cells are located in the islets but are also found scattered among the surrounding acini (see Fig. 12-19). These cells produce a polypeptide that when injected into animals produces increased peristalsis of the gut. Its function in humans is not known.

Actions of Insulin

Insulin is a hormone composed of protein. Once it has entered the bloodstream, it has a relatively short life and is broken down rapidly by tissues, especially the liver. The main action of insulin is to bring about the rapid absorption, storage, and use of glucose in the body (Fig. 16-34). It also has important effects on fat and protein metabolism, however.

Insulin and Carbohydrate Metabolism

Insulin reduces the circulating levels of blood glucose after a meal by stimulating the uptake and storage of glucose in liver cells and the formation of liver glycogen. Furthermore, insulin inhibits the splitting of liver glycogen into glucose. Because it causes the phosphorylation of glucose within the liver cells, any glucose present is trapped and unable to diffuse back into the bloodstream.

Once the blood level of glucose begins to fall

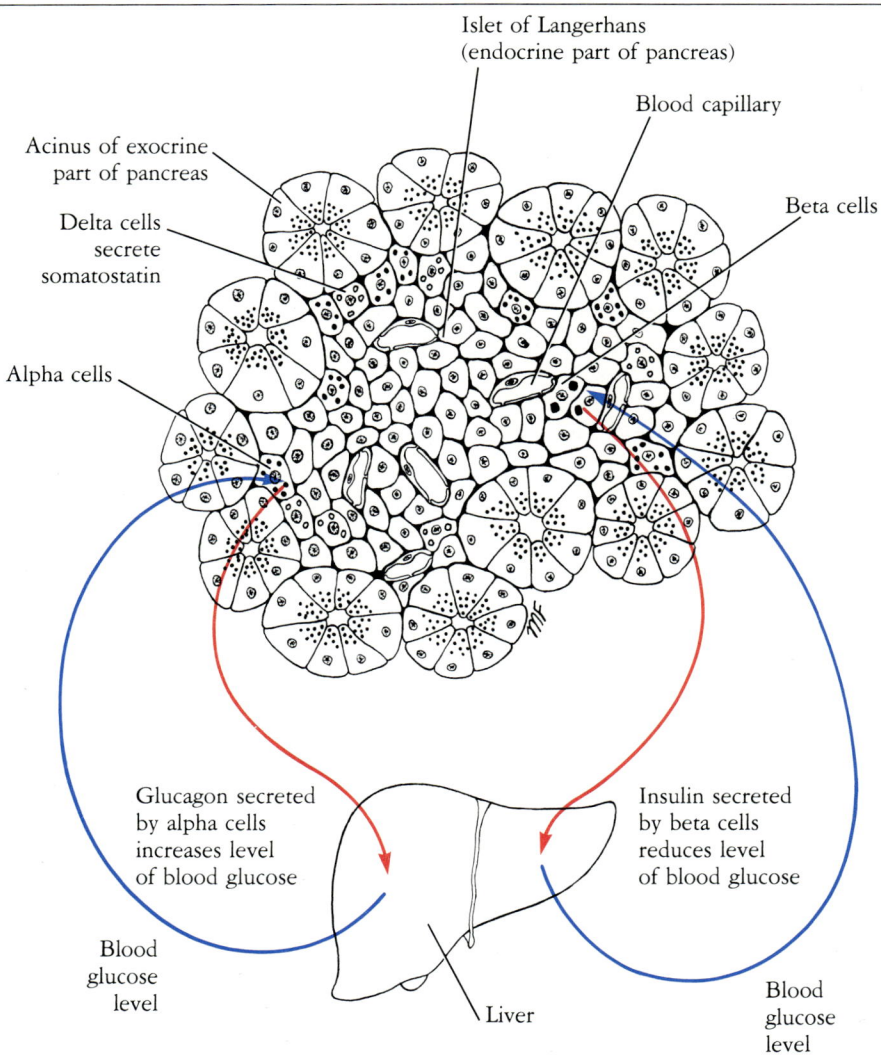

Fig. 16-34. Effects of insulin and glucagon, secreted by the beta and alpha cells, respectively, of the islets of Langerhans, on the blood glucose level. Note the feedback action of blood glucose on the activities of these cells.

between meals, the islets of the pancreas decrease their output of insulin, the whole process within the liver cells is reversed, and glucose diffuses back into the bloodstream.

Insulin also promotes the absorption and storage of glucose in muscle, processes that occur principally during the few hours after a meal and during heavy exercise. Glucose can be stored in muscle as muscle glycogen. In the liver, as we have seen, glucose is trapped within the cells by the process of phosphorylation. It is believed that insulin promotes the absorption of glucose into muscle by stimulating in some way the carrier mechanism responsible for the transport of glucose across cell membranes.

Insulin and Fat Metabolism

Insulin stimulates the conversion of excess glucose in the liver into fatty acids. This process takes place when sufficient glucose has been stored in the liver as glycogen. The fatty acids so formed are carried by the blood from the liver to the adipose tissue cells, where they are stored.

Insulin also stimulates the formation of glycerol in adipose tissue cells. The glycerol then combines with the fatty acids in the adipose cells, so that additional fat is formed and stored within these cells. In addition, insulin inhibits the breakdown of fat by lipase in adipose tissue cells.

In the absence of insulin, the triglycerides of adipose cells are split by the enzyme lipase into fatty acids and glycerol. The fatty acids diffuse into the blood, where they are taken up by the cells of the body as a source of energy. In the liver, the fatty acids are absorbed from the blood and synthesized into triglycerides, cholesterol, and phospholipids. These substances are then excreted into the blood in the lipoproteins. Prolonged excessively high concentrations of cholesterol in the blood, as occur in severe diabetes mellitus, lead to atherosclerosis.

The absence of insulin and the entry of the fatty acids into the liver cells lead to the formation of acetoacetic acid, β-hydroxybutyric acid, and acetone. These substances, commonly referred to as *ketone bodies,* pass into the bloodstream. The presence of excessive amounts of ketone bodies in the blood is a condition known as *ketosis* (see p. 681).

Insulin and Protein Metabolism

Insulin increases the quantity of protein formed in the body. This effect is believed to result from the increased uptake of amino acids into cells and the increased formation of protein from the amino acids; in addition, the breakdown of protein within cells is inhibited.

Control of Insulin Secretion

The normal fasting level of blood glucose is 80 to 90 mg per 100 ml. Under these conditions, the beta cells of the islets of Langerhans are stimulated to secrete increased amounts of insulin immediately, and the blood glucose level rises above normal. As a result, increased amounts of glucose are transported into the liver cells, where they are stored as glycogen, thereby reducing the blood glucose level to normal. This glucose stimulus for insulin seretion is greatly increased by a rise in amino acid concentration in the blood. The gastrointestinal hormones gastrin, secretin, and cholecystokinin also stimulate the production of insulin. It will be remembered that these hormones are secreted in large amounts after a meal, and it is interesting to note in this connection that they participate in insulin production.

Actions of Glucagon

Glucagon is a hormone composed of protein and produced by the alpha cells of the islets of Langerhans. Its main function is to increase the blood glucose concentration; therefore, its effect is opposite that of insulin (see Fig. 16-34). Its action on the glucose level is brought about by stimulating the breakdown of glycogen into glucose and the formation of new glucose from amino acids, both in the liver. To aid in this formation of new glucose, glucagon stimulates the breakdown of tissue protein into its component amino acids and also increases the uptake of amino acids from the blood into liver cells.

Control of Glucagon Secretion

The alpha cells of the islets of Langerhans are stimulated to secrete increased amounts of glucagon immediately when the blood glucose level falls below normal (80–90 mg per 100 ml of blood; compare with the conditions of insulin secretion). Glucagon rapidly mobilizes the glucose from the liver glycogen.

Actions of Somatostatin

Somatostatin is a hormone produced by the delta cells of the islets of Langerhans. It is the same hormone that is produced by the hypothalamus, in which case it is called the growth hormone–inhibiting hormone.

The actions of somatostatin are not understood, although the hormone is known to inhibit the secretion of insulin and glucagon.

INTERSTITIAL CELLS OF THE TESTIS

The testes are paired ovoid organs situated within the scrotum (see p. 539). Each testis is both an exocrine and an endocrine gland. The greater part of each gland is made up of seminiferous tubules, which produce spermatozoa. The spermatozoa constitute the exocrine secretion, which passes via ducts into the urethra (see p. 552).

The endocrine part of each testis consists of groups of interstitial cells (Leydig cells) embedded in loose connective tissue between the seminiferous tubules (Fig. 16-35). The cells are large and polyhedral, with eccentric nuclei and poorly staining cytoplasm. The function of these cells is to secrete androgens, which include testosterone, dihydrotestosterone, and androstenedione; the most important and abundant of these is testosterone.

The interstitial cells are present in large numbers in the fetus but atrophy to some extent after birth. They reappear in large numbers at puberty. In the fetus, the chorionic gonadotropin from the placenta stimulates the interstitial cells of the testis to produce testosterone, which is important in the development of the male genitalia and suppressing the

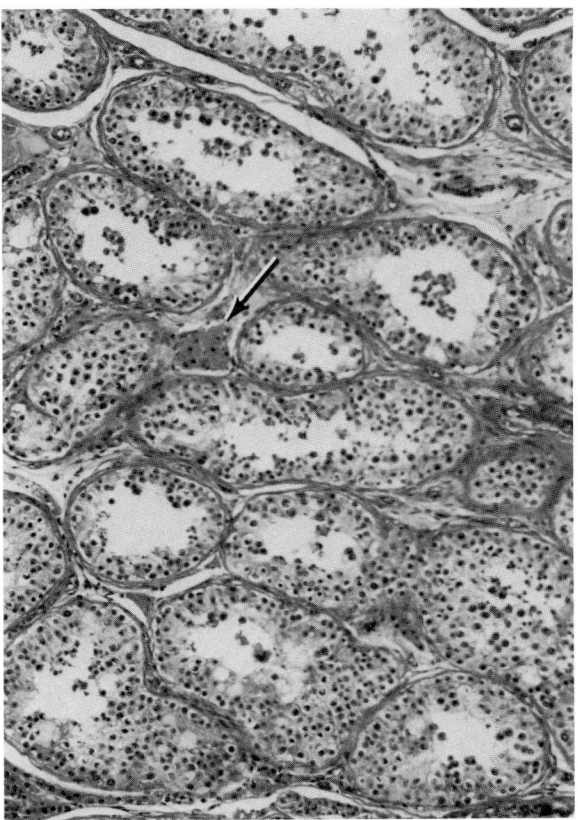

Fig. 16-35. Photomicrograph of a section of the testis, showing cross sections of the seminiferous tubules; a group of interstitial cells (Leydig cells) is also visible (arrow). (H&E; ×100.)

formation of the female genitalia; testosterone also brings about the descent of the testes.

The interstitial cells are less sensitive to heat than are the germinal epithelial cells of the seminiferous tubules. For this reason, testosterone is produced continuously even in individuals with undescended testes (see p. 564).

Actions of Testosterone

Testosterone is a steroid hormone. It plays an important role in the development of the male acces-

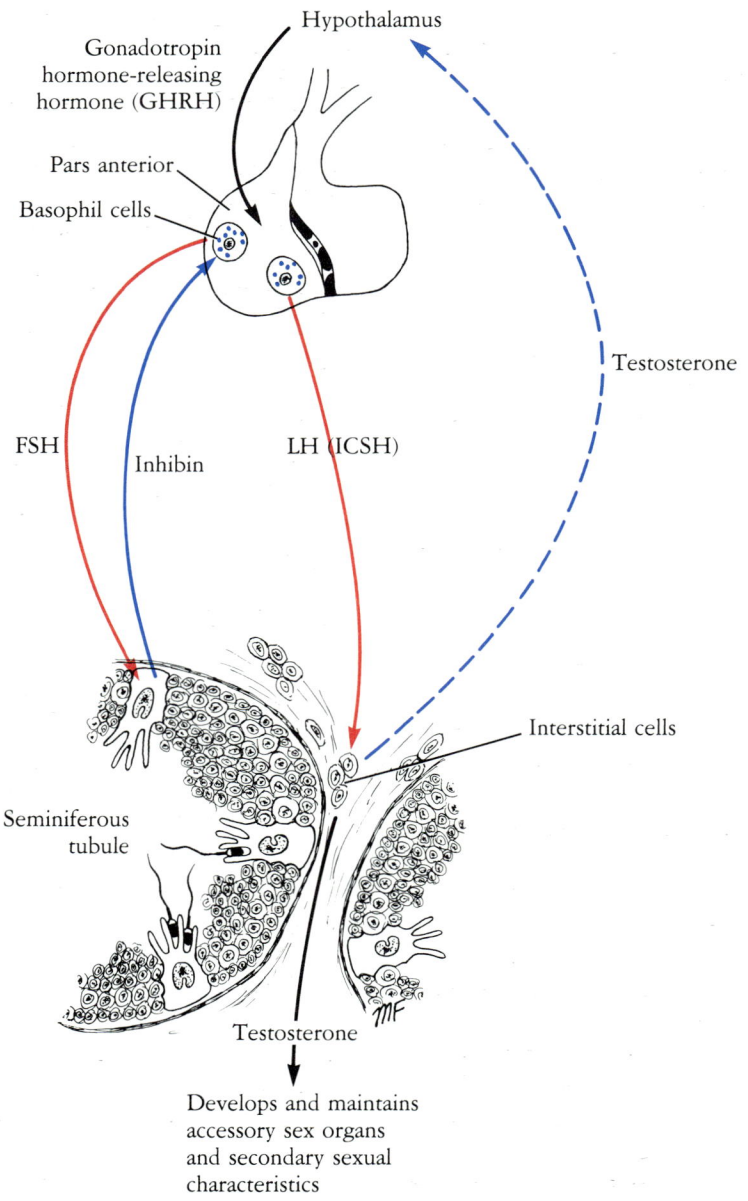

Fig. 16-36. Control of the activities of the testis by the hypothalamus and the pars anterior of the pituitary gland. Note the possible feedback mechanisms provided by inhibin from the Sertoli cells and testosterone from the interstitial cells (Leydig cells).

sory sex organs and the secondary sexual characteristics at puberty and in their persistence through adult life (Fig. 16-36). Small quantities of testosterone are produced in the fetus, practically none is produced in childhood, large quantities are produced at puberty, and thereafter the production slowly diminishes with age.

Actions at Puberty and during Adult Life

At puberty, the testes increase in size, and spermatogenesis and interstitial cell activity commence (see Fig. 16-36). The epididymis, the seminal vesicles, the prostate, and the penis undergo considerable growth, and the following secondary sexual characteristics make their appearance:

Hair growth. Pubic hair develops, which in the male extends upward to the umbilicus. Hair growth occurs on the face and in the axillae. Some hair growth occurs on the chest.

Skin changes. Testosterone increases the thickness of the skin and the secretion rate of the sweat and sebaceous glands; it also stimulates the melanocytes to produce more melanin and thus darkens the skin.

Voice changes. Testosterone causes enlargement of the laryngeal cartilages and lengthening of the vocal cords, thus producing the characteristic bass voice.

Muscle development. Testosterone causes considerable development of the skeletal muscles.

Bone growth. Testosterone stimulates the growth of bone by increasing the amount of matrix and depositing calcium salts.

Metabolic changes. Testosterone increases the basal metabolic rate by stimulating the metabolic activity of tissue cells throughout the body.

Control of Testosterone Secretion

The interstitial cells of the testes are stimulated to produce androgens, especially testosterone, by the luteinizing hormone. In the fetus, as mentioned previously, the chorionic gonadotropin secreted by the placenta has the same effect and is responsible for the production of testosterone by the developing testes.

The level of blood testosterone in the adult influences the production of the gonadotropin-releasing hormone in the hypothalamus. This hormone stimulates the cells of the pars anterior of the pituitary gland to release LH. Testosterone, therefore, provides a feedback mechanism that maintains a constant level of testosterone production by the testes.

Estrogen Production by the Testes

Very small amounts of estrogens are produced by the testes. The site of production is the cells of Sertoli. The function of the estrogens in the male is unknown.

OVARIES

The mature ovaries are paired ovoid organs situated within the pelvis (see p. 571). Each ovary has an outer cortex and an inner medulla, but the division between the two is ill defined. Embedded in the connective tissue of the cortex are the *ovarian follicles* at different stages of development (Figs. 16-37 and 16-38). The medulla consists of very vascular connective tissue (see Fig. 15-3).

Ovarian Hormones

The ovarian hormones are the steroids *estrogen* and *progesterone.*

Estrogens

The estrogens secreted by the ovary are mainly β-estradiol and estrone. They are produced by the theca interna cells, which are the cells found in the stroma of the ovary immediately outside the graafian follicle, and by the cells of the corpus luteum (Fig. 16-39). Once they have completed their physiological functions, these hormones are broken down in the liver into nonactive compounds.

At puberty, the increased estrogen produced by the ovaries is responsible for the development of the uterus and vagina, the external genitalia, the pel-

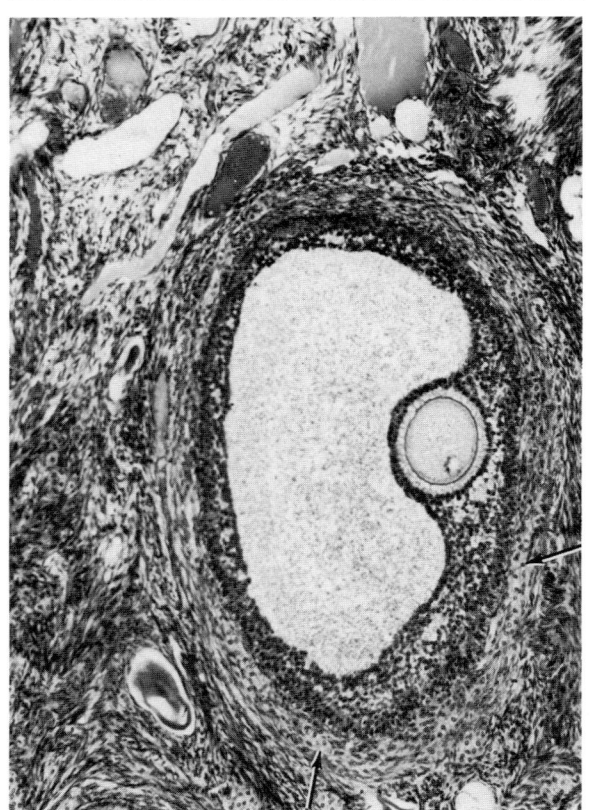

Fig. 16-37. Photomicrograph of a section of the ovary, showing a mature graafian follicle. The cells of the theca interna of the stroma are visible immediately outside the follicle (arrows). (H&E; ×100.)

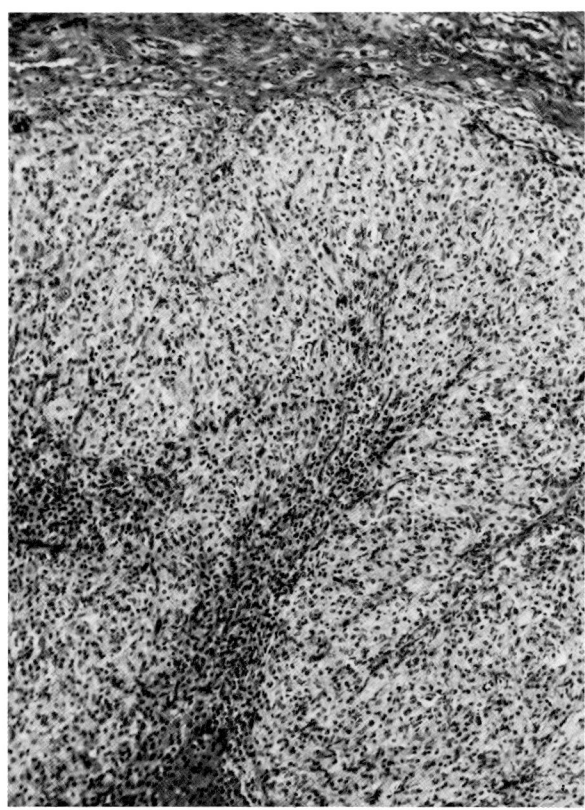

Fig. 16-38. Photomicrograph of a section of the ovary, showing the cells of a corpus luteum. (H&E; ×100.)

vis, the breasts, and pubic and axillary hair. The hair growth is also controlled by the adrenal androgens.

SPECIFIC EFFECTS. *Effect on the Uterus.* In addition to increasing the size of the uterus at puberty, the estrogens cause the repair and proliferative changes in the endometrium following the menstrual period (see p. 588). During the second half of the menstrual cycle, the combined action of the estrogens and progesterone produces the secretory changes in the endometrium (see p. 589). During pregnancy, there is an enormous enlargement of the uterus, caused by the increasing amounts of estrogens and progesterone produced first by the corpus luteum and later by the placenta.

Effect on the Vagina. In addition to increasing the size of the vagina at puberty, the estrogens thicken the lining epithelium, increasing it from a few cells thick to many layers thick. The squamous cells become loaded with glycogen, and, when shed into the vaginal lumen, the glycogen is broken down into lactic acid by bacteria (the Doderlein's bacilli). Lactic acid tends to inhibit the growth of pathogenic organisms within the vagina.

Effect on the Uterine Tubes. In addition to increasing the size of the uterine tubes at puberty, the

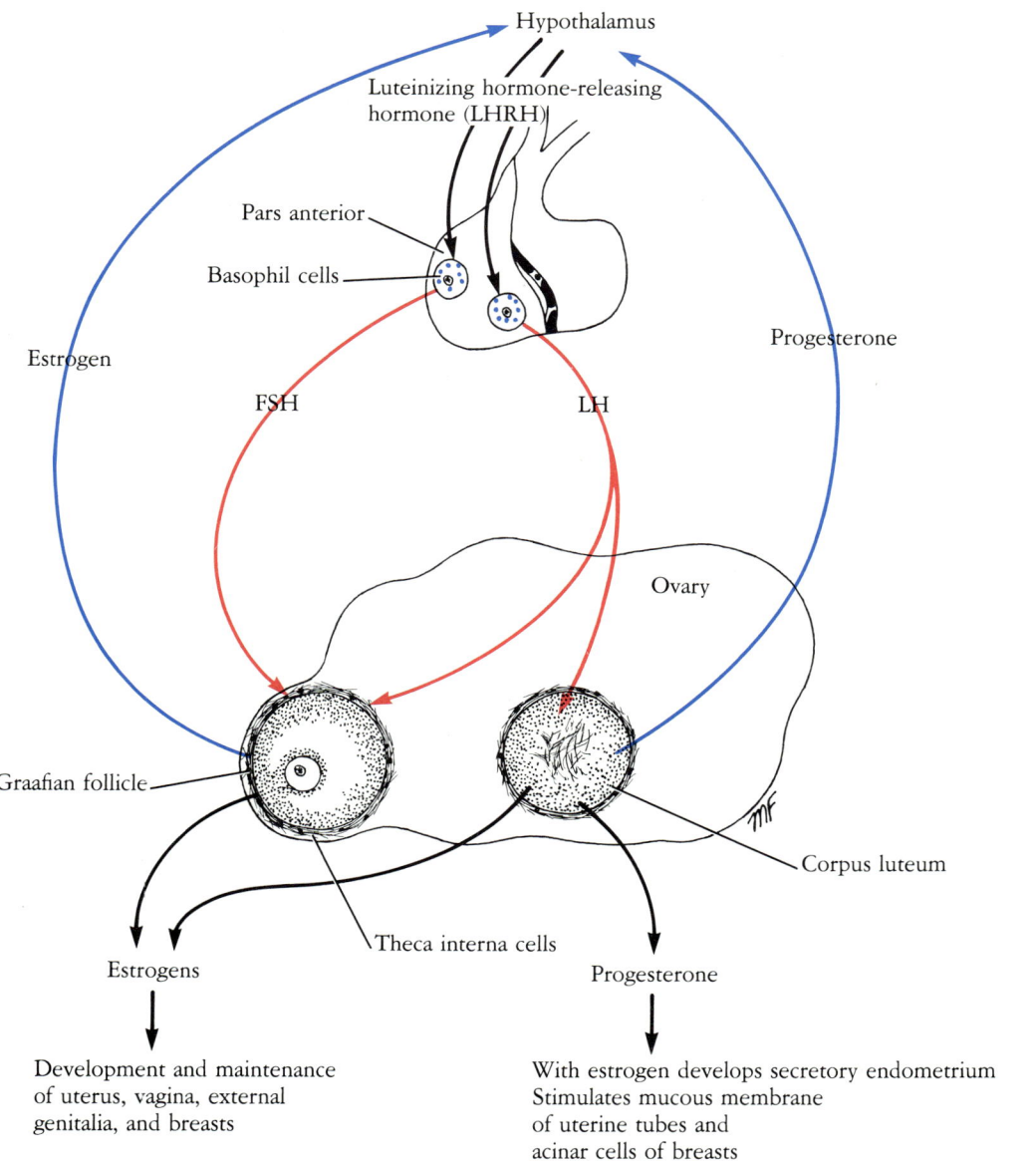

Fig. 16-39. Control of the activities of the ovary by the hypothalamus and the pars anterior of the pituitary gland. Note the feedback mechanisms provided by estrogen and progesterone.

estrogens stimulate the lining secretory cells to increase their activity during the follicular phase of the menstrual cycle.

Effect on the Breasts. The estrogens, at puberty, are responsible for the growth in the size of the breasts that results from the deposition of adipose tissue. Estrogens also cause extensive development of the duct system. During pregnancy, the large amounts of estrogens secreted by the corpus luteum and, later, by the placenta are responsible for the further considerable development of the duct system and the increased vascularity of the connective tissue.

Effect on Bones. At puberty, estrogens stimulate the metabolic activity of the osteoblasts, so that the skeletal growth rate is increased. Later, the estrogens stimulate the union of the epiphyses with the diaphyses in long bones, thus bringing the female's growth in height to an end. The estrogens have a specific effect on the growth of the bony pelvis; the result is a broader pelvis than exists in the male, which allows ease of passage of the fetal head during parturition.

Effect on Hair and Skin. At puberty, the female develops axillary and pubic hair. The pubic hair is limited to the mons pubis. Although originally believed to be under the control of estrogens, this process is now thought to be effected by adrenal androgens as well.

Estrogens also influence the texture and vascularity of the skin. They stimulate the melanocytes of the epidermis to produce more pigment.

Effect on Fat Metabolism and Electrolyte Balance. Estrogens stimulate the deposition of fat in the adipose tissue of the breasts, buttocks, and thighs and are responsible for the development of the rounded figure of the female.

Estrogens also affect the kidney tubules, causing sodium and water retention, especially in pregnancy.

Progesterone

Progesterone is produced by the corpus luteum of the ovary (see Figs. 16-38 and 16-39). After exerting its physiological effects, it is quickly broken down, mainly by the liver.

SPECIFIC EFFECTS OF PROGESTERONE. *Effect on the Uterus.* Progesterone, along with estrogens, is responsible for the secretory phase in the development of the endometrium during the second half of the menstrual cycle (see p. 589). If fertilization occurs, the endometrium undergoes further thickening and becomes known as the decidua. The development and maintenance of the decidua are under the control of progesterone and estrogens. After the fourth month of pregnancy, the production of progesterone and estrogens is taken over from the corpus luteum by the placenta. Progesterone stimulates the cells lining the uterine tubes and causes the release of their secretions. The secretions provide nutrition for the fertilized ovum as it passes along the tube to the uterus, where it is implanted.

Effect on the Breasts. Progesterone may cause some epithelial enlargement in the cells at the end of the duct system during the second half of the menstrual cycle. During pregnancy, progesterone causes extensive alveolar development.

Control of Estrogen and Progesterone Secretion by the Ovaries

The pars anterior of the pituitary gland secretes two gonadotropic hormones that control the secretion of the estrogens and progesterone (see Fig. 16-39). These are the follicle-stimulating hormone and the luteinizing hormone. During each monthly menstrual cycle, there is a cyclic rise and fall in the production of FSH and LH, and these variations bring about the cyclic changes in the rate of production of the ovarian hormones.

The FSH stimulates the development of the ovarian follicles and the production of estrogens by the theca interna cells. The LH assists the FSH in bringing about the final stages leading to ovulation, and then stimulates the transformation of the theca interna and granulosa cells into lutein cells, with the resultant formation of the corpus luteum. The corpus luteum, which is controlled by LH, is responsible for the production of progesterone and estrogens.

During the second half of the menstrual cycle, the

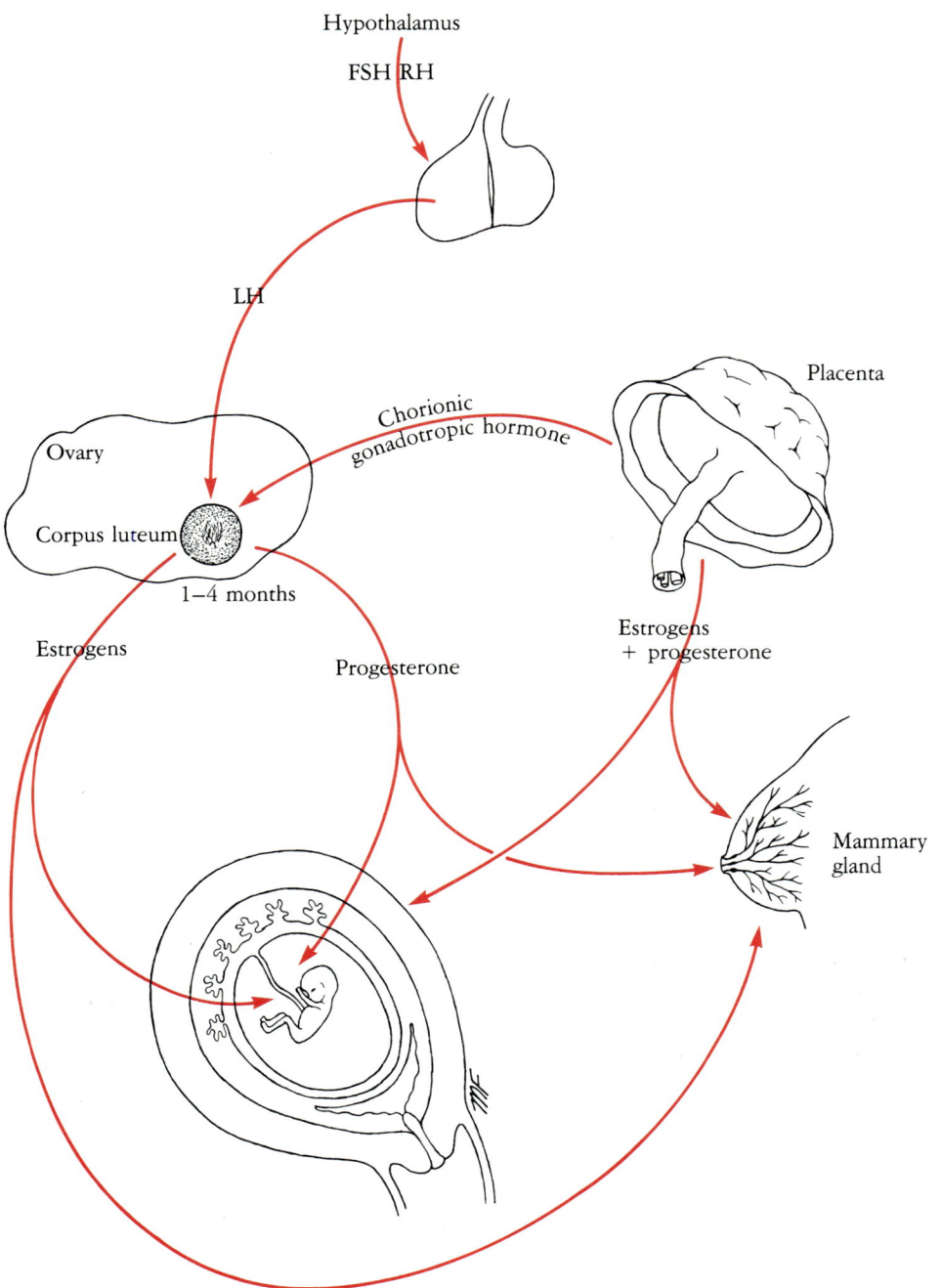

Fig. 16-40. Activities of the placental hormones. The hormones are produced in the syncytiotrophoblast in the fetal part of the placenta.

large amounts of ovarian hormones circulating in the blood inhibit the further production of FSH and LH (negative feedback), and a fall in the blood levels of estrogens and progesterone follows. Toward the end of the cycle, the corpus luteum degenerates and the endometrium suddenly is deprived of the supporting action of estrogens and progesterone. The spiral arteries of the endometrium constrict, and the process leading to menstruation begins.

PLACENTA

The development and function of the placenta during pregnancy have been described fully on page 593. As we indicated, one of its main functions is to serve as an endocrine gland. The placenta secretes estrogens, progesterone, chorionic gonadotropin, and chorionic somatomammotropin (Fig. 16-40). Extraction procedures and histochemical studies have revealed that these hormones are produced in the fetal part of the placenta, in the syncytiotrophoblast.

Function of Placental Estrogens

The placental estrogens are responsible for the continuing enlargement of the uterus, the growth of the glandular ducts in the breast, and the increase in size of the maternal external genitalia. Toward the end of pregnancy, the high concentrations of circulating estrogens bring about relaxation of the sacro-iliac joints and the symphysis pubis, thus enlarging the pelvic inlet and outlet for the passage of the fetus. Estrogen also increases the contractility of the smooth muscle of the uterine wall and thus promotes uterine contractions when labor commences.

Function of Placental Progesterone

The placenta takes over the main production of progesterone from the corpus luteum at about the fourth month of pregnancy. Progesterone is essential for the development and maintenance of the decidua throughout pregnancy. It is also responsible for the further development and growth of the glandular alveoli of the breasts. Progesterone opposes the action of estrogen that increases the contractility of the smooth muscle of the uterus. Toward the end of pregnancy, the amount of estrogen produced increases, whereas that of progesterone does not. The uterine muscle at the end of pregnancy thus becomes more irritable and susceptible to the influence of oxytocin from the posterior lobe of the pituitary and to other factors.

Function of Chorionic Gonadotropin

Chorionic gonadotropin appears in the mother's bloodstream as the fertilized ovum is being implanted in the endometrium. It is responsible for the continued growth and maintenance of the corpus luteum at the end of the menstrual cycle once fertilization has occurred. The corpus luteum, in turn, produces increasing quantities of estrogens and progesterone, which further develop the secretory endometrium, resulting in the formation of the decidua. As we have stated, the corpus luteum starts to degenerate at about the fourth month of pregnancy and the formation of large and increasing amounts of estrogens and progesterone is taken over by the placenta. The corpus luteum becomes progressively smaller but persists until parturition.

Chorionic gonadotropin also enters the fetal circulation and, in the male fetus, stimulates the interstitial cells of the testes to produce small amounts of testosterone, thus causing the fetus to develop male genital organs. Chorionic gonadotropin has no such effect on the development of the female genital organs.

The presence of chorionic gonadotropin in the urine of a woman 12 days after ovulation is a definite indication of pregnancy.

Function of Chorionic Somatomammotropin

Chorionic somatomammotropin is a recently discovered hormone that may influence the carbohydrate and fat metabolism of the mother and make more glucose and fatty acids available for the fetus.

CLINICAL NOTES

In previous chapters, great emphasis has been placed on the maintenance of a constant internal environment within the body (homeostasis) so that normal cellular metabolism can continue without interruption. The hypothalamus, which occupies a central area of the nervous system, exerts a very important control over homeostasis. By means of chemical and nervous feedback mechanisms that affect it via the blood and afferent neurons, the hypothalamus is able to detect the smallest changes in the internal environment of the body. The hypothalamus can restore conditions to normal through the activities of the autonomic and endocrine systems. We have been concerned in this chapter with the endocrine system, which is composed of numerous endocrine glands that produce chemical messengers, the hormones, that are poured into the blood to influence target cells. The hormones adjust the activities of the different systems of the body to meet the needs of changes in the internal and external environments.

Endocrine disease is usually caused by an increase or decrease in hormone secretion, as in hyperthyroidism or hypothyroidism. Blood transport of the hormone may be defective when, for example, the plasma proteins are abnormally low. Such an abnormality would affect the levels of protein-bound thyroxin, for example. The normal chemical breakdown of hormones may be disrupted, as in liver disease, leading to excessively high hormonal levels in the blood. Also, the target tissues may fail to respond to hormonal control or may be excessively sensitive to such action.

Although most endocrine diseases are confined to one endocrine gland, syndromes involving multiple endocrine neoplasias should not be forgotten. In these conditions, the pituitary, the pancreas, and the parathyroid glands are involved simultaneously. The condition tends to occur in families and probably results from a genetic defect. Another pathological condition that may cause confusion is the existence of multihormonal tumors. For example, a tumor of an islet of Langerhans may, in addition to producing insulin and glucagon, secrete ACTH, MSH, and other hormones.

Perhaps the most confusing syndromes occur in a small number of patients with advanced malignant disease. In these cases, the malignant tumor starts to produce a hormone or a hormonelike substance inappropriate to the tissue that has given rise to the tumor. An example is a patient presenting all the signs of Cushing's syndrome, when the abnormalities actually have been brought about by the production of large quantities of ACTH by a carcinoma of the bronchus.

PITUITARY GLAND

Diseases of the Anterior Lobe of the Pituitary
Pituitary Tumors

The most common pituitary tumor is the chromophobe adenoma; this tumor usually produces no hormones. As it expands, it destroys the surrounding pituitary tissue and causes a decrease in the production of the pituitary hormones. This decrease in turn leads to diminished activity of the dependent endocrine glands, leading to other hormonal abnormalities. Large chromophobe adenomas erode the bone of the sella turcica and may extend superiorly to involve the hypothalamus and the optic chiasma. Disturbances of sleep, temperature control, and appetite may follow. Pressure on the optic chiasma may lead to bitemporal hemianopia. Continued growth of the tumor may increase intracranial pressure and produce headache, nausea, and vomiting.

Occasionally, chromophobe adenomas produce hormones; they have been known to secrete GH, ACTH, TSH, and other anterior lobe hormones.

Conditions Caused by
Excessive Secretion of Growth Hormone
GIGANTISM AND ACROMEGALY. Excessive production of the growth hormone by the somatotrope cells of the pars anterior or by tumors of these cells

can produce abnormal growth of the skeleton. Gigantism occurs in the young before the epiphyses in long bones fuse with the diaphysis. The growth hormone stimulates the cartilage cells of the epiphyseal cartilage to continue laying down new matrix, so that fusion of the epiphyses with the shaft of long bones is delayed and the bones lengthen enormously. In this way, giants 9 feet tall have been produced before the epiphyseal cartilage finally stops growing. These patients suffer from muscle weakness and almost always have enlargement of the heart, liver, spleen, and kidneys.

Acromegaly is a form of abnormal skeletal and soft tissue growth that occurs after adolescence, following the fusion of the epiphyses in long bones with the diaphysis. In this disease, the individual cannot grow taller, but overgrowth occurs in the bones and soft tissues of the forehead, nose, lower jaw, hands, and feet. In the fully developed syndrome, the prominent supraorbital ridges and mandible, the very large nose, and the very large, thick hands and feet make the diagnosis relatively easy. Many affected patients suffer from muscular weakness.

One serious complication associated with somatotrope adenomas is the destruction of the surrounding pituitary tissue. This may affect the production of the gonadotropic hormones and lead to impotence, irregular menstrual cycles, or amenorrhea. Hyperthyroidism and diabetes mellitus may also occur in acromegalics.

Conditions Caused by
a Deficiency of Growth Hormone

DWARFISM. A deficiency in the growth hormone secreted by the somatotrope cells of the pars anterior during childhood leads to pituitary dwarfism. Growth does not stop entirely, and the different parts of the body are in relatively normal proportions. The person is of normal intelligence, but the facial skin is often wrinkled and sexual maturation is delayed.

PANHYPOPITUITARISM IN THE ADULT. This condition is defined as a decreased secretion of all the hormones of the pars anterior. The most common cause of destruction of the pars anterior in adult life is a tumor of the pituitary, especially a chromophobe adenoma. Necrosis of the gland, caused by vascular thrombosis of its blood supply following childbirth, can also produce this condition. The effects of the disease are caused by the loss of pars anterior control over other endocrine glands. As a result, the adrenal cortex, the thyroid gland, and the gonads atrophy. The clinical picture in postpartum patients is a failure to lactate and to resume menstruation. Loss of libido and loss of pubic and axillary hair also occur. Patients are strengthless and coldly indifferent to their surroundings.

Diseases of the Posterior Lobe of the Pituitary
Diabetes Insipidus

This syndrome results from a lesion of the supraoptic and paraventricular nuclei of the hypothalamus and a failure of these cells to synthesize the antidiuretic hormone, or from destruction of the hypothalamohypophyseal tract. There are many causes of this syndrome, including cerebral tumors, cerebral abscesses, surgical or radiation damage, and head injuries. The disease does not always occur if the posterior lobe of the pituitary alone is destroyed, because the nerve cells of the nuclei of the hypothalamus may continue to secrete adequate amounts of ADH, which then pass directly into the blood without previous storage in the posterior lobe of the pituitary.

Characteristically, the patient passes large volumes of urine (polyuria) of low specific gravity. The absence of ADH results in a failure to conserve water, which is not reabsorbed in the collecting tubules of the kidneys. As a result, the patient is extremely thirsty (polydipsia) and drinks large quantities of fluids. The condition must be distinguished from diabetes mellitus, in which there is glucosuria.

There is no recognized syndrome involving a failure of the posterior lobe of the pituitary to secrete oxytocin. It will be remembered that this hormone stimulates the contraction of the smooth muscle of the uterus and the myoepithelial cells of the lactating mammary gland.

PINEAL GLAND AND PINEAL CALCIFICATION

As a result of regressive changes with age, calcium and magnesium phosphate and carbonate accumulate within the glial cells and connective tissue of the pineal gland. These deposits, sometimes referred to as *pineal sand,* are useful to radiologists, because they serve as a landmark and assist in determining whether the pineal gland has been displaced laterally by a space-occupying lesion within the skull.

Although the function of the pineal gland is not fully understood, clinical observation of patients with pineal tumors has revealed that the pineal gland may have an antigonadotropic effect. Pinealomas are tumors of pineal cells. As they increase in size, they may obstruct the aqueduct of Sylvius of the midbrain, producing hydrocephalus. Occasionally, the tumor destroys the pineal gland and causes precocious puberty.

THYROID GLAND

The thyroid gland is continuously changing its activity in response to different stimuli. At certain times during life, such as during puberty, pregnancy, lactation, or physiological stress, there is a great demand for the thyroid hormones; at other times, the demand is less great. The structure of the thyroid gland is continuously changing in response to this changing demand. When there is great functional activity, hyperplasia of the follicular epithelium occurs, the colloid is absorbed, and the follicular cells become tall and columnar. When the demand for the thyroid hormones abates, the follicular epithelium involutes, the colloid accumulates, and the follicular cells become cuboidal or squamous. Examination of a histological section of the thyroid gland may show that the follicles are very active in some areas and resting in others. This is quite normal. In pathological conditions, the balance between the hyperplastic and the involuted follicles becomes upset. The thyroid gland may be compared with the mammary gland and the endometrium, in that it is continuously undergoing structural changes in response to changing hormonal control. The hormone responsible for changing the activity of the thyroid gland is the thyrotropic hormone of the pars anterior of the pituitary.

Thyroid Function Tests

Radioactive Iodide Uptake

The thyroidal radioactive iodide uptake (RAIU) test measures the rate of iodide uptake from the blood into the thyroid gland and thus directly measures the glandular function. The patient is given a small dose of radioactive iodide, and the amount that accumulates in the thyroid gland is determined at different time intervals. The test is particularly valuable in the diagnosis of hyperthyroidism.

Hormonal Concentration and Binding in the Blood

The concentration of tetraiodothyronine (T_4) in the blood can be measured by determining the ability of T_4 extracted from the serum to displace labeled T_4 from a protein mixture containing thyroxin-binding globulin (TBG). The result is compared with that obtained with serum containing known quantities of T_4. This test is very specific and has replaced the old test of estimating the serum-bound iodine concentration (PBI). The PBI test measures the iodine content of T_4 and any other iodide that might be present in the blood (for example, from iodine-containing contrast media used in radiological studies) and is therefore not highly specific.

TSH Concentration in the Serum

The measurement of serum TSH is helpful in the diagnosis of hypothyroidism. The serum TSH is measured by radioimmunoassay. The ability of the TSH in the sample of serum to displace labeled human TSH from anti-TSH antibody is compared with that of a standard sample of human serum containing known amounts of TSH.

TSH Stimulation Test

The response of thyroid tissue to the injection of TSH can be measured by estimating the uptake of radioactive iodide from the blood. In a patient with a deficiency of TSH from the pituitary, the radioactive iodide uptake would be greatly increased.

TRH Test

The ability of the pituitary anterior lobe to secrete adequate amounts of TSH can be tested by injecting TRH and measuring the serum TSH levels over a period of time. In patients with anterior lobe failure, the serum TSH remains at a low level, because the pituitary does not respond to the injection of TRH.

Thyroid Scans

Following the injection of radioactive iodide, the thyroid gland can be scanned to detect the amounts of iodide being absorbed from the blood into different anatomical sites in the thyroid gland. The test is useful for finding areas of the thyroid gland where the level of activity is above or below normal.

Basal Metabolic Rate

The basal metabolic rate (BMR) measures the energy output of the body as determined by the amount of oxygen used when the person is at complete mental and physical rest, 12 to 18 hours after a meal. Because the thyroid gland controls the metabolic rate of the body, this test at first would appear to be an ideal means of measuring thyroid activity. Unfortunately, it is now known that there are many nonthyroid factors that influence metabolic activity, and this test is no longer used for this purpose.

Hyperthyroidism

In hyperthyroidism (thyrotoxicosis, Graves' disease), which is most common in middle-aged women, the thyroid gland is diffusely enlarged. The walls of the thyroid follicles are much infolded, and the epithelial cells lining the follicular walls are taller than normal. Production of the thyroid hormones is greatly increased, and the colloid present is usually reduced in volume. The serum TSH level is normal or below normal. In most patients, there is a *thyroid-stimulating immunoglobulin* (TSI) in the blood that is capable of stimulating increased thyroid activity. This substance is believed to be an auto-antibody produced against the thyroid epithelial cells by the lymphocytes. The high levels of thyroid hormone in the blood suppress the production of TSH by the pars anterior of the pituitary in some patients.

Hyperthyroidism may also occur in the multinodular goiter of the elderly. In this condition, the thyroid gland exhibits multiple areas of enlargement, possibly caused by oversensitivity of these areas to circulating TSH.

Symptoms

The symptoms of hyperthyroidism are caused by excessive stimulation of the tissues by the thyroid hormones. There is excessive sweating and loss of weight; increased nervousness, with fine tremor of the extended fingers; intolerance to heat; and muscular weakness. The hair thins, and the eyes may protrude (exophthalmos). The heart rate is increased, and the patient may experience palpitations. Frequent bowel movements may occur, and menstrual periods may be missed or scanty. Hyperthyroidism usually is diagnosed easily from the clinical history and physical examination. Thyroid function tests either confirm the diagnosis or enable the diagnosis to be made in difficult cases.

Cause of Exophthalmos in Hyperthyroidism

The cause of this condition is not known. A possible explanation is that an exophthalmos-producing factor (EPF), which is auto-immune in origin, is produced in affected patients in addition to TSH. The EPF is responsible for the increased volume of the extraocular muscles and the increased deposits of hydrophilic mucopolysaccharides in the retrobulbar connective tissues; both these changes cause the eyeball to be pushed forward.

Treatment

Three forms of therapy for hyperthyroidism are available: (1) surgical excision of thyroid tissue, (2) antithyroid drugs, and (3) radioactive iodine.

Subtotal thyroidectomy is the treatment of choice in many patients. The operation is preceded by a short course of antithyroid drug treatment to suppress the thyroid gland, and iodine is given for 2 weeks before the operation to reduce the vascularity of the gland.

The *antithyroid drugs,* such as *propylthiouracil,* block the uptake of iodine by the thyroid tissue and inhibit the coupling of iodotyrosyl. The disadvantage of this treatment is that during pregnancy the drugs cross the placenta and inhibit the fetal thyroid gland; they also appear in the mother's milk and thus block the activities of the thyroid gland in the newborn.

Radioactive iodine suppresses the activity of the thyroid by its radiation effects on the cell metabolism. It is a very satisfactory form of treatment in many patients, but there is a risk of producing hypothyroidism. Here again, pregnancy and lactation are contraindications to this form of treatment.

Hypothyroidism

Hypothyroidism occurs in two forms, cretinism in infants and myxedema in adults.

Cretinism can occur as a result of a failure in the development of the thyroid gland. The child is born with a normal appearance, caused by the mother's thyroid hormone's having crossed the placenta. Soon after birth, the child shows signs of retarded mental and physical growth. If cretinism is diagnosed early and the child is given adequate, lifelong thyroid hormone therapy, he or she will develop normally and live a normal life. A delay in making the diagnosis results in permanent mental retardation.

Myxedema. There are many causes of hypothyroidism in the adult, ranging from spontaneous degeneration of the thyroid gland to hypopituitarism or hypothalamic failure. About a quarter of the cases follow excessive treatment of hyperthyroidism with drugs or surgery. The majority of the patients are female.

Symptoms

In hypothyroidism, there is a slowing of the mental and physical processes of the individual. There is an increase in body weight and a preference for a warm environment. Constipation is present, and the heart rate is slowed. The skin is dry and cold, and the hair is dry and brittle and tends to fall out. The tongue is enlarged, and the voice is hoarse. Libido is diminished in both sexes, and menorrhagia is common in the female.

The term *myxedema* actually refers to the nonpitting edema of the skin that occurs in this condition. It is caused by the infiltration of the tissue spaces by increased quantities of mucopolysaccharides.

Hypothyroidism can be diagnosed from the history and physical examination, and the diagnosis confirmed by thyroid function tests.

Treatment of Hypothyroidism

The disease may be treated successfully by the daily oral administration of desiccated thyroid tissue in tablet form. Once the correct dosage is determined, the hormone is administered daily for life.

Thyroiditis

Inflammatory disease of the thyroid gland is not common, and in many cases the cause is unknown. Virus infection or auto-immune disease is a possible cause. In the chronic forms of the disease, thyrotoxicosis, followed by myxedema, may occur. In *Riedel's thyroiditis,* the thyroid gland is destroyed and replaced by fibrous tissue that extends into the surrounding tissues of the neck.

Simple Goiter

This is an enlargement of the thyroid gland not associated with hyperthyroidism, hypothyroidism, thyroiditis, or tumor. Iodine deficiency is the most common cause, and the condition occurs more frequently in women. It may be endemic or sporadic. In the endemic form, there is usually a lack of iodine in the water supply and soil, so that foodstuffs contain no iodine. This form is common in the Andes, the Himalayas, and the Alps, where people live far from the sea, which is rich in iodine, and rely on local rain water, which is deficient in iodine. Sporadic cases of simple goiter do occur and may be caused by an inability of the thyroid gland to take up iodine from the blood.

Histologically, the thyroid gland displays hyperplasia in response to the raised levels of TSH in the blood. The gland is moderately enlarged and hyperemic, and there is clearly an attempt to extract the maximum amount of iodine from the blood. In the next stage, the follicles enlarge and involute. The follicles are filled with colloid, and the epithelium becomes cuboidal or even squamous. Later still, the diffuse enlargement of the gland changes into a multinodular condition in which there are areas of colloid-filled follicles, of hyperplastic follicles, of cyst formation, and of scar tissue formation; areas of degeneration and hemorrhage are also common.

The treatment of simple goiter is the prophylactic supply of iodine in the food, such as in bread or salt. Giving iodine to a patient with endemic simple goiter does not remove the swelling of the thyroid gland; it merely converts the hyperplastic goiter into a colloid goiter. Giving iodine in the food prevents the occurrence of simple goiter in others, however.

Tumors of the Thyroid Gland

Benign thyroid tumors occur in the form of adenomas. Carcinoma of the thyroid gland is relatively rare.

PARATHYROID GLANDS

Hyperparathyroidism

This condition is caused by a benign tumor, an adenoma, or a hyperplasia of the parathyroid glands. As a result, there is an excessive secretion of the parathyroid hormone, and the blood calcium level rises to as much as 15 mg per 100 ml from the normal level of 10 mg per 100 ml. The parathyroid hormone stimulates the activity of the osteoclasts in bone and liberates calcium from the bones, which returns to the blood. In severe cases, cysts develop in the bones, a pathological condition known as *osteitis fibrosa cystica*.

The increased hormone secretion raises the rate of reabsorption of calcium in the kidney tubules and increases the excretion of phosphate.

The raised levels of blood calcium in this disease may cause the repeated occurrence of renal stones as a result of the spilling over of the calcium salts into the urine. The renal stones are composed of either calcium oxalate or calcium phosphate. The high blood calcium level also affects the central and peripheral nervous systems. Neurological abnormalities include emotional instability, memory loss, and muscular weakness. The treatment of this condition is surgical removal of the diseased gland.

Hypoparathyroidism

In this disease, there is a deficiency in the secretion of parathyroid hormone, which leads to a reduction in the level of blood calcium. The condition is most commonly caused by injury to or removal of the glands during surgical procedures on the thyroid gland.

The level of blood calcium may fall as low as 5 mg per 100 ml. The lack of parathyroid hormone causes a lowering of osteoclastic activity, and calcium is retained in bone. There is also an increased rate of reabsorption of phosphate from the kidney tubules, leading to a raised level of phosphate within the blood.

The main symptoms and signs of low blood calcium are numbness and tingling in the fingers and toes and cramps of the muscles in the hands and feet. These cramps are called *carpopedal spasms*. The spasm, or tetany, of muscles may also involve the facial and the laryngeal muscles. Spasm of the laryngeal muscles produces a crowing inspiration, dyspnea, and even cyanosis. The central nervous system may also be affected, as evidenced by signs of mental confusion and loss of memory.

The condition is treated by giving the patient calcium gluconate intravenously and large quantities of vitamin D and calcium by mouth.

SUPRARENAL CORTEX

Diseases of the suprarenal cortex usually fall into two groups: those that produce a decreased output of suprarenal steroids, and those that produce an increased output of suprarenal steroids.

Hypoadrenalism

Hypoadrenalism can be caused by disease of the cortex, or can be secondary to the diminished elaboration of ACTH from the pars anterior of the pituitary.

Primary Hypoadrenalism

Primary hypoadrenalism, or Addison's disease, does not present clinical symptoms until the greater part of the suprarenal cortex has been destroyed. In most patients, the cortex is destroyed by tuberculosis or by idiopathic atrophy.

The lowered cortisol production results in increased secretion of ACTH, which stimulates the melanocytes of the skin and buccal mucous membrane to increase their production of melanin. The result is a darkening of the skin and mucous membrane of the mouth that is characteristic of this disease.*

The lack of cortisol secretion lowers the blood glucose level between meals, resulting in a loss of vigor and muscle strength. The patient is unable to withstand minor physical stresses and easily goes into shock. The lowered aldosterone secretion causes the kidney tubules to fail to reabsorb sodium and chloride ions, and the ions are lost in the urine. As a result, extracellular fluid volume and blood volume are decreased, producing a fall in blood pressure. In addition, the potassium level in the blood rises, which interferes with the contraction of cardiac muscle. In women, the decrease in cortical androgen production causes a loss of axillary and pubic hair.

The diagnosis of Addison's disease is established by injecting ACTH intravenously and finding that there is little or no increase in the level of plasma cortisol. Failure to treat this disease will result in death caused by collapse of the circulatory system and hyperkalemic cardiac arrest. The patient is treated by the administration of adequate amounts of cortisol and a mineralocorticoid. In addition, an ample intake of sodium chloride is required.

Secondary Hypoadrenalism

This condition occurs when disease affects the hypothalamus, the hypothalamohypophyseal portal vessels, or the pars anterior of the pituitary. Essentially, the condition is secondary to a reduced output of ACTH. Secondary carcinoma, irradiation, or interference with the blood supply of these regions can be responsible. The syndrome is identical to Addison's disease, except that there is no increased pigmentation of the skin or buccal mucous membrane, because of the reduced secretions of ACTH. The suprarenal cortex is atrophied and reduced in size in affected patients.

Hyperadrenalism

The signs and symptoms of hyperadrenalism, or Cushing's syndrome, are produced classically by the excessive secretion of cortisol by the suprarenal cortex. The most common cause of the syndrome in recent years, however, has been the prolonged use of glucocorticoids, such as prednisone, in the treatment of nonendocrine disorders, such as certain skin diseases.

There are three possible causes for the excessive production of cortisol by the suprarenal cortex: (1) a tumor of the cortex, (2) the production of excessive amounts of ACTH by a pituitary tumor, and (3) the production of excessive amounts of ACTH by *nonpituitary* tumors.

A typical patient with Cushing's syndrome shows a redistribution of fat. There is wasting of the limbs and extreme obesity of the abdomen. The face becomes rounded and moon shaped, and fat pads appear on the back of the neck, forming the so-called buffalo hump. The skin is fine textured, and the underlying blood vessels show through. Purple striae are present over the abdomen and extremities. Hirsutism of the face, chest, and abdomen occurs. The concentration of glucose in the blood is excessively high. There is a thinning of the bones because of a loss of protein matrix. There is often impotence and hypogonadism in the male and amenorrhea in the female.

The finding of high plasma levels of cortisol or of urinary 17-hydroxycorticosteroids establishes the diagnosis. The treatment of Cushing's syndrome is to reduce the high cortisol levels of the blood by removing, if possible, the tumor responsible. In

---

*ACTH has a chemical structure similar to that of the melanocyte-stimulating hormone.

those patients who demonstrate the syndrome secondary to the excessive use of glucocorticoids, the steroid must be drastically reduced in dosage or its use stopped altogether.

Adrenal Virilism

This condition is produced by an excessive production of cortical androgens. The cause may be hyperplasia or a tumor. Adrenal virilism occurs only in children and women, because in adult males, the normal amounts of testosterone have produced and maintained the male secondary sexual characteristics, and the additional cortical androgens produce no recognizable changes.

In the prepubertal male with excessive androgen production, there is a precocious development of the male sex organs and secondary sexual characteristics. In the prepubertal and adult female, there is enlargement of the clitoris so that it resembles a penis; growth of hair, with a male distribution; and deepening of the voice. There is a great increase in muscular growth. The diagnosis is established by finding an increase in the 17-ketosteroid excretion in the urine, which indicates increased androgen production in the body.

Adrenal Feminization

Very rarely, suprarenal cortical tumors secrete estrogen. The result in males is feminization, with atrophy of the testes and penis, enlargement of the breasts, and diminished interest in the opposite sex.

SUPRARENAL MEDULLA

Two types of tumors occur in the suprarenal medulla: the pheochromocytoma and the neuroblastoma.

Pheochromocytoma

This tumor arises from the catecholamine-producing cells of the medulla. Large quantities of norepinephrine and epinephrine are poured into the bloodstream, producing hypertension that is paroxysmal or sustained. Such tumors are responsible for less than 1 percent of all cases of hypertension. The hypertension can be cured by removal of the tumor. The diagnosis is established by finding a raised level of excreted catecholamines in the urine.

Neuroblastoma

Neuroblastoma is one of the most common malignant tumors in childhood. The tumor metastasizes rapidly via the bloodstream to the lungs, liver, and bones. The neoplasm produces large quantities of catecholamines. The prognosis is extremely poor.

ISLETS OF LANGERHANS AND DIABETES MELLITUS

In diabetes mellitus, the beta cell of the islets of Langerhans lose their ability to secrete insulin, or the target cells of the tissues become insensitive to circulating insulin. In juvenile diabetes, there is total absence of insulin, but when the onset of diabetes occurs in adulthood, the plasma levels of insulin may be normal or only slightly below normal. The exact cause of diabetes mellitus is not known. Genetic, metabolic, and auto-immune factors, as well as viral infections, are thought to play an important causative role in many patients. Recently, glucagon excess combined with insulin deficiency has been suggested as a contributing cause of the high levels of blood glucose. It will be remembered that insulin stimulates the uptake and storage of glucose in the liver and muscle, whereas glucagon inhibits this process.

In all patients with diabetes mellitus, the blood glucose level is above normal *(hyperglycemia)*. Once the blood glucose level reaches a certain threshold value, approximately 180 mg per 100 ml, the glucose spills out into the urine *(glucosuria)*. The osmotic pressure exerted by the high concentration of glucose in the urine inhibits the reabsorption of water in the kidney tubules, so an abnormally large amount of water is lost in the urine, causing excessive urination *(polyuria)*. The patient becomes thirsty because the extracellular fluid volume is reduced, and dehydration may occur. The fluid intake is increased in an attempt to compensate for the water loss.

The abnormally high blood glucose level results from reduced permeability of the cell membranes to glucose, caused by insufficient insulin production or insensitivity of the cell membranes to the blood insulin. Because cells (such as muscle and adipose tissue) are unable to take up glucose from the blood as an energy source, they turn to fat. The breakdown of triglycerides is increased, with the liberation of fatty acids and glycerol, which are then metabolized by the cells. In cases of severe diabetes, excessive lipolysis occurs and the free fatty acids accumulate in the blood, causing an acidosis. Acetoacetic acid, β-hydroxybutyric acid, and acetone may accumulate in the blood, a condition called *ketosis*. In extreme ketosis, the same substances may spill over into the urine, a condition known as *ketonuria*. Sometimes the ketone level in the blood is so high that acetone is excreted in the breath and can be smelled.

The lack of glucose within cells reduces the synthesis of intracellular protein. In addition, the amino acids are lost to protein metabolism by conversion to glucose, which also contributes to the hyperglycemia.

The upset of carbohydrate, fat, and protein metabolism in these patients leads to weight loss and lack of energy.

Diagnosis of Diabetes Mellitus

Fasting Blood Glucose Level

At least 8 hours after a meal, the normal range for blood glucose is 70 to 110 mg per 100 ml. An elevated fasting blood glucose level is highly suggestive of diabetes mellitus.

Glucose Tolerance Test

After the fasting blood glucose level has been measured, the patient is given 100 gm of glucose in solution by mouth and the blood glucose level is measured after 30 minutes, 1 hour, 2 hours, and 3 hours. The normal maximum levels of blood glucose are about 170 mg at 30 minutes, 170 mg at 1 hour, 120 mg at 2 hours, and 110 mg at 3 hours. At no time during this test should glucose appear in the urine. The test measures the ability of the patient's insulin to return the blood glucose to a normal level after the ingestion of glucose.

Glucose in the Urine

In the normal individual, only minute, undetectable amounts of glucose are present in the urine. In the patient with diabetes mellitus, small to large amounts of glucose can be detected in the urine using simple chemical tests. The presence of glucose in the urine is highly suggestive of diabetes mellitus, and if such glucose is found, the diagnosis should be established by carrying out the glucose tolerance test.

In patients with *renal glycosuria,* there is a low renal threshold for glucose but the glucose tolerance test is normal.

Complications of Diabetes Mellitus

Vascular Complications

Arteriosclerosis occurs more commonly in the diabetic than in the nondiabetic and commences at an earlier age. The blood cholesterol levels are high in these patients, and the abnormal fat metabolism is thought to be responsible.

Ocular Complications

The hyperglycemia in diabetes often leads to *cataracts* and the development of abnormalities of the retinal blood vessels.

Renal Complications

The increased incidence of infection and the appearance of microscopical changes in the renal blood vessels can result in renal failure.

Infection

There is an increased incidence of infections in patients with diabetes, presumably because of the upset in the general metabolic activities of the body.

Diabetic Coma

Diabetic coma is preceded by headache, nausea, and vomiting. Breathing becomes deep and slow, and consciousness is lost gradually. The underlying physiological causes are (1) accumulation of acetoacetic acid and the development of acidemia and (2) renal and circulatory failure.

Physiology of the Treatment of Diabetes Mellitus

Sufficient insulin is given to the patient, who is maintained on a special diet, so that the carbohydrate metabolism returns to normal. In those with the less severe type of diabetes, the hyperglycemia often can be treated with a low-calorie, low-carbohydrate diet without the administration of insulin.

INTERSTITIAL CELLS OF THE TESTIS

The function of the testes is the production of spermatozoa and the secretion of the male sex hormones, particularly testosterone, by the interstitial cells. The two functions may be interfered with simultaneously by a severe acute infection or by the occlusion of the blood supply during a repair operation for inguinal hernia. Total absence of testosterone follows surgical castration, which may be necessary following severe trauma to the perineum. Testosterone deficiency is not present in patients with incompletely descended or maldescended testes.

If testosterone deficiency occurs before puberty, the accessory organs of reproduction do not develop; the penis, scrotum, seminal vesicles, and prostate remain small. The secondary sexual characteristics do not appear. There is no growth of the hair on the face or trunk or in the axillae. The pubic hair is of the female distribution and develops in response to the suprarenal androgens. The larynx fails to enlarge, and the voice remains high pitched and infantile. The muscles are poorly developed. There is a delay in the fusion of the epiphyses in long bones with the diaphysis. The shoulders tend to be narrow, and excessive fat deposits may occur in the pectoral region, abdomen, and buttocks, and on the hips.

Testosterone deficiency after puberty causes the accessory sex organs to atrophy and the secondary sexual characteristics to regress. Those organs and structures that do not require testosterone for their maintenance are unaffected, however. Thus, the penis remains of normal size, the voice remains unchanged, and facial hair growth may be affected only slightly. Sexual desire and erection may be absent.

Tumors of Interstitial Cells

These tumors are relatively rare and usually are benign. They are of interest in that they may produce androgens, or androgens and estrogens. In the child, interstitial tumors may cause precocious puberty or feminization. In the adult, tumors producing the female hormone may cause gynecomastia.

OVARIES

Menopause

The menopause is the period of life when the ovaries normally cease to respond to the gonadotropic hormones of the anterior lobe of the pituitary. Menopause occurs on the average between age 45 and age 50. The ovaries become smaller, and the graafian follicles atrophy and are replaced by fibrous tissue. The tunica albuginea thickens. The corpora lutea and the ovarian hormones are no longer produced.

As a result of the cessation of the production of ovarian estrogen and progesterone, menstruation ceases and the genital organs atrophy to some extent. Vasomotor changes, in the form of hot flashes, occur in the skin of the face, neck, and chest. The vaginal mucous membrane thins and atrophies. The breasts may enlarge, because of the deposition of fat, or shrink, because of atrophy of the glandular ducts. The patient usually gains weight from a diffuse deposition of fat. The patient often complains of pains in the joints, fatigue, and insomnia. Anxiety, depression, and emotional instability may also be present.

The lack of estrogen also increases protein catabolism. This change reveals itself by an alteration in the texture of the hair and nails, wrinkling of the skin, and osteoporosis.

In the great majority of women, the symptoms of the menopause are slight, but for some, the body changes and emotional disturbances are very severe, requiring considerable patience and understanding from the husband and relatives.

Hypogonadism

Ovarian hypofunction may be associated with lesions of the hypothalamus that impair the release of the gonadotropin-releasing hormone. Via a similar mechanism, emotional strain, such as leaving home and attending college, may change the afferent nervous input to the hypothalamus, causing *amenorrhea*. Hypopituitarism with a failure of FSH and LH secretion, caused by a pituitary tumor, may also cause ovarian hypofunction.

When the ovaries fail to develop, the accessory sexual organs remain infantile and the secondary sexual characteristics do not appear. There is a delay in the fusion of the epiphyses with the diaphysis in long bones, so that the individual is taller than normal.

Removal of the ovaries in the adult results in a premature, artificial menopause. The sexual organs atrophy to some extent, but the symptoms may be more pronounced than in the normal menopause, because the woman has not had time to adjust to a gradual decline in estrogen levels, as occurs in the normal menopause.

Hypersecretion of the Ovaries

A rare granulosa–theca cell tumor may occur in women after the menopause. These tumors produce large amounts of estrogen, which stimulate the endometrium to grow, causing irregular bleeding (see p. 620).

PLACENTA

Pre-eclampsia and Eclampsia

These hypertensive disorders of pregnancy are associated with edema and proteinuria. The exact cause of these conditions is unknown, but uteroplacental ischemia may be the underlying disorder. The spiral arteries of the maternal part of the placenta undergo necrosis; the histological changes are similar to those found in an allograft rejection, suggesting an immunological response. The diminished blood flow leads to the decreased production of placental prostaglandins, which normally produce dilatation of peripheral arterioles. The decreased production of prostaglandins may result in the increased sensitivity of the pregnant woman to angiotensin, causing peripheral vasoconstriction and hypertension.

Hydatidiform Mole

Excessive proliferation of the trophoblast during the early stages of placenta formation may lead to the condition of hydatidiform mole. The trophoblastic outgrowths become converted into masses of vesicles that may be as large as grapes. This condition occurs in about one in two thousand pregnancies. The uterus may become filled with the vesicles, and the fetus dies. Very large quantities of chorionic gonadotropin are produced by the trophoblast, and the gonadotropin appears in the urine. Testing for large quantities of chorionic gonadotropin in the urine can be useful in diagnosis.

Chorionepithelioma

This is a rare disease, and over half the cases follow hydatidiform mole. It presents as persistent or repeated uterine bleeding following abortion, normal pregnancy, or hydatidiform mole. A chorionepithelioma is a malignant tumor of the chorionic villi and produces chorionic gonadotropin in large quantities. The test for this hormone in the urine greatly assists in diagnosis.

CLINICAL PROBLEMS

For the answers to these problems, see page 817.

1. A 17-year-old boy is taken by his parents to a pediatrician because the parents are concerned about his excessive height and his complaints of fatigue and general lassitude. His standing height is 84 inches. Questioning reveals that the boy has grown very rapidly since his thirteenth birthday. As a young child, he excelled in competitive sports, but for the past 3 years, he has experienced weakness and fatigue and has ceased to compete. His nose is broad, and his mandible and facial features appear larger than normal. He has large hands and feet and takes a size 18 shoe. There is no family history of unusual tallness. The patient is of normal intelligence, and the size of his external genitalia is normal

for his age. His secondary sexual characteristics are normal. Using your knowledge of histology and endocrinology, make a diagnosis. Which cell groups are likely to have undergone pathological changes? How do you account for the excessive tallness and the presence of a large mandible, hands, and feet in the same individual?

2. Give a brief account of the different parts of the pituitary gland. Describe the main connections between the hypothalamus and the pituitary gland.

3. Describe the microscopic structure of the pars anterior of the pituitary gland. Name the hormones produced by the different cells, and indicate their function.

4. Homeostasis is controlled by the activities of the autonomic nervous system and the endocrine system. Describe how the hypothalamus controls the activities of the pituitary gland.

5. A 35-year-old man has been in the intensive care unit for a week following a severe automobile accident involving extensive head injuries. His vital signs are stable, and his urine output has been adequate. During the second week, it is noticed that the urinary output is increasing dramatically. The specific gravity of the urine is 1.004 or less. A diagnosis of diabetes insipidus is made. Because the patient complains of extreme thirst (polydipsia) and the repeated urination (polyuria) is interfering with sleep, the physician orders long-acting vasopressin to be given intramuscularly to control the polyuria. Where is this hormone normally produced and stored in the body? What are the normal actions of this hormone?

6. Describe the microscopic structure of the pars intermedia of the pituitary gland. Where in the pituitary is the melanocyte-stimulating hormone normally produced? Name another hormone produced by the pituitary that stimulates the melanocytes of the skin to produce more melanin.

7. A 25-year-old woman has been in labor for several hours. Her uterine contractions are weak, and her labor is not progressing. The obstetrician decides to give her some pitocin, a synthetic oxytocin hormone. What is the effect of oxytocin on the uterus? In which part of the pituitary is this hormone normally released into the bloodstream?

8. A 17-year-old girl is examined by a physician because she has a large swelling in the front of her neck. She is visiting the United States from Switzerland. After taking a careful history and examining the swelling, the doctor makes a diagnosis of simple endemic goiter caused by dietary iodine deficiency. Describe the microscopic structure of the normal thyroid gland, and indicate how iodine is absorbed and used by the gland. What factors control the activity of the thyroid gland? How does the structure of the thyroid gland change when its activity is increased and decreased?

9. A 45-year-old woman is taken to her family physician for a medical check-up. The woman has no complaints, but her husband has noted the following changes in her appearance during the previous year. She has gained a considerable amount of weight and is becoming mentally and physically slow, often falling asleep while talking to friends. Her face is puffy, and her hair is dry and has developed a tendency to fall out. The lateral third of her eyebrows is missing. Her skin is pale and dry, and her voice is becoming deep and her articulation slow. She frequently complains of the cold when others feel warm. Using your knowledge of functional histology, what do you think is wrong with this patient? What do you think would be the appropriate treatment?

10. A 27-year-old woman is admitted to the hospital for diagnostic tests. When initially seen by her physician, she was complaining of weight loss, insomnia, fatigue, and nervousness. On examination, it is noted that her eyes are prominent and her fingers show a fine tremor when her hands are held out in front of her. Her skin is hot and moist, and she is restless. Her pulse rate is elevated. Examination of her neck reveals an enlarged thyroid gland. A diagnosis of thyrotoxicosis with exophthalmos is made. Name the different thyroid hormones, and explain how they are formed within the thyroid

gland. Why has this patient lost weight even though her appetite has increased? Why does this patient have protruding eyes (exophthalmos)? Using your knowledge of functional histology, describe how you would treat this patient.

11. Describe the histological characteristics of the parafollicular cells of the thyroid gland. What is their function?

12. A 25-year-old woman is operated on for thyrotoxicosis. A partial thyroidectomy is performed successfully without incident. The next morning, on awakening from a deep sleep, the patient mentions to her nurse that she is experiencing some numbness around her lips and in her fingers. By the afternoon, the nurse notices that the patient seems excessively irritable and is complaining about what she describes as excessive noise outside her hospital window. On the second postoperative day, the patient says that the numbness of her face and fingers is still present and that the muscles of her arms and legs feel stiff. The resident notes that the patient is tending to hold her fingers flexed at the metacarpophalangeal joints and extended at the interphalangeal joints; the fingers are also adducted with the thumbs. The patient is also holding her ankles plantar flexed. What is your diagnosis? The resident orders an immediate estimate of the serum calcium levels. Why? How would you treat this patient?

13. A 40-year-old man is admitted to the surgical ward with a history of multiple renal stones. Routine blood studies show that the serum calcium level is 16 mg per 100 ml and the chemical analysis of the stones shows them to be calcium oxalate and calcium phosphate. A diagnosis of hyperparathyroidism is made. What hormone is responsible for raising the serum calcium level, and how does it work? What is the normal microscopic structure of the parathyroid glands? Does the structure of the parathyroid gland change with age?

14. The thymus is a lymphatic organ, but it is also now recognized to be an endocrine gland. Explain this statement.

15. A 38-year-old man is admitted to the hospital for laboratory tests. When seen by his physician, he complains of increasing tiredness and muscular weakness over the previous year. He has experienced five attacks of nausea, vomiting, and diarrhea during this period. His reason for visiting his physician is that his friends have noticed that his skin is becoming darker. After a complete physical examination, a diagnosis of Addison's disease is made, and it is confirmed by laboratory tests. What is the cause of Addison's disease? The secretions of which hormones are defective in this disease? What is responsible for the weakness and increased pigmentation of the skin in this condition? Describe the microscopic structure of the suprarenal cortex. Indicate the names and main functions of the hormones produced by the different layers of the suprarenal cortex.

16. A 29-year-old man is examined by an internist because he recently has experienced on three separate occasions attacks of what he describes as severe pounding palpitations. On the first occasion, the attack had occurred after he had taken his dog for a run in the park. The second attack had followed an argument with his next-door neighbor over the erection of a fence, and the third attack had followed going out into very cold weather to visit a friend. The attacks had lasted about 20 minutes each and had been accompanied by severe sweating, headache, and paleness and coldness of the skin. The patient is admitted to the hospital for observation and evaluation. While in the hospital, he has another attack. His pulse rate is 120 beats per minute, and his blood pressure is 240/140 mm Hg. A preliminary diagnosis of pheochromocytoma is made, which is later confirmed by analysis of the urinary content of catecholamines. Describe the structure of the suprarenal medulla. What is rather special about the blood supply to this structure? What hormones are secreted by the cells of the suprarenal medulla, and what is their action?

17. A 51-year-old man is concerned because he has noticed during the past few weeks that he has started to urinate more frequently and is always

hungry and thirsty. He is also worried because he has received treatment for skin infections from his doctors on six occasions during the previous year. On being questioned and examined by his physician, he reveals a family history of diabetes mellitus. The fasting blood sugar level is measured, and a glucose tolerance test is performed. The urine is also examined for glucose. The results show that the patient has diabetes mellitus. What is the normal fasting blood glucose level? What is the object of the glucose tolerance test? Why does glucose appear in the urine in diabetes mellitus? What is the underlying cause of diabetes mellitus?

18. Describe the appearance of a histological section of the pancreas that had been stained with H&E. What are the islets of Langerhans? Describe the electron microscopic appearances of the different cells that form the islets, and indicate the function of each of these cells.

19. Patients with advanced malignant disease sometimes show signs and symptoms indicative of hormonal imbalance. For example, a patient with carcinoma of the bronchus has been known to develop excessive melanin pigmentation of the skin. Can you explain this fortunately uncommon phenomenon?

20. Explain the following in a patient with diabetes mellitus: (a) polyuria; (b) ketosis; (c) loss of weight; (d) the actions of insulin; (e) the importance of a well-regulated diet in the treatment.

21. Using your knowledge of the functional histological characteristics of the suprarenal cortex, explain the following signs found in Cushing's disease: (a) moon-shaped face; (b) hirsutism of the face, chest, and abdomen in the female; (c) high concentration of glucose in the blood; (d) raised urinary 17-hydroxycorticosteroid excretion.

22. A 21-year-old man sustains a severe injury to the perineum in an airplane crash. The surgeon is forced to amputate the scrotum and remove both testes. Using your knowledge of functional histology, describe the changes that will take place in this individual because of the absence of testosterone. Describe the position and structure of the cells within the testes that produce testosterone. What factors control the secretion of testosterone? Is testosterone produced in patients with bilateral undescended testes?

23. In the mature female, the theca interna and the corpus luteum of the ovary are involved in the production of hormones. What is the microscopic appearance of these structures? Name the hormones produced by these structures. What factors control the secretion of these hormones?

24. Describe the microscopic changes that take place in the ovary at the menopause. What are the clinical signs and symptoms of the menopause? What is responsible for the menopause? Is it caused by a cessation of the activity of the hypothalamus, a cessation of the activity of the pars anterior, or a failure of the ovary to respond to hormonal stimulation from the pituitary?

25. The placenta is an endocrine gland. Which part of the placenta produces hormones, and what are the names and actions of these hormones? A patient with chorionepithelioma, a malignant tumor of the placenta, has large quantities of a certain hormone in the urine. Name this hormone.

ADDITIONAL READING

Altschule, M. D. (ed.). *Frontiers of Pineal Physiology.* Cambridge, Mass.: MIT Press, 1975.

Arimura, A. Hypothalamic gonadotropin-releasing hormone and reproduction. *Int. Rev. Physiol.* 13:1, 1977.

Austin, C. R., and Short, R. V. (eds.). *Mechanism of Hormone Action.* New York: Cambridge University Press, 1979.

Axelrod, J. The pineal gland: A neurochemical transducer. *Science* 184:1341, 1974.

Baetens, D., et al. Endocrine pancreas: Three-dimensional reconstruction shows two types of islets of Langerhans. *Science* 206:1323, 1979.

Baker, B. L., et al. Differentiation of growth hormone and prolactin-containing acidophils with peroxidase-labeled antibody. *Anat. Rec.* 164:163, 1969.

Bodian, D. Cytological aspects of neurosecretion in opossum neurohypophysis. *Bull. Johns Hopkins Hosp.* 113:57, 1963.

Bondy, P. K. The adrenal cortex. In Bondy, P. K., and Rosenberg, L. E. (eds.), *Metabolic Control and Disease* (8th ed.). Philadelphia: Saunders, 1980, p. 1427.

Brodish, A., and Lymangrover, J. R. The hypothalamic-pituitary adrenocortical system. *Int. Rev. Physiol.* 16:93, 1977.

Brownstein, M. J., Russel, J. T., and Gainer, H. Synthesis, transport, and release of posterior pituitary hormones. *Science* 207:373, 1980.

Chan, A. S., and Conen, P. E. Ultrastructural observations on cytodifferentiation of parafollicular cells in the human fetal thyroid. *Lab. Invest.* 25:249, 1971.

Christy, N. P. (ed.). *The Human Adrenal Cortex*. New York: Harper & Row, 1971.

Coupland, R. E. Electron microscopic observations on the structure of the rat adrenal medulla. I. The ultrastructure and organization of chromaffin cells in the normal adrenal medulla. *J. Anat.* 99:231, 1965.

Davis, J. C., and Hipkin, L. J. *Clinical Endocrine Pathology*. Philadelphia: Lippincott, 1977.

Dierick, K., and Vandesande, F. Immunocytochemical localization of the vasopressinergic and oxytocinergic neurons in the human hypothalamus. *Cell Tissue Res.* 184:15, 1977.

Dillon, R. S. *Handbook of Endocrinology: Diagnosis and Management of Endocrine and Metabolic Disorders* (2nd ed.). Philadelphia: Lea & Febiger, 1980.

Dumont, E. The action of thyrotropin on thyroid metabolism. *Vitam. Horm.* 29:289, 1971.

Fajans, S. S. Diabetes mellitus: Description, etiology and pathogenesis, natural history and testing procedures. In Degroot, L. J., et al. (eds.), *Endocrinology*. Vol. 2. New York: Grune & Stratton, 1979, p. 1007.

Falkner, S., Hellman, B., and Taljedal, I. B. *The Structure and Metabolism of the Pancreatic Islets*. New York: Pergamon, 1970.

Farquhar, M. G. Processing of secretory products by cells of the anterior pituitary gland. *Mem. Soc. Endocrinol.* (Cambridge) 19:79, 1971.

Fujita, H. Fine structure of the thyroid cell. *Int. Rev. Cytol.* 40:197, 1975.

Gray, J. K., Cooper, G. W., and Munson, P. L. Parathyroid hormone: Thyrocalcitonin and the control of mineral metabolism. In McCann, S. M. (ed.), *Endocrine Physiology*. Woburn, Mass.: Butterworth, 1974.

Guillemin, R., and Burgus, R. The hormones of the hypothalamus. *Sci. Am.* 227(5):24, 1972.

Guyton, A. C. *Textbook of Medical Physiology* (6th ed.). Philadelphia: Saunders, 1981.

Ham, A. W. *Histophysiology of Cartilage, Bone, and Joints*. Philadelphia: Lippincott, 1979.

Harris, G. W., and Reed, M. Hypothalamic releasing factors and the control of anterior pituitary function. *Br. Med. Bull.* 22:266, 1966.

Hedeskov, C. J. Mechanism of glucose-induced insulin secretion. *Physiol. Rev.* 60:442, 1980.

James, V. H. (ed.). *The Adrenal Gland*. New York: Raven, 1979.

McKenzie, J. M., and Zakarija, M. Hyperthyroidism. In Degroot, L. J., et al. (eds.), *Endocrinology*. Vol. 1. New York: Grune & Stratton, 1979, p. 429.

Moriarty, G. C., and Garner, L. L. Immunocytochemical studies of the cells of the rat adenohypophysis containing both ACTH and FSH. *Nature* 265:356, 1977.

Nir, I., Reiter, R. J., and Wurtman, R. J. The pineal gland. *J. Neural Transm.* (Suppl.) 13, 1978.

Notkins, A. L. The causes of diabetes. *Sci. Am.* 241(5):62, 1979.

Nunez, E. A., and Gershon, M. D. Cytophysiology of thyroid parafollicular cells. *Int. Rev. Cytol.* 52:1, 1978.

Nunez, E. A., Whalen, J. P., and Krook, L. An ultrastructural study of the natural secretory cycle of the parathyroid gland of the bat. *Am. J. Anat.* 134:459, 1972.

Pantic, V. R. The specificity of pituitary cells and regulation of their activities. *Int. Rev. Cytol.* 40:153, 1975.

Raisz, L. G., et al. Hormonal regulation of mineral metabolism. *Int. Rev. Physiol.* 16:199, 1977.

Reiter, R. J. Comparative physiology: Pineal gland. *Annu. Rev. Physiol.* 35:305, 1973.

Rhodin, J. A. G. The ultrastructure of the adrenal cortex of the rat under normal and experimental conditions. *J. Ultrastruct. Res.* 34:23, 1971.

Snell, R. S. Effect of the alpha melanocyte stimulating hormone of the pituitary on mammalian epidermal melanocytes. *J. Invest. Dermatol.* 42:337, 1964.

Snell, R. S. Effect of melatonin on mammalian epidermal melanocytes. *J. Invest. Dermatol.* 44:273, 1965.

Snell, R. S. Hormonal Control of Pigmentation in Man and Other Mammals. In *Advances in Biology of the Skin. Vol. 8. The Pigmentary System.* New York: Pergamon Press, 1967, p. 447.

Steinberger, E. Hormonal control of mammalian spermatogenesis. *Physiol. Rev.* 51:1, 1971.

Tapp, E., and Huxley, M. The histological appearance of the human pineal gland from puberty to old age. *J. Pathol.* 108:137, 1972.

Williams, R. H. *Textbook of Endocrinology* (5th ed.). Philadelphia: Saunders, 1975.

Wong, E. T., and Lindall, A. W. Subcellular location of human parathyroid hormone immunoreactive peptides and preliminary evidence for a precursor to human PTH. *Proc. Soc. Exp. Biol. Med.* 148:387, 1975.

17

SKIN AND ITS APPENDAGES

The skin covers the entire surface of the body and is the largest organ of the body. It is continuous with the mucous membranes lining the alimentary, respiratory, and urogenital systems at sites where these systems open onto the surface. At the margins of the eyelids, the skin is continuous with the conjunctiva; at the ear, it lines the external auditory meatus and covers the tympanic membrane.

The skin consists of two distinct layers, the *epidermis* and the *dermis*, which are firmly attached to each other (Figs. 17-1 and 17-2). The epidermis is the outer layer and is composed of a stratified squamous keratinized epithelium; the dermis is the deeper layer and consists of connective tissue. The skin rests on *subcutaneous tissue*, also known as *superficial fascia*, which is made up of loose connective tissue or adipose tissue. The subcutaneous tissue allows the skin to move freely on the deeper structures.

During embryonic development, the epidermis, which is derived from the ectoderm, grows down into the mesenchyma-derived dermis and gives rise to the skin appendages: the *sweat glands*, *hair follicles*, *sebaceous glands*, and *nails*.

Examination of the surface of the skin with the naked eye reveals three types of markings: tension lines, flexure lines, and papillary ridges. The *tension lines* form a network of fine, shallow grooves that join one another at angles, enclosing polygon-shaped areas. They are produced by the attachment of the collagen fibers in the dermis. The *flexure lines* occur in relation to joints and correspond to the folds in the dermis associated with movements of the joints. The flexure lines are produced by the attachment of the dermis to the underlying deep fascia and are conspicuous on the wrists, palms, soles, fingers, and toes.

The *papillary ridges* are responsible for fingerprints. They consist of narrow ridges separated by narrow grooves, and they are organized into curved arrays. They are caused by the raising up of the epidermis by the underlying dermal papillae or ridges (see Fig. 17-2). The pattern of the ridges and grooves forms early in fetal life, and, apart from enlarging with growth, they remain constant in arrangement throughout life. Each person has a slightly different pattern, and for this reason the pattern of papillary ridges of the fingers has been used with success in criminal detection.

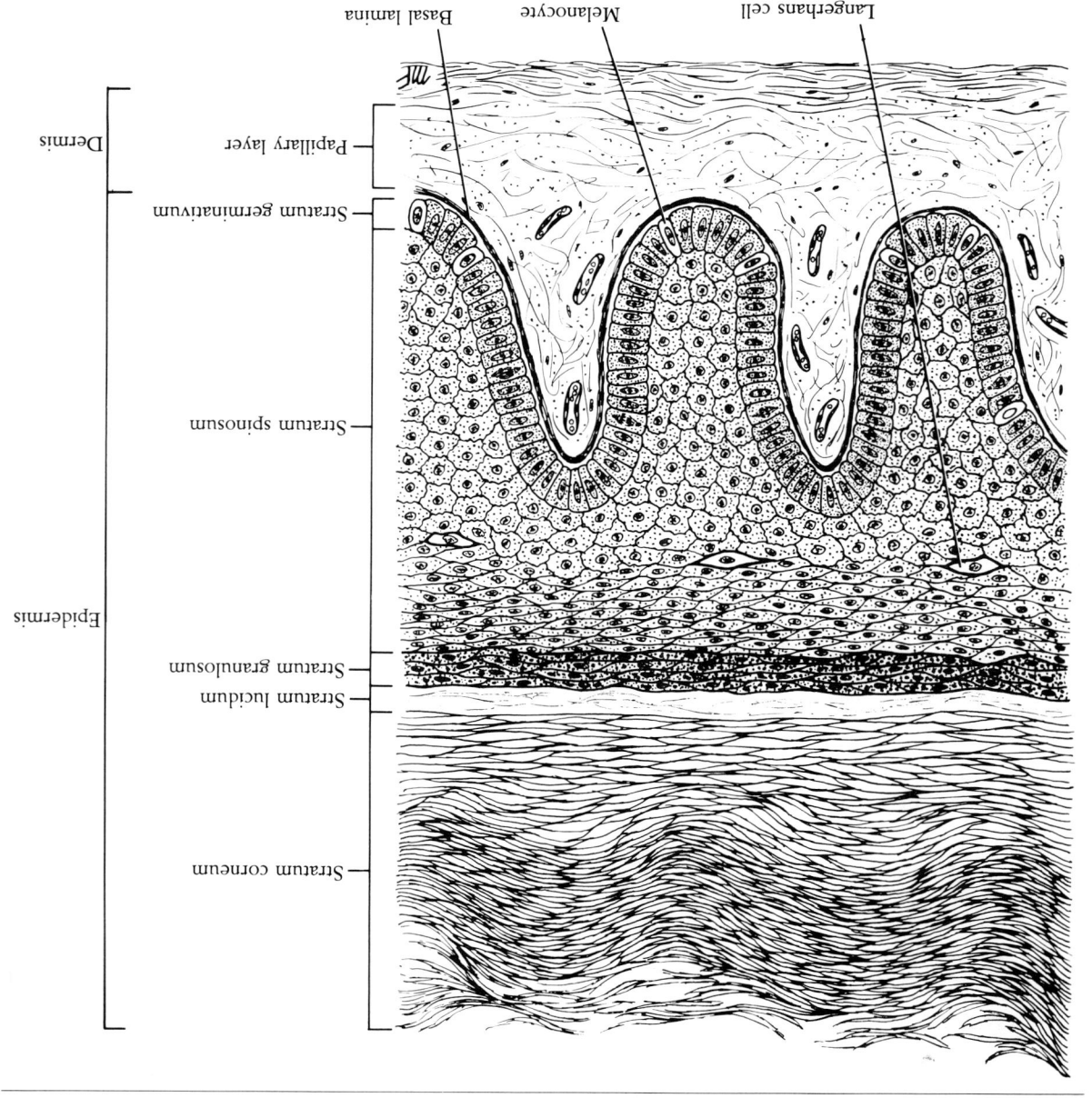

Fig. 17-1. Vertical section of thick skin, showing the general structure of the epidermis and dermis. Note the different layers of the epidermis.

There are two types of skin, *thick skin* and *thin skin* (Figs. 17-3–17-6). These terms refer to the thickness of the epidermis only, not to that of the whole skin, as one might expect (Fig. 17-7). Thick skin covers the palms of the hands and the soles of the feet; the remainder of the body is covered with thin skin.

EPIDERMIS

Cells

The epidermis is a stratified squamous epithelium consisting of three distinct lines of cells: the keratinocyte, the melanocyte, and the Langerhans cells.

A fourth cell, the Merkel cell, may be included in this classification, but it should be considered part of the sensory nerve ending, terminating in the epidermis. It is described in Chapter 7.

Keratinocytes

The keratinocytes make up the major part of the epidermis (Fig. 17-8; see Figs. 17-5 and 17-6). The cells are formed in the deepest layer of the epidermis from columnar cells that continuously undergo mitotic activity. The newly formed cells are pushed to successively more superficial layers by the production of new cells beneath them. As the cells move toward the surface, a protein called *keratin* is formed within their cytoplasm (see Figs. 17-5 and 17-8). As maturation continues, the cytoplasm of the cell is largely replaced by keratin, and the cell

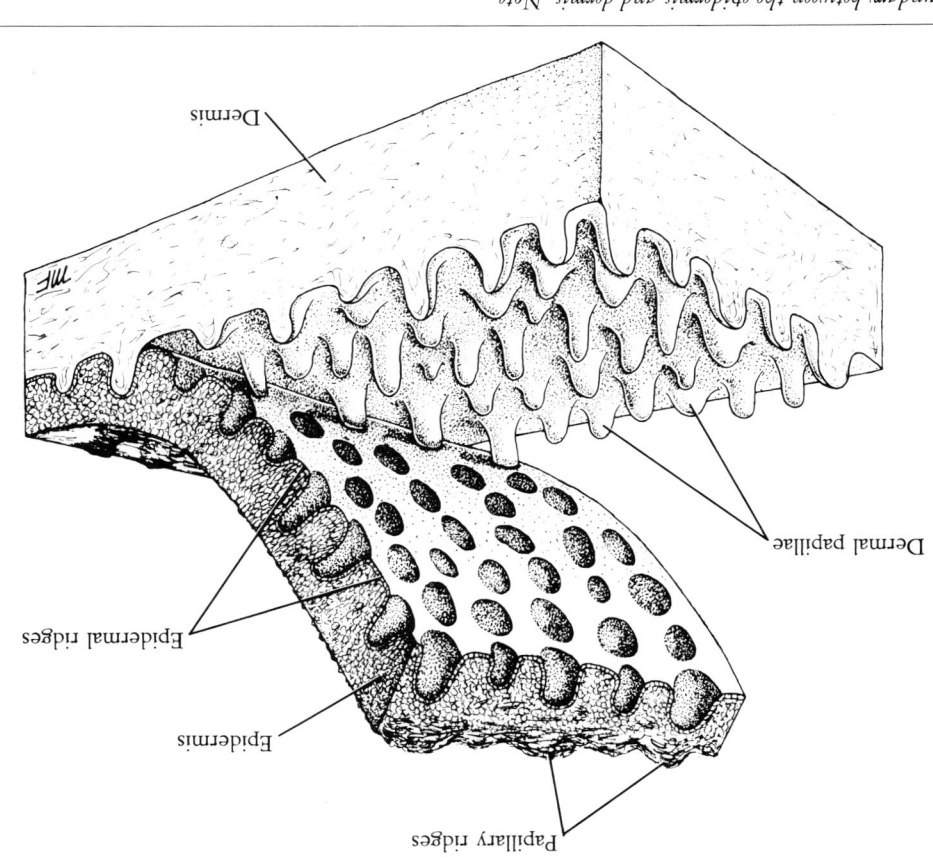

Fig. 17-2. Boundary between the epidermis and dermis. Note how the projections of the dermis, called the dermal papillae, cause infolding of the epidermis. The ridges of the epidermis between the dermal papillae are referred to as epidermal ridges.

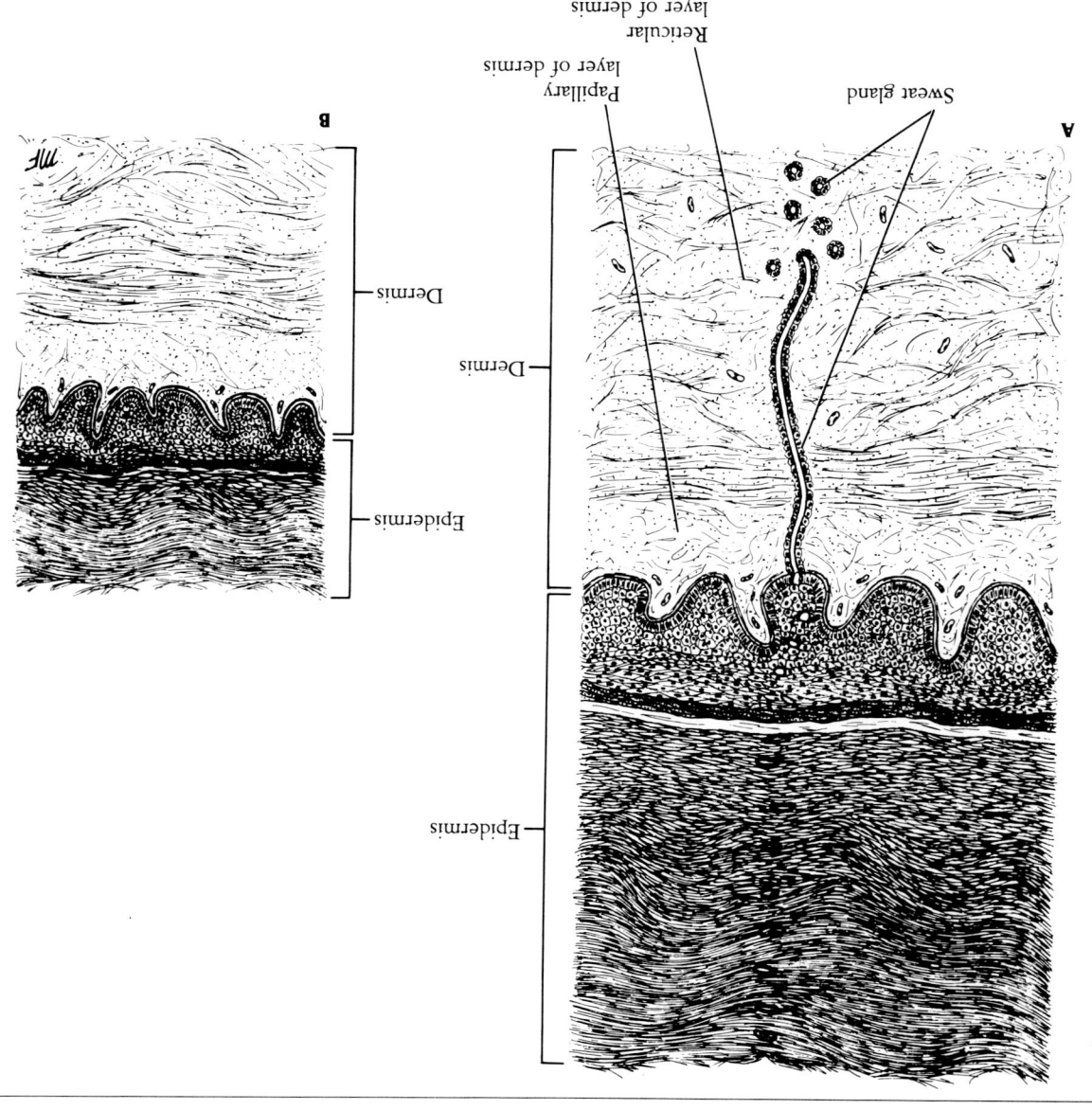

Fig. 17-3. Differences in structure between (A) thick skin, e.g., the sole of the foot, and (B) thin skin, e.g., the anterior abdominal wall. The terms thick and thin refer to the thickness of the epidermis.

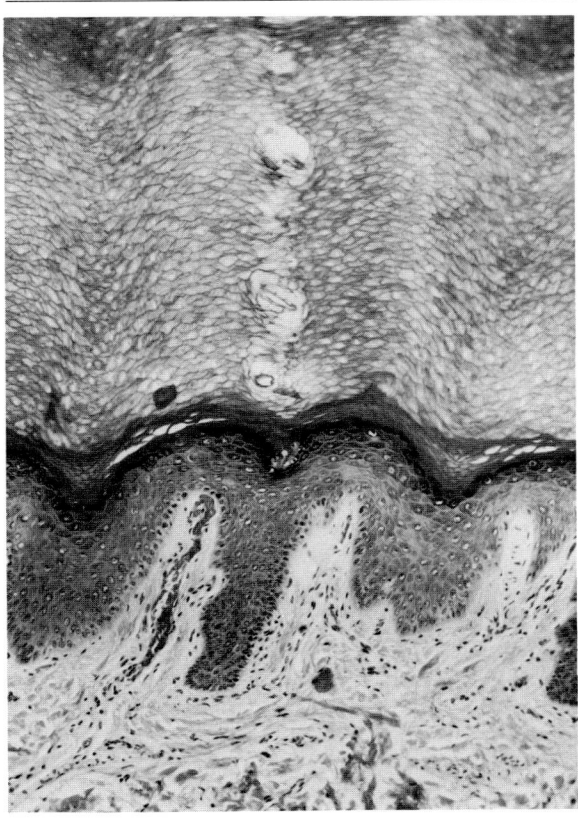

Fig. 17-4. Photomicrograph of a vertical section of skin from the palm of the hand. Note the dermal papillae and epidermal ridges. Note also the different layers of the epidermis and a duct of an eccrine sweat gland. The dermis is shown at the bottom. (H&E; ×100.)

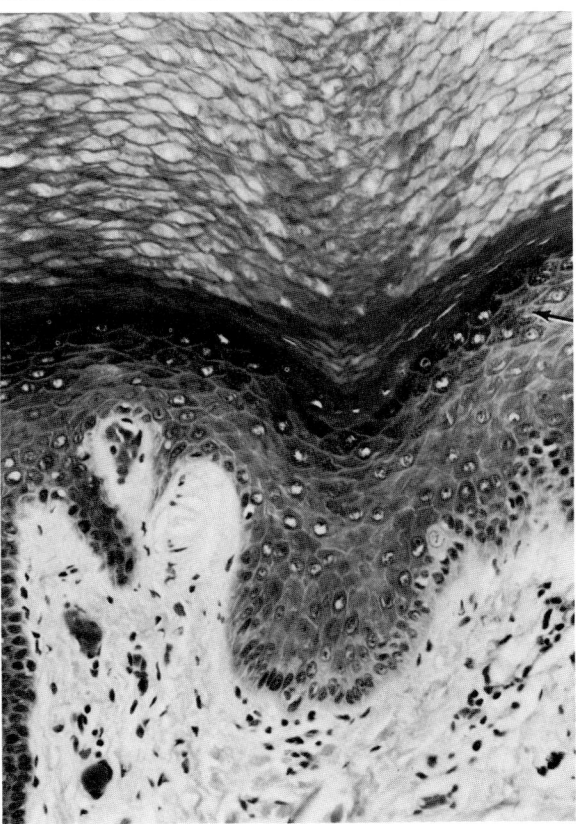

Fig. 17-5. Photomicrograph of a high-power view of a vertical section of skin from the palm of the hand. The different layers of the epidermis are clearly shown; the granules of keratohyalin in the cells of the stratum granulosum can just be identified (arrow). The stratum lucidum is darkly stained in this specimen. (H&E; ×200.)

dies. The nucleus and other cell organelles disappear, and the cell becomes a scalelike structure full of keratin (see Figs. 17-5 and 17-8). Eventually the keratin scales are worn off or desquamated from the surface; they are replaced by underlying cells, which in turn become keratinized and die. The whole process of the formation of a keratinocyte and its maturation as it rises to the surface to be desquamated takes about 1 month.

The degree of keratinization and the thickness of the epidermis in different regions of the body are determined before birth and are under genetic control (see Figs. 17-5–17-7). In the palms and soles, keratinization is extensive, but in the forearm, there is much less. Excessive wear and tear can stimulate the keratinocytes to reproduce more rapidly; as a result, the epidermis becomes thicker and the cells more keratinized. This is an important response of the skin to trauma and clearly is designed to protect the underlying soft tissues.

Melanocytes

Melanocytes are branched epithelial cells that synthesize the pigment melanin (Figs. 17-9 and 17-10).

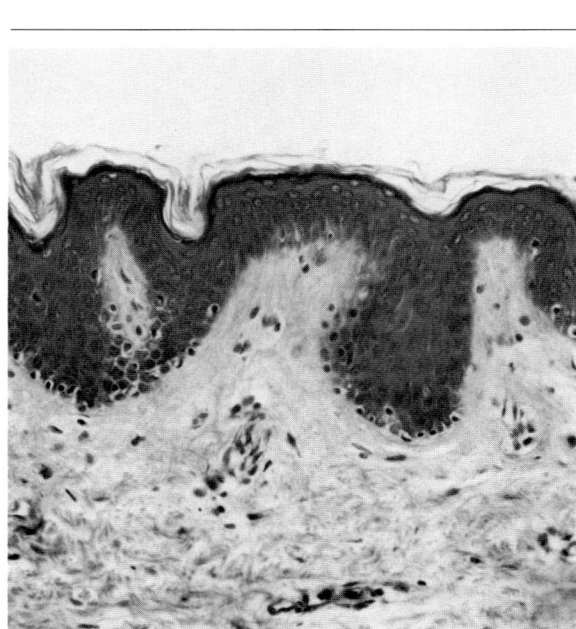

Fig. 17-6. Photomicrograph of a vertical section of thin skin from the thorax. Compare with the thick skin shown in Figure 17-5. (H&E; ×200.)

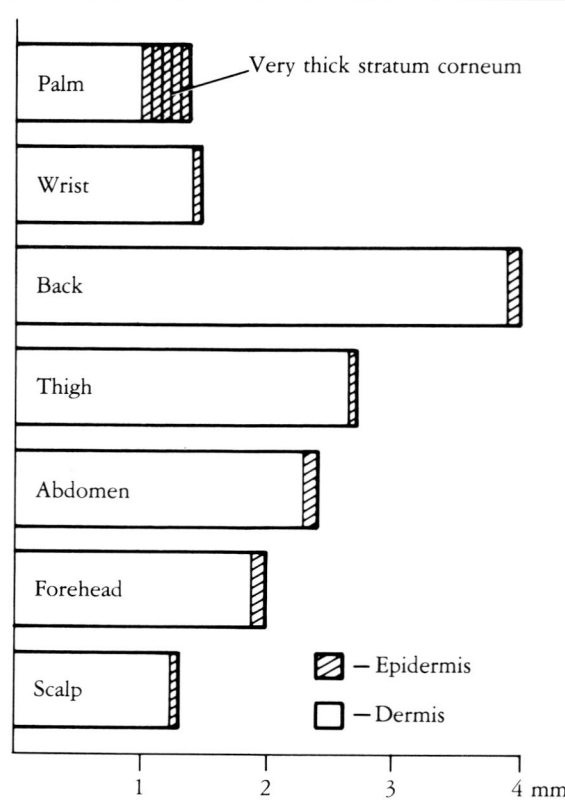

Fig. 17-7. Relative thickness of the epidermis and dermis in skin from different parts of the body. Note that in the examples given, the epidermis is thickest in the palm skin and the dermis is thickest in the skin of the back. (Modified from graph in T. Fitzpatrick, Dermatology in General Medicine. *New York: McGraw-Hill, 1971. Used with permission.)*

The cells are ectodermal in origin and are derived from the neural crest; they migrate to the epidermis early in development. They take up their final position in the deepest layer of the epidermis between adjacent keratinocytes. The melanocytes are less numerous than the keratinocytes, but their branching processes enable them to make contact with all the keratinocytes in the basal layer (Fig. 17-11).

The pigment *melanin* is yellowish, orange, or brown. Chemically, it is a polymer of the amino acid tyrosine and is formed within the melanocytes by the enzyme *tyrosinase* (see Fig. 17-11). The melanin granules, or *melanosomes,* formed within the bodies of the melanocytes pass along the branching processes. Adjacent keratinocytes phagocytose the ends of the branching processes, so that the melanin granules enter the cytoplasm of the keratinocytes; the granules accumulate on the superficial, or "sunny," side of the nuclei (see Fig. 17-11). As the keratinocytes rise to the surface, they carry the melanin pigment within their cytoplasm, so that eventually the melanin is eliminated from the epidermis by desquamation. There are an average of

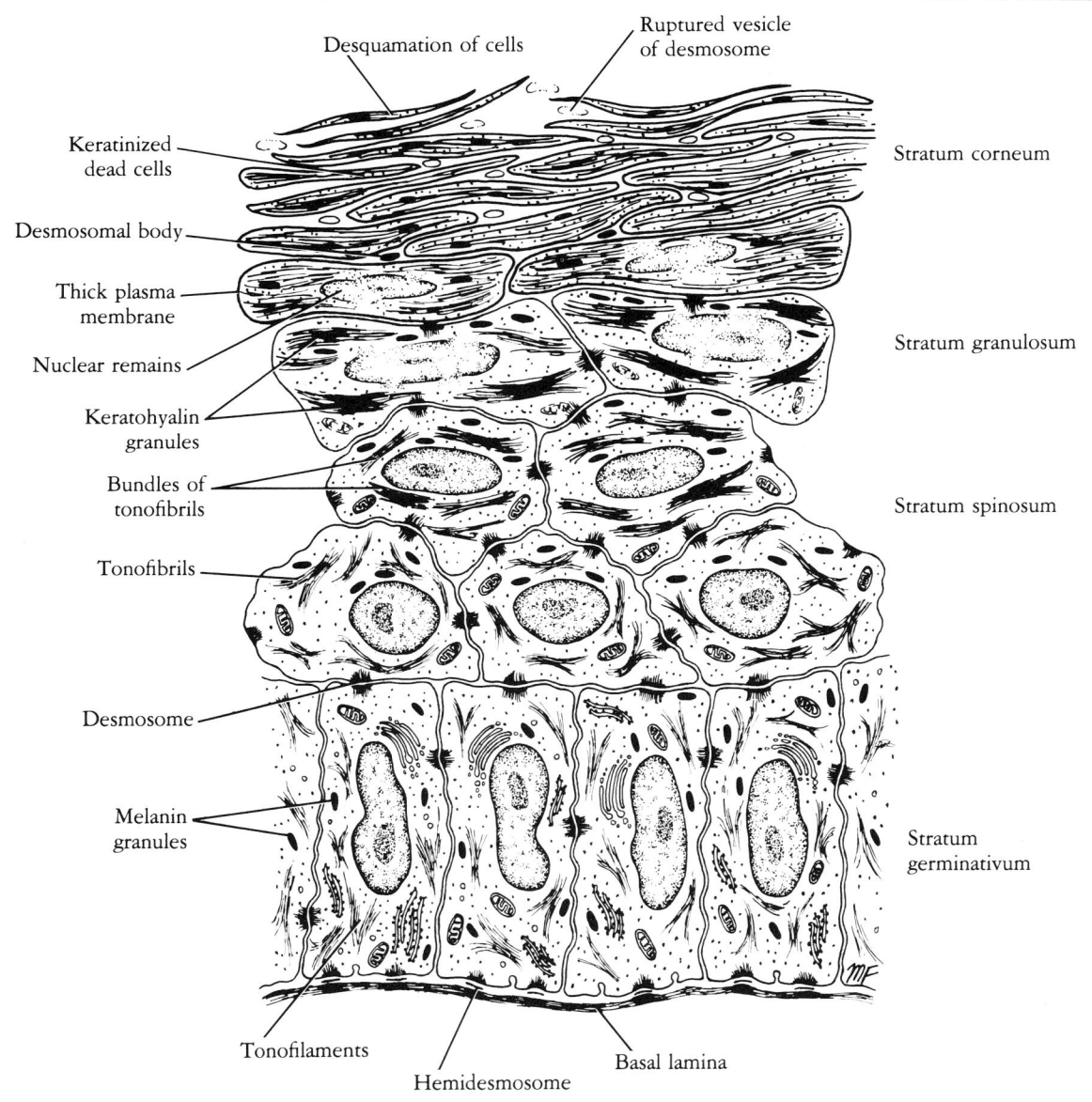

Fig. 17-8. Changes in the structure of keratinocytes as they slowly migrate upward from the stratum germinativum to the stratum corneum. Note also the changes in the desmosomes as the cells rise to the surface.

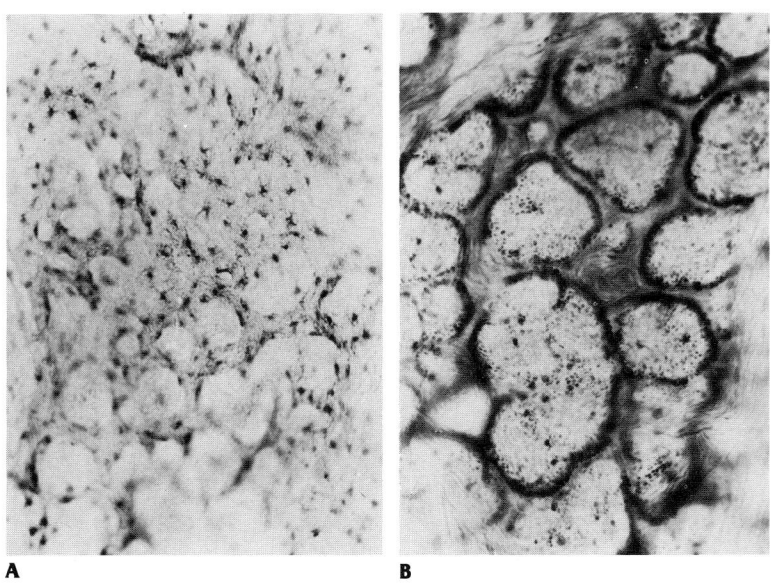

Fig. 17-9. Photomicrograph of epidermal sheets from (A) white and (B) black skin. The epidermal sheets were separated from the dermis by treating the specimens with trypsin. The sheets were then incubated with DOPA reagent to make the melanocytes more visible. Note that in both specimens, the melanocytes are seen as small dark cells with branching processes that contain dark melanin pigment. Note also that there is a much higher concentration of melanin in the black epidermis, especially in the keratinocytes of the epidermal ridges. (×100.)

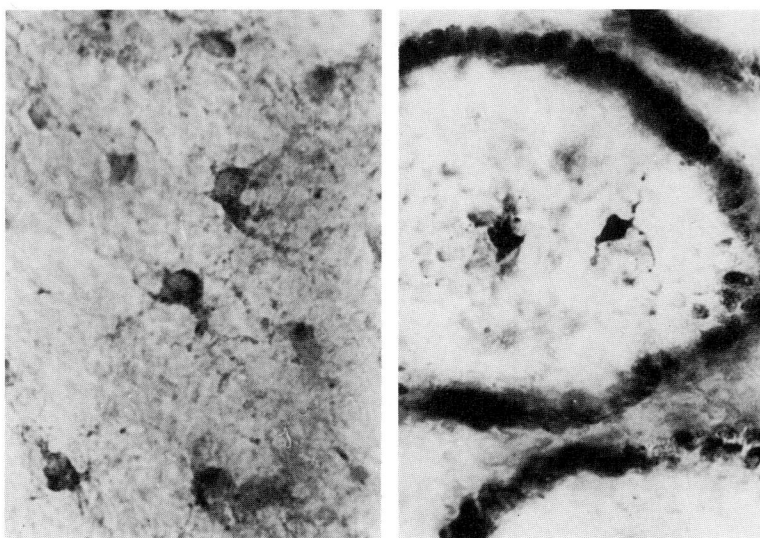

Fig. 17-10. Photomicrograph of high-power view of the white and black epidermal sheets shown in Figure 17-9. Note that the melanocytes have characteristic branching processes containing melanin. Note also the large amount of melanin in the cells of the epidermal ridges in the black skin (right specimen). (Treated with DOPA reagent; ×600.)

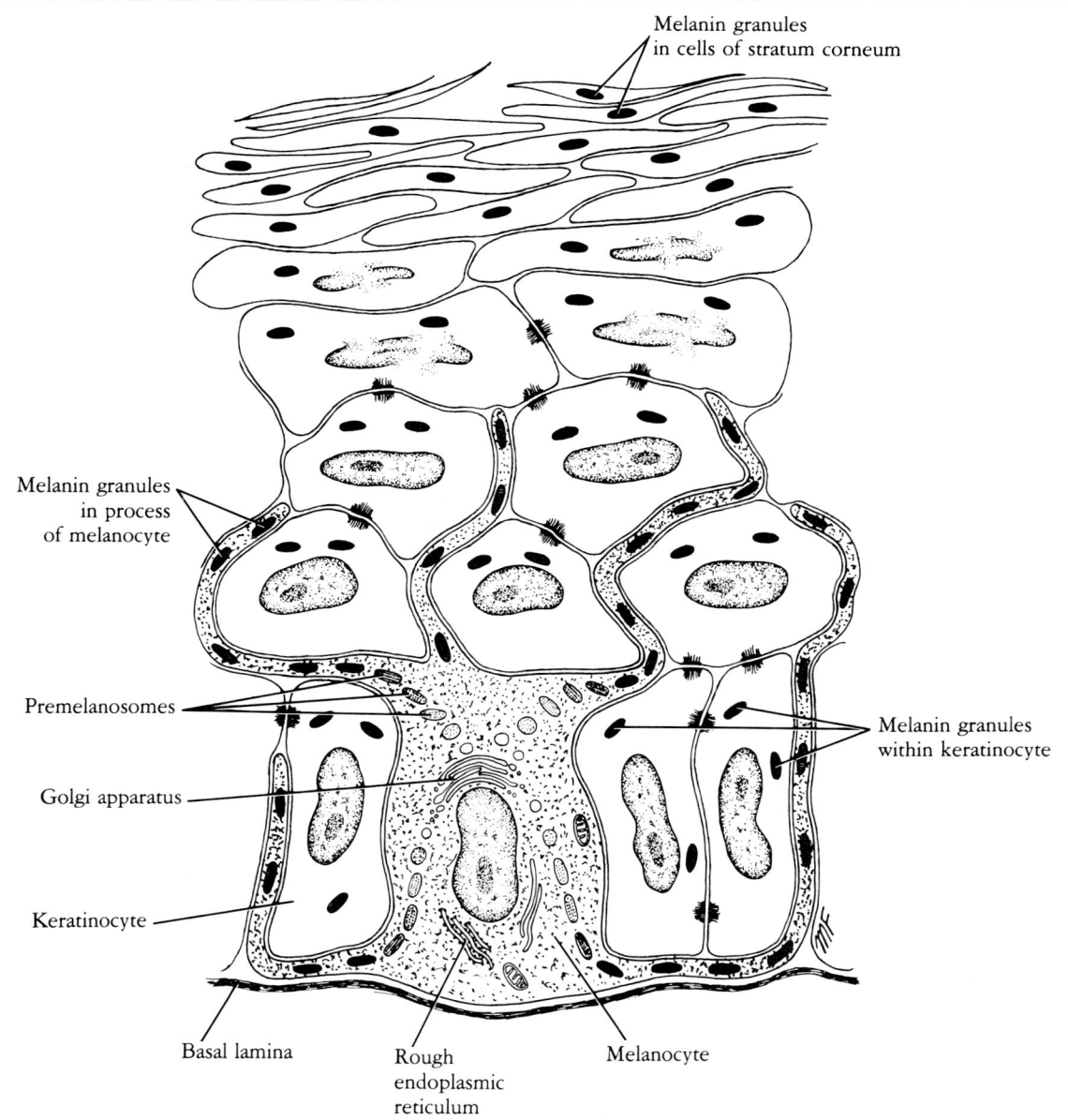

Fig. 17-11. *Relationship between a melanocyte and the adjacent keratinocytes in the epidermis of the skin. Note the changes in the melanin granules as they move away from the Golgi apparatus into the processes of the melanocytes. Note also that the melanocyte processes insinuate themselves between the plasma membranes of neighboring keratinocytes.*

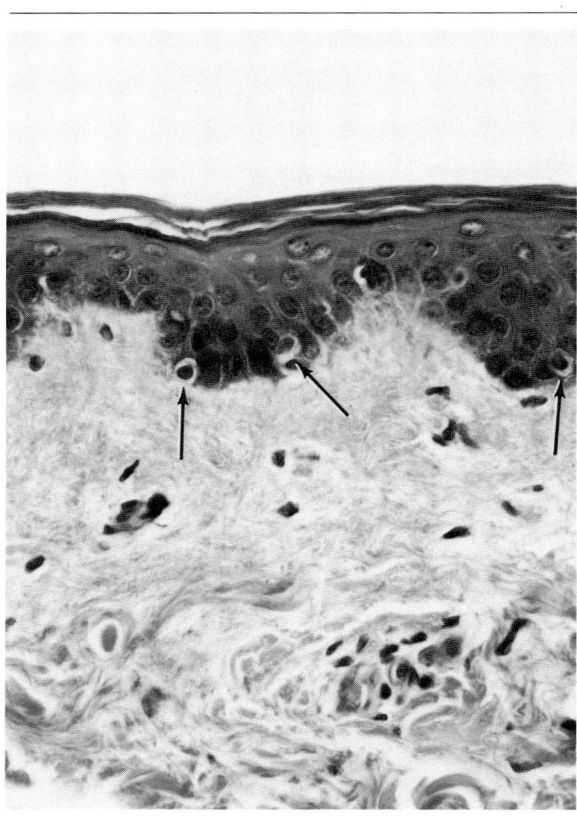

Fig. 17-12. *Photomicrograph of a vertical section of forearm skin of a white individual. The melanocytes (arrows) are seen as clear cells in the stratum germinativum. (H&E; ×400.)*

about 1,500 melanocytes per square millimeter of skin surface. The distribution of melanocytes varies among individuals and bodily regions, with the cells being most numerous in the genital area, less so on the face, and sparsest on the trunk. Although one of the most obvious differences among the various human races is the variation in skin color, the number of melanocytes in the different races is about the same; color differences are caused by differences in the activity of the melanocytes. Black individuals have more active melanocytes in their skin than do whites.

Melanocytes in a vertical section of white skin stained with H&E and examined with a light microscope appear as cells with a clear cytoplasm and cannot be identified readily (Fig. 17-12). If sections of fresh skin are incubated with dihydroxyphenylalanine (DOPA), the tyrosinase within the melanocytes converts the DOPA into melanin, and the black pigment within the cells makes the cells relatively easy to identify (see Figs. 17-9 and 17-10).

Melanocytes are continuously undergoing mitotic activity, although their division is much slower than that of keratinocytes. The newly formed cells are pushed superficially and accompany the keratinocytes to the surface, where they finally are desquamated. As the melanocytes rise to the surface, they lose their ability to form melanin, and they degenerate and die.

Langerhans Cells

Langerhans cells are branching epithelial cells thought to be of mesenchymal origin (Fig. 17-13). They are unrelated to melanocytes, and, whereas there is considerable regional variation in the population density of melanocytes, the number of Langerhans cells is constant in different epidermal areas of the body. Langerhans cells cannot be identified in ordinary skin sections stained with H&E. They can be seen, however, in a suprabasal region of the epidermis if the skin is treated with an acid solution of gold chloride or with supravital stains. When examined with the electron microscope, the cells are seen to lack desmosomes and to contain characteristic tennis racquet–shaped Langerhans granules; the nuclei are greatly indented (see Fig. 17-13). Langerhans cells contain hydrolytic enzymes, and it is believed that they are phagocytic and probably have migrated into the epidermis from the dermis.

Organization of the Epidermis

The epidermis is organized into layers, and as the superficial layers are shed, the deeper layers are repaired by cell division. Each layer represents a stage in the dynamic process of cell division and cell maturation. In the palms and soles, where the epidermis is thick, the maximum number of layers is present (see Figs. 17-3 and 17-4). Elsewhere in the body, the epidermis is thinner, the various layers are thinner,

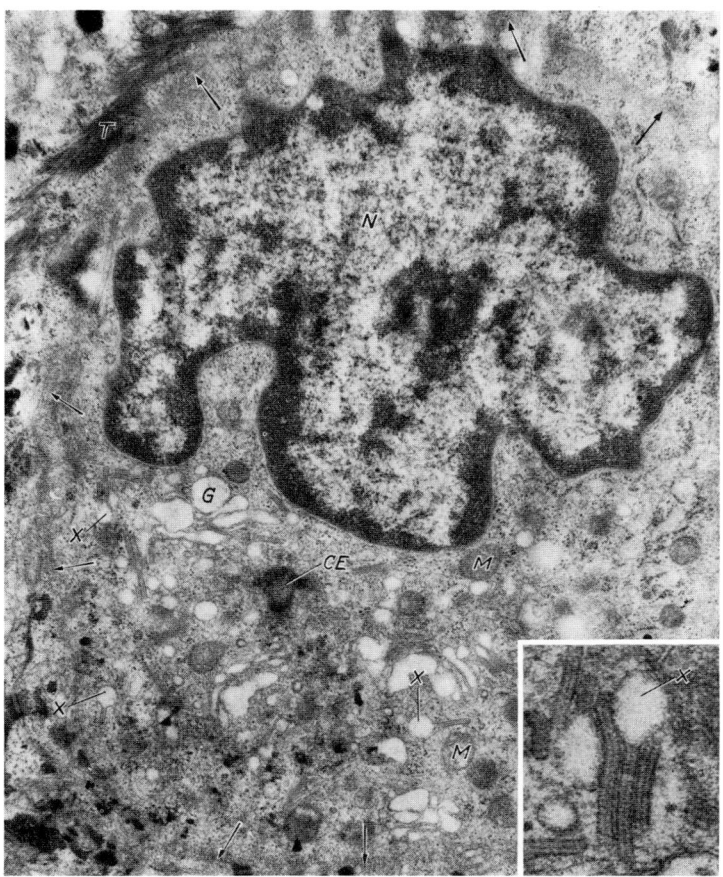

Fig. 17-13. Electron micrograph of a Langerhans cell in the epidermis, showing the typical indented nucleus and numerous racquet-shaped granules in the cytoplasm (X). The plasma membranes are indicated by arrows. A high-power view of the granules is shown in the inset. (T = tonofilaments; N = nucleus; G = Golgi apparatus; CE = centriole; M = mitochondrion.) (×27,270.)

and one layer, the stratum lucidum, commonly is absent.

The various layers of the epidermis can be studied by examining with the light or electron microscope sections of the skin that have been cut perpendicularly to the surface. One first notices that the boundary between the epidermis and the dermis undulates, a pattern caused by the interdigitation of the infoldings of the epidermis, called *epidermal ridges*, with the projections of the dermis, called *dermal ridges* or *papillae* (see Figs. 17-2 and 17-4). In thick skin, the epidermal ridges are deeper, and this depth serves to increase the number of dividing cells in areas exposed to friction and injury. Deeper ridges also increase the area of contact between the epidermis and dermis, important in resisting tangential stresses applied to the skin surface.

The cells of the epidermis receive their nourishment from the blood vessels in the dermis. The food materials pass to the cells in the tissue fluid. Blood and lymphatic vessels thus are absent from the epidermis, and normally, no leukocytes wander between the epidermal cells. Nerve processes extend for a short distance into the epidermis from the dermis (see p. 266).

Layers of the Epidermis

In thick skin (palms and soles) the epidermis consists of five layers, or strata: (1) the stratum germinativum (stratum basale, stratum malpighii), (2) the stratum spinosum (prickle cell layer), (3) the stratum granulosum (granular cell layer), (4) the stratum lucidum (clear layer), and (5) the stratum corneum (cornified or horny layer). In thin skin the stratum lucidum is often absent. As was stated earlier, the great majority of the cells that form each layer are keratinocytes, and also present, in much smaller numbers, are melanocytes and occasional Langerhans cells.

STRATUM GERMINATIVUM. This is the deepest layer and abuts onto the dermis. It consists mainly of a single layer of low columnar cells resting on a basal lamina (see Figs. 17-3 and 17-5). These cells are the keratinocytes that are continuously undergoing mitotic division and forming stacks of new cells that are pushed up to the surface. Mitotic figures are commonly seen in this layer. The cells have large nuclei, with deeply staining basophilic cytoplasm. In dark-skinned individuals, melanin granules are present that have been phagocytosed from adjacent melanocytes.

Electron microscopic examination shows that the keratinocytes are attached to the basal lamina by hemidesmosomes and to neighboring cells by desmosomes (Fig. 17-14). The cytoplasm contains many ribosomes and tonofilaments, occasional mitochondria, and a poorly developed Golgi apparatus. The cells are designed for growth and reproduction, and the formation of tonofilaments is the first stage in the production of keratin (see Figs. 17-16–17-18).

The melanocytes are branched cells situated between the keratinocytes and constitute about a quarter of the cell population of the layer. If they are relatively inactive, they appear as clear cells in an H&E-stained section (see Fig. 17-12). If they are very active, as in dark-skinned individuals or whites who have been exposed to ultraviolet light, the cell bodies and their processes are filled with pigment granules. When adjacent keratinocytes phagocytose the ends of the dendritic processes of the melanocytes, the melanin granules are transferred to the cytoplasm of the keratinocytes. In dark-skinned persons, therefore, melanocytes can be recognized only by identifying cells with melanin-filled processes. In light-skinned individuals, the melanocytes can be identified easily by using the histochemical reaction known as the DOPA reaction, discussed previously. This reaction increases the melanin content of the cells.

Electron microscopic examination of melanocytes shows that they are not attached by desmosomes or hemidesmosomes to surrounding cells or the basal lamina (Fig. 17-15; see Fig. 17-11). A rough endoplasmic reticulum is present and is responsible for the formation of the enzyme tyrosinase. The enzyme is transferred and packaged in the Golgi apparatus, and vesicles known as *premelanosomes* are formed (see Figs. 17-11 and 17-15). Melanin now is formed within the vesicles, which at this point are called *melanosomes*. It is the mature melanosomes or melanin granules that pass into the processes of the melanocytes.

STRATUM SPINOSUM. This layer lies superficially from the stratum germinativum and is several cells thick. The keratinocytes of this layer are somewhat flattened and polyhedral, with their long axes parallel to the surface. The surface of the cells is covered with short dovetailed processes that are attached by desmosomes to similar processes of adjacent cells. In formalin-fixed sections, the processes are accentuated and produce the artificial appearance of prickles, giving the stratum its alternative name, prickle cell layer.

Electron microscopic examination shows that the cytoplasm contains numerous tonofilaments that are grouped together into large compact bundles called *tonofibrils* (Fig. 17-16; see Fig. 17-8). Numerous ribosomes are present, and a few mitochondria are

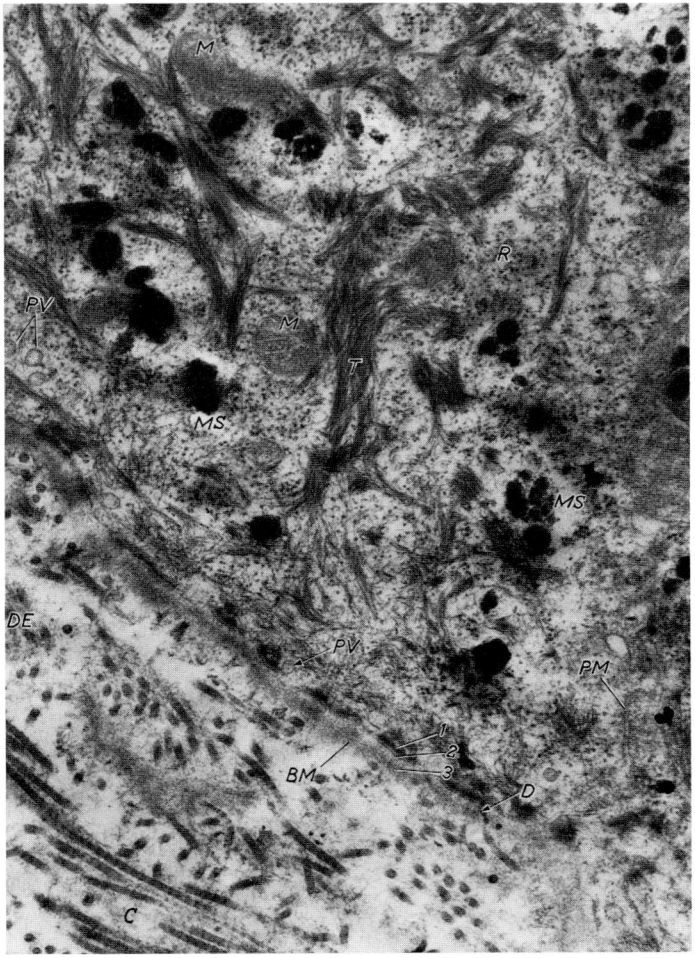

Fig. 17-14. Electron micrograph of the dermoepidermal junctional region, showing part of a keratinocyte above and the superficial part of the dermis below. Note the bundles of tonofilaments (T) and numerous melanin granules, or melanosomes (MS). Note also the electron-dense areas within a hemidesmosome: (1) localized area of thickening of the plasma membrane; (2) thin electron-dense lamina; (3) localized area of increased electron density of the basement membrane. (M = mitochondrion; R = ribosome; PV = pinocytotic vesicles; PM = plasma membrane; BM = basement membrane; C = collagen; DE = dermis.) (×28,500.)

seen; the Golgi apparatus rarely is visible. Melanin granules are present. It is in this layer that Langerhans cells are found.

STRATUM GRANULOSUM. This layer lies superficially from the stratum spinosum and is three or four cells thick (see Figs. 17-4 and 17-5). The cells are flattened, and the nuclei are deeply staining and pyknotic. The cytoplasm contains numerous basophilic granules of *keratohyalin*. The cells stain dark blue with hematoxylin.

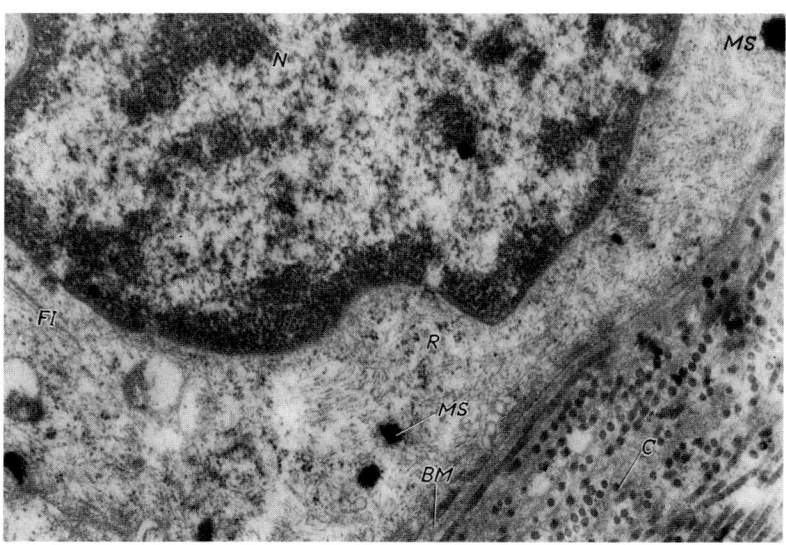

Fig. 17-15. Electron micrograph of the dermoepidermal junctional region, showing part of a melanocyte above and the superficial part of the dermis below. Note the complete absence of hemidesmosomes. (×26,100.)

Electron microscopic examination reveals the irregularly shaped keratohyalin granules, which vary in size from small particles to large masses (Figs. 17-17 and 17-18; see Fig. 17-8). The small particles are situated on a meshwork of tonofibrils, and as the particles enlarge, the tonofibrils fuse. Many ribosomes are present, but the mitochondria and nuclear membranes have degenerated. It is in this layer that the keratinocytes die.

STRATUM LUCIDUM. This layer lies superficially from the stratum granulosum and consists of several layers of flattened anucleate cells (see Figs. 17-1 and 17-5). The cells form a clear, homogeneous band that stains deeply with eosin. Electron microscopic examination shows a disappearance of all the cell organelles and considerable thickening of the plasma membranes. The cytoplasm contains closely packed fibers separated by a small amount of lucent matrix. The keratohyalin material seen in the previous layer probably coats the tonofibrils and increases their electron density.

STRATUM CORNEUM. This is the most superficial layer of the epidermis and in thick skin forms about three-quarters of the thickness of the epidermis (see Figs. 17-1 and 17-4). It consists of many layers of dead cells that are filled with keratin. The cells stain intensely pink with eosin. The deeper cells are closely packed, but on the surface the flattened squamae are continually cast off or desquamated (see Figs. 17-1 and 17-4). The lost cells are replaced by new ones originating from the deeper layers.

Electron microscopic examination shows the cells to be packed with fibers separated by a small amount of lucent matrix (see Fig. 17-18). Most of the fibers run parallel to the long axes of the flattened cells. In the more superficial layers, the fibers appear to be breaking down. The desmosomes show extensive changes. A single oval dense body lying within the intercellular space of each desmosome replaces the original three dense laminae (see Fig. 17-18). In the most superficial zones, the desmosomal body shows evidence of vacuolation. At sites of superficial cell desquamation, the desmosomal vesicles rupture.

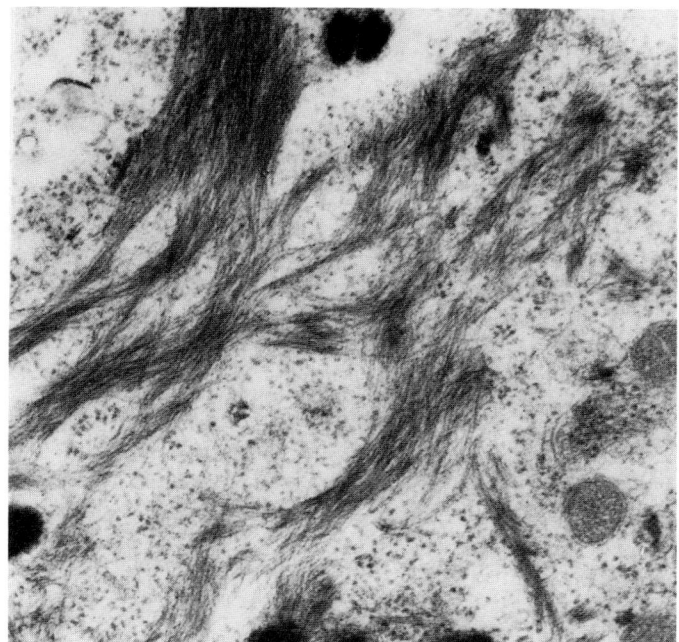

Fig. 17-16. Electron micrograph of a keratinocyte in the stratum spinosum, showing bundles of tonofibrils. A few melanin granules (melanosomes) are also visible. ($\times 45,300$.)

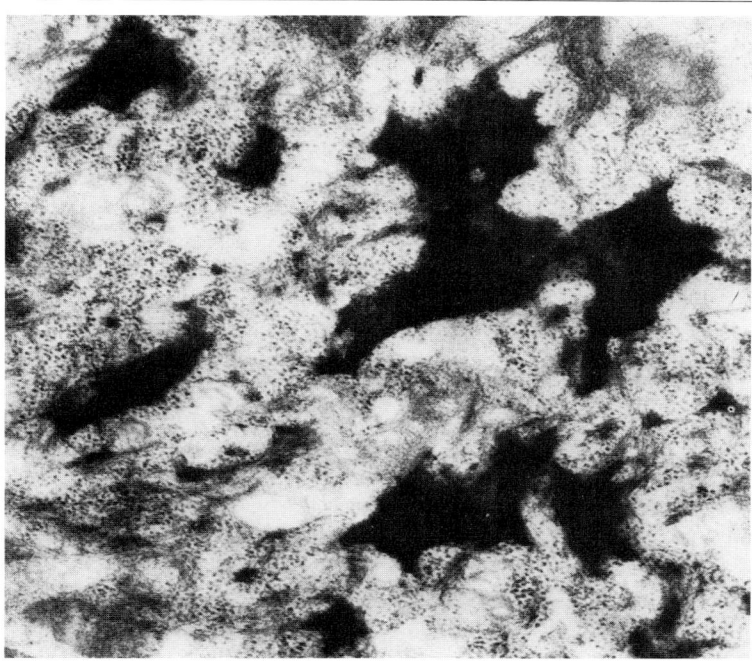

Fig. 17-17. Electron micrograph of a keratinocyte in the stratum granulosum, showing many keratohyalin granules at different stages of development. ($\times 24,400$.)

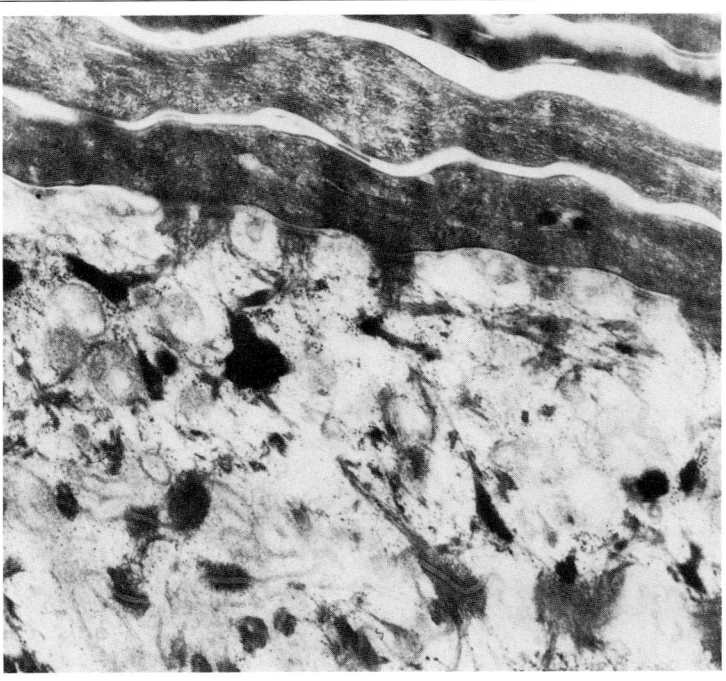

Fig. 17-18. Electron micrograph of superficial layer of stratum granulosum and deeper layers of the stratum corneum, showing cells of the stratum corneum (top) to be closely packed with keratin fibers. ($\times 17,300$.)

Function of the Epidermis

The papillary ridges of the skin surface roughen the skin and improve its frictional properties. These qualities greatly aid manual dexterity and help locomotion by allowing the soles of the feet to grip smooth surfaces.

The stratum corneum, which is composed of dead squamous cells filled with keratin, provides protection for the body against physical and chemical trauma. The continuous self-renewal permits the surface horny cells to be cast off during wear and tear without permanent damage to the skin. The many desmosomes that hold adjacent cells together, especially in the stratum spinosum, successfully resist shearing forces applied to the epidermis. Keratin's impermeability to water prevents desiccation of the body caused by water loss and allows us to bathe in fresh water without becoming waterlogged.

The many layers of interlocking keratinocytes provide a barrier against invasion by microorganisms. The action of ultraviolet radiation on 7-dehydrocholesterol in the keratinocytes forms vitamin D_3, which prevents rickets in children by stimulating the absorption of calcium and phosphate from the intestine.

The melanin pigment in the epidermis protects the underlying tissues from the harmful effects of ultraviolet light. The keratinocytes serve as a carrier, transporting the melanin pigment to the surface. The melanin granules are first dispersed on the "sunny" side of the nucleus within each keratinocyte; together, the many layers of the melanin-containing keratinocytes provide an effective screen for the specialized tissues, such as nerve endings, found in the dermis. The melanocytes, which are situated in the stratum germinativum, are able to supply groups of keratinocytes with pigment via their branching processes. The production of mela-

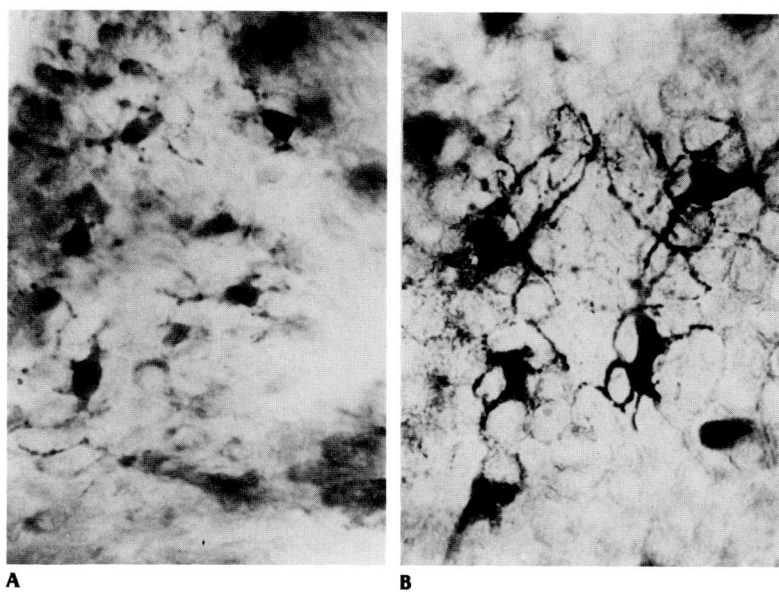

A **B**

Fig. 17-19. Photomicrograph of epidermal sheets of a dark-skinned patient (A) before hormone treatment and (B) after 1 week of treatment with alpha melanocyte-stimulating hormone. The hormone increases the amount of melanin within the melanocytes and causes dispersion of the melanin granules into the processes of the melanocytes. (Treated with DOPA reagent; ×653.)

nin can be increased by stimulating the melanocytes with increasing doses of ultraviolet light. Darkening of the skin in response to ultraviolet light occurs in three stages: (1) the existing melanin darkens rapidly over a period of 1 hour, (2) melanin granules disperse into the dendritic processes of the melanocytes, and (3) after about 2 days of exposure, melanin production increases as a result of increased tyrosinase activity within the melanocytes. Melanocyte activity (Fig. 17-19) is also controlled by the endocrine system (see p. 640).

The function of the Langerhans cells in the epidermis is not known, although they are thought to be phagocytic. The Merkel cells are associated with nerve endings in the epidermis and are believed to have a tactile sensory function (see p. 266).

DERMIS

Organization

The dermis is the thick connective tissue layer that extends from the epidermis to the subcutaneous tissue, also known as the superficial fascia. In the dermis are situated the skin appendages and many blood vessels, lymphatic vessels, and nerves (see Figs. 17-1 and 17-4). The dermis shows considerable variation in thickness in different parts of the body and tends to be thinner in women than in men.

For descriptive purposes, the dermis can be divided into an outer, papillary layer and an inner, reticular layer. The *papillary layer* is the thinner layer and fills in the concavities between the epidermal ridges. It is the papillary layer that forms the dermal papillae, or ridges. The papillary layer is composed of loose connective tissue made up of fine bundles of collagen fibers, reticular fibers, and elastic fibers woven into a loose network. The fibers are surrounded by a gel of glycosaminoglycans (mucopolysaccharides). Embedded in this tissue are capillary loops and nerve endings. The papillary layer is separated from the epidermis by a basal lamina.

The thick *reticular layer* begins just below the level of the epidermal ridges and is composed of dense connective tissue. The tissue is made up of interlacing collagen fibers, together with some elastic and reticular fibers. Most of the fibers run in rows parallel to the skin surface. The rows of collagen form the lines of cleavage (Langer's lines); they tend to run longitudinally in the limbs and circumferentially in the neck and trunk.

In the later months of pregnancy, the collagen fibers of the reticular layer of the dermis of the anterior abdominal wall may rupture because of excessive stretching by the enlarging uterus. The resultant scars show through the epidermis as white streaks known as the *striae gravidarum*. Unfortunately, these scars are permanent. With aging, the elastic fibers of the dermis gradually lose their elasticity, and the skin wrinkles.

Smooth muscle fibers are found in the dermis in relation to hair follicles, where they form the *arrector pili muscles* (see Figs. 17-24 and 17-29).

As does all connective tissue, the dermis contains many different types of cells, including fibroblasts and fibrocytes, tissue macrophages, melanophages, mast cells, and blood leukocytes, particularly neutrophils, eosinophils, lymphocytes, and monocytes. Plasma cells may also be found. The melanophages are seen only in areas of dermis subjacent to heavily pigmented epidermis. In the areola of the nipple, for example, melanin may escape from the epidermis into the dermis and be phagocytosed by dermal macrophages, which then become known as melanophages. The cells of the dermis are most concentrated in the papillary layer.

Melanocytes are found in the dermis in the hair follicles and are responsible for producing the pigment of the hairs. In young children, melanocytes are present in the dermis of the sacral region. The melanin is retained within the cells and produces the bluish or so-called Mongolian spots often seen in that region.

The vascular supply to the skin is confined to the dermis. Small arteries enter the dermis from the subcutaneous tissue and immediately form a sheetlike plexus (see Fig. 17-24). Branches pass from the plexus and ascend to the junction between the papillary and reticular layers to form a second sheetlike plexus. Capillary loops ascend into the dermal papillae and return to the venous plexuses. Arteriovenous communications are common in the reticular layer of the dermis.

The nerve supply to the skin is profuse and consists of myelinated and nonmyelinated nerve fibers. Many of the fibers are sensory and have specialized sensory endings (described in Chapter 7). Many fibers are postganglionic efferent autonomic fibers that supply the sweat glands, blood vessels, and arrector pili muscles.

Function of the Dermis

The dermis provides a firm base for the epidermis and the skin appendages. The collagen fibers give great tensile strength, and the elastic fibers give the skin flexibility and cushion the body against mechanical injury. The vascular plexuses provide blood to the epidermis without actually entering it. The tissue fluid from the capillaries in the dermal papillae diffuses into the basal layers of the epidermis, providing the dividing and actively metabolic cells with nourishment and removing their waste products. It serves a similar function for the skin appendages.

Blood flow in the dermis, and its control via the hypothalamus and the sympathetic nerve fibers, provide the body with a very important thermoregulatory mechanism. In certain areas of the body are specialized vascular shunts, each of which is called a *glomus* (see p. 312); a glomus is under sympathetic control.

The sensory nerve endings in the dermis keep the individual in contact with the environment and together make the skin an important sensory organ. These nerve endings are discussed in detail in Chapter 7.

The dermis of the skin is a very vascular organ and stores a large volume of blood. By constriction and dilatation of the arteries and capillaries, the blood is returned to and taken from the general circulation. By this mechanism, the skin assists in the maintenance of a normal blood pressure.

The relative amounts of oxyhemoglobin and reduced hemoglobin circulating through the capillaries of the dermal papillae substantially contribute to the color of the skin. Melanin and carotene also affect skin color.

Blushing, which is a sudden dermal arteriolar dilatation, is an important emotional response.

The leukocytes and macrophages found in the dermis, principally in the papillary layer, provide a second line of defense against invasion by microorganisms, should they penetrate the epidermis.

SKIN COLOR

Three major pigments contribute to skin color: melanin, hemoglobin, and carotenoids.

Melanin is yellowish, orange, or brown and is produced by the melanocytes in the epidermis. Should it escape into the dermis and be phagocytosed by macrophages, it will appear blue because of the light-scattering effect of the epidermis. The bluish Mongolian spots often found in the sacral region of children are caused by the melanin within melanocytes in the dermis in this region.

Hemoglobin present in the erythrocytes of the dermal capillaries contributes either a red or a bluish color to the skin, depending on the relative concentrations of oxyhemoglobin and reduced hemoglobin.

Carotenoids are yellowish and are present in the stratum corneum. This color is most obvious in the palms and the soles, where the stratum corneum is thickest.

APPENDAGES OF THE SKIN

Nails

The nails are flattened horny plates situated on the dorsal surface of the distal parts of the fingers and toes (Figs. 17-20–17-22). The proximal part of the nail is called the *root;* it emerges from a groove in the skin to form the *body* of the nail, which is exposed. The root of the nail is covered by a fold in the skin called the *proximal nail fold.* The stratum corneum of the nail fold extends out over the body of the nail for a short distance to form the *eponychium.* The lateral borders of the nail body are overlapped by a fold of skin called the *lateral nail fold* (Fig. 17-23). The *nail bed* is the skin beneath the body of the nail, and here the epidermis consists only of the stratum germinativum. Under the proximal part of the body of the nail, the stratum germinativum is thickened and opaque and forms the *lunule.* The stratum germinativum in the lunule is actively proliferative and is responsible for the growth of the nail. This region of activity is known as the *nail matrix.* As the epidermal cells are formed, they become tightly packed keratinized cells that do not desquamate. With continued growth of the nail, the body slides distally over the nail bed. Fingernails grow at the rate of 0.5 to 1.2 mm per week; toenails grow much more slowly.

In the nail bed, the dermis is continuous with the periosteum of the phalanx. The dermal papillae here form longitudinal ridges that run in the long axis of the nail. The dermal papillae are highly vascular, and this produces the pink color seen through the translucent body of the nail. The lunule is white because the dermal papillae in this region are less vascular and the stratum germinativum is thick and opaque.

Hairs

Hairs are present over most of the body surface except the lips, palms, soles, dorsal surface of the distal phalanges of the fingers and toes, glans penis, glans clitoris, labia minora, and the internal surface of the labia majora. Hairs can be divided into those that are short, pale, and fine—the *vellus hairs*—and those that are coarse, dark, and large—the *terminal hairs.*

Hairs are dead epithelial fibers composed of fused keratinized cells that project from the surface of the epidermis (Figs. 17-24 and 17-25). Hairs vary in length, thickness, and color in different parts of the body and in different races. They do not grow continuously but rather have *hair growth cycles.* Growing hairs are said to be in the *anagen phase* (Fig. 17-26). This phase is followed by a short period of involution called the *catagen phase.* A resting phase, or *telogen phase,* follows. At this stage, the hair falls out or is pulled out. The shed hair is called a *club hair,* because of the shape of its root. After a period of rest,

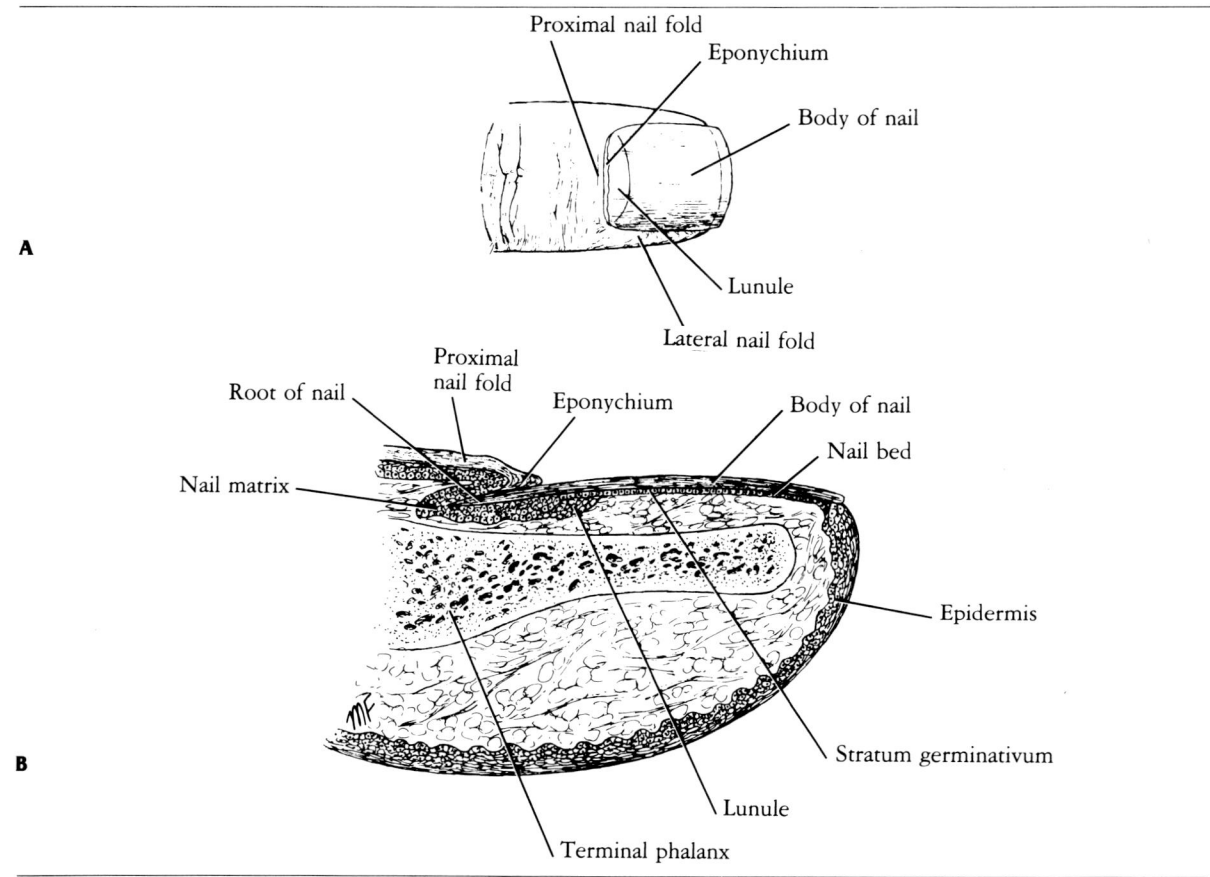

Fig. 17-20. (A) *Nail on the dorsal surface of the finger;* (B) *structure of the different parts of the nail, as seen in longitudinal section of the distal part of the finger.*

a new hair grows to replace the old one, and the hair growth cycle is repeated. The life-span of a single hair varies in different parts of the body, being as long as 4 years in the scalp and as short as 4 months in the axilla. Hairs grow faster between the ages of about 16 and 46 years. After the age of 50, the number of hairs in a given region diminishes. During pregnancy, most hairs continue to grow, but after delivery, there is a temporary increase in hair loss, so that hair density is reduced. This physiological effect is caused by the synchronization of hair cycles during late pregnancy, which results in many hairs entering telogen together and being shed together.

A hair has a *shaft,* which is the part projecting from the skin surface, and a *root,* which is the portion embedded in the skin. The root of the hair arises in a tubular invagination of the epidermis known as the *hair follicle.*

Structure of the Hair Follicle

The hair follicle extends down into the dermis and, in long hairs, may extend into the subcutaneous tissue (Fig. 17-27; see Fig. 17-24). The deep end of the follicle is expanded to form the *hair bulb.* The lower

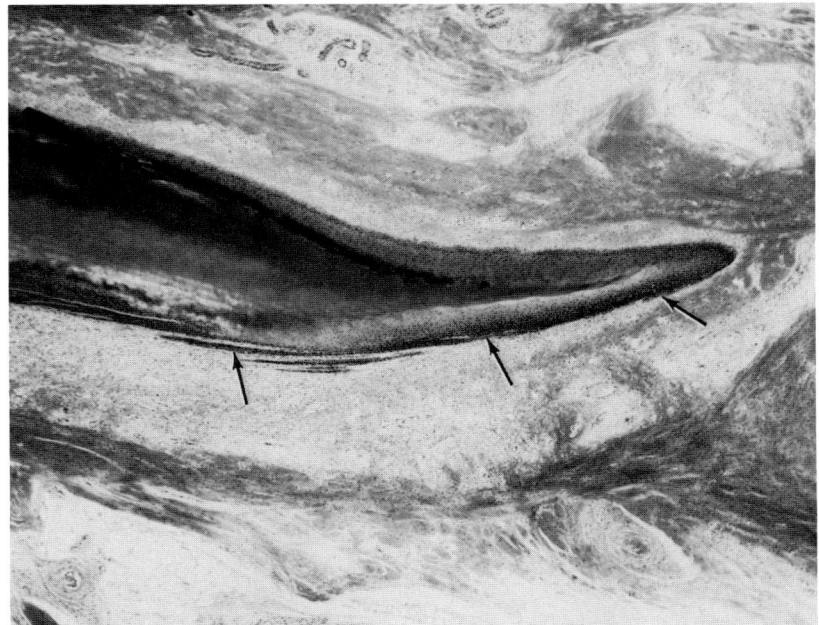

Fig. 17-21. Photomicrograph of a longitudinal section of the root of the nail, showing the nail matrix (arrows). (H&E; ×40.)

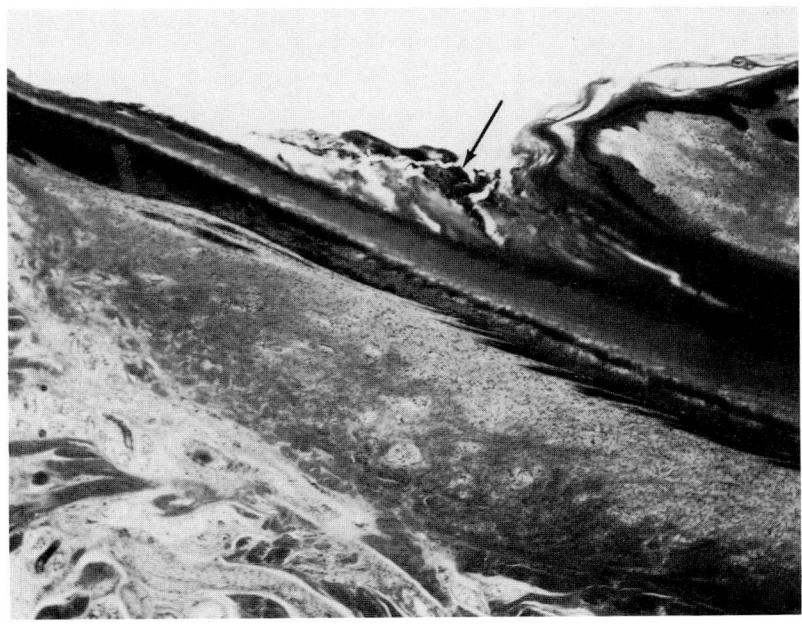

Fig. 17-22. Photomicrograph of a longitudinal section of the root of the nail, showing the proximal nail fold and the eponychium (arrow). (H&E; ×40.)

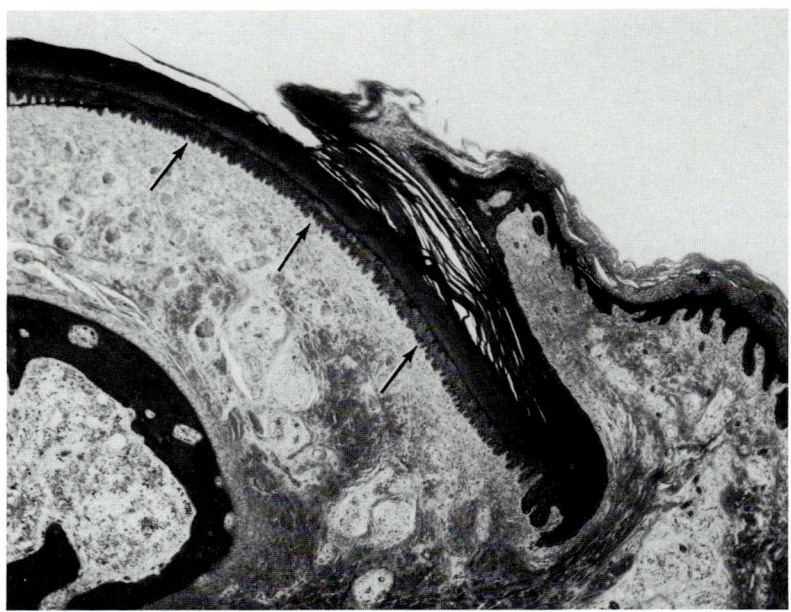

Fig. 17-23. *Photomicrograph of a cross section of the body of the nail, showing the nail bed (arrows) and the lateral nail fold. (H&E; ×40.)*

end of the hair bulb is indented by a connective tissue papilla.

The hair follicle opens onto the surface of the skin by means of a funnel-shaped aperture. The follicle passes down obliquely into the dermis and near its open end receives the duct of one or more sebaceous glands (Figs. 17-28 and 17-29; see Fig. 17-24). The wall of the hair follicle has two coats. The outer coat is made up of connective tissue that is continuous with the dermis. The inner coat is a continuation of the epidermis and is closely related to the hair root; it is known as the *epithelial root sheath* (Fig. 17-30). The epithelial root sheath may be divided into two layers, the outer and inner root sheaths. The *outer epithelial root sheath* is continuous above with the cells of the stratum spinosum of the surface epidermis. The *inner epithelial root sheath* is made up of three distinct layers of cells: (1) an outer layer of cuboidal cells (Henle's layer), (2) one or two layers of flattened cornified cells (Huxley's layer), and (3) the cuticle, which consists of overlapping thin scales, the free edges of which project downward toward the bottom of the follicle and interlock with the upward-projecting scales of the hair cuticle. This arrangement helps to secure the hair within the follicle. The epithelial root sheath is separated from the connective tissue sheath of the follicle by a homogeneous modified basal lamina called the *glassy membrane* (see Fig. 17-30).

Structure of Hair

The shaft of the hair consists of an outer *cuticle*, an intermediate *cortex*, and an inner *medulla* (Fig. 17-31; see Fig. 17-30). The *cuticle* (see Figs. 17-30 and 17-31) consists of a single layer of flat scales that overlap one another from below (see Fig. 17-25). The scales are heavily keratinized with hard keratin and, as mentioned, interlock with the cells of the inner root sheath. The *cortex* forms the main part of the hair and is composed of several layers of flattened elongated cells filled with hard keratin (see Figs. 17-

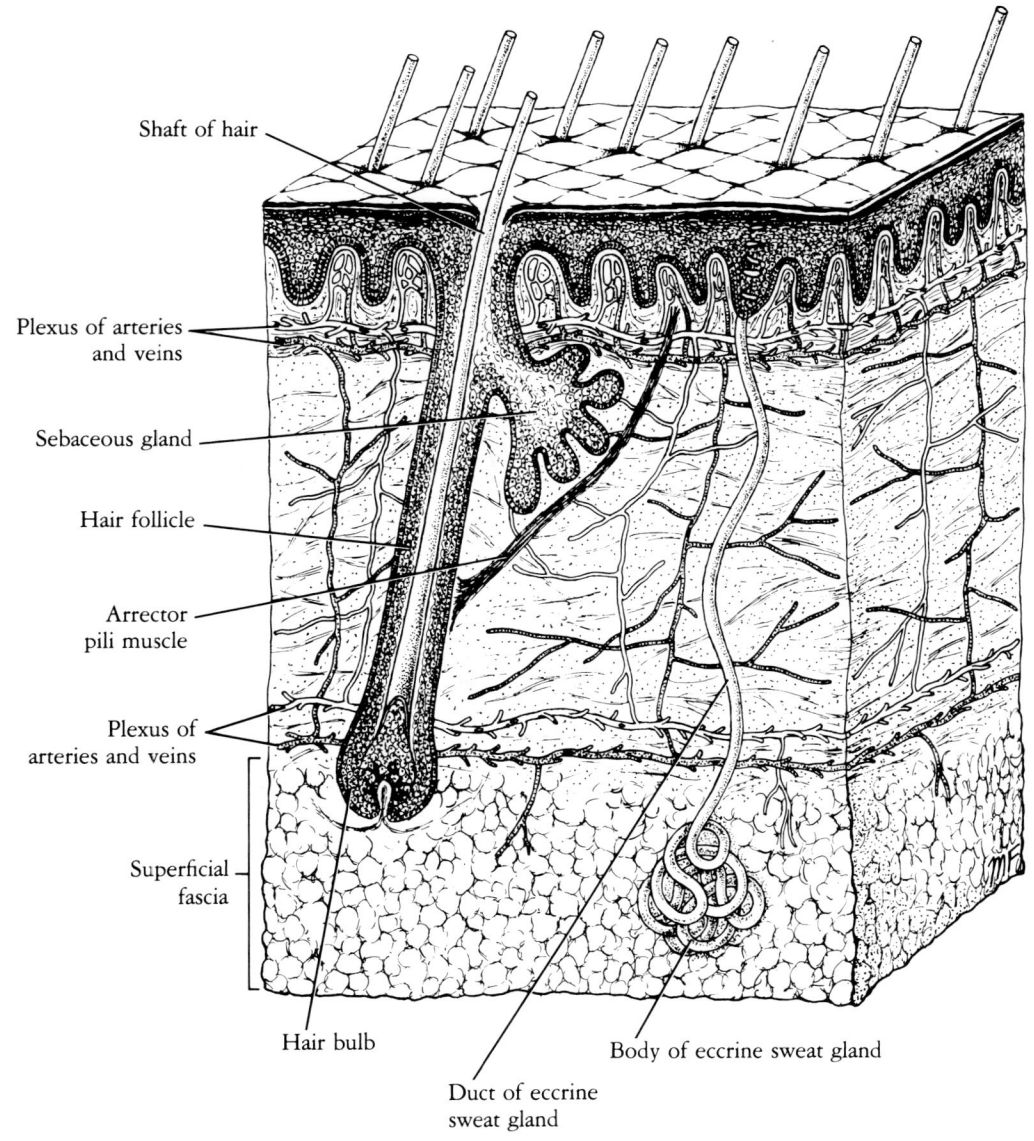

Fig. 17-24. General structure of hairy skin. Note the position of the hair bulb, the sebaceous gland, and the arrector pili muscle. An eccrine sweat gland is also shown. Note that the body of the sweat gland extends deeply into the superficial fascia.

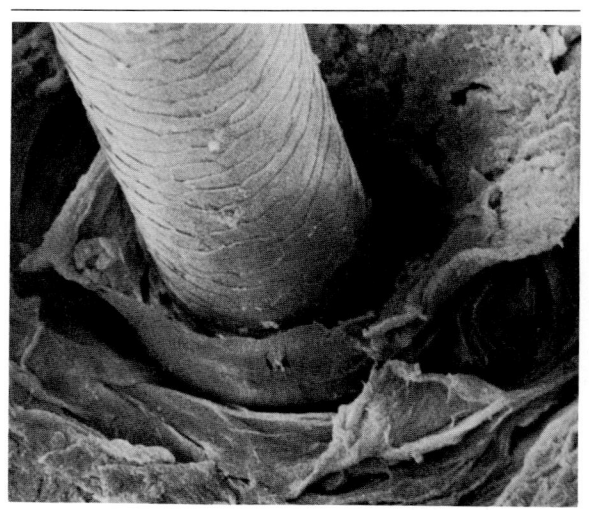

Fig. 17-25. Scanning electron micrograph of the surface of hairy skin, showing a hair shaft emerging from a follicle. Note how the scales of the cuticle of the hair overlap one another. (Courtesy of Dr. T. Fujita.)

Fig. 17-26. Overall shape of the hair follicle during three stages in hair growth. The anagen phase is the growing phase; during the short catagen phase, the hair follicle involutes. The telogen phase is the resting phase; the hair falls out or is pulled out easily.

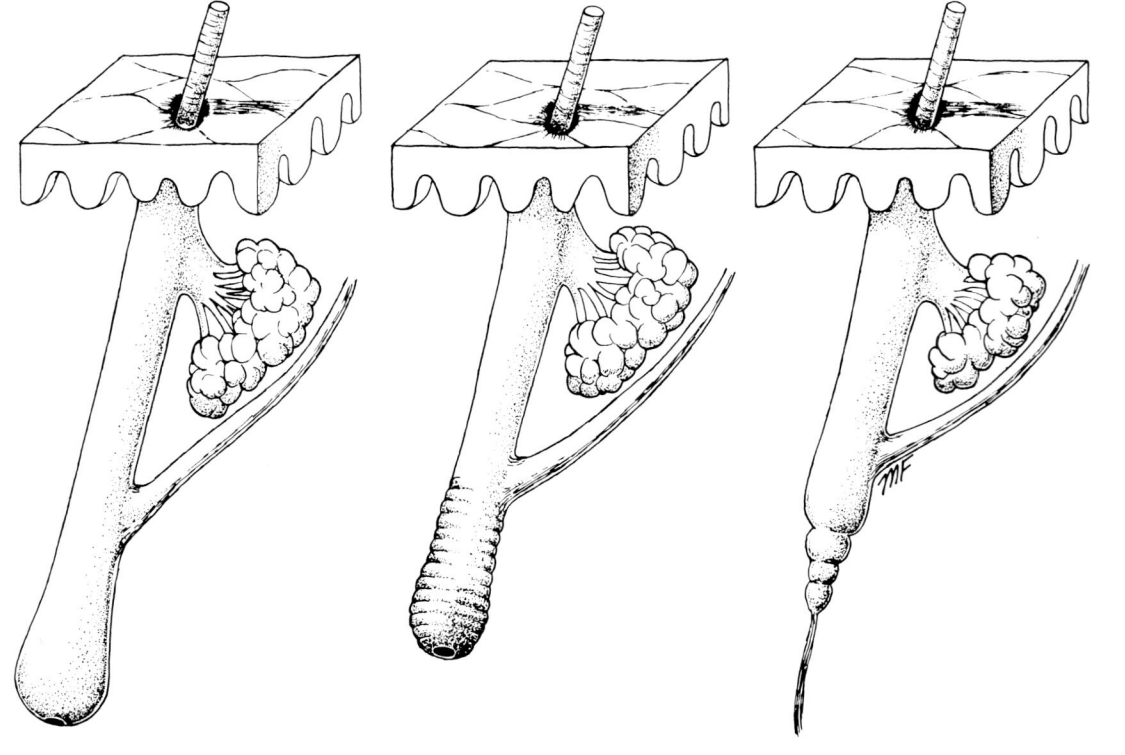

Anagen phase   Catagen phase   Telogen phase

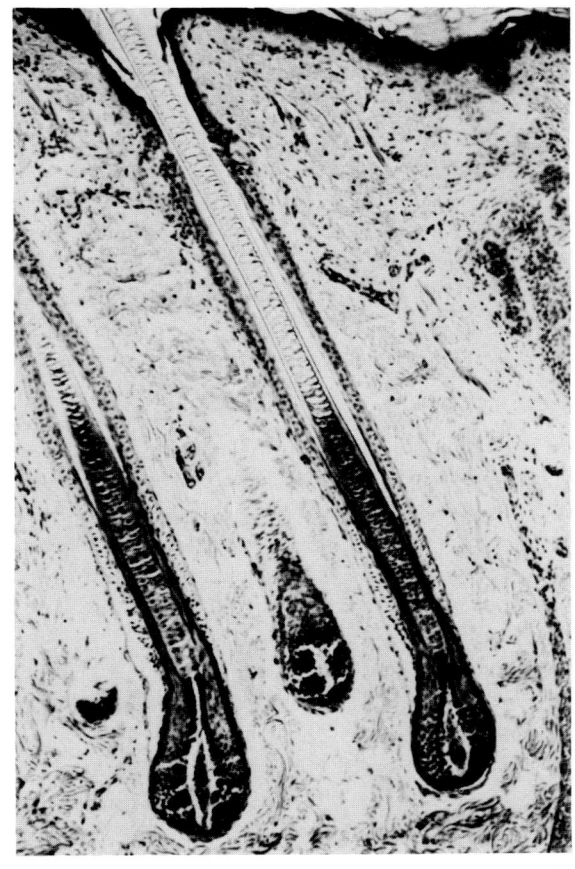

Fig. 17-27. Photomicrograph of a longitudinal section of hairy skin; the hair follicles are clearly visible, but the sebaceous glands are absent. (H&E.)

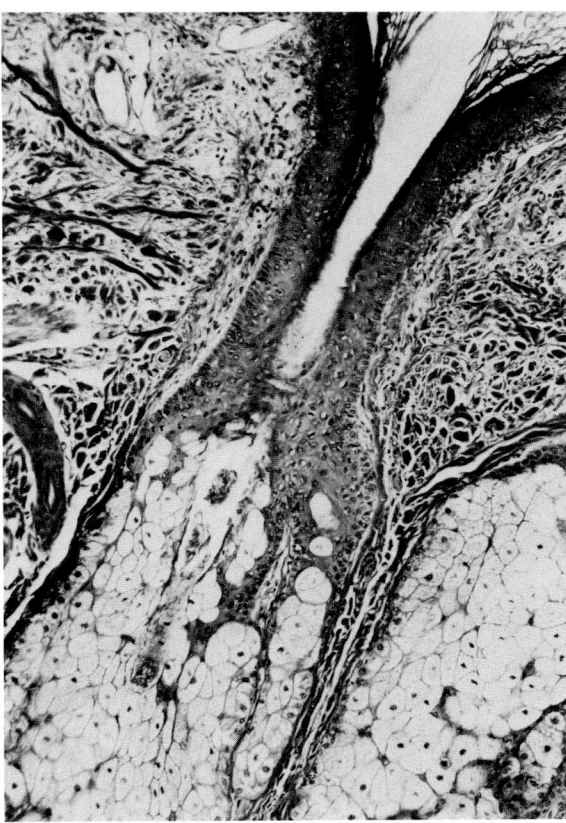

Fig. 17-28. Photomicrograph of a longitudinal section of hairy skin, showing a sebaceous gland opening into a hair follicle. (H&E; ×200.)

30 and 17-31). The cells also contain pigment granules. The *medulla* is absent from the fine hairs covering the surface of the body. It is composed of rows of large vacuolated cells that are separated by air spaces (see Fig. 17-30). The cells contain soft keratin and often possess pigment granules.

Growth of Hair

Hair grows as a result of the mitotic division of the matrix cells in the hair bulb. The cells in this region are nourished by tissue fluid derived from capillaries in the hair papilla. The newly formed cells are forced up the lumen of the outer epithelial root sheath. As the cells ascend, they become keratinized and form the cuticle, cortex, and medulla of the hair shaft.

At the same time, the proliferating cells around the periphery of the hair bulb form a tubular sheath of cells that ascends around the growing hair and separates it from the outer epithelial root sheath. The tubular sheath is called the inner epithelial root sheath and extends upward only as far as the entrance of the sebaceous gland into the follicle (see Fig. 17-24).

The rate of hair growth varies from region to region, as well as with sex and age. It ranges from about 1.5 to 2.2 mm per week.

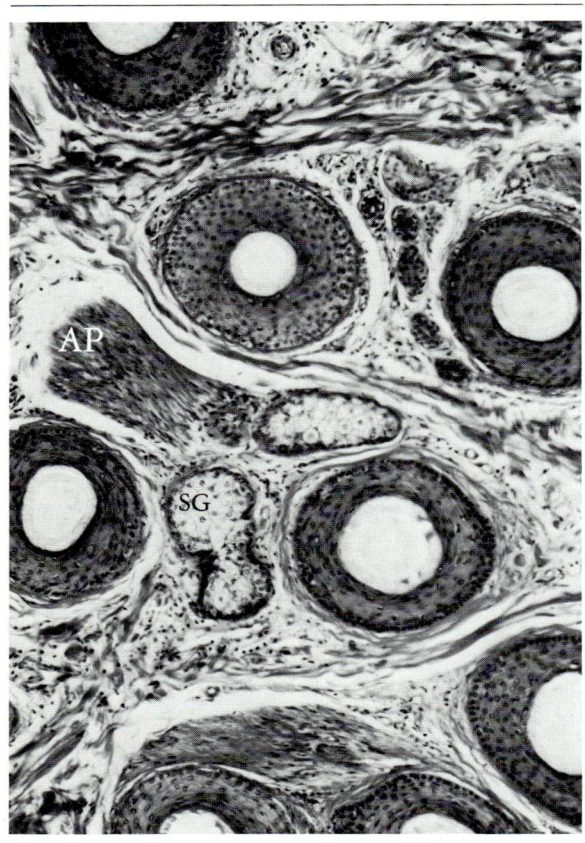

Fig. 17-29. *Photomicrograph of a horizontal section through the dermis of hairy skin, showing several hair follicles cut in cross section. Note the sebaceous glands (SG) and arrector pili muscles (AP). (H&E; ×100.)*

Pigmentation of Hair

The pigment of hair is formed by melanocytes situated in the hair bulb close to the papilla (Fig. 17-32; see Fig. 17-30). The dendritic processes of these melanocytes insinuate themselves among cells that will differentiate into medullary and cortical cells of the hair shaft. The pigment granules then will be transferred to the medullary and cortical cells and later will become embedded in the keratin within these cells (see Figs. 17-31 and 17-32). The melanocytes in the hair bulb replace themselves by mitotic division.

The different hair colors are produced by two pigments, the brown-black melanin and the yellow *pheomelanin*. The brown-black melanin is derived from tyrosine, and the pheomelanin is derived from tryptophan. Graying or whitening of hair with age has two causes: (1) the failure of the melanocytes in the germinal matrix of the hair bulb to continue to form pigment granules and (2) the appearance of small air bubbles in the cortex and medulla of the hair shaft. The reflection of light in the air bubbles is responsible for the glistening or silvery appearance of white hair.

Elevation of Hair

Small bundles of smooth muscle cells called the arrector pili muscle (see Figs. 17-24 and 17-29) arise from the connective tissue of the papillary layer of the dermis and are inserted into the outer coat of the hair follicle below the entrance of the duct of the sebaceous gland. They are located on the side of the follicle toward which the exposed part of the hair slopes (see Fig. 17-24). The smooth muscle is innervated by postganglionic sympathetic fibers. When the muscle contracts, the hair becomes more erect and slightly elevated; the hair follicle is raised slightly, so that the epidermis around the mouth of the follicle is elevated, producing the so-called goose bumps. Because of their position, the sebaceous glands are compressed and sebum is expressed onto the hair.

Sebaceous Glands

Sebaceous glands are found in the dermis of the skin all over the body except the palms and the soles. The great majority discharge their contents via a single duct into the lumen of hair follicles (see Figs. 17-24, 17-28, and 17-29). The remainder of the glands occur independently of hairs and open directly onto the surface of the skin, as, for example, on the margins of the lips, the glans penis, the areola of the breast, the labia minora, and the tarsal glands of the eyelids.

Each sebaceous gland consists of a cluster of alveoli that open into a single duct (see Figs. 17-24 and 17-28). An alveolus is lined with a stratified

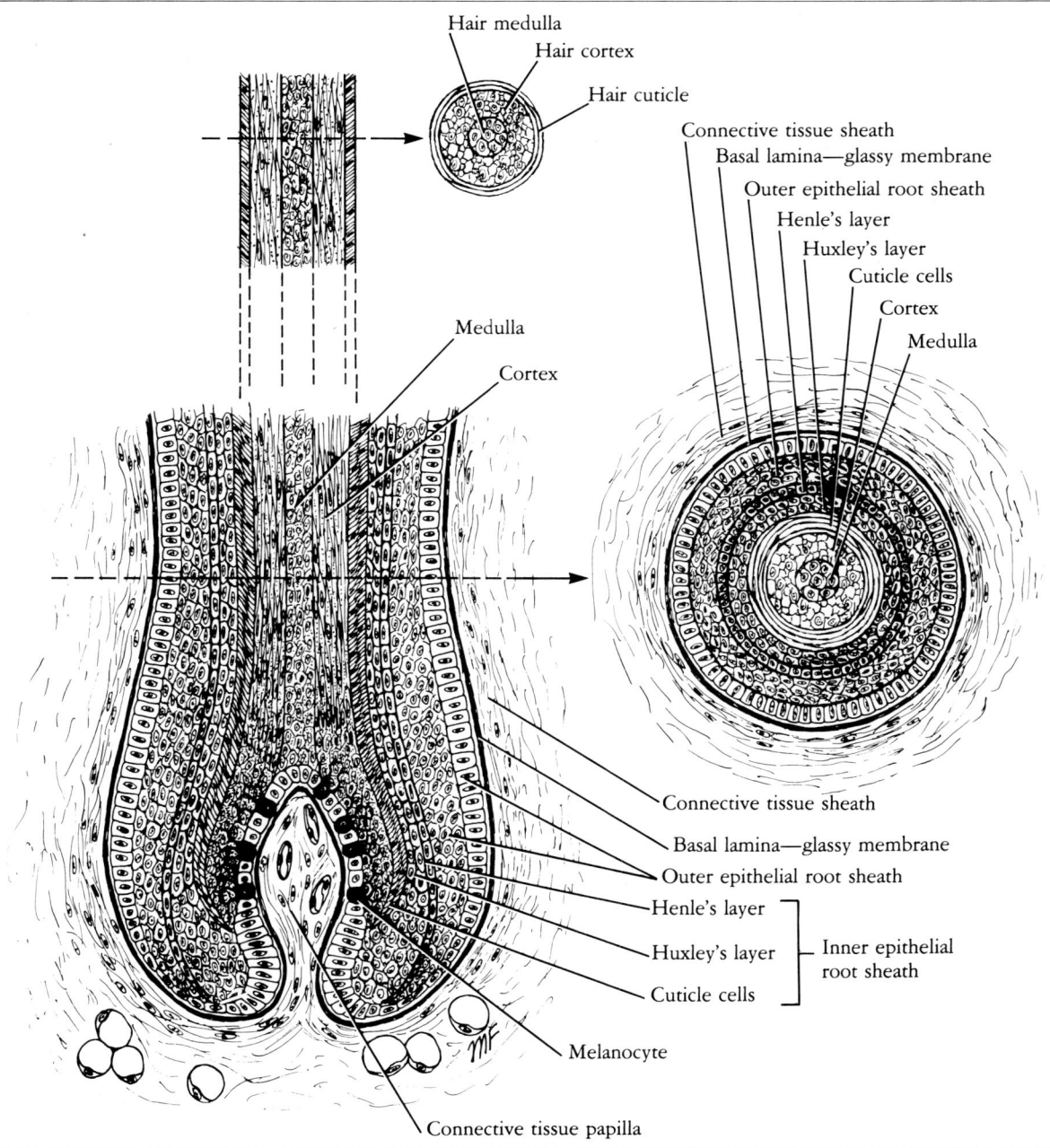

Fig. 17-30. Detailed structure of a hair shaft and a hair follicle in longitudinal and cross sections.

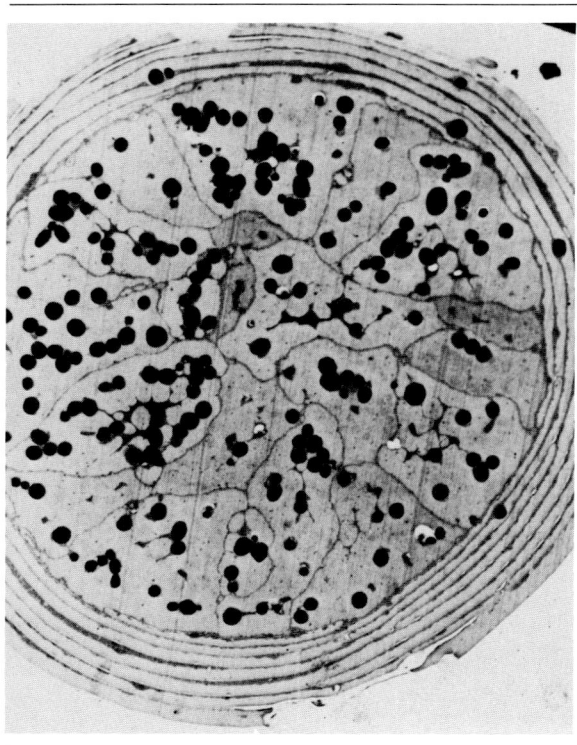

Fig. 17-31. Electron micrograph of a black hair in transverse section, showing a few melanin granules in the concentrically arranged flattened cuticle cells and a large number in the cortical cells in the interior of the hair. No medullary cells are present at this level in the hair.

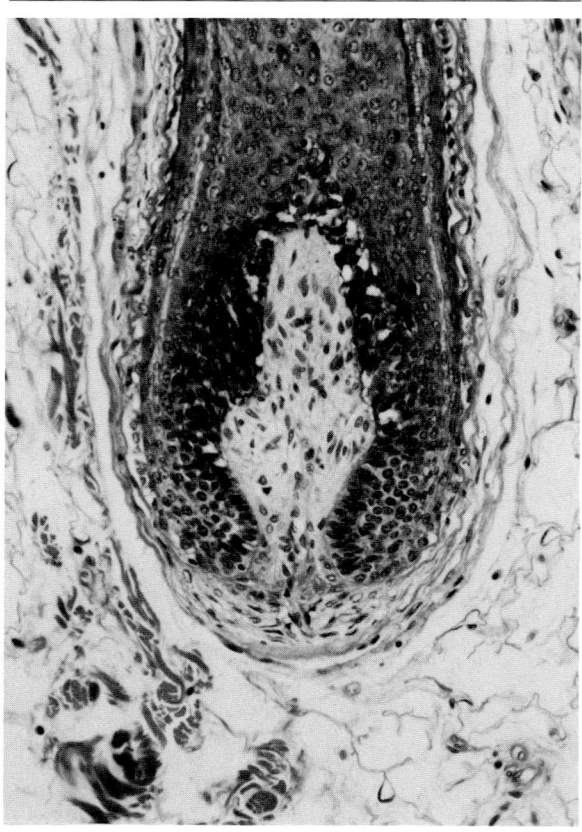

Fig. 17-32. Photomicrograph of a longitudinal section of a black hair bulb, showing the connective tissue papilla, the different layers in the structure of the hair, and the inner and outer root sheaths. Consulting Figure 17-30 should assist you in identifying the main layers. (H&E; ×200.)

epithelium resting on a basal lamina. The lumen of the alveolus is packed with cells containing lipid droplets. The central cells degenerate, die, and disintegrate (holocrine secretion), and the debris (sebum) is discharged into the hair follicle through the duct or onto the skin surface. The dead and disintegrating cells are replaced by deeper cells situated on the basal lamina. The contraction of the arrector pili muscle assists the gland in discharging its contents by exerting pressure on the outer surfaces of the alveoli.

The sebum contains triglycerides, fatty acids, squalene, wax ester, cholesterol, and cholesterol esters. Sebum serves as a natural lubricant of the hair and prevents it from becoming brittle. Sebum also oils the surface of the skin, preventing excessive water evaporation from the stratum corneum when the humidity of the air is low; it also protects the skin against excess surface water. It is believed to have some bactericidal action.

The sebaceous glands are not under nervous control, but they are stimulated by hormones, especially androgens. Before puberty, sebaceous glands are very small, but under the influence of testosterone at puberty, their size and activity greatly increase. In women, the increased activity of sebaceous glands is thought to be caused by adrenal androgens or androgens that may be produced by the ovary. Estrogens depress the activity of sebaceous glands.

Sweat Glands

Sweat glands are distributed throughout the skin of the body except the margins of the lips, the glans penis, and the nail beds. Two types of sweat glands exist, eccrine and apocrine.

The *eccrine glands* are the most common form of sweat glands and are most concentrated in the palms and soles. They are simple tubular glands (Figs. 17-33 and 17-34; see Fig. 17-4). The body of the gland is coiled and situated in the deeper part of the dermis or in the superficial fascia. The duct of the gland is relatively straight and opens onto the free surface of the epidermis by a funnel-shaped aperture.

Microscopically, the tubular gland consists of an outer layer of connective tissue and an inner layer of epithelium (see Figs. 17-33 and 17-34). The connective tissue layer is composed of delicate areolar tissue. The epithelial layer in the body, or secretory part, of the gland consists of cuboidal or polyhedral cells that can be divided into dark and clear cells on the basis of their affinity for stains. Outside the secretory cells but within the basal lamina is an incomplete layer of myoepithelial cells.

The epithelial layer in the duct of the gland is made up of two layers of dark-staining polyhedral cells. On reaching the epidermis, the duct becomes continuous with a spiral intercellular cleft that ascends to the surface between the epidermal cells. The ducts possess no myoepithelial cells.

Eccrine sweat glands are innervated by postganglionic cholinergic (not adrenergic) sympathetic fibers. Glands deprived of their innervation or subjected to anticholinergic drug action cease to be active.

The function of the secretory cells of the sweat glands is to produce a watery secretion. The secretory product of the epithelial cells is modified as it ascends through the duct to the surface. Large amounts of sodium chloride are excreted by this route, as well as urea, lactic acid, and potassium ions. Drugs, proteins, and various antibodies may be excreted by this route.

The primary function of sweat produced by the eccrine sweat glands is to assist in maintaining a normal body temperature. Once the sweat reaches the epidermal surface, it evaporates; the latent heat required for this evaporation is taken from the body. An increase in the temperature of the blood circulating through the hypothalamus increases the activity of the sympathetic nerves, and the body loses heat by sweating and by vasodilatation of the dermal capillaries. Exposure of the body to excess heat causes sweating to begin on the forehead and then spread down over the remainder of the body. In contrast, sweating caused by emotional and mental stimuli starts on the palms and soles and in the axillae and then spreads elsewhere. The contraction of the myoepithelial cells assists in the discharge of the secretion. The hormone aldosterone increases the reabsorption of sodium chloride and the secretion of potassium as sweat passes along the duct of a sweat gland. This process enables the body to conserve sodium chloride in hot climates.

The *apocrine glands* are far less numerous than the eccrine sweat glands and are found mainly in the axilla, scrotum, prepuce, labia minora, and nipple, and the perianal region (see Fig. 17-33). The glands are larger than the eccrine glands and tend to open into the hair follicles just above the openings of the sebaceous glands. They produce a viscous secretion and are innervated by adrenergic postganglionic sympathetic nerve fibers.

The structure of the apocrine sweat glands is similar to that of the eccrine gland, but there are no clear cells in the body, or secretory part, of the gland. The body of the gland is made up of a coiled tube, but many of the coils anastomose to form a network. At one time the apical part of the secretory cell was thought to be lost into the secretion during the formation of sweat by these glands, whence the name apocrine. Now we believe that this occurrence is an artifact and that all sweat glands are merocrine glands.

The secretion of apocrine sweat glands has an oily consistency and sometimes a yellowish color. On reaching the surface, it is odorless; bacterial decomposition is responsible for the musky odor. The secretion is produced continuously and is not con-

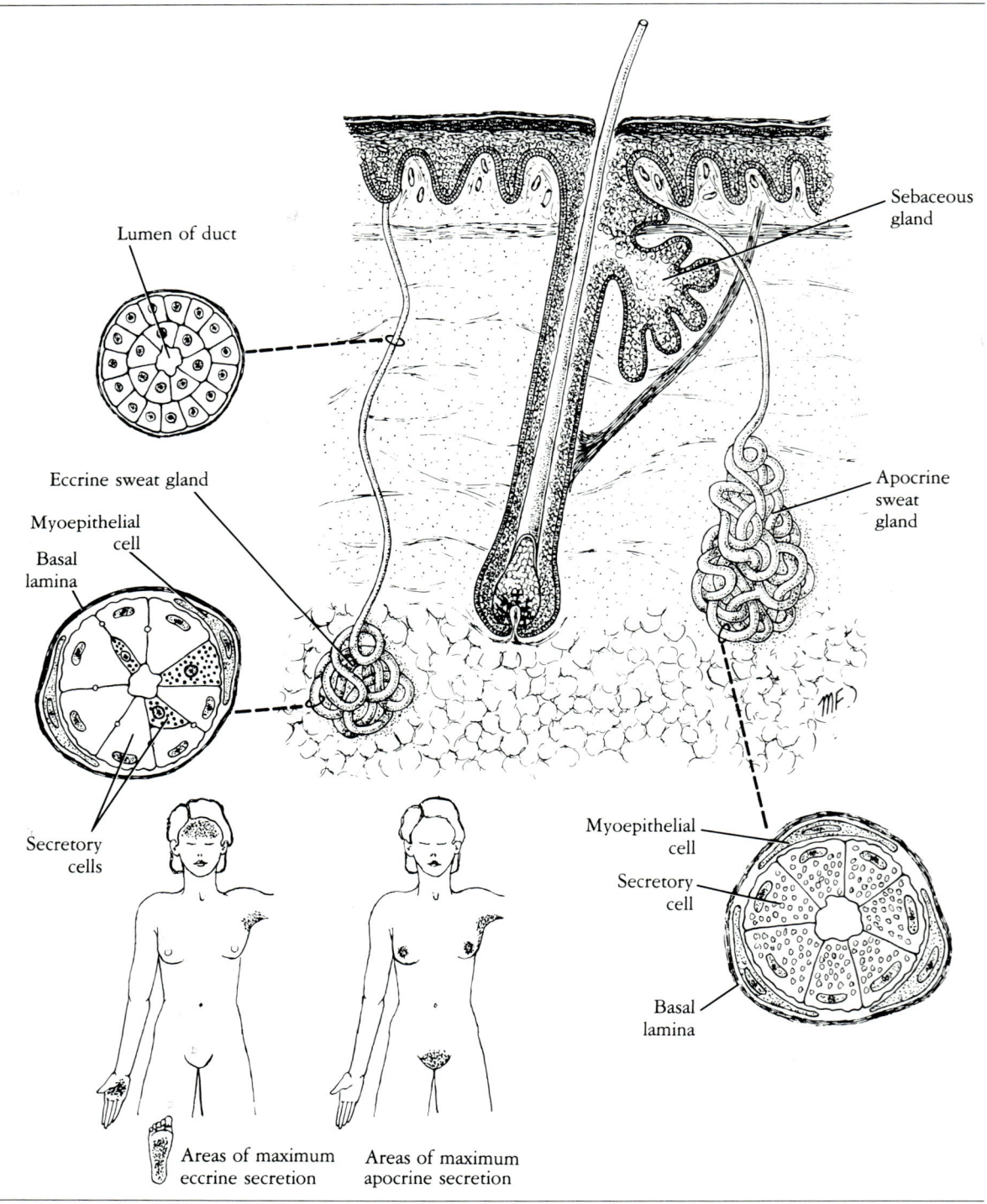

cerned with thermoregulation; the glands may have a sexual function during foreplay. Apocrine glands start to function at puberty and are under the control of the sex hormones; the secretion is increased by emotional stimulation via the sympathetic nerve fibers.

The *ciliary glands (glands of Moll)* are modified apocrine glands that are found at the margins of the eyelids and open into or near the orifices of the eyelash follicles. The *ceruminous glands* are also modified apocrine glands; they are found in the skin lining the external auditory meatus. The ducts of the glands open onto the surface or into the hair follicles. The ceruminous glands secrete ear wax, which protects the skin against maceration and produces a sticky substance to repel insects.

Superficial Fascia

The superficial fascia (subcutaneous tissue, hypodermis) lies beneath the skin and is continuous with the dermis. It is composed of a mixture of loose areolar tissue and adipose tissue and serves to unite the dermis with the underlying deep fascia. In the scalp, the back of the neck, the palms, and the soles, it contains numerous bundles of collagen fibers that hold the skin firmly to the deeper structures. In the eyelids, auricle of the ear, penis and scrotum, and clitoris, it is devoid of adipose tissue. The superficial fascia contains many blood and lymphatic vessels and nerve trunks and nerve endings.

AGING OF SKIN

Generally, skin reaches its optimal appearance during the second and third decades, and then age changes begin to occur. The visible changes in the skin associated with growing old are wrinkling, loss of elasticity, dryness, and spotty pigmentation, particularly on the face and the dorsum of the hands. Depigmentation of the hair and loss of hair are also

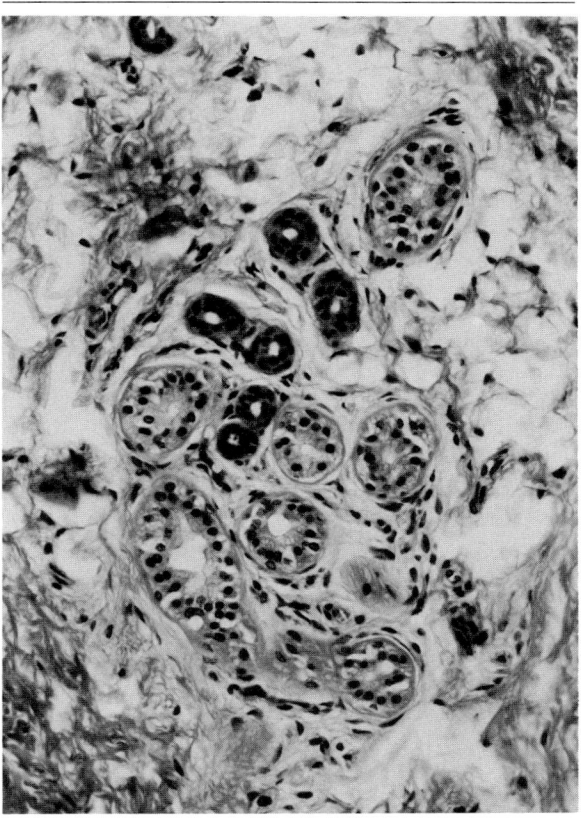

Fig. 17-34. Photomicrograph of a vertical section of the deeper part of the dermis, showing the coiled body and part of the duct of an eccrine sweat gland. Note the clear-staining cells that form the body of the gland and the darker-staining cells that form the duct of the gland. (H&E; ×200.)

Fig. 17-33. Structure of an eccrine and an apocrine sweat gland; note the locations of their duct openings onto the skin surface. The bottom part of the figure shows the skin areas where eccrine and apocrine secretion mainly take place.

signs of aging. In the face, the loss of tone of the facial muscles and loss of subcutaneous fat also add to the senile changes of the face. The whole process can be hastened by prolonged exposure to the wind and sun, as is commonly seen in the skin of farmers and sailors.

The age changes in the dermis are the most obvious. The elastic fibers become fragmented, and the collagen becomes stiffer. More cross links are formed between the collagen fibrils, and they become tougher and less elastic. Females initially have less collagen in their dermis than do males, so they appear to age more rapidly. Red- and fair-haired individuals have less melanin in their epidermis for protection against ultraviolet light, so their exposed dermis ages more rapidly. For the same reason, white skin ages sooner than black skin. There is some flattening of the epidermal ridges with age, but there is no reduction in the number of cell layers. There is a progressive reduction in the number of functioning melanocytes with age. It is generally believed that the number of melanocytes remains unchanged but that the tyrosinase activity of these cells diminishes.

The number of hairs on the scalp is reduced, and there is an associated reduction in the density of hair follicles. The sebaceous glands remain unchanged. Eccrine sweat glands show a reduction in activity and number with age; apocrine glands become less active, and some may atrophy. Nail growth slows with age.

CLINICAL NOTES

The skin is one of the most important organs of the body. It should not be considered merely a covering, for it is made up of a complicated mixture of epithelial, glandular, connective tissue, and neurovascular structures, all of which are important in maintaining body homeostasis. Disease of internal organs commonly reveals itself by changes in the appearance of the skin. A physician can recognize, for example, pallor, cyanosis, jaundice, and changes in melanin pigmentation. A local area of redness, a nodule, or even an ulcer may result from some general pathological process in which the skin is only one of many organs involved. The skin is also subject to a large number of diseases that involve it alone, however.

How, then, are medical students to keep from being overwhelmed by the thousands of different skin lesions that they might come across during a clinical examination of the skin? First, they must have a thorough understanding of the normal appearance, structure, and function of the skin in different parts of the body. Then, they must train themselves to appreciate that a careful examination of the skin, which can be done with the naked eye, will often enable them to detect clues of disease. If the gross examination is insufficient, abnormal cellular changes can often be detected by studying the microscopic appearance of a biopsy specimen. With increasing experience, students will be able to categorize skin lesions into those that involve the skin alone and those that are secondary to disease elsewhere. A good physician knows the normal variations in the appearance of skin in different parts of the body and has trained his or her eye to be receptive to detecting subtle abnormalities of skin structure.

This section will not describe large numbers of skin lesions. Rather, examples of common pathological processes involving the different structures that make up the skin will be discussed briefly to illustrate the importance of knowing the structure and function of normal skin, and how these may be altered by disease.

SURGICAL SCARS, INVASION BY MICROORGANISMS, BURNS AND SKIN GRAFTING

Surgical Scars and Lines of Cleavage

A general knowledge of the direction of the lines of cleavage greatly assists the surgeon in making incisions that will result in cosmetically acceptable scars. This is particularly important in patients to whom physical appearance is of especially great concern and in those areas of the body not normally covered by clothing. A salesman, for example, may lose his job if an operation leaves a greatly disfiguring scar on his face.

A surgical incision through the skin made along or between the lines of cleavage causes the minimum of disruption of the dermal collagen, and the wound heals with minimal scar tissue. An incision made across the rows of collagen disrupts and disturbs the collagen, however, resulting in the massive production of fresh collagen and the formation of a broad, ugly scar. This condition must not be confused with keloid formation. *Keloid scars* occur most often in blacks and are genetically related. In that process, an abnormal production of collagen occurs, leading to a large, unsightly scar.

Potential Sites for Entry of Microorganisms

The nail folds, hair follicles, and sebaceous glands are common sites for the entrance into the underlying tissues of pathogenic organisms, such as *Staphylococcus aureus*. Infection occurring between the nail and the nail fold is called a *paronychia*. Infection of the hair follicle and sebaceous gland is responsible for the common *boil*. A *carbuncle* is a staphylococcal infection of the superficial fascia. It frequently occurs in the nape of the neck and usually starts as an infection of a hair follicle or a group of hair follicles.

Skin Burns

The depth of a burn determines the method and rate of healing. A partial-thickness burn of the skin will heal from the cells of the hair follicles, sebaceous glands, and sweat glands, as well as from the cells at the edge of the burn. A burn that extends deeper than the sweat glands, a full-thickness skin burn, will heal very slowly from the edges only, and there will be considerable contracture caused by fibrous tissue. To speed healing and reduce the incidence of contracture, a deep burn should be grafted.

In a partial-thickness burn, the skin area becomes reddened because the dermal blood vessels dilate. The increased permeability leads to an outpouring of tissue fluid, with the formation of a typical blister. In a full-thickness burn, the connective tissue of the dermis and even the superficial fascia are burned. Massive vasodilatation occurs in the area and surrounding tissues, causing a great loss of fluid and plasma proteins. With large burns, there is a progressive loss of plasma protein and fluid, causing cardiovascular shock.

Burning of the skin sterilizes the area for about 24 hours. Thereafter, pathogenic bacteria, including *Staphylococcus aureus* and streptococci residing on the neighboring skin, quickly invade the area and multiply in the protein-rich exudate. A badly burned patient, therefore, not only has the local injury but, even more important, has to deal with the cardiovascular shock and secondary infection.

Skin Grafting

Skin grafting is of two main types, split-thickness grafting and full-thickness grafting. In a *split-thickness skin graft*, the greater part of the epidermis, including the tips of the dermal papillae, are removed from the donor site and placed on the recipient site. This leaves at the donor site for repair purposes the epidermal cells on the sides of the dermal papillae and the cells of the hair follicles and sweat glands.

A *full-thickness skin graft* includes both the epidermis and dermis and, to survive, requires the rapid establishment of a new circulation within it at the recipient site. The donor site is usually covered with a split-thickness graft. In certain circumstances, a full-thickness graft is made in the form of a pedicle graft, in which a flap of full-thickness skin is turned and stitched in position at the recipient site, leaving the base of the flap with its blood supply intact at the donor site.

CONDITIONS OF THE EPIDERMIS

Conditions of Keratinocytes

Psoriasis

Psoriasis consists of red patches of scaly skin occurring most often on the extensor surfaces. It can occur at any age and its cause is not known; it has been suggested that some patients may have immunological abnormalities. In psoriasis, there is a very rapid turnover time for keratinocytes: 3 to 4 days, compared with 28 days in normal skin. There is incomplete cell differentiation, with decreased formation of tonofilaments and keratohyalin granules. The epidermis is thickened, and the dermal papillary capillaries are dilated. Neutrophils migrate from the capillaries into the epidermis. The treatment of psoriasis is directed to slowing down the mitotic activity of the epidermal cells. Sunlight or ultraviolet light inhibits epidermal mitosis; coal tar applications have a similar effect. Corticosteroids are also effective because of their antimitotic, antimetabolic, and vasoconstrictive properties.

Eczema

Eczema is a very common disorder of the skin involving the epidermis, with edema, exudation, and crusting. It is accompanied by severe itching (pruritus). The dermis shows edema and the presence of lymphocytes, monocytes, and eosinophils. There are many different types of eczema, with different causes. Atopic eczema, for example, starts early in life and is an immunological disorder; contact dermatitis often is caused by an immune hypersensitivity to a foreign antigen.

Benign Tumors of Keratinocytes

Benign tumors of keratinocytes are very common. *Seborrheic keratosis* is a tumor of the cells of the stratum germinativum of the epidermis. Such tumors most often occur after middle age and arise singly or in groups; they grow slowly. They usually require no treatment.

Polyps are soft pedunculated tumors or skin tags that occur most often in middle age. Histologically, a polyp has a core of connective tissue that is continuous with the dermis. The connective tissue is covered with an overgrown epidermis. The lesion is either left untreated or removed for cosmetic reasons.

Malignant Tumors of Keratinocytes

The common tumors are basal cell carcinoma and squamous cell carcinoma. *Basal cell carcinoma* is a tumor that arises from the basal cells or cells of the stratum germinativum of the epidermis. It is locally invasive and is visible as islands of cells that have extended down into the dermis. Clinically, the lesion presents on the sun-exposed parts of the face as a raised area that later has a central ulcer with a beaded edge. Treatment is surgical removal or irradiation. The prognosis is excellent.

Squamous cell carcinoma arises from the cells of the stratum germinativum of the epidermis. It grows rapidly and will spread to local lymph nodes. Chronic exposure to the sun is the most common predisposing factor. The more slowly growing tumors show few mitoses and evidence of keratinization, whereas the more malignant tumors show multiple mitoses and little differentiation. Complete surgical excision or irradiation is the treatment of choice.

Conditions of Melanocytes

Freckles (Ephelides)

Freckles are brown patches of varying size scattered irregularly over white skin that has been exposed to sunlight or ultraviolet light. They contain a group of melanocytes that are capable of forming melanin more rapidly than are the melanocytes in the surrounding, paler skin. Freckles are most often seen in red or blond children and tend to fade with age.

Melasma

Melasma is a hyperpigmentation of the face that occurs commonly in pregnant women (Fig. 17-35). It is a blotchy brown pigmentation of the cheeks, temples, and forehead. Histologically, the melanocytes in this area are producing more melanin than are those elsewhere (except the anterior abdominal wall and genital regions) in response to the increased levels of circulating sex hormones found in pregnancy. The condition fades after parturition.

Vitiligo

Vitiligo is a depigmentation disorder resulting from an inherited defect in the skin and hair that has caused the destruction and disappearance of melanocytes. Clinically, there are scattered, localized patches of white skin or white hairs. The condition occurs at any age. The only treatment available is to apply cosmetics over the affected skin areas or produce depigmentation of the surrounding skin with a cream containing hydroquinone; this drug inhibits melanogenesis.

Albinism

Albinism occurs in two forms, *ocular albinism* and *oculocutaneous albinism*. It is essentially an inherited defect transmitted as an autosomal recessive trait. Melanocytes are present in normal numbers but are

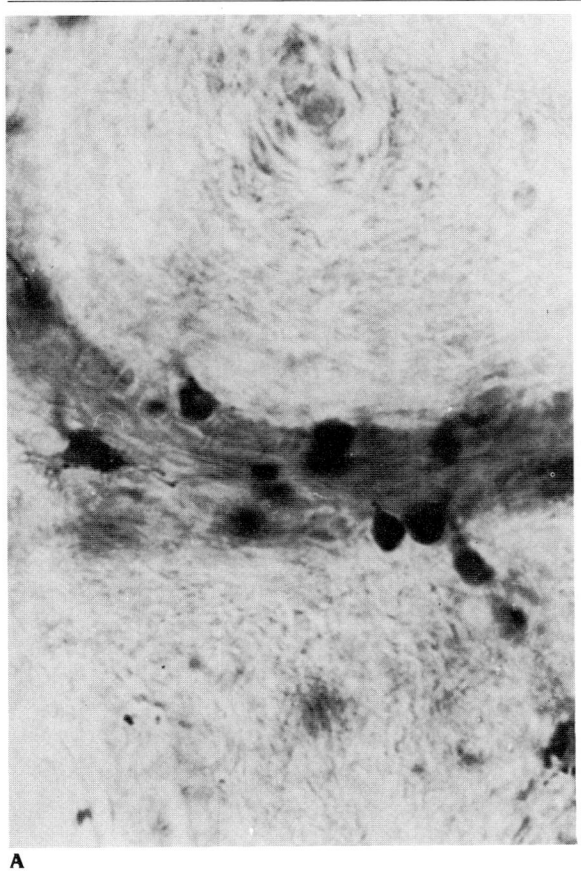 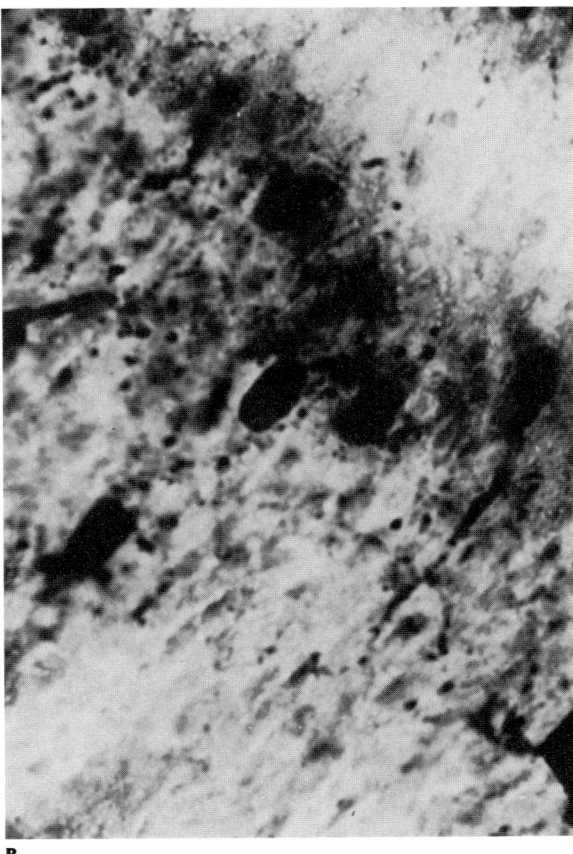

Fig. 17-35. Photomicrograph of epidermal sheets of the anterior abdominal wall skin of women. (A) Nonpregnant woman shows a number of melanocytes containing a moderate amount of melanin situated in an epidermal ridge. (B) Pregnant woman shows many melanocytes packed full with melanin. (Treated with DOPA reagent; ×750.)

incapable of producing normal amounts of melanin. Theoretically, then, the condition could result from (1) a diminished amount of the enzyme tyrosinase within the melanocytes, (2) an inability of the melanocytes to absorb sufficient tyrosine, or (3) the presence of tyrosinase inhibitors. The most probable cause is a deficiency of the enzyme tyrosinase within the melanocytes. In the eye, the lack of melanin pigment in the iris and retina leads to excessive sensitivity to bright light, and visual acuity is impaired. In the skin, there is an increased sensitivity to ultraviolet light, with an increased frequency of malignant disease of the keratinocytes. Affected patients are instructed to apply sunscreen lotions and wear dark glasses; no other treatment is available.

Benign Tumors of Melanocytes

Lentigo is a common lesion found at all ages; it consists of small brown or black pigmented areas. In the epidermis of these areas, the melanocytes have proliferated and are more active than normal. In contrast to freckles, the lesions of lentigo do not darken with exposure to sunlight. Lentigines do not become malignant and require no treatment.

Moles, or *nevi,* are scattered over the body surface in most normal individuals. Moles may be present at birth, although the majority appear in childhood.

They are brown and flat, raised, or even papillary; they may have a few or many hairs emerging from their surface. Histologically, a mole consists of a group of actively proliferating melanocytes. Moles are not premalignant lesions and should be removed only if subject to repeated trauma, such as shaving, or if there is a sudden increase in size or darkening in color.

Malignant Tumors of Melanocytes

Malignant melanoma is a malignant tumor of melanocytes and is responsible for about 1 percent of cancers. Most arise spontaneously, although about 25 percent arise in association with a preexisting nevus. There is an increased incidence of melanoma in whites exposed to excess solar radiation. The rapidly multiplying melanocytes spread deeply into the dermis and invade blood vessels and lymphatic vessels. The treatment is wide local excision and removal of regional lymph nodes. Chemotherapy and regional perfusion with cytotoxic drugs are also employed.

CONDITIONS OF THE DERMIS

The dermis is made up of a large number of different structures, each of which can produce a wide variety of diseases. It is not intended that this section present a synopsis of diseases of the dermis; its purpose is to highlight a few diseases that are important to the physician and to emphasize once again the necessity of knowing the normal structure and function of the skin.

Urticaria

In this condition, there are itchy, pink or white wheals associated with edema of the dermis. Urticaria is produced by a localized increase in capillary permeability, with trapping of the exudate within the connective tissue of the dermis. In most patients, the cause is unknown; in the remainder, there is hypersensitivity to specific substances such as foods, pollens, chemicals, or physical agents. Histamine release is responsible for the local vasodilatation and increased permeability of the capillaries in many patients.

Tumors of the Dermis

Fibrous histiocytoma is a benign tumor involving the proliferation of fibroblasts and dermal macrophages (histiocytes). In a minority of cases, the growth follows trauma to the skin.

A *capillary hemangioma* is a benign vascular tumor of dermal capillaries. It makes its appearance soon after birth, when it is commonly referred to as a strawberry mark or port-wine stain. The majority of these tumors disappear spontaneously within a few years. A *cavernous hemangioma* is a benign lesion composed of large vascular channels that appear in the dermis. These channels produce a raised, red lesion of the skin. The tumors may be removed surgically.

CONDITIONS OF SKIN APPENDAGES

Conditions of the Nails

In *paronychia,* the nail fold becomes infected by bacteria or fungi. The fold becomes tender, swollen, and red. *Brittle nails* are associated with calcium deficiency. *Pale nails* occur in cases of hypoalbuminemia and hepatic disease. The proximal end of the nail appears white because of changes in the nail bed.

Conditions Affecting Hair Growth

Baldness

Baldness occurs in both sexes and is associated with aging. It starts with a gradual recession of the anterior hair line and moves posteriorly over the frontal region to the vertex. The hair loss in women is usually less than that in men. The condition is caused by progressive atrophy of the hair follicles with age. The coarse terminal hairs are replaced with fine vellus hairs. The pathogenesis is related not only to age, but also to genetic factors and the presence of androgenic hormones.

Alopecia

Alopecia may occur following an acute febrile illness, acute metabolic disorders, or acute psychiatric disorders. The cause of the condition is an alteration of the normal hair cycle, so that many anagen follicles are converted into telogen follicles. After the patient recovers from the precipitating illness, the follicles are reactivated and revert to anagen follicles.

Hair loss is seen in endocrine disorders such as hypopituitarism and hypothyroidism. Antimitotic agents used in the treatment of malignant disease may inhibit hair growth, which returns to normal after the drug treatment has ceased. Anticoagulant drugs such as heparin also produce alopecia.

Alopecia areata is a condition in which a patient suddenly notices rounded patches of scalp hair loss. More patches appear over the next 2 months. The hair follicles are surrounded in their lower halves by chronic inflammatory cells, most of which are lymphocytes. The follicles shrink, and the epidermal cells degenerate. The cause of the condition is not known, although autoimmune disease and psychological trauma have been suggested. In most patients, regrowth occurs within a year without treatment.

Hirsutism and Hypertrichosis

Both these conditions involve an excessive growth of hair. The term *hirsutism*, however, is usually used to apply only to excessive hair growth in women and children with a distribution similar to that normally found in men.

In hirsutism, the vellus hairs are converted into large terminal hairs, and in many individuals, the levels of circulating androgens are higher than normal. In female patients, the testosterone may originate in the suprarenal gland or the ovary. Because the general body build remains feminine in many patients, it is thought that in these cases the hair follicles may be excessively sensitive to androgen stimulation.

Hypertrichosis may be localized or generalized and may be caused by a wide variety of diseases. The underlying reason for hypertrichosis in these cases is not always understood. Any condition that increases the local vascularity of the dermis may increase hair growth. For example, chronic trauma or low-grade chronic inflammation may produce localized hypertrichosis.

Conditions of the Sebaceous Glands
Seborrhea
Seborrhea is the production of excess quantities of sebum, which gives the face an oily appearance and makes the hair look lank and greasy. The physiological form of seborrhea starts at puberty and may last until age 25. It is more severe in men. Regular washing of the face and scalp is the most satisfactory treatment.

Acne Vulgaris

This is a chronic inflammatory disease of the hair follicles and sebaceous glands (pilosebaceous follicles) seen in adolescents. It occurs in all races, and more severe lesions are found in the male. The main sites are the face, back, chest, and shoulders, and the lesions are most numerous near the midline. The development of the lesion depends on an increase in sebum production and blockage of the sebaceous gland duct. The cause is multifactorial and includes androgen production and genetic factors.

The combination of increased sebum production and a blocked sebaceous duct leads to a raised, tender area of the skin. Very often, the orifice of the hair follicle is filled with a horny plug of keratin known as a *comedo*. The tip of the plug is dark (a blackhead) because of oxidation. Sometimes, the tip of the comedo is largely covered by the superficial cells of the stratum corneum. Bacterial infection of the follicle by *Corynebacterium acnes* and *Staphylococcus* organisms is nearly always present. It is thought that these organisms break down the trapped sebum, yielding fatty acids that are irritating to the dermis and start the inflammatory response. As the acute and chronic inflammatory reaction progresses, small dermal abscesses form. The process is frequently complicated by the rupture of the upper end of the hair follicle, containing the comedo and the remains of the sebaceous gland; discharge of the sebum into the dermis then occurs, and the inflammatory reaction becomes more intense. The condition is best treated with systemic antibiotics and the temporary use of topical steroids.

Conditions of the Sweat Glands
Conditions of the Eccrine Sweat Glands
Hyperhidrosis is excessive production of sweat. This condition may occur during infective processes, such as tonsillitis, pneumonia, malaria, and tuberculosis. In thyrotoxicosis and obesity, sweating is also an attempt to lose heat. Emotional hyperhidrosis affects primarily the palms, soles, and axillae. The condition is common in the adolescent and the young adult, and, although it may be associated with an emotional disorder, in many patients its cause is unknown. Such patients appear to have a low threshold for physiological mental sweating. The condition usually improves spontaneously.

Anhidrosis is the absence of sweat. There are many possible causes for this condition, ranging from an abnormality of the sweat gland to an interference with its nervous control. The danger of extensive anhidrosis is that it may cause hyperpyrexia when the individual is exposed to heat.

Miliaria is a lesion of the duct of a sweat gland in which the lumen is blocked and sweat production continues. Different kinds of lesions occur, corresponding to the different points of blockage of the duct. *Miliaria rubra,* or prickly heat, is a very common condition occurring in hot, humid climates. The duct is blocked in the midepidermis. The duct becomes dilated proximal to the block just below the stratum granulosum. The secretory part of the gland in the dermis is surrounded by an inflammatory exudate, and capillary dilatation occurs. The patient experiences a prickling, stinging sensation. Examination reveals multiple reddened papules. The treatment is directed to reducing sweating by cooling.

Bromhidrosis is excessive odor emanating from the skin, usually the axillae. In normal individuals, the axillary skin has an odor that starts at puberty and is caused by bacterial decomposition of apocrine sweat. It will be remembered that apocrine glands start to secrete sweat at puberty. Apocrine sweat production is small compared with eccrine sweat production, and on reaching the skin surface, apocrine sweat is sterile and odorless. Within a very short time, bacteria, mainly staphylococci, break down the fatty acids to produce a musty, acrid smell that varies in intensity and quantity in different individuals. The presence of axillary hair increases the surface area for accumulation and evaporation of the apocrine sweat, and the presence of eccrine sweat facilitates the spread of apocrine sweat. The treatment is frequent washing of the axillary region and the application of bactericidal agents, such as aluminum or zinc salts; the latter compounds also reduce to some extent axillary eccrine sweating.

CLINICAL PROBLEMS

For the answers to these problems, see page 821.

1. A dermatologist carefully examines skin markings on the anterior surface of the wrist region of a 35-year-old woman. Name two types of skin markings normally found in this region. What is responsible for these markings?

2. Explain how the skin defends the body against invasion by microorganisms.

3. The depth of a burn determines the method and rate of healing. Explain this statement, using a partial-thickness skin burn and a full-thickness skin burn as examples. If burning the skin sterilizes the area, why is the surgeon so concerned about the possibility of infection? Why is the patient likely to have cardiovascular shock in a severe burn?

4. What is the difference in structure between thick and thin skin? Is the dermis the same thickness in different parts of the body? Is the dermis of equal thickness in both sexes?

5. Describe in detail the process of keratinization. How long does it take for a new keratinocyte to pass from the stratum germinativum to the surface of the skin? Do you think that it is important for a dermatologist to explain the turnover time of keratino-

cytes to a patient who is about to receive steroid cream to be applied daily for contact dermatitis?

6. Name the different layers of cells found in the epidermis in thick skin.

7. Describe the electron microscopic features seen when an epidermal melanocyte is viewed with a transmission electron microscope.

8. What factors are responsible for the color of skin? Are pigment cells present in the dermis? What are Mongolian spots? What are melanophages?

9. Name a dendritic cell present in the epidermis that is not a melanocyte. What is the function of this cell? Is this cell related in any way to the melanocyte?

10. Name three malignant tumors of the epidermis. Identify the cell of origin of each.

11. Describe the structure of a hair follicle. Define each of the following: (a) anagen phase, (b) catagen phase, (c) telogen phase. What is responsible for hair color? Although baldness may occur in the young, it occurs in both sexes and often is associated with aging. What changes take place in the scalp in a middle-aged individual who is going bald?

12. Give a detailed account of the structure of the following: (a) sebaceous gland, (b) eccrine sweat gland, (c) apocrine sweat gland. What factors control the secretions of these glands?

13. A paronychia is a common infection involving the nail fold. Describe the structure of (a) the proximal nail fold, (b) the eponychium, (c) the nail bed, and (d) the nail body.

14. What are the normal changes that take place in the skin with age? Explain the term *striae gravidarum*.

15. Describe the role of the dermal blood vessels and the sweat glands in the thermoregulatory mechanisms of the body.

16. Some sweat glands are cholinergic, and others are adrenergic. Explain this statement.

17. A 25-year-old woman is examined in a mental institution because of excessive hair growth on the back of the index finger of her right hand. While talking to the patient, the physician notices that the woman tends to bite on and chew the dorsal surface of the affected finger. When asked, the charge nurse confirms that the patient often does this, especially in the presence of strangers. Can you explain the cause for the localized hypertrichosis?

18. An 18-year-old woman visits a dermatologist because of the presence of infected spots on her chin, chest, and back. She says she has experienced spots and blackheads in the same regions since she was 13 years old. She has been told by her family doctor that she is suffering from acne vulgaris and will grow out of it. She is now very concerned by the fact that as each lesion resolves, she is left with a scar. What is the cause of acne vulgaris? What course of treatment would you recommend?

19. Billions of dollars are made each year by cosmetic firms throughout the Western world through the sale of antiperspirants. Explain the production of excessive body odor emanating from the axillary skin. What glands are responsible for the secretion? Does the condition occur before puberty? What is the treatment of bromhidrosis?

20. Ultraviolet light can be harmful to the skin. Can you justify this statement? Explain the effect of ultraviolet light on (a) vitamin D metabolism, (b) skin pigmentation, and (c) the reproduction of keratinocytes.

ADDITIONAL READING

Braverman, I. N., and Yen, A. Ultrastructure of the human dermal microcirculation. II. The capillary loops of the dermal papillae. *J. Invest. Dermatol.* 68:53, 1977.

Breathnach, A. S. The cell of Langerhans. *Int. Rev. Cytol.* 18:1, 1965.

Breathnach, A. S. *An Atlas of the Ultrastructure of Human Skin.* London: Churchill, 1971.

Brody, I. Ultrastructure of the stratum corneum. *Dermatology* 16:245, 1977.

Champion, R. H., Gillman, T., Rook, A. J., and Sims, R. T. (eds.). *An Introduction to the Biology of the Skin.* Oxford and Edinburgh: Blackwell, 1970.

Chase, H. B. Growth of the hair. *Physiol. Rev.* 34:113, 1954.

Drochmans, P. On melanin granules. *Int. Rev. Exp. Pathol.* 2:357, 1963.

Ellis, R. A. Fine structure of the myoepithelium of the eccrine sweat glands of man. *J. Cell Biol.* 27:551, 1965.

Epstein, W. L., and Maibach, H. I. Cell renewal in human epidermis. *Arch. Dermatol.* 92:462, 1965.

Fitzpatrick, T. B., and Szabo, G. The melanocyte: Cytology and cytochemistry. *J. Invest. Dermatol.* 32:197, 1959.

Fitzpatrick, T. B., et al. (eds.). *Dermatology in General Medicine* (2nd ed.). New York: McGraw-Hill, 1979.

Guevedo, W. C., Jr. Epidermal melanin units: Melanocyte-keratinocyte interactions. *Am. Zool.* 12:35, 1972.

Halprin, K. M. Epidermal "turnover time": A reexamination. *J. Invest. Dermatol.* 86:14, 1972.

Hashiomoto, K. Ultrastructure of the human toe nail. *J. Ultrastruct. Res.* 36:391, 1971.

Lever, W. F., and Schaumberg-Lever, G. *Histopathology of the Skin* (5th ed.). Philadelphia: Lippincott, 1975.

Matoltsy, A. G. Mechanism of keratinization. In Butcher, E. O., and Sognnaes, R. F. (eds.), *Fundamentals of Keratinization.* Publication No. 70. Washington, D.C.: American Association for the Advancement of Science, 1962.

Mier, P. D., and Cotton, D. W. K. *Molecular Biology of Skin.* Oxford, England: Blackwell, 1976.

Montagna, W. *The Structure and Function of Skin* (3rd ed.). New York: Academic Press, 1974.

Rowden, G. Immuno-electron microscopic studies of surface receptors and antigens of human Langerhans cells. *Br. J. Dermatol.* 97:593, 1977.

Snell, R. S. Effect of the melanocyte stimulating hormone of the pituitary on melanocytes and melanin in the skin of guinea-pigs. *J. Endocrinol.* 25:249, 1962.

Snell, R. S. A study of the effect of chronic irritation on melanogenesis in the skin. *Br. J. Exp. Pathol.* 43:581, 1962.

Snell, R. S. The effect of corticotropin on the activity of mammalian epidermal melanocytes. *J. Endocrinol.* 28:79, 1963.

Snell, R. S. The effect of ultraviolet irradiation on melanogenesis. *J. Invest. Dermatol.* 40:127, 1963.

Snell, R. S. A study of melanocytes and melanin in a healing deep wound. *J. Anat.* 97:243, 1963.

Snell, R. S. Effect of the alpha melanocyte stimulating hormone of the pituitary on mammalian epidermal melanocytes. *J. Invest. Dermatol.* 42:337, 1964.

Snell, R. S. The pigmentary changes occurring in the breast skin during pregnancy and following estrogen treatment. *J. Invest. Dermatol.* 43:181, 1964.

Snell, R. S. Effect of melatonin on mammalian epidermal melanocytes. *J. Invest. Dermatol.* 44:273, 1965.

Snell, R. S. The fate of epidermal desmosomes in mammalian skin. *Z. Zellforsch.* 66:471, 1965.

Snell, R. S. An electron microscopic study of the human epidermal keratinocyte. *Z. Zellforsch.* 79:492, 1967.

Snell, R. S. An electron microscopic study of melanin in the hair and hair follicles. *J. Invest. Dermatol.* 58:144, 1972.

Snell, R. S., and Turner, R. Skin pigmentation in relation to the menstrual cycle. *J. Invest. Dermatol.* 47:147, 1966.

Spearman, R. I. C. *The Integument.* London: Cambridge University Press, 1973.

Szabo, G. The regional anatomy of the human integument, with special reference to the distribution of hair follicles, sweat glands and melanocytes. *Philos. Trans. R. Soc. Lond.* [Biol] 252:447, 1967.

SPECIAL SENSE ORGANS

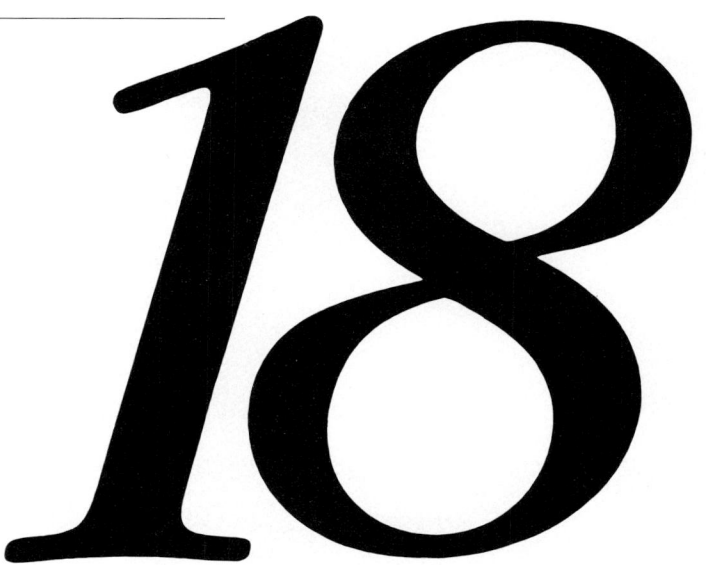

18

An individual receives impressions from the outside world by special sensory nerve endings, or receptors. The eyes are sensitive to changes in light intensity and wavelength, the ears to sound waves, and the olfactory and taste nerve endings to changes in chemical concentrations. The cutaneous sense organs are sensitive to touch, pressure, and changes in temperature. The cutaneous sense organs have been described in Chapter 7. In this chapter, the structure and function of the eye, the ear, and the olfactory and taste nerve endings will be described.

THE EYE

The eyeball is approximately spherical and measures about 2.5 cm in diameter. It is embedded in fat and situated in the cavity of the bony orbit, which protects it from injury. The eyeball is separated from the fat by a membranous sac called the *fascial sheath* of the eyeball, permitting it to move freely. The orbital opening is guarded by two thin, movable folds, the eyelids, which are situated in front of the eye (Fig. 18-1).

Eyelids

The eyelids are thin, movable folds located in front of the eye that protect it from injury and excessive light by their closure. The upper eyelid is larger and more mobile than the lower, and they meet at the *medial* and *lateral angles*. The *palpebral fissure* is the elliptical opening between the eyelids and is the entrance into the conjunctival sac.

The superficial surface of the eyelids is covered by skin, and the deep surface is covered by a mucous membrane called the *conjunctiva*. The skin at the mucocutaneous junction has double or triple rows of *eyelashes*. These are stiff, short, curved hairs situated on the edges of the eyelids (Fig. 18-2). Opening into the eyelash follicles are sebaceous glands (glands of Zeis). The *ciliary glands* (glands of Moll) are modified sweat glands that open separately between adjacent lashes. The tarsal glands (meibomian glands) are long, modified sebaceous glands that pour their oily secretion onto the margin of the lid; their openings lie behind the eyelashes (Fig. 18-3; see Fig. 18-2). This oily material prevents the

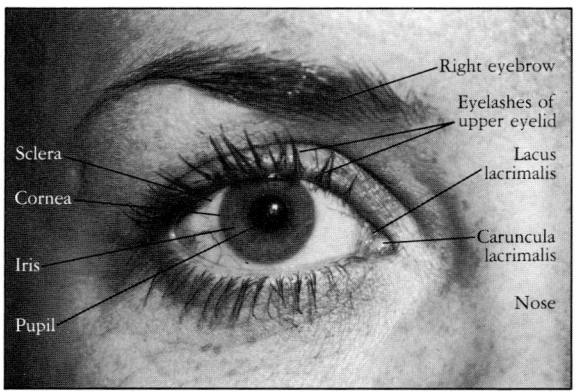
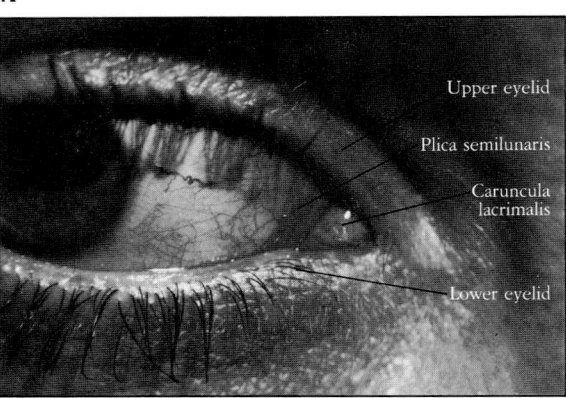
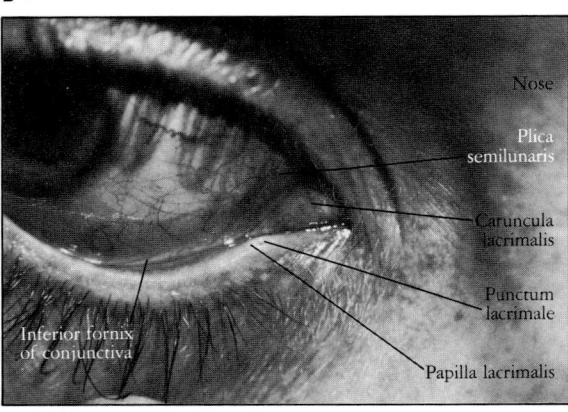

Fig. 18-1. *Right eye of a woman.* (A) Structures of the eye; (B) enlarged view of the medial angle between the eyelids; (C) lower eyelid, pulled downward and slightly everted to reveal the punctum lacrimale.

overflow of tears and helps make the closed eyelids airtight.

The lateral angle of the palpebral fissure is more acute than the medial and lies directly in contact with the eyeball. The more rounded medial angle is separated from the eyeball by a small space, the *lacus lacrimalis*, in the center of which is a small, reddish-yellow elevation, the *caruncula lacrimalis* (see Fig. 18-1). A reddish semilunar fold called the *plica semilunaris* lies on the lateral side of the caruncle.

Near the medial angle of the eye, the eyelashes and the tarsal glands stop abruptly and there is a small elevation, the *papilla lacrimalis*. On the summit of the papilla is a small hole, the *punctum lacrimale*, which leads into the *lacrimal canal* (see Figs. 18-1 and 18-2). The papilla lacrimalis projects into the lacus, and the punctum and canal carry tears down into the nose (see Fig. 18-2).

The *conjunctiva* is a thin mucous membrane that lines the eyelids and is reflected at the *superior* and *inferior fornices* onto the anterior surface of the eyeball (Fig. 18-4; see Fig. 18-2). It is lined with stratified columnar epithelium that rests on a lamina propria composed of loose connective tissue (Fig. 18-5). The epithelium is continuous with that of the cornea. The upper lateral part of the superior fornix is pierced by the ducts of the lacrimal gland. The conjunctiva thus forms a space, the *conjunctival sac*, that opens at the palpebral fissure.

Beneath the eyelid is a groove, the *subtarsal sulcus*, that runs close to and parallel with the margin of the lid (see Fig. 18-2). The sulcus tends to trap small foreign particles introduced into the conjunctival sac and is thus of clinical importance.

The fibrous framework of the eyelids is formed by a membranous sheet, the *orbital septum* (see Fig. 18-2). This is attached to the orbital margin, where it is continuous with the periosteum. The orbital septum is thickened at the margins of the lids to form the *tarsal plates*. These are two crescent-shaped laminae of dense fibrous tissue; the superior tarsal plate is the larger. The lateral ends of the plates are attached by a band, the *lateral palpebral ligament*, to the orbital wall just within the orbital margin. The medial ends of the plates are attached by the *medial*

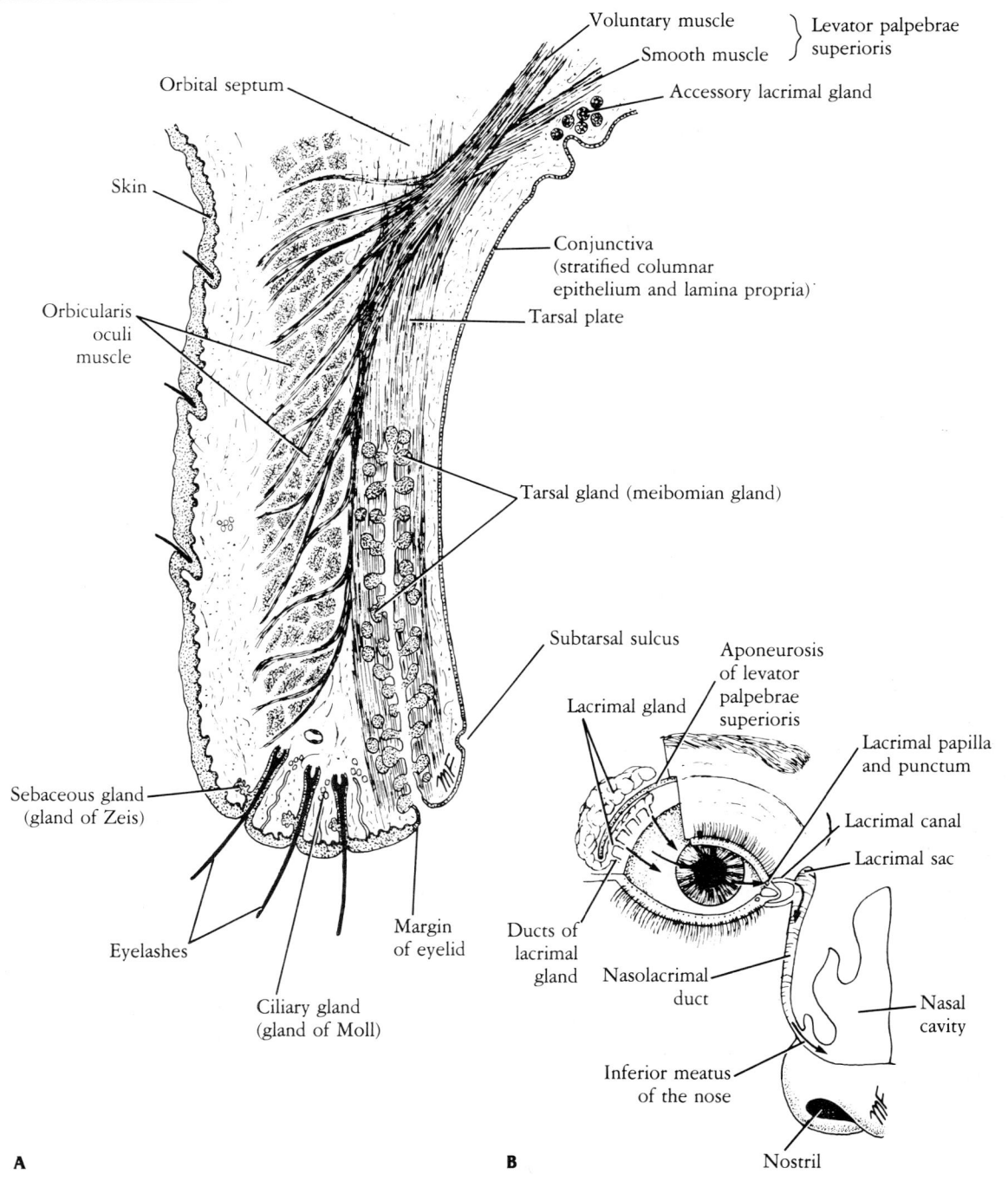

Fig. 18-2. (A) Structure of the upper eyelid as seen in vertical section; (B) formation of tears from the lacrimal gland and their passage across the front of the eye to drain into the nose.

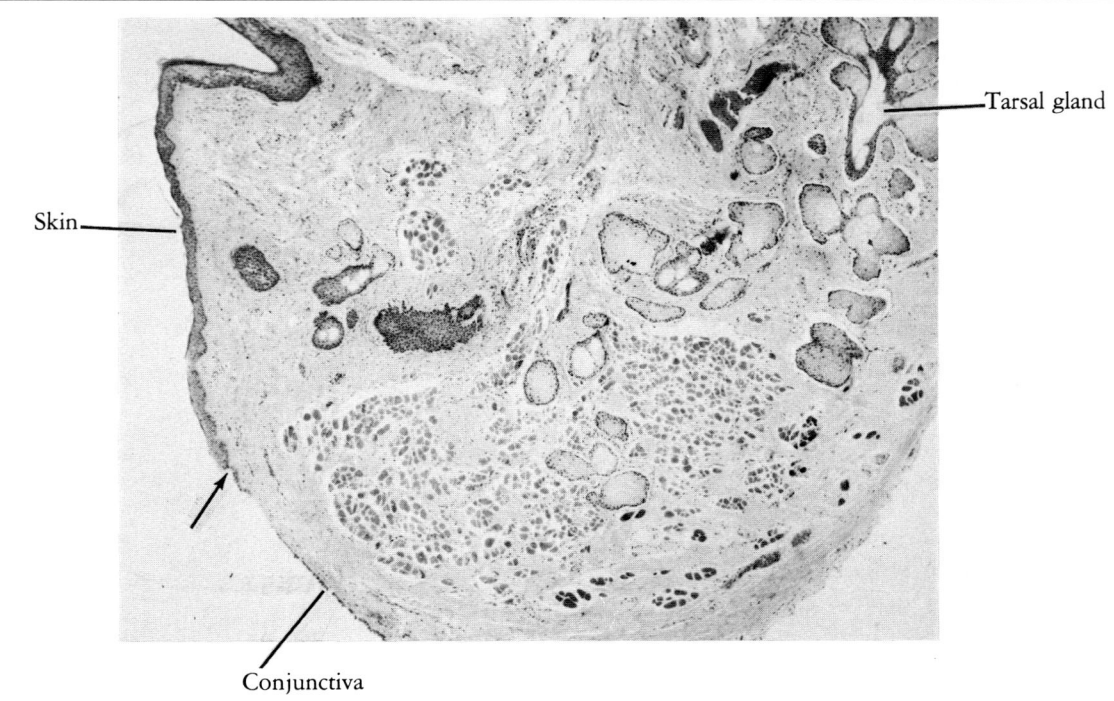

Fig. 18-3. Photomicrograph of a vertical section of the upper eyelid at its free margin, showing the junction of the epidermis of the skin with the conjunctiva (arrow). Portions of an eyelash follicle and its associated sebaceous gland are visible at the left. Portions of a large tarsal gland can be seen on the right. Note the bundles of fibers of the orbicularis oculi muscle. (H&E; ×40.)

palpebral ligament to the crest of the lacrimal bone. The tarsal glands are embedded in the posterior surface of the tarsal plates.

The superficial surface of the tarsal plates and the orbital septum are covered by the palpebral fibers of the *orbicularis oculi muscle* (see Fig. 18-2). This muscle forms part of the muscles of facial expression and is composed of voluntary striped muscle fibers. The aponeurosis of insertion of the *levator palpebrae superioris muscle* pierces the orbital septum to reach the anterior surface of the superior tarsal plate and the skin see Fig. 18-2).

Lacrimal Apparatus

The lacrimal apparatus consists of the lacrimal gland and its ducts and the lacrimal passages, which drain excess tears from the conjunctival sac into the nasal cavity.

The *lacrimal gland* is situated above the eyeball in the superolateral part of the orbital cavity just beneath the conjunctiva. It consists of a large *orbital part* and a small *palpebral part*, which are continuous with each other around the lateral edge of the aponeurosis of the levator palpebrae superioris (see Fig. 18-2). Small accessory lacrimal glands are also present beneath the conjunctiva of the upper and lower eyelids.

The lacrimal glands are tubulo-acinar glands (Fig. 18-6). The acini have relatively large lumina and are lined with columnar cells. Between the bases of the cells and the basal lamina are myoepithelial cells. About twelve ducts open from the lower surface of

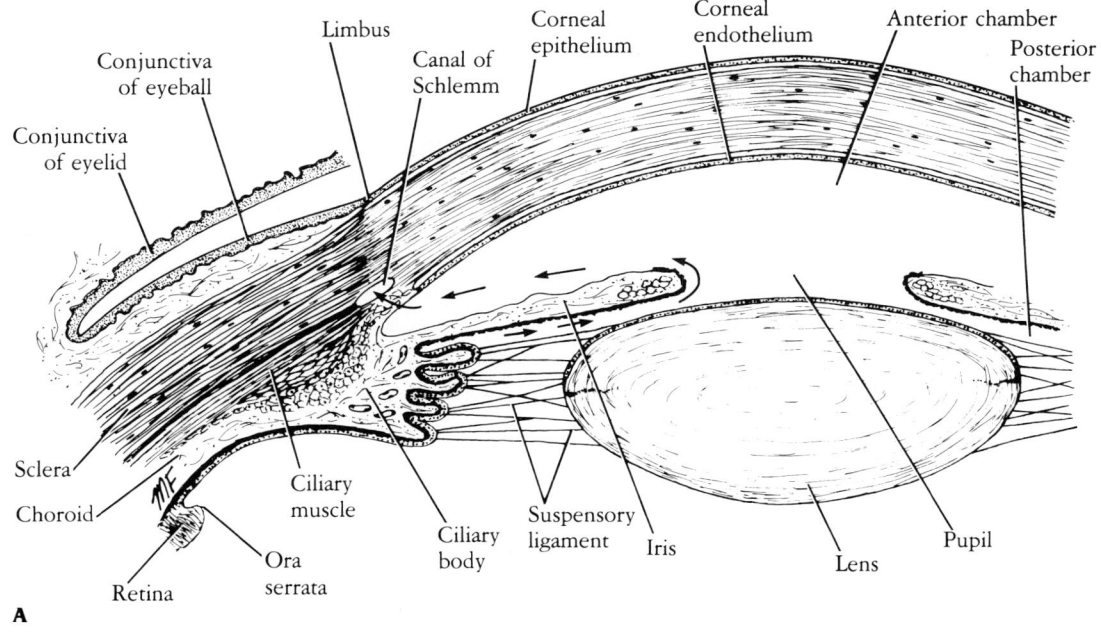
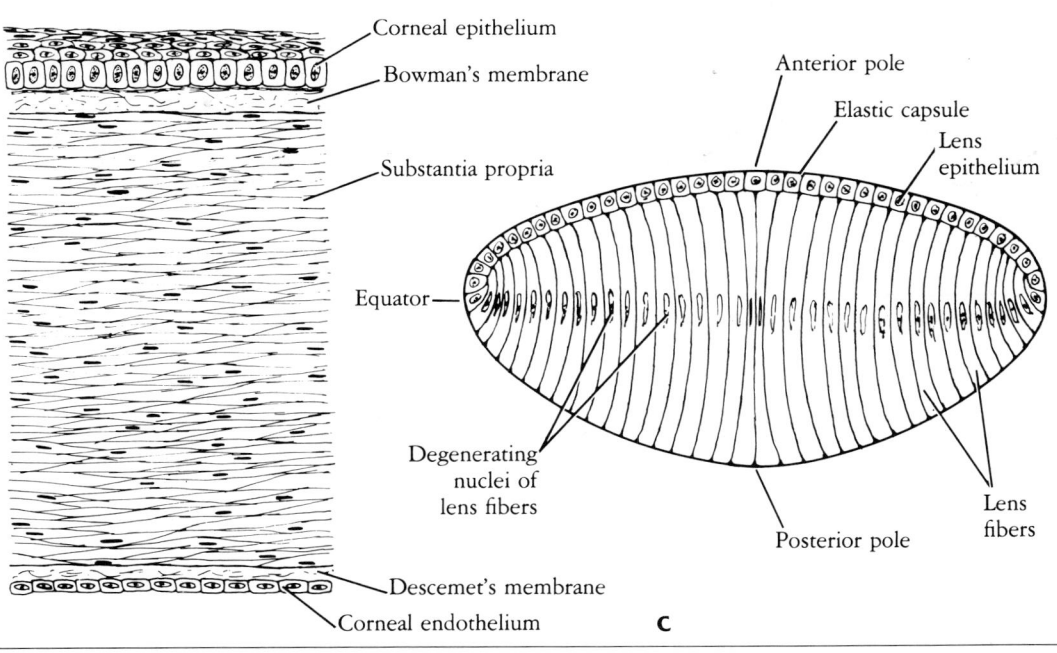

Fig. 18-4. (A) *Structures seen in a section through the anterior portion of the eye; the arrows indicate the pathway taken by the aqueous humor during its circulation.* (B) *Structure of the cornea.* (C) *Structure of the lens.*

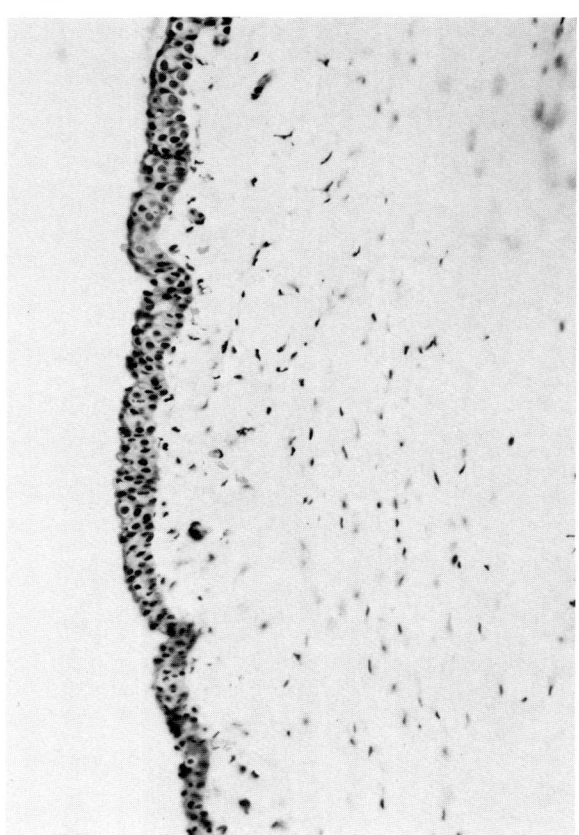

Fig. 18-5. Photomicrograph of a section of the conjunctiva. Note that it is lined with stratified columnar epithelium that becomes stratified squamous epithelium at the edge of the cornea. The epithelium rests on a lamina propria of loose connective tissue. (H&E; ×200.)

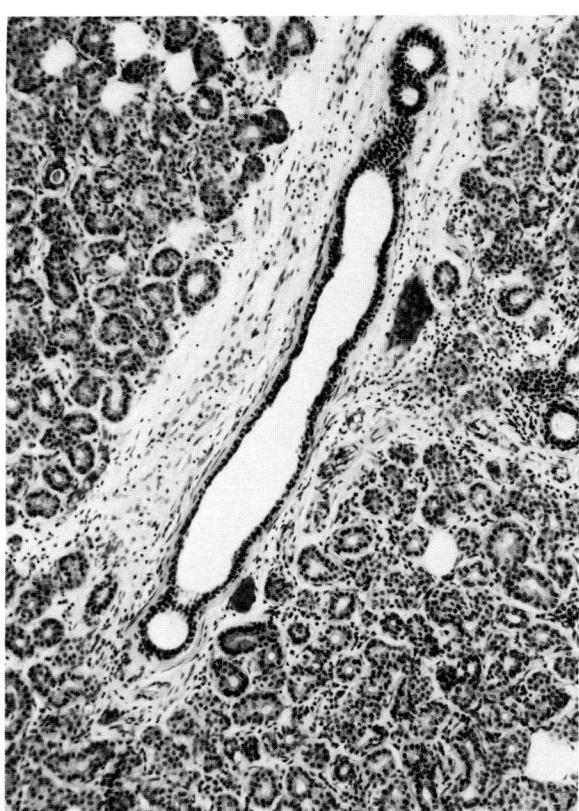

Fig. 18-6. Photomicrograph of a section of the lacrimal gland, showing numerous secretory serous acini and an interlobular duct. (H&E; ×100.)

the gland into the lateral part of the superior fornix of the conjunctiva. The lacrimal gland is innervated by postganglionic parasympathetic secretomotor fibers from the lacrimatory nucleus of the facial nerve; it also receives postganglionic sympathetic nerve fibers.

The *tears* secreted by the lacrimal gland enter the conjunctival sac at its superolateral angle and circulate across the cornea as a result of capillarity that is assisted by the blinking movements of the eyelids. The tears then accumulate in the lacus lacrimalis and from there enter the lacrimal canals through the puncta lacrimalia. The lacrimal canals pass medially and open into the lacrimal sac (see Fig. 18-2). The tears then pass down the nasolacrimal duct into the inferior meatus of the nasal cavity.

The tear fluid is a sterile secretion that keeps the cornea and the conjunctival epithelium moist; it also traps small foreign particles. The secretion contains the enzyme lysozyme, which is bactericidal. The tarsal glands, under normal conditions, prevent the tears from overflowing onto the cheeks from the lid margins; the oily secretion also forms a film that floats on the tears and inhibits evaporation. The continuous evaporation of the tear fluid from the lower end of the nasolacrimal duct ensures that a constant

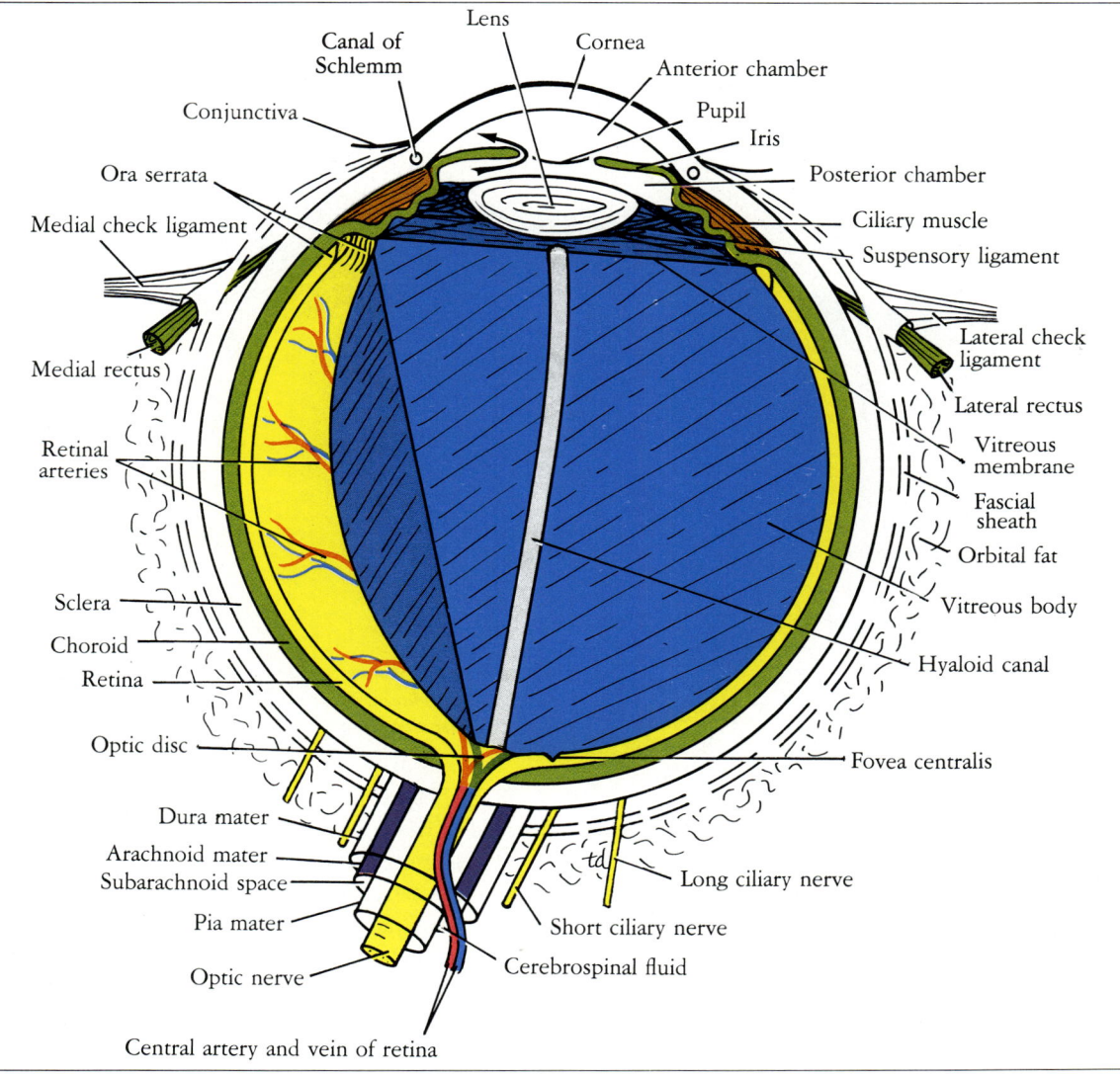

Fig. 18-7. Horizontal section through the eyeball and optic nerve. Part of the vitreous body has been removed to show the retinal vessels. Note that the central artery and vein of the retina cross the subarachnoid space to reach the optic nerve.

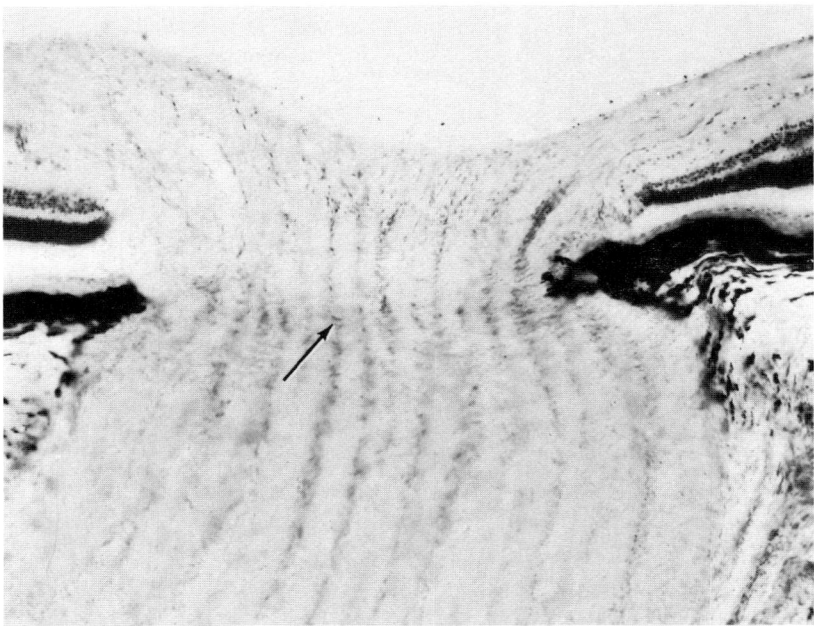

Fig. 18-8. Photomicrograph of a section through the optic disc and the commencement of the optic nerve. The arrow indicates the lamina cribrosa. (H&E; ×100.)

flow of fluid crosses the cornea. This process is furthered by the pumping action of the orbicularis oculi muscle on the lacrimal sac during blinking.

Eyeball

The eyeball consists of three coats, which, moving inward, are: (1) the fibrous coat, (2) the vascular pigmented coat, and (3) the nervous coat.

Coats of the Eyeball

FIBROUS COAT. The fibrous coat is made up of a posterior, opaque part, the sclera, and an anterior, transparent part, the cornea (Fig. 18-7).

Sclera. The *sclera* is composed of dense fibrous tissue and is white. Microscopically, it is seen to consist of bundles of collagenous fibers arranged in many directions; some elastic fibers are also present. Between the bundles of fibers are elongated fibroblasts.

Attached to the outer surface of the sclera are the tendons of the eye muscles. Posteriorly, the sclera is pierced by the optic nerve (Fig. 18-8; see Fig. 18-7), and at that point, it is fused with the dural and arachnoid sheaths of that nerve. The *lamina cribrosa* is the area of the sclera that is pierced by the nerve fibers of the optic nerve. It is a relatively weak area and can be made to bulge into the eyeball by a rise in cerebrospinal fluid pressure in the tubular extension of the subarachnoid space, which surrounds the optic nerve. If the intraocular pressure rises, the lamina cribrosa bulges outward, producing a cupped disc, as seen through the ophthalmoscope.

The sclera is also pierced by the ciliary arteries and nerves and their associated veins, the *venae vorticosae*. The sclera is directly continuous in front with the cornea at the *corneoscleral junction*, or *limbus*.

Cornea. The *cornea* forms the anterior part of the outer, fibrous coat of the eyeball (see Figs. 18-4 and 18-7). It has a smaller radius of curvature than the remainder of the eyeball. The cornea is transparent and devoid of blood vessels and is largely responsible for the refraction of light entering the eye (see Fig. 18-25). Microscopically, the cornea is com-

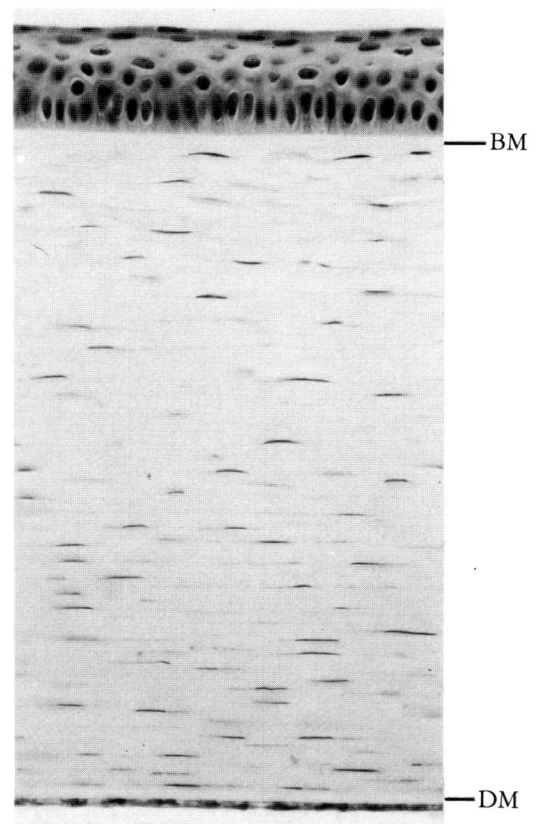

Fig. 18-9. Photomicrograph of a section of the cornea, showing the corneal epithelium (top), the clear Bowman's membrane (BM), the substantia propria, the narrow, clear Descemet's membrane (DM), and the corneal endothelium (bottom). (H&E; ×260.)

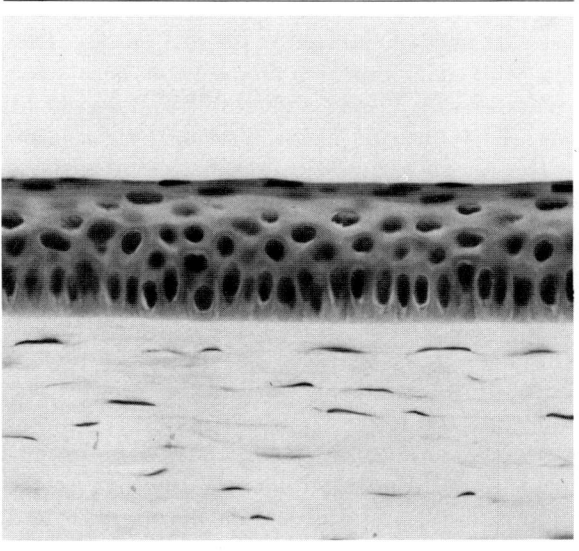

Fig. 18-10. Photomicrograph of a high-power view of the corneal epithelium shown in Figure 18-9. The epithelium is stratified, the deepest cells are columnar, and the superficial cells are squamous and nonkeratinized. Note the clear zone beneath the epithelium that contains Bowman's membrane. (H&E; ×400.)

posed of five layers; from front to back, they are: (1) the epithelium, (2) Bowman's membrane, (3) the substantia propria, (4) Descemet's membrane, and (5) the endothelium.

The *corneal epithelium* is stratified and consists of five layers of cells (Figs. 18-9 and 18-10). The deepest cells are columnar, and the most superficial cells are flattened, nonkeratinized squamous cells. Electron microscopic examination of the outer surfaces of the superficial cells shows microvilli and microplicae (ridges) that are thought to assist in retaining a film of tears on the surface of the cells and thus keeping them moist. Running between the epithelial cells are the naked nerve endings of sensory nerve fibers that are sensitive mainly to pain. Beneath the corneal epithelium is a well-formed basal lamina.

Bowman's membrane lies immediately beneath the basal lamina of the corneal epithelium (see Figs. 18-4 and 18-10). It is acellular and composed of interwoven collagen fibers embedded in intercellular substance. It ends abruptly at the limbus.

The *substantia propria* forms the greater part of the cornea (see Figs. 18-4 and 18-9). It is composed of many lamellae of collagen fibers that run parallel to the surface. The direction of the collagen fibers in any given lamella is the same, but they run at right angles to those of adjacent lamellae. The lamellae are bound together by fibers that pass from one lamella to another. The collagenous fibers are embedded in matrix. Lying between adjacent lamellae are flattened fibroblasts.

Descemet's membrane is composed of small collagenous fibers embedded in matrix (see Figs. 18-4 and 18-9). It appears as a homogeneous layer when examined with the light microscope. It should be regarded as the basal lamina of the endothelial layer.

The *corneal endothelium* is composed of a single layer of cuboidal cells covering the posterior surface of the cornea (see Figs. 18-4 and 18-9).

Because the cornea is devoid of blood vessels, it is nourished by tissue fluid that diffuses in from peripheral blood vessels situated near the limbus and from the aqueous humor.

VASCULAR PIGMENTED COAT. The vascular pigmented coat consists, from back to front, of the choroid, the ciliary body, and the iris (see Figs. 18-4 and 18-7).

Choroid. The choroid lies adjacent to the inner surface of the sclera and can be divided into three layers: (1) the vessel layer, (2) the capillary layer, and (3) Bruch's membrane. The *vessel layer* consists of loose connective tissue containing melanocytes in which are embedded numerous large and medium-sized blood vessels. The *capillary layer* consists of a network of capillaries that are fed by arteries from the vessel layer and drained by veins into the vessel layer. The capillaries are supported by delicate connective tissue containing melanocytes. *Bruch's membrane* is formed by the basal lamina of the capillaries of the capillary layer and the basal lamina of the pigment epithelium of the retina.

Ciliary Body. The ciliary body is continuous posteriorly with the choroid and anteriorly with the peripheral margin of the iris (see Fig. 18-4). Taken as a whole, the ciliary body is a complete ring that runs around the inside of the sclera; it is largely formed of the ciliary muscle. When viewed in section, it is triangular, with its apex pointing toward the interior of the eyeball.

The internal aspect of the ciliary body is divided into an anterior, ridged part called the *pars plicata*, which forms the ciliary processes (Fig. 18-11), and a posterior, flat, smooth part called the *pars plana* (see Fig. 18-4).

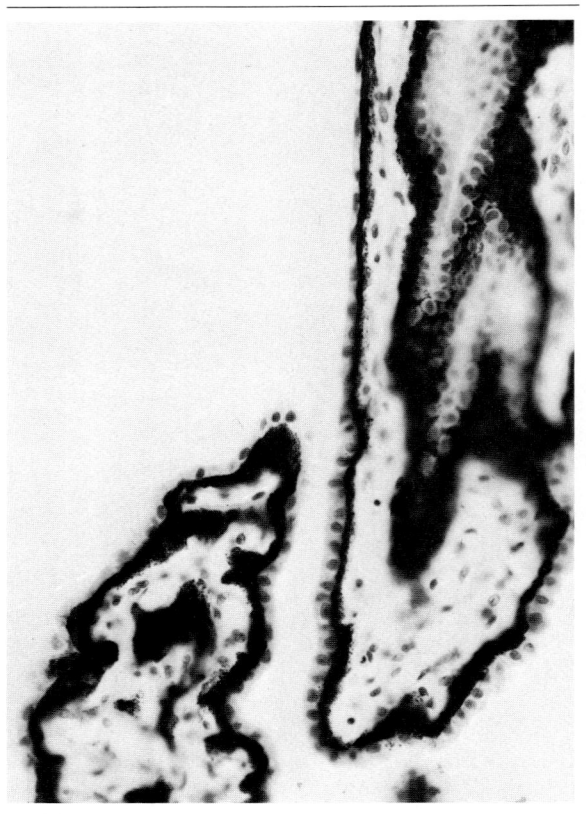

Fig. 18-11. Photomicrograph of a section of portions of two ciliary processes. Note the two layers of cells that cover the processes. The more superficial layer, which is related to the vitreous, is nonpigmented cuboidal epithelium; the deeper layer, comprised of cuboidal cells, is filled with pigment. (H&E; ×200.)

The interior of the ciliary body is made up of loose connective tissue (see Fig. 18-12), rich in blood vessels and melanocytes, in which is embedded the ciliary muscle. Microscopically, the *ciliary muscle* is composed of smooth muscle fibers arranged in three groups. The outer, meridional fibers run backward from the region of the corneoscleral junction to the posterior part of the ciliary body. The radial, or oblique, fibers, which lie internal to the meridional fibers, run backward to the interior of the ciliary body. The circular, or sphincteric, fibers are less numerous and lie internal to the radial

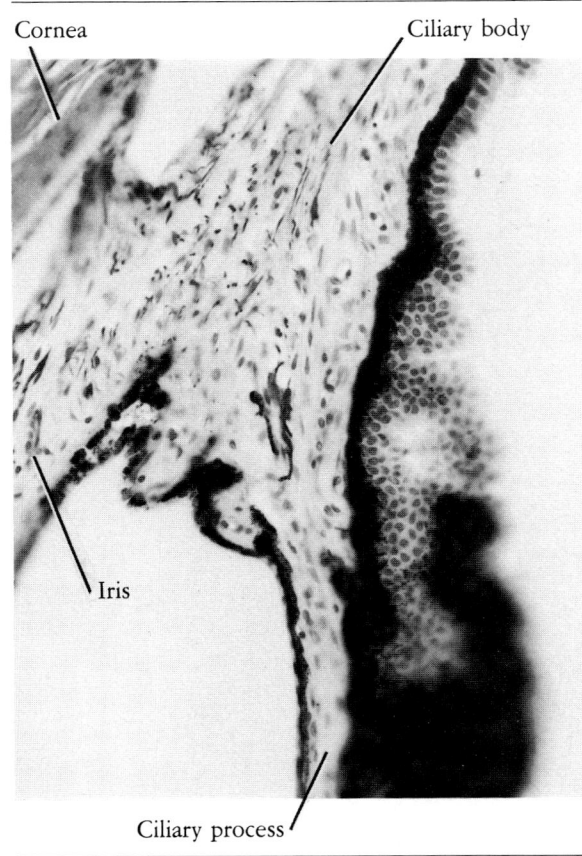

Fig. 18-12. *Photomicrograph of a section of the anterior portion of the eyeball, showing the cornea, the ciliary body, and a ciliary process. (H&E; ×200.)*

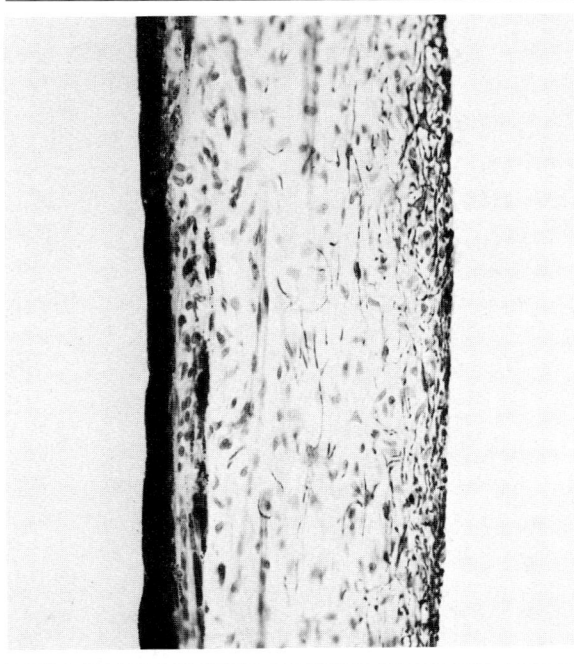

Fig. 18-13. *Photomicrograph of a section of the iris. The anterior surface (right) is formed of connective tissue; the posterior surface (left) is covered by two layers of heavily pigmented cells that form a thick black line in the photograph. The branching melanocytes in the stroma can just be identified. (H&E; ×200.)*

fibers; they are arranged like a sphincter and encircle the eye.

The ciliary muscle is innervated by the postganglionic parasympathetic fibers derived from the oculomotor nerve. Contraction of the ciliary muscle, especially the meridional fibers, pulls the ciliary body forward. This relieves the tension in the suspensory ligament, making the elastic lens more convex and thereby increasing the refractive power of the lens.

The ciliary body is covered by two layers of cuboidal epithelium (see Fig. 18-11). The inner layer, of nonpigmented cells, has a basal lamina and is related to the vitreous; the outer layer, of pigmented cells, also has a basal lamina and is adjacent to the connective tissue of the ciliary body. Each layer of cells has a basal lamina because both are derived from the two layers of the neuroectoderm of the marginal zone of the optic cup.

Iris. The iris is a thin, contractile, pigmented diaphragm with a central aperture, the *pupil* (see Fig. 18-4). It is suspended in the aqueous humor between the cornea and the lens. The periphery of the iris is attached to the anterior surface of the ciliary body. It divides the space between the lens and the cornea into an *anterior* and a *posterior chamber.*

Microscopically, the anterior surface of the iris is formed merely by the anterior part of the connective tissue of the stroma of the iris (Figs. 18-13 and

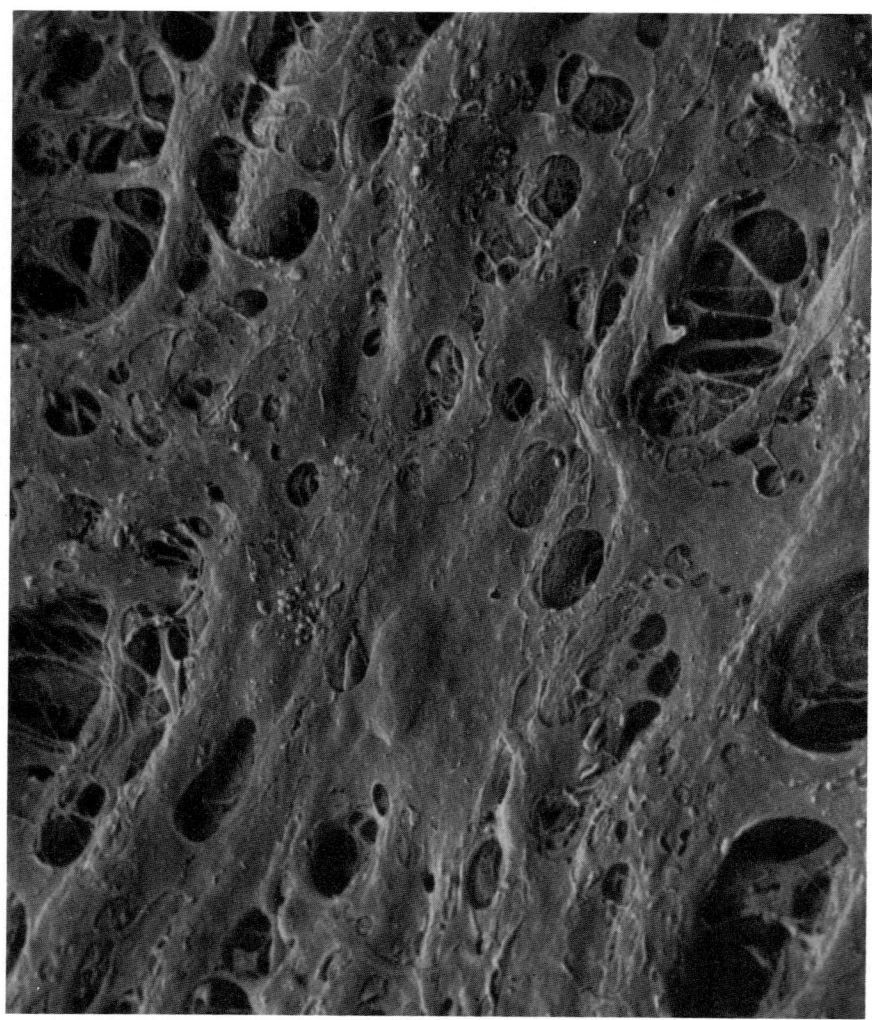

Fig. 18-14. Scanning electron micrograph of the anterior surface of the iris, showing the surface to be covered by an incomplete layer of fibroblasts. In the intervals between the fibroblasts can be seen the branching processes of many melanocytes and bundles of collagen fibers. (×2,300.) (Courtesy of Dr. D. H. Dickson.)

18-14). The posterior surface of the iris is covered by two layers of epithelium that are continuous with the two layers of epithelium covering the ciliary body. Both layers of cells are heavily pigmented, irrespective of the person's skin color. At the pupil, the two layers of pigmented cells extend forward through the aperture and cover the anterior surface of the iris for a short distance, forming a pigmented border.

The stroma of the iris is formed of highly vascular tissue containing fibroblasts, collagen fibers, and melanocytes (see Fig. 18-14). The tissue spaces between the cells are continuous with the anterior chamber. The color of the iris (eye color) depends on the number of melanocytes in the stroma, the amount of melanin pigment within the melanocytes, the position of the melanocytes within the stroma, and the pigment in the epithelium covering the posterior surface of the iris. In individuals with blue eyes, there are few stromal melanocytes, with practically no pigment. The color is caused by the scattering effect of the stroma on the light reflected from the melanin pigment in the cells on the posterior surface of the iris. In gray and green eyes, the light is reflected from the pigment in the deep stromal melanocytes. In individuals with brown or black eyes, large amounts of melanin pigment are present in the melanocytes throughout the iris stroma. In albinos, the iris is pink because of the hemoglobin in the blood capillaries and the total absence of melanin pigment in the iris cells.

The iris is a movable diaphragm and contains two sets of muscle fibers situated within the stroma that alter the size of the pupil. The circular fibers are formed of smooth muscle and are arranged around the margin of the pupil. They constitute the *sphincter pupillae muscle* and are supplied by postganglionic parasympathetic nerve fibers derived from the oculomotor nerve. The radial fibers are formed of myoepithelial cells (i.e., not true smooth muscle cells) and are found close to the posterior surface of the iris. They constitute the *dilator pupillae muscle* and are supplied by postganglionic sympathetic nerve fibers.

The sphincter pupillae constricts the pupil in bright light and during accommodation. The dilator pupillae dilates the pupil in low-intensity light and in the presence of excessive sympathetic activity, such as occurs in fright.

NERVOUS COAT. The nervous coat, or retina, is the internal layer of the eyeball (see Fig. 18-7) and consists of an anterior quarter that is insensitive and a posterior three-quarters that is the photoreceptor organ. The retina consists of an outer, pigmented layer and an inner, nervous layer. Its outer surface is in contact with the choroid, and its inner surface is in contact with the vitreous body (see Fig. 18-7).

The posterior, receptive part of the retina extends forward from the optic nerve to a point just posterior to the ciliary body. Here the nervous tissues of the retina end and its anterior edge forms a wavy ring called the *ora serrata* (see Fig. 18-7). The anterior, nonreceptive part of the retina extends forward from the ora serrata over the back of the ciliary body, with its processes, and the iris; it consists merely of pigment cells, with a deeper layer of columnar epithelium. Recall that on the posterior surface of the iris, both layers of cells are pigmented.

At the center of the posterior part of the retina is an oval, yellowish area, the *macula lutea*, which is the retinal area for the most distinct vision. It has a central depression, the *fovea centralis* (see Fig. 18-7).

The optic nerve leaves the retina about 3 mm to the medial side of the macula lutea by the optic disc (see Fig. 18-8). The *optic disc* is slightly depressed at its center, where it is pierced by the *central artery* of the retina. At the optic disc, there is a complete absence of *rods* and *cones*; it is thus insensitive to light and is referred to as the *blind spot*. On ophthalmoscopic examination, the optic disc is seen to be pale pink, much paler than the surrounding retina.

Pigmented Layer of the Retina. The pigment epithelium is embryologically derived from the outer layer of the optic cup. It consists of a single layer of cuboidal cells situated just internal to the choroid (Figs. 18-15–18-17). At the ora serrata, these cells become the pigmented layer of the epithelium covering the ciliary body. The plasma membrane of the cells is much infolded on their basal surfaces. In the apical region of the cells, the plasma membrane projects between the rods and cones as microvilli (Fig. 18-18). The basal lamina of the cells forms part of the Bruch's membrane of the choroid. The cell nuclei are in the basal part of the cytoplasm, and there are numerous mitochondria and melanin granules. Each cell has a well-developed granular and agranular endoplasmic reticulum and a Golgi apparatus. Lysosomes are present in large numbers, together with residual bodies, or phagosomes. It is believed that the apical mi-

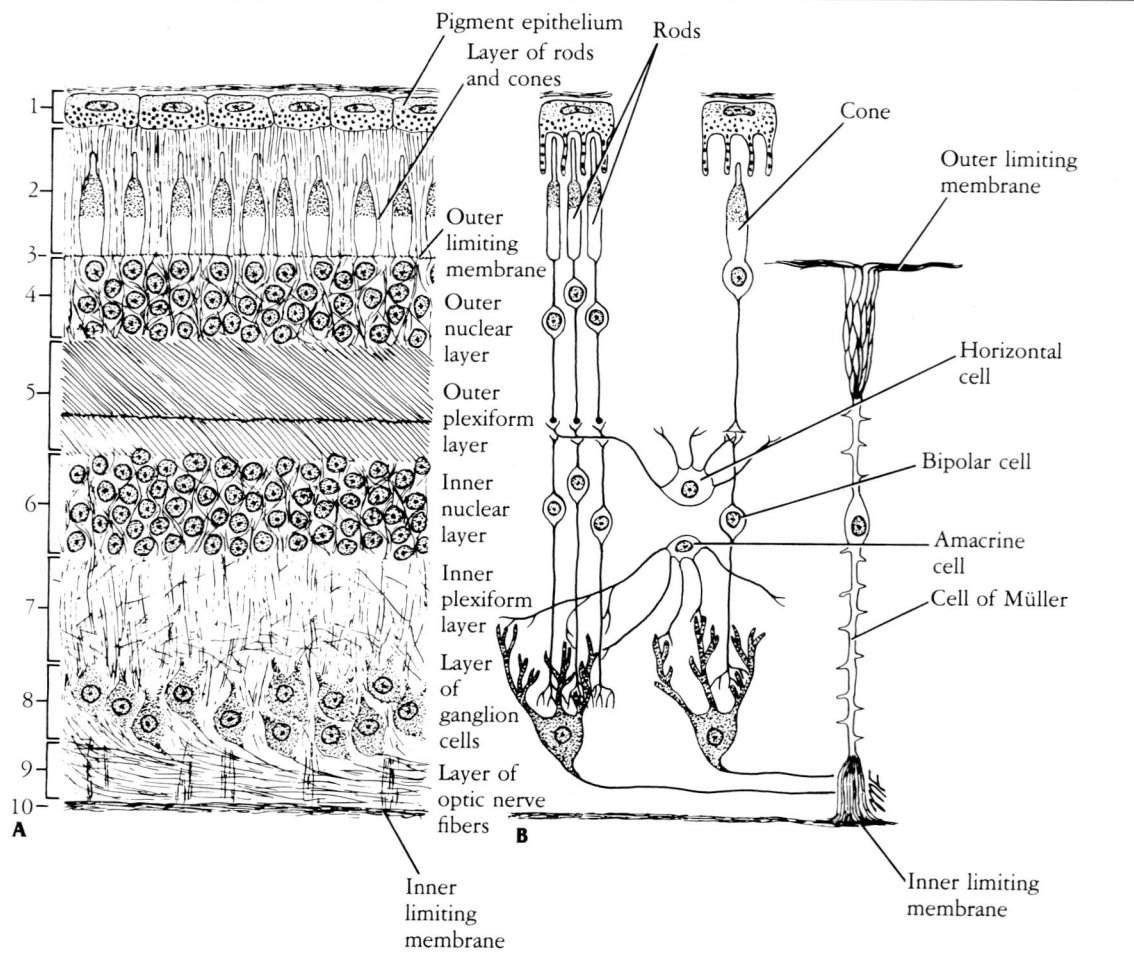

Fig. 18-15. (A) The ten layers of the retina, as seen in an ordinary histological section; (B) arrangement of the nerve cells. Note that the cell processes of the supporting cells of Müller form the outer and inner limiting membranes.

crovilli continuously erode the outer ends of the rods. The pigment cells then phagocytose the debris, which includes the lamellar structures found in the outer processes of the rods. Lysosomes play an active role in breaking down the contents of the phagosomes.

The pigment cells have numerous functions, including the absorption of light, participation in the turnover of the outer segments of the rods, and the formation of rhodopsin by the storage and release of vitamin A, which is a precursor of rhodopsin. These cells also may have a secretory function.

The pigmented epithelium, which is developed from the outer layer of the optic cup, and the rods and cones, which are developed from the inner layer of the optic cup, are separated by a potential space that constitutes the remains of the cavity of the optic vesicle. Although the layers are very close together, they can become separated, a condition referred to as *detached retina* (see p. 772).

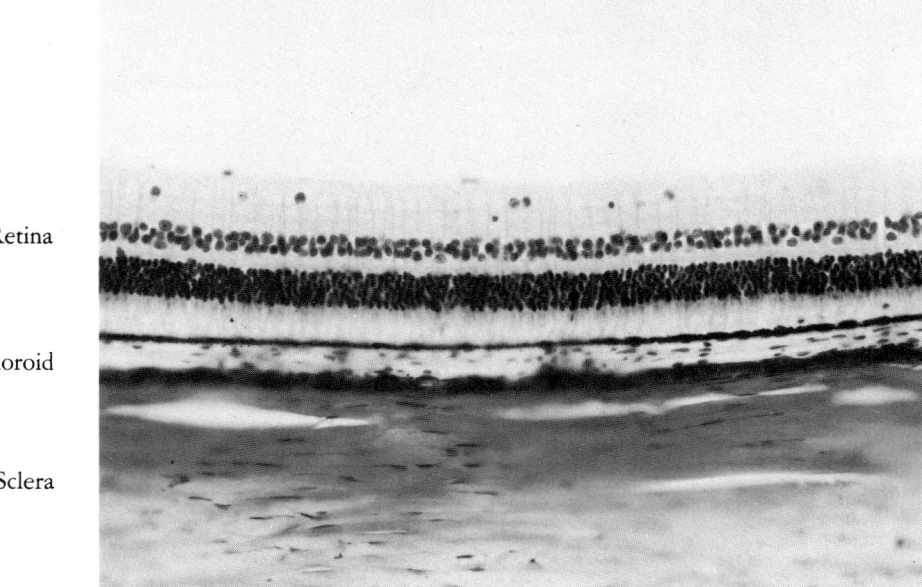

Fig. 18-16. Photomicrograph of a section of the coats of the eyeball, showing the retina, choroid, and sclera. (H&E; ×200.)

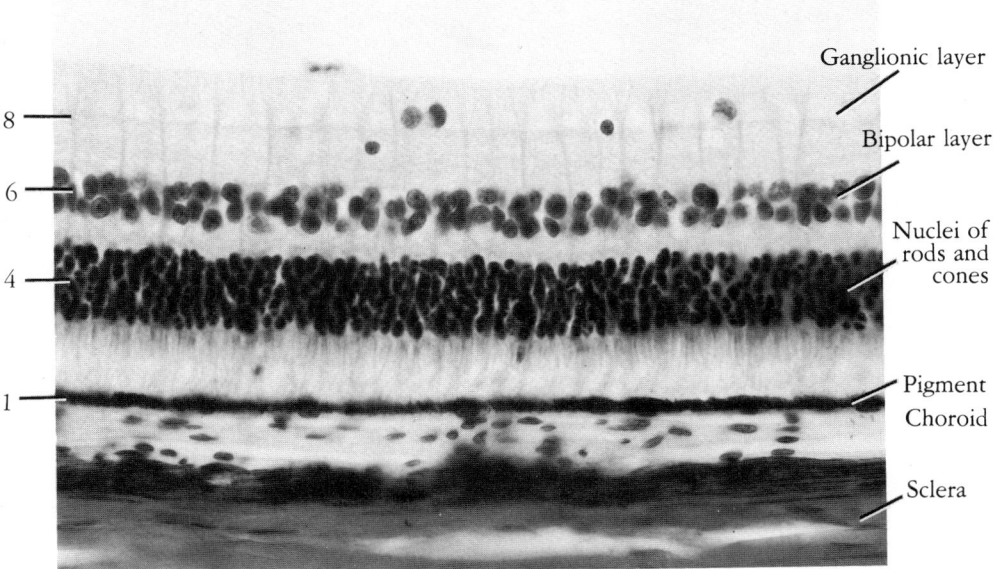

Fig. 18-17. Photomicrograph of a high-power view of a section of the retina shown in Figure 18-16. Identify layers 1, 4, 6, and 8. The numbers signify layers shown diagramatically in Figure 18-15. (H&E; ×400.)

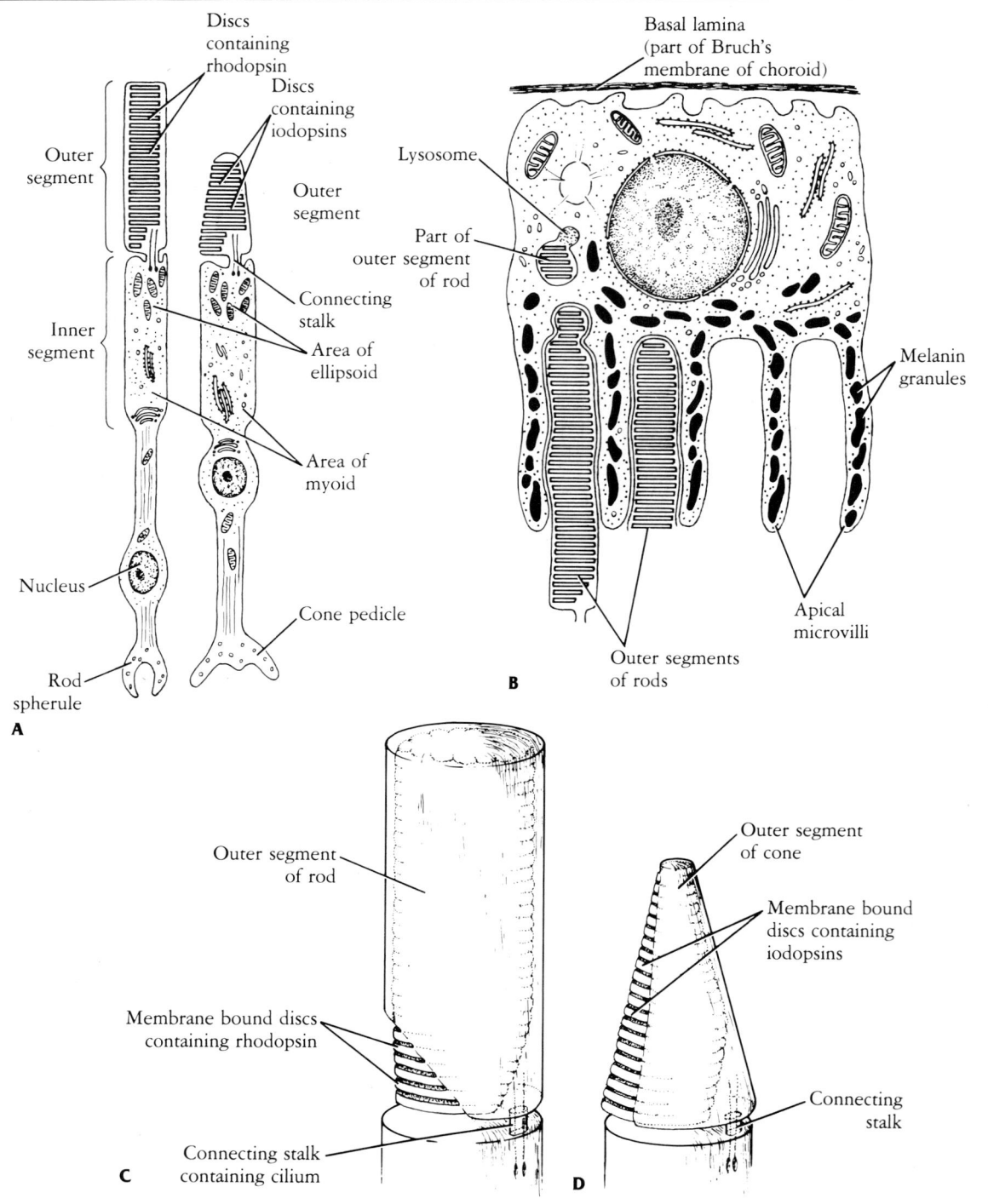

Fig. 18-18. Detailed structure of (A) a rod and a cone; (B) a pigment cell. Note the relationship of the pigment cell to the outer segments of the rods. (C) Outer segment of a rod; (D) outer segment of a cone.

Neural Retina. The neural retina is embryologically derived from the inner layer of the optic cup. It consists of three main groups of neurons: (1) the photoreceptors, (2) the bipolar cells, and (3) the ganglion cells. The photoreceptors are similar to sensory receptors elsewhere in the body. The bipolar cells are similar to the neurons in the posterior root ganglia and form the first-order neurons. The ganglion cells are similar to the relay neurons found in the spinal cord and brain stem and form the second-order neurons. The axons of the ganglion cells are myelinated and form the optic nerve. The myelin sheaths of these axons are formed from oligodendrocytes rather than Schwann cells, because the optic nerve is comparable to a tract within the central nervous system. The optic nerves and the optic tracts conduct their impulses to the lateral geniculate body, where most of the axons terminate by synapsing with nerve cells. The nerve cells of the lateral geniculate body form the third-order neurons, and their axons terminate in the visual cortex. Thus, the number of neurons involved in conducting light impulses from the retina to the visual cortex is the same as that found in other sensory pathways.

Photoreceptors. There are two types of photoreceptors, the rods and the cones (see Figs. 18-15–18-18). Both are long, narrow cells whose names describe the shape of their free ends. The outer ends of the cells interdigitate with the pigment epithelium and are referred to as the *outer segments*. *Connecting stalks* join the outer segments to the cell bodies, or *inner segments*. For these receptors to be stimulated, light must pass through the full thickness of the retina. There are about 120 million rods and about 6.5 million cones. The rods are distributed mainly around the periphery of the retina; the cones are densest in the central retinal areas.

The *rod cells* are slender cells about 100 to 120 μm in length (see Figs. 18-15 and 18-18). The outer segment contains the photosensitive pigment rhodopsin (visual purple). Electron microscopic examination shows that the outer segment contains 600 to 1,000 transversely arranged membrane-bound lamellae, or discs, stacked upon one another like a pile of coins (see Fig. 18-18). The rhodopsin is located within the discs. There is evidence that the discs are formed at the base of the outer segment and are then pushed up to the free end of the outer segment. When the discs reach the tip of the segment, the free end and the contained discs are phagocytosed by the cells of the pigment epithelium.

The connecting stalk, which is eccentrically placed, contains a modified cilium. The cilium possesses the usual nine doublet microtubules but lacks a central pair. It originates in a basal body found in the inner segment.

The inner segment consists of two areas, the *ellipsoid*, situated next to the connecting stalk, and the *myoid*, located near the vitreous. The ellipsoid contains numerous mitochondria, and the myoid contains the granular and agranular endoplasmic reticulum, free ribosomes, and a Golgi apparatus. The remainder of the rod cell contains the nucleus and terminates in a small end knob, the *rod spherule*, which synapses with the dendrites of the bipolar cells.

The *cone cells* are also long, slender cells, measuring about 65 to 75 μm (see Fig. 18-18). They have a structure similar to that of the rods, having an outer segment, a connecting stalk, and an inner segment. The outer segment is conical, and the membranes of the transversely arranged discs are continuous with the outer plasma membrane (see Fig. 18-18); thus, the lumina of the discs, unlike those of the rods, are continuous with the extracellular space. In the cones, there is no movement of the discs toward the pigment epithelium, and the pigment cells do not phagocytose the tips of the cones. Several photochemicals are found in the cones; they are similar in composition to rhodopsin and are known as *iodopsins*. As in the rods, the photosensitive pigments are incorporated into the membranous discs. The inner end of the cone cell terminates as an expanded end called the *cone pedicle*, which synapses with the dendrites of the bipolar cells.

Bipolar Cells. The dendrites of the bipolar cells pass outward to synapse with the photoreceptor cell terminals (see Fig. 18-15). The single axon is directed inward to synapse with ganglion cells and amacrine cells. Two types of bipolar cells exist, those that synapse with two or more photoreceptors and those that synapse with a single cone terminal and only one ganglion cell. The latter arrangement provides a direct pathway from the cone to a single optic nerve fiber.

Ganglion Cells. Ganglion cells are so named because they resemble cells found in nervous ganglia. They are situated in the inner part of the retina (see Fig. 18-15). Their dendrites synapse with the axons of bipolar cells. The ganglion cells have nonmyelinated axons that make a right-angled turn when they reach the inner surface of the retina. The axons then converge at the exit of the optic nerve at the optic disc. The optic nerve fibers pass through the sclera at a site known as the *lamina cribrosa*; it is the weakest part of the sclera. After piercing the lamina, the nerve fibers become myelinated, the myelin sheath being formed from oligodendrocytes.

Other Nerve Cells. In addition to the rod and cone cells, bipolar cells, and ganglion cells, there are two types of neurons called horizontal and amacrine cells. The *horizontal cells* are situated close to the terminal expansions of the rods and cones (see Fig. 18-15). They have long and short processes that run horizontally, synapsing with different photoreceptors. The probable function of the horizontal cells is to integrate visual stimuli. The *amacrine cells* are situated close to the dendrites of the ganglion cells (see Fig. 18-15). These cells have numerous short processes that synapse with the dendrites of the ganglion cells and the axons of the bipolar cells. Although their function is unknown, it is possibly the integration of visual stimuli.

Supporting Cells. Because the neural retina is developed from the optic cup, which is an outgrowth of the central nervous system, it is not surprising that the supporting cells are similar to neuroglial cells. One of these cell types runs radially and is called the *cell of Müller* (see Fig. 18-15). It is long and narrow and pale staining, and long processes extend from it through almost the whole thickness of the neural retina. On the vitreal surface, side branches of the processes of the Müller cells form a meshwork known as the *inner limiting membrane*. Toward the outer surface of the neural retina, the processes of the Müller cells form junctional complexes with the rods and cones; the resulting meshwork is known as the *outer limiting membrane*. Microvilli project from the free surface of the Müller cells into the intervals between the inner segments of the rods and cones. Processes of the cells also make extensive contact with blood capillaries. These cells support the neurons of the retina and possibly also aid in their nourishment.

Layers of the Retina. Traditionally, based on light microscopic findings, the retina was said to be composed of ten layers. Once the retina was examined with the electron microscope, it was found that no real layers exist. Figure 18-15 illustrates the layers of the retina; you might find it helpful in identifying structures seen in a section of the retina with a light microscope.

Macula Lutea and Fovea Centralis. As stated previously, the macula lutea is an oval, yellowish area at the center of the posterior part of the retina (see Fig. 18-7). The nerve cells and fibers of the inner layers of the retina diverge from the middle of this area, leaving the photoreceptors in the center. This arrangement permits incoming light to have greater access to the photoreceptors than elsewhere, and this greater accessibility explains why this central depressed area, called the fovea centralis, has the most distinct vision. There are no blood vessels or rod cells but many cone cells in the floor of the fovea.

Chambers of the Eyeball

The *anterior chamber* of the eyeball is a small cavity lying behind the cornea and in front of the iris (see Fig. 18-4). It is filled with aqueous humor. At the lateral boundary of the chamber, the iris joins the sclera at an acute angle. At the bottom of the angle is a group of anastomosing channels lined with endothelium that encircle the eye. These channels are collectively known as the *canal of Schlemm* (Fig. 18-19; see Fig. 18-4); they drain the aqueous humor from the anterior chamber into the venous system. Guarding the entrance into the canal is a trabecular formation of aqueous humor is believed to be a secretion or transudate from the ciliary epithelium. The *intra-ocular pressure* is maintained by balancing the rate of production and the rate of drainage. The normal intra-ocular pressure is about 12 to 20 mm Hg. The function of the aqueous humor is to support the wall of the eyeball by exerting internal pressure. It also nourishes the lens and removes the products of metabolism; these functions are particularly important because the lens does not possess a blood supply.

Refractive Media of the Eye

The refractive media consist of the cornea, the aqueous humor, the lens, and the vitreous body. The cornea and the aqueous humor have been described.

LENS. The lens is a transparent, biconvex structure enclosed in a transparent capsule (see Fig. 18-4). It is situated behind the iris and in front of the vitreous

AQUEOUS HUMOR. The aqueous humor is a clear fluid that fills the anterior and posterior chambers of the eyeball (see Fig. 18-7). It is constantly in motion and is formed by the ciliary processes of the ciliary body in the posterior chamber. The aqueous humor flows through the pupil into the anterior chamber and is drained away into the canal of Schlemm. The

chamber.

The *posterior chamber* is also a small, slitlike cavity; it lies behind the iris and in front of the lens and the ciliary and vitreous bodies (see Fig. 18-7). The posterior chamber is filled with aqueous humor and communicates through the pupil with the anterior chamber.

Schlemm.

meshwork of connective tissue whose spaces are lined with endothelium; the meshwork filters the aqueous humor before it enters the canal of

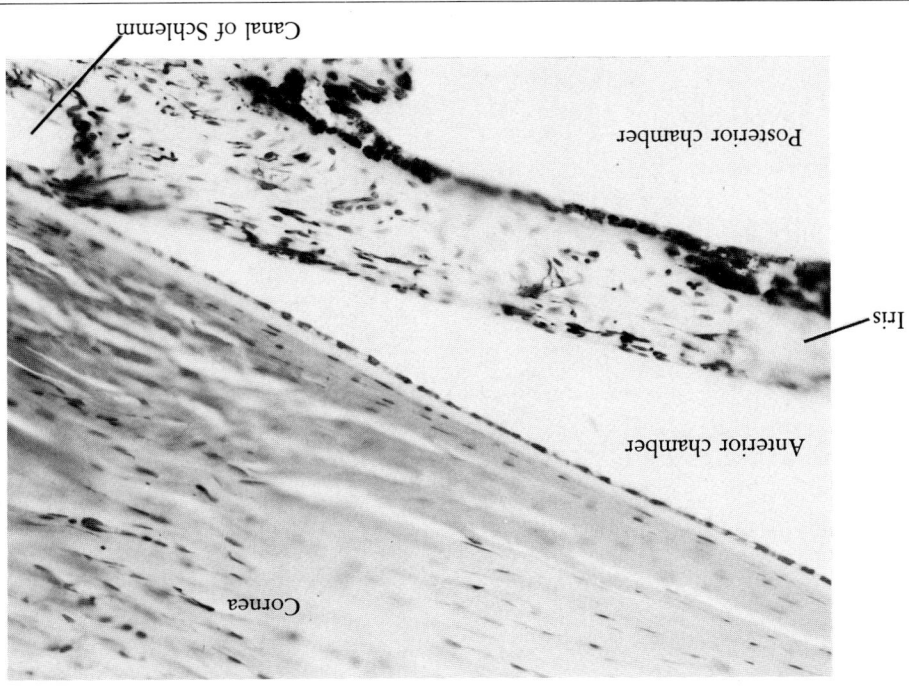

Fig. 18-19. Photomicrograph of the anterior portion of the eyeball close to the corneoscleral junction. Note the cornea, the anterior chamber, the canal of Schlemm, the iris, and the posterior chamber. (H&E; × 200.)

The adult lens is made up of three parts: (1) an elastic capsule; (2) a lens epithelium, which is confined to the anterior surface of the lens; and (3) the lens fibers (see Fig. 18-4).

The *capsule* is an elastic basal lamina that envelops the entire lens (Figs. 18-20 and 18-21; see Fig. 18-4). It is formed by the epithelial lens cells and is composed of reticular fibers embedded in a matrix of glycoproteins and sulfated glycosaminoglycan.

The *lens epithelium* is cuboidal and lies beneath the capsule. It is found only on the anterior surface of the lens. At the equator, these cells elongate and form columnar cells; here, they are transformed into lens fibers (see Figs. 18-4, 18-20, and 18-22).

The dioptric power of the entire eye is about 58 diopters, and the cornea is responsible for most of the lens.

body and is encircled by the ciliary processes. The lens has considerable flexibility. The peripheral edge of the lens is referred to as the *equator*.

The *lens fibers* constitute the main mass of the lens (see Figs. 18-4 and 18-21). The fibers are formed by the multiplication and differentiation of the lens epithelial cells at the equator. The lens cell elongates and turns meridionally (Fig. 18-22). The nucleus disappears, leaving a few microtubules and an occasional mitochondrium in the cytoplasm. As new lens fibers are added concentrically, the lens enlarges. This process continues throughout life. The lens fibers are held together by the interlocking of their adjacent plasma membranes (Fig. 18-23); they extend anteroposteriorly across the entire diameter of the lens.

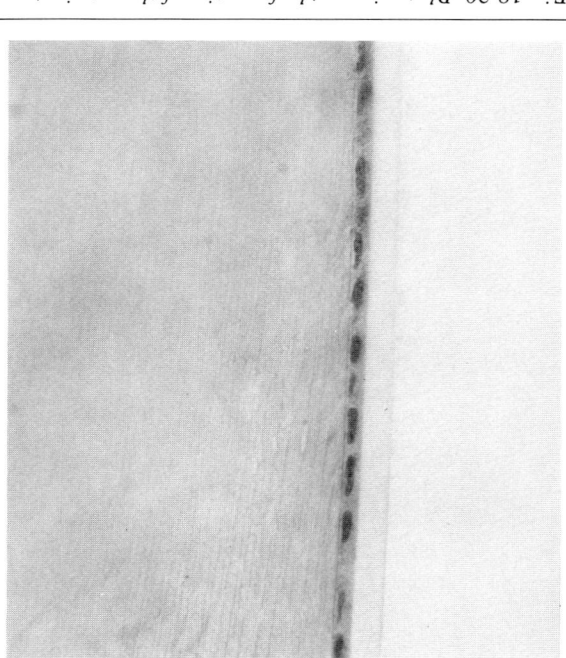

Fig. 18-20. Photomicrograph of a section of the anterior portion of the lens, showing the clear capsule and the underlying lens epithelium (left). The lens fibers, which constitute the main mass of the lens, are also shown (right). (H&E; × 400.)

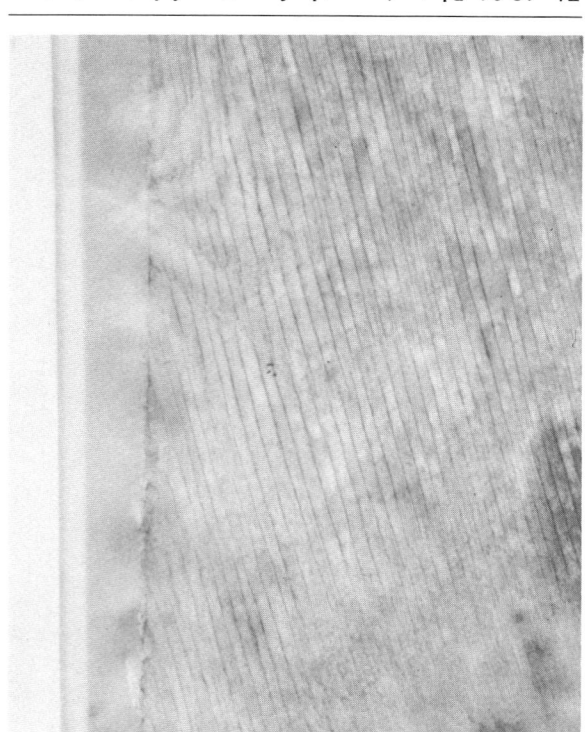

Fig. 18-21. Photomicrograph of a section of the posterior portion of the lens, showing the clear capsule (right) and the lens fibers. (H&E; × 400.)

748   18. SPECIAL SENSE ORGANS

this refractive ability. The lens contributes only about 15 diopters to the total power. The importance of the lens is that it can change its dioptric power, allowing distant and near objects to be focused on the retina.

In adulthood, the lens is transparent and flexible. In old age, it becomes slightly opaque and denser. *Suspension of the Lens.* The lens is held in position by a series of delicate, radially arranged fibers (Fig. 18-24; see Fig. 18-4) collectively known as the *suspensory ligament* of the lens, or *zonule*. The fibers are attached laterally to the ciliary processes and centrally to the capsule of the lens in the equatorial region.

The elastic lens capsule is under tension, causing the lens constantly to endeavor to assume a globular rather than a discoid shape. The equatorial region, or circumference, of the lens is attached to the ciliary processes of the ciliary body by the suspensory ligament, as we have noted. The pull of the radiating fibers of the suspensory ligament tends to keep the elastic lens flattened, permitting the eye to focus on distant objects.

Accommodation. To accommodate the eye for close objects, the ciliary muscle contracts and pulls the ciliary body forward and inward, so that the radiating fibers of the suspensory ligament are relaxed. This process allows the elastic lens to assume a more nearly globular shape. At the same time, the sphincter pupillae muscle contracts, so that the pupil becomes smaller and only the light rays going through the thickest, central part of the lens impinge on the retina.

With advancing age, the lens becomes denser and less elastic, and, as a result, the ability to accommodate is lessened (presbyopia). This disability may be overcome by the use of an additional lens in the form of eyeglasses to assist the eye in focusing on nearby objects.

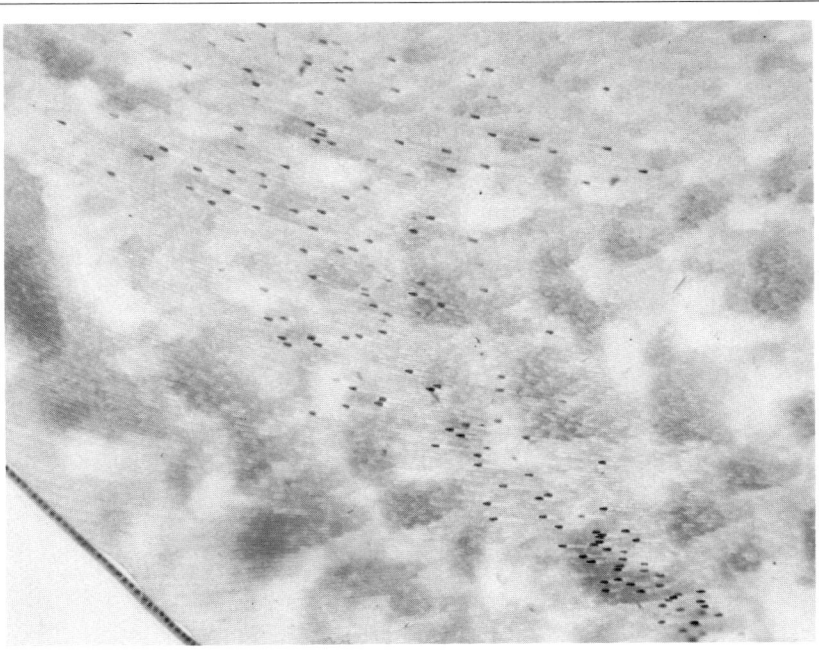

Fig. 18-22. Photomicrograph of a section of the lens close to the equator, showing the anterior lens epithelium (top, right) and the nuclei of the lens epithelial cells. As the lens epithelial cells elongate, the nuclei disappear and the cells become lens fibers. (H&E; × 100.)

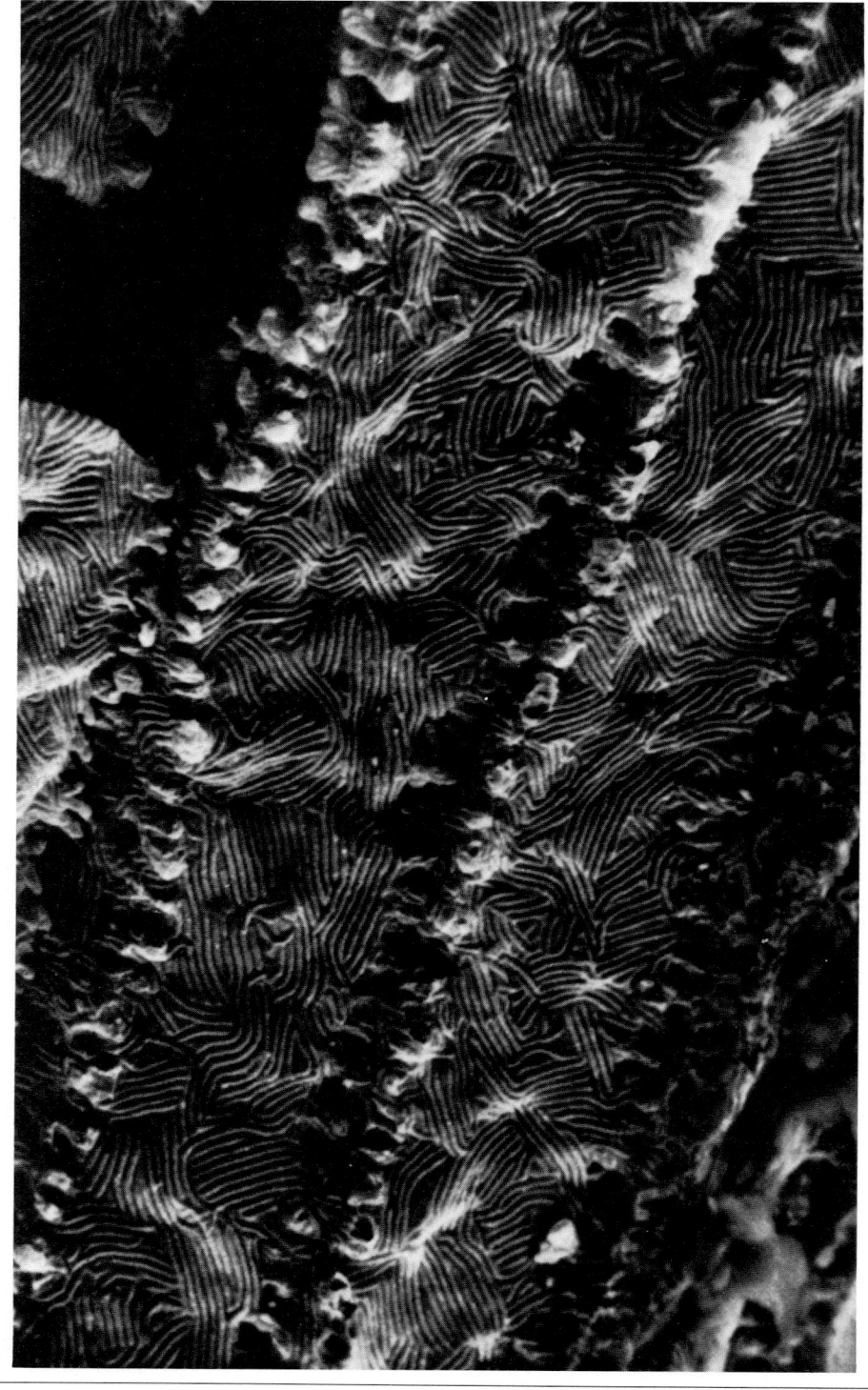

Fig. 18-23. Scanning electron micrograph of a surface view of the lens fibers. Note the fine, interlocking ridges on the surface of the fibers. (×5,500.) (Courtesy of Dr. D. H. Dickson.)

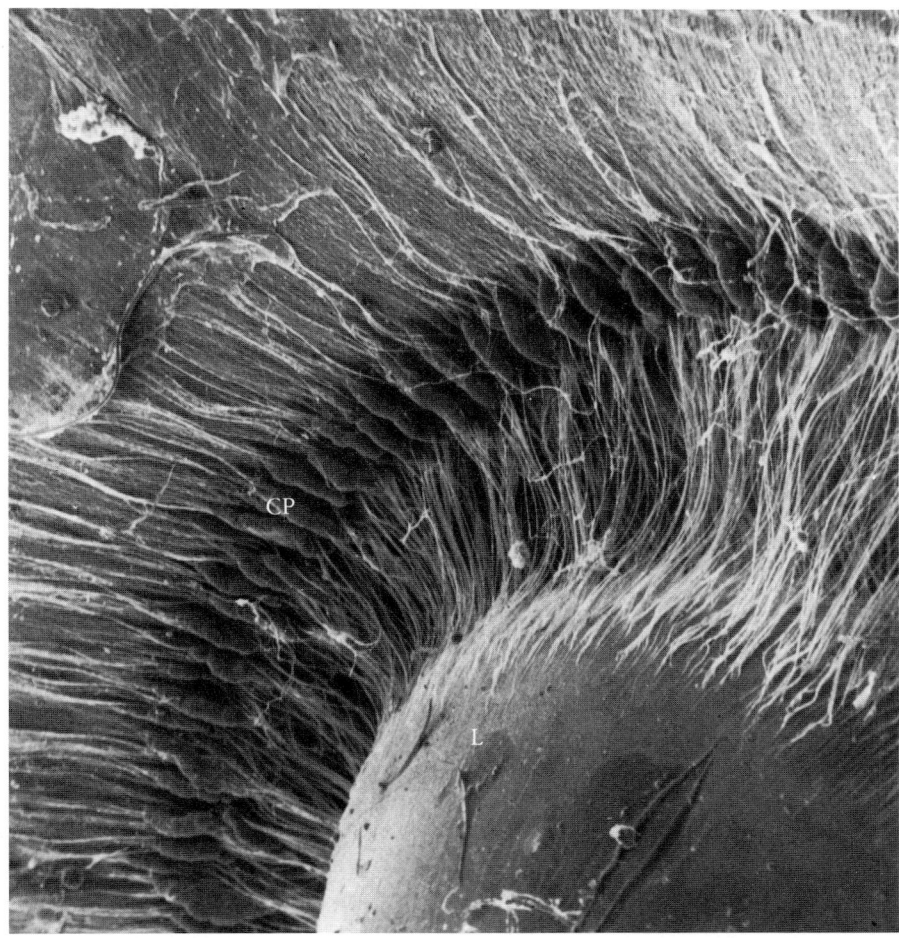

Fig. 18-24. Scanning electron micrograph of the posterior surface of the lens, showing the fibers that form the suspensory ligament, or zonule. The fibers are attached laterally to the ciliary processes (CP) and medially to the capsule of the lens (L) in the equatorial region. (×20.) (Courtesy of Dr. D. H. Dickson.)

VITREOUS BODY. The vitreous body fills the eyeball behind the lens (see Fig. 18-7). It is a transparent gel composed of a network of fine collagen fibrils embedded in a matrix containing hyaluronate. At the periphery, the gel is condensed to form the *vitreous membrane*. Occasional cells called *hyalocytes* are present at the periphery and are thought to be concerned with collagen synthesis. A few macrophages may also be present. The *hyaloid canal* is a narrow channel that runs through the vitreous body from the optic disc to the posterior surface of the lens; in the fetus, it is filled by the hyaloid artery, which disappears before birth.

In front, in the region of the margin of the lens, the hyaloid membrane thickens and becomes closely associated with the suspensory ligament of the lens.

The function of the vitreous body is to transmit light and to contribute slightly to the dioptric power of the eye. It supports the posterior surface of the lens and assists in holding the neural part of the retina against the pigmented part of the retina. It may also play a role in the nourishment of the retina.

Functions of the Eye

The eye closely resembles a camera (Fig. 18-25). The camera contains a variable aperture, and the light rays are bent by the lens and focused on photographic film. The eye also contains a variable aperture, the pupil, and the refracting media include the cornea, aqueous humor, lens, and vitreous humor. The most important of these is the cornea, but the lens, by changing its shape, permits focusing on near and distant objects. This ability to adjust the refracting medium is known as accommodation. In the eye, the retina takes the place of photographic film.

In a camera, the image of an object falls on the sensitive photographic film inverted and reversed from side to side (see Fig. 18-25). In the eye the image is similarly placed on the retina. The conscious brain, however, has been trained to consider the inverted and transposed image as normal, so that the object is perceived in its true position.

Once the light rays have impinged on the retina, the rod cells and cone cells are stimulated, and nerve impulses are conveyed to the brain via the optic nerve.

Function of the Photoreceptors

Light rays impinging on the retina bring about chemical changes in the rod and cone cells, leading to their excitation and the transmission of nerve impulses along nerve fibers leading from the eye. In the discs of the outer segment of the rod cells is the pigment called rhodopsin (visual purple). Rhodopsin is made up of vitamin A aldehyde (retinal) in combination with a protein called rod opsin. On exposure to light, the rhodopsin decomposes and the color bleaches out. This photochemical reaction leads to hyperpolarization of the rod cell plasma membrane, which in turn causes depolarization of the plasma membrane of a bipolar neuron. By this mechanism, light energy is transduced into a membrane potential. The rod cells are concerned with detecting light of low intensity; they are absent from the fovea centralis but concentrated in the periphery of the retina. The rod cells enable us to see only outlines of objects, with no detail or color.

The photochemical mechanisms for the cone cells are similar. The cone pigment is called iodopsin and is a combination of retinal and cone opsin. The light-sensitive chemicals decompose only when exposed to bright light. Cone cells are present in large numbers in the fovea centralis, but few are present at the periphery of the retina. The cone cells enable us to see high-intensity light, in which we see detail and color. The great visual acuity obtained with cone cell stimulation is a result of the synapsing of cone cells on individual bipolar cells.

COLOR VISION. Different types of photochemicals exist in three different types of cones. One type of cone is stimulated primarily by long-wavelength light (such as red light), some by green light, and some by blue light, which has a short wavelength. Stimulation of the three types of cones equally results in the perception of white light.

RELATIONSHIP BETWEEN VITAMIN A AND VISION. The photochemical rhodopsin in the rod cells is a complex made up of the aldehyde of vitamin A (retinal) and a protein called rod opsin (scotopsin). The photochemicals called iodopsins found in the cone cells are complexes made up of the aldehyde of vitamin A (retinal) and proteins called cone opsins (photopsins). The retinal portions are identical in the rod and cone cells.

When the photochemicals decompose on exposure to light, vitamin A is formed and stored in the adjacent pigment cells of the retina. Vitamin A returns to the photoreceptors during dark adaptation.

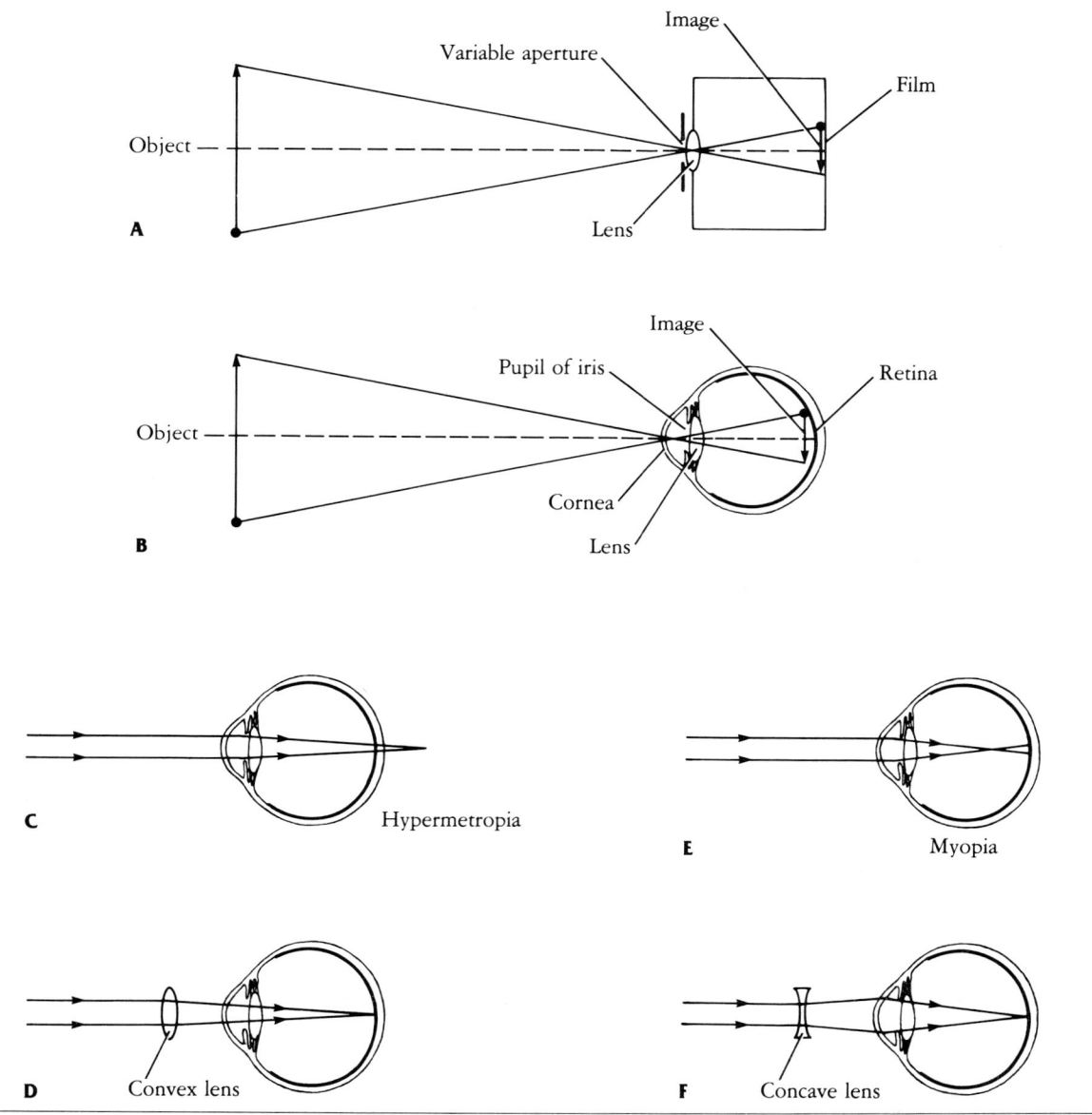

Fig. 18-25. (A) Optics of a simple camera; (B) optics of the eye; (C) parallel light rays focusing behind the retina in hypermetropia; (D) correction of hypermetropia with a convex lens; (E) parallel light rays focusing in front of the retina in myopia; (F) correction of myopia with a concave lens.

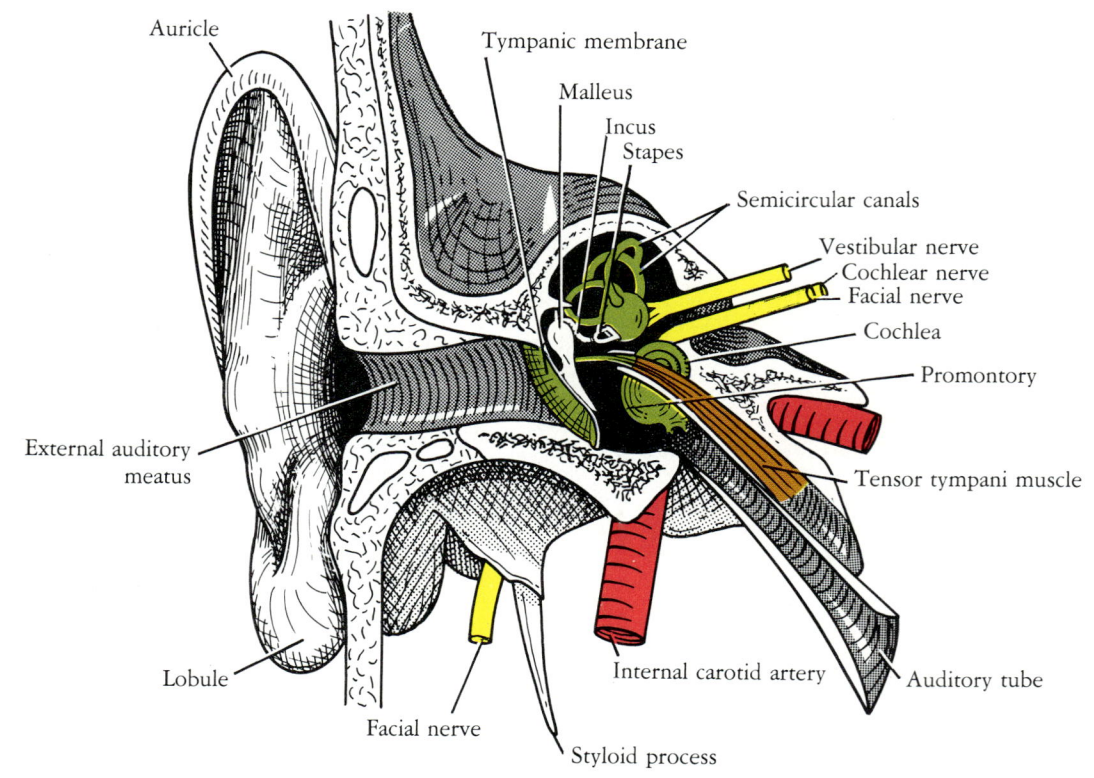

Fig. 18-26. *External, middle, and internal portions of the ear, viewed from the front.*

THE EAR

The ear can be divided into the external ear, the middle ear (or tympanic cavity), and the internal ear (or labyrinth), the last containing the organs of hearing and of balance.

External Ear

The external ear consists of the auricle and the external auditory meatus.

Auricle

The auricle has a characteristic shape (Fig. 18-26) and serves to collect air vibrations. It consists of a thin plate of elastic cartilage (Fig. 18-27) that is continuous with the cartilaginous part of the external auditory meatus. It possesses both intrinsic and extrinsic muscles, composed of voluntary striped muscle. The auricle is covered with thin skin containing hairs and sebaceous and sweat glands.

External Auditory Meatus

The external auditory meatus is a sinuous tube that leads from the auricle to the tympanic membrane (see Fig. 18-26), conducting sound waves along this pathway. The framework of the outer third of the meatus is elastic cartilage, and the inner two-thirds is bone, formed by the tympanic plate of the temporal bone. The meatus is lined with skin, and its outer third is provided with hairs and sebaceous and ceruminous glands (Fig. 18-28). The *ceruminous glands* are modified sweat glands that open directly onto the surface of the meatus or into the ducts of

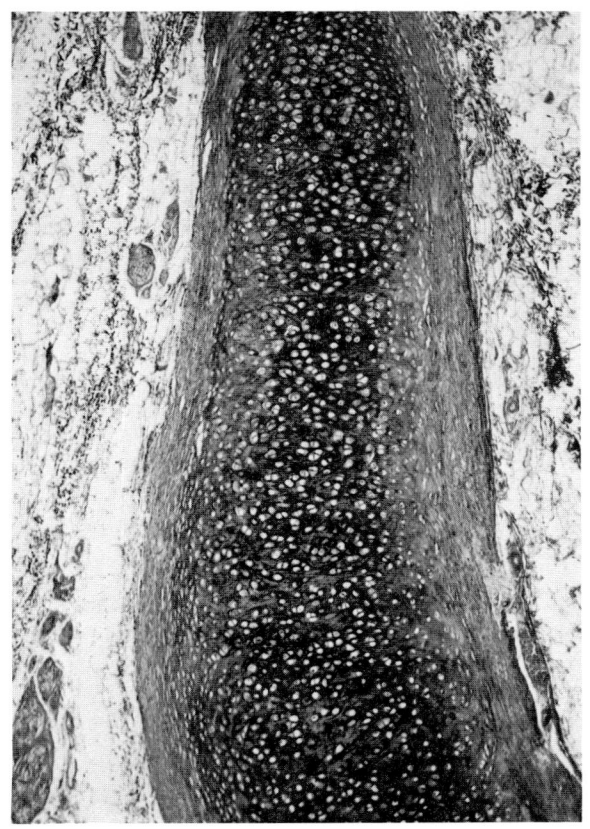

Fig. 18-27. Photomicrograph of a section of the auricle of the external ear, showing the thin plate of elastic cartilage that stiffens the structure and maintains its shape. (Verhoeff's stain; ×40.)

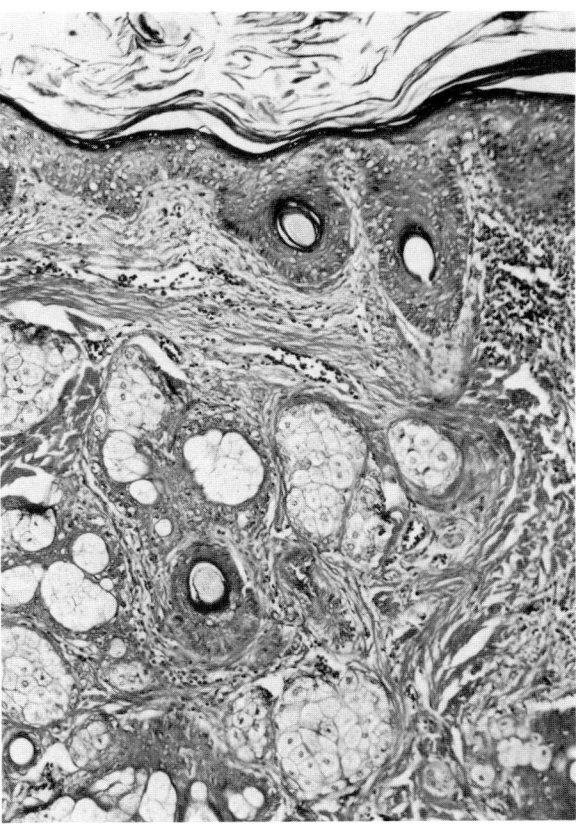

Fig. 18-28. Photomicrograph of a section of the external auditory meatus, showing the meatus to be lined with skin possessing hair follicles and large sebaceous and ceruminous glands. (H&E; ×40.)

the sebaceous glands. The ceruminous glands secrete a yellowish-brown wax called *cerumen*. The hairs and the wax provide a sticky barrier that prevents the entrance of foreign bodies.

Tympanic Cavity

The tympanic cavity, or middle ear, is an air-containing cavity in the petrous part of the temporal bone (Fig. 18-29) and is lined with mucous membrane. It contains the auditory ossicles, composed of compact bone, which transmit the vibrations of the tympanic membrane (eardrum) to the perilymph of the internal ear. The tympanic cavity communicates in front with the nasopharynx through the *auditory tube* and behind with the mastoid antrum.

The mucous membrane of the tympanic cavity is continuous with that of the pharynx through the auditory tube. It clothes the ossicles and muscles in the tympanic cavity and lines the tympanic membrane. The mucous membrane is lined with low columnar epithelium that in many areas is ciliated. There are no glands, but there are goblet cells in the region of the auditory tube. The lamina propria is thin and attached to the underlying periosteum.

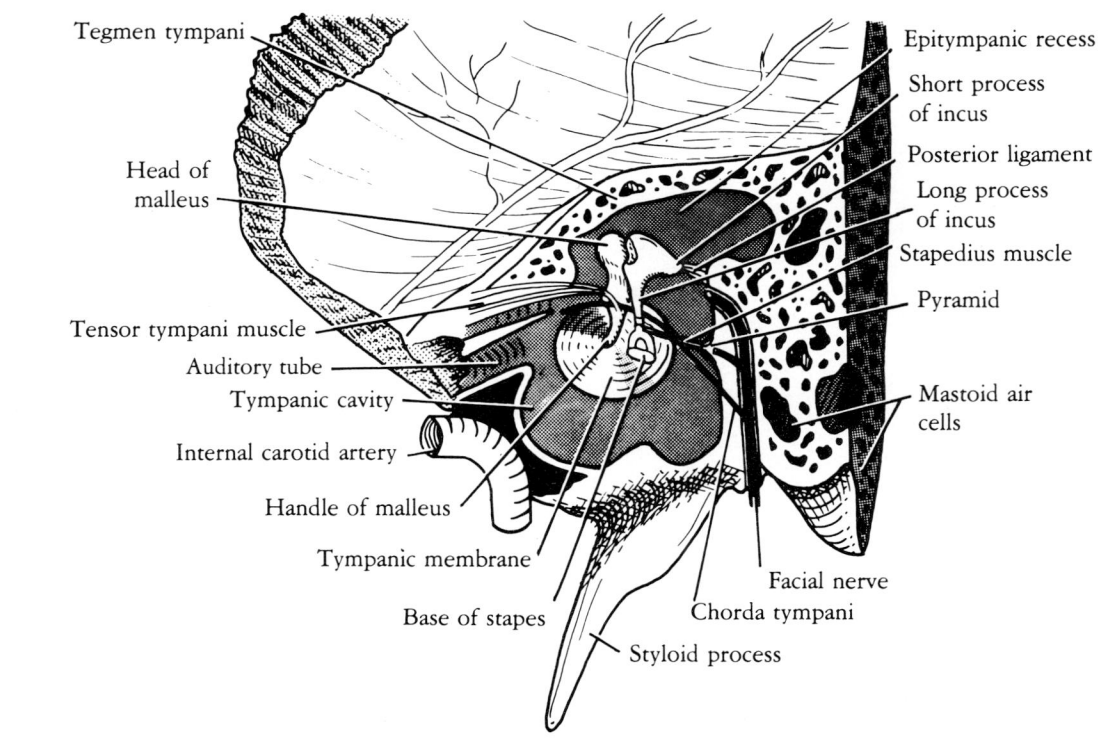

Fig. 18-29. Lateral wall of the right middle ear viewed from the medial side. Note the position of the ossicles on the medial side of the tympanic membrane.

Tympanic Membrane

The tympanic membrane (see Fig. 18-29) is pearly gray and consists of a thin, two-layered fibrous membrane. It is covered on its outer surface by thin skin that is continuous with that lining the external auditory meatus. It is thus covered externally by stratified squamous keratinized epithelium. It is lined on its inner surface with the mucous membrane of the tympanic cavity, which is covered by low columnar epithelium and may be ciliated in part.

The greater part of the circumference of the tympanic membrane is thickened, and this edge is slotted into a groove in the bone. A small triangular area in the superior part of the tympanic membrane, the *pars flaccida*, is devoid of fibrous tissue and is thin and slack; this area is bounded by the *anterior* and *posterior malleolar folds*. The remainder of the membrane is tense and is called the *pars tensa*. The handle of the malleus is bound to the inner surface of the tympanic membrane by the mucous membrane. The tympanic membrane transmits sound vibrations to the ossicles of the middle ear.

Auditory Ossicles

The auditory ossicles are formed of compact bone and are the malleus, the incus, and the stapes (see Figs. 18-29 and 18-30). The *malleus* is the largest ossicle and articulates posteriorly with the incus. The handle of the malleus is attached firmly to the medial surface of the tympanic membrane. The *incus* articulates with the malleus; its long process bends medially and articulates with the stapes. The *stapes* is stirrup-shaped and articulates by a small head with the long process of the incus. The base of the stapes is oval and is attached to the margin of the

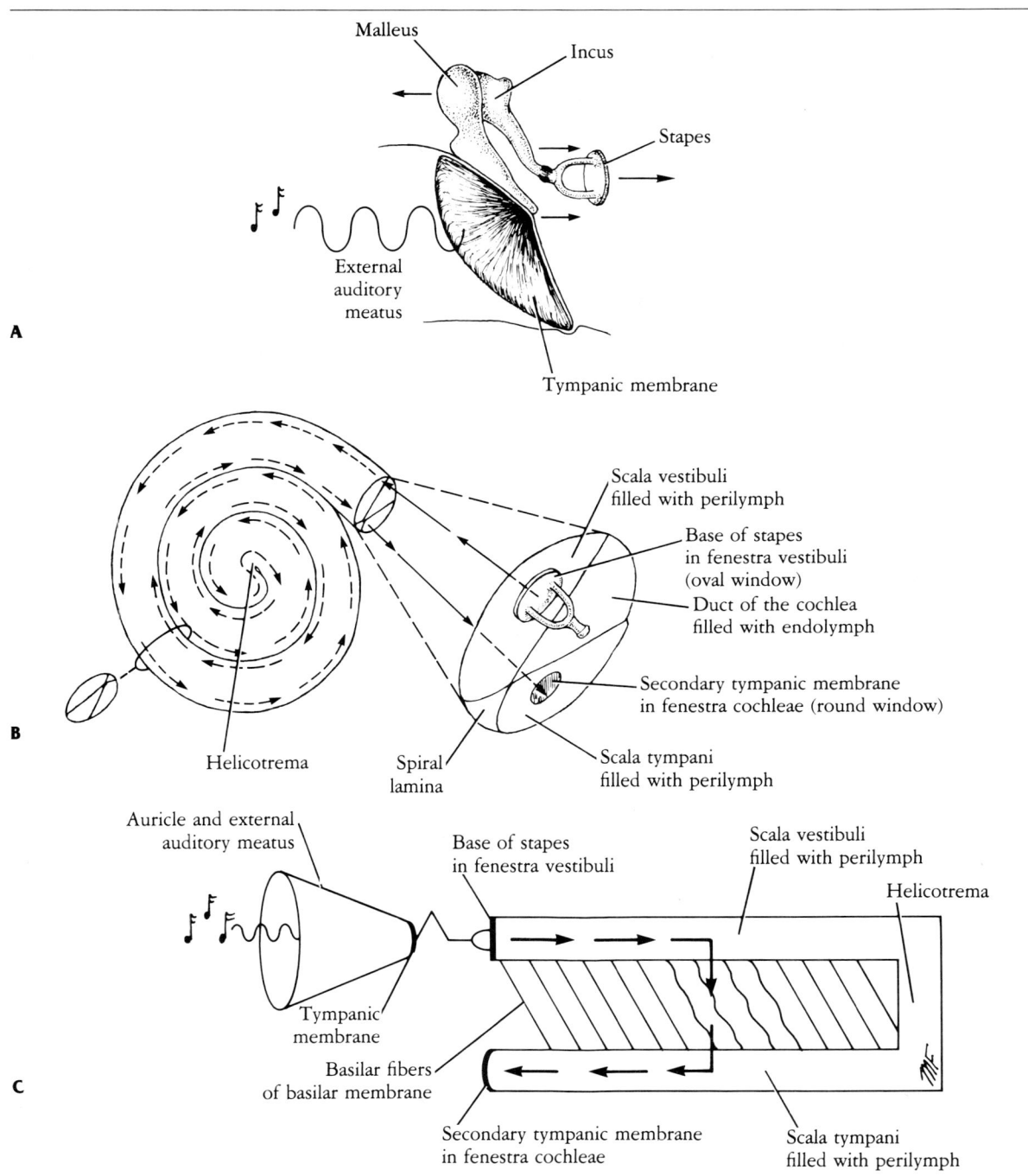

Fig. 18-30. (A) Vibrations of music passing down the external auditory meatus and causing the tympanic membrane to move medially; the head of the malleus and incus move laterally, and the long process of the incus, with the stapes, moves medially. (B) The movement medially of the base of the stapes in the fenestra vestibuli causes motion (arrows) in the perilymph in the scala vestibuli. At the apex of the cochlea (the helicotrema), the compression wave in the perilymph passes down the scala tympani, causing a lateral bulging of the secondary tympanic membrane in the fenestra cochleae. (C) Movement of the perilymph (arrows) following movement of the base of the stapes. Note the position of the basilar fibers of the basilar membrane.

fenestra vestibuli by a ring of fibrous tissue called the *anular ligament*.

MOVEMENTS OF THE OSSICLES. When the tympanic membrane moves medially, the handle of the malleus also moves medially (Fig. 18-30). This causes the malleus and incus to rotate on an anteroposterior plane, so that the head of the malleus and the head of the incus move laterally. The long process of the incus moves medially with the stapes. The base of the stapes is pushed medially in the fenestra vestibuli, and the motion is communicated to the perilymph in the scala vestibuli (see Fig. 18-30). Because liquid is incompressible, the pressure of the perilymph causes an outward bulging of the secondary tympanic membrane in the fenestra cochleae at the lower end of the scala tympani (see Fig. 18-30). These movements are reversed if the tympanic membrane moves laterally. Excessive lateral movements of the head of the malleus cause a temporary separation of the articular surfaces between the malleus and incus, so that the base of the stapes is not pulled laterally out of the fenestra vestibuli.

During the passage of the vibrations from the tympanic membrane to the perilymph via the small ossicles, the leverage increases in a ratio of 1.3:1. Moreover, the area of the tympanic membrane is about seventeen times greater than that of the base of the stapes. These factors together cause the effective pressure on the perilymph of the internal ear to increase by a total ratio of 22:1.

MUSCLES OF THE OSSICLES. The two muscles of the tympanic cavity are the tensor tympani and the stapedius; they are composed of voluntary striped muscle. The tensor tympani is a slender muscle that arises from the cartilaginous wall of the auditory tube and is inserted into the handle of the malleus. It acts to dampen reflexly the vibrations of the malleus by making the tympanic membrane more tense.

The stapedius is attached within the posterior wall of the tympanic cavity and is inserted into the neck of the stapes. It reflexly dampens the vibrations of the stapes by pulling on the neck of that bone.

Fenestra Vestibuli

The fenestra vestibuli, or oval window, is an oval opening on the medial wall of the tympanic cavity; it is closed by the footpiece, or base, of the stapes (see Fig. 18-30). On the medial side of the window is the perilymph of the scala vestibuli of the internal ear. As mentioned previously, the edge of the base of the stapes is attached to the margin of the fenestra vestibuli by a ring of fibrous tissue called the *anular ligament*.

Fenestra Cochleae

The fenestra cochleae, or round window, is a circular opening on the medial wall of the tympanic cavity below and behind the fenestra vestibuli. It is closed by an elastic membrane called the *secondary tympanic membrane* (see Fig. 18-30). On the medial side of this window is the perilymph of the blind end of the scala tympani. When the pressure of the perilymph rises as a result of medial movement of the base of the stapes, the secondary tympanic membrane stretches laterally and bulges into the tympanic cavity to accommodate the increased pressure.

Auditory Tube

The auditory tube extends from the anterior wall of the tympanic cavity downward, forward, and medially to the nasal pharynx. The framework of the posterior third is bone, and that of the anterior two-thirds fibrocartilage. The mucous membrane of the tube is lined with ciliated columnar epithelium, and there are numerous mucous glands. At the pharyngeal opening of the tube, there is an accumulation of lymphoid tissue called the *tubal tonsil* (see p. 357). The function of the auditory tube is to equalize air pressures in the tympanic cavity and the nasal pharynx.

Internal Ear

The internal ear, or labyrinth, is situated in the petrous part of the temporal bone, medial to the middle ear (Fig. 18-31). It consists of (1) the bony labyrinth, comprising a series of cavities within the bone, and (2) the membranous labyrinth, comprising a

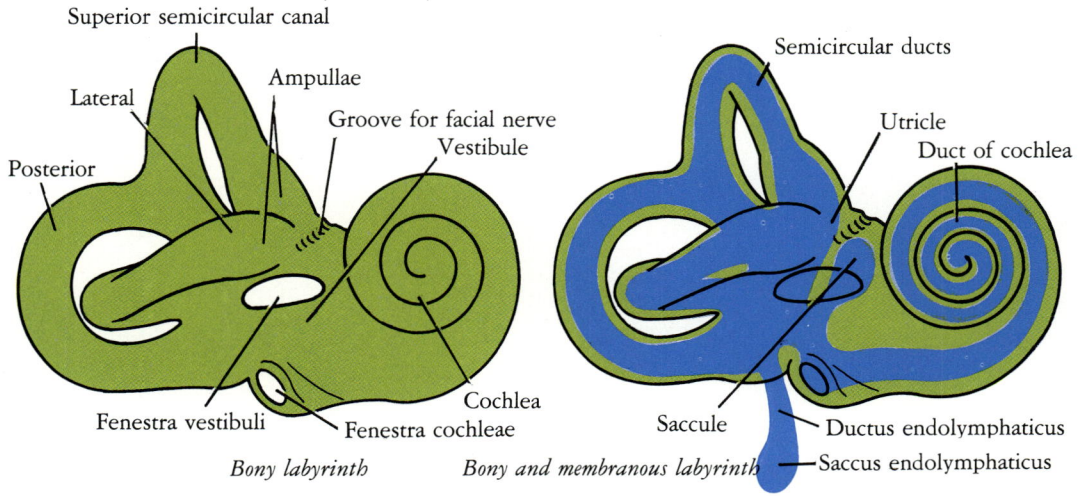

Fig. 18-31. Bony and membranous labyrinths.

series of membranous sacs and ducts contained within the bony labyrinth.

Bony Labyrinth

The bony labyrinth consists of three parts: the vestibule, the semicircular canals, and the cochlea (see Fig. 18-31). These are cavities situated in the substance of dense bone. They are lined with endosteum and contain a clear fluid, the *perilymph*, in which is suspended the membranous labyrinth.

VESTIBULE. The vestibule is the central part of the bony labyrinth and lies posterior to the cochlea and anterior to the semicircular canals. In its lateral wall are the fenestra vestibuli (oval window), which is closed by the base of the stapes and its anular ligament, and the fenestra cochleae (round window), which is closed by the secondary tympanic membrane. Lodged within the vestibule are the saccule and utricle of the membranous labyrinth (see Fig. 18-31).

SEMICIRCULAR CANALS. The three semicircular canals—the *superior* (anterior), *posterior*, and *lateral*—open into the posterior part of the vestibule. Each canal has a swelling at one end called the *ampulla*. The canals open into the vestibule by five orifices, one of which is common to two of the canals. Lodged within the canals are the *semicircular ducts* (see Fig. 18-31).

The superior semicircular canal is positioned vertically and anteriorly (see Fig. 18-31) and lies at right angles to the posterior semicircular canal, which is located vertically and posteriorly. The lateral canal is set in a horizontal position. The lateral canals of the right and left ears are in the same plane, and the superior canal of one side is parallel to the posterior canal of the other (see Fig. 18-34).

COCHLEA. The cochlea resembles a snail shell. It opens into the anterior part of the vestibule (see Fig. 18-31). Basically, it consists of a central pillar, the *modiolus*, around which a hollow, bony tube makes two and one-half spiral turns. Each successive turn is of decreasing radius, so that the whole structure is conical. The apex faces anterolaterally, and the base posteromedially.

The modiolus has a broad base that is situated at the bottom of the internal acoustic meatus. It is perforated by branches of the cochlear nerve. A spiral ledge, the *spiral lamina*, winds around the modiolus and projects into the interior of the canal, partially dividing it (see Fig. 18-36).

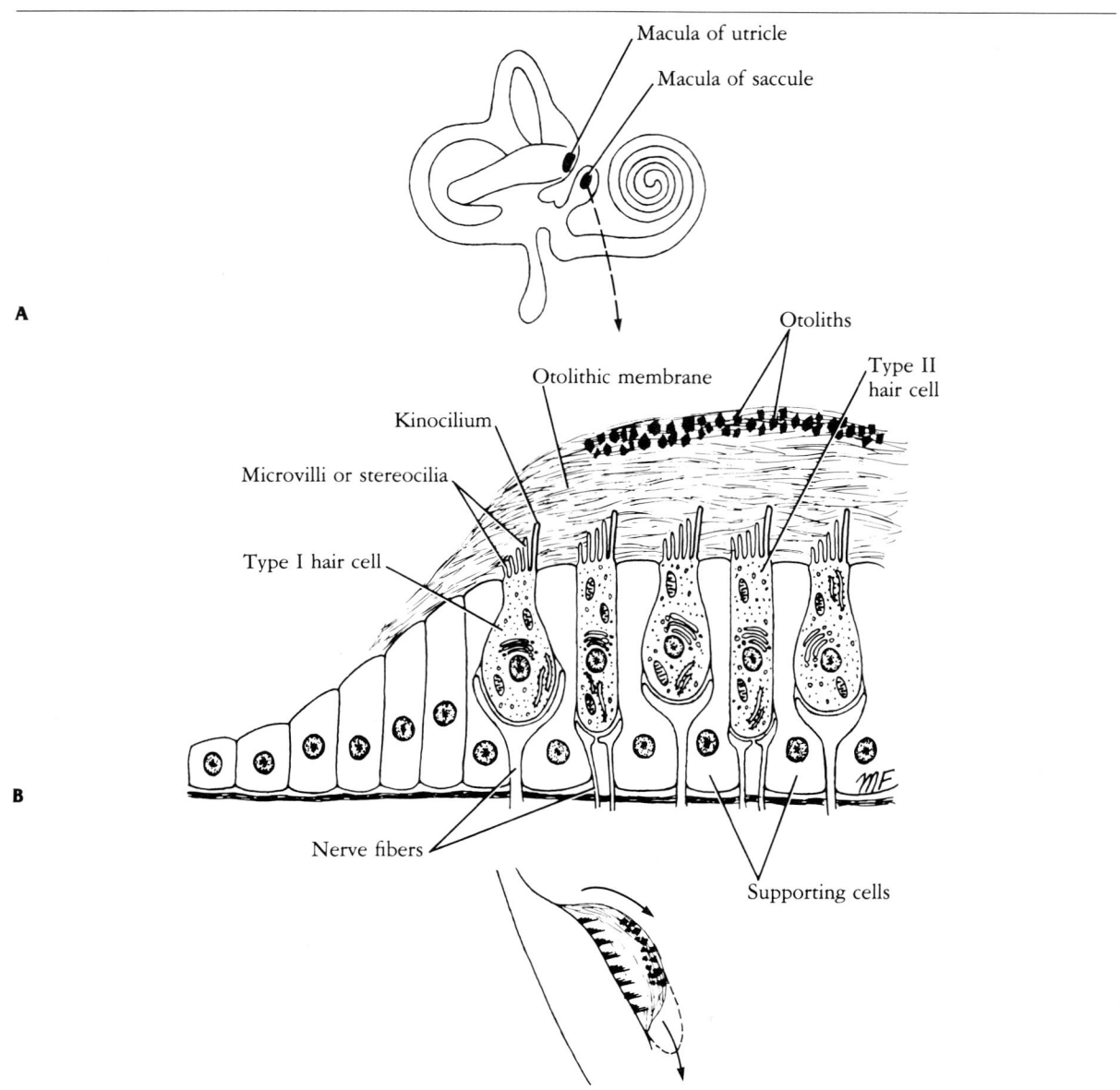

Fig. 18-32. (A) *Locations of the macula of the utricle and the macula of the saccule in the membranous labyrinth;* (B) *structure of a macula.*

Membranous Labyrinth

The membranous labyrinth is lodged within the bony labyrinth (see Fig. 18-31). It is filled with endolymph and is surrounded by perilymph. It consists of the utricle and saccule, which are lodged in the bony vestibule; the three semicircular ducts, which lie within the bony semicircular canals; and the duct of the cochlea, which lies within the bony cochlea. All these structures freely communicate with one another. The membranous labyrinth is lined with epithelium and is connected to the periosteum lining the bony labyrinth by thin strands of connective tissue containing blood vessels. Flowing between the connective tissue strands is the perilymph.

UTRICLE AND SACCULE. The *utricle* is the larger of the vestibular sacs (see Fig. 18-31). It is connected indirectly to the saccule and the *ductus endolymphaticus* by the *ductus utriculosaccularis*.

The *saccule* is globular and connected to the utricle, as we have described. The ductus endolymphaticus, after being joined by the ductus utriculosaccularis, passes to end in the *saccus endolymphaticus* (see Fig. 18-31). This small, blind pouch lies beneath the dura on the posterior surface of the petrous part of the temporal bone. From the lower end of the saccule, a small duct, the *ductus reuniens*, joins the saccule to the duct of the cochlea (see Fig. 18-31).

Located on the walls of the utricle and saccule are specialized sensory receptors called the *macula of the utricle* and the *macula of the saccule*, respectively (Fig. 18-32). These receptors are sensitive to the orientation of the head in relation to gravity or other acceleration forces.

A macula consists of a thickened area of epithelium resting on a basal lamina (Fig. 18-33; see Fig. 18-32). The epithelial cells are of three types: (1) Type I hair cells, (2) Type II hair cells, and (3) supporting cells.

Type I hair cells are flask-shaped; *Type II hair cells* are cylindrical (Fig. 18-32). Each hair cell possesses on its free surface elongated microvilli, or stereocilia, and a single kinocilium; the latter has the microtubular structure of a cilium but is longer than

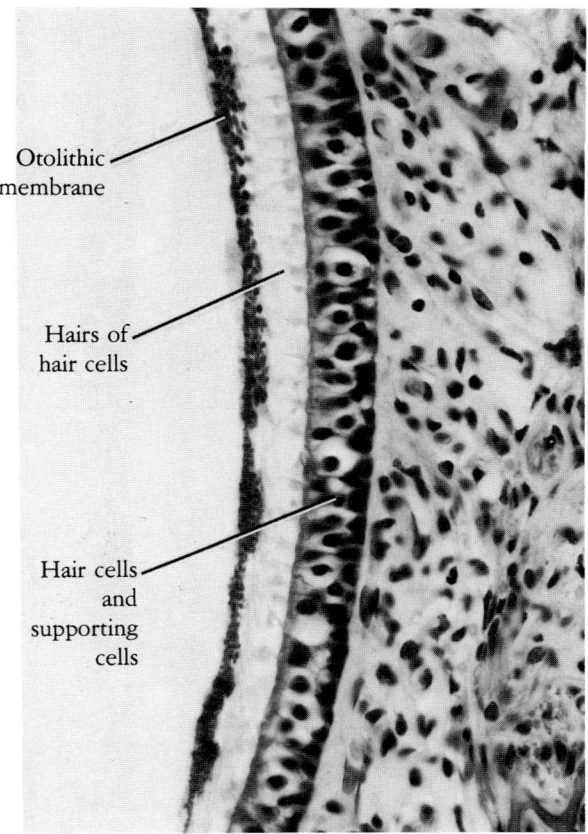

Fig. 18-33. Photomicrograph of the macula of the utricle, showing the hair cells with apical hairs extending into the otolithic membrane. (H&E; ×400.)

the microvilli. The microvilli and the kinocilium constitute the so-called hairs, and they are embedded in a gelatinous membrane called the *otolithic membrane*. Within the membrane are numerous crystalline bodies called *otoliths*, composed of calcium carbonate and associated with protein. When the position of the head is altered in relation to the force of gravity, the otoliths pull on the hairs, which stimulates the nerve endings of the vestibular division of the eighth cranial nerve that are situated between the hair cells. Other forces of acceleration produce the same stimulatory effect on the nerve endings.

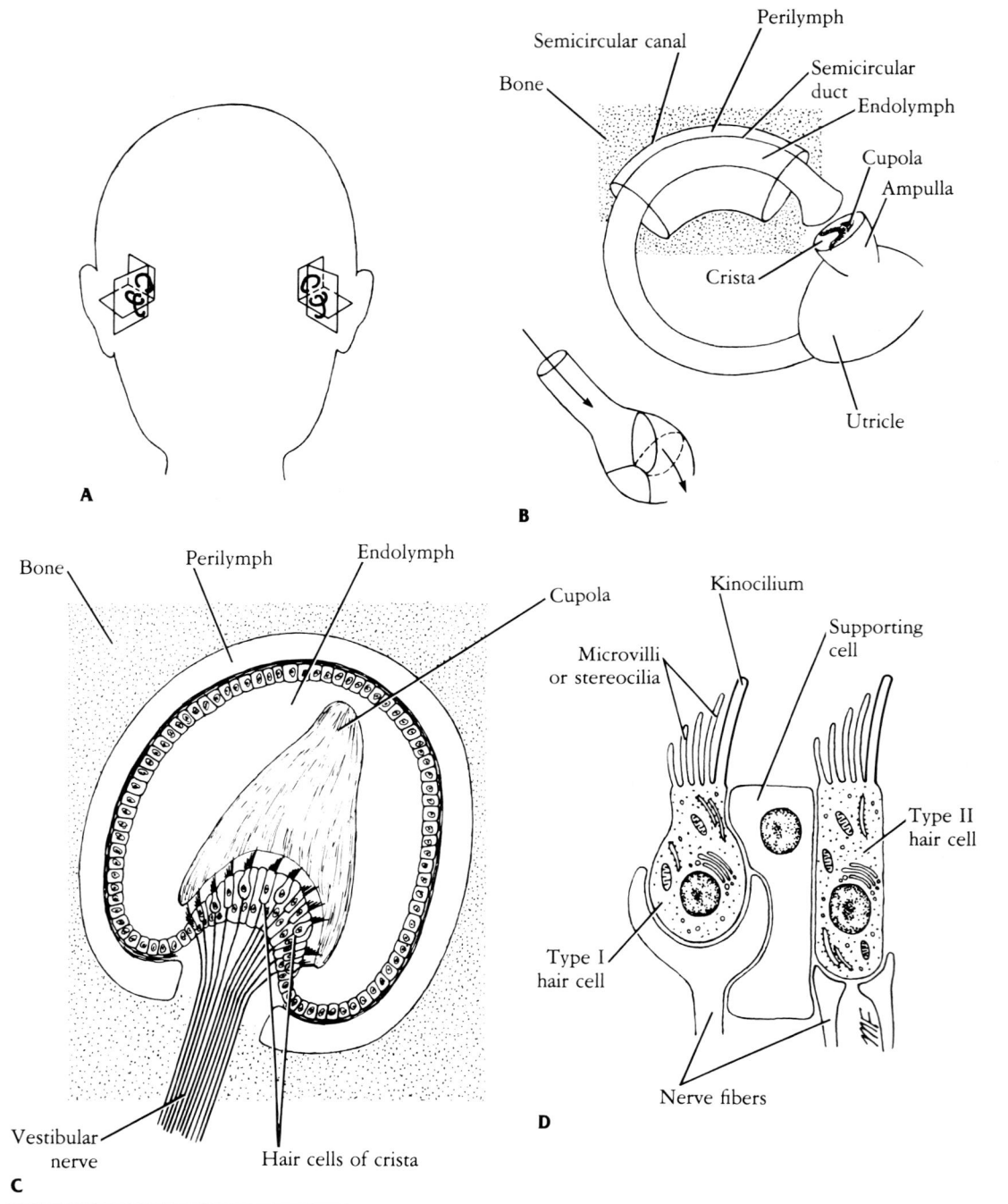

Fig. 18-34. (A) Positions of the semicircular canals relative to one another on the two sides of the head. (B) Position of the crista within the ampulla of a semicircular duct. Note that with movement of the endolymph (arrows), the cupola is forced to move also. (C) Detailed structure of a crista. (D) Arrangement of the hair cells, supporting cells, and sensory nerve terminals in a crista.

The *supporting cells* are elongated and lie on the basal lamina between the hair cells. Each possesses small microvilli on its free surface. The function of the supporting cells is not known with certainty. The cells may assist in the nutrition of the hair cells or modify the composition of the endolymph.

SEMICIRCULAR DUCTS. The three *semicircular ducts*, although much narrower than the bony semicircular canals, have the same configuration. They are arranged at right angles to one another, so that all three planes are represented. Whenever the head begins or ceases to move, or whenever a movement of the head accelerates or decelerates, the endolymph in the semicircular ducts changes its speed of movement relative to that of the walls of the ducts. This change is detected in the sensory receptors in the ampullae of the semicircular ducts (Fig. 18-34).

Ampullary Cristae. Each ampulla contains a transverse ridge in its lining epithelium called a *crista* (Fig. 18-35; see Fig. 18-34). The crista is composed of Type I and Type II hair cells and supporting cells similar to those found in a macula. The microvilli and kinocilia are embedded in a gelatinous membrane without otoliths that is called the *cupola*. Movement of the endolymph in the semicircular ducts, associated with an angular movement of the head, causes the cupola to move and pull on the hairs of the hair cells. These cells are stimulated and in turn stimulate the nerve endings of the vestibular division of the eighth cranial nerve that are situated between the hair cells.

DUCT OF THE COCHLEA. The *duct of the cochlea* is triangular in cross section and is connected to the saccule by the *ductus reuniens*. The duct of the cochlea is a spirally arranged tube lying within the bony cochlea and situated against its outer wall (Figs. 18-36 and 18-37). The sides of the triangular cross section of the duct are made up of the following structures: (1) the basilar membrane, (2) the stria vascularis, and (3) the vestibular membrane.

Walls of the Cochlear Duct. The *basilar membrane* extends from the free edge of the bony spiral lamina

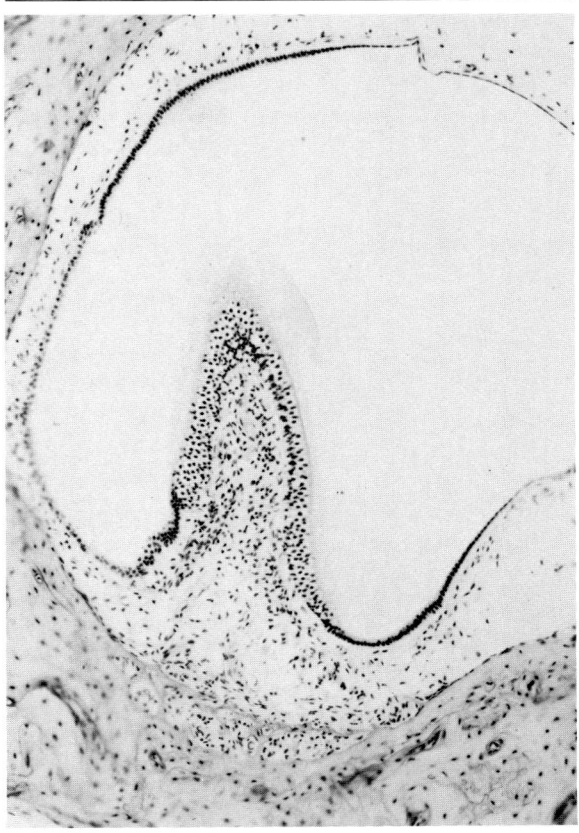

Fig. 18-35. Photomicrograph of a section through the crista of an ampulla; the faintly stained cupola can just be identified. (H&E; ×100.)

to the spiral crest, which is a thickening of the periosteum on the outer wall (Fig. 18-38; see Figs. 18-36 and 18-37). It is composed of collagenous fibers, and some elastic fibers, embedded in matrix. The collagen fibers are collected into compact bundles known as *basilar fibers*. The basilar membrane extends from the base of the cochlea to the apex and gradually widens as it ascends. The highly specialized epithelium that lies on the upper surface of the membrane forms the spiral organ of Corti (see Figs. 18-36 and 18-38). The undersurface is lined with flattened mesothelial cells.

The *stria vascularis* forms the outer wall of the cochlear duct (see Fig. 18-36). It is composed of a

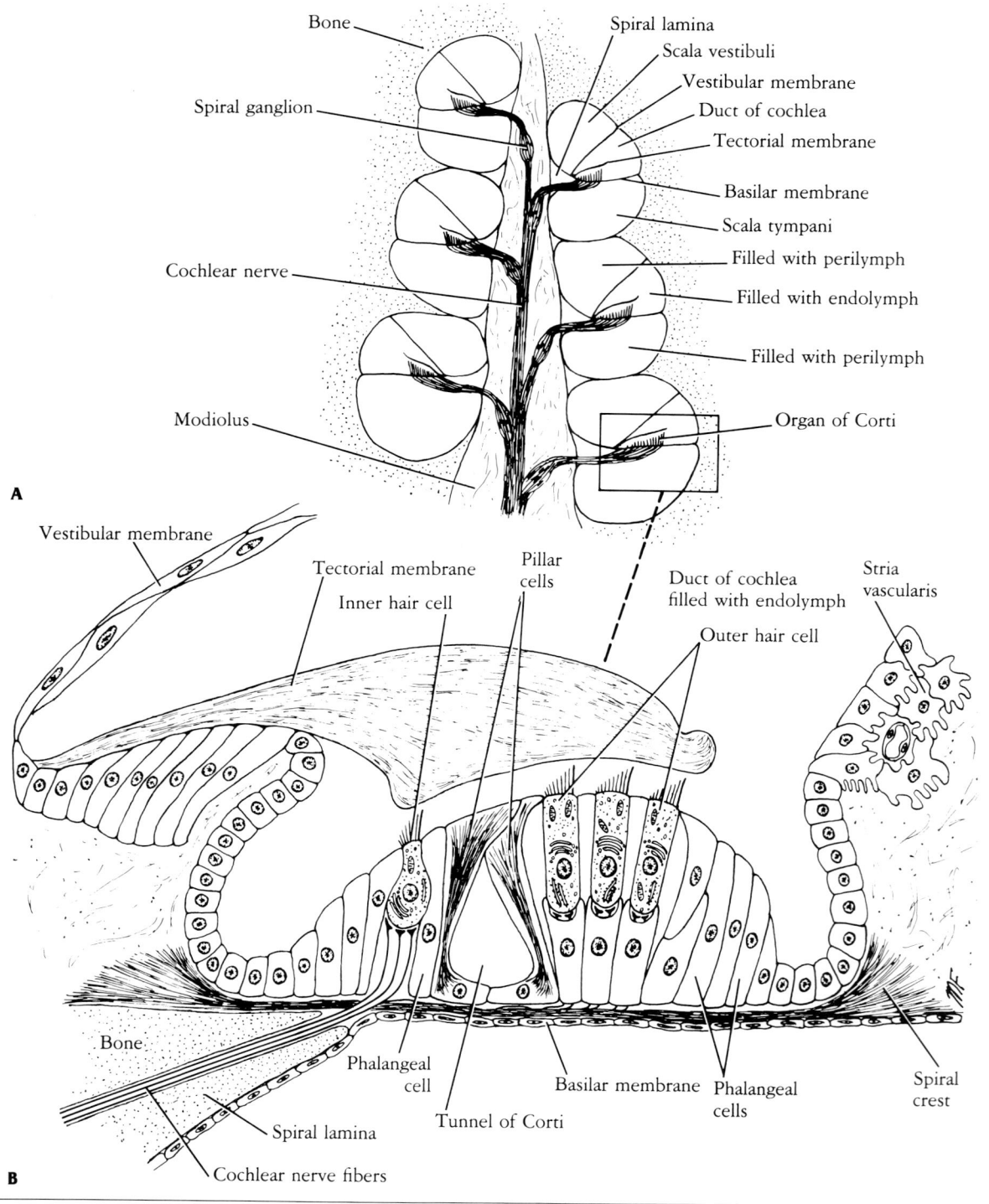

Fig. 18-36. (A) Parts of the cochlea; note the position of the organ of Corti. (B) Detailed structure of the spiral organ of Corti.

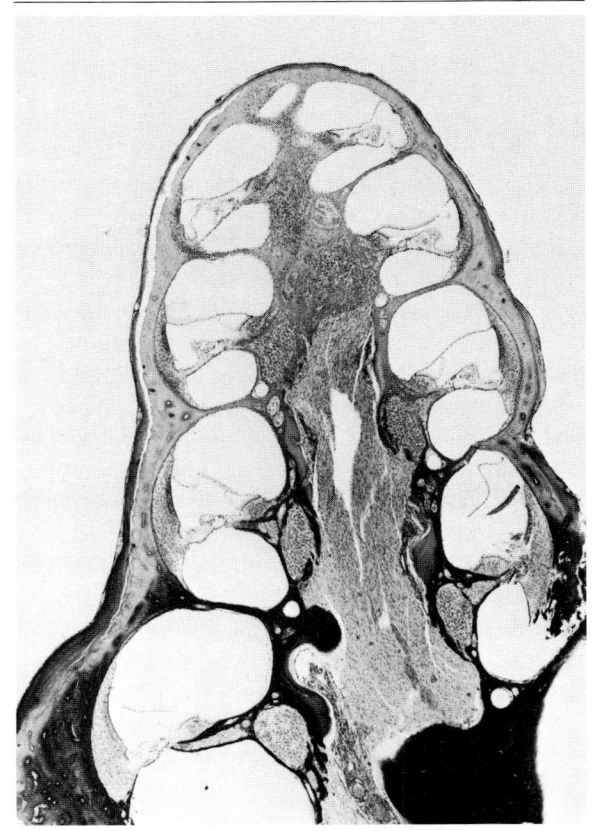

Fig. 18-37. *Photomicrograph of a section of the cochlea; use Figure 18-36A to assist you in identifying the different structures. (H&E; ×25.)*

Fig. 18-38. *Photomicrograph of a section through the spiral organ of Corti; use Figure 18-36B to assist you in identifying the different structures. (H&E; ×200.)*

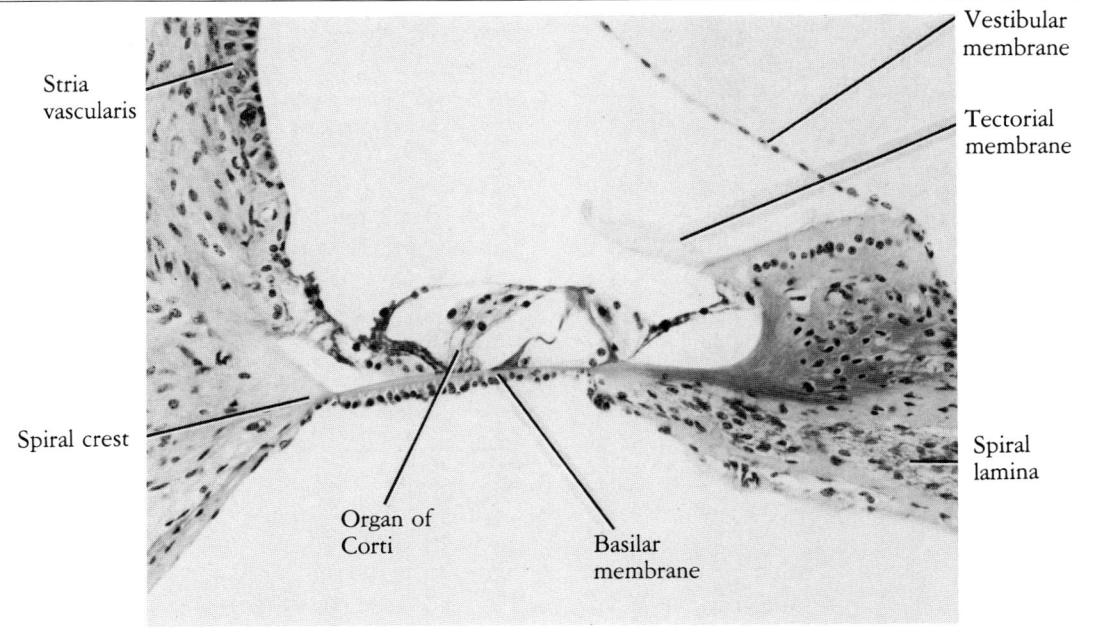

stratified epithelium, between the cells of which runs a rich plexus of capillaries. The stria vascularis is believed to form endolymph.

The *vestibular membrane* (Reissner's membrane) forms the third wall of the cochlear duct. It is composed of two layers of flattened epithelial cells separated by a basal lamina. The cells possess numerous microvilli and may be involved in fluid transport.

Examination of a cross section of the cochlea (see Figs. 18-36–18-38) shows that the basilar and vestibular membranes divide it into three distinct portions: a scala vestibuli above (filled with perilymph), a scala tympani below (filled with perilymph), and the cochlear duct (filled with endolymph). The perilymph within the scala vestibuli is separated from the tympanic cavity by the base of the stapes and the anular ligament at the fenestra vestibuli (oval window). The perilymph in the scala tympani is separated from the tympanic cavity by the secondary tympanic membrane at the fenestra cochleae (round window). The duct of the cochlea (sometimes called the *scala media*) is joined to the saccule by the ductus reuniens and ends as a blind sac at the apex of the cochlea. The *helicotrema* is the point at the apex of the cochlea where the scala vestibuli and the scala tympani become continuous (see Figs. 18-30 and 18-36).

Spiral Organ of Corti. The spiral organ of Corti contains the sensory receptor cells for hearing and is situated on the cochlear duct surface of the basilar membrane. It is composed of hair cells and supporting cells arranged around a space called the *tunnel of Corti* (see Figs. 18-36 and 18-38). The hair cells are classified as outer and inner hair cells according to their position relative to the tunnel. There are from three to five rows of outer hair cells and only one row of inner hair cells. The hair cells are similar in structure to the Type I hair cells of the maculae and ampullae, having many long microvilli, but they lack kinocilia (see Fig. 18-36). The hairs are embedded in a jellylike, proteinaceous material that forms the *tectorial membrane*.

The supporting cells are tall columnar cells known as *phalangeal cells* and *pillar cells* (see Figs. 18-36 and

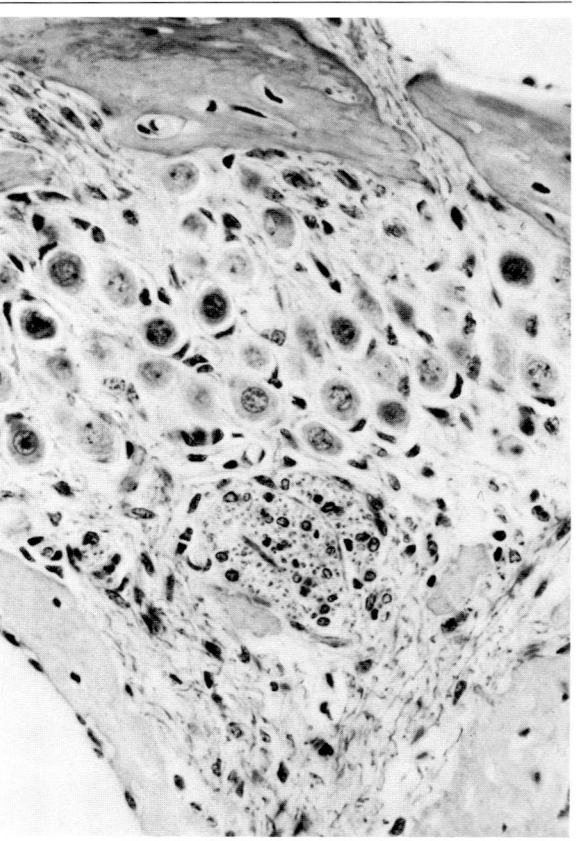

Fig. 18-39. Photomicrograph of a section of the spiral ganglion of the cochlear nerve in the modiolus. Note the numerous ganglion cells. (H&E; ×400.)

18-38). Their function appears to be to support the hair cells and the nerve endings near the bases of the hair cells.

Afferent and efferent nerve endings are present between the inner and outer hair cells. The great majority of the efferent nerve fibers are distributed to the inner hair cells. The efferent nerve fibers reach the brain via the cochlear division of the eighth cranial nerve.

Spiral Ganglion. The efferent nerve fibers from the spiral organ of Corti enter the spiral lamina and converge on the spiral ganglion cells in the modiolus (Fig. 18-39; see Fig. 18-36). The spiral ganglion consists of bipolar neurons whose central processes converge to form the cochlear division of the eighth cranial nerve.

The vestibular division of the eighth cranial nerve, which receives sensory information from the maculae of the utricle and saccule and from the ampullae of the semicircular canals, has a vestibular ganglion situated in the internal auditory meatus.

Mechanisms of the Appreciation of Position and Movement

POSITION SENSE. The specialized areas called maculae in the walls of the utricle and saccule (see Fig. 18-32) are sensitive to the orientation of the head with respect to gravity or other acceleratory forces. As the head changes position, the weight of the otoliths bends the stereocilia and kinocilia of the hair cells, and nervous impulses are transmitted to the vestibular nuclei of the brain stem via the vestibular nerve. Secondary neurons carry the impulses to the cerebellum and to the lower motor neurons in the anterior gray columns of the spinal cord (vestibulospinal tract). By this means, the tone of the muscles of the body can be adjusted so that equilibrium can be maintained.

MOVEMENT SENSE. As we have stated, the three semicircular ducts in each ear are arranged at right angles to one another, so that all three planes are represented. Whenever the head begins to move or stops moving, and whenever a movement of the head accelerates or decelerates, the endolymph in the semicircular ducts changes its speed of movement relative to that of the walls of the ducts. This change is detected in the crista of each ampulla. Alteration in the flow of the endolymph within a semicircular duct will bend the cupola, thus stimulating the hair cells (see Fig. 18-34). This stimulation in turn activates the terminal branches of the vestibular nerve that lie around the bases of the hair cells. Nerve impulses thus pass to the vestibular nuclei and are relayed to the cerebellum and the lower motor neurons in the anterior gray column of the spinal cord. As with position sense, this mechanism brings about adjustment of muscle tone so that posture can be adapted in response to changes in motion in any direction.

Hearing

The external and middle ears collect sound waves and transmit them to the inner ear. The vibrations of the tympanic membrane are transmitted across the middle ear by auditory ossicles, as we have described. The lever action of the ossicles reduces the sound waves in amplitude but increases their force. The inward and outward movements of the base of the stapes in the fenestra vestibuli (oval window) set up corresponding movements in the perilymph of the scala vestibuli (see Fig. 18-30). By this means, pressure waves in the perilymph are conveyed almost at once throughout the length of the basilar membrane. Because fluid is incompressible, the fluid is pushed from the scala vestibuli at the apex of the cochlea through the helicotrema into the scala tympani, causing the secondary tympanic membrane in the fenestra cochleae (round window) to bulge laterally.

The basilar membrane is composed of many thousands of *basilar fibers* that can vibrate. Sounds of high frequency cause the short basilar fibers near the base of the cochlea to vibrate in resonance with the fluid pressure wave, and low-frequency sounds cause the same response in the longer basilar fibers near the apex of the cochlea. Resting on the basilar membrane is the *spiral organ of Corti* (see Figs. 18-36 and 18-38), which is the receptor organ for hearing. When the basilar membrane vibrates, the hair cells, which are supported by the membrane, start to vibrate, and this bends the stereocilia of the hair cells against the rigid tectorial membrane. The stimulated hair cells now initiate nerve impulses that pass to the brain via the cochlear division of the eighth cranial nerve.

Because different regions of the basilar membrane vibrate in resonance with different sound frequencies, the same distinction in response is found among the different groups of hair cells of the organ of Corti. The site along the basilar membrane that

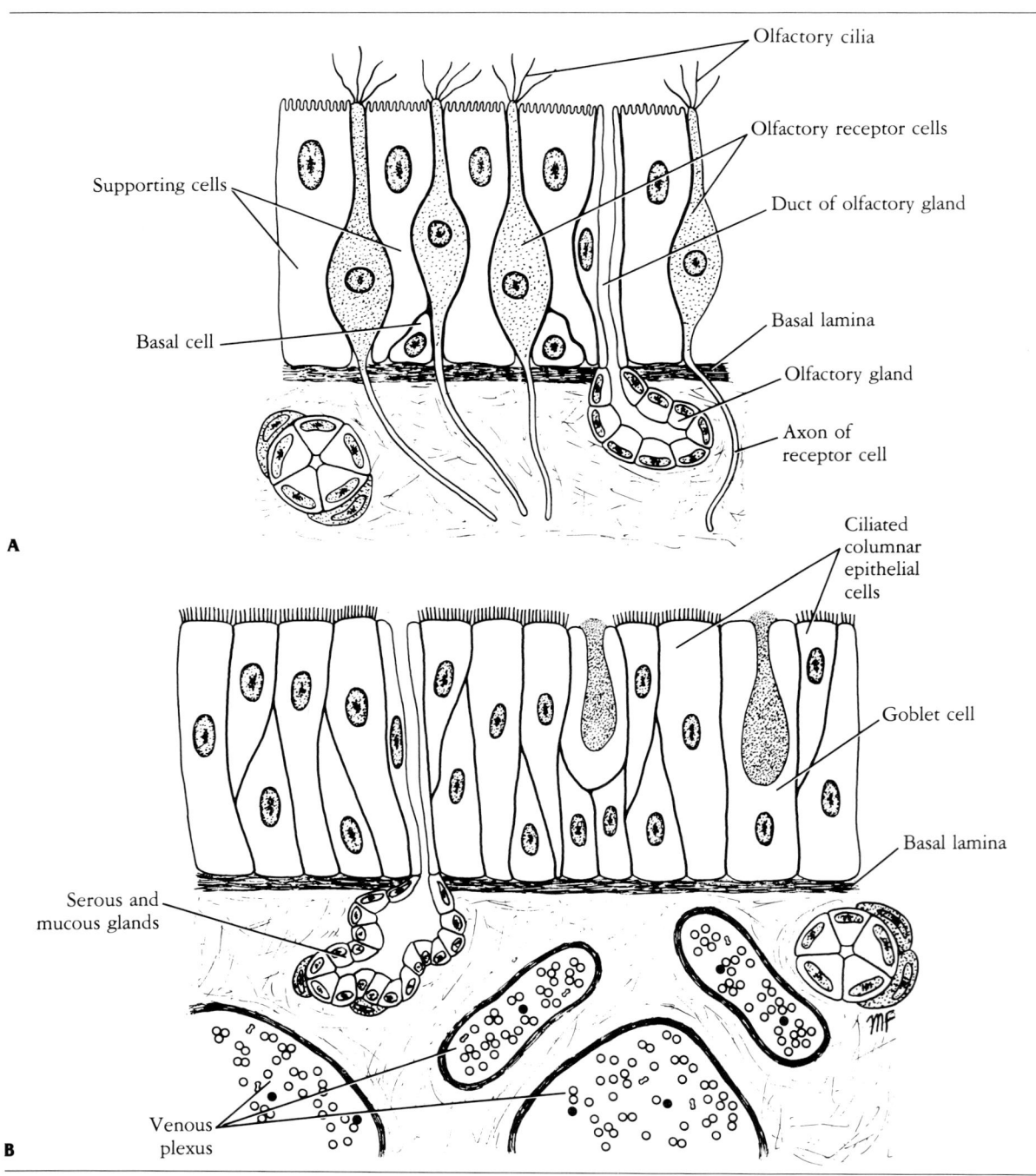

Fig. 18-40. (A) Structure of the olfactory mucous membrane of the nose. Compare with the structure of the respiratory mucous membrane (B).

vibrates in resonance with a particular frequency dissipates all the energy in the fluid pressure wave, so that the wave does not travel farther along the basilar membrane.

The functional distinctions between the outer and inner hair cells are not fully understood. The inner hair cells, with their rich nerve supply, are believed to be the more important. It is possible that the outer hair cells inhibit the inner hair cells during the process of fine tuning for a sound of a particular frequency.

Different parts of the basilar membrane and the organ of Corti are represented in different parts of the cochlear nuclei in the brain stem and in different parts of the auditory area (superior temporal gyrus) of the cerebral cortex. This spatial arrangement enables the individual to detect sounds of different frequencies. The ability to recognize the origin of the sound—for example, a flute or piano—is dependent on the ability of the cerebral cortex to store memories of past sound experiences.

OLFACTORY MUCOUS MEMBRANE

The olfactory mucous membrane lines the upper surface of the superior concha and the sphenoethmoidal recess of the nasal cavity (Figs. 18-40 and 18-41). It also lines a corresponding area on the nasal septum and lines the roof. Its function is the reception of olfactory stimuli, and for this purpose it possesses specialized olfactory nerve cells. The lining epithelium is pseudostratified columnar and consists of three types of cells: (1) olfactory nerve cells, (2) supporting cells, and (3) basal cells that lie on a lamina propria.

The *olfactory nerve cells* are spindle-shaped cells whose dendrites extend to the surface of the epithelium and whose axons run into the lamina propria (see Fig. 18-40). Each dendrite terminates as a rounded end, from which project a number of long *olfactory cilia*. The cilia lie along the surface of the mucous membrane embedded in mucus.

The axon of each olfactory cell is unmyelinated and joins with others in the lamina propria to form bundles of olfactory nerve fibers. The myelinated olfactory nerves pass through the cribriform plate of

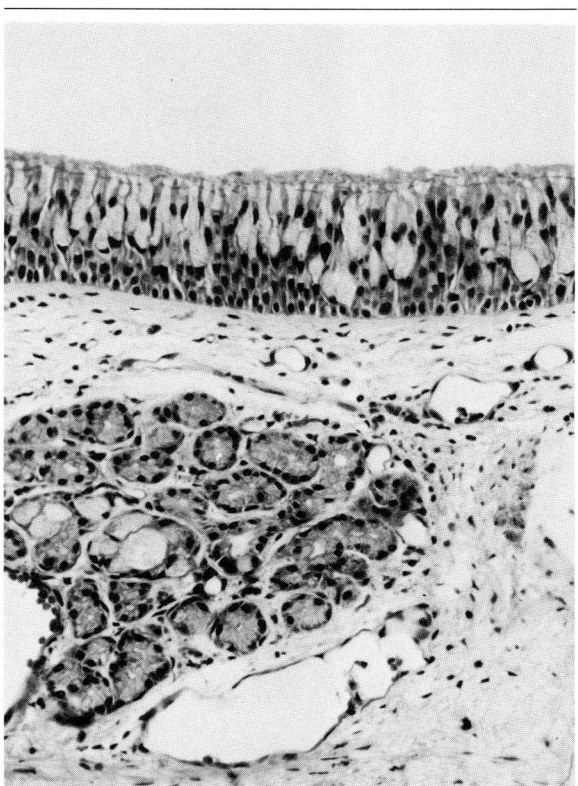

Fig. 18-41. Photomicrograph of a section of the olfactory mucous membrane. Note that the epithelium is pseudostratified columnar and that it rests on a lamina propria. The olfactory cilia are embedded in mucus on the free surface. Note also the olfactory gland in the lamina propria. (H&E; ×200.)

the ethmoid to end on the mitral cells in the olfactory bulb. Here the nervous impulses are relayed to the olfactory areas of the cerebral cortex. Additional neurons relay the information to the thalamus and hypothalamus to be correlated with other sensory information related to eating and sexual activities.

The olfactory cells are stimulated by odorous materials that are inhaled through the nose and dissolve in the mucus covering the cilia.

The *supporting*, or *sustentacular*, *cells* are tall, cylindrical cells that taper toward their bases (see Fig. 18-40). The free surface of these cells possesses many slender microvilli that protrude into the covering of

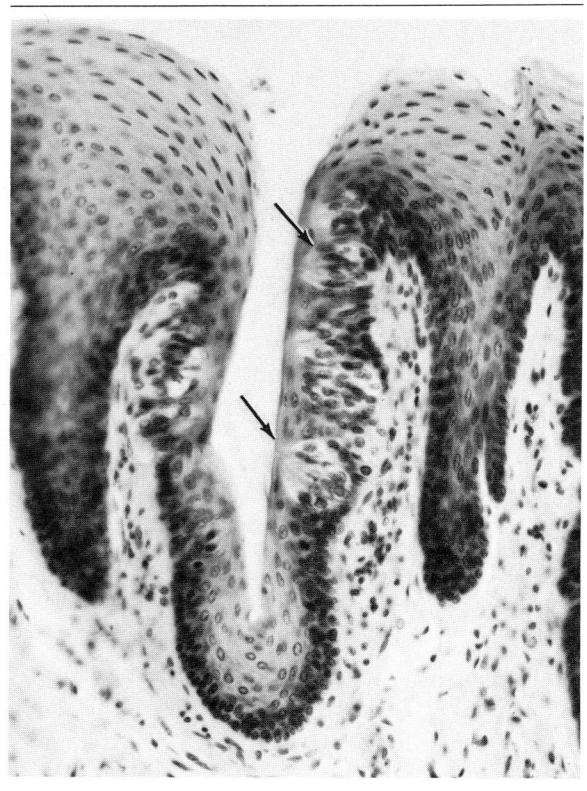

Fig. 18-42. Photomicrograph of a section through portions of two adjacent fungiform papillae of the tongue, showing taste buds (arrows). (H&E; ×200.)

mucus. The cells contain lipofuscin granules, which are responsible for the yellow color of the olfactory mucous membrane.

The *basal cells* are small and conical and lie between the bases of the supporting cells (see Fig. 18-40). They are thought to give rise to new supporting cells.

The *lamina propria* is composed of loose connective tissue in which are found tubulo-alveolar glands (see Figs. 18-40 and 18-41). The thin, watery mucous secretion is carried to the surface of the mucous membrane by narrow ducts. The mucus keeps the mucous membrane moist and serves as a solvent for odiferous substances.

The olfactory function of the nose very rapidly adapts to stimulation. Although this phenomenon is believed to result partly from adaptation by the receptors, adaptation of the central nervous system is also thought to occur.

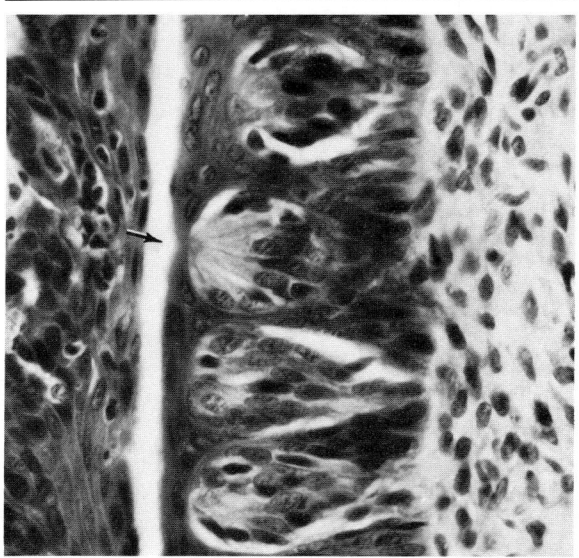

Fig. 18-43. Photomicrograph of a section through several taste buds in the wall of a vallate papilla. Note the light-staining cytoplasm of the taste cells and the taste pore (arrow). (H&E; ×400.)

TASTE BUDS

Taste buds are the sensory receptors for the sensation of taste. They are situated in the walls of the mouth and pharynx, the majority being located on the tongue. Taste buds are found particularly along the sides of the vallate papillae and in the fungiform papillae.

Taste buds are seen with the light microscope as barrel-shaped structures that extend through the full thickness of the surface epithelium (Figs. 18-42 and 18-43). The cavity of the taste bud communicates with the surface through a small opening, the *taste pore*. The taste buds are composed of three types of cells: (1) taste cells, (2) supporting, or sustentacular, cells, and (3) basal cells.

The *taste cells* have a light-colored cytoplasm, are crescent shaped, and possess numerous fine microvilli that protrude through the taste pore as *taste hairs*. Lying alongside the taste cells are branches of the taste nerves.

The *supporting,* or *sustentacular, cells* have a dark cytoplasm and are also crescentic; they are situated between the taste cells. Some of these cells separate the taste cells from the surrounding epithelium. The supporting cells also possess microvilli that protrude through the taste pore (see Fig. 18-43).

The *basal cells* are small and are found between the bases of other cells. They are believed to give rise to the other cells found in a taste bud.

The sensation of taste from the anterior two-thirds of the tongue travels first in the lingual branch of the mandibular division of the trigeminal nerve. It then passes via the chorda tympani nerve to the facial nerve and ends by synapsing on the nerve cells in the *tractus solitarius* in the pons of the brain. The sensation of taste from the vallate papillae and the posterior third of the tongue travels via the glossopharyngeal nerve. The nerve fibers end by synapsing on nerve cells in the *tractus solitarius* in the medulla oblongata.

The four primary taste sensations are *sweet, salty, bitter,* and *acid,* and most taste buds respond to all these stimuli to varying extents. The appreciation of a particular taste—for example, a salty taste—occurs through the stimulation of a taste bud that responds strongly to salty stimuli and gives rise to a stronger series of nerve impulses than does a taste bud that responds only weakly to the salty taste. Other taste buds are particularly sensitive to sweet, bitter, and acid tastes, and the taste mechanisms for these sensations work in a similar manner. There is an almost unlimited number of taste stimuli, and our appreciation of them depends on a varying combination of the four primary taste sensations.

CLINICAL NOTES

THE EYE

Eyelids

The eyelids are thin, movable curtains that protect the eyeball, distribute the tears over the cornea, and control the amount of light entering the eye. They have a complicated structure of skin and mucous membrane and contain striated muscle, connective tissue, hair follicles, and numerous glands. All these structures are subject to disease, but only a few of the more common conditions will be considered here.

Baggy Eyelids

Edema of the eyelids may accompany hyperthyroidism, nephrosis, and angioneurotic edema. Premenstrual edema may cause puffiness of the eyelids. The loose arrangement of the delicate subcutaneous tissue predisposes to the accumulation of edema fluid in this area.

Blepharitis

Inflammation of the eyelid margins may result from seborrheic dermatitis, bacteria, or hypersensitivity reactions.

Hordeolum (Sty)

Acute suppurative infection of the eyelash follicle, the associated sebaceous gland (gland of Zeis), or the associated ciliary gland (gland of Moll) may produce a localized, red swelling of the eyelid margin that ultimately may rupture. The cause is usually a *Staphylococcus* organism.

Chalazion

Acute or chronic inflammation of the tarsal glands (meibomian glands) produces a swelling in the substance of the eyelid. Later, the swelling may point on the inside of the eyelid. Retention of the secretion of the tarsal gland may cause a cystic swelling, sometimes referred to as a meibomian cyst.

Conjunctiva

The conjunctiva is a thin mucous membrane that lines the eyelids and covers the noncorneal portion of the anterior part of the eyeball. The exposed position of the conjunctiva makes it very prone to trauma and bacterial and viral infections. Allergic reactions, as in hay fever, are very common. Inflammation of the conjunctiva (*conjunctivitis*) is very common and is accompanied by vasodilatation of the conjunctival arteries, which become engorged and give the conjunctiva a bright red color.

Lacrimal Apparatus

The lacrimal apparatus consists of the lacrimal glands, which produce the tears, and a drainage system that carries the tears from the eye to the nasal cavity. Diseases of the apparatus include inflammations and tumors of the lacrimal glands, which may produce either excessive or decreased tear formation. Deficient tear formation may be associated with keratinization of the cornea and may cause the loss of an eye. Drainage system blockage may result from congenital blockage of the nasolacrimal duct or may occur secondary to infection. The tears well up over the lower eyelid and drain down the cheek.

Eyeball

Cornea

The cornea forms the transparent anterior part of the eyeball. The central part receives its oxygen for metabolism directly from the atmosphere, whereas the peripheral part receives its oxygen by diffusion from the anterior ciliary blood vessels. This fact is of clinical significance, because leukocytes, in order to combat injury or infection, may have to migrate some distance from the blood vessels at the periphery. In severe infections, new blood vessels invade the cornea in order to bring cellular and humoral defense mechanisms closer to the site of infection. The transparency is compromised, however, and an opacity may develop.

Because a portion of the cornea is exposed, injuries from foreign bodies or abrasions are very common. Damage to the corneal epithelium causes considerable pain and lacrimation. Fortunately, most corneal abrasions heal without treatment.

The cornea, unlike the conjunctiva, is very resistant to infection. It is sensitive, however, to the gonococcus, *Chlamydia trachomatis*, herpes simplex, and herpes zoster.

A *corneal transplant* is the excision of corneal tissue and its replacement by a cornea from a human donor. Full-thickness or partial-thickness grafts can be performed, and the cornea can be replaced entirely or only partially excised. The donor graft is held in position with fine sutures. Corneal implants of nonreactive plastic material can also be used.

Retina

In embryonic life, the optic vesicle is invaginated to form the optic cup. The outer wall of the cup becomes the retinal pigment epithelium, and the inner wall differentiates to form the light-sensitive sensory retina. A potential space remains between these two layers, except at the optic nerve and the ora serrata. Should a hole form in the inner sensory layer, or trauma be applied to the eyeball, fluid may accumulate between the two layers of the retina, resulting in loss of function. This condition is known as *retinal separation* or *detachment*. Treatment of simple retinal detachment is directed toward absorption of the subretinal fluid and closure of the hole in the sensory part of the retina. The closure is accomplished by producing a localized adhesion in the region with a laser beam or by the application of intense cold or intense heat. About 10 percent of patients with retinal detachment in one eye develop the condition in the other eye.

Visual Acuity

The visual acuity of a patient should be tested for near and distant vision. Near vision is tested by asking the patient to read a card with a standard size of type. Each eye is tested in turn, with and without spectacles. Distant vision is tested by asking the patient to read Snellen's type at a distance of 6 m.

Visual Fields

A visual field is the area seen by an eye when it is in a fixed position. The area seen on the side of the nose is called the *nasal field of vision*, and the area seen on the lateral side—that is, toward the temple—is called the *temporal field of vision*. The visual fields are tested as follows: The patient and the examiner sit facing each other at a distance of 2 feet. The patient is asked to cover his or her right eye, and the examiner covers his or her own left eye. The patient is asked to look into the pupil of the examiner's right eye. A small object is then moved in an arc around the periphery of the field of vision, and the patient is asked whether he or she can see the object. The extent of the patient's field of vision is compared with the normal examiner's field. The other eye then is tested. It is important not to miss loss or impairment of vision in the central area of the field (central scotoma).

Circumferential blindness may be caused by hysteria or optic neuritis. *Total blindness* of one eye can follow complete section of one optic nerve. Blindness in one half of each visual field is called *hemianopia*. Lesions of the optic tract and optic radiation produce the same hemianopia for both eyes, i.e., *homonymous hemianopia*. *Bitemporal hemianopia* is a loss of the lateral halves of the fields of vision of both eyes. This condition is produced most commonly by a tumor of the pituitary gland that exerts pressure on the optic chiasma.

Fundi

The ocular fundus (back of the eye) should be examined with an ophthalmoscope. The patient is asked to look at a distant object. When the right eye is examined, the physician should use his or her own right eye and hold the ophthalmoscope in the right hand. The physician should systematically examine the back of the eye, looking first at the optic disc, then at the retina, then at the blood vessels, and finally at the macula.

The *optic disc* is creamy pink, and the lateral margin is seen clearly. The center of the disc is paler and hollowed out. The *retina* is pinkish red because of the blood circulating in the choroidal blood vessels; there should be no hemorrhages or exudates. The *blood vessels* should consist of four main arteries with their accompanying veins. Careful examination of the arteriovenous crossings is important; the veins should not be indented by the arteries. The *macula* is examined by asking the patient to look directly at the light of the ophthalmoscope. It should look slightly darker than the surrounding retina.

Movements of the Eyeball

The muscles that move the eyeball are innervated by the oculomotor, trochlear, and abducens nerves.

The oculomotor nerve supplies all the orbital muscles except the superior oblique and the lateral rectus. It also supplies the striated muscle of the levator palpebrae superioris and the smooth muscles concerned with accommodation, namely, the sphincter pupillae and the ciliary muscle. The trochlear nerve supplies the superior oblique muscle, and the abducens nerve supplies the lateral rectus.

In an examination of the extraocular muscles, the patient's head is fixed and he or she is asked to move the eyes, in turn, to the left, to the right, upward, and downward, as far as possible in each direction. The patient should then be asked to look upward and laterally, upward and medially, downward and medially, and downward and laterally.

In complete oculomotor paralysis, the eye cannot be moved upward, downward, or inward. At rest, the eye looks laterally (*external strabismus*), owing to the activity of the lateral rectus muscle, and downward, owing to the activity of the superior oblique. The patient sees double (*diplopia*). There is drooping of the upper eyelid (*ptosis*) caused by paralysis of the levator palpebrae superioris. The pupil is widely dilated owing to paralysis of the sphincter pupillae and the unopposed action of the dilator (supplied by the sympathetic system). Accommodation of the eye can no longer occur.

In trochlear nerve paralysis, the patient complains of double vision on looking straight downward. This diplopia occurs because the superior oblique is paralyzed and the eye turns medially as well as downward. In fact, the patient has great difficulty in turning the eye downward and laterally.

In abducens nerve paralysis, the patient cannot turn the eyeball laterally. When the patient looks straight ahead, the lateral rectus muscle is paralyzed and the unopposed medial rectus pulls the eyeball medially, causing *internal strabismus*.

Ocular Reflexes

Pupillary Reflexes

If a light is shone into one eye, normally the pupils of both eyes constrict. The constriction of the pupil on which the light is shone is called the *direct light reflex*; the constriction of the opposite pupil is called the *consensual light reflex*.

The afferent impulses travel through the optic nerve, optic chiasma, and optic tract and synapse on nerve cells in the *pretectal nucleus*, which lies close to the superior colliculus. The impulses are passed by axons of the pretectal nerve cells to the parasympathetic nuclei (*Edinger-Westphal nuclei*) of the third cranial nerve on both sides. Here the fibers synapse and the parasympathetic nerves travel through the third cranial nerve to the *ciliary ganglion* in the orbit. Finally, postganglionic parasympathetic fibers pass through the short ciliary nerves to the eyeball and the *constrictor pupillae muscle* of the iris. Both pupils constrict in the light reflex because the pretectal nucleus sends fibers to the parasympathetic nuclei on both sides of the midbrain. The fibers that cross the median plane do so close to the cerebral aqueduct or in the posterior commissure.

Accommodation Reflex

When the eyes are directed from a distant to a near object, contraction of the medial recti brings about convergence of the ocular axes, the lens thickens via contraction of the ciliary muscle and thus increases its refractive power, and the pupils constrict to restrict the light waves to the thickest, central part of the lens. The different impulses travel through the optic nerve, the optic chiasma, the optic tract, the lateral geniculate body, and the optic radiation to the visual cortex. The visual cortex is connected to the eye field of the frontal cortex. From here, cortical fibers descend through the internal capsule to the oculomotor nuclei in the midbrain. The oculomotor nerve travels to the medial recti muscles. Some of the descending cortical fibers synapse with the parasympathetic nuclei (Edinger-Westphal nuclei) of the third cranial nerves on both sides. Here the parasympathetic nerves travel through the third cranial nerve to the ciliary ganglion in the orbit. Finally, postganglionic parasympathetic fibers pass through the short ciliary nerves to the ciliary muscle and the constrictor pupillae muscle of the iris.

Corneal Reflex

Light pressure on the cornea or conjunctiva results in blinking of the eyelids. Afferent impulses from the cornea or conjunctiva travel through the ophthalmic division of the trigeminal nerve to the sensory nucleus of the trigeminal nerve. Internuncial neurons connect with the motor nucleus of the facial nerve on both sides through the medial longitudinal fasciculus. The facial nerve and its branches supply the orbicularis oculi muscle, which causes closure of the eyelids.

Visual Body Reflexes

The automatic scanning movements of the eyes and head made when reading, the automatic movement of the eyes and the head and neck toward the source of a visual stimulus, and the closing of the eyes and even the raising of the arm for protection are reflex actions. In these bodily reflexes, the visual impulses follow the optic nerves, optic chiasma, and optic tracts to the superior colliculi. Here the impulses are relayed to the tectospinal and tectobulbar (tectonuclear) tracts and to the neurons of the anterior gray columns of the spinal cord and cranial motor nuclei.

Pupillary Skin Reflex

The pupil dilates if the skin is painfully stimulated by pinching. The afferent sensory fibers are believed to have connections to the efferent preganglionic sympathetic neurons in the lateral gray columns of the first and second thoracic segments of the spinal cord. The *white rami communicantes* of these segments pass to the sympathetic trunk, and the preganglionic fibers ascend to the superior *cervical sympathetic ganglion*. The postganglionic fibers pass through the *internal carotid plexus* and the *long ciliary nerves* to the dilator pupillae muscle of the iris.

Defects of Refraction

Hypermetropia (Far-sightedness)

In this condition, either the eyeball is too short anteroposteriorly or the lens of the eye is not strong enough to bend the light rays sufficiently (see Fig. 18-25). In either case, parallel light rays entering the eye cannot come into sharp focus on the retina, and the image falls behind the retina. In order to see a distant object clearly, the hypermetropic, or farsighted, person increases the strength of the lens of the eye by accommodation. Only then can the image be focused on the retina. Such an individual thus is unable to focus on a near object and hence is called hypermetropic, or far-sighted. This condition can be corrected by placing a convex lens in front of the eye, as in the use of eyeglasses (see Fig. 18-25).

Myopia (Near-sightedness)

In this condition, the eyeball is too long anteroposteriorly, or, rarely, the lens of the eye is too strong (see Fig. 18-25). In either case, parallel light rays entering the eye cannot come into sharp focus in the retina, and the image falls in front of the retina. Such an individual is unable to see a distant object clearly. If the individual moves close to the object, however, the image eventually comes into sharp focus on the retina; the person is myopic, or near-sighted. This condition can be corrected by placing a concave lens in front of the eye in order to diverge the light rays (see Fig. 18-25).

Presbyopia

With increasing age, the lens loses its elasticity. As a result, the individual is unable to accommodate for near vision because the lens cannot assume a spherical shape. In order for an older person to see both near and distant objects clearly, bifocal glasses frequently are necessary. The upper part of the lens permits focusing on distant objects, and the lower part of the lens, which is stronger, makes it possible to focus on near objects, such as reading material.

Color Blindness

Color is detected by three light-sensitive pigments in three different types of cones. One type of cone is stimulated by light of long wavelength (such as red light), some by green light, and some by blue light, which has a short wavelength. Stimulation of the three types of cones equally results in the perception of white light. A person who is *color blind* has one or more types of cones missing. When an individual has cones that are not functioning to their normal capacity, he or she has *color weakness*.

Cataract

In this condition, the lens becomes opaque. The condition may be congenital or acquired. Eyesight is restored by excision of the lens and replacement with a corrective lens in the form of spectacles or, preferably, a contact lens.

Glaucoma

Glaucoma is caused by an increase in the pressure of the aqueous humor within the eye. The cause is a failure in the drainage of the fluid in the anterior chamber of the eye. The rising intra-ocular pressure causes progressive damage to the retina, with loss of sight. Glaucoma is one of the commonest causes of blindness. In most cases, the cause is unknown. In a few, the drainage of aqueous humor becomes blocked by debris as a result of infection or trauma to the eyeball.

THE EAR

Auricle

Injury to the auricle may result in an extremely painful effusion of blood under the perichondrium of the cartilaginous skeleton. If infection does not occur, the serum is absorbed after a few days, but some permanent thickening usually remains. Boxers and wrestlers commonly suffer from this condition, and at the end of their careers, their auricles often are seen to be greatly enlarged and deformed (cauliflower ear).

External Auditory Meatus

The introduction of foreign bodies, such as beans, erasers, and small toys, into the external auditory meatus is very common in children. Impacted wax, foreign bodies, and exostoses (abnormal bone growths) in the external meatus all will interfere with the conduction of sound waves to the tympanic membrane and produce symptoms of deafness. Diffuse infection of the skin lining the external meatus (*otitis externa*) is very common and is often caused by drying the ears with dirty towels. Infection of the sebaceous and ceruminous glands is also very common and may lead to boils in the canal, which are very painful.

Tympanic Membrane

Otoscopic examination of the tympanic membrane is facilitated in the adult by first straightening the external auditory meatus by gently pulling the auricle upward and backward. In infants, because of the lack of development of the bony part of the external meatus, the auricle should be pulled downward and backward. A speculum should be used in patients with well-developed vibrissae, because these interfere with visualization. Normally, the tympanic membrane is pearly gray, highly polished, and concave. Reddening of the membrane, dilated blood vessels covering the membrane, dullness of the membrane, and loss of concavity indicate infection in the tympanic cavity.

Small openings in the tympanic membrane produced by a surgical incision (*myringotomy*) to drain pus from the middle ear usually heal with scar tissue (fibrous tissue). Large, irregular openings caused by rupture of pus from the middle ear in otitis media, however, may not be closed completely with scar tissue. Such free communication between the external and middle ear not only impairs normal hearing, but also permits pathogenic organisms to enter the middle ear from the exterior.

Tympanic Cavity

Because of the close relationship of the pharyngeal opening of the auditory tube to the nose and pharyngeal lymphoid tissue, infections in these areas easily can spread to the tympanic cavity via the lumen of the tube. Such spread is especially common in young children, in whom the tube is wider and shorter than in the adult. Acute infection of the tympanic cavity (*otitis media*) produces a bulging and redness of the tympanic membrane.

Inadequate treatment of otitis media may result in the spread of the infection into the mastoid antrum and the mastoid air cells (*acute mastoiditis*). Acute mastoiditis may be followed by the further spread of the organisms beyond the confines of the middle ear. The meninges and the temporal lobe of the brain lie superiorly, and spread of the infection in this direction can produce a meningitis and a cerebral abscess in the temporal lobe. Beyond the medial wall of the tympanic cavity lie the facial nerve and the internal ear. A spread of the infection in this direction can cause a facial nerve palsy and *labyrinthitis*.

Otosclerosis

The base of the stapes is fixed to the margin of the fenestra vestibuli by the anular ligament. In a common disease known as *otosclerosis,* the base of the stapes becomes fixed by the formation of new bone. The disorder is more common in women and occurs frequently in early adult life. The symptom is progressively worsening deafness.

Disturbances of Vestibular Function

Disturbances of vestibular function include giddiness (vertigo) and may be investigated with *caloric tests*. These involve the raising or lowering of the temperature in the external auditory meatus, which induces convection currents in the semicircular ducts and stimulates the vestibular nerve endings.

Disturbances of Cochlear Function

Disturbances of cochlear function reveal themselves as deafness and tinnitus (ringing or other noise in the ears).

Deafness

There are two types of deafness, conductive deafness and cochlear nerve deafness. *Conductive deafness* can be caused by any disease that interferes with the conduction of sound waves from the auricle to the organ of Corti. Foreign bodies and excessive wax in the external auditory meatus, otitis media (interfering with the movements of the ossicles), and otosclerosis (because of fixation of the base of the stapes in the oval window) can be responsible. *Cochlear nerve deafness* can be caused by diseases that damage the organ of Corti or the cochlear nerve. Rubella, nerve degeneration, and acoustic nerve tumor may be responsible. The patient's ability to hear can be tested by using a vibrating tuning fork.

HEARING TESTS. In *Rinne's test,* a vibrating fork is first held near the ear. In a normal individual, the air-conducted sound can be heard much longer than if the base of the tuning fork is placed on the mastoid process of the temporal bone and the person hears by bone conduction through the skull. In patients with air conduction deafness, bone conduction lasts longer than air conduction.

In *Weber's test,* the base of a vibrating tuning fork is placed on the forehead in the midline. In a normal individual, the ears hear the sound by bone conduction through the skull equally well. In patients with air conductive deafness, the sound is heard better in the diseased ear, because the sound is not masked by air-conducted extraneous room noise. In patients with severe, unilateral cochlear nerve disease, the ear on the affected side is unable to transmit nerve impulses to the brain. The Weber's test in this condition reveals that the sound is heard only by the normal ear.

Ménière's Disease

This condition is characterized by recurrent attacks of giddiness, tinnitus, and deafness. It is caused by the excessive formation of endolymph, leading to degeneration of the receptor cells in the membranous labyrinth. The cause is unknown.

ORGAN OF SMELL

Olfaction can be tested by applying substances with different odors to each nostril in turn. Loss of the sense of smell is known as *anosmia.* Anosmia can be produced by disease of the olfactory mucous membrane, as in viral invasion accompanying the common cold. Chronic infection of the mucous membrane (*chronic rhinitis*) may produce a permanent loss of smell. Long exposure to industrial odors, which may be neurotoxic, may damage the mucous membrane permanently. Two of the most common causes of permanent anosmia are fractures of the anterior cranial fossa and cerebral tumors of the frontal lobes that produce lesions of the olfactory nerves.

ORGAN OF TASTE

The sensation of taste on the mucous membrane of the tongue can be tested by applying small quantities of sweet, salty, bitter, and acid substances. There are many pathological processes that can affect the sensation of taste, including those that affect the taste buds, such as the common cold, influenza, vitamin deficiencies, and anesthetic agents. Certain diseases affect the conduction of the nervous impulses to the central nervous system, such as interruption of the facial and glossopharyngeal nerves.

CLINICAL PROBLEMS

For the answers to these problems, see page 823.

1. A 10-year-old boy is taken to a pediatrician because he has been complaining of pain and tenderness in the lower lid of the right eye. The discomfort started 24 hours previously, and there is now a discrete red swelling on the outer edge of the medial part of the right lower eyelid. A diagnosis of a sty is made. Describe the different types of glands that are present in the eyelid, and, where possible, indicate their function. What is a meibomian cyst?

2. A 3-month-old baby is taken to a pediatrician because the mother has noticed that tears from the left eye tend to run down the cheek even when the baby is not crying. Examination shows defective

drainage of tears (*epiphora*) from the left eye, and the application of slight pressure over the left lacrimal sac results in pus appearing at the orifice on the punctum of the lower eyelid. A diagnosis is made of congenital obstruction of the left nasolacrimal duct that has resulted in chronic inflammation of the lacrimal passages (*chronic dacryocystitis*). The treatment is the application of antibiotics and the passage of a fine probe down the nasolacrimal duct so that it opens into the inferior meatus of the nose. Describe the structure and function of the lacrimal gland. What mechanisms exist to ensure that the tears circulate over the surface of the cornea?

3. A patient comes to you complaining of a foreign body in the eye. The foreign body has been in the conjunctival sac for several hours, and the patient has been unable to remove it. Where would you look for a foreign body that has been floating around the conjunctival sac? Describe the structure of the conjunctiva. Is the conjunctiva a common site for infection?

4. A 56-year-old man is walking along a street when he passes some workers digging a hole in the road. A gust of wind blows some dirt into the air, and suddenly the man experiences an acute, stabbing pain in the right eye. Although he blinks his eyes vigorously for several minutes, the pain persists. Because of the severity of the pain and excessive lacrimation, the man goes immediately to the emergency room of a local hospital. On examination of the cornea with a slit lamp and a magnifying device, the ophthalmologist can identify a small abraded area where the corneal epithelium is missing. The patient is treated by tightly patching the eye, because small abrasions of the cornea heal quickly and usually require no further treatment. Describe the structure and function of the cornea. How does the cornea receive its nourishment? Is the cornea resistant to most infections?

5. A 42-year-old woman visits her ophthalmologist complaining of intense pain in her left eye. The pressure of the aqueous humor in the anterior chamber of the eye is found to be elevated abnormally. A diagnosis of glaucoma is made. Using your knowledge of the histology and physiology of the eye, describe the formation and circulation of the aqueous humor. What mechanism is responsible for maintaining the normal intra-ocular pressure?

6. A 48-year-old woman is found on ophthalmoscopic examination to have edema of both optic discs (bilateral papilledema) and congestion of the retinal veins. The cause of the condition is found to be a rapidly growing intracranial tumor. Using your knowledge of the histology of the eyeball, explain the papilledema. Why does the patient exhibit bilateral papilledema?

7. A 38-year-old man is referred to an ophthalmologist because of a recent history of headaches that occur especially after he reads extensively. The ophthalmologist, after examining the eyes, explains to the patient that he has reached an age at which he requires glasses for reading. Using your knowledge of the histology, physiology, and physics of the eye, decide whether this man would be advised to wear convex or concave lenses for reading. What media normally exist in the eye for refracting light so that an image can be focused on the retina? Describe the histological structure of each of the refractive media.

8. Explain in detail the mechanisms involved in accommodating the eye.

9. Describe the histological structure of the following: (a) the fovea centralis, (b) the iris, (c) the ciliary body, (d) the ora serrata.

10. A 35-year-old man suffering from extreme nearsightedness notices some flashes of light before his right eye. His immediate reaction is that a thunderstorm is about to take place and that he has observed flashes of lightning. No storm occurs, however, and during the next few days the flashes of light are repeated. He also begins to notice small specks floating across his vision in the right eye and on occasion thinks he sees what he describes as a curtain floating down within his right eye. He consults an ophthalmologist, who diagnoses a retinal detachment in his right eye. Describe the embryological

development of the retina, and explain how retinal detachment can occur. What is the significance of the nearsightedness (myopia) in this patient? What is responsible for the lightning flashes? What forms the curtain that this patient saw?

11. A 15-year-old boy is walking along a country road when a flying insect enters his right ear. The boy tries without success to expel the foreign body by vigorously shaking his head. What structures exist in the external auditory meatus to trap insects? Describe the microscopic structures of the glands that produce ear wax.

12. An 11-year-old girl is suffering from intense left earache and deafness. Her pediatrician makes a diagnosis of acute otitis media, having examined the lateral surface of the tympanic membrane with an otoscope. What is the histological structure of the tympanic membrane?

13. Describe the mechanisms involved in conducting sound waves from the external auditory meatus to the inner ear.

14. Describe the histological structure of the following: (a) the basilar membrane, (b) the stria vascularis, (c) the macula, (d) the ampulla of a semicircular canal, (e) the tectorial membrane.

15. A 25-year-old medical student is able to earn his tuition fees for medical school by tending bar in a local discotheque. After 6 months, he notices that he is having difficulty in hearing high-frequency notes. When asked by his otolaryngologist whether the music is played very loudly, he responds that the volume of the audio system is always turned up to the maximum. Using your knowledge of histology and physiology, state which part of the membranous labyrinth is involved in the hearing process. How is it possible to distinguish between low- and high-frequency sounds? Which part of the ear is most likely to show evidence of disease in this patient?

16. A 30-year-old man visits his otolaryngologist complaining of bilateral gradual hearing loss. He also states that he occasionally experiences ringing noises (tinnitus) in his ears. After careful examination with an otoscope, performing tuning fork tests and audiometric testing, the physician makes a diagnosis of otosclerosis. Describe the stapes and its normal attachment to the oval window. What lies on the medial surface of the foot of the stapes, endolymph or perilymph?

17. A 57-year-old man visits his otolaryngologist because of repeated attacks of giddiness (vertigo). The giddiness is usually rotatory, and the patient is forced to lie down with his eyes closed because any movement worsens the condition. On three occasions, the giddiness has been accompanied by nausea and vomiting. The attack lasts from a few minutes to an hour and is followed by a humming noise in the ears (tinnitus) and deafness. After a thorough examination, the physician makes a diagnosis of Ménière's disease. Although the pathological characteristics of this condition are not fully understood, it is known that there is an increase in the volume of endolymph. What is endolymph, and where is it found in the ear? Where is endolymph normally formed? A common finding in this condition is that the vestibular membrane (Reissner's membrane) is distorted and displaced. What is the vestibular membrane, and what is its structure?

18. Describe the structure of the auricle of the ear. What is a cauliflower ear?

19. Describe the spatial arrangement of the semicircular canals and semicircular ducts, and explain their function.

20. Describe the spiral organ of Corti. What is the possible functional difference between the outer and the inner hair cells?

21. Following a severe automobile accident, a 31-year-old man is treated in the hospital for a fracture of the anterior cranial fossa. During his recovery, it is noted that he has lost the sense of smell in both sides of his nose. Describe the extent and structure of the olfactory mucous membrane. Which cells give origin to the olfactory nerve fibers? What is responsible for keeping the mucous membrane moist in this area of the nasal cavity? Why did this patient suffer from anosmia?

22. Describe the structure of a taste bud. Where are taste buds normally found in the body? What happens to a taste bud if the nerve is sectioned surgically?

ADDITIONAL READING

Allen, E. W. *Essentials of Ophthalmic Optics.* New York: Oxford University Press, 1979.

Carterette, E. C., and Friedman, M. P. *Hearing.* New York: Academic, 1978.

Dick, G. L. *Studies in Ocular Anatomy and Physiology.* Kensington, N.S.W.: New South Wales University Press, 1976.

Engstrom, H., and Ades, H. W. (eds.). Inner ear studies. *Acta Otolaryngol.* (Suppl.) 301, 1973.

Evans, E. F., and Wilson, J. P. (eds.). *Psychophysics and Physiology of Hearing.* New York: Academic, 1977.

Feeney, L. Lipofuscin and melanin of human retinal pigment epithelium. *Invest. Ophthalmol.* 17:583, 1978.

Hodgson, E. S. Taste receptors. *Sci. Am.* 204(5):135, 1961.

Hunter-Duvar, I. M. Hearing and hair cells. *Can. J. Otolaryngol.* 4:152, 1975.

Kavner, R. S., and Dusky, L. *Total Vision.* New York: A & W Publishers, 1980.

Kimura, R. S. The ultrastructure of the organ of Corti. *Rev. Cytol.* 42:173, 1975.

Last, R. J. *Wolff's Anatomy of the Eye and Orbit* (5th ed.). Philadelphia: Saunders, 1968.

Miller, D. *Ophthalmology: The Essentials.* Boston: Houghton Mifflin, 1979.

Moulton, D. G. Spatial patterning of response to odors in the peripheral olfactory system. *Physiol. Rev.* 56:578, 1976.

Murray, R. G. The ultrastructure of taste buds. In Friedman, J. (ed.), *The Ultrastructure of Sense Organs.* New York: North Holland, 1973.

Ohloff, G., and Thomas, A. F. (eds.). *Gustation and Olfaction.* New York: Academic, 1971.

Orzalesi, N., Riva, A., and Testa, F. Fine structure of the human lacrimal gland. *J. Submicrosc. Cytol.* 3:283, 1971.

Raviola, E. Intercellular junctions in the outer plexiform layer of the retina. *Invest. Ophthalmol.* 15:881, 1976.

Records, R. E. *Physiology of the Human Eye and Visual System.* Hagerstown, Md.: Harper & Row, 1979.

Rodieck, R. W. *The Vertebrate Retina.* San Francisco: Freeman, 1974.

Singh, R. P. *Anatomy of Hearing and Speech.* New York: Oxford University Press, 1980.

Sjöstrand, F. S., Kreman, M., and Crescitelli, F. Freeze-fracture analysis of photoreceptor cell outer segment disks after minimal extraction of rhodopsin. *J. Ultrastruct. Res.* 69:53, 1979.

Soudijn, E. R. Scanning electron microscopy of the organ of Corti. *Ann. Otol. Rhinol. Laryngol.* 86:16, 1976.

Spoendlin, H. Innervation densities of the cochlea. *Acta Otolaryngol.* 73:235, 1972.

Young, R. W. The renewal of photoreceptor cell outer segments. *J. Cell Biol.* 33:61, 1967.

Young, R. W. Visual cells and the concept of renewal. *Invest. Ophthalmol.* 15:700, 1976.

ANSWERS TO CLINICAL PROBLEMS

CHAPTER 1

1. Homeostasis is the maintenance of a constant cellular environment that permits the cells to function normally. The respiratory system, the cardiovascular system, the renal system, and the endocrine system are very important in the maintenance of normal homeostasis. Accordingly, severe bronchitis with emphysema, heart failure, or renal failure will alter homeostasis. Endocrine disease, such as diabetes mellitus or Addison's disease of the suprarenal cortex, will also upset homeostasis (see also p. 26).

2. The cells in all epithelial tissue are situated close to one another; in connective tissues, the cells are usually widely separated by large amounts of matrix.

3. Sickle cell anemia, goitrous cretinism, juvenile diabetes mellitus, and cystic fibrosis are examples of genetic cellular defects.

4. Tissues reach their maximum efficiency during young adulthood.

5. Bones become less resilient with age because of increased concentrations of inorganic materials within the matrix (see also p. 25). With age, the red bone marrow recedes up the bones of the limbs and is replaced by yellow marrow. The lymphatic tissues reach their maximum development at puberty; thereafter, they atrophy.

CHAPTER 2

1. A mitochondrion is a vesicular structure of varying shape and size that is bounded by two plasma membranes. The outer membrane is smooth and completely surrounds the mitochondrion. The inner membrane is folded to form cristae. Viruses consist merely of a molecule of nucleic acid, either DNA or RNA, surrounded by a protein envelope. There is no plasma membrane.

Mitochondria are capable of reproducing by simple binary fission. For this, they contain their own supplies of DNA or RNA in the form of closed loops in the mitochondrial matrix. Although mitochondria are known to possess many of the enzymes necessary to carry out a semiautonomous existence, the enzymes and proteins are controlled not by mitochondrial DNA but by nuclear genes and are synthesized by cytoplasmic ribosomes and then passed into the mitochondrion. Therefore, a mitochondrion cannot exist separately from a cell.

Viruses can replicate only within living cells. The viral nucleic acid programs the infected cell to synthesize, by means of its enzymes, specific macromolecules for the formation of new viruses. Viruses can exist in an inert form separately from a host cell.

2. The mitochondrial enzymes that are associated with electron transport and oxidative phosphorylation are situated on the inner mitochondrial membrane and its cristae. Elementary particles are small particles that stud the inner, semipermeable membrane of a mitochondrion. They are the sites of enzymes concerned with oxidative phosphorylation and hydrolysis of ATP.

3. Stereocilia are very long microvilli found on the free surface of columnar cells lining the epididymis. They are formed of extensions of the plasma membrane, and each has a core of cytoplasm. They are nonmotile and serve to increase the surface area of the cell to aid absorption.

Cilia are found on the free surface of columnar cells lining the respiratory system and in parts of the female and male reproductive tracts. They are larger and have a more complex structure than stereocilia. Within the cytoplasmic core are microtubules that extend out from a centriole (basal body) found within the cell close to the base of the cilium. The cilia are immersed in mucus, which is moved in one direction by the bending of the cilia. The movement of the cilia is thought to occur as the result of the microtubules within them sliding upon one another.

4. The processes of passive and active transport across cell membranes are fully discussed on pages 58–60.

5. Gap junctions and tight junctions occur in numerous parts of the body where two cells come into close proximity. A gap junction is a spotlike area where the outer lamellae of adjacent plasma membranes come very close together but are not fused. Minute bridges of protein and lipid have been shown to bridge the gap, passing from one cell membrane to the other and piercing the membranes, so that there is continuous communication between the cytoplasms of adjacent cells.

A tight junction (zonula occludens) is a girdle of fused plasma membranes that surrounds a cell near its free surface. It is formed by the fusion of the outer lamellae of adjacent plasma membranes and prevents the passage of molecules between the cells.

The bridges of gap junctions permit the passage of ions and small molecules from one cell to another. They are found between the cells of smooth muscle and cardiac muscle fibers, where it is important that a wave of excitation pass quickly from one cell to another.

It is probable that the establishment of gap junctions between cells that are actively multiplying in the healing of a wound inhibits excessive growth and reproduction. Cancer cells form fewer and often abnormal intercellular junctions, giving them a greater freedom to invade surrounding tissues.

6. The nonionized form of a drug, which is generally lipid soluble, will diffuse rapidly across the plasma membrane, because the main part of the membrane is formed of two molecular layers of lipid.

7. The smooth endoplasmic reticulum is described on page 44. It is formed from the rough endoplasmic reticulum by the simple loss of the attached ribosomes. In the cells of the suprarenal cortex, its function is to synthesize lipids, lipoproteins, and steroid hormones. In the hepatocytes of the liver, the reticulum also synthesizes glycogen. In skeletal muscle cells, it participates in the binding of calcium and is thus associated with the process of muscle contraction.

8. Lysosomes are essentially membrane-bound bodies found within the cytoplasm of many types of cell; they contain hydrolytic enzymes. Lysosomes exist in three functional states, which are described on page 47.

Lysosomes are important in the destruction and removal of dead cells following cell injury. In polymorphonuclear leukocytes, they bring about the removal of bacteria that have been phagocytosed by these cells. A rare, fatal disease in children is caused by a defect in the lysosomal membrane that prevents the fusion of lysosomes with vacuoles containing bacteria within polymorphonuclear leukocytes.

9. Atrophy, hypertrophy, and hyperplasia are defined on pages 72 and 73.

Some physiological examples of atrophy are: (1) reduction in size of the thyroid and suprarenal glands following removal of the anterior lobe of the pituitary; (2) reduction in size of the ovaries and uterus following the cessation of hormonal stimulation after the menopause; and (3) reduction in size of skeletal muscle cells following immobilization of a limb in a plaster cast. Some pathological examples of atrophy are: (1) reduction in size of skeletal muscle cells following section of the motor nerve; and (2) reduction in neuronal size following a reduction in blood supply resulting from arterial disease (arteriosclerosis).

Some physiological examples of hypertrophy are: (1) increase in size of skeletal muscle cells accompanying an increased workload in athletes in training; and (2) increase in size of the smooth muscle cells in the uterus during pregnancy as the result of increased hormonal stimulation by estrogen. Some pathological examples of hypertrophy are: (1) increase in size of cardiac muscle cells when their workload is increased, as in right ventricular hypertrophy caused by pulmonary hypertension and left ventricular hypertrophy caused by a raised blood pressure in the aorta; and (2) hypertrophy of the bladder muscle following partial obstruction of the urinary flow caused by an enlarged prostate.

Some physiological examples of hyperplasia are: (1) the increase in the number of circulating red cells in the blood that occurs in persons who live at high altitudes and that results from the low oxygen pressure in the atmosphere causing the red bone marrow to produce more red cells; and (2) the increase in the number of smooth muscle cells in the uterus during pregnancy, caused by stimulation by estrogen.

Some pathological examples of hyperplasia are: (1) There is an increase in the number of white cells in the blood (leukocytosis) in a patient with an acute infection. The toxins liberated by the invading organisms stimulate the increased production of, for example, polymorphonuclear leukocytes in the red bone marrow. (2) In wound healing, the fibroblasts of connective tissue are stimulated to multiply in preparation for the laying down of new collagen.

10. Human cells are surrounded by a plasma membrane; they do not possess an outer cell wall as bacteria do. Penicillin, which interferes with the formation of the bacterial cell wall, consequently has no effect on the human cell. Viruses are unaffected by penicillin, because they neither need nor possess a cell wall.

11. Ribosomes are cell organelles. They are described on page 49. Ribosomal RNA is the ribonucleic acid of which ribosomes are composed. Messenger RNA is found in close association with ribosomes. It is formed in the nucleus within the nucleolus, where it receives its genetic coding from the DNA of the chromosomes. The messenger RNA now leaves the nucleus and becomes associated with the ribosomes. It is the messenger RNA that determines the precise synthesis of a specific protein. A third RNA, known as transfer RNA, is present in the cytoplasm and attaches itself to a specific molecule of amino acid, transferring it to the ribosome for incorporation into the new protein in a position determined by the messenger RNA.

12. (a) Membrane pores are sites in a plasma membrane where water and dissolved ions can pass through rapidly. Their existence has not been demonstrated with the electron microscope, but it is thought that the protein molecules that exist within the plasma membrane and cross the lipid layers may be the site of such openings. (b) A drug receptor site is the chemical group(s) present on the cell surface or within the cell involved in the combination of the drug with the receptor. The receptor is the cell structure that is initially involved with the action of the drug. (c) A centromere is the site where two chromatids are attached to each other. (d) Metaplasia is a reversible change in which one type of adult cell is replaced by another type. See page 74

for examples of metaplasia. (e) A prokaryotic cell has no true nucleus, no nuclear membrane, and no cell organelles. A bacterium is an example. (f) The basement membrane connects epithelial cells to underlying connective tissue and serves as a semipermeable membrane. It consists of a basal lamina and a reticular lamina (see p. 71). (g) A desmosome is a form of cell junction where the plasma membranes of adjacent cells do not come into close contact but are held together strongly by a special area of the cell coat formed of protein (for details, see p. 68).

13. The nucleus has two chief functions: (1) it plays the major role in reproducing the cell and in maintaining the hereditary characteristics of the cell; and (2) it controls the metabolic activities of the dividing cell. A mature red cell is an example of a cell that has lost its nucleus and yet is able to carry out vital activities; its functions are associated with the transport of oxygen and carbon dioxide in the blood. Surface epidermal cells of the skin are dead, but, because they are tough and horny and remain attached to one another, they protect the underlying cells from physical trauma, dehydration, and excessive hydration. Osteoclasts, foreign body giant cells, and hepatocytes are examples of cells that may possess more than one nucleus.

14. Cancer cells vary in size; their nuclei vary in shape, size, and staining ability; and the cells show a great increase in the frequency of mitosis. Once the cells become malignant, they multiply rapidly and invade surrounding tissues.

15. When a cell is damaged, there are four sites of biochemical activity that are particularly susceptible to injury: (1) sites of oxidative phosphorylation reactions, (2) the plasma membrane, (3) sites of formation of structural and enzymatic proteins, and (4) nuclear DNA and RNA. Cell injury is described on page 75. Note that if the injury is not too severe, the cell will recover and the morphological changes that reflect the injury will revert to normal. Severe or repeated cell injury, however, will lead to cell death.

16. A solution of 0.9% sodium chloride or 5% dextrose could be given intravenously in this patient, because either is isotonic with the fluid within the blood cells.

17. (a) Cancer cells multiply by the process of mitosis. Vincristine arrests mitosis by damaging the spindle, which is one of the fundamental components of cell division. (b) DNA is the chemical basis of heredity and the carrier of the genetic code. It is also involved in the formation of messenger RNA. Adriamycin, by binding with DNA, blocks the formation of messenger RNA, and cell death results. (c) Cystosine arabinoside inhibits the formation of DNA and therefore blocks the formation of messenger RNA. Cell death quickly follows.

18. Down's syndrome is caused by a chromosomal abnormality in which there is an additional chromosome on the 21 pair; hence the alternate name trisomy 21. Parents of a child with a serious congenital anomaly should have their chromosomes examined and analyzed so that accurate information can be obtained about risks of recurrence.

19. The Papanicolaou smear is a very valuable diagnostic method. All women over 20 years old should have the test annually. The accuracy in diagnosis of cancer of the cervix is approximately 90 percent. The final diagnosis, however, is determined by biopsy. In the Papanicolaou test, the exposed cervix is scraped with a spatula and the cervical cells are smeared on a slide. The specimen is then appropriately stained, and the slide is examined under a microscope. Tumor cells may be detected by this method.

20. Change in adult cell type is called metaplasia. A cilium is a motile, hairlike projection of the plasma membrane from the free surface of a columnar cell. It possesses microtubules within its cytoplasmic core (for details, see p. 66). A flagellum is a very long cilium. The spermatozoon is the only human cell to possess an active flagellum.

The function of the ciliated cells lining the bronchi is to move mucus upward toward the trachea, larynx, and pharynx, where it is swallowed. A loss of ciliated cells as a result of disease is followed by the accumulation of mucus in the lungs, with the likelihood that pathological organisms will infect the lung tissue.

21. The oral or buccal smear is a common test used for identification of sex. The test depends on the identification of the sex chromatin in the female cell nucleus (Barr body) adjacent to the nuclear membrane and the absence of this chromatin in male cells.

CHAPTER 3

1. Epithelial tissue is one of the four main tissues of the body. It covers surfaces, lines body cavities, and forms the secretory cells of many glands. The cells rest on a basal lamina and are held together by a small amount of amorphous intercellular material and by cell junctions.

The simple squamous epithelium that lines the heart and the blood and lymphatic vessels is called endothelium; the lining of the pleural, pericardial, and abdominopelvic cavities is called mesothelium.

2. The cells of the red bone marrow are constantly dividing to replace worn-out red cells and granular white cells in the blood. In the same manner, the cells lining the gastrointestinal tract are rapidly dividing to replace cells that are worn off the surface by the passage of intestinal contents. Because these normal cells are undergoing rapid mitotic activity similar to that seen in malignant tumors, they are also damaged by chemotherapeutic agents.

3. Epithelial tissue differs from connective tissue in that its cells are held close together and rest on a basal lamina. The cells of connective tissue are characteristically separated from one another by large amounts of intercellular material produced by the cells. The intercellular material contains collagen, elastic and reticular fibers, and amorphous material.

The surface types of epithelium can be classified into surface epithelium, glandular epithelium, and special epithelium. The detailed classification is given on page 85, together with examples of locations where they may be found.

4. A squamous cell is a flat epithelial cell commonly found covering the surface of the body and lining the tubes and cavities of the body. A carcinoma is the name given to a malignant epithelial cell.

5. There are three types of specialized columnar epithelial cells: (1) goblet cells, (2) absorptive cells with microvilli, and (3) ciliated cells.

Goblet cells produce a mucous secretion that accumulates in the distal portion of the cell. The cytoplasm is displaced toward the sides of the cell, and the stem of the goblet is formed by the basal portion of the cell, which contains the nucleus and a little cytoplasm. Goblet cells line the respiratory and intestinal systems.

Absorptive cells have microvilli that project from the free surface area of the cell and further absorption. Absorptive cells line the stomach, intestines, and gallbladder.

Ciliated cells have motile processes that project from the free surface of the cell. The cilia move mucus and other fluids that cover the cell surface in a definite direction. Ciliated cells line the respiratory system and the uterine tubes and uterus.

6. Metaplasia is a change in the characteristic structure of a tissue as a result of disease. Normally, the calyces and pelvis of the ureter are lined with transitional epithelium. In this patient, a large stone (calculus) has repeatedly traumatized the lining epithelium, eventually resulting in its replacement by a simpler form of epithelium, a stratified squamous epithelium.

7. Exocrine glands can be classified, according to the means by which they release their secretions, as merocrine, apocrine, and holocrine glands. Exocrine glands can be classified also on the basis of their secretions and the arrangement of their ducts and acini. For details, see page 93.

Exocrine glands possess ducts that convey the glandular secretions to the surface of the body or into the lumen of a hollow organ. Endocrine glands have no ducts and pour their secretions directly into the bloodstream, where they are distributed to different parts of the body. The secretions of endocrine glands contain chemical substances known as hormones that regulate the activities of cells.

8. Irreversible and reversible injuries to cells are discussed on page 75. Epithelial regeneration in labile, stable, and permanent cells is described on page 98.

CHAPTER 4

1. Adipose tissue of the breasts, thighs, and buttocks in the female is under the control of sex hormones and increases in amount in those regions at puberty, producing the characteristic female shape. It follows that it would be undesirable in this 8-year-old girl to transfer subcutaneous fat of the thigh to the hand, because it would increase in amount at puberty.

2. IgE is an antibody produced by lymphocytes and plasma cells in response to the entrance into the body of a foreign antigen. The IgE antibody attaches itself to the plasma membranes of mast cells in connective tissue and basophils in the blood. Histamine is released, which produces the signs and symptoms of anaphylaxis.

3. Reticuloendothelial cells all possess the characteristic of phagocytosis. Examples of these cells are the Kupffer cells of the liver, the monocytes of the blood, the alveolar phagocytes of the lungs, the histiocytes in connective tissue, and the microglial cells of the central nervous system. The macrophages in a healing wound phagocytose red cells that have escaped from blood vessels and cell debris in the blood clot.

4. Long bones receive their blood supply by three routes: (1) the nutrient artery, which perforates the shaft to enter the marrow cavity; (2) periosteal arteries that penetrate and supply the outer part of the compact bone through Volkmann's canals; and (3) arteries that supply the epiphyseal ends of the bone.

5. Healing of a surgical wound is described on page 145. Vitamin C is essential for the formation of normal collagen and for the development of a strong scar (see p. 145).

6. A torn cartilage in a joint does not heal by regeneration. If the cartilaginous tear is severe and interferes with the function of the joint, the entire cartilage should be surgically removed.

7. On entering the body, foreign antigens are engulfed by macrophages, which then present them to the B lymphocytes. The B lymphocytes, often assisted by the T lymphocytes, then proliferate and mature into plasma cells. The plasma cells thus play a major role in the production of humoral immunity to infection.

8. In the embryo, bones are preceded by a membranous or cartilaginous model. Intramembranous ossification takes place in the bones of the vault of the skull and the clavicle; the process is described on page 135.

9. The line of cleavage refers to the direction of the rows of collagen in the dermis. They tend to run circumferentially in the neck. A surgical incision through the skin along or between these rows of collagen causes minimal collagen disruption, and the resulting wound heals with the minimum of scar tissue. Disruption of the collagen rows leads to the formation of broad, ugly scars.

A keloid is an excessive formation of scar tissue in a healing wound. It is more likely to occur in black than white people.

10. The fixed cells of connective tissue include fibroblasts, fat cells, plasma cells, mast cells, histiocytes, and uncommitted mesenchymal cells. The freely mobile cells include neutrophils, eosinophils, lymphocytes, and monocytes.

11. The structure of hyaline cartilage is described on page 127. It is firm because of the presence of the amorphous intercellular substance of the matrix and the presence of collagen and a few elastic fibers. It is flexible because the collagen fibers are flexible and loosely arranged. Collagen fibers are present in large quantities in hyaline cartilage; there are only a few elastic fibers. In elastic cartilage, the elastic fibers predominate over the collagen fibers.

12. Granulation tissue is a pink, soft tissue that has a granular appearance when seen from the surface. It is formed in a wound by the vascularization of the blood clot and the proliferation of fibroblasts (see p. 145). Because the endothelial cells of the blood capillaries of granulation tissue are loosely attached to one another, white blood cells and plasma leak out into the tissue and provide a cellular and humoral defense against infection.

Wound contraction is a phenomenon seen in wounds when there has been a large amount of tissue loss. As the result of the contraction of the fibroblasts and the shortening of the collagen fibers, a surface wound may be reduced in size by as much as 90 percent. Wound contracture is the end result of wound healing in which there has been an excessive shortening of the collagen, often producing deformities. Severe contracture commonly follows the full-thickness skin loss secondary to a severe burn.

13. The fibroblast, the chondroblast, and the osteoblast are the cells responsible for forming collagen. The stages in the formation of collagen are fully described on page 116. Vitamin C is essential for the hydroxylation of proline to hydroxyproline. Nonhydroxylated collagen is unstable and cannot form the triple helix required for normal structure.

14. The diaphysis of a developing long bone is the shaft of the bone.

15. The epiphysis of a developing long bone is the cartilage found at either end of the diaphysis. As development proceeds, one or more secondary centers of ossification appear in each epiphysis.

An epiphyseal plate is a plate of cartilage that persists between the centers of ossification in the diaphysis and the epiphysis. It is the continued growth of the epiphyseal cartilage that causes the bone to increase in length. When bone growth ceases, the epiphyseal plate is ossified and the diaphysis fuses with the epiphysis.

16. The structure of a synovial joint is described on page 143. Its essential feature is that the opposing joint surfaces are separated by a joint cavity that is enclosed by a fibrous capsule. The capsule is lined with synovial membrane, which produces a lubricating fluid called synovial fluid. The shoulder, elbow, wrist, hip, knee, and ankle joints are good examples of synovial joints.

17. Callus is hard, new tissue formed between the fragments of a fractured bone. The formation and structure of callus are described on page 146.

18. Some authorities believe that fat cells are formed during three main periods of life: (a) the last 3 months of fetal life, (b) the first 5 years of life, and (c) the period immediately after puberty. It is thought that these cells in some way influence the feeding centers of the hypothalamus, so that the more fat cells laid down during these periods, the greater will be one's appetite throughout life.

The microscopic structure of a fat cell is described on page 108. Fat in adipose tissue has a calorific value of about 9 calories per gram. Adipose tissue has the following functions: (a) providing energy storage, (b) insulating against heat loss, (c) protecting against trauma, (d) supporting organs, such as the kidney, and (e) contributing to the sexual shape of the individual.

19. The marrow cavity of the shaft of the adult femur is filled with yellow marrow. (The red marrow is restricted to the head of the femur in the adult.) Because yellow marrow is composed largely of adipose tissue, severe injury to the bone may result in fat globules entering the blood circulation, a condition known as fat embolism. Large numbers of fat emboli can obstruct the pulmonary and cerebral circulations and cause death.

20. Vitamin D in adequate amounts is necessary for the absorption of calcium from the small intestine and the reabsorption of calcium in the renal tubules. Calcium is necessary for the normal mineralization of bone matrix. Sunlight brings about photoconversion of sterols in the skin, resulting in the formation of vitamin D.

In rickets, the epiphyseal cartilages or plates are thickened, because there is a failure of mineralization of cartilage matrix. As a result, the cartilage cells continue to grow, producing excessive cartilage.

CHAPTER 5

1. During the process of spontaneous abortion, bleeding sometimes becomes excessive, requiring transfusion with whole blood. At the same time, the uterine hemorrhage is stopped by stimulating the uterus to contract by the injection of ergometrine. The normal blood volume of a healthy adult is about 5,000 ml. The patient's blood group is determined and the blood is cross matched before the transfusion is started.

2. The hematocrit value for a man is normally about 40 and is an expression of the volume of red cells per 100 ml of blood. The hematocrit value is raised in shock (because of the sudden release of red cells stored in the red bone marrow) and following burns (because of the loss of plasma from the circulatory system at the burn site). The hematocrit value is lowered during the recovery phase of severe hemorrhage (when tissue fluid enters the circulatory system to compensate for the diminished blood volume) and when excessive intravenous fluids, other than whole blood, are administered.

Repeated hematocrit readings can be of value in studying the recovery from such conditions as severe burns.

3. Patients with large, untreated hemorrhoids commonly suffer from hypochromic microcytic anemia. The continued loss of small quantities of blood with each defecation slowly reduces the store of iron in the body necessary for the formation of hemoglobin. This patient's breathlessness on exertion is caused by the reduced oxygen-carrying capacity of the blood. The sallow skin and pale conjunctivae result from the low hemoglobin content of the blood. The spoon-shaped nails, which are brittle, are caused by tissue anoxia at the site of nail growth. The blood examinations were ordered to confirm the diagnosis of anemia and to determine its severity. The normal red cell count in an adult male is about 5 million per cubic millimeter. The normal hemoglobin content of blood is 15 gm per 100 ml.

4. At high altitudes, the percentage of oxygen in the air is considerably less than at sea level. To compensate, the low oxygen content of the blood stimulates the red bone marrow to produce an increased number of red cells for circulation in the blood (see erythropoietin, p. 161). When the professor returns to an environment where the oxygen content of the air was higher, the stimulus is diminished, the output of red cells from the bone marrow becomes lower, and his red cell count will return to its original level. His initial breathlessness and tiredness at high altitudes were caused by hypoxia.

5. Exhausted red blood cells are phagocytosed by cells of the reticuloendothelial system, especially those found in the spleen, liver, and bone marrow. The hemoglobin is broken down into an iron-containing pigment called hemosiderin and the pigment bilirubin. The bilirubin is released into the blood and later secreted by the liver into the bile.

6. Lymphocytic leukemia is an abnormal, uncontrolled proliferation of one type of white blood cell and its precursors. Even though the white cell count may be extremely high (in the hundreds of thousands of cells per cubic millimeter), there may be a deficiency of normally functioning neutrophils, which are necessary to defend the body against infection.

7. The determination of a differential white blood cell count is described on page 184. The percentages of the different types of white blood cells are given on page 161. *Neutrophilia* can stem from many acute (especially bacterial) infections, intoxication from physical or chemical agents, acute hemorrhage, leukemia, and other conditions. *Eosinophilia* can be caused by bronchial asthma, hay fever, angioneurotic edema, and parasitic infections such as intestinal worms. *Basophilia* occurs in myelocytic leukemia, polycythemia vera, hypersensitive states, chronic hemolytic anemias, and other conditions. *Lymphocytosis* results from whooping cough (pertussis), viral infections such as infectious mononucleo-

sis, lymphatic leukemia, and other causes. *Monocytosis* occurs in, among other conditions, monocytic leukemia, chronic infections (such as tuberculosis), viral infections, and Hodgkin's disease. *Leukopenia* may occur in such conditions as typhoid fever, viral infections, and aplastic anemia. *Lymphopenia* may follow the administration of adrenocorticotropic hormone or cortisone.

8. At birth, all bone marrow is red and hematopoietic. At 7 years of age, the child begins to develop yellow marrow in the distal bones of the limbs, and it gradually replaces the red marrow in all the limb bones. In the adult, the red marrow is restricted to the bones of the skull, the vertebral column, the thoracic cage, the girdle bones, and the head of the humerus and the femur.

9. The mechanism of blood clotting is described on page 171. In this patient, large amounts of thromboplastin were released from the damaged blood vessel walls and the adjacent tissues. By this means, the process of clotting was initiated, and bleeding from the wound quickly stopped.

10. In polycythemia vera, the number of red cells in the blood is greatly increased, and this increases the viscosity of the blood. Viscous blood flows slowly through small blood vessels and increases the likelihood that platelets will aggregate and thus initiate the clotting process. A thrombus is a small, stationary blood clot that adheres to the wall of a blood vessel. An embolus is a foreign substance, usually a thrombus or a fragment of a thrombus, that has broken loose and is traveling in the bloodstream. It finally becomes lodged in a blood vessel whose diameter is smaller than the embolus.

11. Vitamin K is fat-soluble, and any disease that interferes with the absorption of fat from the intestine will lead to vitamin K deficiency. Vitamin K is necessary for the formation of prothrombin in the liver. A lowered plasma prothrombin level will delay the normal process of blood clotting.

12. Sedormid is a sedative that can be toxic to bone marrow. In hypersensitive individuals, the drug forms a platelet-drug complex that induces the formation of antibodies against the patient's own platelets. The number of platelets in the blood is thus diminished (thrombocytopenia), and the likelihood of spontaneous bleeding is increased. In this woman, the drug was discontinued, the platelet count returned to normal, and the spontaneous bleeding stopped.

13. The part played by neutrophils in acute inflammation is described on page 188. *Margination* is the accumulation of neutrophils along the inside walls of capillaries at the site of acute inflammation. *Diapedesis* is the movement of neutrophils from a capillary through tissue to the actual site of bacterial invasion or tissue destruction. *Pus* is a mixture of dead or dying neutrophils, dead tissue cells, and living and dead pathogenic organisms. It forms a creamy yellow liquid.

14. The cardinal signs of acute inflammation are fully described and explained on page 188.

15. Vitamin B_{12} is essential for the normal formation of red blood cells in the bone marrow. An intrinsic factor secreted by the stomach (see p. 185) combines with vitamin B_{12} in food and allows the vitamin to be absorbed from the small intestine. Because of the previous gastrectomy, this patient lacks the intrinsic factor, and vitamin B_{12} therefore cannot be absorbed.

16. The detection of the presence of Rh antibodies in the mother's serum is important, because these antibodies will cross the placenta and destroy the fetal Rh-positive red cells. A knowledge of the presence of these antibodies will enable the obstetrician and pediatrician to initiate the appropriate treatment, such as premature delivery or exchange transfusion at the time of delivery. The determination of the husband's Rh genotype provides the obstetrician with information helpful in predicting the outcome of subsequent pregnancies. An Rh-negative woman who in the past has been transfused with Rh-positive blood probably already has formed anti-Rh antibodies. She is likely to have increased her susceptibility to stimulation by an Rh-positive fetus.

CHAPTER 6

1. When muscle tissue is sutured together, there is always the danger that the sutures will cut through the tissue if the suture line is subjected to stress. It is more satisfactory to suture together aponeuroses, which are tough and composed of fibrous tissue. Muscle is made up of bundles of muscle fibers supported by connective tissue. The connective tissue layers are called the epimysium, the perimysium, and the endomysium. The connective tissue supports the muscle fibers, together with their nerve supply and blood supply.

2. Skeletal muscle, smooth muscle, and cardiac muscle all show longitudinal striations under the light microscope when appropriately stained. The striations are caused by the myofibrils in the sarcoplasm. Skeletal and cardiac muscle is referred to as striated muscle because of the transverse bands resulting from the arrangement of the contractile proteins present within the cells. Smooth muscle does not show transverse bands, because the contractile proteins are not arranged in the same orderly manner.

3. Skeletal muscle tone is caused by the constant full contraction of a few muscle fibers within a muscle. The mechanisms responsible for muscle tone are described on page 220. Muscle tone is abolished in tabes dorsalis, poliomyelitis, syringomyelia, injury to a spinal nerve or its roots, section of a motor nerve to a muscle, and other conditions.

4. A motor unit is a single motor nerve cell and all the muscle fibers that it supplies. A motor end-plate or neuromuscular junction is the site at which the motor nerve terminates on a muscle fiber. When a nerve impulse reaches a motor end-plate, it causes the release of acetylcholine into the synaptic cleft. The acetylcholine now affects the sarcolemma, making it more permeable to sodium ions and starting a wave of depolarization. The action of acetylcholine is limited by the acetylcholinesterase in the sarcolemma. This enzyme brings about the hydrolysis of acetylcholine.

5. This young, healthy male is experiencing oxygen lack and lactic acid build-up within his leg muscles. The breathlessness (dyspnea) is caused by acidosis.

6. Skeletal muscles increase in size in response to work by increasing the number of myofibrils in each fiber. There is no increase in the number of muscle fibers.

7. For definitions, see the pages indicated: (a) A band, page 197; (b) Z line, page 197; (c) sarcoplasmic reticulum, page 198; (d) T tubule, page 198; (e) white muscle fibers, page 198; (f) intercalated disk, pages 205 and 206; (g) Purkinje fibers, page 206.

8. The specialized cardiac muscle fibers of the sinoatrial and atrioventricular nodes have a higher rate of intrinsic rhythmic contraction and a slower speed of conduction than do ordinary cardiac muscle fibers. The specialized fibers of the atrioventricular bundle and its terminal branches have a higher speed of conduction than do ordinary cardiac muscle fibers.

The specialized fibers of the sino-atrial node and the atrioventricular node are composed of small cardiac muscle fibers and are embedded in connective tissue that is highly vascular and that contains sympathetic and parasympathetic nerve endings. The atrioventricular bundle and its branches are composed of cardiac muscle fibers that are larger than ordinary muscle fibers; they contain fewer myofibrils, and the center of the sarcoplasm contains larger amounts of glycogen. The sarcoplasmic reticulum is poorly developed in the special muscle fibers, and there is no T tubule system.

9. The chemistry of muscle contraction is fully described on page 218. The source of energy for muscle contraction is discussed on page 219.

10. In skeletal muscle atrophy, the nuclei become hyperchromatic and tend to assume a more central position within the muscle fibers. There is a reduction in the number of myofibrils, and the mitochondria break up and disappear. Later, the transverse bands also disappear. The muscle fibers break up

and are replaced by increased connective tissue of the endomysium and perimysium. Clinical examples of muscle atrophy can be found whenever the motor innervation is interrupted or nonfunctional, as occurs in poliomyelitis, polyneuritis, myasthenia gravis, or muscle disease, such as muscular dystrophy. Prolonged immobilization also produces muscle atrophy.

11. Physiologically, the smooth muscle of the pregnant uterus undergoes hypertrophy and hyperplasia in response to the increased production of estrogen during pregnancy. Pathologically, the smooth muscle in the walls of the urinary bladder and intestine undergoes similar changes when the outlet or lumen is obstructed. The smooth muscle in the walls of arteries undergoes hypertrophy and hyperplasia in response to high blood pressure within the lumina of the arteries. The role of smooth muscle in the production of atherosclerosis is described on page 222.

12. The skeletal muscles of the suicide victim underwent contracture soon after death, a condition known as rigor mortis. As a result, the gun became firmly held in his right hand and is difficult to dislodge. Rigor mortis may last several days, depending on the outside temperature. The muscles eventually relax, however, as the muscle fibers are destroyed by enzymes liberated from the intracellular lysosomes. After 5 days, the hands normally would be relaxed.

13. Cardiac muscle fibers do not regenerate after death; they are replaced by fibrous tissue.

14. On cardiac and smooth muscle fibers, the postganglionic autonomic nerve fibers end in a similar manner. The axon rises to the surface of the Schwann cell and becomes naked, permitting the free diffusion of the neurotransmitter substance from the axon to the muscle cell (see also pp. 214 and 215). In a heart that has been transplanted, the cardiac muscle has no nerve supply. The rate of muscle contraction is determined by the inherent rhythmicity of the specialized cardiac muscle fibers present in the sino-atrial node and will be influenced by the norepinephrine circulating in the bloodstream.

CHAPTER 7

1. The radial nerve is made up of nerve fibers derived from motor, sensory, and autonomic neurons. By definition, the nerve fibers, or nerve cell processes, are referred to as neurites. The short neurites are called dendrites, and the long neurites are called axons. It is customary to refer to those neurites that conduct the nervous impulse toward the cell body as dendrites and those that conduct impulses away from the cell body as axons. In the case of the unipolar sensory neurons found in the posterior root ganglia, however, the neurite carrying nervous information toward the cell body has all the structural characteristics of an axon and is referred to as an axon. Thus, the radial nerve, which is composed of sensory and motor fibers, is made up of axons.

The nerve fibers are arranged in parallel bundles, and each fiber is supported by delicate connective tissue called endoneurium. Bundles of nerve fibers are surrounded by a connective tissue sheath called the perineurium. Several bundles are surrounded by a dense connective tissue sheath called the epineurium.

2. The nucleolus in any cell is concerned with the synthesis of RNA. The large size in nerve cells is probably related to the very large volume of cytoplasm possessed by certain neurons. For example, the axons of the motor nerve cells that supply the muscles of the sole of the foot are situated in the lumbar and sacral regions of the spinal cord; thus, the axons may be as long as 4 feet.

3. If the wound is not infected, the best time to perform a nerve suture is about 3 weeks after the injury. Satisfactory results have been obtained after a delay of as much as 14 months, provided that paralyzed muscles have not been overly stretched and joint adhesions have been avoided by passive movement of the joints. In other words, the neuron

retains the ability to regenerate its processes even after 14 months, but the degree of recovery of function will depend a great deal on the care that the denervated structures have received in the intervening time.

4. (a) Nissl substance is composed of vesicles, tubules, or stacks of flat cisternae. Associated with the vesicles are dense granules measuring 10 to 30 nm in diameter and containing ribonucleoprotein. The Nissl substance is responsible for synthesizing protein. (b) Golgi apparatus is composed of clusters of flattened cisternae and vesicles made up of smooth-surfaced endoplasmic reticulum. It is thought to serve as an intracellular storage area and to be active in lysosome production. It may also be involved in the synthesis of cell membranes (see also p. 45). (c) Lysosomes are dense spherical bodies that are membrane bound, measuring about 0.25 to 2 μm in diameter. They contain acid phosphatase and other hydrolytic enzymes. They serve as intracellular scavengers. (d) Other membranous vesicles include some that contain engulfed substances that move through the cytoplasm until they fuse with a lysosome. Such vesicles are often termed phagosomes (see p. 48).

5. The plasma membrane is composed of lipid and protein molecules and has a coat of glycoprotein on its outer surface (see also pp. 55 and 57). When a neuron is excited, the permeability of the plasma membrane to Na^+ ions is increased, and these diffuse from the tissue fluid into the neuron cytoplasm. Local analgesics act as membrane stabilizers and inhibit the increase in permeability to Na^+ ions in response to stimulation. It is not exactly understood how this stabilization is brought about. One theory is that the analgesic agent becomes attached to receptor sites on the protein layer of the plasma membrane, reducing the permeability to Na^+ ions and preventing depolarization. Small-diameter nerve fibers are more readily blocked than are large fibers, and nonmyelinated fibers more readily blocked than myelinated. For these reasons, nerve fibers that conduct pain and temperature are most easily blocked and the large motor fibers are the least easily blocked. The small autonomic nerve fibers are blocked early and account for the rapid appearance of vasodilatation.

6. Tetraethylammonium salts and hexamethonium salts have been used for this purpose. These salts closely resemble acetylcholine in structure and compete with acetylcholine at the postsynaptic membrane. By this means, they successfully block a ganglion, although the amount of acetylcholine released is unaffected.

7. With the electron microscope, it is possible to resolve within the cytoplasm of a neuron small tubules that measure about 20 to 30 nm in diameter; they extend throughout the cell body and its processes. Some researchers have shown that wavelike movements occur along the microtubules, and it is possible that these structures are responsible for axoplasmic flow.

8. Nerve tracts are bundles of nerve fibers found in the brain and spinal cord; the majority are myelinated. Some of the main structural differences between a nerve tract and a peripheral nerve fiber are as follows:

NERVE TRACT	PERIPHERAL NERVE FIBER
Oligodendrocyte	Schwann cell
Mesaxon absent in mature fibers	Mesaxon present in mature fibers
Schmidt-Lanterman incisures present	Schmidt-Lanterman incisures present
Nerve fibers supported by neuroglia	Nerve fibers supported by connective tissue sheaths, endoneurium, perineurium, and epineurium

9. (a) The myelin sheath is not part of a neuron; it is formed by a supporting cell, the oligodendrocyte in the central nervous system and the Schwann cell in the peripheral nervous system. The myelin sheath serves as an insulator and separates the axolemma from the surrounding tissue fluid; it thus plays an

important role in nerve conduction (see p. 266). The sheath is formed from the plasma membrane of the supporting cell (oligodendrocyte or Schwann cell) and consists of a series of laminae of lipoprotein. (For further details, see page 255.) (b) The node of Ranvier is the gap that exists between two adjacent Schwann cells (or oligodendrocytes, in the central nervous system) in a myelinated nerve; nodes of Ranvier do not exist in a nonmyelinated nerve. A myelinated nerve can be stimulated only at a node of Ranvier. (c) Schmidt-Lanterman incisures are seen on longitudinal sections of myelinated nerve fibers. They represent areas of localized persistence of Schwann cell cytoplasm. They involve all the layers of the myelin, and there is thus a continuous spiral of cytoplasm from the outermost region of the Schwann cell to the region of the axon. The cytoplasm may serve as a pathway for the conduction of metabolites from the surface region of the Schwann cell to the axon. Schmidt-Lanterman incisures also occur in myelinated nerve fibers of the central nervous system. (d) Satellite cells in sensory and autonomic ganglia envelop the neuron cell bodies. They should be regarded as modified Schwann cells and probably serve to insulate the neurons from adjacent nervous activity.

10. Myelination is fully described on page 255. Myelin sheaths begin to be formed during the last part of fetal development and during the first postnatal year.

11. Peripheral nerve fibers may be classified into groups according to their size and speed of conduction. Group or type A fibers are 1 to 22 μm in diameter and conduct at the rate of 5 to 120 m per second. They are myelinated, somatic, efferent and afferent fibers. Group or type B fibers are 1 to 3 μm in diameter and conduct at 3 to 15 m per second. They are myelinated, efferent, preganglionic, autonomic fibers.

The resting membrane potential is the potential difference across the axolemma when a nerve fiber is at rest. A typical resting potential is 80 mV.

The absolute refractory period is the short period of time that immediately follows the passage of a nerve impulse when a second stimulus, however strong, is unable to excite the nerve.

Conduction velocity and saltatory conduction are fully explained on pages 265 and 266.

12. (a) *Wallerian degeneration* is the name given to the changes in the distal segment of an axon following its section. The details are fully described on page 280. (b) The band fiber is the endoneurial sheath and the contained cords of Schwann cells that replace the degenerated peripheral nerve following nerve section. The band fiber will serve to guide regenerating axons to their end-organs. A band fiber is not formed in the central nervous system. (c) Transneuronal degeneration occurs in the central nervous system when one group of neurons is injured and a second group, farther along the pathway and serving the same function, undergoes degeneration.

13. Degeneration occurs in the central nervous system in a manner similar to that found in the peripheral nervous system. The axon breaks up into small fragments, and the debris is digested by the neighboring microglial cells. The myelin sheath is broken down into lipid droplets that are also phagocytosed by the microglial cells.

There is an attempt to regenerate the axons, evidenced by sprouting of the axons, but there is no indication that restoration of function ever occurs. The reasons for the failure of regeneration are fully described on page 283.

14. The only sensory receptors in the cornea are free nerve endings. The cornea is sensitive to light, touch, and temperature changes in addition to pain.

15. All hair follicles possess a rich innervation. Free nerve endings occur in a branching network that winds around the follicle below the entrance of the sebaceous duct. Merkel's discs also are found in the epidermis of the follicle. The hair shaft acts as a lever, so that the slightest movement of the hair readily stimulates the nerve endings in the hair follicle. In this patient suffering from trigeminal neuralgia, the temporal region of the scalp is the trigger

area that on stimulation initiates the intense stabs of pain.

16. The cerebral cortex is made up of six identifiable layers. In the motor cortex in the precentral gyrus, there is a lack of granular cells in the second and fourth layers, and in the somesthetic cortex in the postcentral gyrus, there is a lack of pyramidal cells in the third and fifth layers. The motor cortex is thicker than the sensory cortex.

17. The different types of neurons found in the cerebellar cortex are fully described on page 274.

18. Neuroglia composes about half the total volume of the central nervous system. Neuroglial cells outnumber neurons five or ten to one.

19. *Microglia* is the collective name for microglial cells. Microglial cells are smaller than astrocytes and oligodendrocytes. They are scattered throughout the central nervous system and closely resemble connective tissue macrophages in function. Neuroglia consists of several varieties of nonexcitable cells found within the central nervous system. Neuroglial cells, which serve to support the neurons, are of four main types: astrocytes, oligodendrocytes, microglia, and ependyma.

20. The different functions of neuroglia are fully described on page 252. Researchers increasingly believe that neuroglial cells play a far greater role in the function of the central nervous system than has been determined so far.

CHAPTER 8

1. The structure and function of the pericardium are described on pages 294 and 324. The pericardial cavity is lined with mesothelial cells. In normal individuals, the volume of pericardial fluid is about 50 ml, and the fluid is produced by the mesothelial cells lining the serous pericardium. Excessive production of pericardial fluid (150 to 200 ml) or fibrous contraction of the pericardium following chronic infection will cause pressure on the chambers of the heart and seriously interfere with venous filling.

2. The mitral valve has two cusps, each consisting of a double layer of endocardium with a small amount of connective tissue forming the core. The base of each cusp is attached to the fibrous atrioventricular ring of the skeleton of the heart. The margins and ventricular surfaces of the cusps are connected to papillary muscles by a number of tendinous cords, the chordae tendineae.

The aortic valve consists of three semilunar cusps. Again, each cusp consists of a double layer of endocardium with a connective tissue core. The base of each cusp is continuous with the fibrous skeleton of the heart. At the center of the free edge, the connective tissue is thickened to form a fibrous nodule.

The mitral valve closes off the left atrioventricular orifice during left ventricular systole. The pliable, tissue-paper-thin cusps float into position and close the opening. The contraction of the papillary muscles and the presence of chordae tendineae prevents the thin cusps from being forced into the left atrium as the intraventricular pressure rises.

The aortic valve closes the aortic orifice during left ventricular diastole. As the left ventricle begins to relax, aortic blood flows back toward the left ventricle and enters the open mouths of the semilunar cusps, which quickly fill. The delicate, pliable semilunar cusps now bulge into the lumen and come into apposition in the center of the aorta, closing off the aortic orifice.

Rheumatic fever induces an immunological response to infection with group A β-hemolytic streptococci. The valve cusps become red, swollen, and thickened, and this change is often accompanied by a precipitate of fibrin along the line of closure of the cusps. The cusps may stick together. This inflammatory response causes the cusps to malfunction, because they are no longer thin and pliable but, rather, thick and rigid and often stuck together. This condition leads to mitral and aortic regurgitation of blood, because the valves now leak.

Later, especially if repeated attacks of rheumatic fever have occurred, the valve cusps become fibrosed, shrunken, and scarred. The chordae tendineae also become shortened. Fibrous adhesions between the cusps lead to narrowing of the valve orifices, with the later development of mitral and possible aortic stenosis.

3. The structure of cardiac muscle is fully described on page 203. The myocardial layer of the atrial walls is much thinner than that of the ventricular walls, because the workload is far less; in fact, the intra-atrial pressures rise to only about 6 mm Hg when the atria contract. The myocardial layer of the left ventricle is very thick, because it must eject blood into the aorta, where the pressures are high (systolic, about 120 mm Hg; diastolic, approximately 80 mm Hg). The myocardial layer of the right ventricle is about one-third the thickness of that of the left ventricle, and this is because of the smaller workload (about one-sixth the pressure in the pulmonary trunk of that in the aorta).

Cardiac muscle fibers are crossed by *intercalated discs* that are formed by the cell membranes that separate adjacent cardiac muscle cells (see p. 206). The electrical resistance across these discs is very small, allowing action potentials to travel from one cardiac muscle cell to another with minimal delay. Thus, if one muscle cell is stimulated, the action potential spreads to all the muscle cells very rapidly.

The microscopic structure of the specialized cardiac muscles fibers found in the conducting system of the heart is described on page 206. The sino-atrial node is capable of spontaneously giving origin to rhythmical impulses that spread in all directions through the cardiac muscle of the atria and cause the muscle to contract; it controls the rate of contraction of the entire heart. The atrioventricular node picks up the wave of excitation from the atrial muscle, and the wave is conducted to the ventricular muscle via the atrioventricular bundle. The Purkinje fibers of the atrioventricular bundle are fast-conducting. The cardiac impulse travels from the beginning of the atrioventricular bundle to the terminal branches of the Purkinje plexus in about 0.03 second. This rapid rate of conduction through the specialized cardiac muscle fibers, faster than the rate in ordinary cardiac muscle, ensures that the entire myocardium of the ventricles is stimulated to contract at almost exactly the same time. The terms all-or-none law, absolute refractory period, and compensatory pause are all defined on page 300.

4. The external jugular vein can be used clinically as a venous manometer. The zero line is the level of the right atrium in the thorax. Normally, in a person propped up on pillows in bed, the venous pressure is so low that the blood level does not extend above the clavicle. This patient has right-sided heart failure with a backup of venous blood on the right side of the heart. Consequently, the venous pressure is high, and the external jugular vein is engorged with blood throughout its length.

Venous return is the term used to describe the blood flowing into the right atrium of the heart. The Frank-Starling law is fully explained on page 302.

5. The agonizing chest pain is caused by ischemia of the cardiac muscle secondary to blockage of the anterior interventricular branch of the left coronary artery by advanced atherosclerosis. Because of the death of a large area of the muscular wall of the left ventricle, the cardiac output is considerably diminished, accounting for the low systolic blood pressure and weak radial pulse. The irregular pulse wave is caused by the interference with the blood supply to the conducting system secondary to the coronary atherosclerosis.

The pale, cold, moist skin and the tachycardia are caused by the increased activity of the vasoconstrictor and cardioaccelerator centers as they respond to the fall in blood pressure by increasing the peripheral resistance and the heart rate. The increased sweating accompanies the increased activity of the sympathetic nerve fibers.

Although in this patient the fall in blood pressure largely is caused by extensive cardiac muscle damage, some of the reduction in pressure may be secondary to the severe pain. The moist sounds heard with a stethoscope over the lower basal areas of the inferior lobes of both lungs are secondary to left ventricular failure. The blood in the pulmonary circulation is being dammed in the lungs, and excessive amounts of tissue fluid are being formed and entering the alveoli and bronchioles.

Cardiac output is the quantity of blood pumped out of each ventricle per minute; in the young resting man, it averages about 5.6 liters per minute (see p. 301). Stroke volume is the volume of blood pumped out of one ventricle at each beat of the heart. Under resting conditions, it equals 60 to 70 ml (see p. 301).

6. The electrical changes that take place in cardiac muscle when it contracts and an electrocardiogram are described on page 304. The very small electrical resistance that exists between adjacent cardiac muscle fibers at the intercalated discs permits the action potential to travel from one cardiac muscle fiber to another with minimal delay.

7. The basic structure of all blood vessels consists of a tunica intima, a tunica media, and a tunica adventitia (see p. 307). The structure of each of these layers varies with the function of the vessel. In the large conducting arteries, there is a large amount of elastic tissue in the tunica media, which allows the artery to accommodate the blood ejected from the heart during ventricular systole. The wall of the artery then recoils during ventricular diastole; the elastic tissue thus plays a major role in maintaining the diastolic arterial blood pressure.

In the muscular distributing arteries, the large amount of smooth muscle in the tunica media, which is under autonomic nervous control, permits regulation of the flow of blood to different organs of the body.

In arterioles, the tunica media is very thick in proportion to the size of the vessel. Activation of the smooth muscle, as a result of stimulation of the sympathetic innervation, will cause vasoconstriction and increase the peripheral resistance to the blood flow. In this way, the muscle of the arteriole wall assists in maintaining the arterial blood pressure and controls the flow of blood through the tissues.

8. The structure of capillaries, metarterioles, and the precapillary sphincter are described on page 310. The local chemical and nervous control of blood flow in tissues is described on page 323.

9. The coronary arteries are muscular arteries. They have a well-defined tunica intima, tunica media, and tunica adventitia (see p. 308). The right and left coronary arteries arise from the ascending aorta just superior to the anterior and left posterior cusps of the aortic valve. The flow of blood through the coronary arteries is greatest during ventricular diastole, because during systole, the contracting ventricular muscle compresses the terminal branches of the coronary arteries. The coronary arteries are made to dilate by the sympathetic nerve fibers and by the hormones norepinephrine and epinephrine. The vagus does not affect the blood flow.

Functional end arteries are vessels whose terminal branches anastomose with those of adjacent arteries, but the caliber of the anastomoses is insufficient to keep the tissue alive should one of the arteries become occluded.

10. In the young, the tunica intima is thin. With advancing years, the connective tissue of this coat becomes thicker because of the accumulation of mucopolysaccharides and the appearance of myointimal cells, which can synthesize collagen and elastic fibers. These changes have little or no effect on the circulatory system. The elastic fibers in the tunica media of the larger blood vessels degenerate with age and are replaced by bundles of collagen fibers. The loss of elastic tissue causes the vessels to elongate and become more rigid. Increasing rigidity interferes with the ability of the circulatory system to maintain a normal blood pressure (see p. 316).

11. The structure of veins of different sizes are described on page 311. A small venule, like a capillary, provides a site where oxygen and nutrition materials can pass from the blood into the tissue fluid, and carbon dioxide and waste products of tissue metabolism can pass into the bloodstream.

The walls of veins are thinner than those of corresponding arteries; thus, their lumina can be narrowed by external pressure. Bicuspid valves in the medium-sized veins enable changing external pressures to milk the blood along the veins in one direction toward the venous side of the heart, as seen in the thoraco-abdominal pump, the skeletal muscle pump, and the arterial pump.

The small amount of smooth muscle present in the vein walls allows the vessels to adapt its capacity to the volume of blood traveling along the lumen.

12. The various factors controlling arterial blood pressure are fully described on page 316. The arterial blood pressure within the pulmonary arteries is approximately one-sixth that in the aorta and other large systemic arteries. The structures of a blood sinusoid and an arteriovenous anastomosis are described on page 312.

13. Atherosclerosis most often involves the aorta and the coronary and cerebral arteries; other medium-sized arteries, such as the mesenteric artery and arteries of the lower limbs, may be affected. The tunica intima is the principal layer that is diseased, although the tunica media may undergo atrophy. The endothelial cells of the tunica intima are believed to be damaged initially by stress, and the smooth muscle cells of the tunica media migrate into the intima and take part in the pathological process. The smooth muscle cells proliferate and phagocytose the lipoproteins present in the tunica intima. (For further details, see page 328.)

14. The great and small saphenous veins are histologically classed as medium-sized veins. The tunica intima consists of a lining of endothelial cells resting on a thin layer of connective tissue. There are several bicuspid valves along the length of these veins, the leaflets of which are composed of a fold of tunica intima. The tunica media consists of circularly arranged smooth muscle cells mixed with connective tissue. The tunica adventitia is the thickest layer and consists of bundles of collagen fibers, elastic networks, and longitudinally arranges bundles of smooth muscle cells. Many vasa vasorum are present.

The saphenous veins are anatomically poorly positioned, in that they lie in the superficial fascia and consequently are poorly supported externally. They also are situated in the most dependent part of the body and are therefore subject to high hydrostatic venous pressures.

A varicosed vein is one whose diameter is greater than normal and whose length is elongated and tortuous. Prolonged increased venous pressure is responsible for the stretching of the thin walls of the veins. Microscopically, the vein wall usually shows some thickening, caused by increased amounts of connective tissue in the tunica media and additional smooth muscle cells in the tunica media.

CHAPTER 9

1. The immobilization of the patient's arm in a sling reduces the muscular activity and, thus, the rate of lymph flow from the limb. This serves to limit the spread of toxins and bacteria from the site of infection.

2. (a) The auricle of the ear is swollen by inflammatory edema. Edema is an abnormal accumulation of tissue fluid in the intercellular spaces. The fluid dynamics of inflammatory edema are explained on page 188. (b) The right side of the neck is swollen because the bacteria have spread from the right auricle via the lymphatic vessels to the right superficial and deep cervical lymph nodes, which are enlarged as a result of the proliferation of the contained lymphocytes. (c) In the early stages of infection, heat causes arteriolar vasodilatation, which in turn raises the blood flow through the infected skin, hastening the arrival of neutrophils, antibodies, and antibiotics to the site of infection. Once the infection is controlled, the increased vascular and lymphatic flow will help reduce the local accumulation of tissue fluid and cause the swelling of the ear to diminish.

3. (a) *Lymph* is the name given to tissue fluid once it has entered a lymphatic vessel. (b) A reticulocyte is a fusiform or star-shaped cell found in close associa-

tion with reticular fibers. In the thymus, unlike other lymphatic tissue, it is the reticulocytes, not the reticular fibers, that form the basic framework of the organ. In addition to forming reticular fibers, reticulocytes can become phagocytic. (c) The subcapsular sinus of a lymph node is the area of empty spaces in the reticular network found just beneath the capsule. It provides a channel into which the afferent lymphatic vessels to a lymph node empty their lymph. (d) Hassall's corpuscles are whorled, epithelial structures found only in the medulla of a thymic lobule. They are formed of reticulocytes, and their significance is unknown. (e) Red pulp consists of blood circulating through the meshwork of reticular fibers and venous sinusoids in the spleen. Reticulocytes and macrophages are also present in large numbers. (f) T lymphocytes are described on page 339.

4. The factors that aid lymph flow are described fully on page 338.

5. The structure of a lymphatic capillary is described on page 333. The gap that exists between adjacent endothelial cells, the absence of pericytes, and the discontinuous basal lamina enables these small vessels to absorb large molecules, such as proteins and other particulate matter. The lymphatic anchoring filaments possibly prevent the lumina of the vessels from collapsing completely when compressed by surrounding muscles.

The structure of a medium-sized lymphatic vessel is described on page 335. The smooth muscle cells in the wall exert tone on the contents. The presence of bicuspid valves ensures that the lymph passes in one direction toward the large veins in the root of the neck.

The structure of the large lymphatic ducts is discussed on page 335. The relatively thin walls of these vessels, as compared to veins of comparable size, allow them to be compressed by outside pressures, such as that of contracting muscles or increased abdominal pressure. The thoracic duct and the right lymphatic duct serve to channel all the lymph in the body into the large veins in the root of the neck.

6. Cellular and humoral immunity and the parts played by the T and B lymphocytes in these processes are described on pages 339 through 343.

Lymphatic vessels may provide an invasive carcinoma with a pathway for spread from the primary site of the tumor. The malignant cells may grow along the interior of a vessel and be bathed with nourishing lymph, or they may break away and form lymphatic emboli that are rapidly conveyed in the lymph to the regional lymph nodes or to other neighboring tissues.

The lymph nodes temporarily may trap and limit the spread of malignant cells arriving in the afferent lymph vessels. Only too often, however, the carcinoma cells, nourished by the lymph, continue to multiply within the nodes, causing the nodes to enlarge. By this means, a secondary tumor, or metastasis, is formed that can spread further via the lymphatic vessels and even enter the bloodstream by this route.

7. Throughout the alimentary tract, from the mouth to the anal canal, there is lymphatic tissue in the connective tissue of the mucous membrane. Around the junction of the nose and mouth with the pharynx are the tonsils, which are described on page 354. Nonencapsulated lymphatic nodules are scattered along the mucous membrane of the remainder of the gastrointestinal tract. The lymphatic tissue is especially concentrated in the terminal part of the ileum and in the appendix. The aggregations found in the lower part of the ileum are known as Peyer's patches.

8. (a) A lacteal is a single lymphatic capillary that ends blindly within a villus of the small intestine. It is called a lacteal because of its milky appearance after a fatty meal. (b) The fat droplets found in a lacteal are called chylomicrons. (c) Lymphokines are chemical substances released by sensitized T lymphocytes in response to specific antigens; they are toxic to the cells producing the antigen. (d) Lymphatic germinal centers are found in the central area of a lymphatic nodule and are the sites of active lymphocyte production. They are recognized by the lighter-staining central area of the nodule, and they

appear only following the exposure of the nodule to a foreign antigen. (e) Lymphangitis is an infection of a lymphatic vessel (see p. 360).

9. The structure and functions of a lymph node are described on pages 345 through 349. The structure and functions of the spleen, including the open and closed theories of blood circulation through the spleen, are described on pages 349 through 354.

10. The mechanism of allograft rejection is described on page 362. In congenital absence of the thymus, the patient lacks T lymphocytes and, therefore, cellular immunity.

CHAPTER 10

1. The lateral wall of the nose has three projections of bone called the superior, middle, and inferior conchae. The area below each concha is referred to as a meatus. It is not uncommon for young children to push foreign objects up their noses, and these become lodged between the conchae.

The mucous membrane lining the middle meatus of the nose consists of a layer of pseudostratified ciliated columnar epithelium with goblet cells, resting on a basal lamina. Beneath the basal lamina is the lamina propria, which consists of fibroconnective tissue containing numerous mucous and serous glands. The mucus is produced by the goblet cells of the surface epithelium and the mucous glands of the lamina propria.

The blood supply of the respiratory mucous membrane is profuse, and the plexus of veins in the lamina propria normally warms the inspired air.

2. The paranasal air sinuses communicate with the nasal cavities through small apertures in the lateral walls of the nose. Spread of infection from the nose to the sinuses is a common condition and is known as sinusitis. This patient is suffering from a right-sided frontal and maxillary sinusitis.

The mucous membrane lining the paranasal sinuses is covered with pseudostratified ciliated columnar epithelium and contains goblet cells. There is a thin lamina propria attached to the underlying periosteum by a thin layer of connective tissue.

3. The structure of the mucous membrane lining the maxillary sinus, a paranasal sinus, is described under answer 2. The carcinoma in this patient is a columnar cell carcinoma.

4. The vocal folds consist of the vocal ligaments, composed of bundles of elastic fibers with a few collagen fibers. The vocal folds are covered with mucous membrane lined with stratified squamous nonkeratinized epithelium.

The stratified squamous epithelium is able to resist the wear and tear of the vibrating vocal folds better than the pseudostratified ciliated columnar epithelium found lining the remainder of the larynx.

5. Except in the region of the vocal folds, the mucous membrane lining the larynx is loosely attached to the underlying cartilages and fibrous membranes. Consequently, edema fluid will accumulate quickly in the submucosa, causing the mucous membrane to bulge into the cavity of the larynx and thus compromise the airway.

The wall of the trachea is made up of the mucous membrane, the submucosa, and the adventitia. The structure of each of these layers is fully described on page 373.

6. The defense mechanisms that exist throughout the length of the respiratory tract are described on page 402.

Inhaled asbestos fibers settle on the lining of the respiratory bronchioles and the alveoli. Because of the irritating chemical substances (hydrated silicates) within the asbestos fibers, a diffuse reaction occurs. The alveoli become invaded by phagocytic macrophages that sometimes fuse to form giant cells. A fibrous reaction also occurs in the alveolar walls, which thicken. The result is a lowering of the efficiency of the gaseous exchange, and respiratory difficulty. The condition is known as asbestosis; unfortunately, many patients later develop bronchogenic carcinoma.

7. The structures of the trachea, a bronchus, a bronchiole, and a respiratory bronchiole are described on pages 373 through 381. Note the differences in the epithelium lining these passages. Note also how the

cartilaginous content and smooth muscle content in the walls of these tubes change from one area to another.

8. As one traces the respiratory tract downward, one finds that the hyaline cartilaginous tracheal rings are replaced by large, irregular plates of hyaline cartilage. These plates become smaller as the bronchi diminish in diameter until they finally disappear in the bronchioles. The amount of smooth muscle in the wall of the trachea relative to the size of the tube is relatively small and is concentrated mainly in the trachealis muscles. These are situated posteriorly between the ends of each horseshoe-shaped cartilage. As the plates of hyaline cartilage in the bronchial walls diminish in size, the amount of smooth muscle increases. The submucosa of the bronchioles possesses a complete layer of circularly arranged smooth muscle fibers.

Contraction of the trachealis muscle in response to parasympathetic stimulation can modify the diameter of the lumen of the trachea only slightly because of the rigidity of the cartilaginous rings in the tracheal walls. Contraction of the smooth muscle in the walls of the smaller bronchi and bronchioles, however, where there is little or no cartilage, can reduce the size of the air passages greatly.

9. A tuberculous lesion localized to a bronchopulmonary segment can be removed surgically from the lung. A bronchopulmonary segment is pyramid shaped, with its apex pointing toward the root of the lung and its base facing the lung surface. Each segment has its own tertiary bronchus, a branch of the pulmonary artery, and a tributary of the pulmonary vein.

A pulmonary lobule is a subunit of a bronchopulmonary segment. The entering air passage measures less than 1 mm in diameter and is known as a bronchiole. The bronchioles divide into terminal bronchioles, and these divide into respiratory bronchioles. The respiratory bronchioles in turn give rise to the alveolar ducts, alveolar sacs, and alveoli (see p. 381).

10. The instrument used to measure the volumes of air in the lungs is called a spirometer (see p. 402). (a) Tidal volume is the volume of air inspired and expired with each normal breath during quiet breathing. It amounts to about 500 ml. (b) Inspiratory reserve volume is the additional volume of air that can be inspired above and beyond the normal tidal volume when the individual makes the maximum inspiratory effort. It amounts to about 3,000 ml in the young male adult. (c) Expiratory reserve volume is the additional volume of air that can be expired above and beyond the normal tidal volume when the individual makes the maximum expiratory effort. It amounts to about 1,100 ml in the young male adult. (d) Residual volume is the volume of air that remains within the lungs after the individual has made the maximum expiratory effort. It amounts to about 1,200 ml in the young male adult. (e) Vital capacity is the sum of the tidal volume (500 ml), the inspiratory reserve volume (3,000 ml), and the expiratory reserve volume (1,100 ml) and equals about 4,600 ml in the young adult.

11. (a) An alveolar duct is lined with cuboidal epithelium supported by connective tissue containing elastic fibers and a few smooth muscle fibers. (b) An alveolar sac consists of several alveoli opening into a single chamber. (c) The walls of an alveolus are composed of flattened cells supported by delicate connective tissue containing elastic fibers and a rich network of blood capillaries. Scattered among the flattened or squamous cells (type I) through which gaseous diffusion readily takes place are occasional cuboidal cells (type II), which are responsible for secreting surfactant (see p. 381). Bulging into the alveolus or residing in the walls of the alveolus are the alveolar phagocytes. Such cells remove debris, such as carbon particles, from the lumen of the alveolus.

12. The lumen of the alveolus is separated from the lumen of the blood capillary by the following: (1) surfactant-containing fluid produced by the type II alveolar cells, (2) the alveolar squamous epithelium

or type I cell, (3) the epithelial basement membrane, (4) a minute tissue space, (5) the blood capillary basement membrane, which fuses with the epithelial basement membrane in many places, and (6) the capillary squamous endothelium. The combination of these layers is called the respiratory membrane. It measures about 0.5 μm in thickness.

The gaseous exchanges that take place across the respiratory membrane are described on pages 392 through 397.

13. The pressure of oxygen in the blood leaving the lungs in the pulmonary veins is about 100 mm Hg. The oxygen saturation in the blood reaching the tissue is about the same as in that leaving the lungs — that is, about 97 percent — and the pressure of the oxygen is about 100 mm Hg. In the tissues or tissue fluids, however, the oxygen saturation may be as low as 70 percent and the pressure of oxygen is only about 40 mm Hg.

14. Seventy percent of carbon dioxide transported in the blood is in the form of bicarbonate ions. The remaining thirty percent is transported in physical solution or in combination with hemoglobin and plasma proteins.

Carbonic anhydrase is an enzyme within red cells. It catalyzes the combination of carbon dioxide with water to form carbonic acid (H_2CO_3). To maintain electrical neutrality within the red cells, chloride ions rapidly diffuse from the plasma into the red blood cells, a phenomenon referred to as the chloride shift.

15. The respiratory center consists of the groups of nerve cells in the medulla oblongata and pons in the brain that automatically control respiratory movements. The respiratory center can be divided into (1) the medullary respiratory center, (2) the apneustic center, and (3) the pneumotaxic center (for details, see p. 397). Metrazol, caffeine, theophylline, and picrotoxin can stimulate the respiratory center directly, whereas Coramine can stimulate the center indirectly by stimulating the carotid and aortic body reflexes. Intracranial tumors, anesthetics and narcotic agents, and cerebral edema following severe head injuries can depress the respiratory center.

16. (a) Cheyne-Stokes breathing is described fully on page 405. (b) Compliance is the ease with which a hollow viscus may be distended. Compliance of the lungs is reduced if, for example, they are involved in fibrotic disease or the bronchi become blocked. For further examples, see page 392. (c) Pneumothorax is a condition in which air enters the pleural cavity, resulting in partial or complete collapse of the lung. Pneumothorax can be spontaneous or artificial. (d) Surfactant is a lipoprotein material produced by cuboidal cells in the alveolar walls. It reduces the surface tension of the lining cells and permits the alveolar walls to separate from each other as air enters during inspiration.

CHAPTER 11

1. The outer surface of the lip is covered with skin (see p. 409). The epidermis of the skin consists of stratified squamous keratinized epithelium, and among the basal keratinocytes are pigment cells, the melanocytes; there are also Langerhans cells and Merkel cells. The squamous cell carcinoma has arisen from the keratinocytes.

The margin of the lip is red because of the blood in the large capillary loops in the underlying connective tissue of the dermis. The epidermis of the red margin is not heavily keratinized, so that it is translucent and the red hemoglobin in the blood can be seen easily. In patients with heart failure or severe respiratory disease, for example, the hemoglobin exists in the blood as deoxygenated hemoglobin. This form of hemoglobin is dark blue and can be seen easily on the lip margins when present in large quantities. The condition is known as cyanosis.

2. Dental caries is the destruction of the calcified structure of the tooth by a mixture of bacteria and fungi. The bacteria and fungi require the presence of carbohydrate on the tooth surface for their metabolism.

Dental enamel consists of long, thin, calcified enamel rods. Each rod is surrounded by an organic matrix that is destroyed by the bacteria and fungi in caries. Dentin is a calcified connective tissue formed by the odontoblasts. As the dentin is formed, the cell bodies of the odontoblasts recede toward the center of the tooth, each leaving behind an odontoblastic process. Each odontoblastic process is housed in a thin, curved *dentinal tubule* that runs from the pulp cavity to the periphery of the dentin. The odontoblastic processes are sensitive to pain, and it is thought that they transmit the sensory information to the nerve endings in the pulp.

The periodontal ligament consists of bundles of collagen fibers that extend from the cementum of the tooth root to the alveolar bone. The ligament suspends the root within its bony socket.

3. The mucous membrane of the cheek consists of stratified squamous nonkeratinized epithelium lying on the connective tissue of the lamina propria. Small groups of mucous glands, the *labial glands,* are situated in the lamina propria and pour their secretions onto the surface through small ducts. Infection of or trauma to the duct orifices or blockage of the ducts with thick secretion may lead to cystlike distention of the glands.

4. The papillae on the dorsum of the tongue are of three types: (1) filiform, (2) fungiform, and (3) vallate. The structure of these papillae is described on page 414. In deficiency diseases, such as those of iron, vitamin B_{12}, and folic acid, the cells of the papillae are incapable of carrying out normal metabolic activity and die, leaving a smooth-surfaced tongue. This condition therefore may be seen in hypochromic anemia, pernicious anemia, and steatorrhea, where there is a failure of absorption of vitamins. The histological structure of a taste bud is described on page 770.

5. The submandibular salivary gland is a tubuloalveolar acinose gland of the mucous and serous type; the majority of the acini are serous. The ducts are the intercalated and striated ducts. The intercalated ducts lead directly out of each acinus and are lined with cuboidal epithelium. The striated ducts are located distally and are lined with tall columnar cells showing vertical striations. The striated ducts join one another to form interlobular ducts, and these open finally into the excretory duct. The excretory ducts are lined with columnar epithelium. The submandibular gland is surrounded by a fibrous capsule and has fibrous septa that divide it into lobes and lobules.

Calculi are more common in the submandibular than in the parotid salivary gland. The stone is composed of a mixture of calcium phosphate and carbonate; in the center, there are usually desquamated cells or bacteria. The viscosity of the secretion, caused by the presence of mucus, is an important factor in the development of this condition. The parotid secretion is thin and watery and devoid of mucus.

6. The palatine tonsils are situated in the lateral pharyngeal walls. The tonsils are composed of lymphoid tissue lying in the lamina propria of the mucous membrane. The covering epithelium is stratified squamous and nonkeratinized that dips down into the lymphoid tissue, forming deep crypts called the *tonsillar crypts.* The tonsil is covered on its lateral surface by a fibrous capsule that sends trabeculae into the organ. Tonsils reach their maximum development during childhood and at puberty start to atrophy. Both T and B lymphocytes are present in the tonsils.

7. The muscle in the wall of the esophagus is found in the muscularis mucosae and the muscle coat or muscularis externa. The muscularis mucosae consists of a thin layer of smooth muscle fibers having a longitudinal and circular arrangement. The thick muscle coat of the esophagus consists of a circular inner and a longitudinal outer layer. In the upper third of the esophagus, the muscle is skeletal, in the lower third, it is smooth, and in the middle third, there is a mixture of skeletal and smooth muscle. There is no cardioesophageal sphincter recognizable on a histological slide. There is, however, a good possibility that a sphincter mechanism exists at the lower end of the esophagus; this is fully discussed on page 430.

The esophageal cardiac glands at the upper and

lower ends of the esophagus in the lamina propria of the mucous membrane secrete mucus. The esophageal glands of the submucosa also secrete mucus.

8. The apical plasma membrane of the lining cells of the stomach is protected from the acid and pepsin of the gastric juice by the alkaline mucus secreted by the surface cells and the reflux of alkaline duodenal secretions through the pyloric sphincter. The tight junctions that unite the adjacent surfaces of the lining cells effectively prevent leakage of the gastric juices into the underlying tissues.

9. The stomach possesses three types of glands: (1) cardiac glands, (2) glands of the fundus and body, and (3) pyloric glands. The cardiac glands are found around the opening of the esophagus; the columnar cells secrete alkaline mucus. The glands of the fundus and body are simple branched tubular glands with the following secretory cells: (a) chief or peptic cells that secrete pepsinogen, lipase, and amylase; (b) parietal or oxyntic cells that secrete hydrochloric acid and the intrinsic factor; (c) mucous neck cells that secrete alkaline mucus; and (d) argentaffin cells that secrete serotonin and enteroglucagon. The pyloric glands are simple branched tubular glands whose columnar cells secrete alkaline mucus and the hormone gastrin.

10. Gastric secretion is controlled by nervous and hormonal mechanisms. For details, see pages 441 through 442.

11. Situated between the bases of the villi of the duodenum are the openings of the tubular glands known as the crypts of Lieberkühn. The goblet cells in the glands secrete an alkaline mucus. Opening into the lower ends of the crypts of Lieberkühn are the large compound tubular mucous Brunner's glands, which occupy the greater part of the submucosa and add their alkaline secretion to the duodenal lumen. In addition, the alkaline bile and pancreatic secretions are poured into the second part of the duodenum in response to the presence of chyme from the stomach. The pH of bile is about 6 and that of the pancreatic secretion is about 8.2.

12. A summary of the processes of digestion that take place in the small intestine is given on pages 455 and 496. The structure of the columnar absorptive cells is described on page 446.

13. Analysis of samples of intestinal contents aspirated through a nasal tube shows that the jejunum is the main site of digestion and absorption, and that the ileum absorbs the remainder of the digested residue.

The following structures exist in the jejunum that greatly increase the surface area of the mucous membrane, aiding absorption of the luminal contents: (1) the permanent folds of the mucous membrane called the *plicae circulares,* which gradually become smaller and farther apart in the ileum; (2) the fingerlike projections of mucous membrane called villi, which are broader and taller in the jejunum and reach their minimum size at the distal end of the ileum; and (3) the columnar absorptive cells on the surface of the villi, which have closely packed microvilli on their free surface that are present in all absorptive cells of the small intestine.

A person can lose about three-quarters of the small intestine without resultant nutritional defects, provided that adequate amounts of vitamin B_{12} and vitamins A, B, D, E, and K are administered; calcium and iron also should be given.

14. Patients with steatorrhea usually have a deficiency of the vitamin B group, including nicotinic acid, riboflavin, folic acid, or vitamin B_{12}. Vitamins A, B, D, E, and K may also be deficient.

15. Crypts of Lieberkühn are tubular glands situated between the bases of the villi of the mucous membrane of the small intestine. They are also present in large numbers in the mucous membrane of the large intestine. In the small intestine, the neck of each crypt possesses columnar absorption cells, goblet cells, and argentaffin cells. In the lower half of the crypts are undifferentiated stem cells and Paneth cells.

The crypts of Lieberkühn in the large intestine are longer and packed closer together. They have no Paneth cells but possess more goblet cells.

Paneth cells are found in the crypts of Lieberkühn of the small intestine. They are usually found in small groups at the bottom of a crypt. The cytoplasm contains large secretory granules in the apical cytoplasm that stain pink with eosin. The function of the Paneth cells is unknown, but some authorities believe they secrete lysozyme, an enzyme that dissolves bacteria.

A Peyer's patch is a confluent mass of lymphatic tissue found in the mucous membrane of the distal part of the ileum along its antimesenteric border. An argentaffin cell is an endocrine cell found in the glands of the mucous membrane in the stomach and intestine. It contains dense cytoplasmic granules.

Argentaffin cells produce serotonin, secretin, cholecystokinin, and, possibly, somatostatin and endorphin.

16. The appendix is part of the large intestine. Its wall has the usual four layers:

1. Mucous membrane. There are no villi, and the crypts of Lieberkühn possess numerous goblet cells. The lamina propria contains large collections of lymphatic tissue.
2. Submucosa, into which the lymphatic tissue of the mucous membrane usually extends.
3. Muscular coat. Unlike that in the colon, the longitudinal muscle here forms a continuous coat that surrounds the appendix and becomes continuous with the teniae coli at the root of the appendix.
4. Serous coat, which completely surrounds the appendix and leaves as two layers, forming a small mesentery.

For further details, see page 458.

The tissue that dominates the mucous membrane and extends into the submucosa is the lymphatic tissue. It takes the form of lymphatic nodules that surround the lumen and in many areas become continuous with one another.

The appendix has a narrow lumen, and it is common for fecal material to become lodged within it. As water is absorbed from the material through the mucous membrane, the feces become hard and are then referred to as a fecolith. The fecolith may irritate the wall of the appendix, initiating appendicitis. Inflammatory edema of the appendicular wall now leads to swelling of the mucous membrane, so that the lumen closes completely around the fecolith. Rising intraluminal pressure within the distal end of the appendix first causes a compression of the venous outflow and then comprises the arterial flow. The distal end of the appendix has a small blood supply, so it is quite common for this area to become gangrenous and perforate into the peritoneal cavity.

17. The main functions of the large intestine are absorption of water and storage of the undigested food residue that enters the large intestine at the ileocecal junction. The final product that enters the rectum is known as feces. Bacteria in the lumen of the colon have an important function in the formation of certain vitamins and clotting factors (see p. 460).

Absorption of water is carried out by the columnar absorptive cells found on the surface of the mucous membrane and within the neck regions of the crypts of Lieberkühn. The free borders of these cells are closely packed with microvilli, greatly increasing the surface area and furthering absorption. The segmental contraction of the teniae coli serves to mix the luminal contents thoroughly and facilitate absorption of water. The goblet cells of the crypts produce mucus that lubricates the passage of the fecal material.

18. The movements of the large intestine are coordinated by the autonomic nerve plexus, called Auerbach's plexus, situated in the muscular coat. Megacolon is a congenital condition in which the ganglion cells of Meissner's and Auerbach's plexuses in the region of the lower end of the rectum fail to develop. The child is born with a functional obstruction of the distal end of the rectum. The treatment is operative excision of the aganglionic segment of the bowel.

19. The longitudinal layer of smooth muscle in the wall of the colon is not a continuous layer surround-

ing the gut, as it is in the small intestine, but is grouped to form three bands called the teniae coli. These bands come together to form a continuous coat around the appendix and rectum. Blood vessels entering or leaving the submucosa of the colon pierce the circular layer of muscle between the teniae coli. These points are potentially weak sites in the colonic wall, and excessive pressure within the lumen of the colon can cause outpouching of the mucous membrane and submucosa along the paths taken by the blood vessels, producing a condition known as diverticulosis. Unfortunately, the walls of the pouches are devoid of a muscle coat; stagnation of the contents thus tends to occur, followed by inflammation, a condition referred to as diverticulitis.

20. The structure of the anal canal is fully described on page 463. The mucous membrane of the upper half of the canal resembles that of the rectum and is lined with columnar epithelium; distal to the anal valves, the mucous membrane is lined with stratified squamous epithelium. Internal hemorrhoids are dilatations of the tributaries of the superior rectal vein found in the submucosa of the anal columns of the upper half of the anal canal. These veins are the most dependent part of the portal venous system when one is in a standing position. External hemorrhoids are dilatations of the tributaries of the inferior rectal vein as they run laterally from the anal margin. They are covered with skin.

21. Columnar cells line the rectum and upper half of the anal canal. The usual malignant condition in this area is a columnar cell adenocarcinoma. The lower half of the anal canal is lined with stratified squamous epithelium containing melanocytes. Squamous cell carcinoma is the most common form of malignant tumor in this area, although melanomas do occur rarely.

CHAPTER 12

1. There are three classifications for the basic and functional unit of the liver: (a) The so-called classic lobule is hexagonal, with a central vein around which plates of liver cells radiate out to the periphery. On either side of the plates of liver cells are the hepatic blood sinusoids. At the periphery of the lobule are small branches of the portal vein and hepatic artery and a tributary of the bile duct. These vessels are supported by connective tissue and collectively are called the portal canal. (b) The portal lobule is arranged around a bile duct and is limited peripherally by imaginary lines that connect three central veins. (c) The liver acinus consists of liver cells that lie between any two central veins; the branches of the hepatic artery and portal vein lie in the center of the acinus. Pathologists prefer this classification, because liver disease is closely related to the hepatic blood supply. For further details, see page 486.

2. The human liver possesses relatively little connective tissue, explaining its proneness to tearing in traumatic accidents to the abdomen. The liver is surrounded by a thin capsule (Glisson's capsule) that enters the liver at the porta hepatis. Here, the capsule becomes continuous with the small amount of connective tissue that supports the portal triad in the portal canals. Apart from the reticular network and occasional collagen fibers that support the blood sinusoids, there is no other connective tissue in the liver.

Cirrhosis of the liver is a disease in which there is diffuse necrosis of the heaptic cells, a disorganized attempt at regeneration of the hepatic cells, and diffuse fibrosis. The disease is progressive and leads to the obstruction of portal blood flow through the liver. The vessels in the portal canal, the hepatic sinusoids, and the central veins are compressed by the regenerating liver cells and the extensive fibrosis, leading to portal hypertension. The rise in portal venous pressure leads to the excessive production of peritoneal fluid, a condition known as ascites.

3. (a) An intrahepatic bile canaliculus is a minute cleft or channel that runs between adjacent hepatocytes. The cell membrane of the hepatocytes in this channel possesses short microvilli. (b) The space of Disse is a perisinusoidal space between the blood sinusoids and the hepatic cells. The space is in com-

munication with the blood sinusoids through the gaps between adjacent endothelial cells lining the sinusoids and through the fenestrae of the endothelial cells. (c) Kupffer cells are large fixed macrophages that are scattered along the lining of the hepatic blood sinusoids. They are involved in the phagocytosis of worn-out blood cells. (d) The portal triad is found at the periphery of a classic liver lobule. It consists of small branches of the portal vein and hepatic artery and contains a tributary of the bile duct. (e) Glisson's capsule is the thin connective tissue capsule of the liver. (f) Rokitansky-Aschoff sinuses are small, normal outpouchings of mucous membrane of the gallbladder that extend into the muscle coat.

4. Worn-out erythrocytes are phagocytosed by parts of the reticuloendothelial system. The hemoglobin is broken down within the phagocytes into the pigment heme and globin. Heme is converted into biliverdin, which is reduced to bilirubin. The bilirubin is released slowly from the phagocytes into the blood, where it combines with albumin. The hepatocytes absorb the bilirubin complex from the blood. The bilirubin is removed from the albumin within the cells and conjugated with other substances. The hepatocytes finally excrete the conjugated bilirubin in the bile into the canaliculi. A small amount of conjugated bilirubin is returned to the blood. The bile is concentrated in the gallbladder and finally discharged into the second part of the duodenum through the common bile duct.

In the normal individual, the plasma bilirubin consists mainly of the bilirubin albumin complex, that is, unconjugated bilirubin and a small amount of conjugated bilirubin. A rise in the plasma concentration of the conjugated form of bilirubin, which occurs, for example, if there is an obstruction of the common bile duct and escape of the bilirubin into the bloodstream, can be detected by the diazo reaction. This test is called the direct van den Bergh reaction.

In patients with hemolytic anemia, in which there is an excessive breakdown of hemoglobin, the plasma concentration of the unconjugated form of bilirubin rises. This increase can be detected by the diazo test only if the plasma is pretreated with alcohol. This test is called the indirect van den Bergh reaction.

5. The structure of the gallbladder is fully described on page 488. The function of the gallbladder is to store bile, concentrate it, and discharge it into the duodenum when appropriately stimulated by the entrance of fatty foods into the duodenum.

The ability of the gallbladder to concentrate bile can be used radiologically to display the gallbladder. An orally administered or injected iodine-containing compound is excreted by the liver and, when concentrated in the gallbladder, becomes radiopaque (see p. 499).

The mucous membrane of the neck of the gallbladder contains a number of mucus-secreting tubulo-alveolar glands. They are the source of the mucus in a mucocele of the gallbladder.

6. Bile salts aid digestion by emulsifying fat in the intestine and assisting in the absorption of fatty acids, monoglycerides, and lipids. Bile salts are produced by the hepatocytes. About 94 percent of the bile salts is reabsorbed from the intestine and reexcreted by the hepatocytes.

Insufficient concentrations of bile salts in the bile are a leading causative factor in the development of gallstones (see p. 499).

Obese women who have had many children show a high incidence of gallstones. Excessive fat and pregnancy are related to excessive excretion of cholesterol in the bile, which predisposes to gallstones. The symptoms commonly make their appearance in middle age.

7. The mechanisms controlling the delivery of bile to the duodenum are described on page 490. Cholecystokinin is a hormone produced by the argentaffin cells of the mucous membrane of the duodenum. It enters the blood in response to the presence of fatty foods in the duodenum. The hormone causes the gallbladder to contract.

8. The exocrine portion of the pancreas is a compound acinar gland that produces about 1,200 ml of

secretion in 24 hours. The enzymes present in the alkaline secretion are trypsinogen, chymotrypsinogen, procarboxypolypeptidase, lipase, cholesterol esterase, and amylase.

The endocrine portions of the pancreas are the islets of Langerhans, whose structure and microscopic appearance are described on page 493. The hormones insulin, glucagon, and somatostatin are produced by the islets.

The pancreas can be distinguished easily from the parotid salivary gland by the following features: (a) The pancreas possesses islets of Langerhans, which are small groups of pale-staining cells. (b) The pancreas has only a thin connective tissue capsule and septa, which loosely divide the gland into lobules, whereas the parotid gland has a thick fibrous capsule.

9. The structure of the islets of Langerhans is described in detail on page 493. The beta cells show a loss of cytoplasmic granules in diabetes mellitus.

Reflux of bile from the common bile duct or duodenal reflux through the sphincter of Oddi can activate trypsinogen into trypsin. A heavy meal, the consumption of alcohol, or the impaction of a gallstone in the ampulla of Vater can precipitate the condition. Normally, trypsinogen is activated in the duodenal lumen by the enzyme enterokinase.

CHAPTER 13

1. This patient has acute glomerulonephritis. The throat swab taken 2 weeks previously revealed a group A β-hemolytic streptococcal infection, which commonly precedes the development of acute nephritis. The initial edema of the eyelids probably was caused by retention of sodium and water in the blood stemming from blockage of the glomerular filtration barrier with antibody-antigen precipitate (see p. 530). Later, large amounts of protein and red cells escaped into the Bowman's capsule, reducing the plasma protein colloid level of the plasma and allowing additional water to escape into the tissues. Hemolysis of the red cells in the urine and liberation of hemoglobin gave the urine the smoky-brown or even red appearance. Examination of the urine revealed a sediment of red cells (red cell casts) and severe proteinuria. The low back pain was caused by swelling of the kidney substance within the fibrous capsule.

2. (a) A glomerulus is a network of capillaries that indents the Bowman's capsule. It has an afferent and an efferent arteriole. For its function, see page 511. (b) A medullary ray is a striation extending into the renal cortex from the base of a renal pyramid. It is formed by continuations of groups of tubules extending into the cortex from the medulla. For its function, see pages 516 through 519. (c) A renal papilla is the apex of the renal pyramid, which projects into a minor calyx. For its function, see page 519. (d) A nephron consists of four distinct parts: the renal corpuscle, the proximal convoluted tubule, the loop of Henle, and the distal convoluted tubule. They form a continuous tubule. For their functions, see pages 511, 516, 517, and 519. (e) Podocytes are star-shaped cells that cover the outer surface of the glomerulus. For their function, see page 511. (f) A mesangial cell is star-shaped, contractile, and capable of phagocytosis. It lies between the glomerular capillaries and supports them. For its function, see page 509.

3. In patients with myocardial infarction, thrombosis commonly occurs on the inner surface of the heart wall. Sometimes, small thrombi become detached from the wall of the left ventricle and enter the circulation as emboli. Many of these emboli go to the kidney, producing a renal infarction. The renal circulation is always vulnerable because the branches of the renal artery are end arteries and do not anastomose with their neighbors.

A renal infarct signifies the death of an area of kidney supplied by an end artery that has become blocked. Blockage of a segmental or interlobar artery will result in the death of a triangular area of kidney, which becomes white in color. The edge of the surrounding kidney is congested because blood vessels in that area vasodilate in response to the death of the neighboring kidney tissue.

4. (a) A slit pore measures about 25 nm across and is the gap between adjacent foot processes of podo-

cytes. Extending across a slit pore is a thin sheet about 6 nm thick called a slit diaphragm. (b) A filtration barrier in the kidney is a collection of structures that separate the blood in the glomerular capillaries from the cavity of the Bowman's capsule. These structures are: fenestrated endothelial cells of the capillaries, a thick basement membrane, the slit pores of the podocytes, and the slit diaphragms. (c) The juxtaglomerular apparatus consists of the juxtaglomerular cells of the afferent (and, to a small extent, the efferent) arterioles and the macula densa of the distal convoluted tubules (see p. 523). (d) The macula densa is part of the juxtaglomerular apparatus (see p. 523).

5. The countercurrent multiplier and countercurrent exchanger are fully described on pages 517 and 524. These mechanisms play a very important part in the physiological functioning of the renal medulla. The mechanisms keep the tissue fluid around the collecting tubules hypertonic and thus permit the reabsorption of water in the collecting tubules, allowing the formation of a concentrated urine.

6. The kidney produces two important hormones, renin and erythropoietin. Renin is an enzyme in the juxtaglomerular cells that can raise the arterial blood pressure. For details, see page 523. Erythropoietin is a glycoprotein that stimulates the bone marrow to increase red blood cell formation. For details, see page 161.

7. The normal specific gravity of urine is about 1.002 to 1.04. As renal function fails, this range diminishes, resulting in a specific gravity of about 1.01. The kidneys, thus, are unable to respond to varying fluid intake and to the needs of the body. Albumin is the plasma protein that escapes through the filtration barrier in glomerulonephritis. This is not surprising, because it is the plasma protein with the smallest molecular weight. When the glomerular filtration rate falls in severe chronic nephritis with renal failure, the end-products of nitrogen metabolism are retained within the blood and the blood urea and blood creatinine levels rise. Hypertension often accompanies renal failure and is caused by the renin-angiotensin mechanism described on page 523.

8. The structures of the proximal and distal convoluted tubules are fully described on pages 511 and 519. Note the following similarities and differences in their structures:

PROXIMAL CONVOLUTED TUBULE	DISTAL CONVOLUTED TUBULE
Cuboidal cells with numerous microvilli	Cuboidal cells with a few microvilli
Cleft between bases of microvilli	No clefts between microvilli
Plasma membrane on lateral surfaces and base much infolded	Plasma membrane on lateral surfaces and base much infolded
Numerous rodlike mitochondria in basal cytoplasm	A few rodlike mitochondria in basal cytoplasm
No macula densa	Macula dense is present

Note the following similarities and differences in their functions:

PROXIMAL CONVOLUTED TUBULE	DISTAL CONVOLUTED TUBULE
	Reabsorption
65 percent of glomerular filtrate is reabsorbed	*Straight Segment* Impermeable to water
Freely permeable to water and chloride ions	Active transport of chloride ions
Active transport of sodium, glucose, and small protein molecules and amino acids, calcium, potassium, phosphate, and vitamin C	Passive transport of sodium ions *Convoluted Segment* Permeable to water Possibly controlled by ADH Active transport of sodium and passive transport of chloride — controlled by aldosterone

	Secretion
Creatinine	Hydrogen, ammonium,
Dyes — Diodrast	and potassium ions
(iodopyracet)	
Drugs — penicillin	

9. This patient has diabetes insipidus caused by an insufficient production of ADH by the hypothalamus. The operation for the removal of the cerebral tumor has damaged the hypothalamus and thus interfered with the functioning of the hypothalamohypophyseal tract leading to the posterior pituitary. Because of the lack of ADH, the collecting tubules and, possibly, the convoluted part of the distal convoluted tubule are not absorbing water from the glomerular filtrate. The large volume of very dilute urine voided by this woman and the intense thirst that she experiences are the result.

10. In patients with severe vascular collapse following, for example, hemorrhage caused by a ruptured spleen, the blood flow through the kidneys is diminished and the pressure within the glomeruli is reduced. In severe cases, the pressure may be so low that the glomerular filtration rate into the Bowman's capsule is reduced. The output of urine will be reduced. The diminished blood flow through the renal tissue will stimulate the production of renin, which in turn will lead to the formation of angiotensin. The angiotensin will constrict the peripheral blood vessels. (A vicious cycle may be produced, because it also constricts the afferent arterioles to the glomeruli.)

A decrease in the glomerular blood pressure leads to a decrease in the blood pressure in the peritubular capillaries, thereby causing an increase in absorption of sodium, water, and urea. If the capillary blood pressure remains very low over a long period, tubular necrosis may occur.

The initial blood loss may lead to the release of greater amounts of ADH from the pituitary, increasing the absorption of water in the distal convoluted tubules and the collecting tubules. Later, with hemodilution caused by the absorption of water from the tissues back into the blood circulation, this effect is lost.

These effects indicate that the kidney participates with many other reflex mechanisms to restore blood pressure to normal and to provide an effective circulatory volume of blood.

11. Normal daily secretion volumes are: saliva, 1,200 ml; gastric secretion, 2,000 ml; pancreatic secretion, 1,200 ml; and bile, 700 ml. In addition, there is the secretion from Brunner's glands and the crypts of Lieberkühn. Total loss through the suction tube in this patient is therefore about 5,500 ml per day. Intravenous fluid intake per day at least would have to equal the sum of: (a) the volume of gastrointestinal suction; (b) the total urinary output; and (c) the water loss from sweat (100 ml) and lungs (350 ml) and insensible skin loss (350 ml).

12. The patient could be kept alive by dialysis treatment. The procedures of hemodialysis and peritoneal dialysis are described briefly on page 533.

13. Advanced cirrhosis of the liver causes obstruction of the normal circulation of portal venous blood through the liver. The resulting rise in venous pressure produces an excess of peritoneal fluid in the peritoneal cavity. In addition, the plasma colloidal osmotic pressure falls because of a reduction in the formation of plasma albumin in the liver. The different types of diuretics are described on page 532.

The ascitic fluid is an extracellular fluid and contains large amounts of sodium. The production of excess extracellular fluid can be limited somewhat by reducing the salt intake in the diet.

14. An intravenous pyelogram involves the injection of an iodine-containing compound into a subcutaneous arm vein. The compound is secreted by the cuboidal cells at the proximal convoluted tubule and concentrated in the collecting tubules. This renders the urine in the calyces and ureter opaque to x-rays. Eventually, the urinary bladder also becomes filled with radiopaque urine and is thus visualized. The visualization of the urinary tract on each side by this method demonstrates that the kidney is present and functioning. The degree of contrast obtained provides an estimate of the concentrating ability of the collecting tubules.

15. (a) The pain is caused by spasm of the smooth muscle in the wall of the pelvis and ureter as the muscle attempts to move the calculus down the urinary tract. (b) Afferent pain fibers enter the spinal cord in the first and second lumbar segments. The anterior rami of the first lumbar nerves are distributed to the skin in the lumbar region and groin. The painful region is thus extensive. (c) A calculus can be arrested at three sites: at the pelvi-ureteric junction, where the ureter crosses the pelvic brim, and where the ureter enters the bladder.

16. Afferent nerves passing from the bladder to the spinal cord travel in company with the parasympathetic and sympathetic fibers that innervate the bladder. They enter the cord at segments S2, S3, S4, L1, and L2. From these levels, the nerve impulses ascend within the cord to higher centers in the brain, where the stimuli of bladder distention are recognized consciously. (a) A transection of the spinal cord in the midthoracic region would deprive the patient permanently of this sensory information from the bladder. (b) After the patient recovers from spinal shock, his bladder will fill and empty reflexly, and he will have an automatic bladder.

17. The bladder wall has a mucous membrane, a muscle coat, and a fibrous coat. The mucous membrane is lined with transitional epithelium resting on a lamina propria of connective tissue. The muscle coat consists of three layers of smooth muscle fibers: an outer longitudinal layer; a middle circular layer; and an inner longitudinal layer. Near the neck of the bladder, the circular layer is thickened to form the sphincter vesicae. The fibrous coat is formed of loose connective tissue.

Papillomas arise from the transitional epithelium of the mucous membrane. They may be benign or malignant. The benign form is easily removed through an operating cystoscope, because it is attached only to the mucous membrane. Malignant papillomas can be treated by irradiation or removal of the bladder.

18. Cystitis is common in women. The shorter urethra in the female increases the likelihood of bacteria ascending from the vulva. The occurrence of urethral trauma during sexual intercourse also helps explain the high incidence of infection in the female. Numerous mucosal diverticula, with their accompanying mucous glands, provide locations for organisms to reside and cause a urethritis. The infection then may ascend easily to the bladder, causing a cystitis.

19. Inadequate treatment of gonorrhea, either by giving too small a dose of an antibiotic or by continuing the antibiotic for too short a time, often leads to chronic infection of the male urethra. The glands in the prostate, the bulbo-urethral glands, and the numerous small mucous glands of the urethra provide numerous locations for the organisms to lodge and proliferate. It is these organisms that perpetuate the infection and are likely to infect others during sexual intercourse.

20. In the male, the following types of epithelium line the urethra: in the prostatic urethra, transitional; in the membranous urethra, stratified or pseudostratified columnar; in the glans penis, stratified squamous epithelium.

In the female urethra, the lining epithelium is transitional above, pseudostratified columnar in the middle of its course, and stratified squamous at the lower end.

The sphincter urethra, which is situated in the urogenital diaphragm in both sexes, is composed of skeletal muscle.

CHAPTER 14

1. Many men in their eighties and nineties are capable of engaging in satisfactory sexual intercourse. Provided that they are physically fit, there should be no reason normal intercourse should not take place. Those who experience pain because of arthritis or some other disability are usually able, with the cooperation of a loving and understanding partner, to adopt a position that causes minimal discomfort. According to McCary (1967), about one-quarter of men become impotent by age 70. Some at this age believe, or are made to believe, that they are sexually impotent when in fact they are not. Recently,

inflatable intrapenile devices have been constructed that can be implanted by a urological surgeon in patients with genuine impotence and that will produce sexual satisfaction in both partners.

Aging of the testes is a gradual process, and, after age 45, spermatogenesis gradually decreases. The number of Sertoli cells remains unchanged, but fewer spermatogonia are evident. Nevertheless, abundant spermatozoa have been found in the testes of extremely old men, and many such men have fathered children successfully. With our present knowledge, the examination of a masturbation specimen of human semen cannot prove or disprove the fertilizing ability of the spermatozoa.

2. Mumps is a virus infection of the salivary glands, most commonly the parotid, and other tissues, notably the testes, pancreas, and central nervous system. Orchitis usually develops 1 to 2 weeks after salivary gland enlargement and is most common in postpubertal males.

The inflammatory edema within the testes results in pressure on the seminiferous tubules. The tough, fibrous tunica albuginea and the septa within the gland seriously restrict the swelling of the gland, so that the condition is extremely painful and is usually followed by some atrophy of the seminiferous tubules. Fortunately, the condition is commonly unilateral; even if it is bilateral, it is rarely followed by sterility.

3. The process of spermatogenesis is fully described on page 540. The primary spermatocytes divide by meiosis into smaller, secondary spermatocytes, each containing half the number of chromosomes of the primary cell (i.e., 23 instead of 46). Because of the meiotic division, the secondary spermatocyte receives half the chromosomes originally of maternal origin and half those originally of paternal orgin. By this means, the various genes of maternal and paternal origin are well mixed, and this mixing process benefits the human race.

4. The testes are richly innervated with nerve endings, especially ones sensitive to pressure. A blow to the testes causes a mass of impulses to ascend to the renal and aortic sympathetic plexuses. From here, nerve impulses enter the spinal cord at the level of the tenth and eleventh thoracic segments, where considerable neuronal spread occurs. Shock and collapse may follow, because sympathetic vasoconstrictor activity on the blood vessels is inhibited and there is a consequent fall in blood pressure. The general structure of the testes is described on page 539.

5. A Sertoli cell is somewhat columnar in shape. It is tall and extends from the basement membrane to the lumen of the tubule. It possesses an ovoid or indented nucleus, and the cytoplasm contains numerous organelles, including mitochondria, rough and smooth endoplasmic reticulum, a Golgi complex, granules, microfilaments, and microtubules. Adjacent Sertoli cells are held together by gap junctions and multiple tight junctions. The germ cells are closely related to the Sertoli cells and occupy deep recesses in the lateral and, later, the apical surfaces of the supporting cells. For details concerning the blood-testis barrier, see page 549.

The Sertoli cells have the following functions: (1) support, protection, and release of the spermatogenic cells, including their nourishment; (2) phagocytosis of the residual cytoplasm (residual bodies) derived from the spermatids; (3) secretion of fluid into the seminiferous tubules for the transport of spermatozoa; and (4) production of small quantities of estrogens. In addition, they produce the hormone *inhibin,* which inhibits the production of FSH. Because FSH stimulates spermatogenesis, the Sertoli cells provide a feedback mechanism for the control of spermatogenesis.

6. After a careful examination of the external genitalia, testes, and vasa deferentia and prostate (rectal examination), a seminal analysis should be made. A masturbation specimen of semen should be examined for volume, viscosity, sperm count, sperm motility, and sperm structure.

7. If a child's testes remain within the abdominal cavity or in the inguinal canal beyond the age of 5 years, irreversible degenerative changes take place

within the seminiferous tubules. If a testicle is not in the scrotum by the time of puberty, it will be incapable of producing spermatozoa thereafter. An intra-abdominal testis, however, is capable of producing testosterone from its interstitial cells. The temperature within the scrotum (2 to 3°C lower than the intra-abdominal temperature) is sufficiently low to allow normal spermatogenesis to take place. If a testis remains within the abdomen beyond the age of 30, testicular fibrosis may result in diminished testosterone production. Moreover, an undescended testis is very likely to undergo neoplastic change. For these reasons, both testes should be surgically placed in the scrotum in this patient.

8. The structure of the epididymis is described on page 552. The head of the epididymis is composed of several ductules held together by connective tissue, whereas the body and tail are made up of a single duct that is much coiled and held together by connective tissue. The functions of the epididymis are: (1) permit storage and maturation of spermatozoa, (2) reabsorption of water from the seminal fluid, (3) secretion of substances to nourish the spermatozoa, and (4) phagocytosis of fragmented spermatozoa.

The smooth muscle in the wall of the duct of the epididymis propels the sperm onward during ejaculation. Retrograde infection spreads from the urethra, bulbo-urethral glands, prostate, and seminal vesicles.

9. The operation of bilateral vasectomy is a simple procedure performed under local anesthesia. There is minimal postoperative pain, and there are no immediate aftereffects. Spermatozoa may be present in the first few postoperative ejaculations, but they represent simply an emptying process. There is no effect on testosterone production by the testes, and no adverse effect on the prostate or seminal vesicles. There is some evidence that as a result of the back pressure of accumulated spermatozoa in the testes and epididymes, spermatozoa extravasate into the interstitial tissue and enter the lymphatic and blood vessels. This condition could induce an immune response, with the development of serum antibodies against the sperm; there is no evidence that this does in fact occur.

Vasovasotomy, the procedure of joining the vas deferens to the epididymis, has been performed using microsurgical techniques and often has been followed by the return of spermatozoa to the ejaculate; in many cases, successful fertilization has resulted.

The vas deferens has a mucous membrane lined with columnar epithelium. Toward the distal end, the epithelium is pseudostratified and the columnar cells bear stereocilia. The muscular coat is very thick and consists of three layers of smooth muscle. The inner and outer layers are arranged longitudinally, and between them is a well-defined circular layer. There is an outer fibrous coat.

The vas deferens conducts mature spermatozoa from the epididymis to the ejaculatory duct by waves of peristalsis of the smooth muscle in its wall during ejaculation.

10. Enlargement of the median lobe of the prostate will cause it to encroach upon the sphincter vesicae at the neck of the bladder, permitting urine to leak into the prostatic urethra.

The structure of the prostate gland is fully described on page 558. The glands are tubulo-alveolar, and they are embedded in a stroma of smooth muscle and connective tissue.

The prostatic secretion contains citric acid and acid phosphatase and is alkaline in reaction. It provides additional fluid for the transport of spermatozoa and assists in neutralizing the acidity of the vaginal fluid, which inhibits the motility of the ejaculated spermatozoa. The prostate is controlled and maintained by the hormone testosterone.

Benign enlargement of the prostate is common in men over 50 years of age. The cause is unknown but is believed to be an imbalance between estrogen and testosterone. The condition is a hypertrophy and hyperplasia of the prostatic glands and their surrounding fibromuscular stroma. The nodules arise in the inner zone of the prostate, close to the urethra.

The cleavage line is caused by compression of the outer glandular tissue of the prostate by the enlarging nodules in the inner zone. The surgeon is able to insert a finger between these areas and thus enucleate the inner zone of the prostate when performing a suprapubic prostatectomy.

11. A carcinoma of the prostate arises from the columnar secretory cells of the tubulo-alveolae and is an adenocarcinoma. Excess acid phosphatase is produced in this disease, and the serum level rises as a consequence. The peripheral, or outer, zone of the prostate is the common site of origin of carcinoma.

Carcinoma of the prostate is androgen-dependent. The administration of estrogens, bilateral orchidectomy to remove the androgen secretion, or both can inhibit the growth of carcinoma of the prostate even in patients with multiple bone metastases. Such treatment causes the tumor to shrink, which reduces the bone pain, and it can greatly increase the length of survival. This treatment, however, will not cure carcinoma of the prostate.

12. The structure of the penis is described on page 561. Erection of the penis and ejaculation are described on page 561 and 563. Impotence is the inability to obtain an erection of the penis. Infertility is the inability to fertilize an ovum. The causes of infertility and impotence are described on pages 564 and 567.

CHAPTER 15

1. The terms *puberty, menarche, adolescence,* and *menopause* are fully described on page 618. Most girls are anovulatory for the first 12 to 18 months after menarche; the uterine bleeding during this phase results from estrogen stimulation and withdrawal. The uterus is incompletely matured at this time. A girl at this stage is thus usually infertile.

2. No blood-ovarian barrier has been determined to exist. This is surprising because the formation of the mature ovum takes place on the completion of the second meiotic division, which does not occur until after fertilization. The result is that many thousands of immature ova occupy the cortex of each ovary for the entire reproductive life of the female and during this time presumably are exposed to toxic substances that may be circulating in the blood. This may explain the higher incidence of trisomy 21 (Down's syndrome) in infants born to women over 35 years of age.

The reason for the ovary's descent into the pelvis is not known. It is possible that the ovary produces some hormonelike substance that enters the peritoneal cavity and influences the activity of the neighboring tube or its fimbriated opening. It is unnecessary for the ovaries to leave the peritoneal cavity, because oogenesis and hormone production can take place satisfactorily at the temperature of the abdominal cavity.

3. The process of ovulation is fully described on page 577. The hormonal control of ovulation is described on page 578. The clinical tests that might be used in the investigation of ovulation include (a) recording basal body temperature (p. 619), (b) endometrial biopsy (p. 619), (c) examination of cervical mucus (p. 619), (d) vaginal smear (p. 619), (e) plasma and urinary hormonal assay (p. 620), and (f) laparoscopy. Laparoscopy is an examination of the surface of the ovary through an illuminated instrument inserted into the peritoneal cavity through a small incision in the anterior abdominal wall.

4. The use of progesterone-containing pills as an ovulation-inhibiting agent has become an accepted method of controlling conception. It is described on page 623.

5. The normal monthly buildup of the endometrium is carefully controlled by the rise and fall of the plasma levels of estrogens and progesterone. A failure of this hormonal control can lead to excessive buildup of the endometrium, atrophy of the endometrium, or premature shedding of the endometrium. Many of these conditions are accompanied by irregular menstrual bleeding or bleeding between the menstrual periods.

6. The administration of pregnant-mare serum gonadotropins, which have large amounts of follicle-stimulating activity (FSH), followed by the administration of human chorionic gonadotropin isolated from pregnant women's urine and containing large

amounts of LH, has been successful in some cases of anovulation associated with secondary amenorrhea. A greater number of successes have occurred with the use of human pituitary gonadotropin extracts followed by human chorionic gonadotropin. Clomiphene citrate, a nonsteroid substance, also has been used with success. This substance is believed to act on the pituitary or the hypothalamus, causing the release of LH, which in turn stimulates ovulation and corpus luteum development.

The two complications that may follow these two types of therapy are cystic enlargement of the ovary and a greatly increased frequency of multiple births.

7. Normal implantation takes place in the endometrium of the body of the uterus, most frequently on the upper part of the posterior wall. Implantation of the blastocyst outside the uterine cavity is called an *ectopic pregnancy*.

The wall of the uterine tube is made up of three layers: a mucous membrane, a muscular coat, and a connective tissue coat. The mucous membrane is lined with three types of cells: ciliated columnar, nonciliated columnar secretory mucous cells, and intercalated cells. The muscle coat consists of circular inner and longitudinal outer layers of smooth muscle. The connective tissue coat is formed of areolar tissue. For further details, see page 580.

Implantation in the wall of the uterine tube is a serious condition. Because there is no decidua formation in the tube, the eroding action of the trophoblast quickly destroys the wall of the tube. Tubal abortion or rupture of the tube, with the effusion of a large quantity of blood into the peritoneal cavity, is the common result.

8. A detailed description of the structure of the endometrium at different times during the life of the female is given on the following pages: before puberty, page 590; after puberty, page 586; after the menopause, page 590. The hormonal control of the endometrium at these different times is given on pages 588 and 590.

9. The decidua is the name given to the endometrium of the pregnant uterus. As a result of the continued production of progesterone and estrogens by the enlarging corpus luteum, the endometrial stromal cells lying close to the trophoblast enlarge, become polyhedral, and become filled with glycogen and lipid material. The capillaries of the endometrium become congested and dilated, forming intercommunicating sinusoids. The enlarged stroma cells, or decidual cells, first occur in the immediate area of implantation, but they soon are found throughout the lining of the uterus.

Once the blastocyst becomes implanted in the decidua, the syncytial trophoblast starts to secrete the chorionic gonadotropic hormone. This causes the corpus luteum to increase further the output of estrogens and progesterone that are responsible for the maintenance of the decidua.

At the end of the fourth month of pregnancy, the corpus luteum starts to degenerate, and the production of estrogens and progesterone is taken over by the placenta.

10. The structure and functions of the placenta — respiration, nutrition, excretion, protection, and hormonal production — are described fully on pages 597 and 602.

The permeability of the placental membrane reaches its maximum during the thirty-sixth week and then rapidly declines during the last few weeks of pregnancy. This normal physiological change is accompanied by the deposition of fibrinoid material on the maternal surface of the chorionic villi, which tends to thicken the placental membrane. As the placenta undergoes these senile changes, it is still able to meet the fetal requirements during labor. Pre-eclampsia, hypertension, and diabetes may accelerate these senile changes. Placental infarction involving large areas of the placenta can interfere seriously with its function, and death of the fetus may follow.

11. The placenta secretes estrogens, progesterone, chorionic gonadotropin, and chorionic somatomammotropin. All these hormones are produced in the fetal part of the placenta in the syncytiotrophoblast. The functions of these hormones are described on page 603.

12. The placental barrier, or placental membrane, is the structure that separates the fetal blood in the villi from the maternal blood. In the mature placenta, it consists of (a) the very thin syncytiotrophoblast, (b) the mesenchymal stroma, and (c) the endothelial lining of the fetal capillaries. The total area of this barrier corresponds to about 14 square meters.

The placenta serves as a protective barrier against many infecting organisms and drugs. Bacteria are unable to cross the barrier unless the placenta itself becomes involved in the inflammatory process. *Treponema pallidum* (the spirochete of syphilis), tubercle bacilli, protozoa of malaria, and toxoplasmosis can reach the fetal circulation. Rubella virus can pass easily through the barrier and may cause many congenital anomalies if the mother is infected during the eighth to twelfth week. The Rh antigen can cross the placenta. Morphine, barbiturate drugs, and general anesthetics easily cross into the fetal circulation and depress the respiratory center of the fetus. Teratogenic drugs, such as thalidomide, can cross the placental membrane and produce numerous congenital defects.

13. Normally, the placenta is situated in the upper half of the uterus. Should implantation occur in the lower half of the body of the uterus, the condition is called placenta praevia. As the lower half of the body of the uterus dilates toward the end of pregnancy, the placenta is separated from the uterine wall and hemorrhage occurs. The bleeding is painless because the blood escapes through the cervix; the uterus does not contract and is not distended.

14. The cervix of the uterus has a wall composed of three layers: (a) the mucous membrane, (b) a muscular coat and (c) a connective tissue coat. The mucous membrane is lined with ciliated columnar epithelium. In the lower part, the cilia are absent; at the external os, the columnar cells give way to the stratified squamous epithelium that covers the outer surface of the vaginal part of the cervix. The glands of the lining of the cervix are large and branched and secrete a thick, alkaline mucus.

The muscular coat consists of interlacing fibers of smooth muscle mixed with connective tissue. The outer surface of the supravaginal part of the cervix is covered with loose connective tissue.

The majority of carcinomas of the cervix arise from the squamous epithelium near the squamocolumnar junction at the external os. The remainder arise from the columnar cells of the lining of the cervical canal or from the glands.

15. The vagina remains relatively free from infection during the reproductive period of life because of the acidity of the vaginal fluid, which inhibits the growth of pathogenic organisms. The wall of the vagina has three coats: the mucous membrane, the muscular coat, and the connective tissue coat. The mucous membrane is lined with stratified squamous nonkeratinized epithelium. During the reproductive period of life, ovarian estrogens stimulate the production of glycogen within the squamous cells. As the surface cells are desquamated, the glycogen is liberated and fermented by the Doderlein's bacilli, which convert it into lactic acid. By this means, the pH of the vaginal lumen is lowered.

During pregnancy, the lining epithelium becomes thicker in response to the outpouring of placental estrogens.

16. A "Pap smear" is a vaginal smear, the technique for which was described by Dr. George Papanicolaou. The patient should not have had a vaginal examination or a vaginal douche during the preceding 24 hours. A sample of vaginal fluid is sucked up into a glass pipette from the posterior fornix of the vagina. This sample is then smeared onto a glass slide, and the smear is fixed in alcohol to prevent cellular degeneration. The smear is then stained and the cells studied by a cytologist. This technique can be used to study abnormalities in the hormonal control of the epithelium lining the vagina and covering the outer surface of the vaginal portion of the cervix. The technique, however, is most commonly used annually for all women over 20 years of age in detecting the early stages of carcinoma of the cervix. Some gynecologists prefer to take the smear

directly from the cervix in the region of the external os, using a spatula. The cytological changes seen in a vaginal smear during a typical ovarian cycle are as follows: after menstruation, the smear shows few squamous cells but many histiocytes and neutrophils. At midcycle, numerous large squamous cells with pyknotic nuclei occur, because of the influence of the ovarian estrogens; the histiocytes and neutrophils are absent. During the second half of the cycle, the squamous cells are smaller and the nuclei less pyknotic, and neutrophils reappear in large numbers in response to ovarian progesterone. Once menstruation commences, the smear is contaminated with red blood cells and endometrial cells.

17. The greater vestibular glands are a pair of tubulo-alveolar mucus-secreting glands that lie under cover of the posterior parts of the bulb of the vestibule and the labia majora. The glandular cells are columnar. Each gland drains its secretion into the vestibule by a small duct that opens into the groove between the hymen and the posterior part of the labium minus. Infection of the gland leads to edema and swelling of the duct wall, with closure of its lumen. Later, fibrosis and contraction of the duct wall may lead to permanent closure of the duct. The accumulation of secretion leads to distention of the alveoli of the gland and the formation of a large cyst (Bartholin cyst).

18. The outer and inner surfaces of the labia minora are covered by a thin layer of stratified squamous nonkeratinized epithelium. The outer surface of the vaginal part of the cervix is also covered with stratified squamous nonkeratinized epithelium.

19. The structure of the mammary gland at different stages of life in the female has been fully described on the pages indicated: (a) before puberty, page 610; (b) in the adult resting stage, page 610; (c) during pregnancy, page 614; (d) during lactation, page 615; (e) after the menopause, page 617. The hormones responsible for each of these structural changes are described on pages 612, 615, 617, and 618.

20. Fibrocystic disease is believed to be caused by an imbalance between the ovarian estrogens and progesterone in their cyclic control of the mammary gland. Excess estrogen is thought to be the main cause of the connective tissue and glandular hyperplasia; similar changes can be produced by the injection of estrogens into animals.

21. Most carcinomas of the breast arise from the columnar cells lining the ducts of the gland; the remainder arise from the acini. As many of the carcinomas invade the breast tissue, there is an accompanying increase in the fibrous tissue stroma. This gives the tumor a feeling of hardness and tends to fix the tumor to the underlying muscle, the overlying skin, and the neighboring lactiferous ducts. As the fibrous tissue matures and contracts, it pulls on the skin, causing dimpling, and pulls on the lactiferous ducts, causing retraction of the nipple.

22. In the male, the mammary gland consists of fifteen to twenty ducts radiating from the nipple and embedded in connective tissue. The ducts do not extend beyond the margin of the areola. There are no glandular acini. The so-called witch's milk is a milky fluid that sometimes is expressed from the nipples of both sexes during the first week of life. It is caused by the crossing of the placental barrier by the maternal and placental hormones during pregnancy and the resulting stimulation and proliferation in the duct epithelium and the surrounding connective tissue. The condition resolves spontaneously as the maternal hormone levels in the child fall.

23. A mammary abscess should be drained through a radial incision to avoid spreading the infection into neighboring compartments. The compartments or lobes of the gland are separated from one another by fibrous septa that extend from the skin to the deep fascia covering the chest muscles. A radial incision also will minimize the damage to the radially arranged ducts.

24. Although the cause of carcinoma of the breast is not known, it is generally accepted that the repeated, cyclical hyperplasia and subsequent atrophy of the glandular tissue that occur in response to the

ovarian hormones estrogens and progesterone throughout the reproductive life of the female likely make the organ very susceptible to malignant change. It would follow that women who have late menarche, multiple pregnancies, or early menopause have a lower incidence of carcinoma of the breast, and such a low incidence has been observed.

CHAPTER 16

1. This patient has the signs and symptoms of gigantism and acromegaly caused by the excessive secretion of growth hormone by the acidophil cells of the anterior lobe of the pituitary gland. The condition started before the epiphyses of the long bones fused with the diaphysis, hence the gigantism, and continued after the fusion had taken place, hence the acromegalic changes.

2. The classification of the different parts of the pituitary gland is given on page 635. The hypothalamus is connected to the pars anterior of the gland by the hypothalamohypophyseal portal vessels, and to the posterior lobe by the hypothalamohypophyseal tract (see p. 635).

3. The pars anterior of the pituitary is made up of three main cell types, which may be distinguished from one another by the affinity of their cytoplasmic granules for different stains: acidophils, basophils, and chromophobes. The hormones produced by these cells are GH, prolactin, TSH, ACTH, and the gonadotropins (FSH and LH). The cells of origin and the functions of these hormones are described on pages 635 and 637 through 640.

4. The hypothalamus controls the activities of the master endocrine gland, the pituitary, by means of releasing and inhibitory hormones. The two hormones secreted by the posterior lobe are actually produced in the nerve cell bodies in the hypothalamus and descend in the nerve fibers of the hypothalamohypophyseal tract to be released into the bloodstream from the posterior lobe. A detailed description of the influence of the hypothalamus on the pituitary is given on page 635.

5. The head injuries associated with the automobile accident in this patient have damaged the hypothalamohypophyseal tract. Vasopressin, most often referred to as the antidiuretic hormone because antidiuresis is its main action, is produced in the nerve cell bodies in the supraoptic nucleus of the hypothalamus. The hormone is transported in combination with the carrier protein *neurophysin* down the axons in the hypothalamohypophyseal tract to the posterior lobe of the pituitary. The hormone accumulates and is stored in the nerve endings and is then released into the bloodstream. The hormone is released from the nerve endings when nerve impulses from the hypothalamus reach the endings.

ADH conserves body water by increasing the reabsorption of water from the collecting tubules of the kidneys (see p. 520). In patients with severe hemorrhage, this hormone also causes vasoconstriction of peripheral arterioles, hence the alternate name, vasopressin.

6. The microscopic structure of the pars intermedia of the pituitary gland is described on page 640. It is not known whether MSH in humans is produced by the cells of the pars intermedia or by the basophil cells of the pars anterior.

The ACTH produced by the basophil cells of the pars anterior of the pituitary gland, when present in excessive amounts, as in Addison's disease, is capable of stimulating epidermal melanocytes, causing darkening of the skin.

7. Oxytocin stimulates the smooth muscle of the uterus to contract. Normally, it plays an important role in labor and delivery. During the third stage of labor, when the placenta and the fetal membranes have been delivered, it stimulates the uterine muscle to contract and prevents excessive bleeding. In this patient the obstetrician was supplementing the patient's own oxytocin with synthetic hormone in order to increase the force of the uterine contractions.

Oxytocin is produced by the nerve cells in the hypothalamus. The hormone reaches the posterior lobe of the pituitary via the hypothalamohypophyseal tract, where it is stored and later released from the nerve endings.

8. The microscopic structure of the thyroid gland is fully described on page 644. The iodine in the diet is rapidly absorbed from the small intestine and carried in the blood as iodides. Part of the iodine is extracted from the blood and stored in the thyroid gland in organic form; the remainder is excreted by the kidneys in the urine. The formation of the hormones secreted by the thyroid gland is described on page 646.

The activity of the follicular cells of the thyroid gland is controlled by the thyroid-stimulating hormone of the pars anterior of the pituitary. In addition, norepinephrine released from the postganglionic sympathetic nerve endings increases the formation of cyclic AMP, an increase followed by an upsurge in the release of thyroid hormones.

The structural changes seen in the thyroid follicles when the gland increases or decreases its functional activity are described on page 645.

9. This patient has the signs and symptoms of hypothyroidism and myxedema. After confirming the diagnosis by estimating the PBI and serum T_4 levels, which are low in this disease, the doctor should prescribe daily doses of thyroid hormone, and this treatment should be continued indefinitely.

10. The hormones that enter the bloodstream from the thyroid gland are thyroxine (T_4) and triiodothyronine (T_3). The formation of these hormones is explained on page 646.

The weight loss may be explained as follows: The thyroid hormones increase the metabolic activity of most cells of the body, and the appetite of the individual increases also. The supply of food materials may be insufficient to satisfy the metabolic needs, however. In addition, overabundant thyroid hormones cause excessive protein breakdown.

Exophthalmos in hyperthyroidism is produced by an increase in bulk of the extraocular muscles and extraocular connective tissues. There is an increase in the water, mucopolysaccharide, and mucoprotein content of these tissues. The underlying cause of this lesion is not known. A possible explanation is that an exophthalmos-producing factor (EPF), autoimmune in origin, is responsible.

The different forms of treatment applicable to this patient are discussed briefly on page 676.

11. The parafollicular cells are situated singly or in small groups between the thyroid follicles. These cells are oval, and their cytoplasm contains numerous membrane-bound secretory granules. The parafollicular cells produce the hormone thyrocalcitonin, which lowers the level of blood calcium by inhibiting the breakdown of bone by the osteoclasts. The parafollicular cells are stimulated by hypercalcemia and suppressed by hypocalcemia.

12. This patient is manifesting the signs and symptoms of tetany caused by acute hypoparathyroidism secondary to her thyroidectomy. The cause of this condition is probably an interference with the blood supply to the parathyroid glands during the course of the operation. When tetany lasts only a few hours, the cause is possibly manipulation of the thyroid gland, with the excessive release of thyrocalcitonin into the circulation. For this reason, the surgeon usually handles the thyroid gland with care and removes only the anterior two-thirds of the gland, leaving the posterior third behind without disturbing the parathyroids.

In tetany, the level of serum calcium may fall to below 5 mg per 100 ml from the normal level of 10 mg per 100 ml. An estimate of the serum calcium level in this patient will confirm the diagnosis. The treatment is the repeated intravenous injection of calcium gluconate until the functioning of the parathyroid glands returns to normal. The parathyroid hormone should not be given, because the patient becomes resistant to it. Large doses of vitamin D are also given.

13. The chief cells of the parathyroid glands are responsible for producing the parathyroid hormone. This hormone stimulates the osteoclastic cells of bone and mobilizes the bone calcium, thus increasing the calcium level of the blood. The parathyroid hormone also increases the absorption of dietary calcium from the small intestine and the reabsorption of calcium in the proximal convoluted tubules of the kidney.

This patient was later found to have an adenoma of one of the parathyroid glands that was causing an excessive secretion of the hormone. The multiple renal stones resulted from the high levels of calcium excretion in the urine in such patients.

The normal microscopic structure of the parathyroid gland is described on page 648. Until puberty, only the chief, or principal, cells are present. At puberty, the oxyphil cells appear, but they remain in the minority throughout life. The chief cells produce the parathyroid hormone; the functional significance of the oxyphil cells is not known. In the young, the gland is packed with epithelial cells. In the adult, adipose tissue appears in the connective tissue that separates the cells into columns. In the old, the adipose tissue diminishes.

14. The thymus and its function are fully described in Chapter 9. It is recognized as an endocrine organ because a hormone called thymosine is produced by the reticular cells and stimulates the T lymphocytes (see p. 343).

15. Addison's disease occurs as a result of the destruction of the suprarenal cortex by tuberculosis or idiopathic atrophy; it may also occur secondary to a failure of elaboration of ACTH from the pars anterior of the pituitary, which results in atrophy of the suprarenal cortex. Cortisol and aldosterone are the two hormones that are lacking in this disease. The weakness is caused by the absence of cortisol secretion, which causes a fall in the level of blood glucose. The increased melanin pigmentation in the skin and buccal mucous membrane is caused by the increased secretion of ACTH from the pars anterior of the pituitary. (The increased pigmentation does not occur in patients in whom the disease is caused by hypopituitarism.) The ACTH stimulates the melanocytes to increase their production of melanin.

The microscopic structure and function of the different cells forming the suprarenal cortex are fully described on page 651.

16. The suprarenal medulla is composed of groups of epithelial cells supported by a delicate connective tissue that is richly supplied by blood sinusoids. The epithelial cells contain cytoplasmic granules. The electron microscopic appearance of these cells is described on page 657. The epithelial cells synthesize and secrete norepinephrine and epinephrine, and their actions are described on page 657.

The suprarenal medulla receives a double blood supply, one from the cortex and a direct one from the capsular arteries. The cortical blood is rich in glucocorticoids, which are necessary for the synthesis of an enzyme needed for the formation of epinephrine and norepinephrine in the medullary cells. It has been suggested that the activity of the medullary cells could be modified by altering the relative amounts of blood reaching the medulla from the two sources.

17. The normal fasting blood glucose level is about 110 mg per 100 ml. The object of the glucose tolerance test is to measure the ability of the patient's insulin to return the blood glucose to a normal level after the ingestion of a given amount of glucose. Once the blood glucose level in diabetes reaches a certain threshold value, approximately 180 mg per 100 ml, the glucose spills out into the urine. The exact cause of diabetes mellitus is not known (see the discussion on p. 680). In this disease, the beta cells of the islets of Langerhans lose their ability to secrete insulin, or the target cells of the tissues become insensitive to circulating insulin.

18. A histological section of the pancreas is composed largely of the exocrine portions of the gland. These portions consist of many acini whose cells contain numerous acidophilic zymogen granules situated in the apical parts of the cells. The basal parts of the cells are basophilic because of the numerous elongated mitochondria. The spherical nucleus in each cell is situated toward the cell base. Between the acini is delicate connective tissue, blood and lymphatic vessels, nerves, and ducts.

The endocrine portions of the gland are easily recognized as large pale areas among the darker-staining secretory acini. Each pale area consists of irregular clusters of cells known as the islets of Langerhans. The electron microscopic appearances and the functions of the cells of the islets are described on page 662.

19. Why a malignant tumor starts to produce a hormone or a hormonelike substance inappropriate to the tissue that has given rise to the tumor is not known. The condition may cause considerable confusion, especially if the tumor is small and has not been detected.

20. (a) Polyuria, or excessive urination, is caused by the high concentration of glucose in the urine, which inhibits the reabsorption of water in the kidney tubules. (b) Ketosis is a condition in which there is an excess of acetoacetic acid, β-hydroxybutyric acid, and acetone in the blood. It is caused by the excessive breakdown of fat by the liver cells in order to supply energy in the absence of available glucose (see p. 681). (c) Loss of weight is caused by the reduced synthesis and increased breakdown of protein, the breakdown of fat, and the loss of glucose in the urine and the lack of utilization of glucose by the body cells. (d) The main action of insulin is to bring about the rapid absorption, storage, and use of glucose in the body. Insulin reduces the level of circulating blood glucose after a meal by stimulating the uptake and storage of glucose in liver cells and the formation of liver glycogen (see p. 662). (e) The importance of the diet in the treatment of diabetes mellitus is discussed on page 682.

21. (a) The moon-shaped face is caused by the increased deposition of fat in the adipose tissue of the face as a result of stimulation by increased concentrations of cortisol in the blood. (b) The hirsutism is caused by excess cortisol and androgens produced by the suprarenal cortex. (c) The hyperglycemia is caused by the increased formation of glucose from protein. (d) Cortisol is excreted by the kidneys as 17-hydroxycorticosteroids, and this fact provides a useful method of determining whether the production of cortisol by the suprarenal is above normal, as it is in Cushing's disease.

22. Because the testes were removed after puberty, many of the accessory sex organs of this patient will atrophy and the secondary sexual characteristics will regress. For details, see pages 667 and 682.

Testosterone is produced by groups of rounded interstitial cells (Leydig cells) embedded in loose connective tissue between the seminiferous tubules. The cells are large and polyhedral, with a poorly staining cytoplasm.

The interstitial cells are stimulated to produce testosterone by the LH of the pars anterior of the pituitary. The level of testosterone in the blood influences the production of gonadotropin-releasing hormone in the hypothalamus. This hormone stimulates the cells of the pars anterior of the pituitary to release the luteinizing hormone. In the fetus, the chorionic gonadotropic hormone secreted by the placenta stimulates the interstitial cells in the developing testes to produce testosterone (see p. 665).

Testosterone is produced continuously in individuals with undescended testes, because the cells are not as sensitive to heat as are the germinal epithelium of the seminiferous tubules.

23. The detailed structure of the theca interna and the corpus luteum is given on pages 576 and 577. The theca interna produces estrogens, and the corpus luteum produces progesterone and estrogens. The control of the secretion of estrogens and progesterone by the ovaries is described on page 671.

24. At the menopause, the structure of the ovaries shows considerable change. Some primordial follicles are usually present, but growing follicles are absent. The ovarian stroma becomes dense, and the tunica albuginea thickens. There are no corpora lutea. The structures responsible for the production of estrogens and progesterone have disappeared, and there is a decrease in the level of circulating estrogens and progesterone as well.

The menopause is the time when the menstrual periods cease. It usually occurs between the mid-forties and the early fifties. For a summary of the clinical signs and symptoms of the menopause, see page 682.

At the menopause, the few remaining follicles cease to be sensitive to stimulation by the gonadotropic hormones of the pars anterior of the pituitary, even though the blood levels of these hormones rise after the menopause. The hypothalamus-pituitary-ovary hormonal mechanism thus ceases to operate.

25. The placenta is an endocrine gland and produces the following hormones: estrogens, progesterone, chorionic gonadotropin, and chorionic somatomammotropin. These hormones are secreted by the syncytiotrophoblast in the fetal part of the placenta. The actions of these hormones are discussed on page 672.

A patient with a chorionepithelioma excretes large quantities of chorionic gonadotropin in the urine. This fact can be helpful in making the initial diagnosis. It can also be used to determine the success of treatment.

CHAPTER 17

1. Tension lines and flexure lines are normal skin markings found on the skin on the anterior surface of the wrist. Tension lines are fine, shallow grooves that join one another at angles and enclose small, polygon-shaped areas. They are produced by the pull of the attachment of the collagen fibers in the dermis.

Flexure lines are related to the underlying proximal edge of the flexor retinaculum and the wrist joint. Here, again, the collagen fibers of the dermis are responsible and bind the dermis to the flexor retinaculum and the deep fascia. This arrangement permits the wrist joint to perform the movements of flexion and extension while the skin is held in position.

2. The skin defends the body against invasion from pathogenic organisms in the following ways: (a) The keratinocytes of the multilayered epidermis interlock and provide a mechanical barrier against penetration. (b) On the surface of the epidermis, one finds the secretions of the sebaceous and sweat glands, which contain bacteriocidal agents. (c) Leukocytes and macrophages, found principally in the papillary layer of the dermis, form a second line of defense, should the organisms penetrate the epidermis. (d) The dermis has a rich supply of blood vessels that can quickly bring more leukocytes and antibodies to the area of invasion.

3. A partial-thickness skin burn will heal from the cells of the hair follicles, sebaceous glands, and sweat glands, as well as from the cells at the edge of the burn. A full-thickness skin burn extends deeper than the sweat glands and will heal very slowly from the edges of the burn only, and there will be considerable contracture caused by fibrous tissue. To speed healing and reduce the incidence of contracture, a deep burn should be grafted.

A burn sterilizes the skin for about 24 hours. Thereafter, pathogenic bacteria residing on the neighboring skin quickly invade the burned area.

Massive vasodilatation of dermal blood vessels occurs in the burned skin area and surrounding tissues, accompanied by a great loss of fluid and plasma proteins into the tissues. With large burns, the combination of vasodilatation and the consequent loss of peripheral resistance with the loss of large volumes of protein-rich fluid will lead to cardiovascular shock unless corrective measures are instituted.

4. There are two types of skin, thick skin and thin skin. These terms refer to the thickness of the epidermis and not to the whole skin. Thick skin covers the palms and soles; the remainder of the body is covered with thin skin.

The dermis varies greatly in thickness in different parts of the body, tending to be thinner on the anterior than the posterior surface. It is thinner in women than in men.

5. The process of keratinization is fully described on page 691. It takes about 28 days for a new keratinocyte to reach the surface of the epidermis from the stratum germinativum. It is important to explain this fact to a patient, so that he or she will understand that visible improvement in a skin condition cannot be expected for at least 28 days.

6. The epidermis of thick skin consists of five layers: the stratum germinativum, the stratum spinosum, the stratum granulosum, the stratum lucidum, and the stratum corneum. The microscopic and func-

tional significance of each of these layers is described on pages 700 through 704.

7. The fine structure of an epidermal melanocyte is fully described on page 700. Note (a) the premelanosomes and melanosomes in the cytoplasm, (b) the multiple branching processes of the cells, and (c) that the cells lie between keratinocytes in the stratum germinativum and are not attached by desmosomes or hemidesmosomes to surrounding cells or the basal lamina.

8. Skin color is determined by three major pigments: melanin, hemoglobin, and carotenoids (see p. 707).

Melanocytes are present in the dermis in hair follicles, where they produce the hair pigment. In young children, melanocytes are present in the dermis of the sacral region. Because of the light-scattering effect of the overlying epidermis, the melanin has a bluish color. Collections of these melanocytes in this area form what are called Mongolian spots. Unlike epidermal melanocytes, these melanocytes retain the melanin.

Melanophages are histiocytes found in the dermis below heavily pigmented epidermal areas, such as the areola of the breast. Melanin granules in these areas escape into the dermis and are phagocytosed by the histiocytes.

9. A Langerhans cell is a dendritic cell situated in the suprabasal levels of the epidermis. It cannot be identified in ordinary skin sections stained with H&E. Langerhans cells can be demonstrated in sections treated with an acid solution of gold chloride or with supravital stains. Electron microscopic examination shows them to contain the characteristic tennis racquet–shaped organelles and to possess a greatly indented nucleus. Langerhans cells contain hydrolytic enzymes and are thought to be phagocytic. The cells are not related to melanocytes.

10. Basal cell carcinoma arises from keratinocytes of the stratum germinativum (see p. 722). Squamous cell carcinoma also arises from keratinocytes of the stratum germinativum (see p. 722). Malignant melanoma arises from melanocytes of the stratum germinativum (see p. 724).

11. The structure of a hair follicle is fully described on page 708. Hairs grow in cycles. Growing hairs are in the anagen phase; this stage is followed by a short phase of involution called the catagen phase; a resting phase, called the telogen phase, follows. The pigment responsible for hair color is produced by the melanocytes in the hair bulb. The different pigments are the brown-black melanin and the yellow phaeomelanin.

In a middle-aged person who is going bald, there is a progressive atrophy of the hair follicles. The coarse terminal hairs are replaced by fine vellus hairs. The pathogenesis is related not only to age but also to genetic factors and the presence of androgenic hormones.

12. For a detailed account of the structure of the glands indicated, see the following pages: (a) sebaceous gland, page 714, (b) eccrine sweat gland, page 717, (c) apocrine sweat gland, page 717. Sebaceous glands are not under nervous control but are stimulated by hormones, especially androgens. Contraction of the arrector pili muscle assists in the emptying of the sebaceous gland of its secretion. Eccrine sweat glands are controlled by postganglionic cholinergic sympathetic nerve fibers. Apocrine sweat glands are controlled by the sex hormones and by postganglionic adrenergic sympathetic fibers.

13. (a) The proximal nail fold is a fold of skin covering the root or proximal part of the nail. (b) The eponychium is a short extension of the stratum corneum of the nail fold distally over the body of the nail. (c) The nail bed is the skin beneath the body of the nail and consists of the stratum germinativum. (d) The nail body is the exposed part of the nail plate.

14. The age changes that take place in the skin are described on page 719.

The term *striae gravidarum* refers to the appearance in some women of white streaks on the skin of the anterior abdominal wall during the later months of pregnancy. The condition is produced by the excessive stretching of the skin by the enlarging uterus, which causes rupturing of the collagen fibers in the reticular layer of the dermis. Unfortunately, the resulting scars are visible through the epidermis and are permanent.

15. The dermal blood vessels are arranged in two plexuses, one at the junction of the dermis and the superficial fascia and the other at the junction of the reticular and papillary layers of the dermis. From the latter plexus, capillary loops ascend into the dermal papillae. Dilatation of these capillary loops allows the blood to circulate near the body surface and thus facilitates the loss of heat from the body by conduction, convection, and radiation. Constriction of these blood vessels has the opposite effect and results in the conservation of body heat. Arteriovenous communications also assist in this process. The degree of dilatation of the vessels is controlled by vasoconstrictor postganglionic sympathetic fibers, which in turn are activated by the heat-regulating center of the hypothalamus.

The secretion of sweat by the eccrine sweat glands permits the body to lose heat through evaporation. The activity of these glands increases when the body temperature rises. The hypothalamus increases the rate of sweating via the postganglionic cholinergic sympathetic nerves that supply these glands.

16. Most sweat glands are eccrine glands and are innervated by postganglionic cholinergic sympathetic nerves. A minority of sweat glands, the apocrine sweat glands, are found in the axillae and in the genital and perianal regions. These glands are innervated by adrenergic postganglionic sympathetic nerve fibers.

17. Localized hypertrichosis occasionally occurs in response to repeated trauma to the skin. It is assumed that the trauma produces an inflammatory response, with vasodilatation and stimulation of the hair bulbs to increase their mitotic activity. In this patient, the repeated chewing of the skin on the dorsal surface of the finger has stimulated localized hair growth.

18. Acne vulgaris is caused by two basic factors: increased secretion of sebum and the blockage of the duct of the sebaceous gland. Increased activity of the sebaceous glands always occurs at puberty and is stimulated by hormones, especially androgens. The various changes that occur in the sebaceous gland in acne are described on page 725.

The inflammatory reaction may be treated satisfactorily by systemic antibiotic administration and the local topical application of steroids.

19. Apocrine sweat glands are located in the axillary skin. Their secretion is small in amount and is sterile and odorless when it reaches the skin surface. Surface bacteria, mainly staphylococci, quickly break down the fatty acids to produce a musty, acrid smell. Because apocrine sweat glands are controlled by sex hormones, they are inactive until puberty. Bromhidrosis, which is the production of excess odor from the skin, is treated satisfactorily by frequent washing of the axillary skin and the application of bactericidal agents, such as aluminum or zinc salts, to the area.

20. Ultraviolet light in excess is known to be a cause of basal cell carcinoma, squamous cell carcinoma, and malignant melanoma of the skin. White individuals living in the tropics are particularly susceptible to ultraviolet radiation.

Ultraviolet light has several effects: (a) It acts on 7-dehydrocholesterol in the keratinocytes to form vitamin D_3. (b) It increases the pigmentation of skin by first darkening the existing melanin and then causing dispersion of the melanin granules within the melanocytes in the epidermis. Ultraviolet radiation then increases tyrosinase activity within the melanocytes, resulting in the increased production of melanin. (c) It inhibits the mitotic activity of keratinocytes and is thus beneficial in the treatment of psoriasis.

CHAPTER 18

1. A sty is an acute infection of an eyelash follicle, its associated sebaceous gland, or a neighboring ciliary gland. The following types of glands are found in an eyelid: (1) Sebaceous glands (glands of Zeis) secrete sebum to oil the eyelashes and keep them supple.

(2) Ciliary glands (glands of Moll) are modified sweat glands whose function is unknown. (3) Tarsal glands (meibomian glands) are long, modified sebaceous glands that pour their oily secretion onto the margin of the eyelid. The oily secretion prevents the tears from overflowing the edges of the eyelids and, by floating on the tears, inhibits their evaporation and thus conserves a film of moisture over the cornea.

A meibomian cyst is a distended meibomian, or tarsal, gland whose duct is blocked secondary to infection. It is most clearly seen on the inner surface of the eyelid.

2. The main lacrimal gland is wrapped around the lateral edge of the aponeurosis of the levator palpebrae superioris. Small accessory lacrimal glands are present beneath the conjunctiva of the upper and lower eyelids. The lacrimal glands are tubulo-acinar glands. The acini are lined with columnar cells, and myoepithelial cells are present. The main gland opens into the superior fornix of the conjunctiva via approximately twelve ducts.

The tears keep the cornea and conjunctiva moist. They contain the enzyme lysozyme, which is bactericidal. Tears also trap small foreign bodies that enter the eye.

The circulation of tears across the cornea is accomplished by (1) the continuous production of tears by the lacrimal glands and (2) the continuous evaporation of the tear fluid from the lower end of the nasolacrimal duct in the nose, a process assisted by the pumping action of the orbicularis oculi muscle on the lacrimal sac during blinking.

3. Foreign bodies in the conjunctival sac tend to lodge in the subtarsal sulcus of the upper eyelid. The eyelid should be everted, and the foreign body wiped off with a piece of moist cotton. The structure of the conjunctiva is described on page 730. The conjunctiva is very prone to trauma and bacterial and viral infections.

4. The cornea is composed of five layers; moving backward, they are: (1) the epithelium, (2) Bowman's membrane, (3) the substantia propria, (4) Descemet's membrane, and (5) the endothelium. The structure of the cornea is described on page 736.

The cornea receives its nourishment from tissue fluid that diffuses in from peripheral blood vessels situated at the limbus and from the aqueous humor. It also receives oxygen directly from the atmosphere on its outer surface. Normally, there are no blood vessels in the cornea.

The cornea is very resistant to infection; it is sensitive, however, to the gonococcus, *Chlamydia trachomatis*, herpes simplex, and herpes zoster.

5. The aqueous humor is a secretion or transudate from the ciliary epithelium of the ciliary body. It enters the posterior chamber of the eye and then flows through the pupil into the anterior chamber and is drained away at the iridocorneal angle into the canal of Schlemm.

The normal intra-ocular pressure is about 12 to 20 mm Hg, and it is maintained by balancing the rate of production and the rate of drainage of the aqueous humor.

6. The optic nerves are surrounded by sheaths derived from the pia mater, arachnoid mater, and dura mater, and these sheaths fuse with the sclera at the back of the eyeball. There is an extension of the intracranial subarachnoid space forward around the optic nerve to the back of the eyeball. A rise in cerebrospinal fluid pressure caused by an intracranial tumor compresses the thin walls of the retinal vein as it crosses the extension of the subarachnoid space and produces congestion of the retinal vein. The raised cerebrospinal fluid pressure causes both optic discs to bulge forward into the eyeballs, a condition known as papilledema. Because the increased cerebrospinal fluid pressure affects both eyes, the patient exhibits bilateral papilledema.

7. With advancing age, the lens of the eye becomes denser and less elastic, and, as a result, the ability to accommodate is lessened (presbyopia). The lens is unable to assume a more globular shape during ac-

commodation because it has lost elasticity. This disability may be overcome by the use of an additional convex lens, in the form of eyeglasses or a contact lens, to assist the eye in focusing the image of an object, such as printed type, sharply on the retina.

The refracting media consist of the cornea, the aqueous humor, the lens, and the vitreous body; of these structures, the cornea is by far the most important. The histological structure of the cornea is described on page 736, and that of the vitreous body on page 751. The formation and circulation of the aqueous humor are described on page 747.

8. Accommodation is a process by which the eye can focus on near objects. Two changes occur in the eye: (1) The lens assumes a more globular shape as a result of the relaxation of the suspensory ligament. The ligament is relaxed by the contraction of the ciliary muscle, which pulls the ciliary body forward and inward. The ciliary muscle is innervated by parasympathetic postganglionic fibers derived from the oculomotor nerve. (2) The pupil constricts as a result of the contraction of the sphincter pupillae muscle. This constriction restricts the light entering the eye, so that only those light rays that pass through the central, thicker part of the lens will reach the retina. The sphincter pupillae muscle is innervated by the postganglionic parasympathetic fibers derived from the oculomotor nerve. These changes together permit the eye to focus the image of a near object on the retina.

9. (a) The fovea centralis is the central, depressed part of the macula lutea situated at the center of the posterior part of the retina. It is the area of most distinct vision. Here the nerve cells and fibers of the inner layers of the retina diverge, leaving the photoreceptors in the center. This arrangement permits the light to have greater access to the photoreceptors than elsewhere on the retina. In the floor of the fovea, there are no blood vessels or red cells but there are many cone cells. (b) The iris is described on page 739. (c) The ciliary body is described on page 738. (d) The ora serrata is the wavy, anterior edge of the nervous part of the retina. It forms a ring around the interior of the eyeball and is situated just posterior to the ciliary body.

10. The retina is developed in the embryo from the outer and inner walls of the optic cup. The outer wall forms the retinal pigment epithelium, and the inner wall forms the light-sensitive sensory retina. A potential space remains between these two layers, except at the optic nerve and the ora serrata. Retinal detachment occurs as a result of a hole forming in the inner sensory layer of the retina, permitting fluid to accumulate between the two layers and causing loss of function of the sensory layer of the retina.

Trauma applied to the eyeball, either directly or indirectly, or extreme nearsightedness may precipitate the condition. Nearsightedness (myopia) may cause the vitreous to pull on the retina secondary to the elongated shape of the eyeball. In this way, the nervous part of the retina is pulled away from the pigmented part of the retina. The lightning flashes seen by this patient are caused by the retina's being pulled upon by the vitreous body. The curtain seen by the patient is caused by the accumulation of fluid between the two layers of the retina.

11. The outer third of the external auditory meatus is lined with skin provided with hairs, sebaceous glands, and ceruminous glands. The ceruminous glands secrete a yellowish-brown wax called cerumen. The hairs and the wax provide a sticky barrier to insects and other foreign bodies that might enter the ear. The histological structure of ceruminous glands is described on pages 717 and also 754.

12. The tympanic membrane is normally pearly gray and is composed of two layers of fibrous tissue that are covered on the outer surface by skin (stratified squamous keratinized epithelium) and are lined on the inner surface with mucous membrane (low columnar epithelium) that may be ciliated in part. The pars flaccida and pars tensa are described on page 756.

13. The mechanisms involved in conducting sound waves from the external auditory meatus to the in-

ner ear are described in detail on page 758, in the discussion of movements of the ossicles.

14. The basilar membrane and the stria vascularis are described on page 763; the macula is described on page 761, the ampulla of a semicircular canal on pages 759 and 763, and the tectorial membrane on page 766.

15. The highly specialized hair cells of the organ of Corti in the duct of the cochlea are the sensory receptors for hearing. The arrangement of the organ of Corti and its relationship to the basilar membrane are fully explained on page 766. The short basilar fibers of the basilar membrane are situated near the base of the cochlea and resonate in response to sounds of high frequency. The long basilar fibers are located near the apex of the cochlea and resonate in response to low-frequency sounds. By this means, different groups of hair cells are able to respond to different sound frequencies, and they send nerve impulses to different parts of the cochlear nuclei and different neurons in the superior temporal gyrus of the cerebral cortex. As a result, the individual is able to distinguish sounds of different frequencies.

In this patient, the basal part of the cochlea showed evidence of degeneration as a result of the repeated reception of abnormally loud sounds of high frequency in the discotheque.

16. The stapes is formed of compact bone and is stirrup shaped. It articulates by means of a small head with the incus. The base, or foot, of the stapes is oval and is attached to the margin of the fenestra vestibuli (oval window) by a ring of fibrous tissue, the anular ligament. Rocking motions of the stapes transmit sound waves to the perilymph that is situated on the medial surface of the base of the stapes.

17. Endolymph is the fluid that fills the membranous labyrinth. It is therefore present within the utricle, the saccule, the three semicircular ducts, and the duct of the cochlea. Endolymph is believed to be formed by the stria vascularis.

The vestibular membrane forms one of the walls of the cochlear duct. It is composed of two layers of flattened epithelial cells separated by a basal lamina. The cells possess numerous microvilli and may be involved in fluid transport.

18. The auricle of the ear consists of a thin plate of elastic cartilage to which are attached intrinsic and extrinsic muscles composed of voluntary striped muscle. The auricle is covered by thin skin containing hairs, sebaceous glands, and sweat glands.

A cauliflower ear is seen commonly in boxers and wrestlers who during the course of their careers have received multiple traumatic injuries to the auricles. The injuries cause an effusion of blood under the perichondrium of the elastic cartilage. Although most of the blood is absorbed, some thickening remains. Repeated injuries lead to enlargement and deformity of the auricle.

19. The semicircular canals form part of the bony labyrinth of the inner ear and must be distinguished from the semicircular ducts, which lie within the canals and form part of the membranous labyrinth. There are three canals on each side of the head, known as superior (anterior), posterior and lateral canals. The canals are arranged at right angles to one another, so that all three planes are represented.

The detailed structure and function of the semicircular canals and semicircular ducts are described on pages 759, 763, and 767.

20. The spiral organ of Corti is described on page 766. The functional difference between the outer and inner hair cells is not fully understood. The inner hair cells, with their rich nerve supply, are believed to be the more important. The outer hair cells may be capable of inhibiting the inner hair cells during the process of fine tuning for a sound of a particular frequency.

21. The extent and structure of the olfactory mucous membrane are described on page 769. The olfactory nerve cells in the mucous membrane give rise to axons that become the olfactory nerve fibers. Tubulo-alveolar glands in the lamina propria of the

mucous membrane produce a watery mucus that keeps the surface of the mucous membrane moist and serves as a solvent for odiferous substances. This patient sustained a fracture of the cribriform plate of the ethmoid bone that irreversibly damaged the olfactory nerve fibers in their ascension from the olfactory mucous membrane to synapse on the mitral cells of the olfactory bulbs.

22. The structure of the taste bud is fully described on page 770. Taste buds are found in the mucous membrane of the mouth and pharynx but are concentrated on the dorsum of the tongue. The cells of a taste bud atrophy if the nerve supply is sectioned. On regeneration of the nerve fibers, the local epithelial cells differentiate to form taste bud cells, and new taste buds are formed.

INDEX

A bands of myofibrils, 197
Abscess, 190
  peritonsillar, 467
Accommodation, of eye, 749
Acetazolamide, 533
Acetylcholine
  and heart rate, 304
  as neurotransmitter, 210, 247
Acetylcholinesterase, 210, 247
Achalasia of esophagus, 468
Achlorhydria of stomach, 469
Achondroplasia, 76, 149
Acid
  carbonic, 394
  fatty, oxidation of, 487
  hydrochloric, 438, 441, 468
Acidophilic tissue components, 9
Acidophils, pituitary, 635
Acinus
  liver, 486
  mucous, of submandibular gland, 422
  serous
    of parotid gland, 422
    of submandibular gland, 422
Acne vulgaris, 725–726
Acromegaly, 673–674
ACTH, 639, 655
Actin, 52
  acitivity in anaphase, 34

Actin—*Continued*
  in cardiac muscle, 205
  interaction with myosin, 218
  in platelets, 175
  in skeletal muscle, 197
α-Actinin, 52
Actinomycin
  action on bacteria, 79
  action on virus DNA, 79
Acuity, visual, 772
Addison's disease, 679
Adenine, 37
Adenocarcinoma, 100
  of endometrium, 621
Adenohypophysis, 635–641
Adenoids, 467
Adenomas, 100
  chromophobe, pituitary, 673
Adenosine diphosphate (ADP), 42
Adenosine monophosphate, cyclic, 633
Adenosine triphosphate (ATP), 42
  and muscle contraction, 219
  and sodium-potassium pump, 62
Adenyl cyclase, 633
Adhesion, pleural, 401
Adipose tissue, 54, 109
  brown, 109
  in obesity, 148
Adolescence, 618, 626

Adrenal glands, 651–661. *See also*
  Suprarenal glands
Adrenocorticotropin, 639, 655
Adrenogenital syndrome, 76
Adventitia. *See* Tunica adventitia
Afterbirth, 605
Agglutination, erythrocyte, 179
Agglutinogens in red cells, 179–181
Aging
  arterial changes in, 327
  body structure and function in, 25–26
  of cells, 76
  and neuronal degeneration, 285
  of skin, 719–720
Agranulocytes, 161
  formation of, 170–171
Air
  alveolar, 392
  dead space, 392
  volume of, 392. *See also* Volume, of air
Ala, nasal, 365
Albinism, 76, 722–723
  ocular, 722
  oculocutaneous, 722
Aldolase, escape from muscle fibers, 221
Aldosterone, 519, 652, 653–655
Alimentary canal. *See* Digestive tract

Alkaline phosphatase, serum levels of, 498
All-or-none law, 300
Alopecia, 724–725
 areata, 725
Alveoli, pulmonary, 381
 air in lumen of, 392
 pressure in, 391–392
Ameloblasts, 419
Amenorrhea, 683
AMP, cyclic, 633
Amphotericin B, action on bacteria or fungi, 79
Ampulla
 of semicircular canals, 759
  crista of, 763
 of uterine tube, 580
 of vas deferens, 556
 of Vater, 488
Amylase
 in gastric secretions, 436, 441
 secretion in small intestine, 455
Anaphase, in mitosis, 34
Anaphylaxis, 147
Anastomoses, arteriovenous, 312–313
Anatomy
 gross, 21
 microscopic, 21
Androgens, 539, 552
Androstenedione, 552
Anemia, 184–185
 anoxia in, 406
 aplastic, 185
 hemolytic, 185
 hypochromic, 185
 macrocytic, 185
 megaloblastic, 185
 microcytic, 185
 normochromic, 184
 normocytic, 184
 pernicious, 185, 469
 sickle cell, 185
Anesthetics
 local, action on nerve conduction, 285
 and respiratory center depression, 404
Aneurysms, developmental, 327
Angina pectoris, 325
Angiotensin, 523, 653
Angle of palpebral fissure
 lateral, 729
 medial, 730
Anhidrosis, 726

Anosmia, 777
Anoxia, 405
 anemic, 406
 anoxic, 405–406
 histotoxic, 406
Antibodies, 14, 342, 349
 formation of, plasma cells in, 147
Anticoagulants, 184
Antidiuretic hormone, 520, 641
 absence of, 674
Antigens, 14
Antrum, pyloric, 432
Anus, 455, 463
Aorta, 307
 coarctation of, 327
Apatite, 137
Aponeurosis, 124, 195
Apparatus
 Golgi, 45–46
  in neurons, 233
 juxtaglomerular, 523–524
 lacrimal, 732–736
  clinical notes on, 772
Appendicitis, 471
Appendix, 458–460
 clinical notes on, 471
 mucocele of, 471
Arch, aortic, pressor receptors in, 323
Area, bare, of liver, 477
Areola of mammary gland, 610
Arrhythmias, 325–326
 sinus, 302
Arterioles, 291, 310
 glomerular
  afferent, 508, 522
  efferent, 508, 522–523
Arteriolosclerosis, 327
Arteriosclerosis, 327–328
 of coronary arteries, 324–325
Artery(ies), 291, 307–310
 age changes in, 327
 central
  of retina, 741
  of spleen, 351
 clinical notes on, 326–329
 congenital defects in, 327
 coronary, 323
 elastic or conducting, 307–308
 end
  anatomical, 313
  functional, 313
 of endometrium
  basal, 589
  spiral, 589

Artery(ies)—*Continued*
 muscular or distributing, 308–309
 nutrient, 132, 177
 periosteal, 132
 renal, 522
  arcuate, 522
  interlobar, 522
  interlobular, 522
  lobar, 522
  segmental, 522
 splenic, 351
Asbestosis, 404
Ascites, 498
Ascorbic acid. *See* Vitamin C
Asthma, 401, 404
Astrocytes, 248–250
 fibrous, 248
 function of, 252
 protoplasmic, 248–250
 reactions to injury, 286
Astrocytoma, 147, 186
Astrocytosis, 286
Atherosclerosis, 182, 327–328
 development of, 328
 smooth muscle fibers in, 222
ATP, 42
 and muscle contraction, 219
 and sodium-potassium pump, 62
Atria of heart, 291
Atrophy, 72–73
 of skeletal muscle, 220–221
Atropine, 286
Auricle
 of atrium, 291
 of ear, 754
  clinical notes on, 775
Autoradiography, 15–16
Autosomes, 41, 543, 578
Axolemma, 209, 243
Axons, 225, 243
 injuries to, changes in, 280–282
 regeneration of, 283–284
 terminals of, 243
Axoplasm, 243
 flow of, 243–245
Azodye methods for phosphatases, 14

Bacilli, Döderlein's, 606, 668
Bacteria, 78–79
 chemotherapy affecting, 79
 in colon, 460
Baldness, 724

Bands of Baillarger, 279
Bar, terminal, 70
Barrier
 blood-testis, 549
 filtration, of renal corpuscle, 509
 placental, 602
Basophilic tissue components, 9
Basophils, 161, 165
 formation of, 167
 pituitary, 635
Bed, nail, 707
Belly of muscle, 195
Benzoquinonium, 221
Bile, formation of, 486
Bilirubin, 54, 161, 486
 detection in blood, 498
 serum levels in jaundice, 499–500
Biopsy
 in cancer diagnosis, 75
 endometrial, 619
 of liver, 499
 of marrow, 187–188
Bladder, urinary, 526–528
 atonic, 535
 automatic reflex, 535
 autonomous, 535
 clinical notes on, 534–535
 parasympathetic outflow from, 535
 sympathetic outflow from, 535
Blastocyst, implantation of, 591
 abnormal, 623
Blepharitis, 771
Blindness
 circumferential, 773
 color, 775
 total, 773
Blocking agents
 neuromuscular, 221
 synaptic, 285–286
Blood, 155–176
 cells in, 155–171
  counts of, 184
  red, 155, 156–161
  white, 155, 161–171
 clinical notes on, 178–187
 clinical problems on, 190–191
 coagulation of, 171
 composition of, 155–176
 filtration in liver, 488
 gaseous transport in, 394–397
 hematocrit of, 156
 oxygen capacity of, 158
 plasma, 175–176

Blood—*Continued*
 platelets in, 171–175
 pressure of, 316–321
 transfusions of, 178–182
 typing of, 179–182
 volume of, 155
Blood groups, 179–181
 O-A-B, 179–180
 Rh-HR, 180–181
Blood vessels, 307–323
 arteries, 291, 307–310
 arterioles, 310
 capillaries, 310
 control of, 321–323
 hypothalamohypophyseal portal, 635
 of lymph nodes, 347
 renal, 522, 529–530
 of spleen, 351
 suprarenal, 661
 umbilical, 597
 veins, 311–312
 venules, 310–311
Body(ies)
 aortic, 314
  chemoreceptors in, 399
  reflexes in, 323
 basal, 30, 52, 66, 231
 carotid, 314
  chemoreceptors in, 399
  reflexes in, 323
 ciliary, 738–739
 of clitoris, 608
 of epididymis, 554
 foreign
  and giant cell formation, 116
  inhalation of, 401
 of gallbladder, 489
 ketone, 664
 multivesicular, 48
 of nail, 707
 of pancreas, 490, 661
 of penis, 561
 polar
  first, 577
  second, 577
 residual
  enzymes in, 47
  in spermatogenesis, 542
 of spermatozoon, 544
 of stomach, 432
  glands of, 436
 of uterus, 584
 vitreous, 751–752

Boils, 721
Bone, 129–145
 cancellous, 131–132, 137
 classification of, 132
 clinical notes on, 149
 compact, 130–131, 137
 estrogens affecting, 670
 examination of, 134–135
 formation of, 135–141
 fracture repair in, 146
 joints of, 141–145
 macroscopic structure of, 131–132
 marrow in, 131, 132–134, 176–178
 spongy, 131–132, 137
 types of, 130–131
Boutons terminaux, 243
Bradycardia, 302
Breast, 610–618. *See also* Mammary glands
Breathing. *See* Respiration
Bridge, of nose, 365
Bromhidrosis, 726
Bromsulphathalein excretion test, 499
Bronchi, 373, 379
 clinical notes on, 401
 constriction in asthma, 401, 404
Bronchioles, 379
 respiratory, 379, 381
 terminal, 379
Bronchoscopy, 401
Buds, taste, 417, 770–771
Bulb
 hair, 708
 of penis, 561
Bundle, atrioventricular, of His, 206, 296, 325
Burns, 721
Bursae, 143–145, 147
 prepatellar, 145
 suprapatellar, 145

Caffeine
 as diuretic, 532
 and respiratory center stimulation, 405
Callus, 146
Caloric tests of vestibular function, 776
Calyces
 renal, 503
 of ureter, 525

Canal
  anal, 463
  central, of spinal cord, 272
  cervical, 586
  haversian, 131
  of Hering, 483
  hyaloid, 751
  nutrient, 132
  portal, 479
  pyloric, 432
  root, of teeth, 417
  of Schlemm, 746
  semicircular, 759
  Volkmann, 131
Canaliculi
  bile, 481, 483
  in bone, 130
  lacrimalis, 730
Cancer. *See* Tumors
Cap, acrosomal, 542
Capacitation, 548
Capacity, vital, 392, 402
Capillaries, 291, 310, 330
  glomerular, 508–509
  increased pressure in, 360
  lymphatic, 333–335
    lacteal, 336
    pump in, 339
Capsule
  bacterial, 79
  Bowman's, 504, 508–509
  fibrous, of kidney, 503
  Glisson's, 477, 484
  of joints, 143
  of lens, 748
  of organs, 124
  of spleen, 349
  of tonsil, 357
Carbohydrates
  fate in digestion, 497
  metabolism of
    glucocorticoids affecting, 655
    insulin affecting, 662–664
    in liver, 486
  in plasma membrane, 55
Carbon, phagocytosis by macrophages, 54
Carbon dioxide
  and blood flow to tissue, 323
  dissociation curve, 397
  exchange in lungs, 392–394
  exchange in tissues, 397
  and heart rate, 304
  transport in blood, 394–397

Carbon monoxide, poisoning from, 405
Carbonic anhydrase, 394
  in red cell cytoplasm, 157
Carboxyhemoglobin, 405
Carboxypolypeptidase, 496
Carbuncle, 721
Carcinoma, 100
  basal cell, 722
  of breast
    in females, 625–626
    in males, 624
  of cervix uteri, 622
  embryonal, of testis, 565
  of endometrium, 621
  of gallbladder, 499
  in situ, 75
  of pancreas, 500
  of prostate, 567
  squamous cell, 722
  of stomach, 469
Cardiovascular system, 23, 291–331
  blood vessels, 307–323
  circulation, 323–324
  clinical notes on, 324–329
  clinical problems on, 329–331
  heart, 291–307
Caries, dental, 466
Carotene, 65
Carotenoids, 707
Carriers, in cell membranes, 60
Cartilage, 124–129
  arytenoid, 370
  cricoid, 370
  development and growth of, 127–129
  elastic, 127
  fibrous, 127
    in joints, 143
  hyaline, 127
    in joints, 143
  thyroid, 370
Caruncula lacrimalis, 730
Cataract, 775
  congenital, 76
Catecholamines, 657–661
  actions of, 657–659
  as neurotransmitters, 247
  regulation of secretion, 661
Cavity
  marrow, 131, 138
  mouth, 409
  nasal, 365
  pericardial, 294

Cavity—*Continued*
  pleural, 375
    pressure in, 392
  pulp, of tooth, 417
  thoracic, diameters of, 384–386
  tympanic, 755–758
    clinical notes on, 776
  of uterine body, 584
Cecum, 456–463
  function of, 460
Celiac disease, 470, 472
Cells, 21–22, 29–82
  acidophils, pituitary, 635
  aging of, 76
  alpha, of pancreas, 494, 662
  amacrine, of retina, 746
  argentaffin
    in small intestine, 447
    in stomach, 438
  atrophy of, 72–73
  basal
    in duct of epididymis, 554
    in olfactory mucous membrane, 770
    in taste buds, 771
  basement membrane of, 71–72
  basket, 274
  basophil, pituitary, 635
  beta, of pancreas, 493, 662
  Betz, 276
  bipolar, of retina, 745–746
  blood
    counts of, 184
    red, 155, 156–161
    white, 155, 161–171
  cancer, 74–75
  capsular, of ganglia, 262, 264
  centrioles in, 51–52
  chief
    parathyroid, 648
    of stomach, 436
  chromaffin, suprarenal, 657
  chromophobe, pituitary, 635
  clinical notes on, 72–80
  clinical problems on, 80–82
  coat of, 57
  coated vesicles in, 48–49
  columnar
    absorptive, 88, 446
    ciliated, 88
    microvilli of, 88
    specialized, 88, 94
  cone, 745
  in connective tissue, 107–116

Cells—*Continued*
- cytoplasm in, 41–55
- decidual, 591
- delta, of pancreas, 494, 662
- in disease, 26, 72
- division of, 34–35
  - meiotic, 34
  - mitotic, 34
- drugs affecting, 80
- dysplasia of, 74
- endoplasmic reticulum of
  - rough, 43–44
  - smooth, 44–45
- enteroendocrine, 438
- in epidermis, 691–698
- epithelial, 85–104
- eukaryotic, 78
- evolution of, 72
- fat, 108–109, 148–149
- follicular, thyroid, 644, 645
- fusiform, cerebral, 276
- ganglion, of retina, 746
- giant, foreign body, 116
- goblet, 88
  - in small intestine, 447
- Golgi apparatus in, 45–46
- graft rejection, 341
- granulosa, of ovary, 572
- growth and production of, 74–75
- hair
  - of ear, 761
  - of organ of Corti, 766
- histiocyte, 114–116
- in homeostasis alterations, 72–74
- horizontal
  - of Cajal, 278
  - of retina, 746
- hyalocytes, 751
- hyperplasia of, 73
- hypertrophy of, 73
- injuries of, 75–76
- internal environment of, 21
- interstitial, of testis, 539, 552, 665–667
  - clinical notes on, 682
  - stimulating hormone, 639
  - tumors of, 682
- of islets of Langerhans, 493
- junctions of, 68–71
- juxtaglomerular, 523
- keratinocytes, 691–693
- Kupffer, 148, 312, 482
- labile, 98
- Langerhans, 698

Cells—*Continued*
- Leydig. *See* interstitial, of testis
- liver, 482–483
- luteal, 577
- lysosomes in, 47–48
- of Martinotti, 278
- mast, 113–114
- melanocytes, 693–698
- Merkel, 705
- mesangial, 509
- mesenchymal, uncommitted, 116
- metaplasia of, 73–74
- microfilaments and fibrils in, 52
- microtubules in, 34, 51
- mitochondria in, 41–43
- mononuclear phagocyte, 116, 148, 359–360
- of Müller, 746
- myoepithelial, 95
- myointimal, 327
- neck, mucous, of stomach, 438
- nerve, 225
- nucleus of, 29–41
- olfactory nerve, 769
- organelles in. *See* Cytoplasm, organelles in
- oxyntic, 436
- oxyphil, parathyroid, 648
- Paneth, 447
- parafollicular, thyroid, 645–646, 648
- parietal, 436
- peptic, 436
- permanent, 100
- phalangeal, of organ of Corti, 766
- pillar, of organ of Corti, 766
- plasma, 109–113, 342, 349
- plasma membrane of, 41, 55–72
- PP, in pancreas, 494, 662
- principal
  - in duct of epididymis, 554
  - parathyroid, 648
- prokaryotic, 78–79
- Purkinje, 276
- pyramidal, 276
- receptors for drugs, 80
- reticular, 177
- ribosomes in, 49–51
- rod, 745
- satellite, of ganglia, 262, 264
- Schwann, 252, 255
- secretory, 93

Cells—*Continued*
- Sertoli, 548–552, 639
  - follicular stimulating hormone affecting, 552
- stable, 98
- stellate
  - cerebellar, 274
  - cerebral, 276
- stem, 158–159
  - pluripotential, 177
  - undifferentiated, in small intestine, 447
- structure of, 29–72
- supporting
  - of macula of utricle, 763
  - of olfactory mucous membrane, 769
  - of organ of Corti, 766
  - of Sertoli, 548–552, 639
  - of taste buds, 771
- sustentacular
  - in olfactory mucous membrane, 769
  - in taste buds, 771
- synovial, 143
- tactile, 266
- taste, 770
- unipotential, 177

Cementocytes, 419
Cementum, 418, 419
Center
- apneustic, 397, 399
- cardioaccelerator, 302
- cardioinhibitory, 302
- expiratory, 397
- germinal, of lymphatic nodules, 347, 354
- inspiratory, 397
- pneumotaxic, 397, 399
- respiratory, 397
  - depression of, 404–405
  - medullary, 397
  - stimulation of, 405
- vasoconstrictor, 321
- vasodilator, 321
- vomiting, 472

Centrioles, 34, 51–52
Centromere, 34
Centrosome, 51
- in neurons, 238

Cephalosporins, action on bacteria, 79
Cerebellum, 274–276
- granular layer of, 276

Cerebellum—*Continued*
    molecular layer of, 274–276
    Purkinje cell layer of, 276
Cerebrum, 276–279
Cerumen, 719, 755
Cervix of uterus, 584
    carcinoma of, 622
    clinical notes on, 621–622
    inflammations of, 621–622
Chalazion, 771
Chamber of eye
    anterior, 739, 746–747
    posterior, 739, 747
Cheeks, 413
Chemoreceptors, in carotid and aortic bodies, 399
Chemotaxis, 163
Chemotherapy
    action on bacteria, 79
    action on viruses, 79
Chest, barrel, 404
Childhood
    external genitalia in female newborn, 609–610
    mammary gland structure in newborn, 618
    ovaries in, 572
    uterus in, 590
Chloramphenicol, action on bacteria, 79
Chloride shift, 394
Cholecystitis, 499
Cholecystokinin, 447
Cholesterol, 54
    formation in hepatocytes, 487
Cholesterol esterase, secretion in pancreas, 496
Chondroclasts, 138
Chondrocyte, 126, 129, 138
Chondroitin sulfates, 126
Chondroma, 147
Chondromucoprotein, 126
Chondrosarcoma, 147
Chordae tendineae
    of mitral valve, 298
    of tricuspid valve, 296
Choriocarcinoma
    of testis, 565
    of uterus, 75
Chorion, 593
    frondosum, 597
    laeve, 597
Chorionepithelioma, 683
Choroid, 738

Chromatids, 34
Chromatin, 30–31
    and chromosome formation, 35
    sex, 30, 163
Chromatolysis, 233, 279, 282
Chromophobes, pituitary, 635
Chromosomes, 30, 35–41
    abnormalities in, 76
    autosomes, 41, 543, 578
    changes during oogenesis, 578–580
    changes during spermatogenesis, 543–544
    classification of, 39–41
    sex, 41, 543, 578
    X, 41
    Y, 41
Chylomicrons, 336
Chyme, 440
Chymotrypsin, 496
Chymotrypsinogen, 494
Cilia, 66–68
    formation of, 52
    olfactory, 769
    in respiratory system, 402
Ciliated cells, 88
Circulation
    coronary, 323
    hepatic, 324
    placental, 600–602
    pulmonary, 292, 301, 323–324
    systemic, 292, 301
Cirrhosis of liver, 498
    coagulation in, 182
Citrate, as anticoagulant, 184
Clearing agents, for tissue specimens, 8
Cleavage furrow, in telophase, 35
Cleavage lines, 146, 151, 706, 720
Cleft, synaptic, 210, 246
Clitoris, 608–609
    erection of, 609
Clotting of blood, 171
    abnormalities in, 182–184
Clotting factors, 172
Coagulation of blood, 171
    clinical notes on, 182–184
    extrinsic pathway of, 171
    intrinsic pathway of, 171
Coarctation of aorta, 327
Coat
    buffy, of cells, 155
    cell, 57

Coat—*Continued*
    fibrous
        of bladder, 528
        of eyeball, 736–738
        of seminal vesicles, 557
        of ureter, 526
        of uterine tubes, 582
        of vas deferens, 556
    muscular
        of anal canal, 463
        of appendix, 460
        of bladder, 526
        of digestive tract, 427, 429
        of esophagus, 430
        of gallbladder, 489
        of large intestine, 456–458
        of pyloric glands, 439
        of seminal vesicles, 557
        of small intestine, 449, 452
        of ureter, 525
        of uterine tubes, 582
        of uterus, 586
        of vas deferens, 556
    nervous, of eye, 741–746
    serosal. *See* Serosa
    vascular pigmented, of eyeball, 738–741
Cochlea, 759
    clinical notes on, 776–777
    duct of, 763–766
Colitis, ulcerative, 472
Collagen, 107, 116–118
    defect in synthesis of, 149
    in vitamin C deficiency, 149–150
Collagenase, 116
Colloid, in thyroid follicles, 645
Colon, 456–463
    bacteria in, 460
    clinical notes on, 471–472
    functions of, 460
Color
    of eye, 741
    of hair, 714
    perception of, 752
        clinical notes on, 775
    of skin, 707
Colostrum, 615, 617
Columns
    anal, 463
    renal, 503
    of spinal cord
        gray, 272
        white, 274
Comedo, 725

Complex, junctional, 70–71
Compliance, pulmonary, 392
Conchae, nasal, 365
Conduction
　cardiac, 295–296, 300
　　clinical notes on, 325–326
　local anesthetics affecting, 285
　in peripheral nerves, 264–266
　saltatory, 266, 287
　velocity of, 265, 287
Cones and rods, 741, 745
Conjunctiva, 729, 730
　clinical notes on, 771–772
Conjunctivitis, 771–772
Connective tissue, 22, 107–152
　amorphous material in, 122
　cells in, 107–116
　clinical notes on, 145–150
　clinical problems on, 150–152
　fibers in, 116–122
　　collagen, 116–118
　　dense, 122–124
　　elastic, 118–121
　　reticular, 121–122
　of liver, 483–485
　loose, 107–122
　regeneration of, 145–147
　supporting, 124–145
　tumors of, 147
Constipation, 472
Contraceptives, oral, 623
　endometrial changes from, 621
Contractile proteins, 52
Contractility of cardiac muscle, 300
Contraction
　of colon
　　peristaltic, 460
　　segmental, 460
　muscular, 22, 218–219
　of small intestine
　　peristaltic, 454–455
　　segmental, 453–454
　wound, 146
Convolutions, in cerebral cortex, 276
Coramine, and respiratory center stimulation, 405
Cord(s)
　medullary, of lymph node, 347
　spinal, 272–274
　　injuries of, bladder function in, 535
　vocal, 370

Cornea, 736–738
　clinical notes on, 772
Corona radiata, 577
Corpus
　albicans, 578
　cavernosum
　　of clitoris, 609
　　of penis, 561
　luteum, 577
　spongiosum, 561
Corpuscle(s)
　bulbous, of Krause, 271
　colostrum, 615
　Hassall's, 343
　Meissner's, 266, 271
　pacinian, 271
　renal, 504–511
　　function of, 511
Cortex
　cerebellar, 274
　cerebral, 276–279
　of hair shaft, 710
　renal, 503
　suprarenal, 651–657
Corticosterone, 652
Corticotropes, 635
Corticotropin-releasing hormone, 639, 655
Cortisol, 652
Cortisone, 652
Cotyledons, placental, 599
Coughing, 372
Count, cellular, 184
Countercurrent multiplier mechanism, renal, 517
Cowper's glands, 560
Crenation of red cells, 77
Cretinism, 677
Cri du chat syndrome, 76
Cristae
　ampullary, of semicircular ducts, 763
　of mitochondria, 41
Crown, of tooth, 417
Crura
　of clitoris, 609
　of penis, 561
Crypt(s)
　of Lieberkühn, 447
　tonsillar, 357, 473
Cryptorchidism, 564
Cumulus oophorus, 576
Curvatures of stomach, 432
Cushing's syndrome, 679–680

Cuticle, of hair shaft, 710
Cyanosis, 406
Cycle
　cardiac, 301
　hair growth, 707
　menstrual, 588–589
　　suppression during lactation, 617
　ovarian, 576–577
　　suppression during lactation, 617
　termination of, 580
Cyst(s)
　Bartholin, 623
　Meibomian, 771
　of ovary, 620
Cystitis, 534
Cytochemistry, 12–14
Cytology, exfoliative, 75
Cytoplasm, 41–55
　fat storage in, 53–54
　glycogen granules in, 53
　inclusions in, 53–54
　matrix of, 54–55
　of neuron, 231–238
　organelles in, 41–53
　　hypertrophy of, 73
　　membranes of, 57
　pigments in, 54
　of skeletal muscle cells, 197
Cytosine, 37
Cytotrophoblast, 591

Dacryocystitis, chronic, 778
Deaf-mutism, 76
Deafness, 776–777
　cochlear nerve, 777
　conductive, 776–777
Decidua, 591–593
　basalis, 591
　capsularis, 593
　hormonal control of, 593
　parietalis, 593
Defecation, 463
　clinical notes on, 472
Defibrillation, 326
Degeneration
　postmortem, 8
　retrograde, 280
　wallerian, 280
Deglutition, 372, 427
　disorders in, 467
Dehydration of tissue specimens, 8

Demilunes, of submandibular
    glands, 424
Dendrites, 225, 241–243
    spines of, 243
Dentin, 418–419
Deoxycorticosterone, 652, 653
Deoxyribonucleic acid. *See* DNA
Depolarization, 238, 264
Dermis, 689, 705–707
    clinical notes on, 724
    function of, 706–707
    organization of, 705–706
Desmosome, 68
    in cardiac muscle, 206
Development, stages of, 618
Diabetes
    insipidus, 531, 674
        clinical notes on, 674
    mellitus, 500, 680–682
        clinical notes on, 680–682
        complications of, 681–682
        diagnosis of, 681
Dialysis, 77–78, 533
    hemodialysis, 77, 533
    peritoneal, 78, 533
Diapedesis, 77, 188
Diaphragm
    muscular, in inspiration, 386
    slit, of podocytes, 509
Diaphysis, 131, 138, 141
Diarrhea, 472
Diastole, 301
Dicumarol, 184
Diffusion, 58
    facilitated, 60
Digestion, 496–497
Digestive tract, 23, 409–475
    clinical notes on, 466–472
    clinical problems on, 472–475
    esophagus, 429–432
    ileus of, 222
    large intestine, 455–466
    mouth, 409–421
    pharynx, 426–427
    salivation, 422–426
    small intestine, 442–455
    stomach, 432–442
    swallowing, 372, 427
    tube from esophagus to anus,
        427–429
Dihydrotestosterone, 552
Diiodotyrosyl, 646
Diisopropylphosphorofluoridate
    (DFP), 286

Dimethyl tubocurarine, 221
Diploë, 137
Diplopia, 773
Disc
    articular, 143
    intercalated, 205, 206, 300
    Merkel's, 266
Disease
    Addison's, 679
    celiac, 470, 472
    cellular abnormalities in, 26
    Hirschsprung's, 471
    Hodgkin's, 361
    Ménière's, 777
    Milroy's, 360
Disk, optic, 741, 773
Diuretics, 532–533
Diverticulosis of colon, 471
Division
    bacterial, 79
    of cells, 34–35
DNA
    chemotherapy affecting, 79
    in chromatin, 30
    in chromosomes, 37
    Feulgen reaction for, 14
    in mitochondria, 42
    in viruses, 79
DNP (DNA-protein complex), 30,
    37
DOPA reaction, for tyrosinase in
    melanocytes, 14
Dopamine, as neurotransmitter,
    246, 247
Down's syndrome, 76
Drainage, postural, 404
Drugs
    action on cells, 80
    anticoagulant, 184
    chemotherapeutic, actions of, 79
    contraceptives, oral, 623
        endometrial changes from, 621
    passage across cell membranes,
        79–80
    receptor sites for, 80
    transplacental passage of, 624
Duct(us)
    alveolar, 381
    bile, 488
        clinical notes on, 499–500
        clinical problems on, 500–501
        common, 488
        radiography of, 499
    of cochlea, 763–766

Duct(us)—*Continued*
    cystic, 488
    ejaculatory, 556–557
        function of, 558
    endolymphaticus, 761
    of epididymis, 554
    excretory, in male reproductive
        system, 552–557
    hepatic
        common, 488
        left, 488
        right, 488
    lymphatic, 335
        right, 335
    of pancreas, 494
        accessory, 494
        intralobular, 494
    papillary, straight, of kidney, 519
    of parotid gland, 422
        excretory, 422
        intercalated, 422
        interlobular, 422
        intralobular, 422
        striated, 422
    reuniens, 761, 763
    semicircular, 759, 763
    thoracic, 335
    utriculosaccularis, 761
Ductules, efferent, of testis, 539, 552
Dumping syndrome, after gastrectomy, 471
Duodenum, 442
    clinical notes on, 469
Dwarfism, 674
Dysgenesis, ovarian, 618
Dysostosis, cleidocranial, 150
Dysplasia, 74
Dyspnea, 405

Ear, 754–769
    cauliflower, 775
    clinical notes on, 775–777
    external, 754–755
    internal, 758–767
    tympanic cavity in, 755–758
Eclampsia of pregnancy, 683
Eczema, 722
Edema, 370, 531
    cerebral, 404
Effusion, pleural, 401
Ejaculation, 563–564
    premature, 568
    retrograde, 568
Elastase, 116

Elasticity
  of blood vessels, 308
    and blood pressure, 319
  of lungs, 392
    loss of, 404
Elastin, 107, 118
Electrical potential difference, membrane, 62–63
Electrocardiogram, 304–307, 326
  leads used in, 307
Elephantiasis, 360
Ellipsoid, retinal, 745
Embedding of tissue specimens
  in electron microscopy, 11
  in light microscopy, 8
Embolism, 184, 329
  fat, 148
  pulmonary, 329
Emphysema, subcutaneous, 401
Empyema, 401
Enamel, 418, 419
Endocardium, 292–294
Endocrine system, 23, 631–686
  clinical notes on, 673–683
  clinical problems on, 683–686
  hormones, 631–634
  interstitial cells of testis, 665–667
  negative feedback mechanism in, 631–632, 655, 667, 672
  ovarian hormones, 667–672
  pancreatic islets of Langerhans, 661–665
  parathyroid glands, 648–651
  pineal gland, 644
  pituitary gland, 635–643
  placental hormones, 672
  suprarenal glands, 651–661
  thyroid gland, 644–648
Endolymph, 766
Endometriosis, 620–621
Endometrium, 586–590
  adenocarcinoma of, 621
  biopsy of, 619
  cyclical changes in, 588–590
  layers of, 591
  oral contraceptives affecting, 621
Endomysium, 197
Endoneurium, 261
Endorphin production, in small intestine, 447
Endosteum, 132
Endothelium, 86
  corneal, 738
  of endocardium, 292

End-plate, motor, 207, 209, 223
  muscular element of, 209
  neural element of, 209
  potential in, 219
Enteroglucagon, 438
Enterokinase secretion, in small intestine, 455
Enzymes
  in histiocytes, 116
  lysosomal, 47
  mitochondrial, 41
Eosin, 9, 10
Eosinophil(s), 161, 164–165
  formation of, 167
Eosinophilia, 185
Ependyma, 252
  function of, 252
Ephelides, 722
Epicardium, 294
Epidermis, 689, 691–705
  cells in, 691–698
  clinical notes on, 721–724
  function of, 704–705
  layers of, 700–702
  organization of, 698–702
Epididymis, 539, 552–556
  function of, 554–556
  infection of, 565
  structure of, 552–554
Epiglottis, 370
Epimysium, 197
Epinephrine
  and heart rate, 304
  as neurotransmitter, 246
  in suprarenal medulla, 657–661
Epineurium, 261
Epiphora, 778
Epiphyses, 141
Epithelium, 22, 85–104
  clinical notes on, 98–100
  clinical problems on, 100–104
  columnar, 86–93
    pseudostratified, 88
    stratified, 88
  corneal, 737
  cuboidal, 86
  germinal, of ovary, 571
  glandular, 93–98
  lens, 748
  regeneration in, 98–100
  simple, 85
  squamous, 86
    keratinized stratified, 86
    nonkeratinized stratified, 86

Epithelium—*Continued*
  stratified, 85
  surface, 85–93
  transitional, 93
  tumors of, 100
Eponychium, 707
Equator of lens, 748
Erection
  of clitoris, 609
  of penis, 561–563
    and impotence, 567
Erythroblast(s)
  basophilic, 159
  polychromatophilic, 159
Erythroblastosis fetalis, 181
Erythrocytes, 155, 156–161
  abnormalities of, 184–185
  antigens in, and blood transfusions, 179
  clinical notes on, 184–188
  crenation of, 77
  fate of, 161
  formation of, 158–161
    control of, 161
  function of, 157–158
  rouleaux formation of, 157
Erythromycin, action on bacteria, 79
Erythropoiesis, 158
Erythropoietin, 161, 503, 524
Esophagus, 429–432
  achalasia of, 468
  clinical notes on, 467–468
  function of, 430–432
  varices of, 329
Estrogens, 571
  function in pregnancy, 603
  ovarian secretion of, 667–670
    control of, 670–672
  functions of, 580
  placental, 672
  produced by testes, 667
Ethacrynic acid, 532
Euchromatin, 31
Excitability, of cardiac muscle, 300
Exercise, and heart rate, 304
Exocytosis, 46, 48, 64
  and acetylcholine release, 210
Exophthalmos, in hyperthyroidism, 676
Expiration, 384, 391
  forced, 391
  lung changes in, 391
  quiet, 391
Extrasystoles, 300, 325–326

Eye, 729–743
  clinical notes on, 771–775
  functions of, 752
  lacrimal apparatus, 732–736
  refractive media of, 747–752
Eyeball, 736–752
  chambers of, 746–747
  clinical notes on, 772
  coats of, 736–746
  movements of, 773–774
Eyelashes, 729
Eyelids, 729–732
  clinical notes on, 771

Factor(s)
  clotting, 172
  intrinsic, 185, 438, 469
Farsightedness, 775
Fascia(e), 124, 147
  adherens, in cardiac muscle, 206
  deep, 124
  occludens, 68
  perinephric, 503
  superficial, 124, 689, 719
Fat
  fate in digestion, 497
  metabolism of
    estrogens affecting, 670
    glucocorticoids affecting, 655
    insulin affecting, 664
  in liver, 487
  perinephric, 503
  storage in cells, 53–54, 108–109, 148–149
  in space of Disse, 482
  synthesis in liver, 487
Fatigue, muscle, 220
Fecalith, 471
Feces, 460, 497
  and defecation, 463
Feet, of podocyte processes, 509
Female reproductive system, 571–628
  clinical notes on, 618–626
  clinical problems on, 626–628
  external genitalia, 607–610
  mammary glands, 610–618
  ovaries, 571–580
  uterine tubes, 580–584
  uterus, 584–606
  vagina, 606–607
Feminization, adrenal, 680
Fenestra
  cochlae, 758, 766, 767
  vestibuli, 758, 766, 767

Ferritin, in antibody-antigen reaction, 15
Fertility
  in females, disorders of, 623
  in males
    disorders of, 564–565
    and testicular temperature, 548
Feulgen reaction, 14
Fever
  rheumatic, 325
  typhoid, 470
Fibers
  basilar, of cochlear duct, 763, 767
  collagen, 116–118
  in connective tissue, 116–122
  elastic, 118–121
    in cartilage, 127
  lens, 748
  in muscle, 197
    extrafusal, 210
    intrafusal, 210
      annulospiral endings of, 212
    nuclear bag, 210
    nuclear chain, 210
      flower spray endings of, 212
    red, 198
    types of, 198–200
    white, 198
  nerve, 225, 252–261
    afferent, 262
    of cerebral cortex, 279
    efferent, 262
    group A, 287
    group B, 287
    myelinated, 252–255
    nonmyelinated, 255–261
    parallel, cerebellar, 276
    radial, in cerebral cortex, 279
    sensory, 262
    to suprarenal medulla, 321
    tangential, of cerebral cortex, 279
  Purkinje, 206, 296
  reticular, 121–122
  Sharpey's, 132
  vasoconstrictor, 321
    and blood flow to tissue, 323
  vasodilator, 321
Fibril(s), 52
  collagen, 118
Fibrillation
  atrial, 326
  ventricular, 326
Fibrin, 171

Fibrinogen, 156
Fibroadenoma of mammary glands, 625
Fibroblasts, 108
Fibrocartilage, 127
Fibrocytes, 108
Fibroma, 147
  in peripheral nerve connective tissue, 285
Fibrosarcoma, 147
Fibrosis, cystic, of pancreas, 76, 472
Fields, visual, 772–773
  nasal, 772
  temporal, 772
Filaments, lymphatic anchoring, 333
Filariasis, 360
Filtrate, glomerular, 509
Fimbriae, of uterine tubes, 580
Fingers, papillary ridges of, 689
Fissures
  in cerebral cortex, 276
  palpebral, 729
Fixatives
  in electron microscopy, 10–11
  in light microscopy, 7–8
Flagella, 68
Flow
  axoplasmic, 243–245
  blood, control in tissues, 323
  lymph
    control of, 337, 338–339
    procedures affecting, 361
  menstrual, 588
Fluid
  pericardial, 294
  pleural, 375, 392
  seminal, 563
  synovial, 143
  tear, 734
  tissue
    in edema, 360
    formation and reabsorption of, 337–338
    oxygen in, 397
Flutter, atrial, 326
Folds
  junctional, of neuromuscular junction, 209
  malleolar, 756
  nail
    lateral, 707
    proximal, 707
  of rectum, transverse, 458
  vestibular, 370
  vocal, 370

Follicle(s)
  hair, 689, 708
    nerve endings related to, 266
  ovarian, 571, 572
    antrum of, 576
    atretic, 576
    graafian, 576
    primordial, 572
  of thyroid gland, 644
Follicle-stimulating hormone, 639, 670
  affecting Sertoli cells, 552
  releasing factor, 576
Foot, of podocyte process, 509
Foramen
  apical, of tooth, 418
  cecum, of tongue, 414
Foreign bodies
  and giant cell formation, 116
  inhalation of, 401
Fornix, conjunctival
  inferior, 730
  superior, 730
Fossae, piriform, 372, 427
Fourchette, 608
Fovea centralis, 741, 746
Fractures, repair of, 146
Freckles, 722
Freeze-fracture etching, 11
Frenulum, of labia minora, 608
Frequency, of voice, 373
Fundus
  of gallbladder, 489
  ocular, examination of, 773
  of stomach, 432
    glands of, 436
  of uterus, 585
Furosemide, 532

Gallamine, 221
Gallbladder, 488–490
  clinical notes on, 499–500
  clinical problems on, 500–501
  function of, 490
  structure of, 488–490
Gallstones, 499
Ganglion
  autonomic, 262–264
  cervical sympathetic, 774
  ciliary, in orbit, 774
  posterior root, of spinal nerve, 262
  sensory, 262
  spiral, of cochlear nerve, 766
Ganglioneuroma, 285

Gap junction, in cardiac muscle, 206
Gas
  exchange in lungs, 392–394
  exchange in tissues, 397
  transport in blood, 394–397
Gastrectomy, dumping syndrome after, 471
Gastrin, 439
Gastrointestinal tract. *See* Digestive tract
Genes, 37
  abnormalities in, 76
Genitalia, external, in females, 607–610
  clinical notes on, 622–623
  in newborn, 609–610
Giemsa stain, 10
Gigantism, 673–674
Gingiva, 417, 420–421
  disorders of, 466
Gland(s), 93–98
  accessory, in male reproductive system, 557–560
  acinous, 95
  anal, 463
  apocrine, 95, 717
  areolar, 612
  Bartholin's, disorders of, 623
  Brunner's, 449
  bulbo-urethral, 560
  cardiac, 436
    esophageal, 429
  ceruminous, 719, 754
  ciliary, 719, 729
    infection of, 771
  compound, 93–95
  Cowper's, 560
  eccrine, 717
  endocrine, 95–98, 631
  esophageal, 429
  exocrine, 93–95, 631
  holocrine, 95
  labial, 411
  lacrimal, 732
    orbital part of, 732
    palpebral part of, 732
  of Littré, 528
  mammary, 610–618
  Meibomian, 729
    inflammation of, 771
  merocrine, 95
  of Moll, 719, 729
    infection of, 771
  Montgomery's, 612

Gland(s)—*Continued*
  mucous, 95
  parathyroid, 648–651
  parotid, 422
  pineal, 644
  pituitary, 635–643
  pyloric, 439–440
  salivary, 422–424
  sebaceous, 689, 714–717
    of eye, infection of, 771
  seromucous, 95
  serous, 95
  simple, 93
  sublingual, 424
  submandibular, 422–424
  suprarenal, 651–661
  sweat, 689, 717–719
  tubular, 95
  vestibular, greater, 609
  of Zeis, 729
    infection of, 771
Glans
  clitoris, 609
  penis, 561
Glaucoma, 775
Glioblastoma, 286
Gliomas, 286
Gliosis, 286
Globin, 157, 158, 161
Glomerulonephritis, 530
Glomerulus, renal, 508
  conditions affecting, 530
  juxtamedullary, 517
Glomus, 312, 706
Glucagon, 662
  actions of, 664
  secretion in pancreas, 494
  control of, 665
Glucocorticoids, 652, 655–657
  circadian rhythm of, 655
Gluconeogenesis, 486, 655
Glucose
  serum levels in diabetes, 680–681
  tolerance test, 681
Glucosuria, 680, 681
Glutamic oxalacetic transaminase, serum levels of, 498
Glutamic pyruvic transaminase, serum levels of, 498
Glycine, in microfibrils, 118
Glycocalyx, 57
Glycogen
  in neurons, 238
  storage in cells, 53

Glycosuria, 680, 681
  renal, 681
Goiter, 677–678
Golgi apparatus, 45–46
  in neurons, 233
Gonadotropes, 635
Gonadotropin, 639
  chorionic, 75, 593, 672
    function of, 603–604
Grafts
  corneal, 772
  rejection of, 341, 362
  of skin, 721
    clinical notes on, 721
    full-thickness, 721
    split-thickness, 721
Granulation tissue, 145
Granule, acrosomal, 540
Granulocytes, 161
  formation of, 167–170
Graves' disease, 676–677
Ground substance, 122
Growth
  of cartilage, 127–129
    appositional, 129
    interstitial, 129
  of hair, 713
  and stages of development, 618
Growth hormone, 637–638
  deficiency of, 674
  excessive secretion of, 673–674
  inhibitory hormone, 638
  releasing hormone, 637
Guanine, 37
Gums, 417, 420–421
  disorders of, 466
Gyri, in cerebral cortex, 276

H bands of myofibrils, 197
Hair(s), 707–714
  anagen phase of, 707
  catagen phase of, 707
  clinical notes on, 724–725
  club, 707
  elevation of, 714
  estrogens affecting, 670
  follicles of
    nerve endings related to, 266
    structure of, 708–710
  growth of, 713
  pigmentation of, 714
  structure of, 710–713
  taste, 770–771
  telogen phase of, 707

Hair(s)—*Continued*
  terminal, 707
  vellus, 707
Halitosis, 425
Hand, lobster-claw, 76
Haustra of colon, 456, 460
Haversian systems, 131
Head
  of pancreas, 490, 661
  of spermatozoon, 544
Healing
  by first intention, 145
  by secondary intention, 146
Hearing, 767–769
  defects in, 776–777
Heart, 291–307
  blood supply of, 299
  cardiac cycle, 301
  cardiac output, 301
    and blood pressure, 316
  clinical notes on, 324–326
  conducting system of, 205, 295–296
    structure of, 206–207
  congestive failure of, 325
    left-sided, 325
    right-sided, 325
  coronary circulation, 323
  electrical changes in, 304–307
  endocardium, 292–294
  epicardium, 294
  measures of activity, 301–304
  microscopic structure of, 292–299
  myocardium, 294
    ischemia of, 222–223, 324–325
  pericardium, 324
  physiology of cardiac muscle, 300
  rate of, 302–304
    control of, 302–304
  skeleton of, 294–295
  stroke volume of, 301–302
  valves of, 296–299
    diseases of, 325
  venous return to, 302
    mechanisms aiding, 321
  wall of, 292–294
Heidenhain iron hematoxylin, 10
Helicotrema, 766
Hemangioma
  capillary, 724
  cavernous, 724
Hematocrit, 156

Hematopoiesis, 176
  extramedullary, 178
Hematoxylin, 9, 10
Hematuria, 530
Heme, 157, 158
Hemianopia
  bitemporal, 773
  homonymous, 773
Hemidesmosomes, 72
Hemispheres, cerebellar, 274
Hemocytoblasts, 159
Hemodialysis, 77, 533
Hemoglobin, 157, 158
  oxygen dissociation curve, 394
  reduced, 157
  and skin color, 707
Hemolysis, 77
Hemophilia, 76, 182
Hemopneumothorax, 401
Hemorrhage, 178
  external, 178
  internal, 178
Hemorrhoids, 329
  external, 472
  internal, 472
Hemosiderin, 54, 161
Heparin
  as anticoagulant, 184
  in basophils, 165
  in mast cells, 113
Hepatitis, coagulation in, 182
Hepatocytes, 482–483
Heterochromatin, 30–31
Hexamethonium, as synaptic blocking agent, 285
Hillock, axon, 231, 243
Hilus, renal, 503
Hirschsprung's disease, 471
Hirsutism, 725
Histamine
  in basophils, 165
  and gastric secretion, 468
  in mast cells, 114
Histiocytes, 114–116, 148
Histiocytoma, fibrous, 724
Histochemistry, 12–14
Histology, 21
Hodgkin's disease, 361
Homeostasis, 25
  alterations in, 26
    cellular adaptation to, 72–74
Hordeolum, 771
Hormones, 93, 631–634
  action of, 632–633

Hormones—*Continued*
  affecting heart rate, 304
  antidiuretic, 520, 641
    absence of, 674
  chorionic gonadotropin, 75, 593, 603–604, 672
  follicle-stimulating, 639, 670
    affecting Sertoli cells, 552
    releasing factor, 576
  growth. *See* Growth hormone
  inhibitory, 635
  luteinizing, 577, 639, 670
  ovarian, 667–672
  parathyroid, 650–651
  pituitary
    anterior lobe, 637–641
    posterior lobe, 641–643
  placental, 603–604, 672
  releasing, 635
  secondary, 633
  suprarenal
    of cortex, 652–657
    of medulla, 657–661
  thymic, 343
  thyroid, 646–648
Horns of spinal cord, gray
  anterior, 272
  lateral, 272
  posterior, 272
Humor, aqueous, 747
Hyaline cartilage, 127
Hyalocytes, 751
Hydrocephalus, 76
Hydrochloric acid, 438, 441, 468
Hydropneumothorax, 401
Hydrops, fetal, 624
Hydroxyapatite, 130
Hydroxylysine, 118
Hydroxyproline, 118
Hymen, 606
Hyperadrenalism, 679–680
Hyperglycemia, 680
Hyperhidrosis, 726
Hypermetropia, 775
Hyperparathyroidism, 678
Hyperplasia, 73
  of smooth muscle, 222
Hyperpolarization, 241
Hypersensitivity, anaphylactic, 147
Hypersplenism, 362
Hypertension, 328–329
  portal, 498
  in renal disease, 531
Hyperthyroidism, 676–677

Hypertonic solutions, 60
  saline, 77
Hypertrichosis, 725
Hypertrophy, 73
  of cardiac muscle, 222
  of skeletal muscle, 221
  of smooth muscle, 222
Hyperventilation, 405
Hypoadrenalism, 678–679
Hypodermis, 719
Hypoparathyroidism, 678
Hypothalamus, control of pituitary, 635
Hypothyroidism, 677
Hypotonic solutions, 60
  saline, 77
Hypoventilation, 405
Hypoxia, 405

I bands of myofibrils, 197
Ileitis, 472
Ileum, 442–452
  clinical notes on, 469–471
Ileus, 222
  adynamic, 222
  paralytic, 470
  spastic, 222
Immunity
  cellular, 339, 343
  humoral, 341–342
  and splenic function, 354
Immunocytochemistry, 14–15
Immunoglobulin, thyroid-stimulating, 676
Immunology, 147–148
Implantation of blastocyst, 591
  abnormal, 623
Impotence, 567
Impulse
  cardiac, 302
    disorders of, 325–326
  nerve, 241, 264
Incisions, repair of, 145
Incisura angularis, of stomach, 432
Incisures of Schmidt-Lanterman, 255
Inclusions, cytoplasmic, 53–54
Incus, 756
Infarction
  myocardial, 325
  of placenta, 624
Infertility
  in females, 623
  in males, 564–565

Inflammation, 188–190
Infundibulum
  pituitary, 635
  of uterine tube, 580
Inhibin, 552, 639
Insertion, of muscle, 195
Inspiration, 384–391
  forced, 386–391
  lung changes in, 391
  quiet, 384–386
Insulin, 493, 662–664
  actions of, 662–664
  control of secretion, 664
  deficiency in diabetes mellitus, 680
Interferon, 116
Interphase, cellular, 34
Intestine
  large, 455–466
    anal canal, 463–466
    appendix, 458–460
    clinical notes on, 471–472
    functions of, 460–463
    secretions of, 466
    structure of, 456–458
  small, 442–455
    clinical notes on, 469–471
    duodenum, 442
    functions of, 452–455
    jejunum and ileum, 442–452
    malabsorption from, 470
    movements of, 453–455
    secretions of, 455, 497
    short bowel syndrome, 470–471
    structure of, 442–452
Intrinsic factor, 185, 438
  and pernicious anemia, 469
Iodine
  in goiter prevention, 678
  protein-bound, in serum, 675
  radioactive
    thyroid uptake of, 675
    in treatment of hyperthyroidism, 677
  secretion of, 646
Iodopsin, 745, 752
Iris, 739–741
Ischemia, of cardiac muscle, 222–223, 324–325
Islets of Langerhans, 493, 661–665
  clinical notes on, 680
Isotonic solutions, 60
  saline, 77
Isthmus of uterine tube, 582

Jaundice, 499–500
Jejunum, 442–452
  clinical notes on, 469–471
Joints, 141–145
  cartilaginous, 141–143
    primary, 141–143
    secondary, 143
  fibrous, 141
  synovial, 143–145
Juice, gastric, 441
Junctions
  cellular, 68–71
    communicating or gap, 68–70
    in cardiac muscle, 206
    complex of, 70–71
    tight, 68
  corneoscleral, 736
  neuromuscular, 209–210

Karyolysis, 75
Karyorrhexis, 75
Karyotyping, 39
Keloid, 146, 721
Keratin, 86, 691
Keratinocytes, 691–693
  clinical notes on, 721–722
Keratohyalin, 701
Keratosis, seborrheic, 722
Ketonuria, 681
Ketosis, 664
  diabetic, 681
Kidneys, 503–525
  blood flow through cortex and medulla, 524
  blood vessels of, 522–524, 529–530
  Bowman's capsule, 504, 508–509
  clinical notes on, 529–534
  collecting tubules, 519–520
  convoluted tubules
    distal, 519
    proximal, 511–516
  corpuscle of, 504–511
  dialysis of, 533
  disorders of, 529–533
    treatment of, 532–533
  endocrine function of, 524
  failure of
    acute, 531
    chronic, 531–532
  function of, 524–525
  function tests, 533–534
  glomeruli, 508
    conditions affecting, 530

Kidneys, glomeruli—*Continued*
    juxtamedullary, 517
    juxtaglomerular apparatus, 523–524
  loop of Henle, 516–519
  nephrons in, 504–519
  nervous control of, 524
  structure of, 503–504
  tubules of
    collecting, 519–520
    conditions affecting, 530
    convoluted, 511–516, 519
    function tests, 533–534
    uriniferous, 504–522
  urine concentration in, 520–521
Klinefelter's syndrome, 76
Kupffer cells, 148

Labia
  majora, 608
  minora, 608
Labor
  placental separation in, 604–605
  role of uterus in, 605
  uterus after, 606
Labyrinth, 758–767
  bony, 759
  membranous, 761–763
Labyrinthitis, 776
Lactase, secretion in small intestine, 455
Lactation, 615–617
Lacteals, 336
  of villi in small intestine, 446
Lacuna(e)
  in bone matrix, 137
  in cartilage, 126
Lacus lacrimalis, 730
Lamellae
  circumferential, 131
  concentric, 131
  interstitial, 131
Lamina
  basal, of basement membrane, 71
  cribrosa, of sclera, 736, 746
  elastic
    of elastic arteries, 308
    of muscular arteries, 309
  propria
    of appendix, 460
    of digestive tract, 427
    of olfactory mucous membrane, 770
    of small intestine, 447–449

Lamina—*Continued*
  reticular, of basement membrane, 71
  spiral, of cochlea, 759
Laryngitis, 400
Laryngopharynx, 369
Larynx, 370–373
  clinical notes on, 400
  sinus of, 372
  sphincters in, 372–373
Law
  all-or-none, 300
  Frank-Starling, 302
Layer(s)
  basal, of endometrium, 591
  capillary, of choroid, 738
  of cerebellar cortex, 274–276
  compact, of endometrium, 591
  granular, of cerebellum, 276
  Henle's, 710
  Huxley's, 710
  molecular, of cerebellum, 274
  papillary, of dermis, 705
  pigmented, of retina, 741–742
  Purkinje cell, 276
  reticular, of dermis, 706
  of retina, 746
  spongy, of endometrium, 591
  subendothelial, of endocardium, 292
  vessel, of choroid, 738
Lead, as cytoplasmic inclusion, 54
Leads, precordial, in electrocardiography, 307
Leiomyoma of uterus, 621
Lens of eye, 747–749
  suspension of, 749
Lentigo, 723
Leukemia, 185
  lymphatic, 361
Leukocytes, 155, 161–171
  abnormalities of, 185
  clinical notes on, 184–188
  formation of, 167–171
  polymorphonuclear, 161
Leukocytosis, 185
Leukopenia, 185
Leukorrhea, in cervicitis, 621–622
Lids of eye, 729–732
Ligament(um)
  annular, of stapes, 758
  elastic, 124
  falciform, of liver, 477
  fibrous, 122, 143

Ligament(um)—*Continued*
  flavum, 124
  nuchae, 124
  palpebral
    lateral, 730
    medial, 730–732
  periodontal, 417, 420
  round, of ovary, 571
  suspensory
    of lens, 749
    of mammary gland, 610
    of ovary, 571
  vocal, 370
Limbus, 736
Lines
  of cleavage, 146, 151, 706, 720
  flexure, 689
  Langer's, 146, 151, 706, 720
  tension, 689
Lip(s), 409–411
Lipase
  in gastric secretions, 436, 441
  pancreatic secretion of, 496
Lipid
  in neurons, 238
  osmium tetroxide stain for, 14
  in plasma membrane, 55
  Sudan black stain for, 14
Lipocytes, 53–54, 108–109, 148–149
  in space of Disse, 482
Lipofuscin, 54
  in neurons, 238
Lipoproteins, formation in hepatocytes, 487
Liquor folliculi, 576
Liver, 477–488
  bile canaliculi in, 481, 483
  biopsy of, 499
  cells of, 482–483
  circulation in, 324
  clinical notes on, 497–499
  clinical problems on, 500
  connective tissue of, 483–485
  disorders of, 497–498
    clotting in, 182
  function of, 486–488
  function tests, 498–499
  lymphatic drainage of, 485
  regeneration of, 498
  sinusoids in, 312, 324, 479, 481–482
Lobes
  liver
    caudate, 477

Lobes, liver—*Continued*
    left, 477
    quadrate, 477
    right, 477
  of lungs, 379
  of mammary gland, 610
  pituitary
    anterior, 635–641
    posterior, 635, 641–643
Lobster-claw hand, 76
Lobules
  of epididymis, 554
  of liver, classic, 477, 485–486
  of lung, 379
  portal, 486
  renal, 504
  of thymus, 343
Lochia, 606
Loop of Henle, 516–519
Lungs, 379
  air volume measurements in, 402
  bronchopulmonary segment of, 379
  changes on expiration, 391
  changes on inspiration, 391
  circulation through, 323–324
  clinical notes on, 401–402
  compliance of, 392
  defense clearance mechanisms in, 402
  disorders of, 404
  distensibility of, loss of, 404
  elasticity of, 392
    loss of, 404
  gas exchange in, 392–394
  postural drainage of, 404
  segmental resection of, 402
  surfactant of, 381
Lunule, 707
Luteinizing hormone, 577, 639, 670
Lymph, 333
  drainage from liver, 485
  factors controlling flow of, 338–339, 361
  formation of, 338
Lymphadenitis, 361
Lymphangitis, 360–361
Lymphatic system, 23, 333–363
  clinical notes on, 360–362
  clinical problems on, 362–363
Lymphatic vessels, 333–337
  afferent, 347
  arrangement of, 335–337
  bicuspid valves of, 335

Lymphatic vessels—*Continued*
  capillaries, 333–335
  ducts, 335
  infection of, 360–361
  medium-sized, 335
  metastasis through, 361
  obstruction of, 360
  structure of, 333–335
Lymphoblast, 339, 342
Lymphocytes, 161, 165–167, 339–343
  B cells, 167, 341–343
  formation of, 170–171
  in spleen, 354
  T cells, 167, 339–341
    killer, 341
    and tissue grafting, 341, 362
  in thymus, 343
Lymphocytosis, 185
Lymphokines, 148, 339
Lymphomas, 361
Lymphopenia, 187
Lymphosarcoma, 147
Lysosomes, 47–48
  in disease, 76–77
  in neurons, 234
  in neutrophils, 164
  primary, 47
  secondary, 47
Lysozyme, 116, 447

Macrocytes, 185
Macrophages, 114–116
  alveolar, 148
  and immunity development, 147–148
Macula
  adherens, 68
    in cardiac muscle, 206
  densa, 519, 523
  lutea, 741, 746
  occludens, 68
  of saccule, 761
  of utricle, 761
Malabsorption, from small intestine, 470
Male reproductive system, 539–569
  accessory glands, 557–560
  clinical notes on, 564–568
  clinical problems on, 568–569
  ejaculatory ducts, 556–557
  epididymis, 552–556
  excretory ducts, 552–557
  penis, 561–563

Male reproductive system—
Continued
  prostate, 558–560
  testes, 538–552
  vas deferens, 556
Malleus, 756
Mallory's aniline blue collagen stain, 10
Maltase, secretion in small intestine, 455
Mammary glands, 610–618
  after menopause, 617–618
  clinical notes on, 624–626
  disorders of, 624–626
    in females, 624–626
    in males, 624
  estrogens affecting, 670
  in females, 610–613
  fibrocystic disease of, 625
  lactating, 615–617
    regression of, 617
  in males, 610, 624
  in newborn, 618
  palpation of, 625
  in pregnancy, 614–615
  progesterone affecting, 670
  tumors of, 625–626
Mammotropes, 635
Margination, of neutrophils, 188
Marrow, 131, 132–134, 176–178
  biopsy of, 187–188
  clinical notes on, 187–188
  failure of, 188
  hematopoietic, 176
  red, 134, 137, 138, 176
  structure of, 177–178
  yellow, 134, 176
Masson's trichrome stain, 10
Mast cells, 113–114
  and anaphylactic hypersensitivity, 147
Mastoiditis, acute, 776
Matrix
  cytoplasmic, 54–55
  mitochondrial, 41
  nail, 707
  territorial, cartilage, 126
Matter
  gray, 225, 272–274
  white, 225, 274
Meatus
  auditory, external, 754
    clinical notes on, 776
    disorders of, 776
  nasal, 365

Mediastinum, 375
Medulla
  of hair shaft, 713
  of lymph node, 347
  renal, 503
  suprarenal, 657–661
  of thymus, 343
Medulloblastoma, 286
Megacolon, 471
Megakaryocytes, 175, 178
Megaloblasts, 185
Meiosis, 34
Melanin, 54, 694, 707
  in neurons, 238
Melanocyte(s), 693–698
  clinical notes on, 722–724
  tyrosinase in, DOPA reaction for, 14
Melanocyte-stimulating hormone, 640–641
Melanoma, malignant, 724
Melanosomes, 54, 694, 700
Melasma, 722
Melatonin, 644
Membrana granulosa, 576
Membrane
  basement, 71–72, 85
  basilar, of cochlear duct, 763
  Bowman's, 737
  Bruch's, 738
  buccopharyngeal, 370
  cell. *See* plasma
  of cytoplasmic organelles, 41, 57
  Descemet's, 738
  glassy, of hair follicle, 710
  limiting, or retina
    inner, 746
    outer, 746
  mitochondrial, 41
  mucous
    of anal canal, 463
    of appendix, 460
    of bladder, 526
    of digestive tract, 427
    of esophagus, 429
    of gallbladder, 489
    of large intestine, 456
    olfactory, 367, 769–770
      disorders of, 777
    of pharynx, 427
    respiratory, 367–368
    of seminal vesicles, 557
    of small intestine, 444
    of stomach, 433

Membrane, mucous—*Continued*
  of trachea, 373
  of ureter, 525
  of uterine tubes, 582
  of uterus, 586–590
  of vas deferens, 556
  nuclear, 32–34
  otolithic, 761
  placental, 602
    drugs crossing, 624
    structure of, 602
    transport across, 603
  plasma, 21, 41, 55–72
    active transport in, 60–62
    of axon, 209
    bacterial, 78
    carriers in, 60
    defects in, 77
    diffusion in, 58, 60
    electrical potential difference in, 62–63
    in exocytosis, 64
    junctions of, 68–71
    of neurons, 238–241
    osmosis in, 58–60
    passage of substances through, 77–80
    in phagocytosis, 63–64
    physical properties of, 57–64
    in pinocytosis, 63
    pores in, 62
    of skeletal muscle cells, 197
    specializations in, 64–68
    structure of, 55
  postsynaptic, 210, 246
  presynaptic, 209–210, 246
  Reissner's, 766
  respiratory, 381–383, 392
  synovial, 143
  tectorial, 766
  tympanic, 756
    clinical notes on, 776
    secondary, 758
  vestibular, 766
  vitreous, 751
Menarche, 618, 626
Ménière's disease, 777
Menopause, 618, 626, 682
  mammary gland structure after, 617–618
  uterine changes in, 590–591
Menstruation, 580, 588–589
  and dysfunctional uterine bleeding, 621

Mesaxon, 255
Mesentery, of small intestine, 444, 452
Mesoappendix, 460
Mesotendon, 145
Mesothelium, 86
Mesovarium, 571
Metabolism
  basal rate of, 676
  catecholamines affecting, 659
  glucocorticoids affecting, 655
  insulin affecting, 662–664
  in liver, 486–488
Metachromasia, 9
Metamyelocytes, neutrophil, 167
Metaphase, in mitosis, 34
Metaplasia, 73–74
Metarterioles, 310, 323, 330
Metastases, lymphatic, 361
Metrazol, and respiratory center stimulation, 405
Microbodies, 48
Microfibrils
  collagen, 118
  elastic, 118
Microfilaments, 52
  contractile, 52
  in disease, 77
  in neurons, 234
  supportive, 52
Microglia, 250–252, 288
  function of, 252
  reactions to injury, 286
Microorganisms
  eukaryotic, 78
  prokaryotic, 78–79
  viruses, 79
Microscope
  base of, 1
  coarse adjustment of, 3
  compound, 1
  condenser of, 1
  definition of image with, 3
  depth of focus of, 3
  electron
    in cardiac muscle studies, 205–206
    preparation of tissues for, 10–12
    scanning, 7
    in skeletal muscle studies, 197–198
    in smooth muscle studies, 200–203

Microscope, electron—*Continued*
    in synapse studies, 245
    transmission, 5–7
  eyepieces of, 1
  fine adjustment of, 3
  fluorescence, 4–5
  in histochemistry, 13–14
  in immunocytochemistry, 14–15
  interference, 4
  and interpretation of tissue sections, 16–18
  iris diaphragm of, 2
  light, 1–4
    in cardiac muscle studies, 205
    preparation of tissues for, 7–10
    in skeletal muscle studies, 197
    in smooth muscle studies, 203
  light filters of, 2
  magnification of, 3
  mechanical stage of, 2
  mirror of, 2
  nosepiece of, 1
  numerical aperture of, 3
  objective lenses of, 1, 3
  oil-immersion objective of, 3–4
  phase contrast, 4
  pillar of, 1
  polarizing, 4
  in radioautography, 15–16
  resolution of, 3
  simple, 1
  stage of, 1
Microtome, 8
  ultramicrotome, 11
Microtubules, 34, 51, 52
  in disease, 77
  in neurons, 234
Microvilli, 64–66
  of columnar cells, 88
Micturition, 529
Miliaria, 726
  rubra, 726
Milk, witch's, 618
Milroy's disease, 360
Mineralization of bone, defects in, 149
Mineralocorticoids, 652, 653–655
Mitochondria, 41–43
  cristae of, 41
  elementary particles of, 41
  in neurons, 233
Mitomycins, action on bacteria, 79
Mitosis, 34–35
Mitotic figures, 35

Modiolus, 759
Moles, 723–724
  hydatidiform, 683
Mongolism, 76
Monocytes, 148, 161, 167
  formation of, 171
  phagocytic, 116, 148, 359–360
Monoiodotyrosyl, 646
Monosomy, 76
Mouth
  clinical notes on, 466
  in digestion, 496
Movements
  of colon, 460
  of eyeball, 773–774
  of ossicles, 758
  sense of, 767
  of small intestine, 453–455
  of stomach walls, 440–441
Mucocele, of appendix, 471
Mucosa. *See* Membrane, mucous
Mucus, 95
  cervical, 619
  in large intestine, 466
  in small intestine, 455
  in stomach, 441
Multivesicular bodies, 48
Murmurs, cardiac, 325
Muscle, 23, 195–224
  action potential of, 219
  arrector pili, 706, 714
  buccinator, 413
  bulbospongiosus, 561, 607, 608
  cardiac, 203–207, 294
    action potential of, 219
    clinical notes on, 222–223
    conductivity of, 300
    contractility of, 300
    electron microscopic structure of, 205–206
    excitability of, 300
    hypertrophy of, 222
    ischemia of, 222–223
    light microscopic structure of, 205
    nerve supply to, 215–218
    physiology of, 300
    rhythmicity of, 300
  ciliary, 738
  clinical notes on, 220–223
  clinical problems on, 223–224
  constrictor pupillae, 774
  contraction of, 218–219
  detrusor, of bladder, 526

Muscle—*Continued*
  dilator pupillae, 741
  intercostal, 386
  ischiocavernosus, 561, 609
  levatores costarum, 386
  nerve supply of, 207–218
  orbicularis oculi, 732
  orbicularis oris, 409
  of ossicles, 758
  papillary, 296
  serratus posterior
    inferior, 391
    superior, 386
  skeletal, 195–200
    action potential of, 219
    atrophy of, 220–221
    clinical notes on, 220–221
    electron microscopic structure of, 197–198
    fatigue of, 220
    hypertrophy of, 221
    light microscopic structure of, 197
    motor point of, 207
    motor unit of, 220, 223
    nerve supply of, 207–214
    neuromuscular blocking agents affecting, 221
    neuromuscular junctions of, 209–210
    neuromuscular spindles of, 210–212
    neurotendinous spindles of, 212–214
    regeneration of, 221
    rigor mortis of, 221
    tone of, 220
    types of fibers in, 198–200
  smooth, 200–203
    action potential of, 219
    clinical notes on, 222
    electron microscopic structure of, 203
    hypertrophy and hyperplasia of, 222
    in ileus, 222
    light microscopic structure of, 200–203
    nerve supply of, 214–215
    regeneration of, 222
    role in atherosclerosis, 222
  sphincter pupillae, 741
  stapedius, 758
  striated, 195
  tensor tympani, 758

Muscle—*Continued*
  trachealis, 373
  voluntary, 195
Muscular coat. *See* Coat, muscular
Myasthenia gravis, 221, 362
  swallowing difficulty in, 467
Myelin
  formation of, 255
  major dense line of, 255
  minor dense line of, 255
Myelin figures, 47
Myeloblasts, 167
Myelocytes, neutrophil, 167
Myocardium, 203, 294
  ischemia of, 324–325
Myofibrils, 197
  in cardiac muscle, 205–206
Myoglobin, 198
Myoid, retinal, 745
Myometrium, 586
Myopia, 775
Myosin, 52
  activity in anaphase, 34
  in cardiac muscle, 205
  interaction with actin, 218
  in platelets, 175
  in skeletal muscle, 197
Myringotomy, 776
Myxedema, 677

Nails, 689, 707
  brittle, 724
  clinical notes on, 724
  pale, 724
  paronychia, 721, 724
Narcotics, and respiratory center depression, 404–405
Nares, 365
Nasopharynx, 369
Nearsightedness, 775
Neck
  of gallbladder, 489
  of pancreas, 490, 661
Necrosis
  fat, 148
  of liver
    centrilobular, 498
    midzonal, 498
    peripheral, 498
  renal tubular
    ischemic, 530
    toxic, 530
Neoplasms, 74–75. *See also* Tumors

Nephron, 504–519
Nephrosclerosis, arteriolar, 531
Nephrotic syndrome, 530–531
Nerves, 207–218
  abducens, paralysis of, 773–774
  of bladder, 528
  of cardiac muscle, 215–218
  ciliary, long, 775
  cochlear, damage to, 777
  cranial, 262
  fibers of, 252–261
    myelinated, 252–255
    nonmyelinated, 255–261
  of lymph nodes, 347
  motor, 207
  oculomotor, 773
  sensory, 207–209
  of skeletal muscle, 207–214
  of smooth muscle, 214–215
  spinal, 261–262
    anterior root of, 261
    posterior root of, 261
  trochlear, 773
  vagus, and heart rate, 302
Nervous system, 23, 225–288
  autonomic, 214, 225
  central, 225
    myelin formation in, 255
    nonmyelinated fibers in, 261
  clinical notes on, 279–286
  clinical problems on, 286–288
  parasympathetic, 225
  peripheral, 225, 261–272
    conduction in, 264–266
    endings on secretory cells, 271–272
    free nerve endings. 266
    group A fibers in, 261
    group B fibers in, 261
    group C fibers in, 261
    myelin formation in, 255
    nonmyelinated fibers in, 255
    sensory endings or receptors in, 266–271
      encapsulated, 266–271
      nonencapsulated, 266
    tumors of, 285
  sympathetic, 225
    cardiac, 302
Nervous tissue, 22–23, 225–288
  in cerebellum, 274–276
  in cerebrum, 276–279
  in spinal cord, 272–274

Nervous tissue—*Continued*
  staining of, 225–227
  structure of, 225
Neurites, 227
Neuroblastoma, 285, 680
Neurofibrils, in neurons, 234
Neuroglia, 225, 247–252, 288
  astrocytes, 248–250
  ependyma, 252
  function of, 252
  microglia, 250–252
  oligodendrocytes, 250
  reactions to injury, 186
  tumors of, 286
Neurohypophysis, 635, 641–643
Neurolemmomas, 285
Neuroma, 283
Neurons, 225, 227–252
  bipolar, 227
  body of, 231
    injury to, 279
  classification of, 227–231
  cytoplasm of, 231–238
  degeneration of
    in aging, 285
    transneuronal, 284–285
  depolarized, 238
  Golgi type I, 227
  Golgi type II, 231
  hyperpolarization of, 241
  multipolar, 227
  nucleus of, 231
  plasma membrane of, 238–241
  processes of, 241–245
    injury to, 279–282
  reaction to injury, 279–284
  refractory period in, 241
    absolute, 265
    relative, 265
  structure of, 231–245
  summation in, 241
  synapses of, 245–247
  tumors of, 285
  unipolar, 227
Neurophysin, 641
Neurotransmitters, 246–247
Neutropenia, 185
Neutrophil(s), 148, 161–164
  drumstick, 153
  formation of, 167
  margination of, 188
Neutrophilia, 185
Nevi, 723–724
Newborn. *See* Childhood

Nicotine, as synaptic blocking agent, 285
Nipples, 610
  inverted, congenital, 625
  supernumerary, 625
Nissl substance, 231–233
Node
  atrioventricular, 206, 295–296, 325
  lymph, 336, 345–349
    axillary, 336
    blood supply of, 347
    function of, 347–349
    infections of, 361
    inguinal, 336
    neoplasms of, 361
    nerve supply of, 347
  of Ranvier, 252, 255
  sino-atrial, 206, 295, 325
Nodules, lymphatic, 347, 349, 354
Norepinephrine
  and heart rate, 304
  as neurotransmitter, 246, 247
  in pineal gland, 644
  in suprarenal medulla, 657–661
Normoblasts, 159
Nose, 365–369
  clinical notes on, 400
  olfactory mucous membrane, 769–770
  paranasal sinuses, 368–369
Nostrils, 365
Nuclear sap, 32
Nucleolus, 29–30
Nucleus, 29–41
  basal, cerebral, 276
  chromatin in, 30–31
  Edinger-Westphal, 774
  functions of, 34
  membrane of, 32–34
  of neuron, 231
  nucleolus of, 29–30
  pretectal, 774
Nystatin, action on bacteria or fungi, 79

Obesity, fat cells in, 148–149
Odontoblasts, 418
Olfaction, organ of, 769–770
  disorders in, 777
Oligodendrocytes, 250
  function of, 252
  reactions to injury, 286

Oliguria, 530
Oocytes
  primary, 572
  secondary, 577
Oogenesis, chromosomal changes during, 578–580
Oogonia, 572
Opsins, rod and cone, 752
Ora serrata, 741
Orcein elastic stain, 10
Orchitis, 564
Organ(s), 23
  spiral, of Corti, 766, 767
  target, 631
Organelles, cellular, 41–53
  hypertrophy of, 73
  membranes of, 57
Orgasm
  in female, 610
  in male, 563–564
Orifice
  cardiac, 432
  pyloric, 432
Origin, of muscle, 195
Oropharynx, 369
Os of uterus
  external, 584
  internal, 586
Osmium tetroxide, 11, 14
Osmosis, 58–60
Ossicles, auditory, 756–758
  movements of, 758
  muscles of, 758
Ossification, 135–141
  endochondral, 137–141
  intramembranous, 135–137
Osteitis fibrosa cystica, 678
Osteoblasts, 135
Osteoclasts, 137, 138
Osteocytes, 130, 137
Osteogenesis imperfecta, 76, 149
Osteoid, 135
Osteoma, 147
Osteomalacia, 149
Osteosarcoma, 147
Otitis
  externa, 776
  media, 776
Otoliths, 761
Otosclerosis, 776
Ovaries, 571–580
  before puberty, 572
  clinical notes on, 618–620, 682–683

Ovaries—*Continued*
  cysts of, 620
    follicular, 620
    luteal, 620
    multiple, 620
  failure of
    primary, 619
    secondary, 619
  follicles of, 571, 572
  hormones of, 667–672
  hypersection of, 683
  hypofunction of, 683
  malformations of, 618–619
  in menopause, 682
  at puberty, 576–577
  tumors of, 620
Ovulation, 577
  hormonal control of, 578
Ovum, 571
  malformation of, 619
  mature, 577
Oxalate, as anticoagulant, 184
Oxygen
  anoxia, 405–406
    affecting heart rate, 304
    and blood flow to tissue, 323
  capacity of blood, 158
  dissociation curve, 394
  exchange in lungs, 392–394
  exchange in tissues, 397
  hypoxia, 405
  transport in blood, 394
Oxyhemoglobin, 157, 394
Oxytocin, 641–643

P wave, in electrocardiogram, 304
Pacemaker, cardiac
  electronic, 326
  sino-atrial, 206, 295
Pain
  in gallbladder and bile duct disorders, 499
  in labor, 605
  renal, 532
  ureteric, 534
Palate, 421
  hard, 421
  soft, 421
Pancreas, 490–496
  cells of, 493–494
  clinical notes on, 500
  clinical problems on, 501
  cystic fibrosis of, 76, 472
  ducts of, 494

Pancreas—*Continued*
  endocrine portion of, 493
  exocrine portion of, 493
  islets of Langerhans, 661–665
  secretions of, 494–496
  structure of, 490–494
Pancreatitis, acute, 500
Panhypopituitarism, in adults, 674
Papanicolaou test, 622
Papillae
  dermal, 700
  duodenal, 488
  lacrimalis, 730
  renal, 503, 525
  of tongue, 414
    filiform, 414
    fungiform, 414
    vallate, 414
Papillomas, 100
  of mammary glands, 625
Parathyroid glands, 648–651
  clinical notes on, 678
  hyperparathyroidism, 678
  hypoparathyroidism, 678
  inferior, 648
  superior, 648
Parenchyma, 93
Paronychia, 721, 724
Parotid gland, 422
Pars (part)
  anterior, pituitary, 635–640
  flaccida, of tympanic membrane, 756
  intermedia, pituitary, 635, 640–641
  orbital, of lacrimal gland, 732
  palpebral, of lacrimal gland, 732
  plana, of ciliary body, 738
  plicata, of ciliary body, 738
  tensa, of tympanic membrane, 756
  tuberalis, pituitary, 635, 641
Patches, Peyer's, 354, 449
  in typhoid fever, 470
Pause, compensatory, 300
Pedicle, cone, 745
Pelvis, of ureter, 503, 525
Penicillin, action on bacteria, 79
Penis, 561–563
  clinical notes on, 567
  erection of, 561–563
  and impotence, 567
Pepsin, 436, 441, 468
Pepsinogen, 436, 441

Peptidases, secretion in small intestine, 455
Peptidoglycan, in bacterial cell wall, 78
Pericarditis, 324
Pericardium, 324
  fibrous, 294
  serous, 294
Perichondrium, 126
Pericytes, 310
Perilymph, 766
Perimysium, 197
Perineurium, 261
Periodic acid-Schiff reaction, 14
Periosteum, 132, 137, 138
Peristalsis, 430
  in colon, 460
  in small intestine, 454–455
  waves in, 429
Peroxisomes, 48
Phagocytes
  alveolar, 381, 402
  and immunity development, 147–148
  mononuclear, 116, 148, 359–360
Phagocytosis, 48, 63–64, 114–116, 148
Phagosome, 48
Pharynx, 369–370, 426–427
  clinical notes on, 467
  fibrous layer of, 427
  mucous membrane of, 427
  muscular layer of, 427
Phenothiazines, 286
Pheochromocytoma, 285, 680
Pheomelanin, 714
Phimosis, 567
Phlebothrombosis, 329
Phosphatase
  acid, 75
  alkaline, 75, 137
  azodye methods for, 14
Phosphocreatine, and muscle contraction, 219
Phospholipids, 54
Photoreceptors, 745
  function of, 752
Picrotoxin, and respiratory center stimulation, 405
Pigment, in cytoplasm, 54
Pigmentation. *See* Color
Pineal gland, 644
  calcifications in, 644, 675
  clinical notes on, 675
  tumors of, 675

Pinealocytes, 644
Pinocytosis, 63
Pit(s), gastric, 433
Pitch, of voice, 373
Pituicytes, 641
Pituitary gland, 635–643
　anterior lobe of, 635–641
　　diseases of, 673
　clinical notes on, 673–674
　control by hypothalamus, 635
　pars anterior, 635–640
　pars intermedia, 635, 640–641
　pars tuberalis, 635, 641
　posterior lobe of, 635, 641–643
Placenta, 593–605
　abnormalities in, 623–624
　circulation in, 600–602
　　fetal, 602
　　maternal, 600–602
　clinical notes on, 623–624, 683
　as endocrine gland, 603, 672
　establishment of, 593–599
　fetal part of, 597, 600
　functions of, 602
　gross appearance of, 599–600
　maternal part of, 597–599, 600
　praevia, 624
　separation during labor, 604–605
Plaque
　atheromatous, 327
　dental, 466
Plasma, 155, 175–176
　proteins in, 175–176
　seminal, 564
Plasma cells, 109–113, 342, 349
　in antibody production, 147
　neoplasms of, 147
Plasma membrane. See Membrane, plasma
Plate
　epiphyseal, 141
　sole, of neuromuscular junction, 209
　tarsal, 730
Platelets, 171–175
　fate of, 175
　formation of, 175
Pleura, 375
　clinical notes on, 401
　parietal, 375
　pressure in, 392
　visceral, 375
Pleuritis, 401

Plexus
　Auerbach's, 429, 452
　carotid, internal, 775
　Meissner's, 429, 449
　myenteric, 429
　Purkinje, 296
　subendocardial, 206
Plica
　circulares, of small intestine, 444
　semilunaris, 730
Pneumonia, 404
Pneumothorax, 401, 404
　artificial, 401
　spontaneous, 401
Podocytes, 508
Point, motor, 207
Poisoning, carbon monoxide, 405
Polycythemia
　physiological, 185
　vera, 185
Polydipsia, in diabetes insipidus, 674
Polyp(s), 722
Polypeptide, pancreatic, 662
Polyribosome, 49
Polyuria
　in diabetes insipidus, 674
　in diabetes mellitus, 680
Pores
　membrane, 62
　nuclear, 32–34
　slit, of podocytes, 509
　taste, 770
Porta hepatis, 477
Position, sense of, 767
Potassium, in sodium-potassium pump, 62
Potential
　action
　　of cardiac muscle, 219, 300
　　of neurons, 238, 264
　　of skeletal muscle, 219
　　of smooth muscle, 219
　resting, 264, 287
　　of cardiac muscle, 300
P-Q interval, in electrocardiogram, 304
P-R interval, in electrocardiogram, 304
Predentin, 419
Pre-eclampsia, 683
Pregnancy
　disorders in, 683
　ectopic, 620, 623
　mammary gland in, 614–615
　melasma in, 722

Pregnancy—*Continued*
　molar, 683
　striae gravidarum in, 706
　at term, 605
　ureter in, 534
　uterus in, 591–605
Premelanosomes, 700
Prepuce
　of clitoris, 608
　of penis, 561
Preparation of tissue
　in electron microscopy, 10–12
　　embedding in, 11
　　fixation in, 10–11
　　freeze-fracture etching in, 11
　　sectioning in, 11
　　staining in, 11
　in light microscopy, 7–10
　　fixation in, 7–8
　　obtaining specimens for, 7
　　processing in, 8
　　sectioning in, 8
　　staining in, 8–10
Presbyopia, 749, 775
Pressure
　blood, 316–321
　　arterial, 316–321
　　capillary, 321
　　　increased, 360
　　diastolic, 316, 328
　　　pulmonary, 324
　　hypertension, 328–329
　　measurement of, 328
　　pulse, 316
　　systolic, 316, 328
　　　pulmonary, 324
　　venous, 321
　intra-alveolar, 391–392
　intra-ocular, 747
　in pleural cavity, 392
　pulmonary, 324, 391–392
Prickly heat, 726
Procarboxypolypeptidase, 494
Process(es)
　odontoblastic, 418
　of podocytes
　　primary, 508
　　secondary, 508
Proerythroblasts, 159
Progesterone, 571
　function in pregnancy, 603
　ovarian secretion of, 670
　　functions of, 580
　placental, 672

Prolactin, 635, 638–639
Promonocytes, 171
Promyelocytes, 167
Prophase, in mitosis, 34
Propylthiouracil, 677
Prostate, 558–560
  clinical notes on, 565–567
  enlargement of, benign, 565–567
  function of, 560
Prostatitis, 565
Proteins
  contractile, 52
  fate in digestion, 497
  hypoproteinemia, 360
  metabolism of
    glucocorticoids affecting, 655
    insulin affecting, 664
  in liver, 487–488
  plasma, 175–176
    serum levels in liver disease, 499
  in plasma membrane, 55
  regulator, of muscle, 218
Proteinuria, 530
Protoplasm, 21, 29
Psoriasis, 721–722
Ptosis of eyelid, 773
Ptyalin, 425, 496
Puberty, 618, 626
  in males, 667
  ovarian changes in, 576–577
Pulp
  splenic, 349–351
    red, 349–351
    white, 349, 351
  of tooth, 419–420
Pump
  abdominothoracic, 321, 339
  lymphatic capillary, 339
  sodium-potassium, 62
Punctum lacrimale, 730
Pupil, 739
Purple, visual, 752
Purpura, idiopathic thrombocytopenic, 362
Pus, 190
Pyelogram, intravenous, 534
Pyelonephritis, 531
Pyknosis, 75
Pylorus, 432
Pyramids, renal, 503

Q wave, in electrocardiogram, 304
Q-T interval, in electrocardiogram, 304
Quinsy, 467

R wave, in electrocardiogram, 304
Race, and body structure and function, 25–26
Radioautography, 15–16
Rami communicantes, white, 774
Rays, medullary, renal, 504
Reaction, van den Bergh
  direct, 498
  indirect, 498
Receptors
  chemoreceptors in carotid and aortic bodies, 399
  pressor, carotid and aortic, 323
Rectum, 456–463
  clinical notes on, 471–472
  functions of, 460
  transverse folds of, 458
Reflex(es)
  accommodation, 774
  aortic body, 323
  automatic reflex bladder, 535
  Bainbridge, 302
  baroreceptor afferent, and heart rate, 302–304
  cardiac, 302–304
  carotid body, 323
  corneal, 774
  gastrocolic, 460
  gastroduodenal, 460
  Hering-Breuer
    deflation, 400
    inflation, 400
  light
    consensual, 774
    direct, 774
  ocular, 774–775
  pupillary, 774
  vascular, 323
  visual body, 774
Refraction, defects of, 775
Refractory period, 241
  absolute, 265, 300
  relative, 265, 300
Regeneration
  of axons, 283–284
  of connective tissue, 145–147
  of epithelial cells, 98–100
  of liver, 498

Regeneration—*Continued*
  of skeletal muscle fibers, 221
  of smooth muscle fibers, 222
Renin, 503, 523, 524, 653
Reproductive system, 23
  female, 571–628. *See also* Female reproductive system
  male, 539–569. *See also* Male reproductive system
Residual bodies, enzymes in, 47
Resistance, peripheral, in blood vessels, 319–321
Respiration
  abdominal type of, 391
  abnormalities in, 405–406
  artificial, 402–404
  Cheyne-Stokes, 405
  control of, 397–400
    chemical, 399–400
    nervous, 400
  external, 365, 392–394
  and heart rate, 302
  internal, 365, 397
  mechanics of, 384–391
  thoracic type of, 391
  types of, 391
Respiratory system, 23, 365–407
  clinical notes on, 400–406
  clinical problems on, 406–407
  conducting portion of, 365–379
  larynx, 370–373
  lungs, 379
  mediastinum, 375
  nose, 365–369
  pharynx, 369–370
  pleura, 375
  pulmonary pressures in, 391–392
  respiratory portion of, 379–383
  trachea, 373–375
  volumes of air in, 392
Rete testis, 539, 552
Reticular fibers, metallic impregnation of, 10
Reticulocytes, 161
Reticuloendothelial system, 116, 148, 358–360
Reticulum
  endoplasmic
    rough, 43–44
    smooth, 44–45
  sarcoplasmic, 198
Retina, 741–746
  clinical notes on, 772

Retina—*Continued*
  detachment of, 742, 772
  neural, 745–746
  pigmented layer of, 741–742
Retinal, 752
Retinitis pigmentosa, 76
Rheumatic fever, 325
Rhinitis, 400
  chronic, 777
Rhodopsin, 742, 752
Rhythmicity
  of cardiac muscle, 300
  circadian, of glucocorticoids, 655–657
Rib changes, in inspiration, 385–386
Ribonucleic acid. *See* RNA
Ribosomes, 37, 43, 49–51
  attached, 49
  bacterial, 79
  free, 49
Rickets, 149
Ridges
  dermal, 699
  epidermal, 699
  papillary, of fingers, 689
Rifampin, action on viruses, 79
Rigidity, decerebrate, 220
Rigor mortis, 221
Rima glottidis, 370
Ring, terminal, of spermatozoon, 542
RNA
  messenger, 37, 43, 49
    in nucleoli, 29
  ribosomal, 49
    in nucleoli, 29
  transfer, 39, 43, 50
  in viruses, 79
Rods and cones, 741, 745
Root(s)
  canals of teeth, 417
  of clitoris, 608
  hair, 708
  of nail, 707
  of nose, 365
  of penis, 561
Rouleaux formation, 157
Rugae of stomach, 433
Rush, peristaltic, 455

S wave, in electrocardiogram, 304
Sac(s)
  alveolar, 381
  conjunctival, 730
Sacculations, of colon, 456
Saccule
  laryngeal, 372
  of membranous labyrinth, 761
Saline solutions
  hypertonic, 77
  hypotonic, 77
  isotonic, 77
Saliva, 425
  control of secretion of, 425–426
  functions of, 425
Salivary glands, 422–424
  clinical notes on, 466–467
Salivation, 422–426
Salpingitis, 620
Salts, bile, 486
Sand, brain, 644, 675
Sap, nuclear, 32
Sarcolemma, 197
  T tubules in
    in cardiac muscle, 206
    in skeletal muscle, 198
Sarcoma, 147
  osteogenic, 147
  in peripheral nerve connective tissue, 285
Sarcomere, 197
Sarcoplasm, 197
Scab, 145
Scale
  media, 766
  tympani, 758, 766
  vestibuli, 758, 766
Scar, 145
  gliotic, 286
  keloid, 721
  surgical, 720
Schiller's test, 622
Schwann cells, 252, 255
Sclera, 736
Scopolamine, 286
Scurvy, 149–150
Sebaceous glands, 689, 714–717
  clinical notes on, 725
Seborrhea, 725
Sebum, 716
Secretin, 447
Secretions, 93
  gastric, 441–442
  of large intestine, 466
  of pancreas, 494–496
  of small intestine, 455, 497

Sectioning of tissue specimens
  in electron microscopy, 11
  in light microscopy, 8
Segment, rod
  inner, 745
  outer, 745
Semen, 563, 564
Seminomas, 565
Sensation, taste, 771
  disorders in, 777
Sense
  of movement, 767
  of position, 767
Sense organs, 729–780
  clinical notes on, 771–777
  clinical problems on, 777–780
  ear, 754–769
  eye, 729–753
  olfactory mucous membrane, 769–770
  taste buds, 417, 770–771
Septum
  nasal, 365
  orbital, 730
  placental, 599
Serosa
  of appendix, 460
  of digestive tract, 429
  of gallbladder, 490
  of large intestine, 458
  of small intestine, 452
  of uterus, 586
Serotonin
  in pineal gland, 644
  production by argentaffin cells, 438
  in small intestine, 447
  in suprarenal medulla, 657
Serotonin-N-acetyltransferase, 644
Serum, 156
  in blood clot, 171
Sex, affecting body structure and function, 25–26
Sex chromatin, 30, 163
Sex chromosomes, 41, 543, 578
Shaft
  bone, 131
  hair, 708
Sheath
  fascial, of eyeball, 729
  myelin, 252–255

Sheath—*Continued*
  root, epithelial
    inner, 710
    outer, 710
  synovial, 145, 147
Shift, chloride, 394
Shunt, arteriovenous, 312
Silicosis, 404
Silver, as cytoplasmic inclusion, 54
Singing, 373
Sinus
  carotid, 304, 313–314
    pressor receptors in, 323
  of larynx, 372
  marginal, 599
  paranasal, 368–369
    clinical notes on, 400
  renal, 503
  Rokitansky-Aschoff, 489
  subcapsular, lymph in, 347
Sinusoids
  of liver, 312, 324, 479, 481–482
  venous, of spleen, 351
Skeletal system, 23, 129–145. *See also* Bone
Skin, 689–727
  aging of, 719–720
  appendages of, 707–719
  burns of, 721
  clinical notes on, 720–726
  clinical problems on, 726–727
  color of, 707
  dermis, 689, 705–707
  epidermis, 689, 691–705
  estrogens affecting, 670
  grafts of, 721
  thick, 691
  thin, 691
Skull, tables of, inner and outer, 137
Smears, vaginal, 619
Smell, organ of, 769–770
  clinical notes on, 777
Sneezing, 372
Sodium-potassium pump, 62
Solutions
  hypertonic, 60
  hypotonic, 60
  isotonic, 60
  saline, 77
Somatomammotropin, chorionic, 604, 672
Somatomedins, 637

Somatostatin, 638, 662
  actions of, 665
  production in small intestine, 447
Somatotropes, 635
Space
  of Disse, 481, 482
  intervillous, chorionic, 597
  perisinusoidal, hepatic, 481, 482
  retromammary, 610
Spasm, carpopedal, 678
Speech, normal, 373
Spermatids, 540
Spermatocytes
  primary, 540
  secondary, 540
Spermatogenesis, 540–548
  chromosomal changes during, 543–544
Spermatogonia, 539
Spermatozoa, 539, 540
  abnormal, 565
  maturation of, 546–548
  mature, 544–546
  storage and transport of, 563–564
Spherule, rod, 745
Sphincter
  anal, 463
    involuntary internal, 463
    voluntary external, 463
  of Boyden, 488
  gastroesophageal, 432
  ileocecal, 455–456
  in larynx, 372–373
  of Oddi, 488
  precapillary, 310, 323, 330
  pyloric, 432
  urethrae, 528
  vesicae, 528
Sphygmomanometer, 328
Spicules, bone, 137
Spinal cord, 272–274
Spindles
  muscle, 207
  neuromuscular, 210–212
  neurotendinous, 212–214
  nuclear, 34, 52
  tendon, 207
Spines, dendritic, 243
Spirometer, 402
Spironolactone, 532
Spleen, 349–354
  blood circulation through, 351
    closed theory of, 351
    open theory of, 351

Spleen—*Continued*
  disorders of, 362
  functions of, 351–354
  pulp of, 349–351
Spot
  blind, 741
  Mongolian, 706
Sprue, nontropical, 470
Staining of tissue specimens
  in electron microscopy, 11
  in light microscopy, 8–10
  nerve tissue in, 225–227
Stalks, connecting, of retinal rods and cones, 745
Stapes, 756
Steatorrhea, 470
Stercobilin, 497
Stereocilia, 66
  in duct of epididymis, 88, 554
Sterility
  in females, 623
  in males, 564–565
Stomach, 432–442
  body of, 432
    glands of, 436
  clinical notes on, 468–469
  functions of, 440–442
  fundus of, 432
    glands of, 436
  movements of walls in, 440–441
  pyloric glands of, 439–440
  secretions of, 441–442
    control of, 441
    phases in, 442
Stones
  gallstones, 499
  renal, 532
Strabismus
  external, 773
  internal, 774
Stratum
  corneum, 702
  germinativum, 700
  granulosum, 701–702
  lucidum, 702
  spinosum, 700–701
Streptomycin, action on bacteria, 79
Stress, suprarenal gland in, 661
Striae
  gravidarum, 706
  vascularis, of cochlear duct, 763
Stroma, 93
Structure and function of body, factors affecting, 25–26

Sty, 771
Sublingual gland, 424
Submandibular glands, 422–424
Submucosa
  of anal canal, 463
  of digestive tract, 429
  of esophagus, 429
  of pyloric glands, 439
  of small intestine, 449
  of trachea, 373
Substance
  ground, 122
  Nissl, 231–233
Substantia propria, of cornea, 727
Sucrase, secretion in small intestine, 455
Sulcus
  in cerebral cortex, 276
  gingival, 421
  subtarsal, 730
  terminalis, of tongue, 414
Sulfonamide, action on bacteria, 79
Summation, neuron, 241
Suprarenal glands, 651–661
  blood supply of, 661
  clinical notes on, 678–680
  cortex of, 651–657
  medulla of, 657–661
    sympathetic nerve fibers to, 321
    tumors of, 680
  stress affecting, 661
Surfactant, pulmonary, 381
Swallowing, 372, 427
  disorders in, 467
Sweat glands, 689, 717–719
  apocrine, 717
  clinical notes on, 726
  eccrine, 717
Synapses, 23, 245–247
  axoaxonic, 246
  axodendritic, 246
  axosomatic, 246
  blocking agents, 285–286
  neurotransmitters at, 246–247
  ultrastructure of, 245
Syncytiotrophoblast, 591
Syndrome
  adrenogenital, 76
  cri du chat, 76
  Cushing's, 679–680
  Down's, 76
  dumping, after gastrectomy, 471
  Turner's, 76, 618

Synovium, 143
Systems, 23–25
  cardiovascular, 23, 291–331
  conducting, of heart, 205, 295–296
    diseases of, 325–326
    structure of, 206–207
  digestive, 23, 409–475
  endocrine, 23, 631–686
  haversian, 131
  lymphatic, 23, 333–363
  mononuclear phagocytic, 116, 148, 359–360
  muscular, 23, 195–224
  nervous, 23, 225–288
  reproductive, 23
    female, 571–628
    male, 539–569
  respiratory, 23, 365–407
  reticuloendothelial, 116, 148, 358–360
  skeletal, 23, 129–145
  urinary, 23, 503–537
Systole, 301

T tubules in sarcolemma
  in cardiac muscle, 206
  in skeletal muscle, 198
T wave, in electrocardiogram, 304
Tachycardia, 302
Tail
  axillary, of mammary gland, 610
  of epididymis, 554
  of pancreas, 490, 661
  of spermatozoon, 544
Taste buds, 417, 770–771
Taste sensation, 771
  clinical notes on, 777
Tear fluid, 734
Teeth, 417–421
  clinical notes on, 466
  deciduous, 417
  permanent, 417
Telophase, in mitosis, 35
Temperature
  basal, recording of, 619
  and heart rate, 304
  testicular, and fertility, 548
Tendons, 122, 195
Teniae coli, 429, 456
Terminals, axon, 243
Test
  caloric, of vestibular function, 776
  Rinne's, of hearing, 777

Test—Continued
  Schiller's, 622
  Weber's, of hearing, 777
  of vision, 772
Testis, 538–552
  clinical notes on, 564–565
  efferent ductules of, 539, 552
  incomplete descent of, 564
  interstitial cells of, 539, 552, 665–667
    clinical notes on, 682
    stimulating hormone, 639
    tumors of, 682
  maldescent of, 564
  mediastinum, 539
  rete testis, 539
  straight tubules of, 539, 552
  supporting cells of Sertoli, 548–552, 639
  temperature of, and fertility, 548
  tumors of, 565
Testosterone, 552, 639, 665–667
  actions of, 665–667
  control of secretion of, 667
  deficiency of, 682
Tetracyclines, action on bacteria, 79
Tetraethylammonium salts, as synaptic blocking agents, 285
Theca
  externa, 576
  interna, 576
Theophylline
  as diuretic, 532
  and respiratory center stimulation, 405
Thiazide diuretics, 532
Thrombin, 171
Thrombocytes, 171
Thrombocytopenia, 182
Thrombophlebitis, 329
Thromboplastin, 171
Thrombopoietin, 175
Thrombosis, 182
Thymine, 37
Thymomas, 362
Thymopoietin, 343
Thymosin, 343
Thymus, 343–345
  congenital absence of, 362
  function of, 345
  hormone of, 343
  lymphocytes of, 343
  structure of, 343
  tumors of, 362

Thyrocalcitonin, 648
  relation to parathyroid hormone, 651
Thyroglobulin, 646
Thyroid gland, 644–648
  clinical notes on, 675–678
  function tests, 675–676
  goiter of, 677–678
  hyperthyroidism, 676–677
  hypothyroidism, 677
  tumors of, 678
Thyroid-stimulating hormone, 639
  serum levels of, 675
Thyroidectomy, subtotal, 676
Thyroiditis, 677
  Riedel's, 677
Thyrotoxicosis, 676–677
Thyrotropes, 635
Thyrotropin, 639
  releasing hormone, 639
    pituitary response to, 676
  serum levels of, 675
Thyroxine, 646
  and heart rate, 304
  serum levels of, 675
Tide, alkaline, 441
Tinnitus, 779
Tissue, 22–23
  adipose, 54, 109
    brown, 109
    in obesity, 148
  connective, 22, 107–152
  epithelial, 22, 85–104
  gaseous exchange in, 397
  granulation, 145
  lymphatic, 339–357
    types of, 343–357
  muscular, 22, 195–224
  nervous, 22–23, 225–288
  preparation of specimens
    in electron microscopy, 10–12
    in light microscopy, 7–10
  subcutaneous, 689, 719
Tone, of skeletal muscle, 220
Tongue, 413–417
  disorders of, 466
Tonofibrils, 700
Tonsil(s), 354–357
  lingual, 357, 417
  nasopharyngeal, 357
    hypertrophy of, 467
  palatine, 354, 357
    infection of, 467
  tubal, 357, 758

Tonsillitis, 467
Tooth conditions. *See* Teeth
Trabeculae
  of lymph nodes, 345
  of spleen, 349
Trachea, 373–375
  clinical notes on, 401
Tract(us)
  digestive, 409–475
  hypothalamohypophyseal, 635
  nerve, 252
  solitarius, 771
  vestibulospinal, 767
Transfusions, 178–182
  blood typing in, 179–182
  cross matching of blood in, 180
  incompatible blood in, 179
Translocation, chromosome, 76
Transplantations. *See* Grafts
Transport through membranes
  active, 60–62
  facilitated, 60
  in placental membrane, 603
Trauma, and wound healing, 145–146
Triad, portal, 479
Triglycerides, 54
Trigone of bladder, 526
Triiodothyronine, 646
  and heart rate, 304
Trisomy, 76
  13-15, 76
  17-18, 76
  21, 76
Tropocollagen, 118
Tropomyosin, 52, 218
Troponin, 218
Trypsin, 496
  inhibitor of, 496
Trypsinogen, 494
Tube
  auditory, 755, 758
  caudal, of spermatozoon, 542
  from esophagus to anus, 427–429
  uterine, 580–584
    clinical notes on, 620
    estrogens affecting, 668–670
    function of, 582–584
    inflammation of, 620
    pregnancy in, 620
D-Tubocurarine, 221
Tubule
  dentinal, 418

Tubule—*Continued*
  renal
    collecting, 519–520
    convoluted
      distal, 519
      proximal, 511–516
    necrosis of, 530
  seminiferous, 539
    straight, 539, 552
  uriniferous, 504–522
Tubulin, 51
Tumors, 74–75
  benign, 100
  of bladder, 534–535
  of bone marrow, 188
  cancer cells in, 74–75
  carcinoma. *See* Carcinoma
  chorionepithelioma, 683
  classification by tissue of origin, 100
  of colon and rectum, 471
  of connective tissue, 147
  of dermis, 724
  diagnosis of cancer, 75
  of esophagus, 468
  granulosa-theca cell, 683
  of interstitial cells of testis, 682
  intracranial, 404
  of keratinocytes, 722
  of kidney, 532
  lung cancer, 404
  of lymph nodes, 361
  lymphatic spread of, 361
  malignant, 100
  of mammary glands, 625–626
  of melanocytes, 723–724
  of neuroglia, 286
  of ovary, 620
  of penis, 567
  pineal, 675
  pituitary, 673
  plasma cell, 147
  of salivary glands, 466–467
  of suprarenal medulla, 680
  of testes, 565
  of thymus, 362
  thyroid, 678
  of uterus, 621
  of vocal folds, 400
Tunica
  adventitia
    of digestive tract, 429
    of elastic arteries, 308
    of esophagus, 430

Tunica, adventitia—*Continued*
  of lymphatic ducts, 335
  of muscular arteries, 309
  of trachea, 375
  of veins, 311, 312
 albuginea
  of ovary, 571
  of testis, 539
 fibrosa. *See* Coat, fibrous
 intima
  of elastic arteries, 308
  of lymphatic ducts, 335
  of muscular arteries, 308
  of veins, 311, 312
 media
  of elastic arteries, 308
  of lymphatic ducts, 335
  of muscular arteries, 309
  of veins, 311, 312
 mucosa. *See* Membrane, mucous
 muscularis. *See* Coat, muscular
 serosa. *See* Serosa
Tunnel of Corti, 766
Turner's syndrome, 76, 618
Typhoid fever, 470
Tyrosinase, 694
 in melanocytes, DOPA reaction for, 14

Ulcer
 duodenal, 469
 gastric, 468–469
Ultramicrotome, 11
Union
 primary, 145
 secondary, 146
Ureter
 clinical notes on, 534
 function of, 526
 pain in, 534
 pelvis of, 503, 525
 in pregnancy, 534
Urethra, 528–529
 clinical notes on, 535
 female, 528–529
 male, 528
 membranous, 528
 penile, 528
 prostatic, 528
Urinary system, 23, 503–537
 bladder, 526–528
 clinical notes on, 529–535
 clinical problems on, 535–537
 kidneys, 503–525

Urinary system—*Continued*
 ureter, 525–526
 urethra, 528–529
Urine
 composition of, 521–522
 concentration of, 520–521
 examination of, 533
Urobilin, 522
Urobilinogen, 522
Urticaria, 724
Uterus, 584–606
 after menopause, 590–591
 after parturition, 606
 cervix of
  carcinoma of, 622
  inflammations of, 621–622
 in childhood, 590
 clinical notes on, 620–622
 estrogens affecting, 668
 in pregnancy, 591–605
 progesterone affecting, 670
 role in labor, 605
 wall of, 586–590
Utricle, 761
Uvula, 421

Vagina, 606–607
 clinical notes on, 622
 estrogens affecting, 668
 smears from, 619
Valves
 anal, 463
 aortic, 291, 299
 atrioventricular
  left, 291
  right, 291
 bicuspid, of lymphatic vessels, 335
 of heart, 296–299
  diseases of, 325
 ileocecal, 455–456
 mitral, 291, 298
 pulmonary, 298–299
 spiral, of gallbladder, 489
 tricuspid, 291, 296
 of veins, 311
Van den Bergh reaction
 direct, 498
 indirect, 498
Varices
 esophageal, 329
 of hemorrhoidal vein tributaries, 472

Vas deferens, 556
 clinical notes on, 565
Vasa
 recta
  ascending, 523
  descending, 523
 vasorum, 308
Vasectomy, 565
Vasoconstriction, 321
Vasodilatation, 321
Vasopressin. *See* Antidiuretic hormone
Vasovasostomy, 565
Veins, 291, 311–312
 central, of liver, 479
 clinical notes on, 329
 portal, 324
 valves of, 311
 varicose, 329
 vorticose, 736
Velocity, conduction, 265, 287
Venae
 cavae
  inferior, 291, 301
  superior, 291, 301
 vorticosae, 736
Ventilation. *See* Respiration
Ventilators, mechanical, 404
Ventricles
 cardiac
  left, 291
  right, 291
 cerebral, lateral, 276
Venules, 291, 310–311
Verhoeff elastic stain, 10
Vermis, cerebellar, 274
Vertigo, 776, 779
Vesicles
 coated, 48–49
 olfactory, 769
 pinocytotic, 63
 presynaptic, 246
 secretory, in Golgi apparatus, 46
 seminal, 557–558
Vessels
 blood, 307–323
 lymphatic, 333–337
Vestibule
 of labyrinth, 759
  function disorders, 776
 of mouth, 409
 nasal, 365
Villi
 anchoring, 597

Villi—*Continued*
 chorionic
  primary, 593
  secondary, 597
 in digestive tract, 427
 in small intestine, 446
Virilism, adrenal, 680
Viruses, 79
 chemotherapy affecting, 79
Viscosity of blood, and blood pressure, 319
Vision
 color, 752
 fields of, 772–773
  nasal, 772
  temporal, 772
  testing of, 772
 vitamin A affecting, 752
Vitamin A, and vision, 752
Vitamin C
 deficiency of, 149–150
 and wound healing, 145
Vitamin D
 deficiency of, 149
 relation to parathyroid hormone, 651

Vitamin K, deficiency of, 182
Vitiligo, 722
Voice, production of, 373
Volume
 of air, 392
  measurement in lungs, 402
  reserve
   expiratory, 392
   inspiratory, 392
  residual, 392
  tidal, 392
 of blood, 155
  and blood pressure, 316, 319
  stroke, 301–302
Vomiting, 472
Vulva, 607–610

Wall
 of heart, 292–294
 of stomach, movements of, 440–441
 of uterus, 586–590
Water, reabsorption in kidney, 520
Waves, peristaltic, 429
 in large intestine, 460
 in small intestine, 454–455

Weakness, color, 775
Web
 subsynaptic, 246
 terminal, 52
Weigert's elastic stain, 10
Whispering, 373
Window
 oval, 758, 766, 767
 round, 758, 766, 767
Wounds
 contraction of, 146
 healing of, 145–146
Wright, stain, 10

X sex chromosomes, 41

Y sex chromosomes, 41

Z lines, of myofibrils, 197
Zona
 fasciculata, 651
 glomerulosa, 651
 pellucida, 576
 reticularis, 651
Zonula occludens, 68
Zonule, lens, 749